A companion to medical studies

Volume 2

Editorial board

A companion to medical studies

IN THREE VOLUMES

Volume 2

Pharmacology, microbiology, general pathology and related subjects

EDITORS-IN-CHIEF

R. PASSMORE

J. S. ROBSON

SECOND PRINTING

BLACKWELL SCIENTIFIC PUBLICATIONS

OXFORD AND EDINBURGH

First Published February 1970
Reprinted September 1970

Spanish, Portuguese *and* Italian
Editions *in preparation*

SBN
632 04580 9   Cloth
632 05820 x   Limp
For the three-volume set
632 05840 4   Cloth
632 05850 1   Limp

Printed and bound in Great Britain by
William Clowes and Sons Ltd, London and Beccles

Contents

GENERAL PHARMACOLOGY

EFFECT OF DRUGS ON THE SYSTEMS OF THE BODY

ASPECTS OF COMMUNITY MEDICINE

x

Volume 1

Anatomy, biochemistry, physiology and related subjects

Volume 3

Medicine, surgery, obstetrics, therapeutics and social medicine

Contributors to volume 2

H.M. ADAM *Department of Pharmacology, University of Edinburgh*

KATHERINE M.G. ADAM *Department of Zoology, University of Edinburgh*

G.W. ASHCROFT *Department of Pharmacology, University of Edinburgh*

A.G. BAIKIE *Department of Medicine, University of Tasmania*

JOYCE D.BAIRD *Department of Medicine, University of Edinburgh*

R.B. BARLOW *Department of Pharmacology, University of Edinburgh*

J.M. BARNES *Toxicology Research Unit, Medical Research Council, Carshalton*

J.A. CAMPBELL *Department of Zoology, University of Edinburgh*

J.G. COLLEE *Department of Bacteriology, University of Edinburgh*

J.F. COLLINS *Department of Molecular Biology, University of Edinburgh*

T.B.B. CRAWFORD *Department of Pharmacology, University of Edinburgh*

S.H. DAVIES *Department of Medicine, University of Edinburgh*

K.C. DIXON *Department of Pathology, University of Cambridge*

D. ECCLESTON *Department of Pharmacology, University of Edinburgh*

R.B.L. EWART *Department of Medicine, University of Edinburgh*

D.L. GARDNER *The Mathilda and Terence Kennedy Institute of Rheumatology, London*

R.R. GILLIES *Department of Bacteriology, University of Edinburgh*

B.L. GINSBORG *Department of Pharmacology, University of Edinburgh*

E.A. HARRIS *Clinical Physiology Department, Green Lane Hospital, Auckland, New Zealand*

F. HAWKING *National Institute for Medical Research, Mill Hill, London*

W.J. IRVINE *Department of Therapeutics, University of Edinburgh*

P.J.R.JEBSON *Department of Anaesthetics, University of Edinburgh*

D.B. JOHNSON *Department of Physiology, University of Edinburgh*

M.G. KERR *Department of Obstetrics and Gynaecology, University of Edinburgh*

A.H. KITCHIN *Department of Medicine, University of Edinburgh*

ANNE T.LAMBIE *Department of Therapeutics, University of Edinburgh*

J.M. LAST *Department of Social Medicine, University of Edinburgh*

MARY K. MACDONALD *Department of Pathology, University of Edinburgh*

G.E. MAWER *Department of Pharmacology, University of Manchester*

G.L. MONTGOMERY *Department of Pathology, University of Edinburgh*

S.L. MORRISON *Department of Social Medicine, University of Edinburgh*

J.F. PEUTHERER *Department of Bacteriology, University of Edinburgh*

J. RICHMOND *Department of Medicine, University of Edinburgh*

M.H. RICHMOND *Department of Bacteriology, University of Bristol*

K.B. ROBERTS *Department of Physiology, London Hospital Medical College*

M.B. ROBERTS *Institute of Medical Science, Haile Sellassie I University, Addis Ababa, Ethiopia*

B.V. ROBINSON *Department of Pharmacology, Guy's Hospital Medical School, London*

J.M. ROBSON *Department of Pharmacology, Guy's Hospital Medical School, London*

J.S. ROBSON *Department of Medicine, University of Edinburgh*

G. SCLARE *Department of Pathology, University of Edinburgh*

D.J.C. SHEARMAN *Department of Therapeutics, University of Edinburgh*

A.A. SHIVAS *Department of Pathology, University of Edinburgh*

ISABEL W. SMITH *Department of Bacteriology, University of Edinburgh*

R.P. STEPHENSON *Department of Pharmacology, University of Edinburgh*

D.W. STRAUGHAN *Department of Pharmacology, University of Edinburgh*

J.A. STRONG *Department of Medicine, University of Edinburgh*

D.M. WEIR *Department of Bacteriology, University of Edinburgh*

J. WILLIAMSON *Department of Geriatrics, University of Edinburgh*

P.A.G. WILSON *Department of Zoology, University of Edinburgh*

F.W. WINTON *Department of Bacteriology, University of Edinburgh*

I.J. ZEITLIN *Department of Pharmacology, University of Edinburgh*

Preface

The Companion is a comprehensive work written for medical students. The whole work aims to give them an interesting, intelligent and exciting account of modern medicine and the medical sciences. It also aims to set out concisely the scientific achievements on which modern practice is based and indicates important growing points; thus it should prepare its readers for medical practice in the twenty-first century when they will be at the height of their professional careers.

Today there is much criticism of medical education by both teachers and students. A common complaint is that teaching is carried out in various departments whose staff may have little idea of what is being taught in other departments. Throughout this book unnecessary departmental barriers are broken down. The editors, who represent the major medical disciplines, come from the same medical school; it has been possible for them to meet frequently so that together they have been responsible for planning each part and for the detailed editing of the contributions. One important consequence of these arrangements has been a great reduction in the repetition of material which appears inescapable in a series of departmentally orientated books.

We are grateful to the authors who make the Companion possible. Some of them have spent many hours with the editors going over their manuscripts and have patiently acquiesced when sections of their work have disappeared either into the waste paper basket or into another chapter. Many of them have allowed large alterations in their scripts, and the editors must take responsibility for such errors as remain.

We owe much to the publishers. Without Mr Per Saugman's vision and encouragement we should never have begun. Without Mr Nigel Palmer's industry and perseverance we should never have finished two volumes.

The excellent reception of the first volume encourages the belief that the second will also meet a need amongst students and teachers. It is divided into five sections: General Pharmacology; the Effects of Drugs on the Systems of the Body; Topics in Autopharmacology; Microbiology, General Pathology and Related Pharmacology, and Aspects of Community Medicine. These contain much old and established knowledge that new discoveries have not made less important. The last twenty years have seen the development of an enormous number and variety of new drugs and of advances in molecular biology that allow some understanding of how these drugs act. Molecular biology has led also to many new concepts in immunology and the hypersensitivity reactions, which play a role in pathology far wider than was formerly thought. New knowledge of genetics is being applied to disease, the pattern of which has been changing in all countries.

Although there are no chapters dealing specifically with the behavioural sciences or with psychiatric disorders, chapter 5 gives an account of the action of drugs on the central nervous system and on behaviour and mood which serves as an important introduction to the psychiatric disorders that will be discussed in volume 3.

Important subjects that have been held over to volume 3 include the chemical pathology of shock and of disturbances of electrolyte balance, and of the metabolic disturbances associated with atherosclerosis. These subjects, together with the chemical and structural pathology of individual diseases, seem by the editors to be treated most logically in close association with the clinical conditions for which they are responsible, rather than as part of general pathology.

The division between principles and practice in medicine is arbitrary. This volume deals primarily with principles and much of the material has been included to give an understanding of the scope and range of modern medical science which forms the powerhouse of medicine. The practice is considered only incidentally and will be dealt with in volume 3 where the emphasis will be reversed.

We are indebted to Professor B. P. Marmion for assistance with the section on virology, to Mr T. C. Dodds for help in producing many of the colour plates, to the artists, Mrs Yvonne Miller and Mr Martin Miller, who have drawn or redrawn all the illustrations, and to Dr Judith Park, Mrs Esme Passmore, Dr John Clark and Dr M. Q. K. Talukder who have undertaken the onerous task of producing the index. Mr R. Osborn-King has given invaluable aid in checking and preparing the proofs.

Edinburgh   R. Passmore
October 1969   J.S. Robson

Acknowledgements

We wish to thank all publishers, editors and authors who have allowed us to reproduce illustrations, especially: Academic Press, Inc.; George Allen & Unwin Ltd; The American Physiological Society; Baillière, Tindall & Cassell Ltd; Blackwell Scientific Publications Ltd; The British Museum (Natural History); Cambridge University Press; J. & A. Churchill Ltd; English Universities Press Ltd; E. & S. Livingstone Ltd; McGraw-Hill Book Company; The Macmillan Company; Methuen & Co. Ltd; Oliver & Boyd Ltd; Oxford University Press; Pergamon Press Ltd.; Royal College of Physicians; Charles C. Thomas; The Wellcome Trust; The Williams & Wilkins Company; *American Journal of Obstetrics and Gynaecology; American Journal of Physiology; Annals of the New York Academy of Sciences; British Journal of Pharmacology and Chemotherapy; British Medical Bulletin; British Medical Journal; Circulation; Circulation Research; Diabetes; Geriatrics; Gerontologia (Basel); Journal of Clinical Pathology; Journal of Experimental Biology; Journal of Gerontology; Journal of Laboratory and Clinical Medicine; Journal of the National Cancer Institute; Journal of Pathology and Bacteriology; Journal of Pharmacology and Experimental Therapeutics; Journal of Pharmacy and Pharmacology; Journal of Physiology; The Lancet; The New England Journal of Medicine; New Scientist; Pediatrics; Proceedings of the Royal Society; Proceedings of the Royal Society of Medicine; Proceedings of the Society for Experimental Biology and Medicine; Science; Scientific American; Triangle.*

An account of contemporary pharmacology would be difficult to give without reference to *The Pharmacological Basis of Therapeutics*, edited by L. S. Goodman and A. Gilman, published by The Macmillan Company. The editors and authors have used it frequently as a source of information.

Finally, we would like to acknowledge our indebtedness to other publications if through inadvertence this list is incomplete.

Chapter 1
Introduction to pharmacology

To the ancient Greeks the word 'pharmakon' meant not only a curative drug, but also a poison, a charm, a spell or an incantation. Today the word drug still has all these meanings; the pharmacologist is concerned with four types of substances; some are curative, such as penicillin which cures pneumonia, and others are palliative, for instance morphine which relieves pain; there are also poisons like the organic phosphorus compounds which are used as insecticides but because of their widespread use may also poison man; lastly D-lysergic acid diethylamide (LSD) and other chemicals profoundly influence the activity of the mind. In addition, clinical pharmacologists are concerned with the effect of giving a drug which, even when it is inert, causes a reaction in a sample of the population and appears to act as a charm (placebo reactors, vol. 1, p. 3.5).

Nowadays the vast majority of the drugs used in medicines are prepared by commercial pharmaceutical firms, which form a specialized branch of the chemical industry. The pharmaceutical industry, however, is less than one hundred years old. Previously the hedges and fields were the sources of many household remedies and, together with herbal gardens, provided the materia medica for the compound prescriptions of the medical profession. The poet Kipling lists a few of the herbal remedies that were traditional in rural England.

> Alexander and marigold,
> Eyebright, orris and elecampane
> Basil, rocket, valerian, rue,
> (Almost singing themselves they run)
> Vervain, dittany, call-me-to-you-
> Cowslip, melilot, rose of the sun,
> Anything green that grew out of the mould
> Was an excellent herb of our fathers of old.

A Greek physician, Dioscorides, who was a medical officer with the much travelled Roman legions around the year A.D. 60, produced a book in which 600 plant preparations were described and classified, and this became a standard reference work for 1600 years.

At the time of the Renaissance the medical guilds in many city-states produced their own pharmacopoeias. These contained details of remedies considered to be of value and instructions for their preparation. The London Pharmacopoeia, the forerunner of the present British Pharmacopoeia, first appeared in Latin in 1618. It described 1028 simple and 932 compound remedies. The simple remedies included dosages of dried vipers, boar's horn and powders of fox lung for asthma; some of the compounds contained over 20 different ingredients. Although the student of today may be bewildered by the number of drugs which are described in this book and by the complexity of their chemical structure, in some respects he has a much less heavy task than his predecessors 350 years ago.

The vast majority of these mixtures were of no therapeutic value and many were relics of superstitions of the past, but the old pharmacopoeias contained a few powerful remedies which remain in use. The foxglove leaves contain the digitalis glycosides, still employed in the treatment of cardiac failure; the juice of the white poppy of South Asia is the source of the opium alkaloids which remain invaluable in the relief of pain; quinine from Peruvian bark is still used in the treatment of the cerebral form of malaria.

In the second half of the nineteenth century, the new chemical industry produced general anaesthetics, disinfectants, antipyretics and hypnotics. In the early years of the present century, largely owing to Paul Ehrlich and German chemical firms, a number of synthetic drugs became available for the treatment of some infections, notably syphilis and trypanosomiasis. However it was not until after 1935, the year of the discovery of the sulphonamides, that synthetic drugs rapidly replaced the older remedies.

During the last 25 years, pharmacology and therapeutics have made rapid strides. More new drugs have been introduced in this time than in the whole period since drugs first began to be made, about a century ago. Even in the last 10 years, about half of the drugs in the British Pharmacopoeia have been replaced. Not only are drugs being discovered at an ever increasing rate, but the quantity manufactured and deployed for various purposes is also increasing enormously.

Drugs have now assumed a new importance in matters concerning health, population and environment. This is apparent from the use of drugs under the aegis of the World Health Organization for the control or eradication of endemic disease such as malaria, tuberculosis and diseases due to parasitic worms, or schemes for the massive dispersal of pesticides for the protection of crops, and for the improvement of livestock through the addition of antibiotics to the food.

It seems there is virtually no limit to the demand for new drugs, any more than there is a limit to the number that the organic chemist can make. Not only are there many diseases which still lack effective remedies, but patterns of disease continually change. The development of drug resistant strains of pathogenic organisms, exposure to toxic chemicals in air and food and the strained relationship between man and machine are hazards in the environment which, if not new, are becoming more acute in their effects. Implicit in this view is the belief that it will be possible to select or make drug molecules which interfere in an increasingly specific way with functions of cells. In this problem there are at least two approaches. First, the process of discovery is still what it has always been, namely a search based on trial and error; opportunities turn up by chance and, if recognized, can be exploited. This random approach is costly and laborious but is justified by the results, since most important drugs have been discovered in this way. The second or rational method aims at designing drug molecules for their action at specific sites or in known metabolic pathways. There have been notable successes of this policy but in the history of pharmacology they are few in number. These include in particular British antilewisite (BAL, dimercaprol) devised by Peters, Stocken and Thompson to counteract the lethal effects of arsenical poisoning, folic acid antagonists used in the treatment of the leukaemias and, more recently, allopurinol advocated for the treatment of gout.

The old materia medica which consisted of vegetable drugs, extracts of animal tissues and excrement and a few metals, represented the accumulated experience of innumerable trials which man had carried out on himself over thousands of years. Today, and in the same way, organic chemists in the drug houses, in various parts of the world are making thousands of new compounds which are then tested in ways which depend on the expected action of the drug and on the supposition that a few may have the desired action coupled with low toxicity. Some of the pharmacological and toxicological tests employed are described in this volume.

Only when this stage is completed and when the drugs have been tested and evaluated clinically do they become candidates for inclusion in the pharmacopoeias of different countries or in the International Pharmacopoeia published under the authority of the World Health Organization.

One further difficulty concerns the names of drugs.

A compound always has a chemical name but this is often far too clumsy for everyday clinical use. The company responsible for its discovery, manufacture or sale usually bestows upon it a proprietary name which is registered as a trade mark and by which the drug is advertised and promoted. Finally, and only after it has been shown to be of some value in clinical medicine may it be given an approved name which usually consists of some contraction of the chemical name. In Britain this is bestowed by the Pharmacopoeia Commission and published by the General Medical Council. Thus a simple compound may possess a minimum of three names. In many cases, however, several different firms discover the remedy or devise an alternative method of synthesis which does not offend a registered patent so that a simple compound may possess several proprietary names and other countries may approve yet other official names. Such proliferation of titles leads to great confusion. Whenever possible a drug should be referred to by its approved or official name and as far as possible this policy has been adopted in this book, commonly used other names being given in parenthesis.

How drugs act

Understanding of how drugs act depends on knowing how the normal body works. Pharmacologists and physiologists use the same language. Arabian pharmacologists developed Galen's physiology to provide explanations of how the combination of four qualities of a drug, i.e. hot, cold, moist and dry, could affect the four humours of the body, blood, phlegm, black bile and yellow bile. For many centuries this was the language of pharmacologists. Today attempts to explain the fundamental modes of action of drugs are discussed in terms of enzyme activities, neurotransmission and cell structure as revealed by the electron microscope.

Many of the ideas of contemporary pharmacology are extensions of the theory developed at the beginning of this century that the specific effects of a drug could be explained by the reaction between the drug and a particular chemical group in the cells or tissues. The chemical group is conceived as a **specific receptor**. The development of receptor theory arose largely from the work of Paul Ehrlich, director of the Institute for Experimental Therapy at Frankfurt from 1899 to 1915. Ehrlich conceived of living matter as composed of large protoplasmic molecules with peripheral side chains which were unstable. These side chains were considered as receptors, which could combine chemically with nutrients, drugs or poisons and anchor them to the surface of the cell. Receptors were thus the point of contact between the cell and any substances that might reach it through the blood and tissue fluids. The concept of receptors was taken up by Langley, Professor of Physiology at Cambridge from 1903 to 1925, in explaining the function of the autonomic nervous system; to tackle this problem he made extensive use of experiments with drugs which modified the effects of stimulation of autonomic nerves and he spoke of the 'receptive substances' with which e.g. nicotine reacted. Receptor theory is an important part of the background of pharmacology today and is discussed in chap. 3. It is particularly applicable to drugs which modify the behaviour of excitable tissue. However, drug receptors remain at the present, as in the time of Ehrlich, theoretical models for the most part and their nature is speculative; they should not be confused with the sensory receptors of the body, which are definite histological structures.

However drugs may act, one can conceive that many of them at the molecular level modify the functions of cell membranes and the enzyme systems within them.

DRUGS AND MEMBRANES

Drugs acting on the plasma membrane of cells may interfere with excitation and transport. Where cells communicate in systems for the flow of information, they are more excitable than elsewhere. Thus, specialized junctions between cells, as in the nervous system, heart, smooth and skeletal muscle, are highly permeable structures with conductance for ions far greater than in nonjunctional membranes. Many drugs act selectively on these junctional membranes and have been used to analyse the ionic basis of their electrical properties.

Biogenic amines, alkyl or other radical substituted ammonium compounds, amino acids, local anaesthetics and cardiac glycosides are all drugs that are active in low concentration and alter or fix the polarity of membranes. For example, quinidine and certain antagonists of acetylcholine, adrenaline and histamine share a local anaesthetic action with procaine. Such drugs increase the electrical stability of membranes by making them less permeable to sodium ions. Thus, procaine prevents conduction in axons and when applied to motor end plates by iontophoresis, it prevents depolarization. Procaine is assumed to block channels for the entry of Na^+. By contrast, cardiac glycosides interfere with the outward movement of Na^+ from cells and at the same time reduce the entry of K^+, where this is linked to the extrusion of Na^+. This action of cardiac glycosides is seen not only in junctional membranes of nerve and muscle but also in red blood cells, the gastric mucosa and renal tubules. The effect may be metabolic since the glycosides influence the activity of ATPase, an enzyme which is normally activated by Na^+, K^+ and Ca^{++}. Thus the actions of cardiac glycosides have been related to such biochemical concepts as the metabolically driven Na^+ pump and the role of Ca^{++} in the coupling of excitation with contraction in cardiac muscle. Many drugs influence transport in the cells with special functions. In the nephron, for example, organic mercurial compounds, drugs containing

the sulponamyl group (SO_2NH_2), notably acetazolamide, inhibit the reabsorption of filtered Na^+, whereas aldosterone and corticosterone increase it. The glycoside phloridzin blocks the reabsorption of glucose in the renal tubules as well as its absorption from the intestine. Vasopressin does not affect the transport of solutes but increases, by a highly selective action, the permeability of renal epithelium to water. The drug probenecid, however, interferes with the renal tubular secretion of organic acids, but not organic bases, from the blood and at the blood–CSF barrier.

The effects of drugs on the traffic of ions and other solutes in different regions of the renal tubules have far-reaching consequences for acid-base regulation in the body and profoundly influence the actions of other drugs. For example, drugs that promote the loss of Na^+ may also cause the loss of K^+ and a fall in the body stores of K^+ lowers the threshold for the toxic effects of cardiac glycosides.

DRUGS AND ENZYMES

Study of the action of drugs on enzymes (Greek, *zume*, yeast) began at the turn of the century. Yeast cells, digestive juices and later bacteria and soya beans provided a rich source of enzymes. Heavy metals, cyanide and quinine acted in low concentrations to depress fermentation by enzymes in solution and by living cells. The discovery that enzymes as well as cells were sensitive to drugs marked the beginning of biochemical pharmacology. In receptor theory the interactions between drugs and receptors are seen to be analogous to those between substrate and enzyme. Today, in effect, a new pharmacology is being mapped out within the interior of the cell, where drugs are seen to act at numerous sites within the framework of its ultrastructure. The nucleus, ribosomes, mitochondria, lysosomes, storage granules and other organelles are all known sites of drug action. The problem is not only how drug molecules pass through the plasma membrane but what determines their affinity for these components of the cell. For example, alkylating agents such as mustard gas damage chromosomes and produce mutations by their action on DNA; colchicine, an alkaloid from the corm of the autumn crocus, stops mitosis at the spindle stage; chloramphenicol acts on ribosomes and inhibits protein synthesis; barbiturates act on mitochondria and inhibit respiration; cortisone protects lysosomes once named 'suicide bags'; penicillin interferes with the synthesis of bacterial cell walls so causing the rupture of the unsupported protoplast. Although many drugs act by enzymic inhibition, others actually induce the formation of enzymes in the cells. Phenobarbitone, for example, enables hepatic and other cells to destroy some molecules more quickly by inducing the formation of hydroxylating and other enzymes contained in microsomal particles.

Drugs may act at two levels of cellular organization, firstly, on mechanisms that are entirely intracellular, primitive, and self-regulating, such as those required for respiration, division and growth and represented in unicellular organisms and secondly, on controls that are superimposed on the cell from without, as by neurochemical transmitters and general and local hormones or autacoids. In the multicellular organism, these potent molecules not only control specialized activities within the community of cells but also exercise a continuing influence on the metabolic functions of all cells.

The distinction is useful since many drugs that act on the basic metabolic functions of the cell are those that inhibit respiration and growth and so destroy life. Such drugs include chemotherapeutic agents which act selectively on organisms parasitic in man and animals, and also pesticides and disinfectants. In contrast are drugs which interfere with the synthesis, storage, release and destruction of neurochemical transmitters or general or local hormones, or which are the pharmacological antagonists of these molecules. For example, thiourea inhibits the formation of thyroid hormone; the alkaloid reserpine releases pharmacologically active amines from granules in neurones and other cells; metyrapone inhibits 11β-hydroxylation of the steroid molecule and so reduces the output of cortisol. In all these instances, it can be assumed that the drug acts mainly on enzyme systems that control specialized functions of the cell, and not on the systems that are responsible for its survival.

The classical example in pharmacology of an enzyme inhibitor is the alkaloid eserine (physostigmine) from the Calabar bean, an ordeal poison once used by witch doctors in West Africa. Nearly all its actions arise from the accumulation of acetylcholine at neuronal junctions. As an inhibitor of cholinesterase, eserine was the first drug to be used as a biochemical tool for the identification of substrate which would otherwise have been instantly destroyed. But for eserine, the theory of neurochemical transmission of the nerve impulse might have remained untested by experiment. Today, the biochemist and pharmacologist have a large number of drugs at their disposal which inhibit, stimulate or uncouple enzymic reactions. The discovery of such drugs has frequently depended on the synthesis of compounds that are structurally similar to the substrate or product of the enzyme, or that combine with a cofactor or metal activator. Where the substrate is an essential metabolite, such as *p*-aminobenzoic acid in bacterial metabolism, so a drug with the structure of sulphanilamide is assumed to act as a competitive antagonist to the vitamin and so block access to the receptor on the enzyme. Drugs that act in this way are called antimetabolites.

Among the drugs that stimulate cellular metabolism is dinitrophenol, which for a time was used as a nostrum in the treatment of obesity. In low concentration, dinitrophenol acts by uncoupling oxidation from phosphorylation. Unlike other inhibitors of aerobic phosphorylation, dinitrophenol does not depress respiration and the energy so derived is dissipated as heat, instead of being used for the formation of energy rich phosphates. The drug has no therapeutic application but is used to test *in vitro* for the possible role of phosphate bond energy in various biological processes, for example active transport.

NARCOTICS AND CELLS

Although general anaesthetics had been known since the mid-nineteenth century, theories of how they acted were not proposed until much later. In 1899, the German pharmacologists Overton and Meyer observed independently that substances which were common nutrients, such as sugars and amino acids, did not penetrate readily into cells whereas alcohols, ethers, amides, ketones and various hydrocarbons entered rapidly and produced a narcotic effect (Greek; *narcosis*, numbness). Cells that were active and motile rapidly became inactive on exposure to these agents; when they were removed, the cells promptly recovered. In seeking an explanation for this unexpected difference in the penetration of molecules, Overton suggested:

(1) that entry of the foreign molecules depended on a physical property which was common to them all, namely solubility in lipid, and

(2) that entry of nutrient molecules required the cells to perform work, as in glandular secretion.

The work of Overton and of Meyer had important consequences. It led to the view, first, that lipids might be constituents of cell membranes, secondly, that the entry of nutrient molecules depended on some form of active transport and thirdly, that lipid solubility in drugs producing narcosis provided a clue to their mode of action.

As a test of this hypothesis they obtained the lipid-water distribution ratio for a number of polar and nonpolar substances and showed that this was related to the narcotic potency of the substance. For drugs that were soluble in water as well as lipid (polar compounds), the potency was measured as the concentration required to immobilize tadpoles; for substances that were volatile and nonpolar (i.e. chloroform), potency was estimated as the concentration in air which immobilized mice. At the point of narcosis (immobilization), the concentration of drug in the lipid of cells was expected to be the same for the various drugs, irrespective of their chemical structure. Some of these early results are shown in table 1.1, and seem to justify the theory which assumes that the bulk lipid phases (olive oil and tadpoles) are similar.

TABLE I.I. Narcotic potencies of gases and vapours. Values taken from Höber R. (1947) *Physical Chemistry of Cells and Tissues*. London: Churchill.

	Narcotic concentration for mice volume per cent in air	Solubility coefficient olive oil 37°C	Calculated narcotic coefficient mol/l lipid
Methane	370·0	0·54	0·08
Ethylene	80·0	1·3	0·04
Acetylene	65·0	1·8	0·05
Diethylether	3·4	50·0	0·07
Chloroform	0·5	265·0	0·05

Traube, in 1904, advanced an alternative hypothesis of narcotic action. It was based on the correlation between narcotic potency and the fall in surface tension between two phases. On this view, drug molecules were assumed to be packed in cell lipids in much the same way that they are concentrated at an interface. The hypothesis was not only based on evidence limited to homologous series of hydrocarbons but failed to explain the absence of narcotic activity in many surface active compounds. Nevertheless, it focused attention on the cell membrane as the probable site of narcotic action.

In 1939, Ferguson pointed out that these earlier theories could be unified by applying the thermodynamic concept of chemical potential. Thus, when a drug is distributed between various phases (external phase and biophase) and equilibrium is reached, the chemical potential of the drug in each phase is the same. Chemical potential may be defined as the partial molal free energy of the drug ($\bar{F}$) referred to a standard state (F_0). In the ideal case:

$$\bar{F} - F_0 = RT \ln a$$

where a is thermodynamic activity expressed as the natural logarithm, R the gas constant and T the absolute temperature (vol. 1, p. 14.9).

In practice an approximate value for the activity is given by the ratio p_t/p_s, where p_t is the partial pressure at the narcotic concentration and p_s the saturated vapour pressure at the temperature of the experiment, or by the ratio s_t/s_0, where s_t is the molar concentration for narcosis and s_0, the molar solubility of the drug. Such correlations of physical properties with narcotic activity, however, do no more than restate in more precise terms the conditions under which narcosis may be expected to occur.

More recently, it has been suggested that narcosis occurs when a constant fraction of a highly polar nonaqueous phase of the cell is occupied by molecules of the narcotic. The volume and mass of the molecules are then

important and may, for example, explain the greater potency of halothane ($CF_3CHClBr$) as compared with chloroform ($CHCl_3$). Such molecules might, by obstructing aqueous channels in the membrane, interfere with the movement of Na^+.

Apart from organic narcotics, there are the inert gases of which xenon is the most potent. Both nitrogen and argon produce anaesthesia when given under high partial pressure, but xenon is effective at normal atmospheric pressure. Atoms of the rare gases are incapable of forming covalent, ionic or hydrogen bonds with constituents of cells. However, they may form complex hydrates and these have been implicated in mechanisms underlying narcosis. The atoms of gas are seen either as nuclei for the formation of microcrystals of water, or as providing 'ice cover' at a membrane or surface of a protein, or as being absorbed into cellular interfaces, where they may change the effective dielectric constant and permeability of the membrane.

Polar narcotics, such as ethyl alcohol, are metabolized by cells; nonpolar narcotics, such as ether and chloroform, more closely resemble the inert gases and leave cells unchanged. Although these substances may have other pharmacological effects, the evidence suggests that their narcotic action is more readily explicable in biophysical than in biochemical terms. There is so far no convincing evidence that ether, chloroform, cyclopropane, nitrous oxide or xenon and similar narcotics act through selective inhibition of enzyme systems or by combining with receptors.

FURTHER READING

ALBERT A. (1968) *Selective Toxicity*, 4th Edition. London: Methuen.

CAMPBELL P.N. ed. (1968) *The Interaction of Drugs and Subcellular Components in Animal Cells*, Biological Council Symposium. London: Churchill.

GADDUM J.H. (1954) Discoveries in therapeutics. *J. Pharm. Pharmacol.* 6, 497.

HOLLAND W.C., KLEIN R.L. & BRIGGS A.H. (1964) *Introduction to Molecular Pharmacology*. London: Macmillan.

MONGAR J.L. & REUCK A.V.S., eds. (1962) *Enzymes and Drug Action*, Ciba Foundation Symposium. London: Churchill.

NORTHCOTE D.H., ed. (1968) Structure and function of membranes. *Brit. med. Bull.* 24.

ROBSON J.M. & STACEY R.S., ed. (1968) *Recent Advances in Pharmacology*, 4th Edition. London: Churchill.

SEXTON W.A. (1963) *Chemical Constitution and Biological Activity*, 3rd Edition. London: Spon.

WOLSTENHOLME G.E.W. & O'CONNOR CECILIA M., eds. (1959) *Regulation of Cell Metabolism*, Ciba Foundation Symposium. London: Churchill.

Chapter 2
The administration and fate of drugs

All drugs, apart from those applied superficially to skin or mucosal surfaces for purely local action, must be introduced into the body at some site. After this procedure, known as **administration**, there follows **absorption** from the site of administration and **distribution** by the blood stream to other parts of the organism. The drug then begins to disappear slowly or quickly from the body by **metabolism** and **excretion**, a process collectively called **clearance**; the term here is not to be confused with renal clearance. Fig. 2.1 illustrates these various factors, which constitute the study of pharmacodynamics.

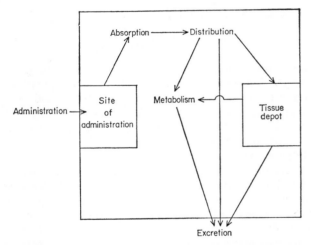

FIG. 2.1. Interrelationships of the various factors involved in the absorption and fate of drugs in the organism.

The main omission in this figure is the **site of action**, at which, naturally, a drug must arrive in order to produce its pharmacological or therapeutic effect. What happens there forms the subject matter of chap. 3. For present purposes, it is assumed that the drug reaches its site of action at some time during its sojourn in the body. This chapter, although emphasizing general principles underlying a drug's journey from administration to clearance, includes important practical aspects of drug administration. It describes the methods by which drugs may be given and how rates of absorption and duration of action

may be altered for specific therapeutic purposes. It underlines the clinical importance of studying the fate of drugs in the body.

Any chemical substance entering or leaving the organism must pass across at least one cell membrane. More commonly, several cell membranes have to be crossed. It is, therefore, necessary to consider the physicochemical mechanisms involved in the passage of drugs and other molecules across cell membranes before the various factors outlined in fig. 2.1 are considered.

FACTORS INFLUENCING PASSAGE OF DRUGS ACROSS CELL MEMBRANES

Nature of the membrane and passive diffusion

The semipermeable membrane surrounding cells consists of a bimolecular layer of lipid material sandwiched between layers of protein, the whole being about 8 nm thick (vol. 1, p. 13.6). If a substance which is readily soluble in lipid is applied to one side of such a membrane, it dissolves freely in the lipid material and establishes a bridgehead on the other side. Transfer then occurs across the membrane at a rate proportional to the concentration gradient. This process is purely passive and does not require the expenditure of energy.

Water, inorganic ions like sodium and chloride, and other small molecules which are not lipid soluble may also penetrate cells. This has led to the concept that the cell membrane is not continuous but is perforated by small pores or channels filled with water. Experiments, on the rat jejunum for instance, suggest that these pores have an effective radius of about 0·4 nm and let water-soluble molecules through up to a molecular weight of about 100. There are, of course, modifications of this fundamental structure in various parts of the body to cater for specialized function. Transport of certain essential nutrients and vitamins would be too inefficient by such purely passive processes, and specialized mechanisms have been evolved to facilitate their absorption from the gastrointestinal tract. The rare occurrence of specialized transport in the absorption of drugs is discussed on p. 2.3.

FACTORS INFLUENCING PASSIVE DIFFUSION OF LIPID-SOLUBLE SUBSTANCES

Diffusion of molecules through the lipid cell membrane depends on factors which render an organic compound soluble in fat or oil rather than water. This property may be measured in terms of its **partition coefficient** between an aqueous and an immiscible non-aqueous phase, e.g. olive oil or heptane, after equilibrium has been reached:

$$\text{partition coefficient} = K = \frac{\text{concentration in olive oil}}{\text{concentration in water}}$$

In general, water solubility of an organic substance is related to what physical chemists call the **polarity** of its molecules. In a polar molecule, at least one of the electron pairs forming a chemical bond between two atoms is displaced by the greater electron-attracting properties of one of the atoms in the bond, thereby disturbing the electrical symmetry of the whole molecule. Hence a definite dipole is produced, although the molecule is in no sense ionized (fig. 2.2). Such distortion of electrical

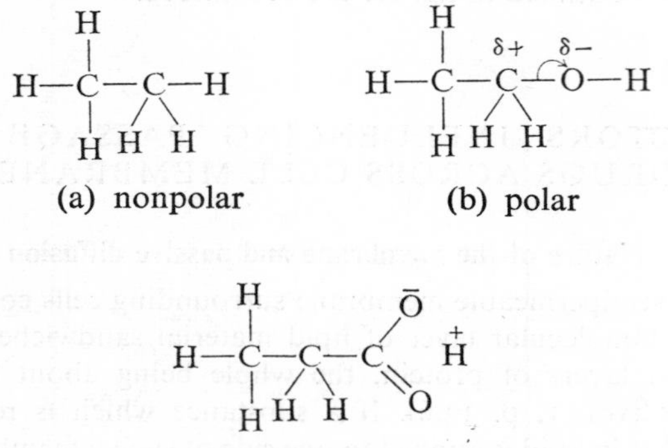

(a) nonpolar   (b) polar

(c) highly polar

FIG. 2.2. The effect of introducing polar groups (hydroxyl and carboxyl) into the nonpolar, lipid-soluble, water-insoluble hydrocarbon ethane (a). In ethyl alcohol (b), the high electronegativity of the oxygen atom causes displacement of the electron pair binding C to O towards the O atom. The O carries, therefore, a fractional negative charge ($\delta-$) and the C a fractional positive charge ($\delta+$). The polarity conferred on the molecule in this way is partly responsible for altering its solubility properties. Propionic acid (c), which can ionize under suitable pH conditions to a molecule with a full negative charge on the O, is even more highly polar.

neutrality is absent or minimal in molecules like the hydrocarbons, but is enhanced by the introduction of strongly electronegative atoms like oxygen, sulphur or halogen. Hydroxyl (OH), carboxyl (COOH), nitro (NO_2) and others are typical polar groups, and the compounds in which they occur are said to be polar. When a substance is in an ionized form, the molecule is even more highly polar. As a general rule, polar substances are soluble in polar solvents such as water or alcohol and insoluble in

nonpolar solvents like the hydrocarbons. The reverse is true of nonpolar substances.

In the case of weak organic acids and bases, a complication arises which is of great importance in understanding drug absorption. These compounds exist simultaneously in both ionized and un-ionized forms in a ratio dependent on the pH of the medium in which they are dissolved. Thus the un-ionized molecule is less polar, and therefore more lipid soluble than the ionized form. Consequently a weak acid or base most readily penetrates the lipid membrane of the cell at the pH at which it is least ionized. Certain strong organic acids or bases, sulphonic acid derivatives or quaternary ammonium bases, are, on the contrary, ionized over a wide range of pH, have low lipid solubility and so are poorly absorbed across cell boundaries.

THE pK_a OF DRUGS

Because most drugs are either weak acids or bases, it is useful to know their strength, which is expressed in terms of their pK_a (vol. 1, p. 6.4). There it was shown that for a weak acid HA,

$$pK_a = pH + \log \frac{[HA]}{[A^-]} \tag{1}$$

and for a weak base BOH,

$$pK_a = pH + \log \frac{[B^+]}{[BOH]} \tag{2}$$

Since the stronger an acid or base is, the more completely it ionizes in solution, it follows from equations (1) and (2) that a high pK_a indicates a weak acid or a strong base, and that a low pK_a indicates a strong acid or a weak base. Fig. 2.3 shows the pK_a values of a number of well-known acidic and basic drugs.

Equations (1) and (2) show also that at a pH equal to the pK_a of a drug, the ratio of ionized to un-ionized molecules is unity. For an acid, a shift of pH to the acid side of the pK_a reduces the degree of ionization, and raising the pH to the alkaline side of the pK_a increases ionization. The converse is true for a basic drug. For an acidic drug with a pK_a of about 4, e.g. the familiar aspirin or acetylsalicylic acid, it can be calculated from equation (1) that, at a pH of 2, $\log [HA]/[A^-] = 4-2 = 2$, and therefore only about 1 per cent of the aspirin is ionized at that pH. On the other hand, it can be shown that, at pH 7, only 0·1 per cent of the aspirin is in the un-ionized form. Since the un-ionized molecules of a drug are more lipid soluble and cross the cell membranes more readily, the pH at the site of administration, as well as the pK_a of the drug, is important in determining its absorption and distribution in the body.

Processes involving specialized transport

Since many of the essential metabolites and nutrients consist of lipid-insoluble molecules, their rapid transfer across gastrointestinal membranes is believed to occur with the help of **carriers**. A carrier can be regarded as a membrane component capable of forming a complex with the substance to be conveyed, the substrate. The

system is that high concentrations of the transported substance saturate the carrier so that the amount which can be conveyed is limited. This contrasts with the process of passive diffusion across lipid membranes, or through

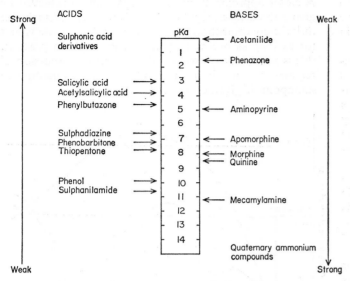

FIG. 2.3. The pK_a values of some acidic and basic drugs. From Brodie B.B. (1964) *Absorption and Distribution of Drugs*, ed. T.B. Binns. Edinburgh: Livingstone.

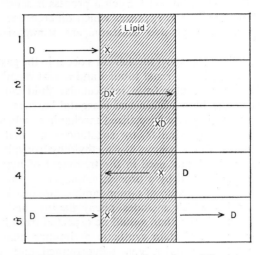

FIG. 2.4. Schematic representation of specialized transport of a drug (D) across a lipid membrane by means of a carrier (X). Serial steps 1 to 5 are illustrated.

complex moves across the membrane and releases the substrate on the other side (fig. 2.4). Simple passive diffusion of the substrate itself may, of course, occur simultaneously with carrier transport.

A characteristic property of a carrier-aided transport

pores, where the amount conveyed increases proportionally with its concentration.

Two types of carrier-aided transport may be distinguished. In **facilitated diffusion**, the physicochemical properties of the carrier–substrate complex speed up passage across the membrane, but the final osmotic equilibrium is not appreciably different from that which

TABLE 2.1. Comparison of passive diffusion and active transport. Modified from Milne M.D. (1964) *Brit. med. J.* **1**, 328.

Parameter	Passive diffusion	Active transport
(a) Concentration	Movement only from high to low concentrations	Transport from low to high concentration occurs
(b) Size of molecule	Smaller molecules in general diffuse at a greater rate	Speed of transport not necessarily related to molecular size
(c) Stereospecificity	Rate of transfer of stereoisomers is the same	Often the naturally occurring isomer is more effectively transported
(d) Saturation of system	Rate of transfer proportional to concentration gradient with no limiting maximal rate	Rate of transfer not proportional to concentration gradient and approaches a limiting maximal value
(e) Competitive inhibition	Rate of transfer unaffected by presence of closely related compounds	Rate of transfer reduced by simultaneous transport of a related compound sharing the same carrier system
(f) Noncompetitive inhibition	Rate of transfer not affected unless obvious cellular damage occurs	Transport reduced by metabolic poisons, e.g. dinitrophenol

would be attained theoretically by passive diffusion. In short, there is no transfer against a concentration gradient ('uphill'). In **active transport**, the substrate is taken up against a concentration gradient, and expenditure of energy is involved. Such a process is sensitive to metabolic inhibitors. Features which differentiate active transport from passive diffusion are summarized in table 2.1.

Specialized transport mechanisms occur in the gastrointestinal tract, in the renal tubules and across membranes dividing extracellular from intracellular fluid compartments at the blood–brain and placental barriers. Drugs are involved in these specialized mechanisms when they are structurally similar to substances of metabolic importance. For example, L-α-methyldihydroxyphenylalanine (methyldopa), used in the treatment of hypertension, is transported by a process employed by the organism for a large group of L-monoamino-monocarboxylic amino acids which includes phenylalanine, and so is absorbed far better than would be expected from its low lipid solubility. Certain synthetic pyrimidine analogues with cytotoxic activity, e.g. 5-fluorouracil and 5-bromouracil, are absorbed by the active mechanisms for uracil and thymine. Drugs known to be absorbed in this way are, however, few in number. Another effect to be borne in mind is that some drugs may suppress or impair these specialized gastrointestinal absorption mechanisms. For example, the antibiotic neomycin, when given orally, may induce malabsorption with histological changes in the jejunal mucosa.

ADMINISTRATION AND ABSORPTION OF DRUGS

The objectives of drug administration

Drugs must be given in such a manner that they reach their site of action as rapidly as possible and in adequate concentration. A therapeutic regime should ensure maintenance of the necessary concentration at the site of action for as long as is required. Then the drug should disappear rapidly from the body. Needless to say, this ideal is difficult to attain, but there are good clinical reasons for attempting an approximation to it (thick line in fig. 2.5). Therapeutic levels are needed quickly in an emergency and then the correct choice of route of administration is particularly important. If an inadequate dose of drug is given, the concentration may rise slowly and never attain the therapeutic level (curve 1, fig. 2.5). This may be dangerous, e.g. in treating a bacterial infection with antibiotics, concentrations too low to kill all the micro-organisms may encourage the development of antibiotic-resistant strains. Trying to overcome this problem by giving a large dose ensures an adequate therapeutic level for the time interval AB, but there is

danger that for a short period CD a toxic level of drug may occur (curve 2, fig. 2.5). An intermediate dose may be selected which avoids toxic effects but which provides therapeutic concentrations for a shorter time than AB. A closer approximation to the ideal can be achieved by giving the drug at regular intervals in doses of such size that the concentration remains at near therapeutic values for as long as necessary (curve 3, fig. 2.5). In practice, this is nearly always what is done. Further discussion of regimes of drug administration from a more quantitative standpoint is given on p. 2.17.

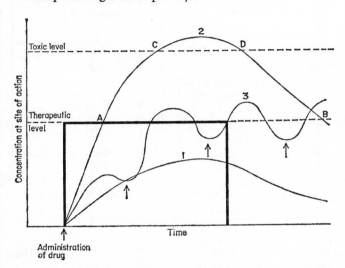

FIG. 2.5. Possible time–concentration curves after administration of drugs. ↑ = administration of drug dose. Thick line, ideal; curve 1, inadequate dose; curve 2, excessive dose; curve 3, showing how repeated dosage can keep drug at more or less therapeutic levels for as long as required.

Routes of drug administration

The most rapid way to introduce a drug into the circulation is to inject it directly into a vein; the simplest is to ask the patient to swallow a pill. Between these two extremes are many other methods, all with their advantages and disadvantages (table 2.2).

ORAL AND ENTERAL ADMINISTRATION

The oral method is convenient, safe and economical and is preferred by patients so long as the drug is palatable. However, a drug given in this way has to survive a number of possible hazards before reaching the circulation. Quite apart from the unpredictable vagaries of absorption to be discussed later, the drug is likely to become mixed with food and water and is exposed to the potentially destructive action of strong hydrochloric acid in the stomach and of a variety of enzymes. If it is irritant to the gastric mucosa it may be vomited, or if it has purgative properties it may pass too rapidly down the gut for efficient absorption. Even after absorption, the drug has

TABLE 2.2. Possible routes of drug administration.

Enteral	Parenteral	Mucosal (other than gastrointestinal)	Percutaneous	Local
Sublingual	Subcutaneous (sc)	Nasal	Inunction	Skin
Oral	Intramuscular (im)	Bronchial	Iontophoresis	Conjunctiva
Colonic	Intravenous (iv)	Urethral		Pleura
Rectal	Intra-arterial (ia)	Vaginal		
	Intraperitoneal (ip)			
	Intrasternal			
	Intrathecal			
	Intracardiac			
	Intra-articular			

to run the gauntlet of the liver and its metabolizing enzymes. The oral route is too slow for emergencies and obviously cannot be used when the patient is vomiting or moribund. Drug manufacturers have used their ingenuity to overcome some of these problems. Acid-sensitive drugs are enclosed in capsules of gelatin or other resistant materials which do not dissolve until they reach the duodenum ('enteric-coated' drugs). On a more sophisticated level, synthetic antibiotics closely related to penicillin have been introduced which, unlike benzylpenicillin, are not destroyed by gastric acid.

Some drugs are absorbed rapidly through the oral mucous membranes, especially from the highly vascular sublingual area, and so escape the hazards of stomach and liver. Drugs such as glyceryl trinitrate for angina pectoris, isoprenaline for bronchial asthma, and ergotamine for migraine, which have high lipid solubility and low ionization at salivary pH, effectively penetrate oral mucous membranes. Raising the pH of the saliva, as is done by Peruvian Indians when they chew euphoriant coca leaves with lime, depresses the ionization of a basic drug, in this case cocaine, and promotes its mucosal absorption. The main disadvantage of **sublingual administration** is a liability to produce mucosal ulceration if used repeatedly. Rectal and colonic mucosa may also be used for the rapid absorption of drugs. A drug can be given rectally in solid form as a **suppository**, e.g. aminophylline for the relief of bronchoconstriction, or in solution as an **enema**, e.g. paraldehyde for sedation.

PARENTERAL ADMINISTRATION

If a drug cannot be given by mouth, it is usually necessary to inject it, using a sterile syringe and an aseptic technique. A choice of routes is available, depending on the speed of absorption desired and the site where therapeutic action is required. Absorption from a **subcutaneous** site on the forearm, shoulder or leg is slow owing to the relatively low vascularity. This may be useful for ensuring a prolonged action. Irritant drugs are liable to induce necrosis and sloughing if given subcutaneously, and are

safer by deep **intramuscular** injection. Absorption from muscle, e.g. the gluteal and deltoid muscles, is more rapid than from a subcutaneous site. The most rapid route is, of course, **intravenous** injection which distributes a drug throughout the body within the circulation time, i.e. about 15–20 sec.

Intravenous injection of drugs in aqueous solution has many advantages. The rapidity of action and the control of plasma concentration made possible by this procedure are important in emergencies. Many irritant and hypertonic solutions should not be given by any other route, e.g. the alkaline (pH 10–11) sodium thiopentone used for general anaesthesia. Fortunately, vein walls, unlike arterial walls, are relatively insensitive structures, and the drug, if injected slowly over a period of at least 1 min, is diluted and buffered by the flow of blood. Sometimes the dose need not be decided beforehand, but can be titrated to the response of the patient, e.g. sodium thiopentone can be injected slowly until unconsciousness is produced. For prolonged action, drugs may be given by continuous intravenous infusion in isotonic saline or dextrose solution. At the same time, intravenous injection may be hazardous, and once the drug is given it cannot be retrieved; a high concentration of drug suddenly reaching the heart or brain may produce an untoward response and there is a much greater chance of a severe hypersensitivity reaction, including anaphylactic shock (p. 23.1). Serious tissue damage may follow accidental extravenous injection, especially with irritant drugs. Accidental intra-arterial injection with irritant drugs may lead to spasm of the artery and distal gangrene in limb or digit. Repeated intravenous injections depend on a good supply of veins, not always readily available in the shocked, old or obese patient, and thrombophlebitis may develop if the same vein is used repeatedly.

Other parenteral routes are of limited application. **Intra-arterial** injection of radio-opaque substances for arteriograms, and intra-arterial perfusion of cytotoxic drugs in treatment of local cancer are performed in hospitals. **Intraperitoneal** injection, utilizing the large absorbing surface of the peritoneal cavity, is seldom used because of the danger of introducing infection and producing adhesions, but is occasionally valuable, for example when giving radioactive gold for malignant effusions in the abdomen. Injections into the bone marrow of the sternum (**intrasternal**) or of the tibia and femur, in children, ensure rapid entry of the drug into the circulation, and may be useful in infants or in adults with poor veins due to circulatory collapse, extensive burns, etc. Injections into the subarachnoid space (**intrathecal** or **intraspinal**) are often necessary for treating meningeal infections, as drugs given intravenously do not always penetrate well into the cerebrospinal fluid. Spinal anaesthesia also involves this route of administration. **Intra-articular** injections are occasionally used in patients with arthritis. **Intracardiac** injections are sometimes given in cardiac arrest.

MUCOSAL SURFACES, OTHER THAN ORAL AND GASTROINTESTINAL

Drugs may be absorbed through mucosal surfaces other than the oral and gastrointestinal. The richly vascular **nasal mucosa** can readily absorb vasopressin, nicotine from snuff or cocaine from 'snow' used by addicts. The extensive surface of the **bronchioles** and **alveoli**, excellent for drug absorption, is best reached by gaseous or volatile drugs which can be inhaled, e.g., the general anaesthetic ether or the volatile amyl nitrite used for angina pectoris. Solutions of nonvolatile substances can be converted in a nebulizer to give an **aerosol spray** containing particles small enough to penetrate to the alveolar wall. Adrenaline, ephedrine or isoprenaline for asthma, and ergotamine for migraine, are examples of drugs which can be given in this way (p. 9.6).

PERCUTANEOUS AND LOCAL ADMINISTRATION

Very few drugs can penetrate intact healthy skin, but those which do may present a hazard. An example is di-isopropylfluorophosphonate (Dyflos), a potent anti-cholinesterase; this and similar organophosphates are used as insecticides in agriculture and are liable to poison the careless farmworker. Some drugs can be intentionally rubbed in; Henry VIII and many other famous men in the sixteenth and seventeenth centuries received mercury by **inunction** for syphilis, but this procedure is not used today. Another technique of percutaneous injection is **iontophoresis**, in which the drug in ionized form is made to migrate through the skin under the influence of a suitably oriented electric potential.

Finally, it should be remembered that drugs are sometimes not intended to be absorbed but to remain localized for therapeutic action. Examples are local anaesthetics, antibiotics for the treatment of wounds or ulcers, and drugs used in the treatment of skin diseases.

Factors influencing rate of absorption

Apart from its route of administration, the rate of absorption of a drug depends mainly on the following:

(1) concentration of the drug at the site of absorption,
(2) molecular weight of the drug,
(3) physicochemical properties of the drug, especially its solubility and pK_a, and
(4) vascularity and area of absorbing surface, and the pH at the site of administration.

The concentration of the drug at the site of absorption is important since a strong solution of a drug is likely to diffuse passively across lipid membranes faster than a more dilute solution. Other things being equal, therefore, the rate of absorption is increased by increasing the dose of the drug.

Drugs of molecular weight greater than 20,000 tend to be absorbed into the lymphatics rather than the blood capillaries and so take longer to reach the general circulation.

At the time of administration a drug need not be in solution. A drug in solid form may dissolve in tissue fluids, and its rate of absorption is then directly related to its rate of solution. Here, physical properties of a drug play a part. A fine amorphous powder dissolves more quickly than do crystals of the same substance, and colloidal preparations dissolve slowly. This principle is used to delay the absorption of insulin from subcutaneous sites. Insulin zinc suspensions prepared in amorphous powder form (semilente) are absorbed quite rapidly, but a crystalline form (ultralente) is absorbed more slowly (p. 6.17).

Some drugs can be compressed into pellets and given subcutaneously as **implants**. A pellet goes into solution slowly, and a fine connective tissue capsule, through which the drug has to diffuse, may form round it. Certain hormones used in endocrine replacement therapy, e.g., testosterone or deoxycorticosterone may be given as implants, and their effects may last for several months. Their absorption tends to be unreliable.

It is sometimes possible to retard the absorption of a soluble drug by making a more insoluble complex or chemical derivative which is slowly broken down to the active principle at the site of administration. Insulin may be combined with protamine or globin to form the more slowly absorbed protamine zinc insulin or globin zinc insulin. Diphtheria toxoid used in immunization may be precipitated with alum, so that the injected complex provides a low but sustained level of toxoid in the circulation. Procaine penicillin is a salt less rapidly absorbed than penicillin itself. Esters of certain hormones, e.g. testosterone propionate, are broken down in the tissues quite slowly to the active substance. Another similar method is to inject a solid drug suspended in olive oil, arachis oil or propylene glycol.

Few fat-soluble drugs are given for their systemic

effects, but anthelminths and insecticides, e.g. hexyl-resorcinol and DDT, are absorbed in small quantity in the small intestine, probably in micelles formed during the digestion of dietary fat. Fat-soluble vitamins are also absorbed in this way.

As already mentioned, the pK_a of a drug affects the rate of absorption, since the un-ionized form of a molecule is less polar, more lipid soluble and, therefore, more readily transported across the cell membrane. Thus strongly basic or acidic drugs are poorly absorbed, and the pH at the site of absorption determines the rate of absorption of drugs of weaker acidity or basicity.

Sites of administration differ in their vascularity and area of absorbing surface, and these factors greatly influence the speed of absorption. For example, intramuscular sites are more vascular than are subcutaneous. The pulmonary epithelium has an especially large absorbent surface for inhaled drugs. It is also possible to a certain degree to vary these factors intentionally at a particular site of administration, and thereby influence rate of absorption. Heat and massage increase vascularity and accelerate absorption of a drug; conversely, cold, or keeping the site of injection immobile, retard absorption. The addition of a vasoconstrictor substance like adrenaline delays absorption, or even prevents it completely. This is why procaine is injected with adrenaline for local anaesthesia, where systemic absorption of the procaine is undesirable. The enzyme hyaluronidase (hyalase), which breaks down the ground substance mucopolysaccharide, hyaluronic acid, is sometimes used to accelerate the absorption of drugs. Hyalase, by opening up the tissue planes, increases the area available for absorption. An example is ergometrine and hyalase given intramuscularly for controlling post-partum haemorrhage.

The pH at the site of administration influences the rate of absorption since on it depends the degree to which most weakly acidic or basic drugs are ionized. The pH at most parenteral sites differs little from the pH of plasma (7·4), at which very few weak bases or acids are highly ionized. The pH in the gastrointestinal tract, however, varies widely from one region to another, and the relationship of absorption to pH and pK_a has been studied carefully in recent years.

In general, it can be predicted that weak acids are well absorbed from the stomach (pH 1·0) because their ionization is suppressed, and less well absorbed from the duodenum and upper small intestine (pH 6·6). The converse is true of weak bases.

Fig. 2.6 illustrates these principles for the absorption of two drugs, a very weak base phenazone (pK_a 1·4) and a weak acid phenylbutazone (pK_a 4·4), from acid gastric juice (pH 1·0) across the gastric mucosa into plasma (pH 7·4). The degree of ionization at the two pH values can be calculated from equations (1) and (2), given on p. 2.2. Since only un-ionized molecules pass the lipid membrane of the gastric mucosa, the concentrations of un-ionized drug are the same on both sides at final equilibrium. Here these concentrations are taken as unity in both gastric juice and plasma. With phenazone, for example, out of seven molecules in gastric juice five are ionized and two un-ionized (giving a ratio of 2·5 : 1), but in plasma only one-millionth (10^{-6}) is in ionized form. Hence, at equilibrium, when the concentration of un-ionized drug is equal on both sides, the ratio of total phenazone in gastric juice to that in plasma is $1 + 2·5$: $1 + 10^{-6}$, or about 3·5. Similarly for phenylbutazone, the concentration ratio between gastric juice and plasma is $1 + 10^{-3·4}$: $1 + 10^{3}$, or about 10^{-3}. In short, for practical purposes phenylbutazone should be completely absorbed from the stomach, whereas only about 22 per cent of phenazone should enter the plasma. Experiments on dogs with Heidenhain pouches in fact confirm 100 per cent absorption for phenylbutazone, and about 19 per cent absorption only for phenazone, figures in close agreement with the theoretical. Of course, this static model of gastric absorption is oversimplified as it ignores clearance by blood flow as the drugs permeate the gastric mucosa.

Some experimental studies with the rat stomach, ligated at both ends, have been carried out to compare drug absorption at pH 1·0 with that after raising the gastric pH to 8·0 with sodium bicarbonate. These results are

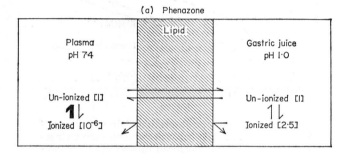

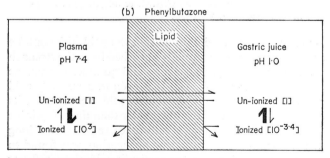

FIG. 2.6. Mechanism of distribution of (a) a very weak base phenazone (pK_a 1.4) and (b) a weak acid phenylbutazone (pK_a 4.4) between gastric juice and plasma. Figures in square brackets represent relative concentrations of ionized and un-ionized species, the concentration of un-ionized molecules being taken always as unity. Data of Brodie B.B. (1964) *Absorption and Distribution of Drugs*, ed. T.B. Binns. Edinburgh: Livingstone.

TABLE 2.3. Comparison of gastric absorption at 1 hr of 1 mg of drug in 5 ml of solution, at pH 1·0 and pH 8·0 in the rat. From Brodie B.B. (1964) *Absorption and Distribution of Drugs*, ed. T.B. Binns. Edinburgh: Livingstone.

Drugs	pK_a	Absorption at pH 1·0 (%)	Absorption at pH 8·0 (%)
Acids			
5-Sulphosalicylic acid	fully ionized	0	0
Salicylic acid	3·0	61	13
Thiopentone	7·6	46	34
Bases			
Aniline	4·6	6	56
Quinine	8·4	0	18

shown in table 2.3 and confirm that acidic drugs are better absorbed at low pH and basic drugs at high pH. This was shown to be equally true in three volunteer scientists to whom a number of drugs was administered in 0·1 *N* hydrochloric acid. The percentage absorption from the stomach was measured over a period of 40 min (fig. 2.7).

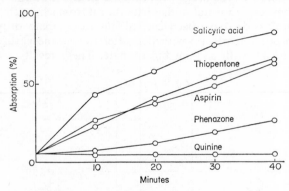

FIG. 2.7. Human gastric absorption of drugs from 0.1 *N* hydrochloric acid. The per cent concentration changes due to absorption are the mean values from three individuals. Data of Hogben C.A.M. *et al.* (1957) *J. Pharmacol. exp. Ther.* **120**, 540.

As expected, the acidic drugs salicylic acid, thiopentone and aspirin were more rapidly absorbed from the stomach than the basic drugs phenazone and quinine. Phenazone is so weak a base (pK_a 1·4) that even in a strongly acid medium it is not completely ionized; this accounts for its absorption being appreciably greater than that of quinine (pK_a 8·4). Ethyl alcohol, a substance regarded for long as the exemplar of gastric drug absorption, was found to be less rapidly absorbed than salicylic acid, though faster than aspirin.

These considerations have led in recent years to a better appreciation of the important role of the stomach in drug absorption. Furthermore, if a drug is partially absorbed through the gastric mucosa, local factors in the stomach may need to be taken into account in assessing how much

is absorbed in specific cases. For example, the low gastric acid secretion rate common in feverish illness, or the achlorhydria of pernicious anaemia, diminishes the absorption of acidic drugs. Since most drugs are given after meals to avoid gastric irritation, the presence of food in the stomach may also alter absorption by modifying pH or gastric emptying time. Reversible combinations of the drug with some constituent of the food may produce a relatively insoluble complex which is slowly absorbed. All these factors may be added to those mentioned on p. 2.4 which make oral administration of drugs unreliable.

Finally, intentional alteration of stomach pH may sometimes be used to increase or decrease gastric absorption of drugs. Giving the drug with sodium bicarbonate decreases the absorption of a weak acid, e.g. salicylate (p. 5.55), and increases absorption of weak bases.

DISTRIBUTION OF DRUGS

Once absorbed into the circulation, a drug in most cases has to gain access to extravascular tissues in order to reach its site of action. To do this, it has to pass through another lipid membrane, the capillary endothelium. The distribution of a drug, therefore, is again related to molecular size and lipid solubility and to an additional factor, binding to plasma components. Substances of high molecular weight, like proteins or the polysaccharide dextran, diffuse only slowly, if at all, across the capillary endothelium. For this reason, solutions of dextran given intravenously may be used in cases of severe blood loss when plasma or blood is not immediately available. If a drug becomes bound to plasma proteins it also remains in the blood stream. For this reason the dye Evans Blue can be used for the estimation of plasma volume.

Binding of drugs is predominantly to albumin, and has important consequences. In the first place, only the unbound drug possesses pharmacological activity and the protein–drug complex is inactive.

Drug (active) + protein $\rightleftharpoons$ drug–protein (inactive)

So although drugs which are strongly protein-bound tend to stay for a long time in the circulation, this is not necessarily an advantage as the level of therapeutic activity is liable to be low. However, once the plasma proteins have become saturated with a drug, further administration may lead to a sudden and unexpected increase in pharmacological effects due to a rise in the concentration of unbound drug molecules. In states of hypoalbuminaemia the patient may be surprisingly sensitive to small doses of such drugs. Another danger arises when a second drug, with even stronger binding power than the first, is given to the patient. The displacement of the first drug can enhance unexpectedly its pharmacological effect or elevate the free drug concentration to toxic levels. This may happen with dicoumarol, an anticoagulant which is displaced from its protein by certain long-acting sulphonamides; this leads to danger of haemorrhage from the increased activity of the dicoumarol.

$$\text{Dicoumarol} + \text{protein} \rightleftharpoons \text{dicoumarol–protein}$$

$$\text{Dicoumarol} - \text{protein} + \text{sulphonamide} \rightleftharpoons$$
$$\text{sulphonamide–protein} + \text{dicoumarol}$$

Extracellular and intracellular compartments

Drugs that enter the interstitial fluid may be sufficiently lipid soluble to penetrate tissue cells. In general, drugs which are strongly ionized at body fluid pH and therefore relatively lipid insoluble tend to remain in the extracellular fluid compartment. Also un-ionized molecules like inulin, small enough to get out of the blood stream but too large to enter cells, and inorganic ions which are actively kept out of cells (Cl^-, Br^-, CNS^-), are confined to the extracellular space. On the other hand, weak acids and bases, which constitute the majority of drugs, are distributed throughout the total body water.

Drugs do not penetrate quite so freely to certain fractions of the extracellular water, such as cerebrospinal, lymphatic, synovial, pericardial, peritoneal and pleural fluids. These normally constitute less than 5 per cent of the extracellular water, but may be increased in inflammatory disease. The CSF must be considered in more detail, as many drugs penetrate there poorly from the systemic circulation. This phenomenon has led to the concept of the blood–brain barrier (vol. 1, p. 24.86).

The blood–brain barrier

Drugs in the blood stream may reach the brain through the brain capillaries, or appear in the CSF via the choroid plexus. A small molecule of high lipid solubility such as urea penetrates into brain and CSF at a much slower rate than it does into nonnervous tissue like muscle (fig. 2.8). There is, therefore, some sort of barrier to rapid equilibrium across the two boundaries, i.e. blood–brain and blood–CSF. From CSF to brain, on the other hand, diffusion is known to take place quite freely. What actually causes these barriers is not clear. The brain capillaries under the electron microscope are not different from capillaries elsewhere in the body, but they are surrounded by glial processes which may possibly alter their permeability. None the less, it is still lipid solubility which is the most important factor determining passage into the CSF, as is shown in fig. 2.9.

Other factors may help to explain the blood–CSF barrier. The choroid epithelium actively secretes organic ions from CSF to blood by mechanisms similar to those operating in the proximal tubules of the kidney. Thus,

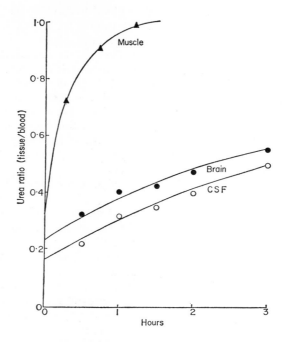

FIG. 2.8. Entry of urea into muscle, whole brain and CSF of the rabbit. Blood urea was raised to 300 mg/100 ml before the experiment, and kept constant at that level. Data from Kleeman, Davson & Levin (1962) *Amer. J. Physiol.* **203**, 739.

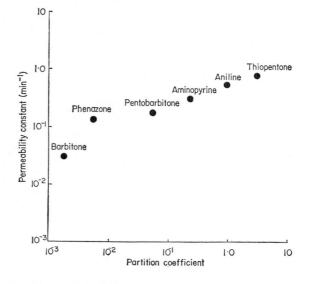

FIG. 2.9. Rate constants for entry of drugs into the CSF, expressed in reciprocal minutes. Partition coefficients are between heptane and water for the un-ionized drug. Data from Brodie, Kurz & Schanker (1960) *J. Pharmacol. exp. Ther.* **130**, 20.

penicillin is rapidly returned to blood from CSF, just as it is efficiently secreted by kidney tubules (p. 11.10). This could account for the apparently poor penetration of this antibiotic into the CSF. Further, substances injected into the CSF intracisternally are often quickly excreted back to the general circulation through the arachnoid villi. This process tends to make CSF concentrations of a drug lower than plasma concentrations. There may also be carrier systems for certain amino acids and sugars required for brain metabolism. However, knowledge of how chemical substances are transported from the circulation to the brain is fragmentary.

In clinical practice two types of drug are required to cross the blood–brain barrier:

(1) chemotherapeutic agents and antibiotics given for the treatment of meningeal and CNS infections, and

(2) drugs used to modify CNS activity.

For severe infection it may be preferable, or even essential, to give the drug, e.g. penicillin, intrathecally. However, it should not be forgotten that the infection itself may render the CNS more accessible to systemic drugs by altering the permeability of the blood–brain barrier. Factors influencing the penetration of drugs acting on the CNS itself are still incompletely understood, though lipid solubility plays an important role here as elsewhere.

The placental barrier

The transfer of potentially harmful drugs from mother to foetus has been highlighted by the thalidomide tragedy. As with the brain, ignorance of the processes involved has been veiled by coining the term placental barrier. Again, un-ionized lipid-soluble substances of low molecular weight, e.g. thiopentone, cross to the foetus more readily than ionized molecules or compounds of high molecular weight. The placenta is a metabolizing tissue, and may inactivate endogenous substances like histamine or 5-HT. The placenta, therefore, acts partly as a protective organ for the foetus. However, drug metabolites formed by placental enzymes might on occasion be more toxic than their precursor, and harm the foetus. Certain polar metabolites of thalidomide, produced in the placenta or the foetus, are now thought to be responsible for the teratogenicity of this drug. It is becoming widely appreciated that as few drugs as possible should be given in pregnancy for fear of adverse reactions on the foetus (p. 12.17).

Tissue binding and redistribution

Just as some drugs are bound to plasma proteins, others have a special affinity for certain tissues, where they are bound in relatively high concentrations. This means that the initial distribution leads immediately to a **redistribution,** and to partial or complete disappearance of the drug from the circulation. In these cases, an attempt to calculate the volume of distribution of the drug from the ratio, dose/concentration in plasma, produces an absurd figure in excess of total body volume. The site at which a drug acts is not necessarily the site at which it achieves its highest concentration. Digoxin, for example, acts mainly on the heart but is present in greatest concentration in the liver. However, mercurial diuretics are concentrated in the renal cortex, where they act. Drugs may be bound in adipose tissue, liver, connective tissue and bones. They may also be taken up by an active process, e.g. the thyroid gland takes up iodine against a concentration gradient.

Drugs that are bound by a tissue may disappear so quickly from the blood as to arouse the suspicion that they are being rapidly metabolized or excreted. An example is the barbiturate anaesthetic thiopentone. After intravenous injection, the drug crosses the blood–brain barrier and reaches the CNS in sufficient concentration to produce unconsciousness within 30 sec. However, redistribution to body fat, which even in an apparently thin woman constitutes 15 per cent of the body mass, is so rapid that concentrations in brain and blood fall precipitously and the patient soon recovers consciousness. Hence the drug is short-acting, not because, as was once thought, of rapid metabolism, but due to its redistribution to adipose tissue. If body fats are saturated with thiopentone by repeated dosage, this barbiturate becomes a relatively long-acting drug. The persistence in fat depots of lipid-soluble substances may become a problem in this age of chemical insecticides such as DDT (p. 32.6).

The binding of certain drugs in the liver can be exploited for therapeutic purposes; for example, chloroquine combines with nucleoproteins in the liver to reach a concentration 200–700 times greater than in the plasma. Although primarily an antimalarial drug, chloroquine is for this reason effective in amoebic hepatitis.

Bone takes up a variety of elements like lead and other heavy metals, fluoride and radiostrontium (^{90}Sr) from radioactive fall out. Tetracycline antibiotics given in pregnancy are liable to stain the infant's first teeth an unsightly brown colour. Phosphorus is taken up by bone marrow and concentrated in the white cells and so ^{32}P may be used for treatment of leukaemia.

CLEARANCE OF DRUGS

The **clearance** of a drug may occur in two ways:

(1) metabolism to another compound or compounds, and

(2) excretion.

A drug may undergo both processes and be excreted partly unchanged and partly as the products of its metabolism.

METABOLISM

Enzymes which metabolize drugs may be classified into three main groups.

ENZYMES OF INTERMEDIARY METABOLISM

Firstly, there are the normal enzymes of intermediary metabolism. Some drugs are sufficiently like normal body metabolites that they are acted upon by these enzymes. The drug L-α-methyldihydroxyphenylalanine (methyldopa) is converted to α-methylnoradrenaline by enzymes involved in the metabolic pathway of DOPA to adrenaline via dopamine and noradrenaline. It is the formation of this false transmitter at sympathetic nerve endings which is thought to be responsible for part of the therapeutic activity of the drug (p. 15.31). Apart from antimetabolites such as mercaptopurine, which were devised for the purpose, however, relatively few drugs compete with substrates of normal metabolic pathways, possibly because the modern synthetic chemist makes so many compounds containing structures quite unfamiliar to mammalian metabolism.

CONJUGATING ENZYMES

The next category consists of enzymes which are located principally in the liver, but also in a few other tissues, and act on substances containing hydroxyl, amino or other suitably reactive groups. This process, known as **conjugation**, involves the condensation of the substance with glucuronic acid, acetic acid, sulphuric acid, glycine or ribose among others. Such reactions require energy, usually derived from ATP. The resulting compound is as a rule more water soluble and therefore more rapidly excreted in the urine. Many hormones and steroids are metabolized in this way, which is a physiological mechanism whereby the organism disarms and then excretes these substances; e.g. progesterone is reduced to pregnandiol and excreted largely as the glucuronide (table 2.4 for further examples). Not only is the conjugate more water soluble, it often has little or none of the biological activity of the unconjugated precursor (vol. 1, p. 31.11). Conjugating enzymes are on the whole not very specific and commonly act upon a variety of drugs. These tend to fall into the general categories listed in table 2.4, i.e. they are phenols like salicylic acid, or amines like the sulphonamides. In the case of drugs, the conjugate may be more insoluble than the drug and less readily excreted in the urine. Some of the acetylated sulphonamides may crystallize out in the kidneys and cause renal damage. A term which has often been applied to this type of drug metabolism, **detoxification**, may therefore be misleading. The metabolites are not necessarily less active or less toxic than the drug itself.

NONSPECIFIC ENZYMES OF THE LIVER MICROSOMES

The enzymes so far mentioned act only on drugs which resemble intermediary metabolites or which have a suitable group for conjugation. It is a matter for some surprise, therefore, that many of the synthetic drugs containing bizarre and unphysiological chemical structures made in the chemical laboratory are none the less actively metabolized in the body. The microsomes of liver cells in zone 3 contain active, nonspecific enzymes, which can metabolize a wide range of compounds. They are especially active on substances of high lipid solubility,

TABLE 2.4. Examples of conjugation of chemical substances (endogenous and exogenous).

Class of compound	Example	Conjugated with	Product
Phenols, alcohols, carboxylic acids	Salicylamide	Glucuronic acid (*O*-glucuronyl transferase)	Salicylamide glucuronide
Phenols	Oestriol	Glucuronic acid and sulphuric acid	Glucuronide and ethereal sulphate
Aromatic acids	Benzoic acid	Glycine	Hippuric acid
Phenolic compounds	Noradrenaline	Methyl groups (*O*-methyltransferase)	Normetanephrine
Amines	Sulphanilamide	Acetic acid (acetyltransferase)	Acetyl derivative
	Histamine	Ribose	Riboside of imidazole acetic acid

which readily penetrate the lipid membrane of the endoplasmic reticulum. These enzymes are unusual in being dependent on $NADPH_2$, cytochrome P-450 and cytochrome reductase which catalyse the direct incorporation of molecular oxygen. Hence they often add hydroxyl groups and so make their substrates more polar and more water soluble. Being less lipid soluble, the metabolites tend to penetrate less readily to sites of action in the body and so are less active pharmacologically and also less

toxic. They are more rapidly excreted in the urine, being less well reabsorbed by the tubular epithelium of the kidneys (p. 2.16). Apart from hydroxylation, the microsomal enzymes may reduce some compounds, substitute oxygen for sulphur and hydrolyse certain esters and amides (fig. 2.10). Following metabolism, the products may be in a form suitable for conjugation with glucuronic acid, sulphuric acid, etc. In fact, the glucuronide-forming enzymes are also located in the microsomes.

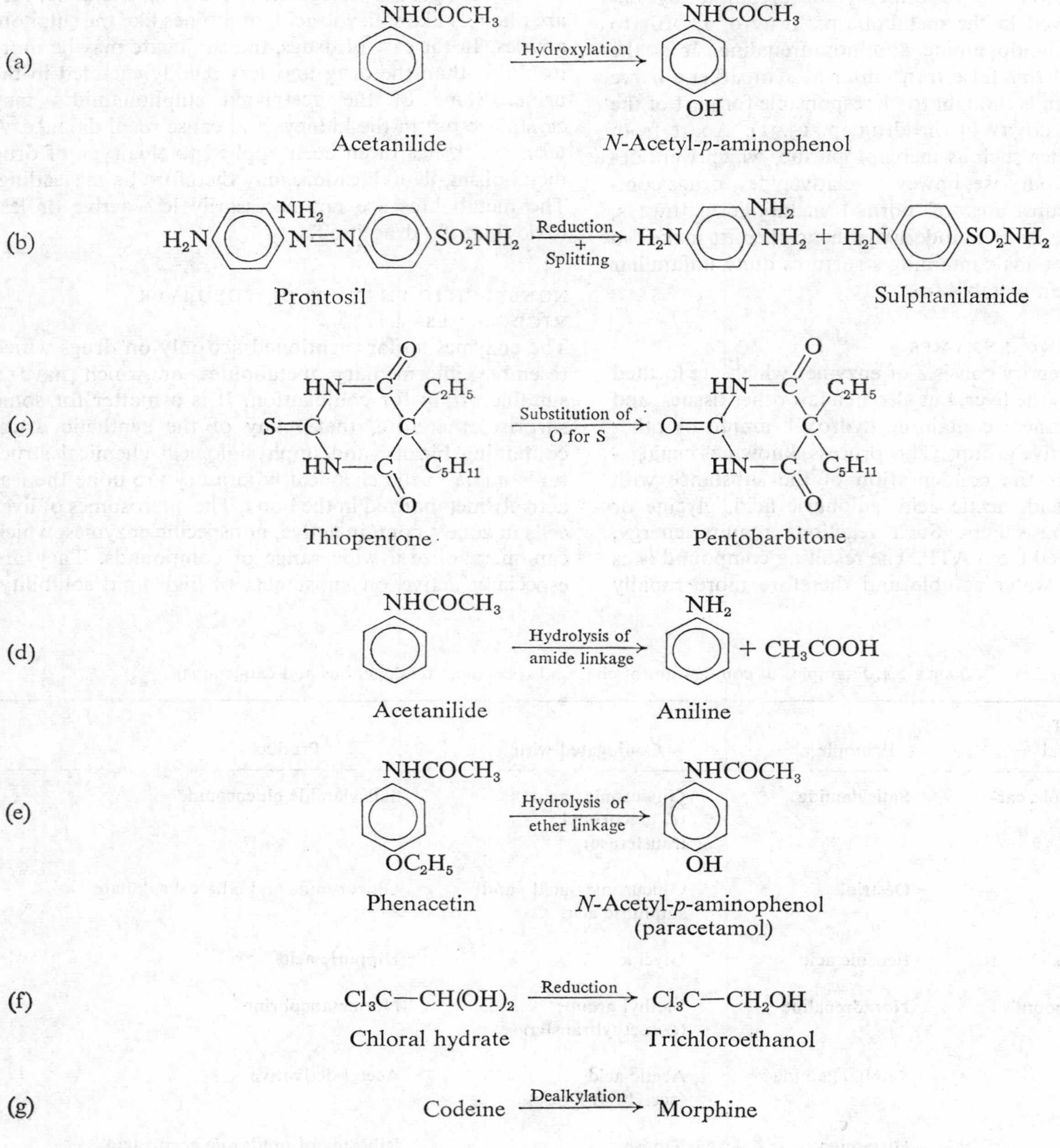

FIG. 2.10. Some examples of chemical changes produced by liver microsomal enzymes.

As mentioned above, the products of microsomal enzyme activity tend to be less active and less toxic, but this is not always true. The examples in fig. 2.10 are chosen to illustrate certain exceptions to this rule, in which the metabolite is just as active as its precursor or where an inactive drug is converted to an active metabolite before therapeutic activity occurs. The classical example of the latter is the discovery by Domagk in Germany (p. 20.2) of an azo-dye, prontosil, which proved to be a very effective agent against β-haemolytic streptococci. Prontosil by itself is inactive but is rapidly metabolized to the potent compound sulphanilamide (fig. 2.10b), which is the parent substance of the sulphonamide group of drugs. The barbiturate, thiopentone, is altered in the body to another active barbiturate pentobarbitone by replacement of sulphur with oxygen (fig. 2.10c). Acetanilide, a substance with mild analgesic and antipyretic properties, is hydrolysed to some extent to aniline (fig. 2.10d), which has toxic effects. In man, however, the main conversion of acetanilide is via hydroxylation to N-acetyl-p-aminophenol or paracetamol (fig. 2.10a). The well-known analgesic, phenacetin, is metabolized rapidly in man also to paracetamol (fig. 2.10e) which accumulates in the plasma and is probably partly responsible for the efficacy of phenacetin (fig. 2.11). As a result of this obser-

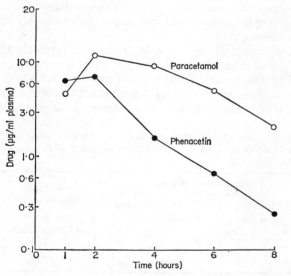

FIG. 2.11. Human plasma levels of ●, phenacetin and ○, paracetamol after 1.8 g phenacetin by mouth. Mean values from nine volunteers. Data of Prescott L.F. (1966) *J. Pharm. Pharmacol.* **18**, 331.

vation, paracetamol itself is now used as an analgesic. This is one example of how measurements of plasma levels of a drug and identification of its metabolites may lead to therapeutic advances. Another example is oxyphenbutazone, first identified as a metabolite of phenylbutazone, which is used in chronic joint disease.

Normal variations in drug metabolism

Species variation may be a source of error in evaluating new drugs in experimental animals. For example, the human liver is much richer in enzymes which conjugate drugs with glucuronic acid than cat liver. Tests for duration of activity of a new drug in cats may, therefore, be misleading. Brodie relates the story of a new barbiturate which had a very brief action in dogs. It could be given by intravenous infusion for continuous deep anaesthesia, since on stopping the infusion the dog recovered within a few minutes. When tried on a human volunteer, the results were disconcerting. After stopping the infusion, 'we sat back and waited for signs of anaesthesia to disappear. Two days later we were not really concerned except that the subject was not yet awake and was expected home to dinner. Plasma levels told us that we had discovered the most long-lasting barbiturate of all time...in man'. Experience has led to the general rule that man metabolizes lipid-soluble drugs more slowly than the majority of animals, the cat being a notable exception. This means that a drug which has little activity in an experimental animal owing to rapid metabolism may be valuable clinically in man. The variability is due to the differences in liver microsomal enzymes which may have had their origin in evolution. Hence one might expect that those species most closely related to man, i.e. the primates, would show the greatest similarities in drug metabolism. This has been more or less confirmed by investigations of comparative pharmacology, which show that Old World monkeys resemble man biochemically more closely than New World monkeys. But even if patterns of drug metabolism are roughly similar, rates of metabolism can vary too widely for therapeutic conclusions to be safely drawn from experiments on primates. This difficulty of finding a species, or even a strain within a species, metabolically similar to man has led some to advocate that drugs should be first tested for therapeutic activity in man, in spite of the risks of adverse effects and the ethical problems involved.

Many of the enzyme systems in the liver do not develop their full activity until a few weeks after birth, and this makes the newborn, and above all the premature, unusually sensitive to the actions of drugs. Infants are defective in enzymes for conjugating substrates with glucuronic acid, and this affects their disposal of drugs. Thus the antibiotic chloramphenicol, even when given in doses adjusted to body weight, reaches blood levels ten to fifteen times greater in premature infants than in adults. Again, in the very old, drugs may be less effectively metabolized and this may lead to toxicity.

Genetic differences may also lead to individual variations in drug metabolism. In man, these are often minor, but on occasion can be large enough to be clinically important. This is the science of **pharmacogenetics**. For example, in man there is a big range in the speed of inactivation of the anticoagulant drug ethyl biscoumacetate; similarly isoniazid, used in the treatment of tuberculosis, is acetylated at rates which vary widely from one patient to another. These facts are important clinically since patients who are 'slow inactivators' of isoniazid are more likely to develop peripheral neuritis if given the usual dose. Fortunately, most drugs do not show such a wide range of inactivation rates, but the clinician should be aware of the possibility of individual variations in drug response. Pharmacogenetics is discussed in greater detail on p. 31.9.

Patients with inborn errors of metabolism lack enzymes which are essential in intermediary metabolism. A deficiency in certain enzymes of lesser physiological importance may not, however, become apparent until a drug is given which is normally acted on by those enzymes. Unexpected adverse reactions may then occur. This is one possible cause of the phenomenon of **idiosyncrasy**, in which a drug produces an effect not met with in the normal person even with large doses. For example, the absence of glucose-6-phosphate dehydrogenase in the red cells, an apparently harmless enzyme deficiency, renders the individual liable to develop haemolysis on the ingestion of certain drugs like sulphanilamide and the antimalarial, primaquine (p. 31.10).

There is good reason to suppose that, as the numbers of potent drugs increase in the years to come, many more of these genetic defects in enzyme activity will be revealed.

Alterations in activity of drug-metabolizing enzymes

The level of activity of metabolizing enzymes in the individual is not fixed and may be altered by pathological states, especially those involving the liver, and by administration of drugs.

Depression of liver microsomal enzyme activity may be produced by malnutrition and starvation, and by diseases leading to an impairment of liver function; this tends to prolong the action of many drugs. Table 2.5 demonstrates the effect of damaging the livers of mice with carbon tetrachloride on the duration of the hypnotic action of two barbiturates. Pentobarbitone is thirty-nine times more soluble in oil than in water and it readily penetrates the microsomal membranes and is metabolized

TABLE 2.5. Effect of liver damage in mice on the duration of action of pentobarbitone and barbitone.

Drugs	Partition coefficient oil/water	Sleeping time in minutes. Normal mice (mean of 5)	Mice with liver damage (mean of 5)
Pentobarbitone (60 mg/kg)	39	60	236
Barbitone (60 mg/kg)	1	212	229

there. Liver damage prolongs its duration of action. Barbitone is much more water soluble and is excreted virtually unmetabolized; liver damage does not significantly influence its duration of action. This emphasizes the important clinical point that lipid-soluble drugs should be given cautiously to patients with impaired liver function, as duration of action may be disconcertingly prolonged.

Long-term administration of drugs such as barbiturates, analgesics, tranquillizers, antihistamines, etc., may stimulate the activity of the liver microsomal enzymes with unexpected clinical consequences. The duration of action of a drug, such as phenobarbitone, diminishes with repeated dosage; this is one possible mechanism of rapidly developing tolerance to the same dose of drug (**tachyphylaxis**). Also, since microsomal enzymes are nonspecific, in a patient receiving regularly one drug (phenobarbitone), the duration of action of an unrelated drug (dicoumarol) may be diminished. So a larger than average dose of the latter will be required to produce an anticoagulation effect. If the phenobarbitone is suddenly stopped, the level of metabolizing enzymes returns to normal, the dose of dicoumarol becomes relatively too high and the patient may suffer severe haemorrhage. This is one possible mechanism for the increasingly important clinical phenomenon of **drug interaction**. In experimental pharmacology, the use of enzyme-stimulating substances like methylcholanthrene is proving a valuable technique in the elucidation of drug metabolism.

Conversely, there are substances which inhibit the activity of liver microsomal enzymes, e.g. iproniazid and β-diethylaminoethyl-diphenylpropylacetate (SKF 525-A). The striking effect of SKF 525-A on the duration of action of hexobarbitone in rats is shown in table 2.6. By

TABLE 2.6. The effect of the liver microsomal enzyme inhibitor SKF 525-A on the duration of action of hexobarbitone in rats.

Drugs given (mg/kg)		Sleeping time in minutes
SKF 525-A	Hexobarbitone	
25	—	no hypnotic action
—	110	19
25	110	117

itself, SKF 525-A exerts no obvious pharmacological action but is a useful experimental tool. So far it has no application in clinical medicine. The effect of drugs on the liver microsomal enzymes is discussed in greater detail on p. 10.9.

EXCRETION

The most important route of excretion for a drug or its metabolites is the urine, but before discussing this in detail some of the other routes are briefly reviewed.

Drugs which appear in the faeces may not have been fully absorbed after oral ingestion or may have been excreted into the **large** or **small bowel**. Some chemotherapeutic agents are very water insoluble (phthalylsulphathiazole), or too polar to pass through the intestinal mucosa (streptomycin and neomycin). For this reason they are given orally for gut infections or to sterilize the bowel before operations on it. Some drugs are absorbed from the jejunum, but are re-excreted into the colon unchanged or as their metabolites. For example, after absorption the anthracene purgatives are partly re-excreted into the colon and broken down there to the active principle emodin. Re-excretion in the bile is quite common, and this may produce recycling of a drug with prolongation of its action, e.g. the purgative phenolphthalein.

Anaesthetic gases and vapours like nitrous oxide or diethyl ether, which are absorbed through the lung alveoli, are very largely eliminated by the same route. Drugs of a volatile nature, e.g. ethyl alcohol, or the sedative paraldehyde, also appear in the **breath** but only a small proportion is excreted by this route.

Drugs may appear in many other secretions, such as the **saliva**, where they may cause a disagreeable taste or irritate the oral tissues, and those of the **sweat** and **bronchial glands**. The passage of drugs across the **placenta**, or secretion into the **milk**, may be a hazard to the foetus or the breast-fed infant. For all these routes of excretion, the general principles enunciated throughout this chapter apply. Un-ionized drugs of low molecular weight and high lipid solubility are more likely to cross the cell membranes involved than drugs of low lipid solubility.

Excretion into the **gastric juice** also occurs, but owing to the great difference between the pH of plasma (7·4) and of gastric juice (1·0–2·0) the elimination of basic drugs is favoured by this route. As explained earlier (p. 2.7 and fig. 2.6), weak bases like phenazone are poorly absorbed from the stomach, and on precisely the same grounds it follows that weak bases pass more readily from plasma to gastric juice than acidic drugs.

Some drugs, e.g. mecamylamine, pass readily from the blood into the stomach where they are 'trapped' owing to ionization in the acid medium. Morphine is also 'excreted' into the stomach as Hitzig (1870) showed by chance. He was demonstrating to a class the effects of morphine in a dog. Soon after the drug had been injected, the dog vomited. A second dog which happened to be standing by consumed the vomit and promptly died of morphine poisoning.

Excretion of drugs into the urine

Mechanisms of the renal excretion of drugs are shown in fig. 2.12. The rate of excretion is influenced by the extent to which the drug is filtered by the glomerulus and reabsorbed or secreted by the renal tubules. In general, the rate of excretion of drugs in the urine is correlated

with the level of glomerular filtration. Since the molecular size of most drugs is well below the functional pore size of the glomerular membrane, the extent to which drugs pass the glomerular barrier depends upon the degree to which they are bound to plasma proteins. Cycloserine, for example, readily passes into the glomerular filtrate and is rapidly excreted. At the other extreme suramin, used to treat trypanosomiasis, persists for several months in the circulation after its administration because it is firmly bound to plasma proteins. Variations in the degree of protein binding between different sulphonamides are largely responsible for differences in their duration of action. Sulphadiazine is rapidly absorbed from the gastrointestinal tract and rapidly excreted in

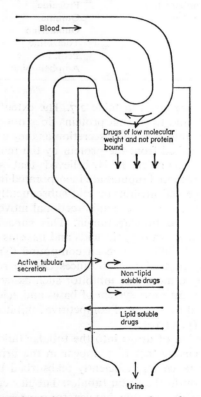

FIG. 2.12. Schematic representation of renal excretion of drugs. From Brodie B.B. (1964) *Absorption and Distribution of Drugs*, ed. T.B. Binns. Edinburgh: Livingstone.

the urine. It is bound to plasma proteins to the extent of about 50 per cent at usual therapeutic concentrations. On the other hand, sulphamethoxypyridazine is a 'long-acting' sulphonamide as it is slowly excreted by the kidney. This is mainly because about 85 per cent of it is bound to plasma proteins and does not pass into the glomerular filtrate.

Tubular function greatly influences the rate of excretion of those drugs which are organic acids or bases. Clearance studies have shown that separate excreting mechanisms exist in the proximal tubules for these two groups of substances. Both processes depend upon energy derived from tubular cell metabolism but they are independent of each other. Commonly used drugs which are excreted

TABLE 2.7. Some drugs which are secreted by the renal tubules. In accordance with the theory of non-ionic diffusion the renal excretion of these substances is influenced by the pH of the urine.

Organic acids	Organic bases
Salicylic acid	Levorphanol
p-Amino salicylic acid	Pempidine
Phenol red	Mecamylamine
Chlorothiazide	Hexamethonium
Phenobarbitone	Procaine
Penicillin	Quinine
	Quinacrine
	Tolazoline
	Pethidine
	Amphetamine

in this way are given in table 2.7. The extent to which drugs are bound to plasma proteins does not greatly influence their rate of tubular secretion as they are capable of being detached from the protein by the renal tubular cell before excretion. It is believed that substances secreted by the renal tubules are incorporated into a complex near the cell membrane and subsequently released in such a way as to achieve unidirectional movement and passage into the tubular lumen. This capacity of the tubules to transport organic acids and bases is limited to a value which differs for each compound (Tm). While tubular transport of all substances can be reduced or abolished by a metabolic inhibitor such as cyanide, the independent transport system of bases and acids may be demonstrated by the use of competitive inhibitors such as probenecid (p. 11.10).

The filtration of drugs into the tubular fluid does not necessarily ensure that they appear in the urine. Lipid-soluble substances are efficiently reabsorbed by passive back diffusion in the distal tubules. Tubular epithelium, however, is an effective barrier to most polar compounds of low lipid solubility. The kidney is, therefore, highly specialized for the elimination of water-soluble drugs, a property enhanced by proximal tubular secretion of strongly ionized substances into the lumen of the tubules. These mechanisms have been developed, presumably, for the rapid disposal of toxic endogenous substances. Active reabsorption of substances which the body needs to conserve, such as amino acids and glucose, also operates in the tubules. Methyldopa is actively reabsorbed by mechanisms utilized by a group of amino acids, and competition between the drug and these normal metabolites can lead to marked amino aciduria.

It follows then that if a drug exists predominantly in the un-ionized form in the filtrate and has high lipid solubility, tubular reabsorption will be favoured and its excretion in the urine retarded. Conversely, water-soluble drugs of high polarity, especially if ionized at urine pH, are rapidly excreted. As already mentioned, metabolizing enzymes tend to convert lipid-soluble drugs to more polar derivatives. These metabolites are not reabsorbed in the tubules and may even be actively secreted if strongly ionized.

Methods of altering renal excretion of drugs

Unlike most body fluids, urine has a pH which can be varied over a wide range by administration of sodium bicarbonate or ammonium chloride. Since most drugs are weak acids or bases, changing the pH alters their degree of ionization and adjusting urinary pH offers a way of retarding or accelerating excretion. Making the urine alkaline retards the excretion of basic drugs by suppressing their ionization and increasing their lipid solubility, but accelerates the excretion of acidic drugs. Making the urine acid retards the excretion of acidic drugs but hastens excretion of basic drugs. Such manipulations are useful clinically for:

(1) prolonging the desirable therapeutic action of drugs which tend to be excreted too rapidly, and

(2) accelerating the excretion of ingested poisons.

For example, the actions of the acidic analgesic phenylbutazone (pK_a 4·4) can be prolonged by making the urine more acid. After an overdose of acetylsalicylic acid (pK_a 3·5) or phenobarbitone (pK_a 7·2) their excretion can be accelerated if the urine is kept at about pH 8·0. The renal clearance of salicylates, which are actively secreted, is greater than the GFR when the urine is alkaline, but falls below it when the urine is acid, as absorption then exceeds secretion in the tubules.

Amphetamine on the other hand is excreted most effectively if the urine is highly acid. The recognition of amphetamine addiction by analysis of urine is successful only if the urine is first rendered acid.

The excretion of certain drugs can be altered by interfering with the active processes of tubular secretion. These may be depressed or blocked by competitive administration of substances which themselves are excreted by these mechanisms. The acidic drug probenecid was synthesized for the purpose of depressing tubular secretion of acidic drugs. It has been suggested that probenecid blocks active transport mechanisms without being itself transported (p. 11.10).

Normally 80 per cent of a dose of benzylpenicillin is actively secreted by the tubules, and this can be much reduced by simultaneous administration of probenecid. This device was used in the days when penicillin was a rare and costly drug, and is still sometimes employed when high plasma levels of the antibiotic are required, for example, in bacterial endocarditis. Probenecid also decreases the tubular secretion of PAH and salicylic acid. Compounds are known which block the active mechanisms for excreting bases but they are too toxic for clinical use.

Renal disease may diminish excretion of drugs and so prolong their duration of action and increase the likelihood of adverse reactions. There are also specific renal defects involving the reabsorptive mechanisms for amino acids and sugars, which, of course, affect only those drugs with structural similarities to these substances.

'Purpose' of drug metabolism and excretion

All that has been said about drug metabolism and excretion may provoke the following fundamental question. Why does man metabolize and excrete with remarkable efficiency so many of the bizarre chemical substances inflicted on him by the medical practitioner? Studies in comparative pharmacology have indicated that fish do not possess liver microsomal enzymes, which first appear in the phylogenetic scale in reptiles living permanently on dry land. Observations such as these have led Brodie and his school to make the fascinating suggestion that non-specific microsomal, as well as conjugating, enzymes have developed *pari passu* with the need to conserve water. Fish can easily get rid of water-soluble substances, and even lipid-soluble compounds pass sufficiently rapidly by simple diffusion through the lipid gill-membranes into the virtually infinite volume of water in which the fish swim. Adaptation to land living has necessitated the development of a waterproof skin and of complex mechanisms for conserving water by tubular reabsorption. Some simple calculations show that in the absence of enzymes capable of making substances more polar, many lipid-soluble compounds would stay in the body for a very long time, especially if they were also bound to plasma protein. A drug which was almost completely reabsorbed in the tubules, at a renal clearance of 1 ml/min, would be half-cleared from the body in 24 days. If the drug was also strongly bound to plasma proteins, half-clearance time could theoretically be as long as 90 years.

The hypothesis, then, is that the drug-metabolizing enzymes in the liver were developed in the course of evolution for the rapid disposal of possibly toxic substances of high lipid solubility present in food. The fact that they also metabolize lipid soluble drugs is due fortuitously, but fortunately, to their lack of specificity. Without them, therapeutics would be a more difficult and dangerous art than it is now.

QUANTITATIVE FACTORS

Rates of clearance of a drug

Two theoretically possible patterns of drug clearance are illustrated in fig. 2.13. Linear clearance (fig. 2.13a), in which the amount of drug cleared in unit time is constant, is uncommon. An example is ethyl alcohol which is oxidized to carbon dioxide and water at a rate of roughly 100 mg/kg/hr in a healthy man. In exponential clearance (fig. 2.13b), the amount of drug cleared in unit time is

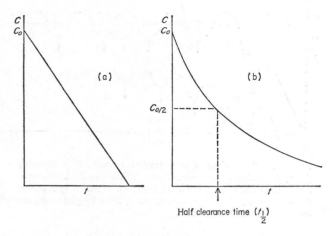

FIG. 2.13. Rates of drug clearance; c, concentration of drug in body; t, time after administration; c_0, initial drug concentration. (a) Linear clearance: $c = c_0 - kt$. (b) Exponential or logarithmic clearance: $c = c_0.10^{-kt}$.

proportional to the amount remaining in the body. The great majority of drugs follow more or less approximately this exponential pattern. For such drugs, clearance is theoretically never complete and it is therefore more convenient to measure the time to clear one-half of the drug from the body ($c_0/2$). This measurement is referred to as the **half-clearance time** or the **half-life** of the drug ($t_{\frac{1}{2}}$).

The half-clearance time of any drug is not, of course, constant, since it may be modified by many of the factors already outlined. But a knowledge of the approximate half-life of a drug, which may range from less than 1 hour for benzylpenicillin to several days for digoxin, is valuable in deciding appropriate dosage regimes in therapeutics. For most drugs, the half-life lies between 8 and 24 hours, which explains why their concentrations can be maintained at more or less therapeutic levels by regular 4–6 hourly administration.

Dosage regimes: loading and maintenance

From the half-clearance time ($t_{\frac{1}{2}}$), it is possible to calculate the loss of drug from the body during any specified time x from the equation:

$$\text{Fraction cleared} = 1 - 0.5^{\frac{x}{t_{\frac{1}{2}}}}$$

Once a drug has reached its therapeutic concentration in the plasma, the amount cleared in 4 hours is obviously

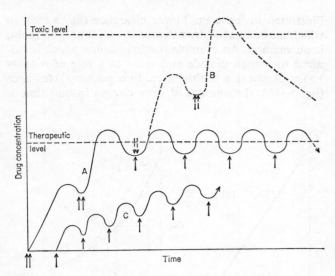

FIG. 2.14. Time–drug concentration curves. ↑↑, loading dose; ↑, maintenance dose. Curve A, loading dose followed by maintenance dose; curve B, result of continuing loading dose; curve C, slow rise to therapeutic level by giving maintenance dose from the start.

the amount needed as a **maintenance dose** every 4 hours to allow therapeutic effect to continue (fig. 2.14, plateau part of curve A).

For a drug like digoxin which has the long half-clearance time of about 4 days, it can be calculated that roughly one-sixth of the amount present in the body is eliminated in 24 hours. Hence, once the therapeutic level is attained, only one-sixth of the amount present requires to be given every day as a maintenance dose. However, if this quite small dose (about 0·5 mg) was given at the start, it would take several days to reach the necessary therapeutic level (fig. 2.14, curve C). Since digoxin is a drug given for cardiac failure, often a serious medical emergency, this is usually far too slow an onset of action. It is usual to give orally a **loading dose** (or **digitalizing dose**) of 2–4 mg which hastens the attainment of the therapeutic level. Once this is achieved, a much smaller maintenance dose is given (fig. 2.14, curve A).

The danger, however, with a drug of this kind is that if the loading dose is not stopped in time, the level of drug within the body may rise to the toxic concentration (fig. 2.14, curve B). For this reason a drug like digoxin needs to be given with some finesse; once toxic levels are established, it takes a relatively long time for the drug to be excreted and for levels to return to the therapeutic value. This introduces the topic of **drug cumulation.**

Cumulation of drugs, and of drug effect

Cumulation is the build-up of a drug in the body when intake exceeds clearance. Theoretically, this may happen with a large enough dose of any drug, however rapidly excreted, but is obviously more likely to occur with drugs having a long half-clearance time. Cumulation is, of course, intentionally brought about during therapeutic regimes involving drug loading. More dangerous, however, is the unintentional cumulation following long-term administration of small doses of drugs with long half-clearance times, since eventually concentrations may reach the toxic level and **cumulative toxicity** develops. Drugs very liable to give cumulative toxicity are those whose clearance is slowed by binding, e.g. digoxin and thyroxine (plasma protein-bound) and heavy metals like lead (bound to bone). This is how the ingestion of incredibly small amounts of a poisonous substance, e.g. two parts per million of lead in tap water, may lead over a sufficiently long period of time to the attainment in the body of toxic levels. A situation of this kind may pose a diagnostic problem to the clinician and is a challenge to the public health expert (p. 32.5).

A rather different type of cumulation has been suggested in recent years, sometimes called **cumulation of drug effect**. A drug may seem to disappear rapidly from the body and yet its pharmacological actions may persist for several weeks. Brodie has graphically called this a 'hit-and-run drug'. Such drugs are believed to act by prolonged inhibition of enzyme systems, and by depleting stores of active transmitters at nerve endings or impairing their repletion. Since regeneration of enzyme or transmitter store may be slow, the pharmacological effects of the drug outlast the period during which the drug is detectable in the body. Examples are reserpine, a drug which impairs amine storage mechanisms and may lead to prolonged central depressive reactions, monoamine oxidase inhibitors of the hydrazine type, and the anticoagulant, ethylbiscoumacetate, which affects liver enzymes involved in the synthesis of plasma coagulation factors. However, the extent to which this effect is due to persistence of the drug in the tissues in amounts which cannot be so far detected is unknown.

The moral of this and indeed of much of this chapter, is that the physician of today and tomorrow, armed with drugs increasingly potent, increasingly subtle in their modes of action and interaction and capable of insidious toxicity, must remain intellectually on his toes if he is to avoid poisoning his patients with the products of the modern pharmaceutical industry.

FURTHER READING

ALBERT A. (1968) *Selective Toxicity and Related Topics*, 4th Edition. London: Methuen.

BINNS T.B., ed. (1964) *Absorption and Distribution of Drugs*. Edinburgh: Livingstone.

BRODIE B.B. & ERDOS E.G., eds. (1962) *Proceedings of the First International Pharmacological Meeting*, Vol. 6.

Metabolic Factors Controlling Duration of Drug Action. Oxford: Pergamon Press.

BRODIE B.B. (1967) Physicochemical and biochemical aspects of pharmacology (The 1967 Albert Lasker Award Lecture). *J. Amer. med. Ass.* **202**, 600.

FINGL E. & WOODBURY D.M. (1965) General principles, in *The Pharmacological Basis of Therapeutics*, 3rd Edition, ed. L.S. Goodman & A. Gilman. New York: Macmillan.

SCHANKER L.S. (1964) Physiological transport of drugs in *Advances in Drug Research*, Vol. 1 ed. Harper and Simmonds. London : Academic Press.

WEINER I.M. (1967) The renal excretion of drugs and related compounds. *Ann. Rev. Pharmacol.* **7**, 39.

WILLIAMS R.T., GILLETTE J.R., SMITH C.C., BRODIE B.B. & REID W.D. (1967). Symposium on comparative pharmacology. *Fed. Proc.* **26**, 4.

Chapter 3
Concepts of drug action, quantitative pharmacology and biological assay

The mechanism of drug action constitutes one of the fundamental aspects of pharmacology but is known in only a few cases. Understanding of the action of drugs is frustrated by ignorance of details of cellular biochemistry. In spite of this, important general concepts of drug action and the relationships of chemical and physical structure to pharmacological effects have been formulated. These general concepts are described in this chapter.

Receptors and drug specificity

It is remarkable that minute amounts of some drugs produce profound effects and that their actions are extremely selective, being confined to certain parts of the body or to certain organisms. Digitalis glycosides, for example, affect mainly heart muscle and apomorphine stimulates a single small area in the brain stem. In the peripheral nervous system, decamethonium blocks transmission at the neuromuscular junction but has little action elsewhere; hexamethonium blocks transmission in ganglia and affects the neuromuscular junction only in much higher doses and atropine blocks the effects of parasympathetic stimulation but has little effect on ganglia or elsewhere in the peripheral nervous system. Many drugs are also remarkably selective in that they affect some micro-organisms but not others and have little effect on man. Penicillin, for instance, prevents some bacteria from growing but has little effect on others, on protozoa or helminths. Further examples of substances which act selectively are weed killers. This specificity parallels the specificity of action of endogenous chemical substances, e.g. hormones and local hormones.

The simplest explanation of these findings is that selective drugs affect only particular groups of cells, probably because they react with particular chemical groups, which are called **receptors** (p. 1.2). Calculations by Clark suggested that receptors for acetylcholine form only a minute part of the cell surface. It was found, for instance, that the rate of beating of the frog heart was slowed to half by a dose of acetylcholine as small as 0.02 µg/g tissue. This dose contains about 10^{14} molecules of acetylcholine and, from the dimensions of the cells, it was calculated that these could cover only about 1/6000th of their surface area. From what is known about enzymes, substrates and inhibitors, it is very likely that some receptors are the active centres of enzymes.

However, whatever the nature of a receptor, its reaction with a drug is presumably chemical and can be described by the Law of Mass Action. The effects produced by a drug would therefore be expected to be related to the **active mass** of drug present. This is best expressed in moles or ideally as a thermodynamic activity; since most drugs are effective in dilute solutions (10^{-3} to 10^{-5} M) and some in very dilute solutions, e.g. atropine is effective in concentrations as low as 10^{-8} to 10^{-9} M, the activity coefficients are likely to be close to unity even in blood. Logically, therefore, all doses of drugs should be expressed in terms of moles and all concentrations in molarity. In a few instances this is not possible because the compound has not been obtained chemically pure. The molecular weights of most drugs are known and can be found in *The Extra Pharmacopoeia* and similar works of reference.

If the dose or concentration is not expressed in molarity but in grammes or some concentration based on weight, it is necessary to use different doses, or concentrations, of different salts to produce the same molar concentration of the active material. Usually the differences are small but sometimes they are quite big; compare for example, suxamethonium chloride, $2H_2O$, (mol. wt. 397), suxamethonium bromide, $2H_2O$ (mol. wt. 478) and suxamethonium iodide (mol. wt. 544). The dose of drugs is not usually expressed in moles in clinical practice; this would involve an additional calculation in dispensing. In pharmacological studies of drug action and in comparison of the relative potencies of different substances, it is proper to think in molar terms.

Types of drug action: agonists and antagonists

Drugs produce a wide variety of effects and these can be classified in several different ways. One drug may cause a gland to secrete, another stop a gland secreting; one may cause smooth muscle to contract whereas another causes the muscle to relax. Some drugs slow the heart and some cause it to beat faster. In fact, drugs can usually be classed either as **stimulant drugs,** which produce an increase in activity, or as **depressant** or **inhibitory drugs** which diminish activity. The appropriate classification may not always be the most obvious; for example, ethyl alcohol is often described as a stimulant because of its effect in certain doses; the loquacity and change in behaviour which it produces are the result of a depression of higher centres rather than direct stimulation of the central nervous system, such as that produced by caffeine or amphetamine. This simple classification is not always easy to apply, particularly to drugs with central actions, and does not reveal much about the way in which they produce their effects; more useful for this purpose is the classification into **agonist** and **antagonist.** Acetylcholine causes several kinds of smooth muscle to contract, i.e. it has a stimulant action. This effect is prevented by atropine which thus has an inhibitory effect. However, acetylcholine also slows the heart and this depressant action is also prevented by atropine. Administered to a resting animal, whose heart is under vagal control, atropine accelerates the heart, i.e. a stimulant action. In both instances atropine produces no observable effect in the absence of acetylcholine and its only effect is as an antagonist of acetylcholine. Substances such as acetylcholine and its synthetic analogues, which initiate cellular changes, are known as agonists. Other examples of agonist–antagonist pairs are histamine and mepyramine (p. 14.18), adrenaline and phentolamine and adrenaline and propranolol. Adrenaline is mentioned twice because it is thought to act on two different activating mechanisms which are blocked by two different groups of antagonists. Each activating mechanism produces both stimulating and inhibitory effects (p. 15.16 & 22).

Some confusion may arise because the term antagonism is applied also to the mutual opposition of some of the actions of acetylcholine and adrenaline. However, the classification of both these substances as agonists is valid. In smooth muscle acetylcholine alters membrane permeability and decreases the membrane potential; adrenaline alters membrane permeability in a different way and increases the potential. The effects thus tend to cancel each other out but the action is not one in which either substance blocks the primary action of the other. Atropine has no effect of its own on membrane permeability but it prevents acetylcholine causing a change. A piece of isolated guinea-pig ileum contracts if either acetylcholine or histamine is added to the bathing fluid and both contractions are reduced in the presence of adrenaline. The fact that both responses are reduced contrasts with the selective action of mepyramine against

histamine and of atropine against acetylcholine; this is another pointer to the difference in the underlying mechanisms. Propranolol reduces the inhibitory action of adrenaline on both the histamine and acetylcholine induced contractions, thereby indicating that it is a single action of adrenaline which affects both histamine and acetylcholine and confirming that the adrenaline effect is the action of an agonist.

Acetylcholine is of course a normal body constituent and when released by nerves produces a wide range of effects. Many substances have been synthesized which have some similarity of structure to acetylcholine and which produce similar effects because they exert the same agonist action, e.g. acetyl β-methylcholine (mecholyl) and carbamylcholine (carbachol) which are used clinically (p. 4.7).

Atropine is racemic hyoscyamine which also occurs naturally but only in plants; the ingestion of these plants results in poisoning by the hyoscyamine. The chemical structure of atropine has features in common with acetylcholine (p. 4.11); again many substances have been synthesized which are similar to acetylcholine in action and structure. This similarity is one reason why it is usually supposed that atropine and related compounds act by occupying acetylcholine receptors.

The idea that similarities in chemical structure between compounds lead to interference with the action of naturally occurring substances is a familiar concept from biochemical studies of substrate inhibition and many drugs act on enzymes in this way. Malonic acid antagonizes the oxidation of succinic acid by succinic dehydrogenase; sulphonamides interfere with the incorporation of p-aminobenzoate into folic acid in certain bacteria (p. 20.2), while penicillin interferes with enzymes involved in the production of the cell wall in others (p. 20.12). Physostigmine may not look very much like acetylcholine but it seems to be sufficiently similar to inhibit some cholinesterases and thereby enhance the effect of endogenous acetylcholine (p. 4.6).

Analysis of how drugs act

One of the main purposes of pharmacology is to elucidate the mechanisms by which drugs produce their effects; this has to be done successively at different levels. Physiological procedures and analysis are first used to find out which parts or organs of the body are affected, and where the effect originates. This is usually comparatively simple, though errors have often been made; the pursuit of knowledge beyond this point is very difficult and for the great majority of drugs there is little or no knowledge of their action at the molecular level.

Digitalis was introduced into medicine in 1785 for the treatment of 'dropsy' of which the main clinical features are breathlessness and oedema of the lower extremities. Its beneficial action has been variously ascribed to an effect exerted by the kidney, the veins and the heart, and a great deal of effort was expended before it was attributed finally to the heart. The fact that the effect is exerted by the heart does not necessarily mean that digitalis acts on the heart; indeed an action on the medulla, modifying the extent of vagal influence on the heart, has been suggested. It is now clear that the most important and perhaps the only significant action of digitalis is exerted directly on the muscle cells of the heart which are made to contract more powerfully. As indicated on p. 1.3 this effect is probably due to an action of the drug on the cell membrane and is further discussed on p. 8.3. Here, as elsewhere, the fundamental action of digitalis is likely to be better understood in step with increased knowledge of the fundamental processes of the cell.

The analysis of drug action is often assisted by the use of other 'specific' drugs. The action of drugs can for instance be differentiated from acetylcholine or histamine by the use of atropine and mepyramine respectively. Use is also often made of the ganglion blocking agent hexamethonium to identify the action of drugs which stimulate ganglia and sometimes use is made of nicotine or dimethylphenylpiperazinium (DMPP) as specific ganglion stimulants to identify a blocking action at ganglia. This kind of analysis has its limitations, because specificity is usually relative rather than absolute and many drugs are not as specific in their actions as is often supposed. Further, it may not indicate exactly at what stage in a sequence a drug is acting. For example, a piece of intestine contracts if acetylcholine is applied to it, and it also does so if nicotine is applied; both effects are antagonized by atropine (not necessarily by the same dose), but whereas the atropine blocks the same receptors as are activated by acetylcholine, it does not block the receptors activated by nicotine. Nicotine stimulates receptors in ganglia and it is the endogenous acetylcholine subsequently released from the postganglionic nerve endings which is antagonized by the atropine. Thus, the use of 'specific' agonists and antagonists is a useful means of checking a physiological analysis of how a drug is acting; although not always satisfactory, it is sometimes the only means available.

In addition to the types of antagonism already mentioned, it is possible for one drug to antagonize another by combining with it chemically. Congo Red, for example, prevents the actions of (+)-tubocurarine chloride because it forms a complex with it. Sulphate ions antagonize the toxic effects of barium ions because they form a precipitate of barium sulphate. Protamine, which is cationic combines with heparin anions. Toxic ions such as As^{+++} and Hg^{++} and organic compounds containing these metals form stable complexes with dimercaprol and so are rendered inactive (pp. 1.2 & 11.5), and many other ions, such as Pb^{++}, form stable complexes with chelating agents, such as ethylenediamine tetraacetic acid (sodium calcium edetate, EDTA, p. 10.12).

COMBINED EFFECTS OF DRUGS

When two drugs which produce similar effects are given simultaneously, the size of the combined effect is not always related in a simple way to the size of the effects of the individual drugs. If the drugs act by the same mechanism, and possibly if they are acting entirely independently, one might expect them to act **additively**. This does not imply that the effects will be additive but rather that the doses will be additive. If a particular effect is produced by a dose X of substance X and also by a dose Y of substance Y, then $X/2$ given together with $Y/2$ should produce the same effect, as should $3X/4$ together with $Y/4$. Often drugs having similar effects do not behave in this way. For example, physostigmine enhances parasympathetic effects and so does acetylcholine. If the two are given together the effect observed is much greater than would be expected from simple addition. This is because the effect of physostigmine is due to the preservation of endogenous acetylcholine; it also protects the added acetylcholine from destruction and so the combined effect is greatly enhanced. Such a situation is described as **potentiation**. In this instance, the physostigmine is potentiating the action of acetylcholine. Another term sometimes used to describe such effects is **synergism**, but this word is better used in a more general sense to describe the acting together of two drugs without specifying addition or potentiation and it may even mean something less than addition. Such vagueness may be necessary due to a lack of information or because the relationship is complex, and the direction of the interaction may be different at different levels of effect. When the effects of two agonist drugs given together fall short of what might be expected, a possible reason is that one of them may be only a partial agonist (p. 3.10).

Some information about the molecular actions of drugs can be obtained by using drugs which reputedly block only certain specific enzymes, such as amine oxidase. As with the use of 'specific' agonists or antagonists in the physiological analysis of drug action, however, this method is not wholly reliable. Iproniazid, for example, inhibits other enzymes besides monoamine oxidase, and although tranylcypromine is demonstrably more specific, there is always some uncertainty attached to results obtained in this way. Another source of information about molecular pharmacology comes from quantitative pharmacological experiments and it is useful to discuss this here.

QUANTITATIVE PHARMACOLOGY

Quantitative pharmacology has evolved over the last 40 years and began because of the need to standardize different batches of drugs, such as digitalis glycosides, hormones, toxins and antitoxins, which could not be obtained chemically pure and the activity of which had to be estimated biologically. With improvements in chemical techniques, many drugs originally standardized **by bioassay** are now obtainable chemically pure and can be assessed by chemical means. Nevertheless, new active materials continue to be discovered and there are always likely to be substances whose potency can be estimated only biologically.

The effects produced by a drug can be divided into two types, **graded responses** and **all or none responses**. If the drug is being tested for its ability to cause a piece of smooth muscle to contract, the response observed may be anything between no contraction and the full contraction of which the muscle is capable; this is a graded response. If the drug is being tested for its liability to produce death, only two results are possible, life or death; this is an all or none response. The methods used for assays in which graded responses are produced are necessarily different from those in which the response is all or none.

Graded responses

As the dose of drug increases, the response also increases but not in proportion, i.e. there is a diminishing return. As the response increases, a further increase in response can be produced only by a greater increment in dose. However, over a certain range of response, the increase is often related to the proportion by which the dose is increased, each doubling of the dose producing the same increment of response. If the response is plotted against the logarithm of the dose, a more or less straight line is produced over a limited range. Since there is a maximum to the response the size of the response cannot go on increasing indefinitely. A point is reached where a further increase in dose does not produce a greater response and may indeed produce a smaller one. There is also usually curvature at low responses (fig. 3.1).

BIOASSAY OF AGONISTS USING PREPARATIONS WHICH GIVE GRADED RESPONSE

If a volume, *A*, of a standard solution of a drug pro-

duces exactly the same response as a volume *B* of an 'unknown' solution, it is reasonable to suppose that there is the same amount of drug present and that the concentration of the unknown solution is, therefore, *A/B* times the concentration in the standard solution. In performing an assay, however, an exact match is seldom obtained between the responses to standard and unknown doses. In fact it is not sufficient to obtain an exact match since the ability of the tissue to discriminate between different sizes of dose would not be established. At least two different doses of one of the solutions, usually the standard solution, must be tested.

Almost invariably the response produced by the dose of the unknown solution does not match either of the responses to the doses of the standard solution. If it lies between the two responses, the amount of drug in the unknown solution lies between the limits of the standard doses. By repeating the experiment with other doses of the standard solution it is possible to narrow the limits further. The value of this process is restricted by lack of reproducibility of repeated responses to the same dose. There is little point in trying to distinguish between two doses when their effects differ by an amount which is less than the range of responses obtained by giving the same dose several times. Accuracy can be improved, however, by repeating the test dose and the standard doses several times and calculating the mean size of the responses. The dose of standard which matches the dose of the unknown can then be interpolated either graphically or algebraically. The interpolation is usually based on the assumption that the response is proportional to the logarithm of the dose (fig. 3.1), and if the assay is to be accurate the slope of the log dose response curve must be known accurately. This can be achieved only if the dose range is fairly wide so that the variation of individual responses is small compared with the difference in response between the two standard doses.

When responses are measured and the assay result obtained by calculation, the accuracy of the assay can be stated in statistical terms. It is best, however, to apply statistical considerations at the outset to the design

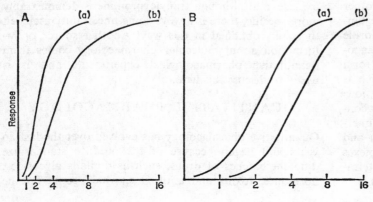

FIG. 3.1. Dose response curves and log dose response curves. The lines in B represent the same responses as shown in A. The lines marked (b) can be regarded as being produced by doses of a solution with half the strength of the solution used to produce (a), in which case the units are units of volume. Alternatively (b) can be regarded as the result of testing a substance which is only half as effective as the substance whose responses are shown by the lines (a), in which case the units are units of weight. Note that in A points on line (b) are always twice as far from the ordinate as the corresponding points on (a). In B there is a constant horizontal distance between the lines; they are in consequence often said to be parallel.

of the experiment. This leads to the use of a symmetrical design so that two doses of the test solution are used as well as the two doses of the standard with which it is being compared. In this way the unknown solution is also used to obtain information about the slope of the log dose response relationship; in addition this provides a check that the two solutions behave in the same way. If they do not do so, the comparison cannot be regarded as valid. This kind of assay is known as a **2 and 2 dose assay** or as a **4 point assay.** The calculation of potency depends on the assumption that the log dose response line is straight, an assumption usually justified from prior knowledge. By complicating the assay to include three doses of each solution, direct evidence about linearity can be sought. Thus in a **6 point** or **3 and 3 dose assay** more information about the shape of the log dose response relation is obtained; even if this turns out to be curved there are techniques by which a valid estimate of potency can still be made.

An analysis of variance (vol. 1, p. 3.12) is used first to determine if the assay is valid. To be valid the responses to the high doses must be significantly different from the responses to the low doses, and the slopes of the log dose response lines must not be significantly different for the two solutions. If these conditions are satisfied, it is permissible to calculate the accuracy of the estimate of the potency of the unknown solution; the variation in the responses which cannot be ascribed to known causes is the only source of error, and the probable extent of this can be estimated in such a way that a range of values for the potency can be specified with the assurance that 95 times out of 100 the actual potency would lie within that range. The limits of this range, calculated in the appropriate way, are referred to as the **fiducial limits.** Clearly a narrow range shows that the assay is accurate; a wide range indicates that it is inaccurate.

When conditions are suitable a surprisingly accurate estimate can be obtained. The assay of acetylcholine on guinea-pig ileum is an example. Doses can be applied at intervals of 1·5 min or even less, so that many responses can be obtained in a relatively short time. Table 3.1 gives the sizes of forty-eight contractions measured in mm on a kymograph record produced by four concentrations of acetylcholine, each tested twelve times. The doses were not applied in a random order; each group of four successive contractions contained each of the four concentrations, and the order in which the concentrations occurred was different in each of the twelve groups. The sum of the contractions (in mm) for each group of four contractions is also shown and indicates that the tissue became less sensitive with time. Because of the grouping of the doses this change in sensitivity does not affect the result and the effect can be eliminated from the estimation of error. Fig. 3.2 shows the way in which the relative strengths of the solutions may be found graphically. Also shown is an interpolation of the $2x$ dose on the 6 ng–12 ng line which indicates how to obtain

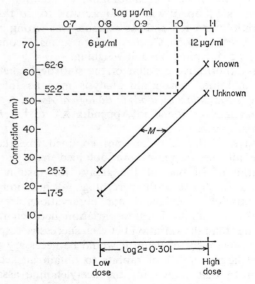

FIG. 3.2. Bioassay of a solution of acetylcholine. The graph shows the mean responses from table 3.1 plotted against dose. The horizontal scale at the bottom shows points only for 'low doses' and 'high doses', the distance between them representing log 2. The distance, M, separating the lines for the known and unknown solutions, therefore represents the logarithm of the ratio of strengths of the known and unknown solutions. The horizontal scale at the top of the graph is the log acetylcholine concentration and the points plotted for the known solutions correspond to this scale. The mean response produced by the $2x$ concentration can be read off this line on to the scale of log concentration. Note that the points plotted for the unknown solutions have no relevance to the top scale.

TABLE 3.1. Responses (mm) on a kymograph of guinea-pig ileum to varying concentration of acetylcholine chloride (ng/ml).

	6 ng/ml	12 ng/ml	x ng/ml	$2x$ ng/ml	Total for 4.
	29·5	66·5	20·0	57·0	173·0
	28·0	67·0	22·0	55·0	172·0
	27·0	64·0	20·0	55·0	166·0
	26·0	67·0	20·0	53·5	166·5
	27·5	62·0	16·5	54·0	160·0
	29·5	61·0	20·0	51·0	159·5
	26·5	63·0	15·0	51·0	155·5
	22·5	61·5	19·0	52·0	155·0
	26·0	59·5	17·0	51·0	153·5
	23·0	60·5	14·0	51·0	148·5
	22·5	59·5	12·0	50·5	144·5
	18·0	60·0	14·5	45·5	138·0
Mean	25·333	62·625	17·500	52·208	

the result of a 3 point assay. The results can be obtained also by calculation.

For the 1 and 2 dose assay

$$\log 2x = \log 6 + \frac{52 \cdot 208 - 25 \cdot 333}{62 \cdot 625 - 25 \cdot 333} \times 0 \cdot 301$$

$$= 0 \cdot 9951$$

$$\therefore \ 2x = 9 \cdot 880.$$

The calculation for the 2 and 2 dose assay is

$$M = \frac{(62 \cdot 625 + 25 \cdot 333) - (52 \cdot 208 + 17 \cdot 5)}{(62 \cdot 625 + 52 \cdot 208) - (25 \cdot 333 + 17 \cdot 5)} \times 0 \cdot 301$$

$$= 0 \cdot 0763$$

$$\text{antilog } M = \text{the ratio } \frac{6}{x} = 1 \cdot 192$$

thus the estimate of x is 5·034 ng/ml and of $2x$ is 10·067 ng/ml. Statistical analysis of the 2 and 2 dose assay shows that the fiducial limits ($P = 0 \cdot 95$) of the ratio 1·192 are 1·16 and 1·22. The narrowness of these limits is unusual and reflects the favourable circumstances. In fact in this experiment the 'unknown' solutions were known and were diluted from the same standard solution as the 'known' solution. x was 5 and $2x$ was 10, so that the true ratio was 1·200 and the estimate was wrong by less than 7 parts in 1,000. Greater errors may arise from poor techniques for pipetting and weighing.

An authoritative account of the statistical considerations and the appropriate analysis may be found in Finney's *Statistical methods in Biological Assay*. A simple account may be found in Appendix XV to the *British Pharmacopoeia*.

Assays of this kind are not confined to situations where all the responses are obtained from a single preparation. In one of the assays for insulin given by the *Pharmacopoeia* the percentage fall in blood sugar concentration is measured, and observations are made in different rabbits. Because variation between rabbits is greater than the variation between successive responses of the same piece of ileum it would be necessary to use a very large number of rabbits to obtain an accuracy similar to that shown for the acetylcholine assay on guinea-pig ileum. The same rabbits can be used again after an interval of a day or two; in a **cross-over test** each rabbit is used twice, once for a dose of standard and once for a dose of unknown insulin.

BIOASSAY OF ANTAGONISTS USING PREPARATIONS WHICH GIVE GRADED RESPONSES

When the substance being assayed is an antagonist it is necessary to expose the test preparation to an appropriate agonist. This may be endogenous but better control is achieved if a constant dose of agonist is applied to the preparation at regular intervals. Application of antagonist then reduces the effect of the agonist and the percentage reduction is used as the response in comparing known and unknown concentrations of antagonist. Much of our knowledge of the role of adrenaline and noradrenaline in the sympathetic nervous system is the result of using tissue perfusates and nerve extracts to inhibit carbachol-induced contractions of isolated rat uterus and colon preparations, and comparing the degree of inhibition with those produced by known solutions of adrenaline or noradrenaline.

All or none responses

In many tests, the response is all or none, e.g. when an animal is given a drug in a toxicity test it either dies or survives. The system on which the drug is being tested is a unit which either shows a response or does not and, since units vary in sensitivity, quantitative comparisons can be made only by using a number of units. Since the individual units vary in their sensitivity to the action of the drug, different doses of the drug kill different proportions of groups of animals; similarly, different concentrations of drugs block different proportions of the nerve fibres in a nerve trunk. In these circumstances an apparently graded response is obtained, but in reality it is **quantal**, i.e. made up of units. If five animals are used in a toxicity test, the only responses possible are 0, 20, 40, 60, 80 or 100 per cent mortality. The graded nature of the response arises solely from the variation in the sensitivity of the individuals in the group. If this variation is small, it may be difficult to find a dose which neither kills all the animals nor is without effect on all the animals, i.e. the graph of log dose against response (percentage mortality) is very steep. On the other hand, if the variation in sensitivity is great, the log dose response curve is flat.

The variation in sensitivity can be observed by infusing drug slowly into each animal until an effect is obtained, thereby learning the **individual effective doses.** If individual lethal doses are grouped in small increments and a histogram in which the number killed is plotted against the dose, the distribution of sensitivity can be seen. This usually approximates fairly well to the normal distribution (vol. 1, p. 3.4). It is often assumed that there is some reason why this should be so, or even that it is mathematically established to be so. In fact all that is known is that most values group around the mean and that doses further from the mean occur progressively less frequently; but there is no *a priori* reason for expecting any mathematically derived curve to be valid. The advantage of assuming that data fit a normal distribution curve is that rigorous deductions about probability can then be drawn and this forms the basis of many statistical calculations. Fortunately the calculations are not likely to go far astray even if the distribution is not strictly normal.

The normal curve is symmetrical so that the mean

effective dose is also the most frequently effective dose (the mode) and the frequency falls away at the same rate on each side of the mean; thus if the mode dose is x then the two doses $x - \delta x$ and $x + \delta x$ occur with the same frequency. It also follows from the symmetry of the curve that if the fixed dose $x - \delta x$ is given to a group of animals it will kill the same proportion of the group as $x + \delta x$ will allow to survive. If δx is the standard deviation (s) of the population, the dose $x - s$ will kill one-sixth (16 per cent) of the population and $x + s$ will kill five-sixths (84 per cent) of the population. If the variation extends over a wide range of dose, it often appears that it is the logarithm of the dose rather than the dose itself which is normally distributed; thus, if the mode dose is x then $\frac{1}{2}x$ will kill the same proportion that $2x$ leaves alive. A distribution which is log normal is of course an example of a skew distribution (vol. 1, p. 3.4).

Assays based on all or none responses can be conducted by measuring either individual effective doses or the percentage responses to fixed doses. Preparations are used most economically if individual effective doses can be measured. An example is the guinea-pig assay of digitalis. A dilution made from a standard extract of digitalis is infused slowly into a vein of an anaesthetized guinea-pig until the heart stops beating. The volume of solution required is recorded. This is repeated in other animals and simultaneously another group of guinea-pigs is tested with a dilution made from the digitalis extract which is being compared with the standard. The assay is thus analogous to the comparison of two solutions of an acid by titrating each of them against the same alkali, but in that case there should be a very small difference between duplicate titrations. Guinea-pigs, however, vary so much that duplicates do not agree very well and the mean dose from about five animals for each preparation has to be found. The accuracy of the estimate of potency depends on how lucky or unlucky the experimenter is in getting sensitive and insensitive animals divided equally between the standard and test preparations. The probability of a given level of accuracy can be calculated from the variability of the individual results.

Because the error depends on how well the two samples of animals represent the whole population of animals, the error is often referred to as the **sampling error.**

If it is not possible to measure individual effective doses, and if many animals are available, fixed doses are injected into groups of animals and the percentage mortality at each dose level determined. The percentage can then be treated as a response and curves comparable with those in fig. 3.1 and 3.2 obtained. A line which is more likely to be straight over a greater dose range can be obtained by converting the percentage mortality into **normal equivalent deviations** or into **probits** (probability units). Every percentage corresponds to a given distance

from the mean on the dose scale. This distance can be measured in units of the standard deviation. Thus 16 per cent is one unit less than the mean (50 per cent), and 84 per cent is one unit greater than the mean. The numbers −1, 0 and +1 are thus equivalent to 16, 50 and 84 per cent; other percentages also have equivalents defined by the equation to the normal curve. Such numbers are known as normal equivalent deviations. Probits are more commonly used and are obtained by the arbitrary process of adding five to the normal equivalent deviation. This avoids negative numbers since −5 standard deviations from the mean corresponds to an extremely small percentage, never likely to be met in practice (vol. 1, p. 3.15).

The straight line relating log dose to probit enables 2 and 2 dose assays to be performed in a way similar to those based on graded responses.

A widely used test of this kind is an insulin assay described in the *British Pharmacopoeia*. In this test two groups of mice are given doses of a standard insulin and two groups receive doses of the unknown preparation. In each case one dose is twice as big as the other. The mice are selected to have a narrow range of weight and are put in a constant temperature environment. They are allotted to the four groups randomly. After subcutaneous injection of the insulin the mice are observed for 1·5 hr. If the doses are in the right range, somewhere between 25 per cent and 75 per cent of the mice in each group will have hypoglycaemic convulsions. The percentage in each group is noted, converted to a probit and the values of the log potency ratio and the potency ratio are calculated in the same way as for a graded response assay. The statistical analysis, however, takes a different form since at any one dose there is only one value, a percentage, or probit available. The accuracy of the assay still depends on the variability of the population, the greater the variation, the lower the accuracy. In this kind of assay, as in one based on graded responses, it is important to have responses not too far from the middle of the range. In this case it is not so much the danger of non-linearity that is the problem, but rather that percentages near to zero or to a hundred can be estimated with any accuracy only if very large groups are tested. The statistical analysis indeed recognizes this by giving less weight to responses the further away they are from 50 per cent.

For the insulin assay the *Pharmacopoeia* recommends the use of twenty-four mice per dose, i.e. ninety-six mice for the assay, and this usually gives an estimate with the required accuracy.

DISGUISED ALL OR NONE RESPONSES

In many tissues an apparently graded response is really the sum of a large number of all or none responses. An example is the neuromuscular junction. Transmission at a single neuromuscular junction is an all or none phenomenon, but different concentrations of curare alkaloids produce varied degrees of neuromuscular blockade in a rat phrenic nerve–diaphragm preparation. The reduction in the size of the response of the muscle to nerve stimulation clearly depends upon the proportion of the neuromuscular junctions which have been blocked in an all or none manner and it is logical in such an experiment to plot log dose against the probit of the percentage reduction in the height of the twitch, rather than against the percentage reduction itself. Since factors such as diffusion affect the results and since each concentration can be tested several times the appropriate form of statistical analysis is that for graded responses.

We have discussed the use of graded responses for the assay of agonists and antagonists and the use of all or none responses for the assay of agonists. It is possible to use all or none responses for the assay of an antagonist by comparing the frequency of a response to an agonist in subjects protected by one preparation of antagonist with the frequency in other subjects protected by a different preparation of the antagonist. The technique is used little, if at all, for bioassay but the analogous procedure is used to compare the effectiveness of different antagonists.

Comparison of the activities of different drugs

The comparison of the activities of different drugs is a more involved problem than the comparison of the amounts of the same drug present in different solutions. Provided the same material is present in the standard and unknown solutions, the nature of the effect and the way it is brought about are irrelevant to its bioassay.

When different drugs are compared, however, the situation is different. Unless both drugs act in the same way, attempts at a comparison of potency will have no absolute validity.

It is difficult to show that two drugs act in exactly the same way; this can only be inferred if they behave in the same way. Drugs seldom produce effects which have exactly the same time courses and intrinsically it is impossible to compare quantitatively the activity of two drugs, one of which acts slowly and the other rapidly. Likewise if the log dose response curves, or log dose probit curves, for the two drugs are not parallel, it is impossible to make a quantitative comparison which has any general validity, because the result depends upon the size of the response at which the comparison is made.

It might be thought that if a dose of one compound produces a response which is twice that of the same dose of another, it is twice as active; this is not so. With preparations which give graded responses, differences in the size of the response depend not only upon the activity of the drug but also upon the steepness of the log dose response curve; this varies not only from one type of preparation to another but also between individual preparations of the same type. In order to multiply the size of the response by two it is necessary to increase the dose very much more when the preparation has a flat log dose response curve than when it has a steep one. With preparations which give all or none responses the same situation is found. The slope of the log dose probit line depends on the variability of the population of units. This varies from population to population as well as from drug to drug.

In order to compare the concentrations of two drugs which produce similar responses, comparisons similar to the assays described earlier can be used. If it is found that x ml of an S molar solution of the standard produce the same response as y ml of a T molar solution of the second drug, then the activity of the second drug is xS/yT times that of the first. If the test drug is more active than the standard, y or T will be small and the ratio will be high. The result is often expressed the other way up, yT/xS, when it is called **equipotent molar ratio**. This indicates the number of molecules of the second compound which produces the same response as one molecule of the reference compound. If the second compound is feeble, y or T is large and the value is high; if it is much more active than the reference compound the value is a small fraction.

A one and two dose assay is the simplest method for estimating the concentrations of two different drugs which produce comparable responses, but it does not reveal whether the log dose response curves have the same slope. For this reason it is better to use a 2 and 2 dose comparison in which the slopes of the log dose response curves for both drugs are measured and can be compared. If, within the limits of error of the experiment, the slopes of the lines in a four-point assay appear to be the same, the comparison is meaningful, at least for the particular conditions of the test. If the lines are significantly divergent, the effects of the two compounds are not capable of being compared quantitatively.

In addition it may be important to check that the experiment is capable of revealing differences in the time course of the effects. Many test methods for comparing the activities of different drugs are evolved in order to screen large numbers of new drugs. Ideally such methods must be simple so that they do not require highly skilled staff and also so that many compounds can be studied rapidly using the minimum amount of each compound. It is inevitable that sometimes the test can be made simple only by procedures which greatly reduce the value of the result; the effects of drugs may be compared only at their peak or, more usually, only after a fixed time interval; often only one dose level of the test drug is studied. Such tests can lead to meaningless estimates of relative potency and this, unfortunately, is not apparent because the test does not itself supply the necessary information which would show that they are meaningless.

Only a full comparison of the time course of the effects and of the slopes of the log dose response curves would do this.

All that has been said about the comparison of the activities of drugs which are agonists is applicable to the comparison of the activities of drugs which are antagonists. The methods which are used to assay solutions of antagonists are easily adapted to compare the activities of different antagonist drugs, provided that the time course of the antagonism and the relationship between antagonism and dose of antagonist is studied for each drug.

Values of the activity ratios or equipotent molar ratios of different drugs are of great practical value. They give some idea as to which drugs are worthy of further study and in some circumstances may indicate what dose of the new drug might be useful clinically. In addition the comparison of the activities of a number of drugs leads to the discovery of empirical relationships between activity and chemical structure, which may indicate what further compounds are likely to be active. The results also immediately raise two fundamental questions: 'why is one drug more active than another?' and 'is there any means of expressing activity in absolute terms or can it be expressed only relative to another (standard) drug?' The answers to both these questions are directly related to the more general question: 'how do drugs affect cells?'

LAW OF MASS ACTION AND DRUG-RECEPTOR INTERACTION

Agonists and receptors

Theories of heterogeneous catalysis and of enzymic catalysis have been evolved by studying the effects of altering the concentrations of different reactants on the rate of the reaction. The results can be analysed mathematically and the information used to interpret how the reaction occurs. The interaction between the receptors in a tissue and an agonist drug, however, is not so easily studied experimentally. There are two obstacles; first there is the fact that results often cannot be obtained with sufficient precision. The accurate measurement of biological responses is often difficult and there is a limited range of suitable experimental procedures. One of the most convenient responses to follow is the contraction of smooth muscle, the mechanical shortening of which is easy to record, and a great deal of theoretical discussion has been based on experiments with isolated pieces of guinea-pig ileum or other kinds of smooth muscle. But the size of the response is affected by the treatment the tissue has already received, e.g. whether it has been recently exposed to a high dose or a low dose of drug, or left quiescent for a period of time. Whereas an enzyme or a metal catalyst can be maintained in

more or less standard conditions throughout an experiment, a tissue is far more complex and the dynamic processes within it are likely to vary from moment to moment. Clark pointed out many years ago (1933) that a single set of experimental results for dose and response could be made to 'fit' an exponential curve, a parabola or a hyperbola. Indeed the shape of the dose response curve depends on the characteristics of the recording system, e.g. whether the lever is isotonic or isometric. This is one aspect of the second and major obstacle standing in the way of a quantitative interpretation of the action of drugs, which is that the observed response is unlikely to be related in any simple way to the initial action of a drug at its receptor. However, the first stage in the process, the interaction between drug and receptor, can be dealt with in the same way as interaction of enzyme and substrate and may be written:

$$\text{Drug} + \text{receptor} \underset{k_{-1}}{\overset{k_{+1}}{\rightleftharpoons}} \text{complex} \longrightarrow \text{response}$$

The rate of formation of the complex is $k_{+1}[A](1-y)$ where $[A]$ is the concentration of drug, y is the proportion of receptors occupied by drug, and k_{+1} is a rate constant; the rate of dissociation of the complex is $k_{-1}y$, where k_{-1} is a second rate constant. At equilibrium the rate of complex formation equals the rate of break down, therefore:

$$k_{+1}[A](1-y) = k_{-1}y$$

and

$$\frac{k_{+1}}{k_{-1}} = K_A = \frac{y}{[A](1-y)}$$

or

$$[A]K_A = \frac{y}{1-y} \tag{1}$$

or

$$y = \frac{[A]K_A}{1+[A]K_A} \tag{2}$$

where K_A is the equilibrium or affinity constant. The various forms of the equation are convenient for different purposes. Equations 1 and 2 correspond to different forms of the Michaelis–Menten equation. For instance equation 2 corresponds to

$$v = \frac{V[S]}{K_m + [S]}$$

which is equation 2 in vol. 1, p. 7.8 dealing with enzyme kinetics; in equation 2 above, y, the proportion of receptors occupied, replaces v/V, where v is velocity and V is the maximum velocity of substrate breakdown; $[A]$ replaces the substrate concentration $[S]$, and K_A is the reciprocal of K_m. The rate of substrate breakdown, v, is proportional to the amount of enzyme-substrate complex and is equal to $k_{+2}[ES]$, where k_{+2} is a further rate constant. It has often been assumed that, in a similar way, the size of the effect produced by a drug on a tissue varies directly with the proportion of receptors occupied but this assumption leads to improbable conclusions.

When one thinks of the complexity of the biological changes which result from, for example, the action of acetylcholine on smooth muscle, such a simple relation seems extremely improbable. The problem posed by the intermediate stages in the production of the effect of a drug can be side-stepped; if r is used to represent the size of response we can write

$$r = f(s) \qquad (3)$$

where $s = ey$ and e is a constant called efficacy which is rather analogous to k_{+2}, the constant which determines the speed of enzyme action. Just as a high rate of substrate breakdown can occur because either ES or k_{+2} is large, so one can get a high value of s either because y or e is large. s is a rather hypothetical entity which has been called the stimulus. Its value might increase almost indefinitely and at some point further increases produce no detectable increase in the response (fig. 3.3). All substances for which e is large enough to give such values of s, bearing in mind that y cannot be greater than 1, produce the same maximum response, which can be

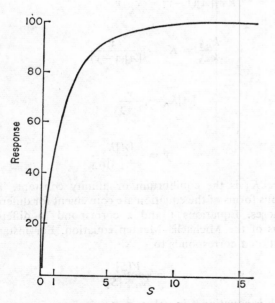

FIG. 3.3. Curve relating the response to the stimulus $s = ey$ based on effect concentration curve for analogues of acetylcholine acting on guinea-pig ileum. The effect is plotted against concentration but the concentration scale is replaced by the scale of s with $s = 1$ corresponding to 50 per cent of the maximum response.

regarded as the true maximum response. If e is not big enough, the response levels off before the true maximum is reached. For compounds where e is large, s reaches a value corresponding to the true maximum response when y is appreciably less than 1, and a whole range of values of e, or efficacy, give the same maximum response from the tissue. There will be different proportions of unused receptors depending on the efficacy of the drug. The unused receptors have been called **spare receptors**, emphasizing the fact that not all the receptors are required to produce the maximum response. The word spare has given rise to misunderstanding and it does not imply that there is any variation in the characterization of the population of receptors. With a compound of high efficacy there are many spare receptors, perhaps 99 per cent; for a compound with a lower efficacy there are fewer spare receptors and with a still lower efficacy it is not possible to obtain the true maximum response even when all the receptors are occupied, and none are spare. A compound with zero or negligible efficacy produces no response, but excludes other drugs and is therefore itself an antagonist. The compounds which have low efficacy also reduce the effect of other agonists because they are occupying many of the receptors. Such compounds, therefore, have properties intermediate between agonist and antagonist and are in consequence called **partial agonists** or competitive dualists.

For compounds with high efficacy which produce effects when the proportion of receptors occupied is small, i.e. when $y \ll 1$, and $(1-y) \to 1$, equation 1 reduces to

$$[A]K_A = y$$

and therefore the stimulus is given by

$$s = e[A]K_A \qquad (4)$$

Thus the stimulus produced by an agonist with high efficacy is directly proportional to its concentration. Hence the relationship between response and stimulus is the same as that between response and concentration.

It is therefore possible by measuring the responses produced by different concentrations to plot a graph of response against stimulus and this is how fig. 3.3 was obtained. It will be observed that quite small changes in stimulus produce large changes in small responses, but that much larger changes in stimulus are needed to increase responses which are already large.

A RATE THEORY OF DRUG ACTION

In the foregoing discussion it has been assumed that the continuing existence of a drug receptor complex is necessary for the action of the drug, and that the magnitude of a drug effect at a given moment is determined by the number of receptors which are combined with drug. This assumption is sometimes given the distinction of being referred to as **occupation theory** to contrast it with an alternative assumption known as **rate theory**. Rate theory starts with the postulate that it is only the act of combination of drug with receptor which initiates action and that a prolonged combination makes no further contribution. If the receptor is some unknown enzyme (if it were known it would not be necessary to call it a receptor) then a drug acting according to occupation theory would be analogous to a prosthetic group which, by modifying the enzyme or receptor, increases the speed of some reaction leading to the observed response. One way in which a drug could act as required by rate theory would be for it to act as a coenzyme which was itself modified by the action of the enzyme or receptor, so that only a single molecular event would be catalysed by one interaction between a drug molecule and the receptor.

If agonist action is associated with the act of combination of drug and receptor then the effect is determined by the rate at which such combinations occur, i.e. $k_{+1}[A](1-y)$; when equilibrium is reached this rate must of course equal $k_{-1}y$. The fact that an effect dependent on the rate of association should be thus related to the dissociation rate constant follows from the fact that the act of combination can continue only if receptors are made re-available by the breakdown of the complexes. If the breakdown is slow, as appears to be the case with antagonists, the equilibrium rate of combination must also be low and this in itself might be sufficient to account for the difference between agonists and antagonists.

Because rate theory predicts that the equilibrium effect is dependent on $k_{-1}y$, i.e. on y, it is difficult to distinguish between the two assumptions, since according to occupation theory also, the effect is dependent on y. In non-equilibrium conditions, i.e. immediately after a drug is applied to or removed from tissue, the two theories make different predictions; while some evidence has been obtained which supports a rate theory, the experiments can be interpreted in other ways and there is no general acceptance that one or other theory is right. Nor is it necessary that there should be; in some instances it may be the continuous occupation which is important while in other situations the rate of interaction may determine the size of the response.

One clear pointer which exists is the difference in the effective concentrations of agonists and antagonist drugs. If agonists act continuously while sitting on receptors then a high affinity would be one way of achieving a high activity and if agonists produce an effect when very few receptors are occupied, while competitive antagonists must occupy many receptors, it would be expected that agonists would be effective at lower concentrations than antagonists. In fact this does not seem to happen; acetylcholine, for example, produces effects in concentrations of about 10^{-8} or 10^{-7} M and atropine exerts a significant blocking action at 10^{-9} M. This fits better with rate theory, which asserts that a drug becomes an antagonist if it does not quickly leave a receptor so that it is difficult for an agonist to have a high affinity.

A feature of rate theory of which William of Occam would have approved is that the separate constant for efficacy (e) becomes redundant since the equilibrium response would be dependent on $k_{-1}y$, and the value of k_{-1} would determine whether a substance is agonist, partial agonist or antagonist, just as the value of e would determine the kind of action according to occupation theory. The fact that e and k_{-1} are interchangeable in this way makes it possible to use K and e for the discussion of drug action without prejudging the nature of the underlying interaction.

In some situations it is found that repeated application of an agonist produces **tachyphylaxis**, i.e. the responses to constant doses become progressively smaller; the tissue has become refractory or **desensitized**. One mechanism by which tachyphylaxis is known to occur depends on the fact that the administered drug does not produce the observed effect directly, but owes its action to the release of an active agent from bound stores. As the stores are depleted less is available for release and tachyphylaxis develops.

A more general explanation of tachyphylaxis would be provided by rate theory; it has been argued that the reduced response is the result of a reduced rate of drug-receptor combination, because the receptors are still occupied by the drug molecules which, by combining, produced the previous response. There are instances where this explanation has been shown to be wrong and one must fall back on undefined metabolic changes, or even more vaguely on fatigue, to account for tachyphylaxis. In experiments aimed at elucidating receptor mechanisms it is necessary to avoid fatigue.

A variation of occupation theory, which has been suggested to explain the quite rapid desensitization which occurs at the neuromuscular junction postulates, the conversion of the normal receptor to a refractory receptor, R', with the following interactions.

$$A + R \underset{k_{-1}}{\overset{k_{+1}}{\rightleftharpoons}} AR \rightarrow \text{response}$$
$$\Big\Updownarrow k_{-2} \quad \Big\Updownarrow k_{+2}$$
$$A + R' \rightleftharpoons AR'$$

If k_{-1} were larger than k_{+2}, desensitization due to this cause would not be likely. If k_{+2} were bigger than k_{-1} desensitization could well occur.

Whatever explanation is given for the way in which agonists act, it is clear that their activity depends upon at least two possibly unrelated properties, i.e. their ability to become bound to the receptors and their ability to activate them. At some sites the ability to desensitize receptors may be involved as well. All this information cannot be obtained merely by comparing concentrations which produce comparable responses and expressing the results as an activity ratio or equipotent molar ratio. Further, a change in chemical structure which leads to a change in activity may do so because it affects any or all of these properties. It is, therefore, unreasonable to expect to be able to correlate chemical structure directly with the biological activity of agonists; attempts must be made to assess separately the effects of chemical structure on affinity, on efficacy and perhaps on ability to desensitize. If a compound does not cause appreciable desensitization, its activity could, in fact, be defined by its affinity constant and its efficacy. Methods for measuring these depend upon the use of antagonists and are described on p. 3.15. There is, as yet, very little experience in the application of such methods.

Antagonists and receptors

Although antagonists produce an effect only in the presence of an agonist, their mode of action is often easier to interpret than that of agonists and theory can be used to predict experimental results. Many antagonists combine reversibly with the receptors, and if the reaction between agonist and receptors is written

$$A + R \rightleftharpoons AR \rightarrow \text{response},$$

that for a competitive antagonist, B can be written

$$B + R \rightleftharpoons BR$$

If the agonist and the antagonist are present simultaneously they will compete with each other for the receptors. With the notation which was used in deriving equation 1, and if the proportion of receptors occupied by the antagonist is z, we can write for the equilibrium condition

$$k_{+1}[A](1 - y - z) = k_{-1}y \tag{5}$$

Combining the two rate constants into the equilibrium or affinity constant as before gives

$$[A]K_A = \frac{y}{1 - y - z} \tag{6}$$

If the affinity constant of the antagonist is K_B, then

$$[B]K_B = \frac{z}{1 - y - z} \tag{7}$$

Dividing these two equations we get

$$\frac{z}{y} = \frac{[B]K_B}{[A]K_A} \quad \text{or} \quad z = \frac{y[B]K_B}{[A]K_A} \tag{8}$$

so that, combining (6) and (8)

$$y = [A]K_A\left(1 - y - \frac{y[B]K_B}{[A]K_A}\right)$$

or

$$\frac{y}{1 - y} = \frac{[A]K_A}{1 + [B]K_B} \tag{9}$$

or

$$y = \frac{[A]K_A}{1 + [A]K_A + [B]K_B} \tag{10}$$

Equations 9 and 10 are forms of Gaddum's equation.

If we compare equation 9 with that for agonist alone (equation 1) we see that the introduction of $[B]$ has the apparent effect of decreasing the agonist affinity constant by dividing it by the factor $1 + [B]K_B$; the effect of the antagonist can therefore be overcome by increasing the agonist concentration by the same factor. This can be expressed algebraically. If we write $[A]_0$ for the concentration of agonist which causes the proportion y^* of the receptors to be occupied by agonist when no antagonist is present, and $[A]_B$ for the agonist concentration producing the same receptor occupancy when antagonist is present, we have from equations 1 and 9

$$[A]_0 K_A = \frac{y^*}{1 - y^*} = \frac{[A]_B K_A}{1 + [B]K_B}$$

or

$$\frac{[A]_B}{[A]_0} - 1 = [B]K_B \tag{11}$$

The ratio of the two concentrations of agonist which produce the same effect with and without the antagonist, $[A]_B/[A]_0$, is usually called the **dose ratio**.

The fact that K_A does not appear in equation 11 indicates that the dose ratio will be the same whatever agonist is used, provided that it acts on the same receptors as the antagonist. The fact that y^* does not appear in the equation indicates that the relationship is true for all values of y so that the dose ratio for a particular concentration of antagonist is independent of the size of response at which the comparison is made.

If the only action of the antagonist is to occupy the receptors, it will not modify the relationship of r to s and the graph of log dose or log concentration of agonist against response will remain the same shape but will be displaced to the right by an amount equal to the logarithm of the dose ratio (fig. 3.4). If a series of concentrations of the antagonist is tested, a series of parallel lines should be obtained and the extent of their displacement will be determined by equation 11. This is a description of the way in which **competitive antagonists** behave. At one time it was thought that evidence of this kind was enough to prove that an antagonist was acting competitively, but it is now realized that other blocking mechanisms could give similar results for dose ratios up to about 100 (p. 3.14). However, when a parallel shift and agreement with equation 11 is obtained over a wider range of concentration it is difficult to avoid the conclusion that the antagonism is competitive.

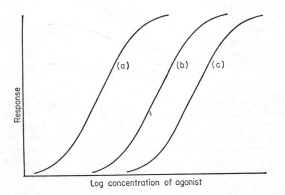

FIG. 3.4. Response plotted against log concentration of agonist. The curve (a) represents the normal response, i.e. when no antagonist is present. Curve (b) represents the behaviour when a competitive antagonist is present and curve (c) when a higher concentration of antagonist is used.

A number of antagonists give results which are consistent with competitive antagonism. Clark found that a 1.0×10^{-6} M solution of acetylcholine slowed the rate of beating of the frog's heart to half its original value; when atropine was present a higher concentration of acetylcholine was needed to produce this effect (table 3.2). From the increase in concentration of acetylcholine required with 10^{-5} M atropine, Clark calculated the affinity

TABLE 3.2. Antagonism of acetylcholine by atropine in the frog heart. The observed value of acetylcholine in the presence of 10^{-5} M atropine was used to calculate K_B for atropine. The concentration of acetylcholine required at the other concentrations of atropine was then calculated from this value of K_B.

Atropine concentration (M)	Acetylcholine concentration (M) which reduced the rate of beating to half	
	Observed	Calculated
0	1.0×10^{-6}	
10^{-8}	1.6×10^{-6}	1.3×10^{-6}
10^{-7}	3.6×10^{-6}	4.0×10^{-6}
10^{-6}	2.5×10^{-5}	3.1×10^{-5}
10^{-5}	3.0×10^{-4}	3.0×10^{-4}
10^{-4}	3.5×10^{-3}	3.0×10^{-3}
10^{-3}	4.7×10^{-2}	3.0×10^{-2}

constant and predicted the concentrations of acetylcholine which would be necessary to produce the effect in the presence of other concentrations of atropine. These agreed quite well with the experimental results over the whole range of concentrations tested, from 10^{-8} M to 10^{-3} M atropine. More recently Schild has performed experiments with acetylcholine and atropine on the isolated guinea-pig ileum and shown that equation 11 is obeyed over a wide range from 3×10^{-9} M to 3×10^{-6} M. Other examples where the results have been shown to be consistent with a competitive mechanism are the antagonism of histamine by some antihistamine drugs and the antagonism of *p*-aminobenzoic acid by sulphonamide drugs.

ABSOLUTE ACTIVITY OF COMPETITIVE ANTAGO-NISTS AND MEASUREMENT OF AFFINITY CONSTANT

When antagonism is competitive, the potency of the antagonist is best represented by the affinity constant and there is no need to rely on comparison with another similar substance, as is usually the case with agonists. The affinity constant can be measured only when the equilibrium effect of a known concentration of the antagonist can be observed. In practice this means that such observations are restricted to isolated tissues bathed in prepared solutions. The experiments of Clark and Schild, mentioned above, are of course appropriate ways of measuring values of K. When there is a number of substances to be tested a formalized procedure is useful and what are essentially variants of 2 and 1 or 2 and 2 dose assays may be used.

Responses r_1 and r_2 are obtained with two concentrations of agonist, $[A]_1$ and $[A]_2$. The antagonist B is then added and responses are obtained in the presence of this concentration of antagonist with an increased concentration of agonist. Since it may take some time before the responses are regular because the antagonist has to come into equilibrium with the tissue, the antagonism may appear to increase with time. When the responses are steady, however, it should be possible to find a concentration $[A]_B$ of agonist which produces a response r intermediate between r_1 and r_2. The concentration of agonist, $[A]_0$, which would have produced the response r in the absence of antagonist can be estimated by interpolation (p. 3.5), the dose ratio calculated and hence the affinity constant found from equation 11. In this modified 2 and 1 dose assay it is assumed that the log dose response curve for the agonist in the presence of the antagonist has the same slope as when the antagonist is absent. It is really better to use a modified 2 and 2 dose assay, with two concentrations of agonist in the presence of antagonist to check that the slope of the log dose response curve for the agonist is not altered by the presence of the antagonist. If the lines are parallel, the dose ratio can be calculated by a procedure similar to that shown on p. 3.6, and the affinity constant can again be calculated from equation 11. If a series of concentrations of antagonist is tested, the graph of (dose ratio − 1) can be plotted against the concentration of antagonist. If the antagonist is competing with the agonist for the receptors, this graph should be a straight line passing through the origin and having a slope of K_B.

NONCOMPETITIVE ANTAGONISM

Although many useful drugs are competitive antagonists, several act by mechanisms which are not competitive, though in certain circumstances they may appear to do so. In some instances the antagonist could block by a mechanism other than combination with the receptor, and so the agonist cannot enter into competition with it. In other instances the antagonist is known to form a very strong bond with the receptor and there are cases where it seems that drugs become attached at a site adjacent to the actual receptor. In these situations the agonist cannot replace the antagonist, though the antagonist either prevents the agonist from combining with the receptor or prevents any subsequent response. We have therefore:

$$[A]K_A = \frac{y}{1-y-z} \qquad (6)$$

but

$$[B]K_B = \frac{z}{1-z} \quad \text{instead of} \quad \frac{z}{1-y-z} \qquad (7)$$

The equation connecting y, $[A]$, $[B]$, K_A and K_B becomes

$$y = \frac{[A]K_A}{1+[A]K_A}\left(\frac{1}{1+[B]K_B}\right) \qquad (12)$$

instead of

$$y = \frac{[A]K_A}{1+[A]K_A+[B]K_B} \qquad (10)$$

As before, when $B = 0$,

$$y = \frac{[A]K_A}{1+[A]K_A}$$

but the situation is quite different from a competitive antagonism. In the latter, increasing $[A]$, the term $[A]K_A$ can always be made $\gg [B]K_B$ and so $y \to 1$; in the noncompetitive situation, even quite low concentrations of antagonist will make $1/(1+[B]K_B) < 1$, and although increasing A will make $[A]K_A/(1+[A]K_A) \to 1$, the whole expression for y will $\to 1/(1+[B]K_B)$ which is < 1. The effect which might thus be anticipated for a noncompetitive antagonist is illustrated in fig. 3.5.

This difference between the results expected from competitive and noncompetitive block has been discussed by pharmacologists for many years, and, though examples of competitive block are well known, no good examples

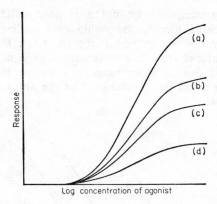

FIG. 3.5. Noncompetitive antagonism. The curve at (a) is the normal dose response curve and those at (b), (c) and (d) represent the curves expected in the presence of increasing concentrations of a noncompetitive antagonist. The expectation is based on the assumption that the response is directly related to the proportion of receptors occupied.

which would match fig. 3.5 seem to have come to light. There were other reasons for thinking that some drugs blocked noncompetitively. For instance papaverine (a nonanalgesic alkaloid from opium) reduces contractions of smooth muscle to the same extent whether the stimulus is provided by acetylcholine, histamine or barium ions. Thus one must suppose either that papaverine combines equally readily with the different receptors, or that it is acting at a site where the actions of the agonists have converged to a common path. If the second alternative is accepted, and it seems more likely, the antagonism cannot be competitive. But the dose response curves do not look like fig 3.5; there is usually some shift to the right before the maximum response is reduced. The size of the maximum is reduced but only with high concentration of papaverine; smaller concentration produces a parallel shift of the dose response curve. The effect of papaverine thus corresponds neither to that illustrated in fig. 3.4 nor to that illustrated in fig. 3.5, but is somewhere between the two.

The discrepancy between fact and expectation became more acute with the discovery of antagonist drugs which appear to form stable covalent bonds with receptors. These are usually called **irreversible antagonists**, though the bonds do in fact break down at a slow rate. In experiments with isolated tissues which have been treated with such antagonists and in which agonists can produce a full response in less than 1 min and often in 5–10 sec, very few of the covalent bonds break down in the time available, so that there can be no effective competition. Yet it was observed that a parallel shift of dose response lines up to dose ratios of about a hundred could nevertheless be obtained; only with greater degrees of block was the maximum response reduced. For a time there was a tendency to believe that two different processes were occurring, that there was a phase of competitive block before the covalent link was established and the block became noncompetitive. Then it was realized that a better explanation was provided if it was accepted that the maximum response did not need all the receptors. This concept has already been discussed on p. 3.10. If a maximum response requires only one per cent of the receptors to be occupied by the agonist then the size of the maximum which can be attained will not be reduced by an irreversible block until more than 99 per cent of the receptors are blocked. There will be some flattening of the dose response curve before this stage is reached. This action of irreversible antagonists provides one of the strong reasons for believing in spare receptors and a means of estimating their extent.

The degree of irreversible block which can be produced before an agonist dose response curve shows a reduced slope and diminished maximum varies with the agonist. This is one of the reasons for believing that agonists differ in their efficacy, i.e. in their ability to activate receptors. A substance with low efficacy, which therefore has to occupy an appreciable fraction of the receptors, has its maximum response reduced when the degree of block is quite small. An agonist with higher efficacy is still able to produce the original maximum and more block is required before its maximum is reduced. It is apparent that experiments of this kind make it possible to evaluate the separate contributions of efficacy and affinity to the overall activity of agonists for which irreversible antagonists are available.

AFFINITY CONSTANT AND EFFICACY OF PARTIAL AGONISTS

Because a true agonist occupies a very small proportion of the receptors the dose response curve contains no information about how the law of mass action applies to the interaction between drug and receptor. A partial agonist on the other hand occupies a lot of receptors and so its dose response curve contains information about the mass law interaction. The mass law information can be obtained by comparing the responses of true agonist and partial agonist. This involves the comparison of the concentrations of the two drugs required to produce given responses. For any given response the product of efficacy (e) and proportion of receptors occupied is the same for the two drugs, i.e.

$$s = e_A y \quad \text{and} \quad s = e_P p$$

(where p is the proportion of receptors occupied by the partial agonist) so that from equation 2,

$$\frac{e_A K_A [A]}{1 + K_A [A]} = \frac{e_P K_P [P]}{1 + K_P [P]} \qquad (13)$$

where $[A]$ and $[P]$ are the concentrations of agonist and

partial agonist producing responses of the same size. We have seen that for an agonist of high efficacy where the proportion of receptors occupied is small, the left side of this equation reduces to $e_A K_A [A]$ so that,

$$e_A K_A [A] = \frac{e_P K_P [P]}{1 + K_P [P]}$$

Taking the reciprocal of both sides and multiplying by $e_A K_A$ gives

$$\frac{1}{[A]} = \frac{e_A K_A}{e_P K_P} \cdot \frac{1}{[P]} + \frac{e_A K_A}{e_P} \qquad (14)$$

It will be seen that this is the equation of a straight line, $y = ax + b$ where the two variables are $1/[A]$ and $1/[P]$. By finding experimentally a series of matching concentrations of the agonist and partial agonist, one can plot the straight line corresponding to equation 14 (fig. 3.6).

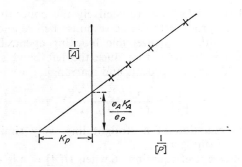

FIG. 3.6. Reciprocal plot of equiactive concentrations of a partial agonist and a true agonist. The abscissa is the reciprocal of partial agonist concentration and the ordinate is the reciprocal of the true agonist concentration. In practice the two ordinates would have very different scales to accommodate the fact that agonists are effective in much lower concentration than partial agonists. The straight line represents equation 14 and the intercept with the abscissa gives the affinity constant of the partial agonist.

Extrapolating to $1/[A] = 0$ the line meets the abscissa at a point where $1/[P] = -K_P$. That is, we have found the affinity constant of the partial agonist.

Values of e have to be given on an arbitrary scale; the scale can be determined by putting s equal to 1 for a response which is 50 per cent of the maximum. If the concentration of A which produces 50 per cent of the maximum response is $[A]_{50}$, and remembering that

$s = e_A K_A [A]$, we have $e_A K_A [A]_{50} = 1$ or

$$e_A K_A = \frac{1}{[A]_{50}} \qquad (15)$$

Now the intercept of equation 14 with the ordinate, when $1/[P] = 0$, corresponds to a value of $1/[A]$ equal to $e_A K_A / e_P$; substituting in equation 15, e_P can be calculated.

AFFINITY CONSTANT AND EFFICACY OF AGONISTS

As was pointed out above, the response curve for agonist does not normally contain any information about the mass law constant; by treatment with irreversible antagonists the number of available receptors can be reduced to a point where the maximum response can no longer be produced and with increasing concentrations of agonist the remaining receptors are increasingly saturated. A comparison of the normal dose response curve with that obtained after blocking most of the receptors allows information about the mass law interaction to be extracted. If z is the proportion of the receptors blocked irreversibly we can write an equation corresponding to equation 13

$$\frac{e_A K_A[A]}{1 + K_A[A]} = \frac{e_A(1-z).K_A[A]_I}{1 + K_A[A]_I}$$

where $[A]$ and $[A]_I$ are respectively the concentrations of A which produce the same response before and after treatment with the irreversible blocking agent. In this case there is no need to reduce the left hand side to $e_A K_A[A]$. Taking reciprocals and rearranging, we obtain

$$\frac{1}{[A]} = \frac{1}{1-z}.\frac{1}{[A]_I} + \frac{zK_A}{1-z} \qquad (16)$$

again an equation of a straight line, very similar to equation 14 (fig. 3.7).

The intercept of equation 16 when $1/[A] = 0$ is $-zK_A$. Since the slope of the line is $1/(1-z)$, z can be found and hence K_A. With K_A known e_A can be found from equation 15.

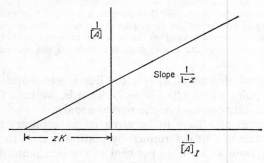

FIG. 3.7. Reciprocal plot of concentrations of agonist before and after treatment with irreversible antagonist to reduce available receptors (equation 16).

DRUGS AS CHEMICALS

When considering how the activity of drugs can be measured it has been supposed that they interact with receptors by some chemical process. While it is not clear how receptors function, some consideration must be given to the chemical properties of drugs, about which, in contrast to those of receptors, information should be readily available.

The chemical properties of drugs depend upon the arrangement of the atoms within the molecule, i.e. its size and shape, and hence the arrangement of electric charge within the molecule, i.e. the electron distribution.

The systematic chemical name of a drug gives an unambiguous description of the arrangement of the atoms of which it is made. The molecular formula may be drawn on paper but, because the molecule is a three-dimensional structure, this may not convey much idea of the shape and may even be entirely misleading. A more complete picture is obtained by studying a scale model of the molecule. Ideally, such a model is based on mathematical analysis of X-ray or electron diffraction patterns obtained with a crystal of the drug. This provides accurate information about bond lengths and bond angles and gives a complete picture of the arrangement of the atoms in the molecule in the crystalline state. Crystallographic analysis, however, is time consuming and expensive and has not been performed except in the case of a few drugs. Atomic models are available commercially which are based on average bond lengths and bond angles and a model of the drug made from these is likely to be approximately correct. Some models attempt to give some idea of the space occupied by the atoms and the drug is represented as a solid, others, stick models, indicate only distances between atoms and the drug is represented as a wire skeleton. Both types have their advantages and disadvantages. With the space-filling models there is always uncertainty as to whether the atoms can really be represented as solid lumps; the size of the lump as a rule depends on the Van der Waals radius for the atom, and this is not as clearly defined as the distance between atoms. The advantage of this type of model is that it may reveal steric hindrance, i.e. a situation when the groups in a molecule obstruct each other and so cannot assume positions which they might be expected to do from a drawing or a stick model. Stick models have the advantage that it is much easier to see the main arrangement of the atoms, e.g. in buckled rings, and to measure the distances between them.

The importance of the use of molecular models is illustrated by studying the antihistamine drug triprolidine (fig. 3.8). In spite of what might be expected from the molecular formula, or from examination of stick models, the benzene and pyridine rings cannot lie in the same plane; there is not enough room. In triprolidine itself, in which the pyridine and pyrrolidine rings are in the *trans* position, the pyridine rings and the double bond are in the same plane and the benzene ring is forced to be at 90° to this plane; the ultraviolet absorption spectrum resembles that of a vinylpyridine. In the isomer in which the pyridine and pyrrolidine rings are *cis*, it is the benzene ring which is in the same place as the double bond and the ultraviolet absorption spectrum resembles that of a styrene. The different arrangements of the groups in the two forms is important; the *trans* compound is a much more potent antihistamine than the *cis*.

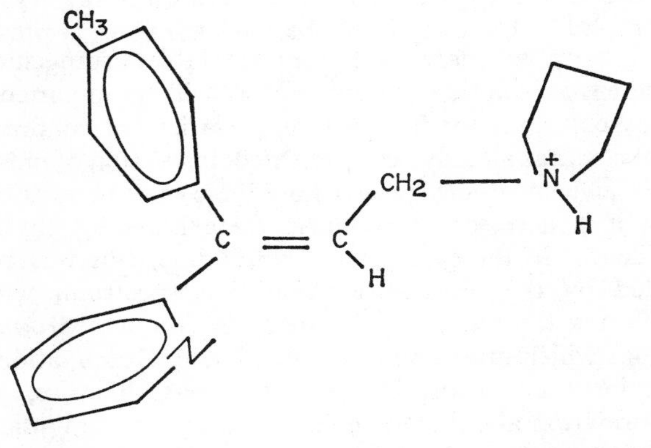

Fig. 3.8. Triprolidine, *trans* form in which the pyridine and pyrrolidine rings lie on either side of the double bond.

The existence of isomeric forms can often, of course, be deduced from a drawing of the molecular formula but it is usually very much easier to appreciate by studying models. When the isomerism exists because of the asymmetrical arrangement of groups about an atom, usually a tetra-covalent carbon atom, the isomers are optically active. The solutions of these compounds rotate the plane of polarization of light clockwise (dextrorotatory +), or anticlockwise (laevorotatory −). The degree of rotation and even the sign of rotation is a function of the wavelength of the light.

The direction of rotation in itself gives no indication of the arrangement of the groups about the asymmetric atom. For example, the (+) form of glyceraldehyde can easily be oxidized to glyceric acid; this has the same arrangement of groups about the asymmetric carbon atom but it is laevorotatory (−). To indicate that the relative configuration is the same in both, the symbol D is sometimes used. In 1891, Fischer proposed that the groups (+) in glyceraldehyde should be assumed to be arranged as in fig. 3.9a; all compounds in which the arrangement of the H, HO, and CH_2OH groups is the same can be referred to by this symbol D, though they will not all be (+) compounds, as has already been shown. For amino acids the reference standard is (−) serine, which is described as L and in which the groups are assumed to be arranged as in fig. 3.9b. All compounds in which the arrangement of these groups is the same can be referred to by the symbol L. The arrangement

of the H, H_2N, and CH_2OH groups in this form of serine is the same as that in the L form of glyceraldehyde.

It is now known that Fischer's assumption is correct and that the groups in (+) glyceraldehyde really are arranged as shown. It is possible, therefore, to describe absolutely the configuration of these compounds,

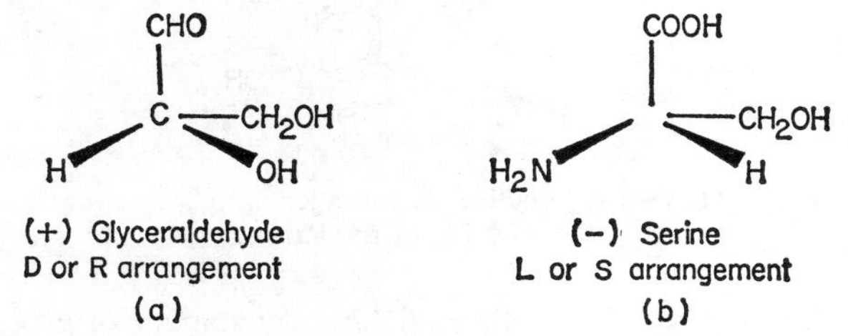

Fig. 3.9(a) (+) glyceraldehyde, D or R arrangement, (b) (−) serine, L or S arrangement. See p. 3.18 for the meaning of R and S.

and that of many others related to them. For sugars or amino acids the absolute configuration can usually be deduced fairly simply from the relative configuration but there is often considerable difficulty and confusion with drugs which do not clearly fall into either class. The configuration of the (+) form of tartaric acid, for example, is ambiguous, and it was this compound which was used to establish the correctness of Fischer's assumption. The absolute configuration of this compound is shown in fig. 3.10. If it is regarded as a sugar, with the

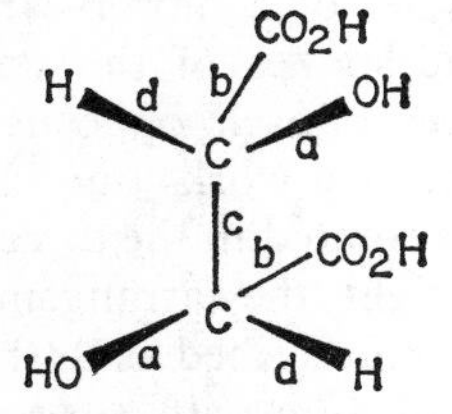

Fig. 3.10. (+) Tartaric acid, R arrangement. See p. 3.18 for the meaning of the letters.

COOH in place of CH_2OH, the arrangement at both asymmetric carbon atoms is L; if it is regarded as an amino acid with HO in place of H_2N, the arrangement is D. It is necessary to describe it as L_g or D_s. The compound adrenaline is likewise difficult to describe. The (−) form, which is much more active biologically than the (+) form, is known to have the configuration shown in fig. 3.11. If this is regarded as a derivative of glyceraldehyde in which the CH_2OH is replaced by CH_2NHCH_3, the arrangement is L; if it is regarded as an amino acid derivative in which the CH_2NHCH_3 replaces the COOH the compound would be a substituted glycine and the arrangement is D. The ambiguity arises because the sugar chemist and the amino acid chemist look at the arrangement of three different groups (vol. 1, p. 9.5); drugs which are neither sugars nor amino acids have to be classified by imaginary replacement of groups, which can often be ambiguous.

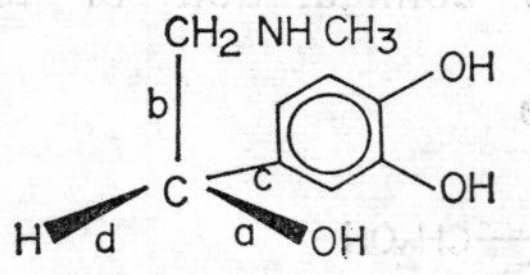

FIG. 3.11. (−) Adrenaline, R arrangement. See below for the meaning of the letters.

An absolute description of the arrangement of groups about an asymmetric atom can be given simply and unambiguously by the convention of Prelog in which the bonds are assigned priority depending on the atomic number of the atoms attached to them. (+) Tartaric acid and (−) adrenaline will serve as illustrations. In (+) tartaric acid each asymmetric carbon atom is attached to a hydrogen atom, an oxygen atom and two carbon atoms. The atomic number of oxygen is greater than that of carbon, which is greater than that of hydrogen, so the carbon–oxygen bond carries greatest priority (a) and the carbon–hydrogen bond least (d). Of the carbon–carbon bonds, one is further attached by three bonds to oxygen, the other by one bond to oxygen, one to carbon and one to hydrogen. The former carries greater priority (b), the latter less (c). Bond (d) is regarded as the steering column of a motor car of which bonds a, b, and c are the spokes of the steering wheel; the observer, who places himself opposite and away from the steering column, then works out what will happen if the steering wheel is rotated in the direction a–b–c. If the car turns to the right the arrangement is described as R, if to the left it is described as S (these symbols were chosen to avoid confusion with D or L). For (+) tartaric acid the configuration at both asymmetric atoms is R (the RS compound is the *meso* form). For adrenaline it is easy to assign greatest priority to the C—O bond and least to the C—H, but the two other bonds are both to carbon atoms. Of these two, one is further bound to nitrogen, and takes precedence over the other which is bound only to carbon, which has a lower atomic number than nitrogen. Even though the latter has three bonds to carbon atoms, this does not compensate for a single bond to an element of higher atomic number. The arrangement is therefore R. This convention is an unambiguous way of describing absolute configuration, and is therefore important in describing the arrangement of groups for drugs which are optically active and are not clearly either sugars or amino acids. Its one disadvantage is that it does not indicate configurational resemblances at first sight; compounds may have the same relative configuration but one may be R and the other S because the groups of atoms which are different may differ in atomic number.

Although it is possible to make a scale model of a drug which should indicate its size and shape with a high likelihood of correctness, it is more difficult to predict how the bonds in the compound can rotate and what arrangements are more likely to be stable than others. This is true even if the model is based on X-ray crystallography of the drug itself, because the drug is present in the crystal only in the most stable arrangement, whereas in solution enough energy will be imparted to it by collisions for it to assume a variety of conformations. As has already been indicated, inspection of models may give some ideas about how these may be restricted but it is necessary to confirm these ideas by physical evidence. In the example of triprolidine, this was provided by the ultraviolet absorption spectrum, which indicated the presence of systems of conjugated double bonds which must lie in the same plane. Examination of the infra-red absorption spectrum may, likewise, give information about steric effects in drugs in the liquid or solid state, but unfortunately this method is not really suitable for studying drugs in solution because water itself absorbs very strongly. One of the most promising new methods of studying the preferred conformations of molecules is that of nuclear (particularly proton) magnetic resonance. With this, drugs can be examined in solution in D_2O.

Electron distribution

Although the size and shape of a drug is important, it is not a homogeneous solid as models sometimes suggest, and its properties depend upon the distribution of electric charge within the molecule. Polar substances, for example, do not dissolve readily in lipids, and non-polar substances are not adsorbed at receptors by electrostatic attraction, though such forces might well bind polar drugs, or ions, to charged groups in a receptor.

From the chemical formula it should be possible to gain a general idea of the distribution of charge within the molecule, although precise information may be very hard to obtain. Quaternary ammonium groups always have a positive charge and strongly acidic groups have a negative charge. As described on p. 2.2, at blood pH an acidic drug with a pK_a of 4 is almost 100 per cent in the ionized form; a basic drug with a pK_a of 10 is almost 100 per cent ionized. Weaker acids or bases are less ionized; one with a pK_a of 7 is roughly 50 per cent ionized. If the pK_a is known, the degree of ionization can be predicted accurately at any pH. The pK_a of an acid or base can quite easily be measured, though the calculations may be complicated if the drug contains more than one acidic or basic group. Even if it has not been measured, it is possible to predict the pK_a of an acidic or basic group with a high likelihood of accuracy, because the pK_a values of so many acids and bases have been measured.

It is more difficult to assess differences of electron distribution which do not involve whole units of charge. This arises when a bond is formed between two atoms which differ in their electronegativity. The electron distribution in the bond between carbon and chlorine, for instance, is not uniform; the electron 'cloud' is pulled towards the more electronegative chlorine atom and the bond is therefore slightly polarized with the chlorine atom slightly negative and the carbon atom slightly positive. The distribution of electrons in the double bond between carbon and oxygen in a carbonyl group is likewise not uniform and the oxygen atom carries a partial negative charge, whereas the carbon atom carries a partial positive charge. From experience of the chemical behaviour of groups and from knowledge of how molecules become oriented in electric fields (measurement of dipole moments), the chemist can make a reasonable guess at the groups which are likely to be polarized in a compound. In some instances, with simple compounds, it is possible to make quantitative predictions about charge distribution. To test the correctness of the guess for a particular drug, however, it is necessary to undertake physical measurements of the properties of the drug. If it is an acid or base the pK_a often indicates the polarization of groups which are in a position to affect the dissociation. Measurements of dipole moments also gives an indication of the polarizations of groups in the molecule, though these sometimes cancel each other

out for geometrical reasons; the C—Cl bond is polarized but CCl_4 has no dipole moment. Unfortunately trouble again arises with ionic compounds; the usual method of obtaining dipole moments depends upon measuring the refractive index and the dielectric constant and is really convenient only for organic liquids.

Although an extensive account of methods used for determining electron distribution is out of place here, sufficient has been said to indicate what is involved and why it is relevant to the actions of drugs. The chemical properties of drugs are responsible for their pharmacological properties and this branch of pharmacology cannot be ignored.

FURTHER READING

BARLOW R.B. (1964) *Introduction to Chemical Pharmacology*, London; Methuen.

CAHN R.S., INGOLD C.K. & PRELOG V. (1956) *Experimentia*, **12**, 81.

FINNEY D.J. (1964) *Statistical Methods in Biological Assay*, 2nd Edition. London: Griffin.

GILL E.W. (1965) Drug receptor interactions, in *Progress in Medicinal Chemistry*, vol. 4, ed. G.P. Ellis & G.B. West. London: Butterworth.

PULLMAN B. & PULLMAN A. (1963) *Quantum Biochemistry* pp. 679–844. New York: Interscience.

WAUD D.R. (1968) Pharmacological receptors. *Pharmacol. Rev.* **20**, 50.

Chapter 4
Drugs and neurochemical transmission

Neurochemical transmission is discussed briefly in vol. 1, pp. 14.23–9, but as drugs play a large part in the experimental study of the phenomenon a fuller account of the subject is now given. The pharmacological properties and clinical uses of many of the drugs mentioned here are given in greater detail in chapters devoted to the systems of the body and in chap. 15 devoted to the catecholamines. Fig. 4.1 is an *aide-mémoire* to the elementary physiological aspects of the subject.

Although there are important differences between the processes involved in transmission at different sites, they possess many common features. The transmitter is synthesized and stored in the prejunctional nerve terminals; it is released as a result of invasion of the terminals by an action potential. Molecules of the transmitter reach the postjunctional cell membrane by diffusion and there react with receptors. The reaction usually results in a brief alteration in the permeability of the membrane to various ions, and as a consequence there is a change in potential difference across the membrane. If the transmitter is **excitatory**, the change is a depolarization which in turn leads to an action potential. If the transmitter is **inhibitory**, a change in permeability counteracts the effect of the excitatory disturbance on the membrane. The effect of the transmitter on the postjunctional membrane is brief because its concentration is quickly reduced both by diffusion and by inactivation.

A large number of substances are useful or dangerous because they interfere with neurochemical transmission and they act in a variety of ways; they may affect the synthesis, storage or inactivation of the transmitters; they may alter the amount of transmitter released by the prejunctional action potential or they may themselves combine with postjunctional receptors and thereby mimic or prevent the action of the transmitter. Some substances have more than one of these actions and different types of junction are affected by different substances.

CHOLINERGIC TRANSMISSION

Although acetylcholine was synthesized in 1867, its physiological effects were not studied in detail until 1914 when Dale showed that, depending on the amounts used, it had actions resembling two substances which had previously been studied extensively. When a small amount was injected into an anaesthetized cat, there was a fall in blood pressure due to vasodilation, slowing of the heart, contraction of smooth muscle in many organs and copious secretion from exocrine glands. Dale called these effects of acetylcholine **muscarinic** because they resembled those of muscarine, a poison found in the mushroom *Amanita muscaria*. The effects of small amounts of acetylcholine, like those of muscarine, were abolished by atropine (p. 4.11). In fact after giving atropine, larger amounts of acetylcholine caused a rise in blood pressure rather than a fall. Dale correctly deduced that this effect was due to the stimulation of sympathetic ganglion cells by acetylcholine, and he called this effect **nicotinic** since

$(CH_3)_3\overset{+}{N}CH_2-$

Muscarine   Nicotine

it was then known that nicotine stimulated autonomic ganglion cells. The term muscarinic is still often used to refer to actions of acetylcholine on cells innervated by postganglionic autonomic cholinergic nerves and to its other actions which are blocked by atropine. The term nicotinic refers not only to the action of acetylcholine on autonomic ganglion cells but also to its action on skeletal muscle fibres and to other actions which are blocked by ganglion- or neuromuscular-blocking agents.

The effects of injected acetylcholine are brief as compared to those of muscarine or nicotine, and Dale rightly guessed that this was because it was rapidly broken down in the body. At neutral and alkaline pH, acetylcholine is hydrolysed to choline and acetic acid spontaneously; in the body hydrolysis is greatly accelerated by a group of enzymes, the **cholinesterases**, which are present in plasma and on the membranes or within the cytoplasm of many cells. Acetylcholinesterase has the greatest activity against acetylcholine; when released from cholinergic nerves it is very rapidly destroyed at its site of action and there is no circulating acetylcholine. The drugs known as **anticholinesterases** (p. 4.6) inhibit the enzymic hydrolysis of acetylcholine.

Transmission between motor nerve and skeletal muscle
The classical evidence that acetylcholine is the trans-

mitter at the neuromuscular junction may be summarized as follows:

(1) Motor nerves contain acetylcholine and also choline acetyltransferase which can synthesize acetylcholine from choline and acetylcoenzyme A.

(2) When the motor nerve to a muscle, perfused with a physiological solution to which an anticholinesterase

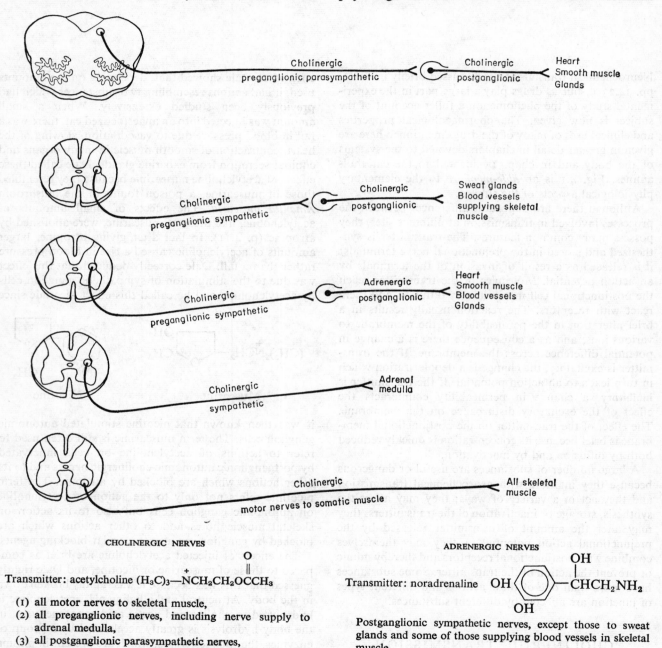

CHOLINERGIC NERVES

Transmitter: acetylcholine $(H_3C)_3 \overset{+}{-}NCH_2CH_2O\overset{O}{\overset{\|}{C}}CH_3$

(1) all motor nerves to skeletal muscle,
(2) all preganglionic nerves, including nerve supply to adrenal medulla,
(3) all postganglionic parasympathetic nerves,
(4) postganglionic sympathetic nerves to sweat glands,
(5) some postganglionic sympathetic nerves to blood vessels in skeletal muscle.

ADRENERGIC NERVES

Transmitter: noradrenaline

Postganglionic sympathetic nerves, except those to sweat glands and some of those supplying blood vessels in skeletal muscle.

FIG. 4.1. Classification of neurochemical transmission.

has been added, is stimulated, an active substance appears in the perfusate. There is too little to identify by chemical methods but the substance is indistingishable from acetylcholine in its effects on biological preparations. If the anticholinesterase is omitted from the perfusing fluid, choline appears in the perfusate. Control experiments show that the acetylcholine is liberated by the nerve and not by the muscle. The acetylcholine released evidently plays a significant part in transmission; when the amount released is reduced, for example by lowering $[Ca^{++}]$ in the perfusing solution, the contraction of the muscle is also reduced.

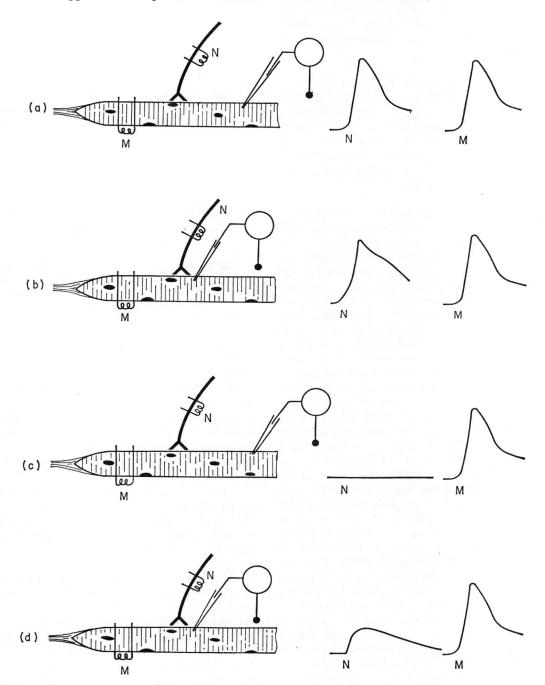

FIG. 4.2. Studies of processes involved in neuromuscular transmission with intracellular microelectrode. N, response to stimulation of motor nerve; M, response to direct stimulation of muscle. For explanation see text.

(3) When acetylcholine is injected into an artery close to its point of entry into the muscle, the muscle twitches in the same way as in response to a short train of electrical stimuli applied to the motor nerve. All the drugs which abolish this effect of acetylcholine also abolish the effect of nerve stimulation.

(4) The effect of the acetylcholine is on the muscle and not the nerve since muscles are still sensitive to acetylcholine after chronic denervation; in fact such muscles are abnormally sensitive.

BIOLOGICAL TESTS FOR ACETYLCHOLINE

Since the amount of acetylcholine collected in the perfusate is too small to be identified by chemical methods, the identity of the active substance has to be established by bioassay (p. 3.4). Suitable tests are the contractions of the dorsal muscle of the leech and the rectus abdominis of the frog, the reduction in rate of the frog heart and the reduction in blood pressure of the cat.

INVESTIGATIONS ON SINGLE MUSCLE FIBRES

The processes involved in neuromuscular transmission have been studied by recording the electrical activity of single muscle fibres with intracellular electrodes (fig. 4.2).

In (a) a recording microelectrode has been inserted into a muscle fibre at a point distant from the neuromuscular junction. When the motor nerve is stimulated the action potential recorded by the muscle is indistinguishable from the action potential which is seen in response to direct stimulation of the muscle fibre. In (b), however, when the microelectrode is close to the neuromuscular junction, the rising phase of the action potential has a component, the **end plate step**, which is not present in the direct response. Suppose that the amount of acetylcholine released by a nerve stimulus is now reduced by lowering $[Ca^{++}]$ in the bathing fluid. If the reduction is sufficient to prevent the muscle fibre twitching in response to a nerve stimulus, no response at all is seen with the electrode distant from the neuromuscular junction (c). Close to the neuromuscular junction, however, a response is still seen (d), now called an **end plate potential**, and it differs from the action potential in several ways. It is smaller in amplitude, has a different time course and is not all or none but is graded according to the amount of acetylcholine released. It seems, therefore, that the primary action of the transmitter is to cause some local effect on the muscle fibre which, if sufficiently intense, gives rise to an action potential. This can be confirmed directly by applying acetylcholine iontophoretically to the muscle fibre. In this method a micropipette is filled with a concentrated solution of the drug which can then be expelled by the passage of a current through the pipette. The amount expelled depends on the amplitude and duration of the current. If progressively increasing amounts are ejected in the end plate region of the muscle

fibre, graded responses are seen at the end plate, until finally the depolarization is suprathreshold and triggers off an action potential (fig. 4.3). With the recording electrode distant from the end plate, no response is seen until the action potential occurs. The conclusion drawn

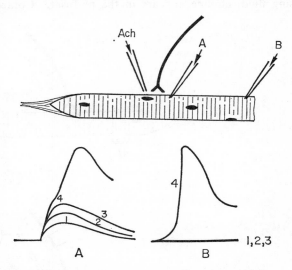

FIG. 4.3. Increasing amounts of acetylcholine (Ach) 1, 2, 3 and 4 are ejected from micropipette on to the end plate of muscle fibre. (A) Graded response in region of end plate; (B) No response with electrode distant from end plate until depolarization is suprathreshold, i.e. 4.

from these results is that the primary action of the acetylcholine is to cause a local depolarization at the end plate, which in turn gives rise to a propagated action potential. If the acetylcholine pipette is moved away from the end plate, no responses occur anywhere in the muscle fibre. Evidently therefore, the acetylcholine receptors are confined to the end plate region. Furthermore, they are apparently present on the outer surface of the membrane since there is no response to acetylcholine when it is applied from within the cell.

Something is also known of the way in which the change in membrane potential is brought about by the acetylcholine. The immediate cause is a simultaneous increase in the permeability to Na^+ and K^+ ions, but how this is brought about is as yet unknown.

SPONTANEOUS RELEASE OF ACETYLCHOLINE

Acetylcholine is released from nerve endings not only when they are invaded by action potentials but also spontaneously. The quantities released are too small to stimulate muscle fibres, but they do have some effect on the muscle fibre membrane. With a microelectrode inserted into a fibre close to the end plate and a sensitive electrical recording system, small depolarizations can be seen from time to time. They have the same time course as end plate potentials, and a number of tests show that they are due to the action of packets of acetylcholine, probably of many hundreds of molecules, combining simultaneously with the receptors. The **miniature end plate potentials**, as they are called, are increased in amplitude when physostigmine (p. 4.6) or some other anticholinesterase is added to the bathing fluid, and they are reduced in size by tubocurarine (p. 4.7) and by other substances which reduce the sensitivity of the end plate to acetylcholine. These results show that acetylcholine causes the miniature end plate potentials. Since they are seen only at the end plate and not elsewhere in the muscle fibre, and as they disappear after denervation of the muscle at the time when the motor nerve endings degenerate, the source of the spontaneously released acetylcholine must be the nerve endings.

The packet of acetylcholine appears to be a basic unit of the transmission process. Normally when an action potential reaches the nerve ending several hundred packets are released simultaneously; it is the joint effect of these which gives rise to the end plate step of the action potential at the neuromuscular junction. The reason for the release of acetylcholine in the form of multimolecular packets, or quanta as they are called, is not known for certain but it is generally believed that the acetylcholine is stored in the vesicles that can be seen in EM pictures of the nerve endings. If this is so, the quantal nature of the release would be explained by supposing that vesicles discharged their contents into the space separating nerve and muscle in an all-or-none way. Whether or not this is true, there is good experimental evidence to show that the agents which interfere with the release of acetylcholine in response to action potentials alter either the number of packets released or the number of molecules of acetylcholine that a packet contains.

ACTIONS OF CALCIUM, MAGNESIUM AND BOTULINUM TOXIN

The presence of calcium ions is essential for the release of acetylcholine by the action potential and if the extracellular $[Ca^{++}]$ is reduced, the number of packets released is also reduced. On the other hand, Mg^{++} inhibit the release of acetylcholine; magnesium appears to do this by competing with calcium for some site in the nerve terminal. Botulinum toxin (p. 25.20) also inhibits the release of acetylcholine but it differs from the effects of a reduction in Ca^{++} or increase in Mg^{++} in that it also abolishes the spontaneous release of acetylcholine. EM studies with ferritin-labelled toxin suggest that the toxin molecules may obstruct the site of acetylcholine release.

HEMICHOLINIUM, TRIETHYLCHOLINE AND MYASTHENIA GRAVIS

In muscles paralysed with **hemicholinium** or **triethylcholine**, or in those taken from patients with myasthenia gravis, an uncommon disease in which the skeletal muscles become readily fatigued, the miniature end plate potentials are abnormally small. The sensitivity of the end plate to applied acetylcholine is not very different from that in normal muscle, so that it must be supposed that the number of molecules in the packets of acetylcholine is less than normal. With hemicholinium and triethylcholine, this has been shown to be due to a failure in the synthesis of acetylcholine; this failure of synthesis is not due to inactivation of choline acetyl transferase but is probably due to competition for the entry into the nerve cell of choline which is therefore not acetylated. These substances cause a slowly developing neuromuscular blockade which is more pronounced during exercise or during rapid motor nerve stimulation because the preformed store of acetylcholine is more rapidly exhausted. In 'myasthenic' muscle, there is no failure of synthesis and the defect perhaps lies in the process which packages the acetylcholine ready for release. As with hemicholinium and triethylcholine, there appears to be no abnormality in the process whereby the action potential releases the transmitter, since a nerve stimulus releases the usual number of packets.

Hemicholinium

$$(C_2H_5)_3\overset{+}{N}CH_2CH_2OH$$

Triethylcholine

ANTICHOLINESTERASES

When a muscle is treated with an anticholinesterase, **a** maximal stimulus to the motor nerve may be followed by a contraction which is larger than in the untreated muscle. This is because some of the treated muscle fibres twitch repetitively in response to a single stimulus. In a normal muscle, the concentration of acetylcholine around the end plate following the nerve action potential is high for just long enough to produce a single action potential in the muscle fibre. When the cholinesterase is inhibited and the acetylcholine is no longer rapidly hydrolysed, its concentration is reduced by diffusion only and remains high for longer. Since normally the cholinesterase is intermingled with the receptor molecules on the outer surface of the membrane and its action is very rapid, not all the acetylcholine that is released is available for reaction with the receptors. Therefore, when the cholinesterase is inhibited, not only is the action of acetylcholine prolonged but there is also an increase in the number of acetylcholine–receptor complexes and the action of the transmitter is intensified. Where too little transmitter is released to cause a suprathreshold end plate potential, as in myasthenia gravis, or where the end plate potential is subthreshold because the sensitivity to acetylcholine has been reduced with neuromuscular blocking agents, anticholinesterases can restore transmission.

Some of the anticholinesterases, **physostigmine (eserine) neostigmine (prostigmine)** and **edrophonium** for example, have been shown by biochemical methods to be competitive inhibitors. Others however, like **di-isopropylfluorophosphate,** (DFP) and **phospholine** which are organophosphorous compounds, form stable bonds with cholinesterase and their action is virtually irreversible. The chemical formulae of these anticholinesterases are shown in fig. 4.4.

POSTJUNCTIONAL BLOCKING AGENTS (table 4.1)

Depolarizing drugs

At first sight it may seem paradoxical that acetylcholine, the neuromuscular transmitter, is also a neuromuscular blocking agent. The fact that this is so may be demonstrated quite simply on an isolated nerve muscle preparation, such as the rat phrenic nerve-diaphragm. If neostigmine is first put into the bath to inhibit the muscle cholinesterase, and acetylcholine then added, the twitches in response to nerve stimuli are soon abolished. Experiments made with microelectrodes show that at first the added acetylcholine depolarizes the muscle fibres at the end plate and produces a train of action potentials followed by twitches. But a depolarized muscle fibre does not continue to produce action potentials indefinitely; in fact a sustained depolarization leads only to an initial short burst of action potentials and after this the muscle fibre is refractory to any form of stimulus. Transmission is therefore said to be blocked by depolarization. As time goes on, however, even though the acetylcholine is left in the bath, the membrane potential reverts to its original value. Clearly the end plate must have become insensitive to acetylcholine and it is therefore not surprising that the muscle will not respond to nerve stimulation. In this state, however, the muscle gives a normal twitch in response to direct stimulation and transmission is said to be blocked by desensitization. Since no other changes in the properties of the muscle fibres in this state have been found, it seems that prolonged exposure of the receptors to acetylcholine changes their properties. This explanation, admittedly incomplete, is supported by the fact that after the acetylcholine is washed out of the bath, it is some time before the muscle regains its full responsiveness to acetylcholine.

During the period in which acetylcholine is present it is obvious that an anticholinesterase will not reverse the neuromuscular block of either depolarizing or desensitizing varieties. After the acetylcholine has been washed away the receptors do not all revert to their responsive state simultaneously; for a time there may be a sufficient number of normal receptors to respond to a nerve stimulus with an end plate potential, but not one sufficiently large to generate an action potential. At this stage, therefore, an anticholinesterase enhances transmission.

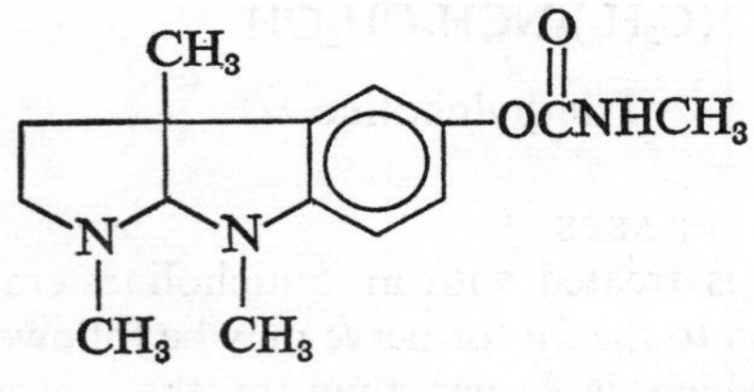

Physostigmine (eserine)

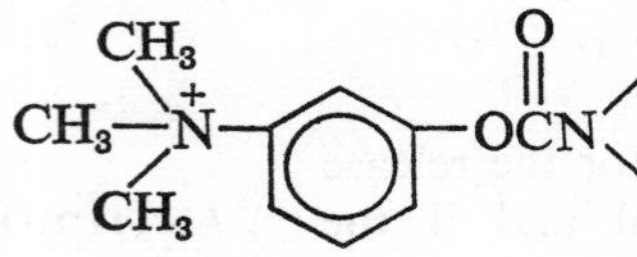

Neostigmine

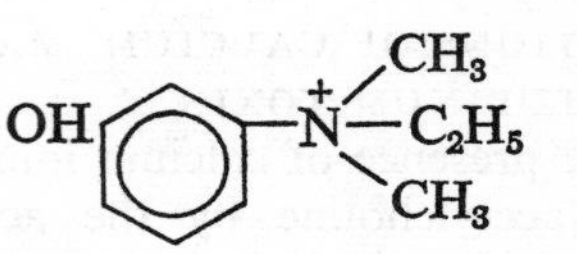

Edrophonium

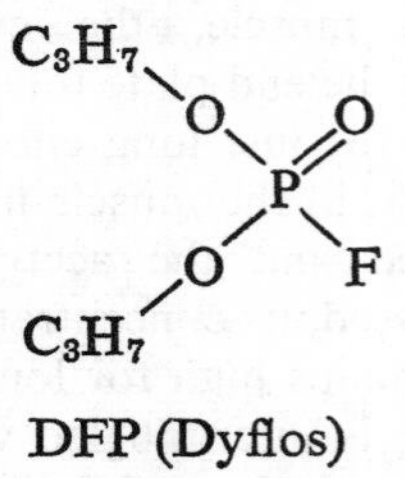

DFP (Dyflos)

Di-isopropylfluorophosphate

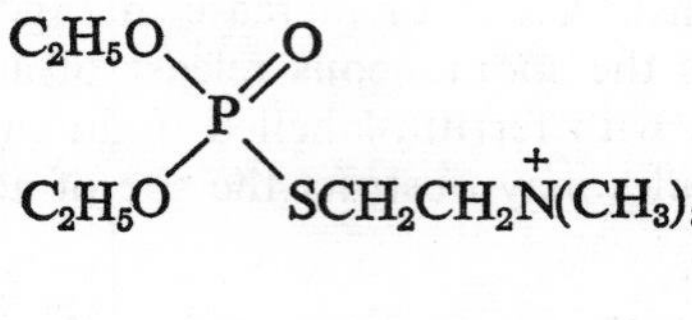

Phospholine

FIG. 4.4. Anticholinesterases.

A number of agonists imitate the action of acetylcholine on the end plate. They include **nicotine, carbamylcholine, decamethonium** and **suxamethonium**. Of these, only suxamethonium which is equivalent to the combination of two molecules of acetylcholine is hydrolysed by cholinesterase. The hydrolysis occurs in two stages and is slower than that of acetylcholine.

TABLE 4.1. Neuromuscular blocking agents.

Substances which first stimulate skeletal muscle and then block neuromuscular transmission:

Acetylcholine $(CH_3)_3\overset{+}{N}CH_2CH_2O\overset{\overset{O}{\|}}{C}CH_3$

Nicotine

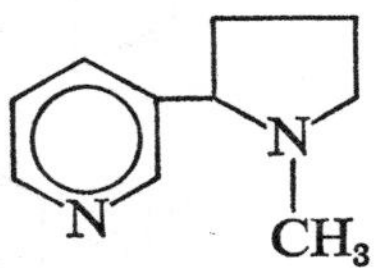

Carbamylcholine (carbachol) $(CH_3)_3\overset{+}{N}CH_2CH_2O\overset{\overset{O}{\|}}{C}NH_2$

Suxamethonium (succinylcholine)
$(CH_3)_3\overset{+}{N}CH_2CH_2O\overset{\overset{O}{\|}}{C}CH_2$
$(CH_3)_3\overset{+}{N}CH_2CH_2O\overset{}{C}CH_2$

Decamethonium $(CH_3)_3\overset{+}{N}(CH_2)_{10}\overset{+}{N}(CH_3)_3$

Substances which block neuromuscular transmission without prior stimulation:

Tubocurarine

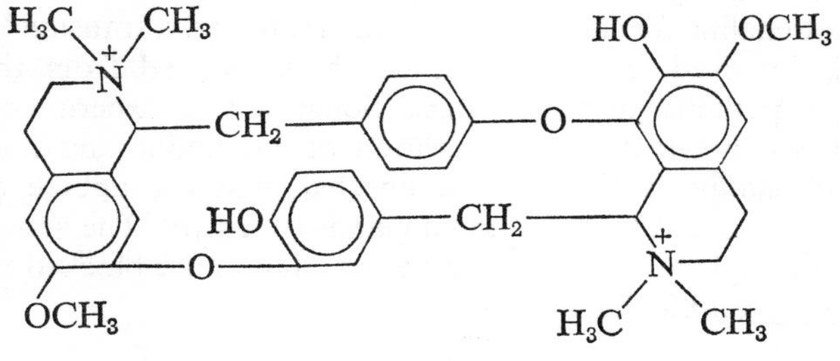

Gallamine

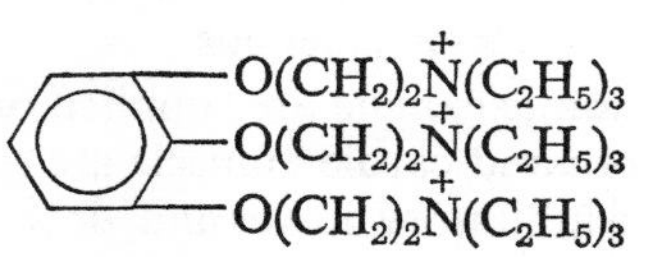

Non-depolarizing blocking agents
Reference has already been made to **tubocurarine** as a neuromuscular blocking agent. It is the most important alkaloid isolated from curare. It does not reduce the amount of acetylcholine released from nerve endings or have any action on acetylcholine itself. It does not alter the properties of resting muscle, nor does it prevent the action potential followed by twitch in response to a stimulus applied directly to the muscle. It blocks neuromuscular transmission by reducing the sensitivity of the end plate to acetylcholine. There is evidence that it combines with the same receptors as acetylcholine, thus making them unavailable to the acetylcholine released from the nerve terminal. The block may be antagonized by anticholinesterase drugs such as neostigmine and, temporarily, by drugs which depolarize the moter end plate, e.g. acetylcholine, suxamethonium or decamethonium. Toxiferine I is another naturally occurring alkaloid with longer action that tubocurarine. The difficulty in obtaining pure natural alkaloids has led to the synthesis of many substances with similar actions; the most important of these is **gallamine** (table 4.1).

Transmission through autonomic ganglia
The evidence that acetylcholine is the transmitter at the ganglionic synapse is of much the same nature as has already been described for the neuromuscular junction. Thus acetylcholine has been collected in the perfusate from ganglia during stimulation of the preganglionic nerves; in addition, the postganglionic cells have been shown to respond to acetylcholine either injected or applied by iontophoresis. By recording from single ganglion cells, it has also been shown that the primary effect of the acetylcholine is to produce a graded depolarization, the synaptic potential, which is the analogue of the end plate potential. If the synaptic potential is suprathreshold it leads to an action potential which is propagated along the postganglionic axon.

The amplitude of the synaptic potential depends on the amount of acetylcholine released by the preganglionic nerve endings and this is affected by the same factors which influence the amount released from motor nerve fibres. Rather surprisingly, the cholinesterase in ganglia does not have such an intimate relation to the receptors as it does in muscle and, as a consequence, anticholinesterases do not significantly enhance transmission through ganglia.

GANGLION BLOCKING DRUGS
Just as acetylcholine is both the transmitter and a blocking agent at the neuromuscular junction so it is at the ganglionic synapse. Fig. 4.5 shows how a single ganglion cell reacts when it is exposed to acetylcholine added to the bathing fluid. At first the cell is depolarized and action potentials are propagated along the postgangli-

onic axon. After a short period the action potentials stop; then the depolarization disappears, but transmission is still blocked. Initially, transmission is blocked by depolarization and subsequently by desensitization, just as in the case of muscle. That ganglion cells could behave in this way when exposed to a drug was discovered by

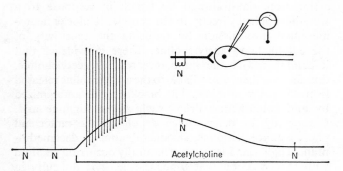

FIG. 4.5. Action of acetylcholine on single sympathetic ganglion cell. At N, stimulus is applied to preganglionic nerve.

Langley and Dickinson in 1889. They applied nicotine to ganglia with a small paint brush and found that this initially produced effects similar to those obtained when either the pre- or postganglionic nerves were stimulated; shortly afterwards these effects subsided and stimulation of the preganglionic nerves then had no effect. It is of interest that suxamethonium and decamethonium which first stimulate at the neuromuscular junction and then block neuromuscular transmission, block only the ganglionic synapse. This shows that the acetylcholine receptors of ganglion cells and muscle fibres are different, although they must be sufficiently alike to react to acetylcholine.

NON-DEPOLARIZING BLOCKING AGENTS (table 4.2)
A number of substances block ganglionic transmission in exactly the same way as tubocurarine blocks neuromuscular transmission. They do not affect the amount of acetylcholine released by nerve stimulation or alter in any way the response of ganglion cells to direct stimulation; their action is confined to reducing the sensitivity of the ganglion cells to acetylcholine. Presumably they do this by combining with the receptors, thereby making them unavailable to the acetylcholine released by the preganglionic action potentials. Tubocurarine itself does this in about the same concentration as it paralyses neuromuscular transmission. However, **hexamethonium, mecamylamine** and **pempidine** are effective ganglion blocking agents in concentrations many times smaller than are required to block neuromuscular transmission.

Tetraethylammonium chloride was first shown to act in this way and later bisquaternary ammonium com-

TABLE 4.2. Ganglion blocking agents.

Tetraethylammonium	$(C_2H_5)_4\overset{+}{N}$
Pentamethonium (C_5)	$(CH_3)_3\overset{+}{N}(CH_2)_5\overset{+}{N}(CH_3)_3$
Hexamethonium (C_6)	$(CH_3)_3\overset{+}{N}(CH_2)_6\overset{+}{N}(CH_3)_3$

Pentolinium

Mecamylamine

Pempidine

pounds, **pentamethonium** and **hexamethonium** were synthesized and were among the first effective drugs to be used in the treatment of high blood pressure. Later, **pentolinium** was developed and was found to be even more potent. Mecamylamine is a secondary and pempidine a tertiary amine which cause ganglion block in the same way as the methonium compounds but which in addition may affect transmitter release. Their use in the treatment of hypertension is now limited (p. 8.8).

TRANSMISSION IN THE ADRENAL MEDULLA
Stimulation of the sympathetic supply to the adrenal medulla causes the liberation of adrenaline and noradrenaline from chromaffin cells. However, a transmitter is involved, acetylcholine, which is released from the sympathetic nerve endings. Some recent experiments have shown that the liberation of adrenaline and noradrenaline is intimately connected with the uptake of calcium ions by the adrenal glands (p. 15.10). The action of acetylcholine and of nerve stimulation are blocked by ganglion blocking agents.

Cholinergic transmission at autonomic neuro-effector junctions
Skeletal muscles and autonomic ganglia are supplied only by excitatory nerves; smooth and cardiac muscle are supplied by both excitatory and inhibitory nerves and, depending on the site, acetylcholine is either an excitatory or an

inhibitory transmitter. There is no evidence to suggest that the postjunctional receptors of cells which are excited are different from those which are inhibited by acetylcholine. Thus pilocarpine, mecholyl and carbachol (table 4.4) which imitate the excitatory effects also imitate the inhibitory ones and atropine blocks both types of action indiscriminately. The different types of response, therefore, probably depend on processes which intervene between the combination of acetylcholine with the receptors and the excitation or inhibition to which it leads.

There is, however, a clear distinction between the receptors responsible for the nicotinic effects of acetylcholine (p. 4.1) and for those responsible for its muscarinic effects. Acetylcholine produces muscarinic effects in much lower concentration than those in which it produces nicotinic ones, and the muscarinic receptors may not be so easily subject to desensitization. Different substances imitate the nicotinic and muscarinic actions of the transmitter and different substances block these actions. At first it was not appreciated that the properties of the receptors at the neuromuscular junction were different from those at the ganglion. It must, however, be borne in mind that, although the term muscarinic refers to what is probably a homogeneous group of receptors, the term nicotinic refers to two distinct groups, at any rate as far as their pharmacology is concerned.

EVIDENCE FOR CHOLINERGIC TRANSMISSION IN THE AUTONOMIC NERVOUS SYSTEM

The sites at which transmission is believed to be cholinergic are shown in table 4.3. They include all the postganglionic parasympathetic junctions and two types of sympathetic junction.

The belief is based on the following evidence.

(1) Acetylcholine can be demonstrated in the perfusion fluid from the heart, stomach and salivary glands when the parasympathetic nerves are stimulated and when acetylcholine is protected from hydrolysis with an anticholinesterase. It is true that some of the acetylcholine comes from the preganglionic nerve terminals. Since the parasympathetic ganglia are generally intimately connected with the effector organs it is not feasible to stimulate only the postganglionic fibres. The effects of ganglion blocking agents, however, show that not all the acetylcholine comes from this source. In their presence the amount of acetylcholine appearing in the perfusate is reduced. Since they do not reduce the amount of acetylcholine released by the preganglionic nerve endings in sympathetic ganglia, it seems reasonable to suppose that the deficit in the acetylcholine collected represents the amount released by the postganglionic nerve endings. Acetylcholine has also been collected in the perfusion fluid from sweat glands which are innervated by sympathetic nerves, when these nerves were stimulated.

(2) At all the sites listed, acetylcholine produces effects similar to those of nerve stimulation.

(3) The effects of both nerve impulses and applied acetylcholine are enhanced by anticholinesterases.

(4) Drugs such as atropine which diminish the response to acetylcholine also diminish the response to nerve stimulation. There are a few exceptions to this and there is no satisfactory explanation for them.

TABLE 4.3. Autonomic cholinergic sites.

Effector	Action of acetylcholine
PARASYMPATHETIC	
Smooth muscle	
Wall of gut and bladder (detrusor muscle)	
Circular muscle of iris	Excitation
Ciliary muscle	
Bronchioles	
Sphincters of gut	
Arterioles of erectile tissue	Inhibition
Arterioles of salivary glands	
Heart	
Cells of sinuatrial node	Inhibition
Glands	
Lachrymal	
Salivary	
Respiratory tract	Secretion
Gastrointestinal tract	
SYMPATHETIC	
Smooth muscle	
Arterioles of skeletal muscle	Inhibition
Glands	
Sweat	Secretion

PROCESSES INVOLVED IN PARASYMPATHETIC TRANSMISSION

Excitation of smooth muscle

Like skeletal muscles, smooth muscles contract when they are activated by action potentials. In spontaneously active smooth muscle like that of the intestine which contracts in the absence of nerve impulses, it seems that the cell membrane is inherently unstable and generates pacemaker potentials which in turn lead to action potentials. These action potentials are propagated from cell to cell, so that not all cells in a particular smooth muscle are necessarily endowed with pacemaker properties. Each action potential is followed by a muscle contraction; if the intervals between the action potentials are short, the individual contractions merge and steady tension or shortening develops, which increases with increasing frequency of action potentials. Simultaneous records of tension and electrical activity have been made from muscle in the gut wall and the effect of stimulating the parasympathetic nerve supply has been observed. At low frequencies each stimulus evokes a slow depolarization which then leads to one or a few action potentials accompanied by a contraction. The slow potential is presumably the analogue of the end plate potential in skeletal muscle. At higher frequencies of nerve stimulation, or when acetylcholine is applied to the muscle, the membrane is continuously depolarized and develops steady tension. In some muscles this depolarization is accompanied by a continuous train of action potentials but in others, although a steady tension is maintained, no action potentials are observed. Detailed studies of the ion movements involved in the depolarization suggest that the primary effect of acetylcholine is to increase the permeability of the smooth muscle membrane to Na^+, K^+ and Cl^-.

Actions on the heart

The heart consists of spontaneously active striated muscle and the chief action of parasympathetic stimulation is to slow its rate of contraction. When the vagus is stimulated the sinuatrial node and to a lesser extent the atrium is hyperpolarized and the spontaneous pacemaker potentials no longer reach the threshold for setting off action potentials. Acetylcholine applied directly to the sinuatrial node produces exactly the same effect. The underlying change caused by the acetylcholine is an increase in the permeability of the membrane to K^+.

Action on gland cells

Although electrical changes are observed when the parasympathetic nerves to salivary glands are stimulated and when they are exposed to acetylcholine, the relation between these changes and the process of secretion remains mysterious.

Substances mimicking the action of parasympathetic nerve stimulation

ACETYLCHOLINE-LIKE SUBSTANCES (table 4.4)
Apart from acetylcholine, two groups of substances imitate the action of parasympathetic stimulation. The first group consists of drugs which combine with the receptors to produce the same effects as acetylcholine itself. One of these is **carbachol**, the carbamic acid ester of choline. Its actions resemble those of acetylcholine very closely. In low concentrations its effects are muscarinic and in higher concentrations it has the additional nicotinic actions. It is not, however, hydrolysed by cholinesterases and is, therefore, more stable than acetylcholine. Other substances with parasympathetic effects are **mecholyl** (acetyl β-methyl choline), **pilocarpine**, obtained from the

Pilocarpus and, of course, **muscarine**. Of these, only acetyl β-methyl choline is hydrolysed by acetylcholinesterase.

TABLE 4.4. Parasympathomimetic drugs.

ANTICHOLINESTERASES
The second group of drugs which appear to be parasympathomimetic are the anticholinesterases (p. 4.6). The parasympathetic system is presumably continuously active even if, at some sites, only at a low level. If the acetylcholine released from the nerve endings is protected from hydrolysis, its concentration in the neighbourhood of the receptors is increased and the tonic activity of the parasympathetic system is therefore enhanced. The evidence for this mode of action of the anticholinesterases is that they do not have parasympathomimetic effects on tissues which have been denervated.

Drugs that block cholinergic transmission at postganglionic junctions

The release of acetylcholine from postganglionic nerve terminals is diminished by a decrease in the external $[Ca^{++}]$ or increase in the external $[Mg^{++}]$ and by hemicholinium and botulinum toxin. These agents therefore affect postganglionic cholinergic nerve terminals in the same way as they affect motor and preganglionic nerve endings.

However, the action of acetylcholine on the postjunctional muscarinic receptors is not affected by the agents which reduce the sensitivity of the nicotinic end plate or ganglion cell receptors. For example, tubocurarine has no effect on the direct response to acetylcholine of the gut or the heart in concentrations many times that which blocks neuromuscular transmission. It will of course be appreciated that ganglion-blocking agents depress or abolish parasympathetic activity, but this is not due to a direct action on the effector cells. There are, however, a number of drugs which block transmission by reducing the sensitivity of these cells to acetylcholine. The prototype of this class of drugs is **atropine**, a naturally occurring substance found in deadly nightshade and various other plants. Atropine is a racemic mixture of (+) and (−) **hyoscyamine**; its blocking action is almost entirely due to the (+) isomer. Atropine probably has no effect on the

Atropine

amount of acetylcholine released from cholinergic post-ganglionic nerves; like tubocurarine at the end plate, it competes with the acetylcholine for the postjunctional cholinergic receptors. Its effects on the body are in general those that would be predicted to result from blockade of autonomic cholinergic transmission, but there are some additional effects probably due to actions on neurones in the central nervous system; furthermore some autonomic sites are particularly resistant to its blocking action. The expected effects are reduction of secretion in the mouth and bronchial tree and of sweat, reduction of peristaltic movement in the gut, increase in heart rate due to the release of vagal inhibition, dilation of the pupil and paralysis of accommodation. One paradoxical effect is that small doses of atropine may initially cause a fall in heart rate. This is supposed to result from the stimulation of neurones in the nucleus of the vagus. Very large doses are required to reduce the gastric secretions and in any case, as would be expected, only the vagal component of gastric secretion is affected; vasodilation in erectile tissue and in salivary glands is also particularly resistant to atropine, and large doses are required to reduce the tone of smooth muscle of the bladder and urinary tract. In large doses atropine causes restlessness and insomnia in some patients, and in severe atropine poisoning convulsions occur which are followed by coma and central respiratory paralysis. For this reason atropine is sometimes described rather loosely as a drug which first stimulates and then depresses the central nervous system. Another effect of atropine which

cannot be explained by its autonomic blocking action is the reduction it causes in the rigidity of Parkinson's disease (p. 5.61). Atropine causes vasodilation in the skin partly as an indirect effect of the inhibition of sweating. An additional process must, however, be involved since an immediate flushing reaction is sometimes seen, presumably before any temperature regulating mechanism would come into play. Hyperpyrexia may occur.

ADRENERGIC TRANSMISSION

Stimulation of sympathetic nerves has a variety of effects (table 4.5). For example, the rate and force of the heart

TABLE 4.5. Effects of impulses in adrenergic sympathetic nerves.

(1) Blood vessels are constricted.
(2) Heart rate and force of contractions are increased.
(3) Motility and tone of gut are decreased.
(4) Smooth muscle in non-gravid uterus and bronchioles is inhibited.
(5) Smooth muscle is contracted in ductus deferens and seminal vesicles, radial muscle of iris (this causes enlargement of the pupil), and capsule of the spleen (in animals also the nictitating membrane).
(6) Submandibular gland secretes viscous saliva.

beat are increased, smooth muscle in the visceral arterioles is contracted and smooth muscle in the wall of the gut is relaxed. These effects can be produced also by noradrenaline. Since it has been shown that noradrenaline is present in sympathetic nerves and that it is released into the circulation when they are stimulated, it is reasonable to believe that noradrenaline is the transmitter for these nerves. Another reason for this belief is that substances which diminish the responses of tissues to noradrenaline also diminish the effects of sympathetic nerve stimulation.

The tissues are also exposed to circulating adrenaline and noradrenaline released from the chromaffin cells of the adrenal medulla and this gives rise to a complication which has no counterpart in the cholinergic system. The responses to adrenaline, which makes up about 80 per cent of the output of the adrenal medulla in man, and to noradrenaline are not identical and the agents which affect the functioning of the adrenergic nerves do not always affect the adrenal medulla in the same way.

The effect of the transmitter and of the circulating adrenaline and noradrenaline is excitatory at some sites and inhibitory at others. As with acetylcholine, this is not because there are separate kinds of receptor for inhibition and excitation, but because different processes result from the combination of the transmitter with the receptors at the different sites. There are, however, different kinds of receptor, just as there are nicotinic and muscarinic receptors for acetylcholine; how they are distinguished is described briefly in the following section. A fuller account is given on p. 15.11.

A large number of substances mimic or interfere with adrenergic transmission. Some react with the receptors either to produce the same effects as noradrenaline or to form inert complexes. Others cause or prevent the release of the transmitter, and finally some affect the rate at which the transmitter is inactivated.

Nature of postjunctional effects

The excitatory effect of sympathetic nerve stimulation has been most extensively studied on the ductus deferens muscle of the guinea-pig, which contracts in response to nerve impulses from the pelvic plexus. When a single stimulus is applied to the nerve, the response recorded with an intracellular electrode consists of a depolarization very much like the end plate potential of skeletal muscle fibres. This depolarization is not accompanied by contraction. When, however, repetitive stimuli are applied, the successive depolarizations are larger and summate, until finally the depolarization becomes suprathreshold and gives rise to an action potential which is accompanied by a contraction. *In vivo*, presumably smooth muscle, when not spontaneously active, is made to contract by trains of impulses propagated along sympathetic nerves.

Even in the absence of nerve activity, small spontaneous depolarizations can be recorded, which are analogous to the miniature end plate potentials of skeletal muscle and are probably due to the spontaneous release of multimolecular packets of noradrenaline from the nerve terminals. The depolarization caused by noradrenaline, which is responsible for the excitatory effect on smooth muscle, is very probably due to an increase in permeability of the muscle fibre membrane to Na^+ and other ions. The other excitatory actions such as that on the heart or on the gland cells which are made to secrete by noradrenaline are poorly understood.

In contrast to the effect of parasympathetic stimulation, sympathetic stimulation diminishes the activity in intestinal smooth muscles. Experiments in which tension and electrical activity of single cells have been recorded simultaneously show that relaxation is associated with the reduction in frequency of action potentials and hyperpolarization of the membrane. These electrical effects are probably the result of an increase in the permeability of the membrane to K^+, brought about by the transmitter and mediated via α-receptors. There is evidence, however, that additional processes are involved in adrenergic inhibition mediated via β-receptors. There are also postganglionic inhibitory nerves to the gut which are neither adrenergic nor cholinergic.

α- AND β-RECEPTORS (table 4.6)

There are at least two kinds of receptor involved in the response to noradrenaline and adrenaline. The grounds for distinguishing between them are analogous to those for distinguishing between nicotinic and muscarinic receptors for acetylcholine. Firstly, different substances imitate the action of the naturally occurring transmitters at different sites. Consider for example the cutaneous blood vessels and the heart. The constrictor effect of nerve stimulation on the blood vessels can be duplicated by the action of the substance **phenylephrine** (fig. 4.6); this, however, has no effect on the heart. On the other hand the effect of nerve stimulation on the heart is mimicked by **isoprenaline** which has no effect on the cutaneous blood vessels. Clearly the receptors at the two sites cannot be identical, although they must be sufficiently alike to react with noradrenaline. Secondly, different substances block the action of the transmitter and transmitter-like drugs at the different sites. For example, the effect of sympathetic nerve stimulation on the heart is prevented by **propranolol** (p. 4.14), but this drug does not prevent vasoconstriction in the skin; this however is blocked by **phenoxybenzamine** which does not diminish the effect of noradrenaline or isoprenaline on the heart.

A list of the sites of α- and β-receptors is shown in table 4.6. Two points may cause confusion. The first is that the smooth muscle in the wall of the intestine and in the blood vessels supplying voluntary muscle have

TABLE 4.6. Distribution of α- and β-receptors.

α-RECEPTORS MEDIATING EXCITATION
Smooth muscle
    Blood vessels
    Radial muscle of iris
    Ductus deferens and seminal vesicle
    Sphincters of gut
    Capsule of spleen
    Nictitating membrane of cat

Glands
Submandibular

α-RECEPTORS MEDIATING INHIBITION
Smooth muscle
    Wall of gut

β-RECEPTORS MEDIATING EXCITATION
Heart

β-RECEPTORS MEDIATING INHIBITION
Smooth muscle
    Bronchial tree
    Wall of gut
    Blood vessels in skeletal muscle* and heart

---

* Insensitive to noradrenaline.

both α- and β-receptors. In the gut both mediate inhibition, i.e. relaxation of the muscle. In the blood vessels the α-receptors mediate vasoconstriction and the β-receptors mediate inhibition. The second is that both noradrenaline and adrenaline activate both kinds of receptor (adrenaline is the more potent substance) with the one exception that noradrenaline has no effect on the β-receptors in the smooth muscle of the blood vessels that supply the voluntary muscles.

Sympathomimetic substances (fig. 4.6)

The more important of the substances which mimic the actions of sympathetic adrenergic nerve stimulation may be regarded as derivatives of β-**phenylethylamine**. Those that are also derivatives of catechol are known as **catecholamines** (p. 15.1).

The catecholamines have a direct action on the tissues mediated via the adrenergic receptors. This was shown in effect as long ago as 1899 by Lewandowsky. He sectioned

the postganglionic nerves to the iris and allowed them to degenerate. When he then tested the effect of an extract of the adrenal medulla, which as we now know contains a mixture of adrenaline and noradrenaline, he found that the pupil dilated, indeed to an even greater extent than in the normal animal. Experiments of a similar kind have been made on many other adrenergically innervated tissues with similar results. Evidently, therefore, these substances act on the cells in the effector organ and not on the nerve endings. The reason for the 'supersensitivity' discovered by Lewandowsky is discussed on p. 4.15.

All the catecholamines and in addition phenylephrine have such a direct action. However, the degree to which α- and β-receptors is affected varies. Thus phenylephrine activates only α- and isoprenaline only β-receptors.

The effects of the other sympathomimetics listed in fig. 4.6 are not enhanced by chronic denervation; they are in fact reduced. This suggests that part of their action depends on their causing the release of the transmitter

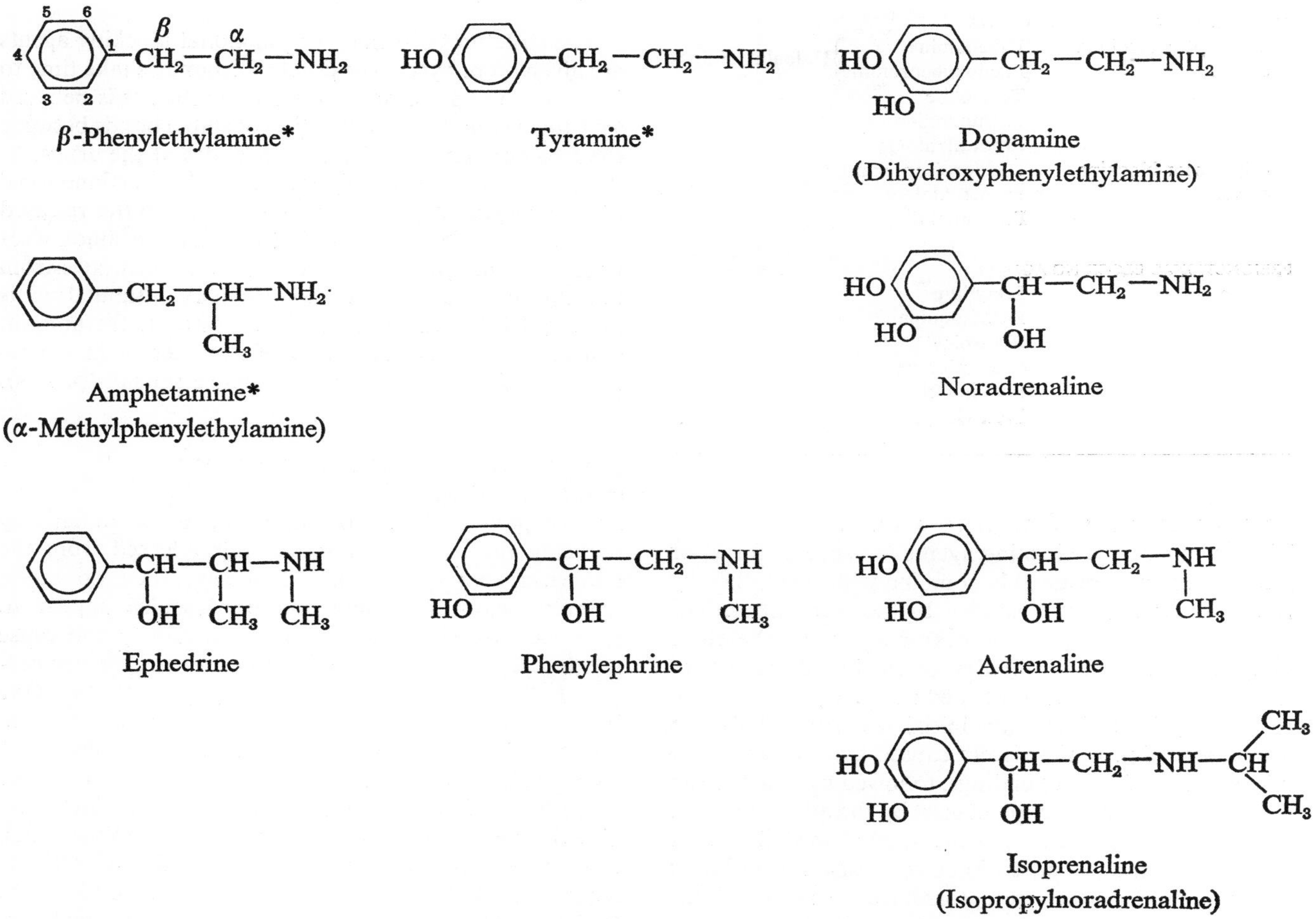

FIG. 4.6. Important sympathomimetic drugs arranged according to the number of hydroxyl substitutions in the benzene ring. The catecholamines and phenylephrine have direct effects via adrenergic receptors. The substances indicated by * have mainly indirect effects via the release of noradrenaline. Ephedrine has mixed effects.

from the adrenergic nerves. This idea is supported by other experiments (p. 15.17).

Adrenergic blocking agents (table 4.7)

There are basically two different types of agents which diminish the effects of sympathetic adrenergic nerve impulses. One kind also diminishes the responses to catecholamines applied artificially or released from the adrenal medulla and may conveniently be described as **postjunctional blocking agents**. The second kind reduces the amount of noradrenaline released from the adrenergic nerve terminals and may be described as **prejunctional blocking agents**.

TABLE 4.7. Drugs which prevent **the actions of adrenergic** nerve stimulation.

Category	Drug
POSTJUNCTIONAL BLOCKING AGENTS	
α-Receptor blocking agents	Dibenamine
	Phenoxybenzamine } Haloalkylamines
	Tolazoline
	Phentolamine
	Ergot alkaloids
β-Receptor blocking agents	Dichloroisoprenaline
	Pronethalol
	Propranolol
PREJUNCTIONAL BLOCKING AGENTS	
	Bretylium
	Debrisoquine
	Reserpine
	Guanethidine
	Bethanidine
	Methyldopa

POSTJUNCTIONAL BLOCKING AGENTS

The postjunctional blocking agents are specific for α- or β-receptors and presumably combine with them, thereby reducing the number available to the transmitter. The action of **dibenamine**, an α-blocking agent, on the effect of splanchnic nerve stimulation on the blood pressure of an anaesthetized cat is illustrated in fig. 4.7. The normal response (A) consists of an initial fast rise (a), due to vasoconstriction in the viscera caused by the transmitter released from the nerve endings, followed by a slower rise (b) due to vasoconstriction caused by the adrenaline and noradrenaline released from the adrenal medulla. After dibenamine, the response (B) consists of a fall in blood pressure. Since all the α-receptors have been blocked, the residual response must be due to the activation of the β-receptors in the skeletal muscle blood vessels by the circulating adrenaline.

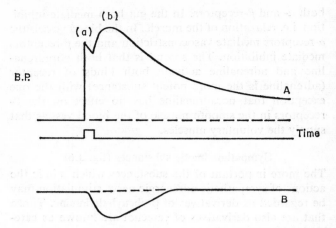

FIG. 4.7. The action of dibenamine on the effect of splanchnic nerve stimulation on the blood pressure (BP) of an anaesthetized cat. (A) normal response, (B) after dibenamine.

The structures of some postjunctional blocking agents are given on p. 15.23. The β-haloalkylamines take time to be effective and are only slowly reversible. It is believed that this is due to the formation of stable bonds between the receptors and reactive intermediates of the drugs.

There is no direct evidence that the postjunctional blocking agents affect the amount of transmitter released from adrenergic nerves. It is true that the amount of noradrenaline which can be collected in perfusates from the spleen as a result of splenic nerve stimulation is increased by phenoxybenzamine. However, the amount collected is increased because of a reduction in the re-uptake of the transmitter by the nerve terminals (p. 4.15).

PREJUNCTIONAL BLOCKING AGENTS
(table 4.7 and fig. 4.8)

All the prejunctional blocking agents act essentially by reducing the amount of transmitter released from the adrenergic nerve terminals. However, they do so in different ways. **Bretylium** and **debrisoquine** appear to have the most simple action; they act rapidly and cause no change other than the diminution of transmitter output. It has been suggested that they prevent the nerve impulse invading the nerve terminal, but there is no direct evidence in favour of this. On the other hand **guanethidine**, **bethanidine** and **reserpine** deplete the nerve terminals of their store of transmitter. With reserpine this appears to be the mechanism of blockade which develops slowly and with an intensity which mirrors the depletion. With guanethidine the blockade develops rapidly, although depletion is slow, so that the depletion is certainly not the sole cause. The action of **methyldopa** represents another variant. This substance is converted

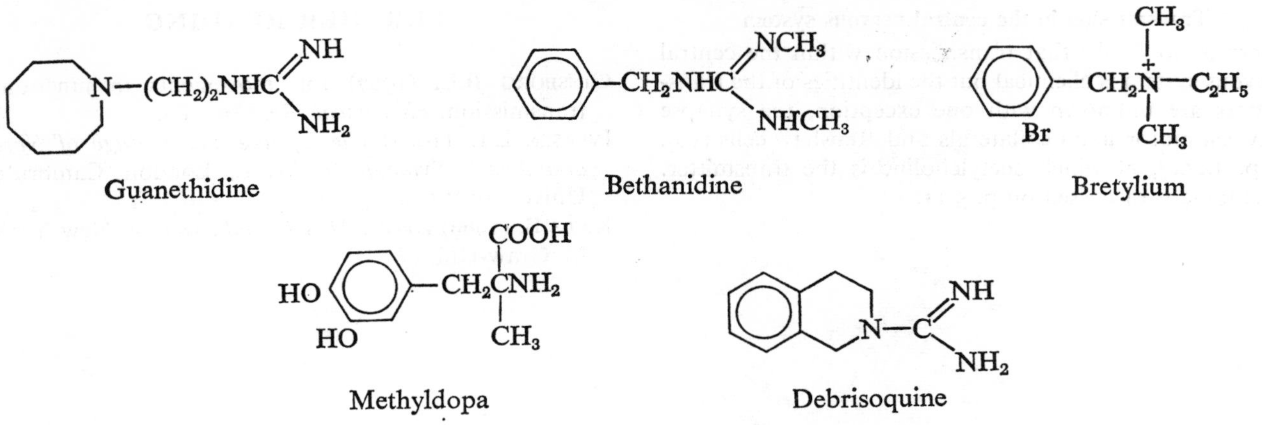

FIG. 4.8. Prejunctional blocking agents.

into α-methyldopamine and α-methylnoradrenaline by the enzymes which normally convert DOPA to noradrenaline; these substances then act as 'false transmitters', which are very much less potent than noradrenaline (p. 15.31).

None of the prejunctional blocking agents reduce the response to injected or circulating catecholamines. In fact, the tissues may become supersensitive. The depleting agents have little effect on the chromaffin cells of the adrenal medulla.

The fate of the transmitter

Two enzymes, monoamine oxidase and catechol-O-methyl transferase, are known to break down noradrenaline (p. 15.7). It was once thought that these enzymes were the equivalent of cholinesterase at cholinergic junctions and that they limited the duration of the effects of adrenergic nerve stimulation. If this were so, drugs which inhibited these enzymes would be expected to enhance the effect of nerve stimulation like the anticholinesterases. Except in very special circumstances this does not happen and the theory has been abandoned (p. 15.29). Some process, however, in addition to diffusion from receptors, limits the action of the transmitter and this appears to be uptake by the nerve terminals from which it has been released. Evidence for this has been obtained by the use of tritium-labelled noradrenaline. When small amounts are infused or injected in normal animals, it disappears rapidly from the plasma and is taken up by tissues with a large number of adrenergic nerves (e.g. heart and spleen). That it is taken up by the nerves is shown by the following:

(1) it can be released into the circulation again by nerve stimulation, and

(2) little uptake occurs in tissues which have been denervated and in which the nerves have degenerated.

The process of inactivation of noradrenaline by uptake provides the basis for the explanation of the enhancement of the effects of adrenergic nerve stimulation caused by a number of drugs which are discussed on p. 15.20. A classical example is cocaine, which has long been known to enhance the effect both of adrenergic nerve impulses, e.g. it causes dilation of the pupil via contraction of the radial muscle of the iris, and of the catecholamines. It is now known that this is due to blockade of the uptake mechanism.

Many other drugs also have this action, and most of them affect adrenergic transmission in other ways as well. This sometimes makes their pharmacological actions seem paradoxical. Phenoxybenzamine for example, which is an α-receptor blocking agent, potentiates the effect of sympathetic nerve stimulation on the heart. This can now be explained by the facts that cardiac receptors are of the β-variety, and that phenoxybenzamine affects the uptake mechanism. Other drugs which block uptake are tyramine (p. 15.19) and guanethidine (p. 15.22).

The existence of this mechanism for the inactivation of catecholamines also explains at least in part, the supersensitivity of denervated tissues first noted by Lewandowsky. There may, however, be an additional factor. There is no reuptake of acetylcholine by cholinergic nerves and yet cholinergically innervated cells also become supersensitive to acetylcholine after denervation. The cells which have been most closely studied are skeletal muscle fibres; for these it is known that after denervation the acetylcholine receptors, normally confined to the small end plate region, spread over the whole surface of the fibre. It may therefore be that a similar process occurs in adrenergically innervated tissues, although there is at present no evidence for this.

Transmission in the central nervous system

There is no doubt that transmission within the central nervous system is chemical but the identities of the transmitters are unknown with one exception, the synapse between motor axon collaterals and Renshaw cells (vol. 1, p. 14.28), at which acetylcholine is the transmitter. This topic is discussed on p. 5.11.

FURTHER READING

GINSBORG B.L. (1967) Ion movements in junctional transmission. *Pharmacol. Rev.* **19,** 289.

IVERSEN L.L. (1967) *The Uptake and Storage of Noradrenaline in Sympathetic Nerves.* London: Cambridge University Press.

KATZ B. (1966) *Nerve, Muscle and Synapse.* New York: McGraw-Hill.

Chapter 5
Drugs that act on the central nervous system

Since time immemorial man has used drugs to alter his state of mind and behaviour, to treat pain, insomnia, epilepsy, various forms of insanity and other diseases arising from disturbance of the central nervous system. Many of these drugs, as the dried plant or extract, were known to ancient China, India, Egypt, Greece and Rome, and passed into Arabian medicine before reaching Europe in the twelfth century. The great navigations of the sixteenth and seventeenth centuries enriched the herbals and drug formularies of the time with new drugs from the Malayan archipelago and the American continent.

Up till the end of the eighteenth century, materia medica was still a department of botany but, with the rise of chemistry, crude vegetable preparations began to be replaced by their active principles. For the most part, these were potent alkaloids of which the first was morphine, from opium. Hyoscine and hyoscyamine likewise were the alkaloids of poisonous solanaceous plants such as mandrake (*Mandragora*) or deadly nightshade (*Atropa belladonna*), and accounted for their narcotic effect. Indeed, opium, alcohol and mandragora were used to stupefy patients requiring drastic surgical treatment, such as amputation of limbs. Opium reduced sensibility to pain and made the patient indifferent to it; alcohol, which was also a food, enhanced this effect; hyoscine dulled the memory of an unpleasant experience and, together with hyoscyamine, it dried up the external secretions.

Apart from their medical uses, traditional remedies provided an escape from the ills of life; they also promoted social activity and enhanced the effect of rituals or religious experiences. Thus, in the Far and Middle East opium and flowers of hemp (cannabis) are to this day widely consumed in a manner similar to alcohol in other parts of the world.

In Peru, natives use the coca leaf to increase their sense of well-being (euphoria) and their powers of endurance. Again, in Mexico, the top of a small cactus plant, *peyotl*, is consumed for its bizarre effects on perception at the time of ritual or festival. The action is due to mescaline, a drug which in structure resembles adrenaline. Tobacco (*Nicotiniana*) which contains the alkaloid nicotine, was known to American Indians and brought to Europe in the sixteenth century; tea and the coffee bean, in which caffeine is the active substance, followed later. Both nicotine and caffeine, which is a purine, act on the brain.

Whereas some of these drugs were harmless, the more powerful euphoriants such as opium and cocaine, induce physical dependence or addiction. For many years, interest in drugs that affect the mind and behaviour lay mainly in the pharmacological and social problems of addiction. Exciting developments followed the discovery, in 1943, that D-lysergic acid diethylamide (LSD) in minute dose (about 1 µg/kg), reproduced all the effects of transient mental disorder, including vivid hallucinations. On the strength of this highly specific action on the brain, it was called a **psychotomimetic**. However, the true significance of this observation did not become apparent until about 10 years later, when it was discovered that the brain contained not only acetylcholine but also amines, namely, noradrenaline and 5-hydroxytryptamine (5-HT). At this point, experiments showed that LSD was a powerful antagonist of the effect of 5-HT on the isolated rat uterus. Hence it was proposed that LSD might act centrally by opposing the actions of 5-HT in the brain. Although this hypothesis could not be sustained, it promoted further studies of amine metabolism in brain. Noradrenaline, 5-HT (monoamines) and later histamine were found to have similar patterns of distribution in the brain and their concentrations could be altered by treatment with **psychotropic drugs**, notably reserpine.

In India, a climbing plant had long been used as a remedy for madness, snake bite and other ailments, and was originally mentioned in the *Ayur-Vedas*, a book on health written in Sanskrit and used by Brahman (priest) physicians. In the eighteenth century, a French botanist brought the plant to Europe and named it *Rauwolfia serpentina*, after Rauwolf, a German traveller and botanist of an earlier time. Although previous efforts had been made to purify the active principle, it was only in 1952 that reserpine and related alkaloids were isolated from the plant. Because reserpine quietened maniacs without clouding consciousness and tamed wild animals, it was called a **tranquillizer**. In the brain, these effects were associated with a drastic fall in the concentration of monoamines and histamine but not of acetylcholine. At about the same time chlorpromazine, which was first used as a drug for lowering the body temperature in patients requiring cardiac surgery, was discovered to be a powerful tranquillizer. However, chlorpromazine, unlike reserpine, did not deplete the brain of amines. It was developed from the potent antihistamine, promethazine which is a derivative of phenothiazine (p. 14.16). Finally, iproniazid, when used with other drugs to treat tuberculosis, was also found to promote a sense of wellbeing and was used in the control of mental depression. In the brain, iproniazid inhibits monoamine oxidase and so alters the metabolism of monoamines.

Thus, for the first time, changes in behaviour in animals and man were linked to biochemical changes in the brain. LSD made it possible to induce temporary psychotic states in healthy subjects, but its mode of action remains obscure. Conversely, in patients with psychoses, reserpine, chlorpromazine or iproniazid facilitated the return of rational behaviour. These findings prepared the way for a new approach to the treatment of psychiatric disorders and to the investigation of functions of the brain. Today, **psychopharmacology** includes the study of animal behaviour, neurophysiology, neurochemistry and observations on the ultrastructure of the brain. These disciplines, allied to those of information theory and the computer sciences, are making it possible to devise models of the brain which will provide insight into how drugs may influence functions of the CNS.

In addition to these recent developments, the achievements of the nineteenth century remain equally important. The discovery of **general anaesthesia** not only revolutionized the practice of surgery but represented the first use of synthetic drugs. Nitrous oxide, ether and halogenated hydrocarbons, e.g. chloroform, have now been in use for more than a century. Chloral hydrate was the first of the synthetic **hypnotics** and salicylic acid the first of the **antipyretics** and **analgesics**. Later, knowledge of the structure of cocaine served as a model for the synthesis of **local anaesthetics** and the study of drugs based on the structure of urea (ureides) led to the discovery of barbiturates. Among these, phenobarbitone was not only sedative and hypnotic but the first effective drug for the control of epilepsy (Greek, *epileptikos*, seizure). Many of these earlier drugs are still in use.

METHODS OF INVESTIGATION AND PHARMACOLOGICALLY ACTIVE SUBSTANCES IN BRAIN

Although many drugs affect the central nervous system (CNS) relatively little is known about how and where they act. The methods used to obtain this information include behavioural, neuropharmacological and bio-

chemical and other techniques. It is difficult to interpret the results of behavioural experiments in biochemical or pharmacological terms, or to relate the activity of single neurones with the function of groups of nerve cells.

Some of the sources of difficulty in experimental work are as follows:

(1) the brain is not easily accessible to study;

(2) it is sensitive to surgical interference and to hypoxia; thus circulatory impairment and loss of excitability may follow damage;

(3) it is difficult to study any particular region in neuronal or vascular isolation;

(4) the blood–brain barrier tends to isolate the brain from the rest of the body; thus it influences the penetration of drugs and metabolic precursors and is an obstacle to the study of their effects after administration;

(5) biochemical analysis of post-mortem material gives valuable information about stable compounds, but it is of limited value in the investigation of substances that are metabolized rapidly;

(6) although information can be obtained *in vitro* from studies on brain slices, cells in culture, tissue homogenates and their subcellular fractions, e.g. synaptosomes, these methods of preparation are likely to damage cellular components, and the results obtained are difficult to interpret in terms of the function of organized neurones. Furthermore, the number of cell types in any one area makes it difficult to define the features of neuronal metabolism from that of glial or vascular cells (p. 5.15).

Drugs and behaviour

There are two approaches to the study of drugs on behaviour; one is to define how a particular behavioural response is modified by drugs; the other is to determine the activity of drugs in a range of tests of behaviour. Whatever the approach, the design of experiments and the interpretation of results depend on a knowledge of pharmacological principles and of the properties of the drugs being studied. For example, a drug which acts on the CNS might be less potent than another because it disappears more rapidly from the body or penetrates less readily into the brain; or its action might be delayed because it is slowly converted into an active form. The point can be illustrated by the behaviour of a strip of guinea-pig's intestine suspended in Ringer's solution which in some ways resembles that of the intact animal. Each is a complicated system which can be only partially defined; each is responsive to environmental change and to drug molecules which activate receptors; in a statistical sense, each is one of a population in which susceptibility to the effects of drugs is assumed to be normally distributed. In short, the concepts and quantitative methods which are used in pharmacology to study the actions of drugs in physiological and biochemical terms are also applicable to the study of behavioural effects. For example, in the rat, an intravenous injection of amphetamine raises the blood pressure; over a longer period, the same dose might depress hunger and improve conditioned avoidance (p. 5.5). Feeding and avoidance are behavioural; the first expresses the desire for food, the second, recognition of some hostile feature in the environment. Fundamentally, both have to do with survival. Each, however, can be transformed into physical values which are measurable, hunger by the amount of work performed to obtain food, and avoidance by the number of successful escapes made from danger, e.g. an electric shock. Each response is the outcome of information retrieval and of programmed action in which orientation, timing and speed are the essential features.

Nevertheless, the question remains to what extent does the measured parameter really represent the complexities of the behavioural response?

In the present context behaviour is the continuing activity of a conscious animal, as may be seen or recorded by a trained observer. The animal is not only alert and responding to minute changes in its immediate environment but is impelled through its own physiological rhythms to search for food and water and to act in other ways.

Behaviour can be measured when input from the environment is controlled and the animal is placed in situations which are designed to evoke characteristic and reproducible responses. Since drugs may affect the response by acting outside the CNS their general effects should be noted before more complicated tests of behaviour are carried out.

DIRECT OBSERVATION

The simplest method is to inject different doses of a drug into rats or mice and to observe general, behavioural, neurological or other effects for which a score is entered on a standard chart (table 5.1).

In this way drugs may not only be screened for CNS activity, but they may reveal peripheral effects which could be misinterpreted as being of central origin. Thus an animal might be less active because a drug has a curare-like action. By contrast in mice, erection of the tail (Straub phenomenon), increased motor activity and diminished response to pain, suggest that the action of the drug is central and like that of morphine. More precise information is obtained by defining and measuring selected parameters of behaviour which fall into two groups, **innate** and **conditioned behaviour**.

INNATE BEHAVIOUR
Spontaneous motor activity
In a rat this is made up of walking, running, rearing on hind legs, sniffing, scratching, gnawing and much else

TABLE 5.1. Neurological and behaviour assessment chart. Observations are scored as slight, moderate or marked. After Everett G.M. & Wiegand R.G. (1962).

General observations	Autonomic responses	Reflexes	Behaviour
Increased motor activity	Salivation Lachrymation	Tendon reflexes	Sociability Contentment
Decreased motor activity	Vomiting Defaecation Urination	Withdrawal Righting Ear twitch Corneal	Defensive Aggressive Stereotyped actions
Altered muscle tone	Miosis Mydriasis		
Ataxia	Ptosis		Disorientation
Tremors	Light reflex		Restlessness
Convulsions	Relaxation of nictitating membrane		
Sleep Coma Catatonia	Piloerection Vasodilation Vasoconstriction		
Response to pain	Heart rate Respiration Temperature		

besides. The activity, which is repetitive, rises and falls during the day and is influenced by light, temperature, noise and the physiological state of the animal. The activity is commonly measured by placing the rat in a jiggle cage which is connected to a gramophone pick-up. This provides a sensitive method for recording movements of the cage which are taken to represent the total motor activity of the animal. Another method is to record with a counter the number of times the animal interrupts infrared beams of light directed across the cage on to photoelectric cells.

Exploratory behaviour
When a rat is placed alone in a new cage it might defaecate as an expression of alarm, pause and then begin to explore its surroundings; it might sniff, rear on its hind legs and gnaw the bars of the cage. This display of exploratory behaviour can be turned into a quantitative test by placing the animal at the centre of a Y-shaped corridor and counting the number of complete entries it makes into each arm (fig. 5.1).

These methods make it possible to study not only the effect of drugs which enhance or reduce spontaneous activity but, equally important, the combined effects of drugs. Thus, treatment with amphetamine increases motor activity and the effect is further increased in rats that have been pretreated with a monoamine oxidase (MAO) inhibitor.

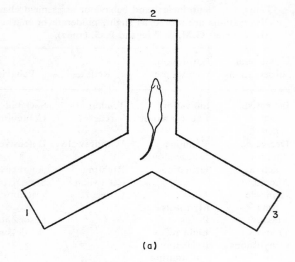

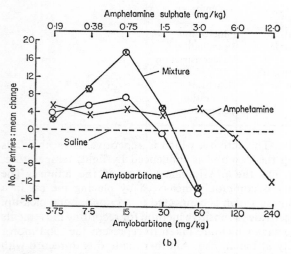

FIG. 5.1. (a) Y-shaped box to determine exploratory behaviour. (b) Effect of the administration of amphetamine and amylobarbitone and a 1:20 mixture of the two drugs at different dose levels compared with saline. The vertical axis represents the mean change in activity of the animals as expressed by the number of entries into the arms of the box in 5 min from that of the control. After Rushton & Steinberg, H. (1963) *Brit. J. Pharmacol.* **21**, 295.

Choice of food and drink
When satiated rats are offered a choice of drinks as in a cafeteria, they usually prefer weak solutions of alcohol, sucrose or even salt, to water. Preference for sucrose holds over a wide range of concentrations but can be reduced by adding quinine to the solution. To the human palate, quinine is a substance with a bitter taste and presumably rats reject it for the same reason. In these tests, the volume of solution consumed and the concentration of solute provide a measure of palatability or hedonic response (Greek, *edone*, pleasurable). The higher the proportion of quinine in the mixture, the lower the intake

of sucrose. Rats that have been deprived of water show less aversion to solutions containing quinine, which confirms the well-known fact that palatability is influenced by physiological need.

Deprivation of hormones or vitamins alters behaviour. After adrenalectomy rats soon develop hunger for salt and prefer more concentrated solutions of NaCl than before the operation. The volume of solution consumed daily depends on the concentration of NaCl. This behavioural response, which is probably due to the effect of sodium depletion on the hypothalamus, is reversed by treatment with DOC (p. 6.11). In the same way, wild rabbits deficient in sodium in the Snowy Mountains of S.E.Australia lick pegs impregnated with NaCl or $NaHCO_3$, in preference to pegs containing other substances.

When rats are deprived of vitamins or amino acids they learn to prefer diets which contain these substances and may even supplement them from bacterial sources in their faeces. So far, little is known about how drugs influence preferences for food and drink.

Behaviour in wild life
Animals are placed in as normal an environment as possible and their complex behaviour such as grooming and their responses to other animals is recorded. Drugs which act on the CNS alter the patterns and frequency of such behaviour in much smaller dose than they do in animals in laboratory conditions.

Species with highly characteristic patterns of behaviour have been used particularly to detect drugs that sedate or tranquillize (p. 5.29). Many animals in the natural state are liable to react in a hostile way to man and other predators but can be tamed with drugs. This effect has been demonstrated in the deer, lynx, dingo, baboon, and such powerful animals as the tiger, kangaroo and sea lion. It may, however, be more conveniently observed in smaller animals such as male Siamese fighting fish (*Betta splendens*) which assume characteristic postures and change in colour before giving combat. The jerboa, a jumping rodent which inhabits sandy plains and dwells in burrows, instinctively digs for safety when placed in a sandpit. On these tests, drugs that tranquillize diminish or annul patterns of behaviour which express hostility, either as fight or flight, but do not interfere with other activities such as eating, drinking or sleeping. A curious exception is the spider which, after treatment with LSD, spins its web with even greater geometrical perfection.

CONDITIONED BEHAVIOUR
More information is gained in tests where the animal learns to avoid punishment or to obtain a reward. Such tests can be elaborated by confounding the reward with obstacles or punishments, so disrupting the learned

response. The animal may then become aggressive or 'frozen' and, in this state of emotional conflict, displays autonomic responses, such as piloerection, urination and defaecation. These methods therefore make it possible to test drugs which protect against the effects of emotional conflict and which may assist in restoring learned behaviour after it has been disrupted.

Avoidance conditioning

Rats it seems, like men, learn more easily to avoid punishment than to earn rewards. A rat may be placed in a cage, the floor of which is a grid of metal bars that are connected to electrodes. The cage may be divided into two compartments or contain a pole in the centre (fig. 5.2).

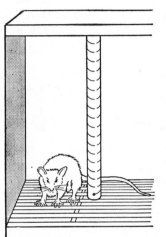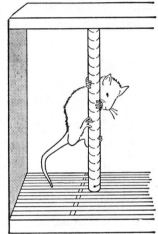

FIG. 5.2. Cage to test avoidance conditioning. The floor of the cage is electrified and the pole provides a safe haven. From *Triangle (En.)* (1960) 4, 245.

One compartment or the pole provides a safe haven from the noxious stimulus delivered from the floor as an electric shock. The conditioning stimulus, which may be a buzzer or a metronome, is coupled with the shock and the rat quickly learns to move into the safe compartment or climb on the pole at the sound of the signal alone. A box which contains two compartments, each of which is alternately safe and unsafe, is called a shuttle box.

Drugs can be tested for their abilities to impair learning and to extinguish it. In the developed response, the test discriminates between two effects; first, avoidance of the shock (response to the auditory signal) and second, escape by the same route after the shock has been received. The responses, whether to the signal or the shock, are counted automatically and the result is expressed as the percentage of the score obtained before treatment with a drug. Thus while 10·5 mg/kg of chlorpromazine

reduces the climbing response of rats to the buzzer, about four times this dose is needed to reduce the response to the shock. Barbitone differs from chlorpromazine in that the dose which halves the response to the auditory stimulus also diminishes the response to shock by about the same amount. Chlorpromazine is therefore more selective in its action than barbitone in suppressing avoidance behaviour.

Reward conditioning

The method attempts to measure the strength of natural drives such as hunger, thirst and sex, and is called **operant** because the animal can achieve its goal only by performing work (vol. 1, p. 24.92).

In **lever pressing** tests, rats learn to work for a reward (food or water) by pressing down a lever to obtain a pellet of food in a cup. After measuring performance, the test can be complicated by making it difficult for the rat to obtain food. For example, the drive for food shown by hungry rats can be combined with avoidance conditioning in which electric shocks increase in strength the nearer the rat gets to the lever. Untreated rats then run more slowly and less often to obtain a reward, but the performance of rats treated with amylobarbitone is virtually unimpaired. It might be supposed that amylobarbitone abolishes fear, or interferes with memory or in some way blocks perception of stimuli applied in the test. Since the rats are able to discriminate between small differences in auditory tone and in distances safe from electric shocks, it can be concluded that amylobarbitone does not affect perception but acts in some other way as yet unknown.

A **maze** may be defined as an intricate structure of passages that communicate with one another, and through which it is difficult to find one's way without a clue. Rats, like humans, vary in their ability to traverse a maze where success depends on learning from mistakes (fig. 5.3). At first the number of mistakes is large, but with repeated trials the mistakes fall off rapidly. The tests can be refined by using a graduated system of mazes. It is a matter for regret that although many drugs are known to interfere with learning, few, if any, are seen to enhance it.

In the pigeon, the **pecking response** provides many useful parameters for measurement. The pigeon is placed in a ventilated, sound-proofed box, and directly in front of its beak is an illuminated dial (fig. 5.4). When the pigeon pecks at it, a brightly illuminated food tray appears for 5 sec. Hence the pigeon learns to operate a device (the response) and obtains a reward for doing so. By coupling reward to response in this way, the process of learning is continually reinforced. The rate of pecking is shown graphically on an ink writing recorder or is counted with digital counters.

Not every response, however, need be rewarded, and

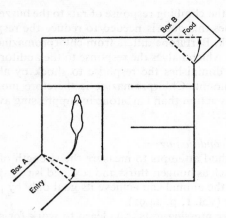

FIG. 5.3. Animal maze to test ability to learn from experience. The rat is placed in box A and has to find its way to box B to obtain a reward.

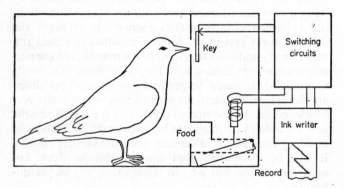

FIG. 5.4. Skinner pigeon box, not to scale. After Dews P.B. (1955). *J. Pharmacol. exp. Ther.* **113**, 393.

it is open to the experimenter to vary the ratio of responses to rewards, and the time lapse between the response and appearance of the reward. For example, the pigeon quickly learns to peck rapidly when the reward is obtained at only every fiftieth peck; or, having pecked once at the dial, to wait for a given period of time until the food appears. Again, the experiment can be elaborated to test the effect of drugs on sensory discrimination and memory, as when the pigeon learns to peck in response to a variety of signals, such as shapes or colours. Pentobarbitone more readily affects the discrimination of the lapse of time than it does the rate of pecking to obtain a reward.

The results of conditioning experiments should always be interpreted with care since drugs which are assayed for this purpose may impair the physiological expression of the drive.

TESTS ON MAN
Methods that have been developed for animals are in principle also applicable to man. Clinical observations,

whether in healthy subjects or mentally ill patients, can give valuable clues about the action of a drug. In addition to drugs which are used for their effects on the brain, many drugs which are taken for their peripheral effects also have direct central actions. For example, antihistamines in doses which control urticaria may cause loss of attention and drowsiness (p. 14.16). The consequences may be important when the person is in charge of machinery whether in the factory, the roads or elsewhere.

Tests are designed to measure different kinds of performance such as physical endurance, manual skills, learning, memory and judgement. One such method involves pressing a morse key and measures the maximum rate of tapping. When this is done at intervals over a period of time, the rate tends to fall off mainly because of boredom. Treatment with amphetamine can be shown to improve the performance (fig. 5.5). Performance also

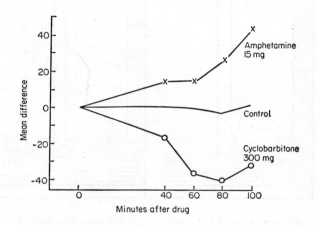

FIG. 5.5. Maximum rate of tapping a morse key. The results are expressed as the mean difference between the control rate and that achieved with amphetamine and cyclobarbitone. After Steinberg H. (1964). *Readings in Psychology*. London: Allen & Unwin.

improves when several subjects compete with one another (fig. 5.6). In this new situation, performance reaches a maximum which coincides with that obtained after treatment with amphetamine. In the same test, treatment with cyclobarbitone had a depressant effect, but when it was combined with amphetamine in a single oral dose, the performance was similar to the value obtained before treatment. The antagonism between barbiturates and amphetamine is seen elsewhere, as on the respiration.

Much remains to be discovered about the effects of drugs on acuity of perception. The methods include measurement of threshold frequencies at which discrete visual or auditory flutter stimuli become fused into a single train. The **tachistoscope** is a device which shows

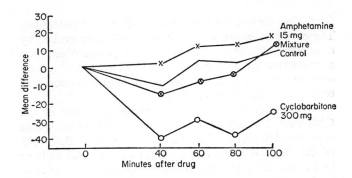

Fig. 5.6. Maximum rate of tapping morse key as in fig. 5.5. for four groups of subjects who were told each other's score rates. Under these competitive circumstances there was little difference between the amphetamine and control groups, but amphetamine countered the effect of the barbiturate. After Steinberg H. (1964). *Readings in Psychology*. London: Allen & Unwin.

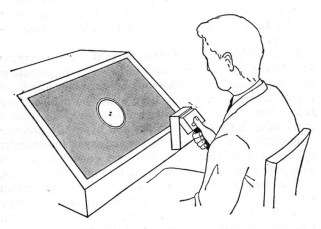

FIG. 5.7. Apparatus for studying performance in tracking a moving target. A moving spot is followed on an oscilloscope screen by another spot, controlled by the observer. After Wilson A. & Schild H.O. (1968) *Applied Pharmacology*, 10th Edition. London: Churchill.

images of numbers, letters or objects for a fraction of a second in order to see how quickly they can be identified. Strychnine enhances acuity of the special senses and enlarges the fields of vision. Skilled movements demanding strict coordination between hand and eye, can be tested in an apparatus for tracking a moving target (fig. 5.7). Effects of small doses of alcohol and barbiturates can be detected in this way.

Other tests are based on mental performance only and require reasoning with words or numbers. Drugs that improve performance in these tests do so by removing effects of anxiety, not by improving the intellect.

Some indication of the effects of drugs on emotions can be obtained by introspection. Various states of feeling

TABLE 5.2. Example of form to record subjective feelings while under the influence of cyclobarbitone (300 mg). From Wilson A. & Schild H. O. (1968). *Applied Pharmacology*, 10th Ed. London: Churchill.

Subjective feeling	Min after drug				
	0	40	60	80	100
Calm	✓				
Clear-headed	✓				
Normal	✓				✓
Warm					
Relaxed	✓				
Distracted		✓		✓	
Dreamy		✓			
Drowsy			✓		
Difficulty in concentration			✓	✓	
Tired					✓

are coded into words which are set out on a standard form. Scores are entered at different time intervals after taking the drug (table 5.2).

The most informative introspective study of a psychotropic drug in the English language is, to this day, that described by Thomas de Quincey in 1822 under the title of *Confessions of an English Opium Eater*, which every medical student should read.

Electropharmacological methods

Apart from altering behavioural responses, drugs that act on the CNS produce a wide range of other effects; these include catatonia, sleep, fits, tremors, ataxia and changes of posture and muscle tone. There may also be disturbances in responses arising from stimulation or inhibition of the nuclei and central connections of the autonomic nervous system. In investigating these effects it can be assumed that there are many sites at which drugs act within neuronal systems of the brain and that they have different affinities for drugs. For example, the convulsant leptazol (pentylenetetrazol) produces loss of consciousness accompanied by electrical discharge from the thalamus and cerebral cortex. By contrast, with strychnine electrical discharge occurs from the brain stem, cerebellum and spinal cord; the thalamus and cerebral cortex are completely spared and consciousness is retained.

Information on the site and mode of action of drugs in the CNS has depended not only on the development of delicate methods of recording potentials but on the perfection of stereotactic techniques which provide controlled access to the particular targets in the brain. The first stereotactic apparatus was introduced by Horsley and Clark in 1890, as an aid to brain surgery.

It is a rigid frame in which the head of the animal is fixed. By taking points of reference on the skull, a locus in the brain is defined in terms of three planes or co-ordinates (fig. 5.8). When many such measurements are made, the solid structure of the brain can be represented in a series of maps. Hence it is possible to place micro-electrodes, micropipettes, cannulae, implants or other instruments deeply in the substance of the brain so that the tip or point coincides with the required locus to within 100 μm. In this way, many experimental procedures

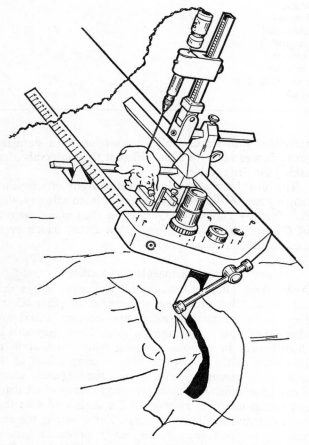

FIG. 5.8. Stereotactic apparatus. From Jasper H.H. & Ajmone-Marsan C. (1954). *A Stereotaxic Atlas of the Diencephalon of the Cat.* Ottawa: The National Research Council of Canada.

previously used to study neurochemical transmission and the action of drugs in the sympathetic ganglion and at the neuromuscular junction, were applied to the study of the CNS.

DRUGS AND BRAIN POTENTIALS

The effects of drugs may be studied on cerebral cortical activity, on subcortical centres which form parts of neuronal systems and on single neurones. Much in-

formation derives from recordings of surface potentials. These may be spontaneous, as in the EEG, or evoked by a sensory stimulus such as a loud click. When fine microelectrodes are placed among neurones (extra-cellular recording) spontaneous or evoked action potentials can also be measured.

Intracellular recordings from single neurones in the CNS were first achieved in motor neurones of the spinal cord and later in single cells elsewhere, as in Betz cells of the cerebral cortex. Recordings of neuronal activity in the cerebral cortex can be related to consciousness and, in the single neurone, to polarization of membranes and the mechanism of firing.

Cerebral cortical electrical activity

Drugs that alter this activity are those that annul consciousness, cause convulsions or heighten awareness. Recordings may be obtained from electrodes on the scalp (electroencephalogram vol. 1, p. 24.47) or on the surface of the brain (electrocorticogram). The effects of drugs on the EEG can thus be related to their effect on behaviour.

In the waking aroused state, cortical activity appears as a totally irregular sequence of low voltage potentials and is said to be asynchronous or desynchronized. At the other extreme, during deep sleep, cortical activity is synchronized and appears as slow waves of greater amplitude. General anaesthetics and hypnotics produce synchronization by depressing the activity of the reticular system of the brain stem. Cerebral convulsants, such as leptazol and picrotoxin cause loss of consciousness, and a hypersynchronous spike-like discharge occurs during the convulsion. Amphetamine, however, and other drugs that produce arousal, promote desynchronization. Cortical activity is compounded of complex rhythms which are poorly understood and drugs may change cortical activity by acting indirectly on subcortical centres in the thalamus, hypothalamus and elsewhere.

Neuronal systems

Many homeostatic and behavioural responses are under the control of the phylogenetically older parts of the brain. These include the olfactory, the limbic, the extra-pyramidal and the reticular systems of the brain stem (vol. 1, p. 24.20, 47, 49, and 65).

The effects of drugs on these systems can be explored by implanting in the brain recording or stimulating electrodes. A study of the actions of barbiturates and chlorpromazine on the reticular activating system provides a good example of this type of investigation. A representation of the system is shown in fig. 5.9. The reticular formation is seen as a polysynaptic network which receives short collaterals from the sensory pathways. Cranially, the formation connects with the hypothalamus and medial thalamic nuclei and from then on it

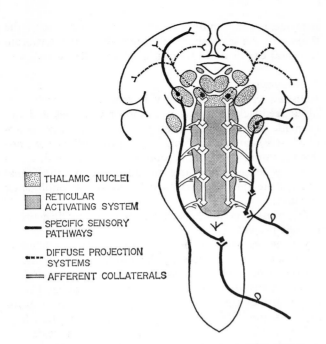

THALAMIC NUCLEI

RETICULAR ACTIVATING SYSTEM

SPECIFIC SENSORY PATHWAYS

DIFFUSE PROJECTION SYSTEMS

AFFERENT COLLATERALS

FIG. 5.9. Representation of the reticular activating system containing a polysynaptic network. From Root W.S. & Hofmann F.G. eds. (1963) *Physiological Pharmacology*, vol. I, *Nervous System*, part A. New York: Academic Press.

is believed, on physiological evidence, to project to all parts of the cortex. On this view, sensory information converging on the midbrain reaches the cerebral cortex by two routes:

(1) the main sensory pathways to the specific area for sensation, and

(2) through the reticular formation and eventually to the entire cortex.

When the reticular formation of the cat is disconnected from the cortex by a transverse cut through the midbrain between the colliculi (*cerveau isolé*), the animal becomes comatose and cannot be aroused by electrical or other stimulation and the EEG becomes synchronized. When, however, the reticular formation is spared by section of the spinal cord at C2 (*encéphale isolé*) and respiration is maintained artificially, the head shows signs of alternating between sleep and wakefulness, despite the enormous loss of sensory information. The sleeping head, as judged by closure of the eyes and the typical EEG pattern, can be easily awakened by electrical stimulation of the reticular formation in the midbrain or by an external sensory stimulus, such as a click; the EEG then shows desynchronization and the click is transduced into an evoked potential in the auditory area of the cortex. The eyes open and follow a moving object; the vibrissae twitch in response to an olfactory stimulus. In this preparation, chlorpromazine (2–4 mg/kg iv)

abolishes arousal by the external sensory stimulus (the click) but not by electrical stimulation; the evoked potential in the auditory cortex is unaffected. Chlorpromazine is thus presumed to limit sensory input to the reticular formation, without impairing consciousness or sensation. In contrast, pentobarbitone blocks arousal both by direct electrical stimulation and external stimuli; again, the evoked potential in the auditory cortex is unimpaired. Unlike chlorpromazine, therefore, pentobarbitone depresses the reticular activating system, an action which also might explain its hypnotic effect.

Single neurones

Studies on single neurones provide the main evidence for neurochemical transmission in the CNS. The recording microelectrode coupled with the technique of iontophoresis makes it possible not only to identify receptors but to analyse the action of drugs in terms of electrical parameters of the nerve cell membrane. As compared with similar studies on the micropharmacology of the neuromuscular junction or sympathetic ganglion, central neurones and synapses are more complicated and may be under the control of several transmitters.

At least two criteria for transmission can be tested by micropharmacological methods. In the first, presynaptic connections are stimulated electrically and the rate of discharge is recorded. The drug under test is then applied to the neurone and if the effect is similar to that of presynaptic stimulation, the drug is presumed to share properties with the natural transmitter. The second criterion is fulfilled when the effects of presynaptic stimulation and of the drug are modified in the same direction by other drugs, which might inhibit or potentiate the effects or act in other ways.

The study of the combined actions of drugs at central synapses came with the development of the multibarrelled microelectrode (fig. 5.10). Four or more glass micropipettes are fused to a central pipette which is filled with a concentrated solution of NaCl and is used for recording. The outer barrels contain solutions of drugs. The tip of the assembly is a cluster of capillaries with a total diameter of 4–8 μm. Since the orifices lie in the same plane, this type of electrode is only suitable for recording extracellular potentials and information is limited to the effect of drugs on the rate of firing. An electrical current which is too small to affect the activity of the neurone, carries a quantity of drug on to the surface of the neurone. In the interval between the doses, a braking current is applied to prevent diffusion of the drug from the tip of the pipette. The dose is measured in coulombs or gramme equivalents passed per second for each nanoampere; for acetylcholine this dose is about 5×10^{-15} gramme equivalents.

For intracellular recording, the recording pipette is parallel with and glued to the pipettes containing drugs,

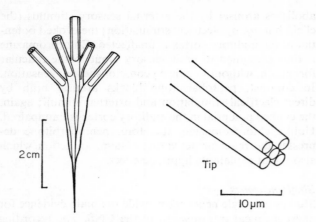

FIG. 5.10. Multibarrelled micropipette. From Robson J.M. & Stacey R.S. ed. (1968) *Recent Advances in Pharmacology*, 4th Edition. London: Churchill.

and projects 50 μm beyond them to impale the cell. Intracellular recording gives more precise information but is technically more difficult, except in the snail where neuronal cell bodies are exceptionally large and easily impaled under direct vision. In mammals, intracellular recording is restricted to parts of the brain with large cells, as in the cerebral cortex or the hippocampus.

With intracellular recording, it is possible to say whether the action of a drug is pre- or postsynaptic and, if postsynaptic, whether the effect arises from depolarization or hyperpolarization of the membrane. With further refinements of the method, the equilibrium potential can be determined for synaptic activation and for drugs placed on the membrane by iontophoresis. The parameters which define the equilibrium potential are:

(1) the concentration gradient of ions carrying membrane charges, and

(2) the relative permeability of the membrane to each species of ion, e.g. Na^+ and K^+.

Hence changes in these values provide a test for the identity between hypothetical neurotransmitters and molecules of known structure. Finally, by devising an internal microelectrode with two parallel channels, ions such as Na^+ and Cl^- can be introduced directly into the neurone, so altering its internal ionic environment. Measurements of the various electrical parameters both for the synaptic process and the effect of a drug applied externally, may then be repeated and compared in further tests of identity.

Most of our information on the action of drugs applied to neurones has been obtained by recording outside cells. Substances that have been tested include organic acids and bases that are extractable from brain, on the assumption that some are concerned with neurochemical transmission. Their effects have been recorded on neurones in the spinal cord (Renshaw cells, interneurones and motor

neurones), the midbrain (reticular formation), the thalamus, the cerebellum (Purkinje cells), the forebrain (cerebral cortex and hippocampus) and elsewhere.

Interneurones

Renshaw cells are inhibitory interneurones which supply a feedback from axons of motor neurones and can be made to fire in response to an electrical stimulus applied to a ventral root (vol. 1, p. 14.28). When the antidromic impulse reaches the motor axon collateral, transmitter is released and acts on the Renshaw cell. Transmission at this synapse is believed to be cholinergic because:

(1) the axon collateral stems from a cholinergic neurone (Dale's principle),

(2) the response of the Renshaw cell to acetylcholine is similar to that induced by the antidromic stimulus,

(3) eserine potentiates both of these responses, and

(4) dihydro-β-erythroidine, a curare alkaloid and weak antagonist of the action of acetylcholine at the neuromuscular junction, blocks them (fig. 5.11). The Renshaw cell, however, is also sensitive to other drugs; it fires in response to nicotine and tetramethylammonium, the effects of which, like those of acetylcholine and electrical

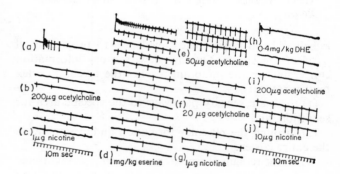

FIG. 5.11. Responses of a Renshaw cell recorded by an extracellular microelectrode. There was no spontaneous discharge. (a) The response to a single antidromic volley; (b) and (c) show responses evoked by intra-arterial injection of acetylcholine and nicotine. Several minutes after the intravenous injection of eserine, the response evoked by an antidromic volley (a) is changed to the enormously increased and prolonged response (d), while (e), (f) and (g) show, respectively, records of the responses then evoked by the intra-arterial injections of acetylcholine and nicotine; as expected there is a greatly increased sensitivity to acetylcholine but no change for nicotine. Records (h), (i) and (j) were obtained during the maximum of the depression produced by the intra-venous injection of dihydro-β-erythroidine (DHE); (h) shows the depressed response evoked by the antidromic volley and (i) and (j), the responses to intra-arterial injections of acetylcholine and nicotine respectively, showing that the sensitivity of the Renshaw cell is reduced to about one-tenth. After Eccles J.C., Eccles R.M & Fatt P. (1956). *J. Physiol.* **131**, 154.

stimulation, can be blocked with hexamethonium and tetraethylammonium. Even when receptors for acetylcholine are blocked with the drugs mentioned, others are free to respond to acetyl-β-methylcholine and can be blocked with atropine. Thus the Renshaw cell contains nicotinic and possibly muscarinic receptors for acetylcholine but their identification and role in synaptic transmission is far from simple. In contrast to Renshaw cells, spinal motor neurones are probably insensitive to acetylcholine and drugs that potentiate or block its actions.

Interneurones are seen as forming part of a negative feedback from sensory to motor neurones (fig. 5.12). These synaptic connections are important as the probable

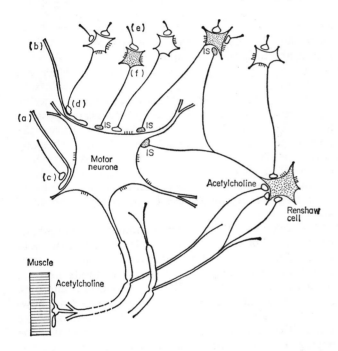

FIG. 5.12. Schematic drawing of motor neurone, Renshaw cell and other interneurones; shaded interneurones form inhibiting synapses (IS). Unshaded interneurones are excitatory. Two primary afferent fibres (a) and (b) end on the motor neurone. Synapses (c) and (d) are shown on the synaptic terminals of (a) and (b) and account for presynaptic inhibition. A primary afferent fibre (e) activates an inhibitory interneurone (f). The areas of pallisade markings on the surface of the motor neurone represent possible receptor sites for the action of amino acids. From Eccles J.C. (1963) *Physiology of Synapses*. Berlin : Springer.

sites of convulsant drugs which act by removing inhibition. Thus, strychnine and tetanus toxin act on the postsynaptic membrane of the motor neurones, block the effects of an inhibitory transmitter, and excitatory actions, therefore, predominate on the motor neurone. Interneurones differ in their functions; some excite or inhibit

motor neurones and even other interneurones; others act on terminals of primary afferent fibres which form a synapse with the motor neurone (fig. 5.12c, d). By depolarizing afferent terminals (fig. 5.12a, b) the interneurones damp down the excitory effect which the terminals exert on the motor neurone. Thus the effect of these interneurones is inhibitory because their site of action is presynaptic. Picrotoxin is an example of a drug that blocks this presynaptic inhibition, whether in the spinal cord or elsewhere in the CNS.

Elsewhere in the CNS, many neurones can be fired by the application of acetylcholine but the evidence is inconclusive that they are cholinergic. In the cerebral cortex, however, Betz cells in layer 5 are excited by electrical stimulation of the ventrolateral thalamus (thalamocortical neurones) and by the local application of acetylcholine; atropine blocks both of these effects. Betz cells, however, are insensitive to nicotine, and the curare alkaloids block neither the effect of electrical stimulation nor of acetylcholine. The evidence suggests:

(1) that thalamocortical neurones may be cholinergic, and

(2) that receptors for acetylcholine on Betz cells are muscarinic.

Again, in the ventrolateral thalamus, thalamocortical neurones can be excited in two ways:

(1) by the iontophoresis of acetylcholine, and

(2) by electrical stimulation of the medial lemniscus.

Whereas atropine and dihydro-β-erythroidine suppress the effect of acetylcholine, neither blocks the effect of electrical stimulation. Thus, it would seem that the major sensory pathway is not cholinergic though the ventrolateral thalamus may receive an input of cholinergic neurones that have still to be identified.

Although acetylcholine acts at many sites to excite neurones, at some, such as the olfactory bulb, it causes hyperpolarization of the membrane and so inhibits firing. This effect is reminiscent of the action of acetylcholine on the pacemaker cells of the heart.

Other biogenic substances

Similar studies have shown that noradrenaline, dopamine, 5-HT and histamine excite some cells and depress others. Nevertheless, identification of the receptors is uncertain for the lack of specific antagonists. In the cerebral cortex and brain stem the catecholamines and 5-HT both excite and depress the activity of sensitive neurones. Peripheral antagonists such as phentolamine for noradrenaline (p. 15.26), and methysergide for 5-HT (p. 13.7) prevent the excitatory effects of these amines more frequently than the inhibitory. In the rabbit olfactory bulb, however, α-receptor antagonists inhibit the depressant action of noradrenaline and of electrical stimulation. In the spinal cord, motor neurones are much less sensitive to the monoamines than are Renshaw cells and other interneurones which may be excited or depressed.

In an entirely different category are various amino acids which excite or depress neurones, when applied iontophoretically as anions. Acidic amino acids such as glutamic acid excite neurones and in their action and potency resemble acetylcholine. In contrast, neutral amino acids are inhibitory; the best known example is GABA and, more recently, glycine.

Results obtained using micropipettes for intracellular recording and iontophoresis (p. 5.9) suggest that glycine is the inhibitory transmitter released by the Renshaw cells on to spinal motor neurones. The evidence for this includes the following:

(1) glycine potentials and IPSPs are hyperpolarizing;

(2) glycine potentials and IPSPs have similar ionic equilibrium potentials;

(3) intracellular injection of Cl^- converts both into depolarizing potentials, suggesting that similar conductance changes are provoked by glycine and the IPSPs, and

(4) strychnine readily blocks the effects of glycine and the IPSPs (vol. 1, p. 14.27) but is less effective against the inhibitory effects of GABA.

Similar studies with intracellular electrodes and the local iontophoresis of GABA in the cortex suggest that GABA is the main inhibitory transmitter in the cerebral cortex.

The high concentrations of free amino acids in the brain are difficult to reconcile with their remarkable potency; as little as 10^{-15} moles of glutamate excites a cortical neurone. The amino acids are not known to be removed by an enzymic action after they have acted on the cell, nor is their activity annulled by any known antagonist.

Although amino acids are unspecific in their actions, they nevertheless pose the problem of how they bring about changes in membrane potential. Study of their structure and potency has led to the discovery of derivatives which are more potent and in which optical isomerism appears to be important. *N*-methyl-D-aspartic acid is 100 times more potent than L or D glutamate; but *N*-methyl-L-aspartic acid is of the same potency as glutamate. The further study of these amino acids may indicate that they share structural properties with the natural transmitter, and so provide important clues.

Pharmacological and biochemical methods

Many of the substances that are regarded as possible transmitters or modulators of the nerve impulse at central synapses were first identified in brain by their pharmacological activity, and doubtless other substances will continue to be discovered in this way. Whether as esters, amines or polypeptides, their presence as chemical con-

stituents of the brain naturally led to questions about their formation and storage in cells, the conditions for their release, their actions and subsequent fate. Thus classical neurophysiological methods of investigating the brain came to receive powerful support from the results of pharmacological, biochemical and histochemical investigations. Information from these sources has done much to strengthen the theory for neurochemical transmission at central synapses.

STUDIES AT THE SURFACE OF THE BRAIN
Pharmacological methods are used to detect and measure the active substances released in different parts of the brain when nerves are stimulated or after treatment with drugs. Detection, however, may be difficult as the quantity released is usually of the order of 2–5 picomoles; unless protected by an inhibitor, enzymes may destroy it and membrane barriers intervene between the site of its release and the point of sampling. Some of the difficulties can be overcome by using biological assays which are highly sensitive to the active substance but insensitive to impurities in the sample; the assay can be made specific by the use of suitable antagonists. Where it is not possible to protect the active substance from destruction, the metabolites are sought instead. Since these are usually devoid of pharmacological activity, their assay depends on chemical methods of assay. For example, a rise in the output of 5-hydroxyindole acetic acid may be taken as a measure of the release or increased turnover of 5-HT.

The technique of vascular perfusion of the sympathetic ganglion *in situ* or of skeletal muscle, made it possible to obtain direct evidence for neurochemical transmission at peripheral synaptic junctions. Such methods are not readily applicable to the CNS which soon fails and dies. Evidence for the release of active substances may, however, be obtained by collecting fluid at the surface of the brain. Cortical or ventricular surfaces present large aggregates of neurones, synapses and glia; in the cortex, pia mater intervenes between nervous tissue and the CSF; in the ventricles it is the ependyma. CSF bathes the entire surface and is in equilibrium with the extracellular fluid of the brain. Substances released from neuronal or other cells might then be expected to accumulate and pass into the CSF or other fluid in contact with the brain.

Studies on acetylcholine illustrate some of these methods. In the brain, as in other tissues, acetylcholine is held mainly in a bound form; some, however, is continually being released and destroyed; normally, none is detectable in the CSF. When cholinesterase in brain is blocked with eserine, acetylcholine appears in the CSF in sufficient concentrations to be measurable by assay on the dorsal muscle of the leech. This preparation, when suspended in Locke's solution containing eserine, is sensitive to concentrations in the test of 1 ng/ml.

PERFUSION OF THE CEREBRAL VENTRICLES

When serial samples of CSF are needed, it is convenient to perfuse the ventricles with artificial CSF containing eserine. Perfusion is made from one lateral ventricle through the aqueduct to cisterna magna and the perfusate is collected from a cannula that pierces the atlanto-occipital membrane (fig. 5.13). With cannulae suitably placed in the skull, perfusion can be restricted to smaller parts of the ventricular system, such as the anterior horn of the lateral ventricle or the third ventricle. It is then possible to monitor electrical activity in the region and to measure the output of acetylcholine in samples of perfusate in response to stimulation of sensory nerves, tracts, or neuronal pathways. Such methods have been used to demonstrate the presence in perfusates not only of acetylcholine but of metabolites of dopamine, which pass out of the caudate nucleus during electrical stimulation of cells in the midbrain (nigrostriate tract).

Cortical cups and push–pull cannula

The cortical surface is more easily accessible than the ventricular and the rise of acetylcholine in response to nervous stimuli may be shown in a simple way. Small plastic cylinders or cups are applied to the surface, and are filled with artificial CSF containing eserine. The fluid is tested periodically for activity and replaced. Subcortical regions of the brain can be explored with the aid of a push–pull cannula which is placed stereotactically (fig. 5.14). Artificial CSF flows through a central cannula

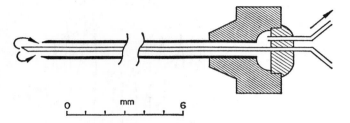

FIG. 5.14. Push–pull cannula in section. Gaddum J.H. (1961) *J. Physiol.* **155**, 1.

and makes contact with a minute area of brain tissue; it returns by syphoning through an outer cannula and is collected in tiny fractions. The rate of flow, the inflow pressure at the tip and the drop size depend on the relative diameters of the cannulae and on the distance between their tips; the latter can be adjusted by pushing or pulling the inner cannula. The samples are tested on leech muscle suspended in a micro-bath. Since the volume of the bath is about 25 μl, activity can be estimated in a sample the size of a large drop, which may contain less than 1 ng. of acetylcholine (fig. 5.15).

Experiments with cups placed on the sensory cortex or with the push–pull cannula in the caudate nucleus, have shown that the output of acetylcholine increases with electrical stimulation of neuronal paths that end in these regions. Such results strengthen the evidence for neurochemical transmission but do not by themselves prove that acetylcholine is a central neurochemical transmitter; under the experimental conditions neither the origin of acetylcholine nor the relationship of the output to nervous activity is known.

Cannulation of the cerebral ventricles is used not only to detect the release of substances formed in the brain but also to study the effect of drugs which do not penetrate the blood–brain barrier. In the cat, D-tubocurarine is convulsant after injection into the cerebral ventricles and is believed to act on the hippocampus. In man, the intraventricular injection of acetylcholine (~1 mg) produces flushing, lachrymation, salivation, bradycardia, vomiting, defaecation and micturition followed by sleep; the same dose injected intravenously is rapidly destroyed and virtually inactive. Atropine by the intraventricular route abolishes the central effects of acetyl-

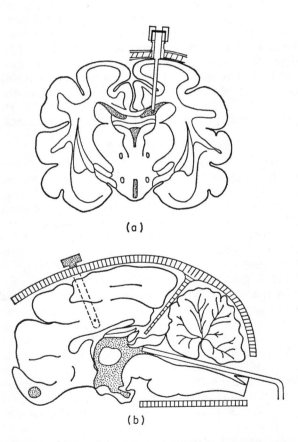

FIG. 5.13. Perfusion of the ventricular system. (a) Coronal section showing cannula tip in lateral ventricle; (b) sagittal section showing cannula in aqueduct sampling the perfusate. After Carmichael, Feldberg & Fleischhauer (1964). *J. Physiol.* **173**, 354

choline; eserine potentiates them. The precise site of action of drugs injected into the cerebral ventricle is not known but might be on subependymal nuclei of the hypothalamus which form part of the lateral walls and floor of the third ventricle.

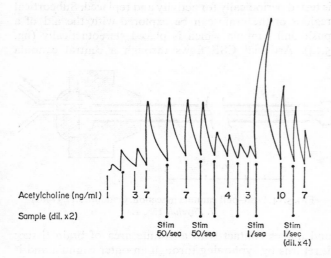

Acetylcholine (ng/ml)   1   3 7   7   4 3   10   7

Sample (dil. x2)

Stim 50/sec   Stim 50/sec   Stim 1/sec   Stim 1/sec (dil. x 4)

FIG. 5.15. Estimates of acetylcholine activity in samples obtained from a push–pull cannula inserted into the medial part of the caudate nucleus. Samples obtained without stimulation contained 2–7 ng acetylcholine/ml. During stimulation of the premotor cortex at 50/sec the output was 14 ng/ml and during stimulation at 1/sec the output rose to about 34 ng/ml. Assays on the dorsal muscle of the leech in a microbath. After Szerb J.C. & Mitchell J.F. (1962) *Abstracts XXII Int. Physiol. Cong.* p. 819.

Recirculation of CSF

In the dog, if a permanent cannula is placed in a lateral ventricle and another in the 4th ventricle and the two are joined, the CSF can be made to circulate outside the brain with the aid of a roller pump. Samples can be withdrawn from the system and substances introduced into it; the arrangement makes it possible to study in the conscious animal exchanges between the CSF and brain, and between the CSF and blood. For example, organic acids that are produced in the brain, appear in the CSF and are rapidly transferred via the choroid plexuses into the blood.

IMPLANTATION OF DRUGS

Drugs may also be applied to the brain by implantation. A pellet of drug is fixed to the tip of a stainless steel needle which is then placed in the brain under stereotactic and radiological control. Spayed female cats refuse the attentions of males but after an implant of oestrogen in the hypothalamus they accept them. Oestrogen molecules acting locally have in some way activated a pattern of sexual behaviour.

PHARMACOLOGICALLY ACTIVE SUBSTANCES IN BRAIN

Acetylcholine was first detected in brain by its effect on the eserinized dorsal muscle of the leech; later, it was isolated as the pure ester and identified chemically. Noradrenaline was recognized in parallel assays on the rat blood pressure and on the isolated rat colon; 5-HT stimulated the rat uterus, histamine and substance P (p. 17.4) the isolated guinea-pig's ileum; finally, prostaglandins acted not only on smooth muscle, but when injected in the chick, caused sedation and changes in postural tone through a central action (vol. 1, p. 25.47). Such tests of activity are not only highly sensitive but can be made quantitative and specific when combined with chromatographic methods of purification and the use of antagonists. However, where the substance is of known structure, the earlier biological methods of assay have been largely replaced by chemical methods which are less tedious to perform and provide more information. Assay by spectrophotofluorimetry has made it possible to estimate in a single sample not only the endogenous amine but also its precursors and known metabolites. If a newly discovered substance is a chemical constituent of the brain and not an artefact made in the course of extraction, two questions arise; first what is the regional distribution of the substance in the brain and secondly how is it formed and destroyed? Answers to such questions may provide a clue to its possible functions.

Regional distribution (fig. 5.16)

The regional distribution of acetylcholine in dog's brain was the first to be studied; others followed for noradrenaline, 5-HT, substance P, dopamine, GABA, and eventually for histamine. The concentrations of amines in brain are generally low (<2 μg/g) in comparison to those found in peripheral nerves or other cells. All the substances mentioned occur mainly in the grey matter of the phylogenetically older parts of the brain, i.e. the diencephalon and remainder of the brain stem. This finding is in accord with the high concentrations, particularly of acetylcholine, dopamine and 5-HT, in the cerebral nuclei of members of different phyla, e.g., the octopus, worm, snail and the common house-fly.

Acetylcholine is widely distributed in the brain but occurs chiefly in the corpus striatum (caudate nucleus). Noradrenaline, 5-HT, and histamine share a characteristic distribution, the concentrations being highest in the hypothalamus, intermediate in the medial thalamus and midbrain, and lowest in the pons and medulla; in the cerebellum, the concentrations of all amines are often too low to be detectable.

Although dopamine is a precursor of noradrenaline, its regional distribution is different, as may be seen from the high concentrations in the corpus striatum and tegmental

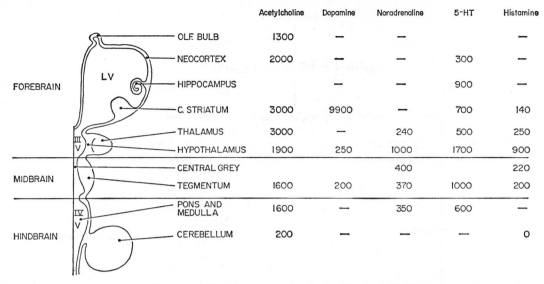

FIG. 5.16. Distribution of acetylcholine and amines in mammalian brain (dog or cat). The mean estimates of concentration expressed as ng/g; (—) concentration < 100 ng/ g; ○, not detected (< 50 ng/g). From Adam H.M. (1969) *Metabolism of Amines in the Brain.* London: Macmillan.

parts of the midbrain. Between these two parts of the brain is the nigrostriatal tract which is believed to be dopaminergic.

Noradrenaline, 5-HT and histamine are all present in the area postrema (canine); this consists of two symmetrical tufts of highly vascular glial tissue which lie on the lower part of the floor of the fourth ventricle. The area postrema, although covered with ependyma and bathed in CSF, is nevertheless outside the blood–brain barrier and, therefore, readily accessible to drugs, for example, apomorphine which causes vomiting. Since removal of the area postrema abolishes the effect of apomorphine, it is believed to contain chemoreceptors which trigger the vomiting response. It may, therefore, be the site of action of some anti-emetic drugs.

In the spinal cord, acetylcholine and the amines are present in low concentrations; acetylcholine occurs in the ventral spinal nerve roots but is not detectable in dorsal roots. Conversely, substance P is found only in dorsal nerve roots and can be traced into the dorsal columns of the cord.

In vertebrates, GABA occurs exclusively in the CNS and more is found in the grey matter than the white. The concentration in different parts of the brain and spinal cord lies between 250 and 500 μg/g and is highest in the diencephalon.

The pituitary gland contains histamine but hardly any 5-HT or noradrenaline; nevertheless the adenohypophysis may remove these and other amines from the blood. In the dog and cat, and probably in man, the highest concentration of histamine is in the pars tuberalis and is contained in numerous mast cells. A portal system of capillaries connects this part of the gland to the median eminence (vol. 1, p. 25.10), an area of the brain which is also rich in dopamine.

Prostaglandins occur in most parts of the CNS (vol. 1, p. 25.47).

Localization in cells

There are two approaches:

(1) the separation of subcellular particles of brain homogenates by differential centrifugation, and

(2) the identification of amines in neurones by fluorescence histochemistry.

These methods are outlined in fig. 5.17, and some results are given in table 5.3.

DIFFERENTIAL CENTRIFUGATION

After removal of nuclei and debris from the homogenate, there remains the crude mitochondrial fraction. When this fraction is applied to a density gradient made of successive layers of sucrose (0·3 M) and centrifuged for an hour at 25,000 g, three fractions are obtained, mitochondria, synaptic nerve endings (synaptosomes) and microsomes (vol. 1, p. 24.85). Under the electron microscope the synaptosomes are seen as fragmented particles and indeed were at first called pinched-off nerve endings. In fact, the particle is a synaptic junction shorn of its connections and is made by the shearing action of the homogenizer. When the active substance is extracted from each fraction, the amount can be expressed as a percentage of the activity in the whole fraction. Table 5.3 shows that acetylcholine and the amines are partly free and partly held in particles. Since particles may be damaged in the homogenizer, the proportion of free substance is probably less than the data suggest.

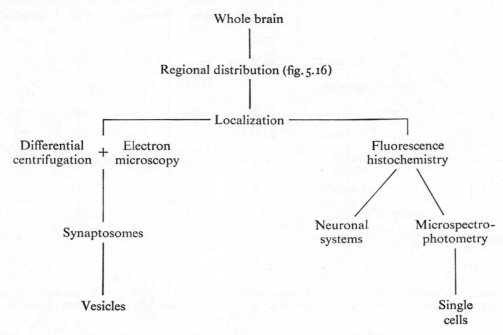

FIG. 5.17. Outline of the method used to determine the distribution of brain amines.

TABLE 5.3. Amines in subcellular fractions of brain homogenate. Modified from Whittaker V.P. (1964) *Progress in Brain Research* vol. 8, Biogenic amines (Ed. Himwich H.E. & Himwich A.W.) Amsterdam: Elsevier.

		Total activity recovered in fractions (%)					
						Histamine in	
$g \times min$	Fraction	Acetylcholine in whole brain	Dopamine in caudate N	Noradrenaline in hypothalamus	5-HT in whole brain	hypothalamus	pituitary
	Supernatant	28	56	32	54	27	} 14
$10^5 \times 120$	Microsomal	6	6	7	0	19	
$1\cdot2 \times 10^4 \times 60$	Mitochondrial and synaptosomal	55	22	43	41	39	5
$10^3 \times 10$	Nuclear	11	16	18	5	15	81

In the brain, particles which contain histamine are of the same density as those which contain 5-HT and noradrenaline; but in the pituitary (dog) most of the histamine is in large dense mast cell particles which sediment with the nuclear material.

Differential centrifugation of synaptosomes that have been disrupted in hypotonic media, yields the following fractions, soluble cytoplasm, synaptic vesicles, membrane fractions and mitochondria of the nerve endings. Most of the acetylcholine is contained in the synaptic vesicles. The number of vesicles in a gramme of cerebral cortex is estimated to be $3\cdot2 \times 10^{13}$ and each vesicle has been calculated to contain about 2000 molecules of acetylcholine. The vesicles, which have a mean diameter of 47 nm, contain various enzymes which are discussed later.

FLUORESCENCE HISTOCHEMISTRY

Catecholamines are only faintly fluorescent, in contrast to indole compounds which show intense fluorescence. Imidazoles do not fluoresce, but when they are condensed with some other molecule, such as O-phthalaldehyde, the product is highly fluorescent. Fluorometric methods have not yet been developed for acetylcholine. When a solution of adrenaline is made alkaline, the molecule undergoes autoxidation to yield a fluorescent compound, as may be seen by placing the solution in the path of UV light; the emitted visible light is of a bright green colour.

The conversion of catecholamines, 5-HT and more recently histamine into highly fluorescent compounds (fluorophors) has made it possible to demonstrate the locus of these amines in nervous and other cells. The fluorophors can be distinguished, and their concentrations obtained, by methods which depend upon analysis of their excitation (activation) and emission spectra.

When freeze-dried sections of nervous tissue are exposed to formaldehyde vapour, the catecholamines and 5-HT are not only fixed *in situ*, but are transformed respectively into highly fluorescent dicyclic and tricyclic compounds. The derivatives of the catecholamines are 3,4-dihydroxyisoquinolones which have an intense, green fluorescence; those of 5-HT and certain other hydroxyindoles are 3,4 dihydronorharmans, which fluoresce a bright yellow. The sections are studied in a fluorescence microscope, or better still, in a microspectrophotofluorimeter. The emission spectrum is determined for the given fluorophor at the wave length which gives peak excitation of the molecule. For example, when the fluorophor for 5-HT shows maximum excitation at 295 nm, fluorescence is maximum at 550 nm; it can be distinguished from the fluorophor for tryptamine for which the corresponding values are 285 nm (excitation) and 360 nm (fluorescence).

These methods have revealed neuronal cells and pathways that were previously unrecognized by conventional methods of neuroanatomy. They have provided convincing evidence that pharmacologically active substances extractable from the nervous system are formed and distributed within neurones, and that the amines might, therefore, act as transmitters or modulators of the nerve impulse.

Fluorescence in a nerve cell, axon or dendrites has been estimated to correspond to a fraction of a picogram of the original amine. By far the brightest fluorescence is seen in the form of varicosities which represent stores of amines at nerve terminals and are presumed to be presynaptic. In neurones containing catecholamines, the green fluorescence is less intense in the remainder of the neurone, but in neurones containing 5-hydroxyindoles, the yellow fluorescence is more or less uniform.

When tracts containing these amines are cut, fluorescence is lost as the fibres undergo degeneration; after transection of the spinal cord (C8), the fine varicose fibres that represent catecholamines and 5-HT lose fluorescence in 6–8 days.

On the basis of this and similar evidence for the brain, it has been suggested that the CNS contains neurones that act through the release of noradrenaline, dopamine and 5-HT. Owing to the difficulty in applying histochemical methods to histamine, the cellular distribution of this amine in brain is not yet known.

Metabolism of acetylcholine and biogenic amines

The identification of potent substances found in regions, cells or particles in the CNS, raises the question not only of their function but of how they are formed and destroyed. Thus the static picture of minute quantities of substances in localities is transformed into one of enzymic reactions which control the production, storage, release and subsequent catabolism of the active substance. These reactions are linked to the transport of precursors and metabolites across cell membranes and ultimately to the release of the active substance in response to a physiological stimulus. The general pathway is depicted in fig. 5.18. Methods of investigation have depended on the use of isotopic, fluorometric, cytochemical and

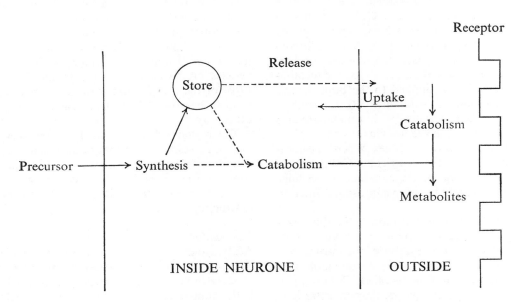

FIG. 5.18. General metabolic pathway of pharmacologically active substances in brain.

pharmacological techniques; more recently those of gas chromatography have become increasingly important.

Details of the pathways for acetylcholine, noradrenaline, 5-HT, histamine and GABA are given elsewhere; at present little is known about the formation of pharmacologically active polypeptides or prostaglandins in brain.

Knowledge of the formation and destruction of pharmacologically active substances in brain derives mainly from the study of model systems *in vitro*. Precursors are incubated under suitable conditions with cell free extracts, subcellular particles or thin slices of brain and products of enzymic reactions are measured. These methods make it possible to search for new potent inhibitors of the enzymes, to map out the distribution of enzymic activities in different parts of the brain or in different fractions of brain homogenate.

In vivo, amino acid precursors may be given by slow intravenous infusion to conscious or anaesthetized animals. As the concentration of free amino acid rises in the blood so more of the amino acid enters the brain until a limiting value is reached. Under these conditions, amine is formed at a faster rate; some may enter stores but much of it is destroyed, as may be seen from the increased production of metabolites.

The transport of amino acids across the blood–brain barrier is selective and presumed to depend on carrier systems for acidic, neutral and basic groups of amino acids. Amino acids may compete for entry into the brain; for example, a high concentration of phenylalanine in the blood leads to a fall in the concentration of tryptophan and 5-HT in the brain and eventually to a fall in the stores of 5-HT.

Another *in vivo* method of investigation is to perfuse the cerebral ventricles with artificial CSF containing a radioactive labelled precursor which, after passing through the ependyma, is taken up by brain cells and metabolized; this method bypasses the blood–brain barrier. The perfusate is collected and analysed for metabolites. When ^{14}C-histidine is applied to the brain in this way, ^{14}C-histamine and its metabolite ^{14}C 1,4 methylhistamine appear in the perfusate; ^{14}C-histamine can also be extracted from parts of the ventricular system, such as the grey matter of the third ventricle. When ^{3}H-noradrenaline is injected into the ventricular CSF, part of the dose is metabolized but part also enters intracellular stores and is found mainly in the synaptosomal fraction (fig. 5.19).

Drugs that act in low concentration to inhibit enzymic reactions *in vitro* are important in the analysis of metabolic pathways *in vivo*. The effect of such drugs may be inferred from the accumulation of substrate molecules or from the altered pattern of metabolites. For example, after treatment with MAO inhibitors, the concentrations of amines rise in the brain from the block in oxidation of

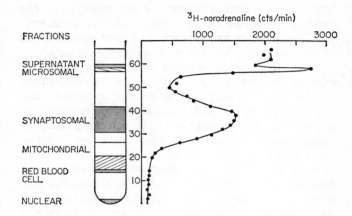

FIG. 5.19. Subcellular distribution of ^{3}H-noradrenaline in rat corpus striatum homogenate obtained 4 hours after the injection of ^{3}H-noradrenaline into the lateral ventricle. Most of the ^{3}H-noradrenaline is localized in a fraction of pinched-off nerve endings (synaptosomes) and some is present in the supernatant fluid and in microsomal particle fraction. After Glowinski J. & Iversen L.L. (1966) *Biochem. Pharmacol.* **15**, 977.

the side chain. The rise of noradrenaline, however, is small because the amine can be inactivated by methylation in the ring (3-OH); hence the main effect of MAO is seen as an increase in the concentration of 3-methoxynoradrenaline and its conjugates.

ACETYLCHOLINE
Formation
Choline acetyltransferase (choline acetylase) occurs in the cytoplasm of cells and especially in synaptosomes. It catalyses the transfer of acetyl radicals from acetylCoA to choline. Since pyruvate is the main source of acetylCoA, the formation of acetylcholine is closely linked to the oxidation of glucose. From sites of synthesis in the cytoplasm, acetylcholine is presumed to pass to sites where vesicles are formed, probably in the Golgi apparatus. Most of the acetylcholine in brain is pharmacologically inactive because it is held in vesicles or bound in some other way.

The regional distribution of choline acetyltransferase in brain coincides with that of acetylcholine; the highest activity is in the caudate nucleus. Acetylcholine is formed continuously in brain where its concentration at any moment depends on the balance between formation and destruction (table 5.4).

Inactivation
Acetylcholinesterase in brain can be studied by cytochemical methods or by measuring the rate of hydrolysis of acetylcholine *in vitro*. The enzyme is widely distributed in the brain and is highly active in parts, such as the cerebellum, which contain little acetylcholine or choline

TABLE 5.4. Acetylcholine (Ach) synthesis and hydrolysis in dog brain (μmoles Ach produced g/hr). From Quastel J.H. (1962) *Neurochemistry*, 2nd Edition, ed. K.A.C. Elliot *et al.* Springfield, Ill.: Thomas.

Part of brain	Choline acetyl transferase (acetylase) activity	Acetyl cholinesterase activity	Benzoylcho- linesterase (pseudocho- linesterase) activity
Cerebral cortex	1·3–3·7	60–100	2–4
Cerebellar cortex	0·09	460	0·5
Caudate nucleus	13·0	1900	2
Thalamus	3·1	220–310	5
Hypothalamus	2·0	190	11

acetyltransferase. When synaptosomes are ruptured and the particles separated on a density gradient, choline acetyltransferase appears in the cytoplasmic fraction, but acetylcholine is in the fraction containing fragments of external membrane. Cytochemical methods show the enzyme is present mainly in the postsynaptic portion of the synaptosome. An isoenzyme, benzoylcholinesterase (pseudocholinesterase), also hydrolyses acetylcholine and is found in walls of blood vessels, the plasma and some glial cells. The prevalence of acetylcholinesterase in brain probably accounts for the numerous central actions of anticholinesterases.

THE AMINES
Formation
Only a minute fraction of the amino acid pool of the brain is destined for the formation of biogenic amines. Both tyrosine and tryptophan are first hydroxylated in the ring, a reaction which limits the rate of their subsequent decarboxylation. By contrast, the decarboxylation of histidine is direct. The regional distribution of the enzymes for ring hydroxylation, or the removal of carboxyl groups, is highly correlated with the distribution of the amines. In brain homogenates, the enzymes and the amines are localized in the synaptosomal fraction.

A tetrahydropteridine, probably dihydrobiopterine, is a necessary co-factor for the hydroxylation of tyrosine and tryptophan; pyridoxal phosphate is necessary for decarboxylation. Aromatic L-amino acid dicarboxylase has a high affinity for DOPA and 5-hydroxytryptophan but not for tyrosine, tryptophan or histidine. Whether it consists of one or several enzymes remains a matter for debate (pp. 14.11 & 15.5).

Whereas noradrenaline, 5-HT and histamine are highly active on pharmacological tests, dopamine is not.

The distribution of β-hydroxylase for dopamine in brain is closely related to that of noradrenaline. The enzyme is a copper protein for which ascorbate, as an electron donor, is a cofactor. It is sensitive to CO and to the diethyldithiocarbamate (p. 15.5) and disulfiram which is used in the treatment of alcoholism (p. 5.72). Treatment with disulfiram in experimental animals increases the concentration of dopamine in brain and at the same time lowers that of noradrenaline.

Inactivation
The brain is rich in monoamine oxidase (MAO) and in methyltransferase so that when amines are released from cellular stores or injected into the brain, they are rapidly destroyed or inactivated. MAO, a mitochondrial enzyme, oxidizes aromatic amines in the side chain so converting them to aldehydes which are in turn oxidized to yield acids.

Methyltransferases are cytoplasmic enzymes and are important for the methylation of noradrenaline and histamine in the brain. Their activity can be studied *in vitro* by incubating supernatant containing the enzymes with substrate, in the presence of ^{14}C-methyl-*S*-adenosylmethionine as the source of methyl groups. Catechol-*O*-methyltransferase inactivates noradrenaline by methylation in the ring to give 3-methoxynoradrenaline. Similarly, imidazole-*N*-methyltransferase methylates histamine in the ring and reduces its activity on the guinea-pig ileum by about 300-fold in comparison with histamine. In the brain, methylhistamine is believed to be the principal metabolite of histamine, since only a small proportion is oxidized by MAO to methylimidazole acetic acid. 5-HT is oxidized without prior methylation to yield 5-hydroxyindole acetic acid (p. 15.7 and p. 14.9).

A nonenzymic process is involved in the inactivation of released noradrenaline by re-uptake into presynaptic nerve endings (p. 15.7). The blood–brain barrier which prevents free access of noradrenaline into brain tissue has made it difficult to demonstrate such active neuronal uptake in the CNS. However, after injection of ^{3}H-noradrenaline into the cerebral lateral ventricles, a proportion of the dose appears in the subcellular fraction that contains endogenous noradrenaline (fig. 5.19).

CLASSIFICATION OF DRUGS

The drugs which are described in this section are classified partly on the basis of their mechanism of action and partly on their most prominent effect as judged by their clinical value. The order in which they are described is as follows:

(1) monoamine oxidase inhibitors,
(2) tricyclic drugs, imipramine and related compounds,

(3) psychotomimetic drugs,

(4) tranquillizing drugs,

(5) general CNS stimulants,

(6) general CNS depressants (excluding anaesthetics and alcohol),

(7) analgesics and antipyretics,

(8) anticonvulsants,

(9) centrally acting muscle relaxants and antiParkinsonism drugs, and

(10) anaesthetics and alcohol.

MONOAMINE OXIDASE (MAO) INHIBITORS

The destruction of amines in the body by oxidative deamination has long been a subject of interest to biochemists and pharmacologists. In 1928, tyramine oxidase was the first enzyme to be identified with this reaction and was later found to be identical to an enzyme oxidizing aliphatic amines and adrenaline. The enzyme received the general name of monoamine oxidase (MAO) to distinguish it from diamine oxidase (DAO p. 14.9). MAO occurs in many tissues of the body and its activity is high in brain, liver, kidney and gut; it is further discussed on p. 15.7.

In 1951 isoniazid (isonicotinoylhydrazid) and later its more potent derivative iproniazid (isopropylisonicotinoylhydrazid) were employed in the chemotherapy of tuberculosis. At about this time, compounds containing the hydrazine group ($-NHNH_2$) were also shown to be potent and irreversible inhibitors of MAO. Early in the use of iproniazid, it was noticeable that the drug produced euphoria in patients which was not matched by improvement in their physical condition. Thus in 1957 iproniazid, introduced as a tuberculostatic agent, came to be tested for its effect in the treatment of mental depression. Although the drug was not curative it brought remission of symptoms in a proportion of patients. These clinical findings, together with the known biochemical properties of the drug, led to the view that mental depression might be the result of a disorder of amine metabolism in which the concentration of monoamines in the brain was reduced. This hypothesis has led to the search for new MAO inhibitors which act more selectively on the brain and which are less toxic than isoniazid. The MAO inhibitors are discussed here at greater length than is warranted by their clinical use today. As a group, they are important for their pharmacological, if not therapeutic, effect for without them knowledge of amine metabolism in brain would not have advanced, nor would so much have been learned about adverse effects arising from the combined effect of drugs.

The main groups of these compounds are shown in fig. 5.20. The usual daily oral dose in the adult is given to indicate the relative potencies of the various compounds.

Pharmacological effects of MAO inhibitors

The effects are discussed under two headings, those directly attributable to the inhibition of MAO and those unrelated to inhibition of the enzyme.

PERIPHERAL EFFECTS RELATED TO MONOAMINE OXIDASE INHIBITION

Amine content of tissues

These drugs increase the concentration of catecholamines in the heart and that of 5-HT in platelets and the gut. The concentrations of amines, e.g. tyramine and octopamine, which are not normally present in tissues also

HO—⬡—$CH_2CH_2NH_2$

p-Tyramine

HO—⬡—$\overset{\displaystyle OH}{\underset{\displaystyle}{C}}HCH_2NH_2$

Octopamine

rise. Tyramine is normally converted to *p*-hydroxyphenylacetic acid. In the presence of inhibitors of MAO tyramine accumulates and is available as a substrate for dopamine β-hydroxylase with the production of octopamine. Octopamine is then taken up into noradrenaline stores in sympathetic nerve endings but is released again during nerve stimulation, so acting as a false transmitter (p. 15.32).

Amines and metabolites in urine

In human subjects given MAO inhibitors, the daily urinary output of tryptamine, tyramine, 5-HT, noradrenaline and normetanephrine rises. Increased excretion of amines is taken as a more sensitive sign of MAO inhibition than a fall in the excretion of the corresponding acid metabolites. Various tests have been devised to assess the degree of MAO inhibition induced by these drugs. One test depends on the measurement of urinary excretion of tryptamine, another on the urinary excretion of 5-hydroxyindolacetic acid (5-HIAA) after an oral dose of 5-HT. In the latter method conversion of 5-HT to 5-HIAA is reduced in patients taking MAO inhibitors; with the hydrazine group of drugs, however, urinary 5-HIAA excretion is not a satisfactory index of inhibition since these drugs also act directly on the kidney to inhibit the tubular secretion of organic acids.

HYDRAZINES AND RELATED COMPOUNDS

Hydrazines

Phenelzine $\langle\text{ring}\rangle$—CH$_2CH_2$NHNH$_2$ 15–45

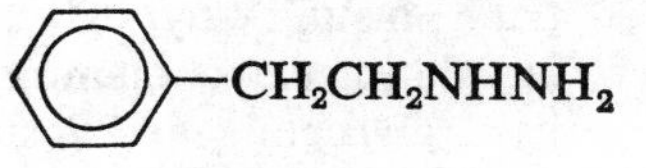

Pheniprazine $\langle\text{ring}\rangle$—CH$_2$CH(CH$_3$)NHNH$_2$ not in clinical use

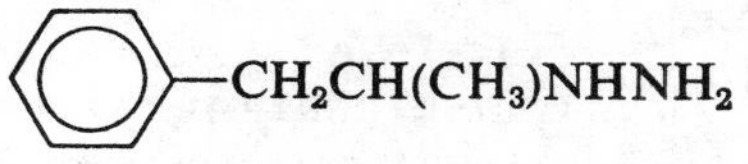

Hydrazides

Iproniazid N$\langle\text{ring}\rangle$—CONHNHCH(CH$_3$)$_2$ 50–100 (not in clinical use in U.S.A.)

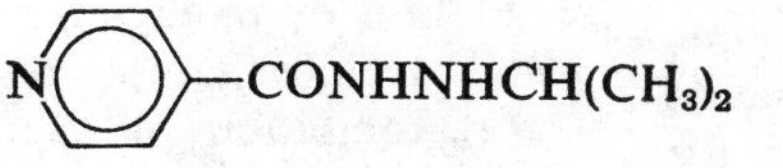

Nialamide N$\langle\text{ring}\rangle$—CONHNHCH$_2CH_2$CONHCH$_2$ $\langle\text{ring}\rangle$ 50–200

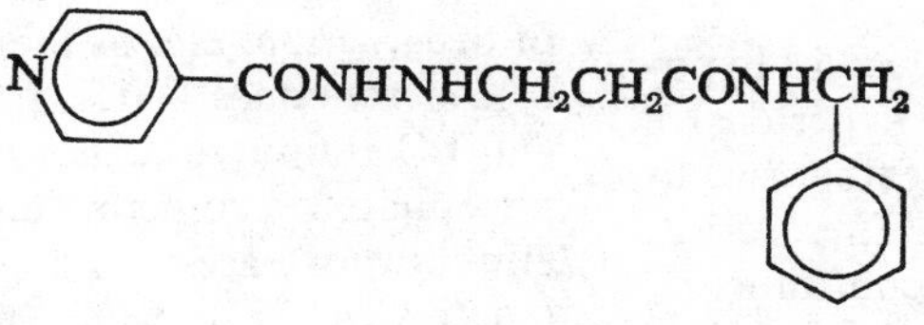

Isocarboxazid $\langle\text{ring}\rangle$—CH$_2$NHNHC(=O) ... CH$_3$ 10–30

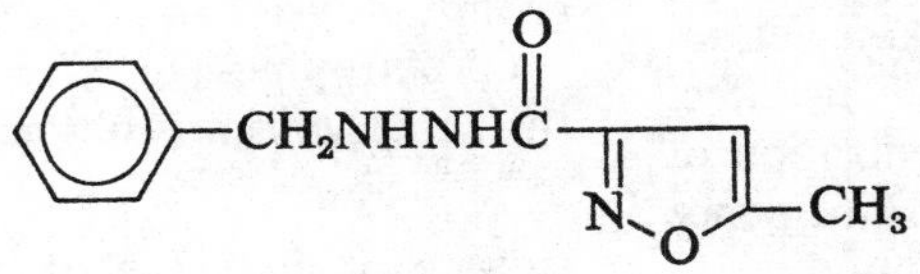

INDOLALKYL AMINES

α-Methyltryptamine $\langle\text{indole}\rangle$—CH$_2$CH(CH$_3$)NH$_2$ not in clinical use

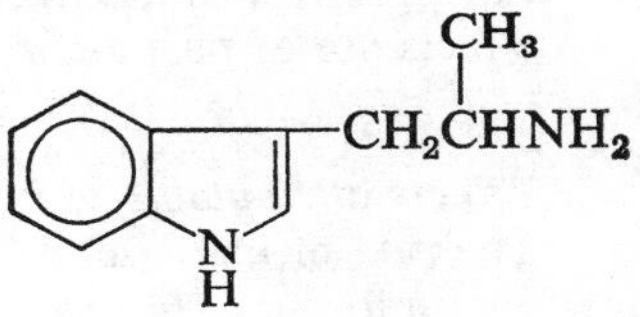

α-Ethyltryptamine $\langle\text{indole}\rangle$—CH$_2$CH(C$_2H_5$)NH$_2$ not in clinical use

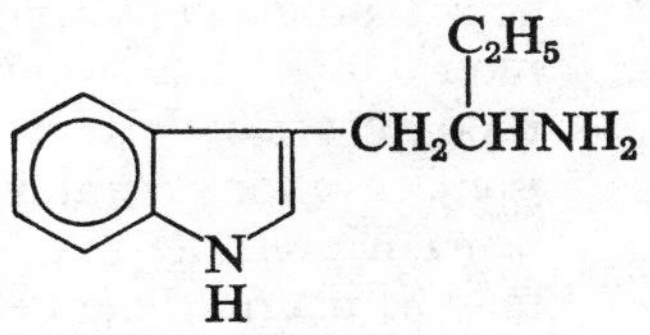

HARMALA ALKALOIDS

Harmine CH$_3$O—$\langle\text{harmine ring}\rangle$—CH$_3$ not in clinical use

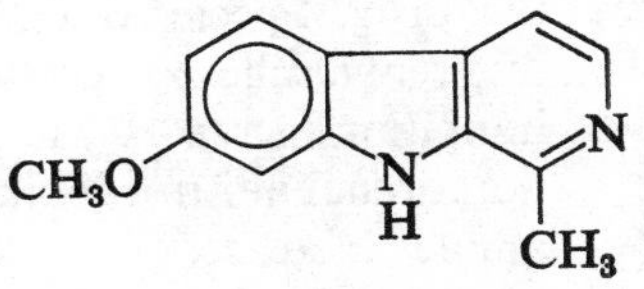

CYCLOPROPYLAMINES

Tranylcypromine $\langle\text{ring}\rangle$—CH—CHNH$_2$ / CH$_2$ 10–20

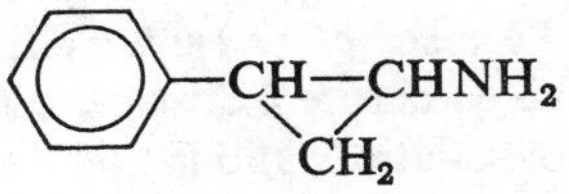

PROPARGYLAMINES

Pargyline $\langle\text{ring}\rangle$—CH$_2NCH_2$C≡CH / CH$_3$ 10–50

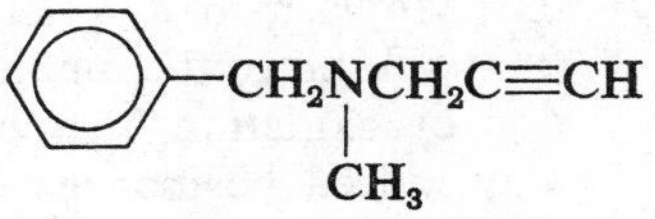

Usual adult daily dose mg

FIG. 5.20. Some monoamine oxidase (MAO) inhibitors.

Effects on the cardiovascular system
Hypotension. In patients undergoing long-term treatment with hydrazine and nonhydrazine inhibitors, there is usually a fall in blood pressure, which may be severe. The cause of this effect is not understood. Possibly the drugs block transmission in sympathetic ganglia, but the concentration which is necessary for this effect in isolated perfused ganglia is high and unlikely to be achieved by doses used in man. Alternatively, the absorption of tyramine from the gut and its accumulation in adrenergic neurones might lead to the formation of octopamine. As a false transmitter, this would displace noradrenaline from stores and so reduce the amount available for release by the nerve impulse.
Hypertensive crisis. Although the usual effect is hypotension, patients may experience acute hypertensive crises with headache and vomiting, and deaths due to cerebral haemorrhage have been reported. These crises are most likely to occur in the following circumstances.

(1) Certain MAO inhibitors, e.g. tranylcypromine, have a sympathomimetic (amphetamine-like) action, liberating noradrenaline from nerve endings. This effect interacts with MAO inhibition and the concentration of noradrenaline at receptor sites rises. The highest incidence of spontaneous hypertensive attacks is found with tranylcypromine; the hydrazine drugs produce hypertension only in the presence of pressor agents that would normally be metabolized.

(2) When MAO inhibitors are given together with sympathomimetic agents, e.g. amphetamine or phenylephrine, noradrenaline is liberated at nerve endings, its subsequent inactivation being impaired by the enzyme inhibitor. Phenylephrine is a particular danger as it is found in proprietary cold cures which are readily available and may be regarded as innocuous by the patient.

(3) MAO inhibitors interact with various foodstuffs. Typical of such effects is the **cheese reaction** in which patients may develop severe hypertension due to the tyramine content in the cheese (Greek, *tyros*, cheese). Tyramine is a sympathomimetic agent normally inactivated after oral ingestion in the liver, but in the presence of MAO inhibition it reaches the general circulation to produce hypertension. Other tyramine-containing foods include wines, strong beer and yeast extracts (Marmite). Yeast extracts also contain histamine. Broad beans can produce reactions because of their high content of DOPA which is decarboxylated in the body to give dopamine.

(4) MAO inhibitors interact with drugs which block other routes for the inactivation of catecholamines, in particular with drugs which inhibit reuptake of amines by sympathetic nerve endings, e.g. the tricyclic group of antidepressants. Such an interaction may increase free catecholamines at receptor sites.

Effects on carbohydrate metabolism
After prolonged administration MAO inhibitors potentiate insulin hypoglycaemia. Increased tissue and circulating catecholamines would be expected to produce hyperglycaemia and insulin antagonism, but paradoxically hypoglycaemia occurs and is so far unexplained.

OTHER PERIPHERAL EFFECTS
(1) Hydrazine type MAO inhibitors inhibit the oxidation of methylhistamine and so reduce histamine catabolism (p. 14.9).
(2) Inhibition of liver microsomal enzymes by the hydrazine group may result in dangerous potentiation of drug action, e.g. of the strong narcotic analgesics and of general anaesthetics (p. 10.9).
(3) Certain hydrazines inhibit enzymes with pyridoxal phosphate as cofactor, e.g. amino acid decarboxylases, aminotransferases and dehydrases. The hydrazine inactivates the cofactor by reacting with the aldehyde group of pyridoxal.
(4) Atropine-like effects and oedema also occur but their mechanism is obscure.

CENTRAL EFFECTS OF MAO INHIBITORS
The main clinical value of these drugs is in the treatment of depression and experimental studies of their central effects are of particular interest.

Effects attributable to inhibition of cerebral MAO
The rate of increase in brain amines varies with the type of inhibitor. The harmala alkaloids are the shortest acting, producing a rapid increase in brain amines which return to normal within a few hours. The hydrazines produce a slow rise in brain amines but a single dose is effective for several days, the inhibition of the enzyme being irreversible (fig. 5.21). The effect of tranylcypromine is intermediate between the other two groups; the amines increase rapidly in concentration and return to normal over a period of 5–12 hours after a single dose of the drug. Species differences are seen when effects of different amines are considered. In the dog and cat, MAO inhibition increases 5-HT and dopamine in brain, but not noradrenaline. In rabbit, rat and mouse brains all three amines increase.

Reversal of reserpine effect. All the MAO inhibitors, if given before a dose of reserpine, prevent the development of sedation, and in some species actually reverse the effect to produce excitation. Reserpine releases the amines into the cytoplasm of the neurone from the granular stores (p. 5.30). Since the amines are protected from destruction by oxidation, the concentration does not fall, and may indeed be increased.

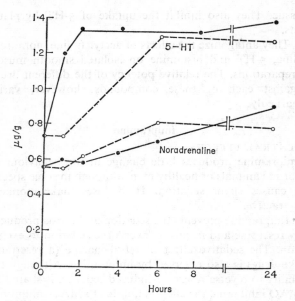

FIG. 5.21. Concentration of 5-HT and noradrenaline in rabbit brain stem after subcutaneous doses of iproniazid, 100 mg/kg (○) and pheniprazine, 2 mg/kg (●). After Spector S. *et al.* (1960). *J. Pharmacol*, **130**, 256.

Potentiation of effects of precursors of the amines. Pretreatment with a MAO inhibitor potentiates the excitatory effects of a large dose of DOPA or of 5-HT. 5-HT, in particular, accumulates in the brain and may lead to fatal hyperthermia (p. 16.5).

Direct sympathomimetic effects are seen with some inhibitors, e.g. tranylcypromine, phenelzine and ethyltryptamine; these may contribute to the efficiency of tranylcypromine in depressive illness.

Potentiation of the central sympathomimetic effects of amphetamine-like compounds results also in increased excitation and hyperthermia.

Effects apparently unrelated to inhibition of MAO
Potentiation of the effects of barbiturates, anaesthetic agents and narcotics is due to the decreased rate of inactivation of the drugs by liver microsomal enzymes (p. 10.9).

Anticonvulsant and convulsant effects are seen with the hydrazine inhibitors. Anticonvulsant effects may be due to increase in the cerebral concentrations of GABA, whilst convulsant effects may occur with compounds which inhibit pyridoxal-containing coenzymes.

Clinical uses of MAO inhibitors

MAO inhibitors have been used mainly to treat depression but are less effective than electroconvulsive therapy or the tricyclic (imipramine) group of drugs. They may be specially useful when anxiety is prominent.

MAO inhibitors have also been employed in the treatment of hypertension, the drug of choice being pargyline (p. 8.10). Their potential toxicity makes it important for clinicians to be aware of their pharmacological actions and of how these may interact with the effects of other drugs. As a precaution patients should carry a card indicating the drugs they are receiving.

Iproniazid is no longer available for clinical use in the USA, because of the occurrence of hepatocellular damage. The newer hydrazine inhibitors may also induce liver damage but do so much less frequently. Pheniprazine was withdrawn from use because it induced red-green colour blindness and α-ethyltryptamine because of agranulocytosis.

MAO inhibitors are given by mouth and readily absorbed. Little is known of their metabolism in man. In rats a dose of isopronazid is eliminated in the urine within 48 hours mainly as isonicotinic acid. Tranylcypromine is also absorbed from the gastrointestinal tract in rats within 24 hours and its metabolites are excreted in the urine. The fate of tranylcypromine in man is unknown.

TRICYCLIC DRUGS—IMIPRAMINE AND RELATED COMPOUNDS

Besides MAO, two other mechanisms are concerned in the inactivation of noradrenaline released at peripheral postganglionic sympathetic nerve endings; these are inactivation by catechol-*O*-methyltransferase and the active reuptake into nerve terminals. The evidence for the presence of reuptake mechanisms in peripheral tissues and an account of drugs affecting these mechanisms is given on p. 15.7. Hydroxylated amines have a low fat solubility and do not readily cross the blood–brain barrier. After intravenous infusion of radioactive 5-HT or catecholamines, activity is not found in the brain except in two areas, the hypothalamus and area postrema, where the blood–brain barrier is incomplete. Cerebral uptake of ³H-noradrenaline, however, occurs after injection into the lateral ventricle (p. 5.18).

In the rat heart cocaine, imipramine, chlorpromazine, phenoxybenzamine, tranylcypromine, amphetamine and many structural analogues of the catecholamines inhibit uptake of noradrenaline. Of these drugs, those without adrenergic blocking action increase sensitivity to circulating catecholamines. Interference with uptake increases the amount of free amines at the adrenergic receptor sites and thus potentiates sympathomimetic effects. A similar uptake mechanism probably operates in the brain and a group of compounds which inhibit this has achieved considerable success in the treatment of depression.

In the mid 1950s in a search for new tranquillizers, an iminodibenzyl compound, now known as **imipramine**, was tested in chronic schizophrenic patients. Instead of sedation the symptoms were intensified in a proportion of patients. A trial was then begun in depressed patients and an apparently specific effect in the relief of depressive symptoms was evident. An earlier pharmacological investigation had already suggested a possible basis for the antidepressant effects.

The chemical structure of tricyclic compounds and of chlorpromazine is shown in fig. 5.22; the difference from chlorpromazine is that the S is replaced by the CH_2-CH_2 group. These drugs are readily absorbed when given by mouth. The usual daily dose indicates their relative potency.

PHARMACOLOGICAL ACTIONS

Imipramine and related compounds inhibit the uptake of catecholamine by peripheral sympathetic nerves and brain tissue. They also inhibit the uptake of 5-HT by platelets.

They antagonize the effects of acetylcholine, noradrenaline, 5-HT and histamine on isolated smooth muscle preparations. The relative potency of the different drugs against each of these compounds, however, varies markedly.

Imipramine

CENTRAL EFFECTS

Imipramine produces little change in the behaviour of normal animals or healthy man, although in some species it causes slight sedation. High doses make monkeys overactive.

Imipramine prevents the sedation and ptosis produced by reserpine and in rats, converts the sedation to excitation. The sedative effect of tetrabenazine (a reserpine-like drug) is also reversed by imipramine. Although the ability to reverse reserpine-induced sedation is shared by MAO inhibitors, the effect is not due to MAO inhibition; this test is used by the drug industry in animals to screen drugs for possible antidepressant activity. A drug

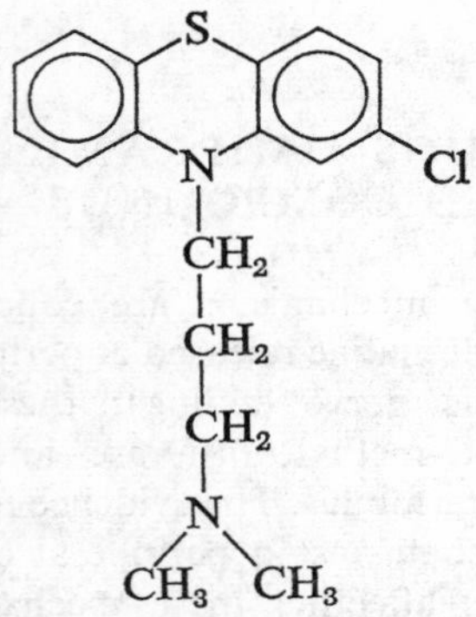

Chlorpromazine (50–200 mg) 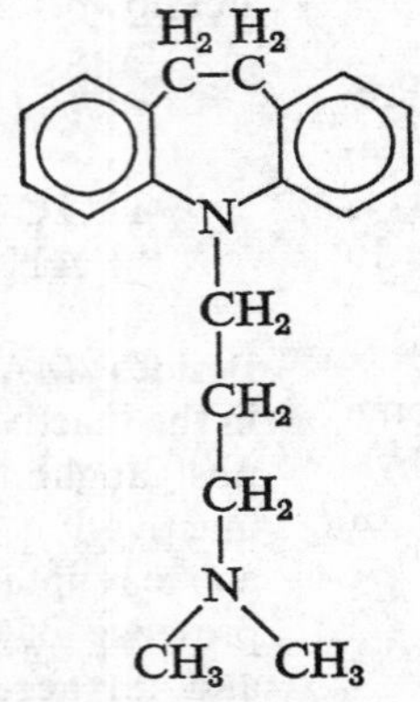   Imipramine (tofranil 75–150 mg) 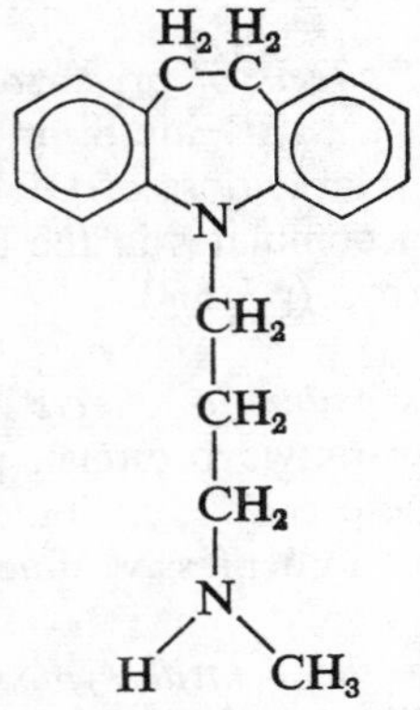   Desipramine (pertofran 75–150 mg)

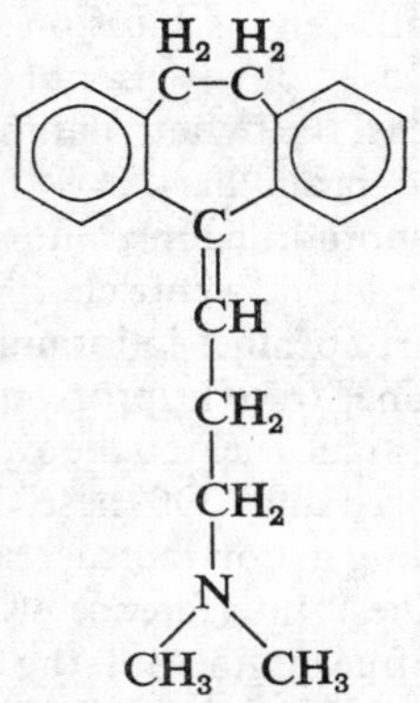

Amitriptyline (tryptizol 75–150 mg) 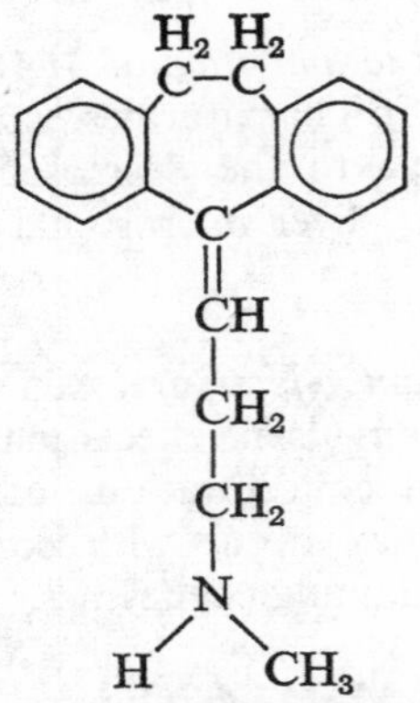   Nortriptyline (allegron 30–75 mg)

FIG. 5.22. Chlorpromazine and commonly used tricyclic compounds.

which conserves amines released at receptor sites either by inhibiting their enzymic destruction or by blocking neuronal reuptake may exert its antidepressant action by potentiating their effect.

Brodie has suggested that before it can affect the brain, imipramine undergoes demethylation. As evidence he found that the onset of reversal of reserpine sedation in rats coincided with the presence in brain of desmethylimipramine rather than imipramine. The suggestion that desmethylimipramine might be more rapidly effective in depressed patients has not been confirmed.

Imipramine has little of the hypothermic or antiemetic activity of the phenothiazines but potentiates the excitation produced by central stimulants such as amphetamine and methylphenidate. Central atropine-like effects occur and may account for the delirium that occasionally occurs and for its beneficial effect in Parkinsonism.

PERIPHERAL AND AUTONOMIC EFFECTS
In the intact animal, treatment with imipramine potentiates the pressor effect of an injection of noradrenaline and the contraction of the nictitating membrane of the cat.

CLINICAL USES
In the treatment of depression imipramine has to a large extent replaced the MAO inhibitors. Its effect in the depressed patient is similar to a spontaneous remission and occurs usually a few weeks after the treatment begins. It is used in Parkinsonism and carbamazepine, a drug related to imipramine, has been shown to be of value in trigeminal neuralgia.

Adverse effects and contraindications
Autonomic effects include atropine-like actions, i.e. dry mouth, disturbance of accommodation and in the elderly urinary retention. Syncope ('drop' attacks) in elderly patients may be a result of transient episodes of hypotension.

Central effects include the production of tremor and of convulsions in epileptics. Acute psychotic episodes may also occur, with visual hallucinations and paranoid delusions. Libido is also occasionally increased.

Other adverse effects include obstructive jaundice, ECG changes similar to those induced by chlorpromazine and agranulocytosis.

ALTERNATIVE DRUGS
The other drugs of this series differ mainly from imipramine in their ability to antagonize the catecholamines, a property shared by chlorpromazine. There is some correlation between this effect and their efficacy in reducing anxiety, hence amitriptyline is preferred to imipramine in the treatment of agitated depression.

DRUG INTERACTIONS
Adverse reactions may be precipitated if imipramine is combined with MAO inhibitors or sympathomimetic agents. Interaction may cause hypertensive reactions, excitement and hyperpyrexia, which are attributed to potentiation of the effects of released catecholamines. As might be expected from its nonspecific antagonism to noradrenaline, amitriptyline is less likely to produce these reactions than imipramine, and has been used together with MAO inhibitors in cases of resistant depression, but only under close supervision in special units.

Since the tricyclic drugs antagonize the hypotensive action of adrenergic blocking drugs such as guanethidine, they should not be used in patients being treated with these antihypertensive agents.

PSYCHOTOMIMETIC DRUGS

In many societies interest has been aroused by drugs which produce changes in perception, in thought and in the emotional states. Such drugs usually of plant origin have found a place in many primitive religions; in the hands of the mystic they have been used in attempts to extend the boundaries of human perception and in the search for new experiences.

Examples of such compounds include *Cannabis sativa* (p. 5.28), mescaline found in the head of the Mexican dumpling or *Peyotl* cactus, and psilocybin found in a Mexican mushroom. The crude extracts often contain more than a single psychotomimetic compound and refined extracts may fail to mimic exactly the effects of the original.

In our society there is a surge of interest in the psychotomimetic or psychedelic drugs. The use of the compounds by students and others reflects once again the attempts of the human species to break out of the confines imposed by our rigid perceptual and conceptual framework. That the escape achieved by drugs is mainly an illusion does not deter the followers of this modern cult. It is important, however, that society does not deny the use of these compounds on emotional grounds only, and it is necessary to examine seriously the claims of both amateur mystic and abolitionist. These claims are best assessed by controlled pharmacological studies of the drugs in animals and man.

The varied description of this group of drugs as hallucinogens, psychotomimetics, psychodysleptics and psychedelics points to the confusion regarding their place in society. Are they to be considered as inducers of model psychosis (psychotomimetic) or of mystical states (psychedelic)? Differences in interpretation of the actions in man have been stated by Giarman and Freedman in discussing the effects of D-lysergic acid diethylamide, as follows.

INDOLALKYLAMINES

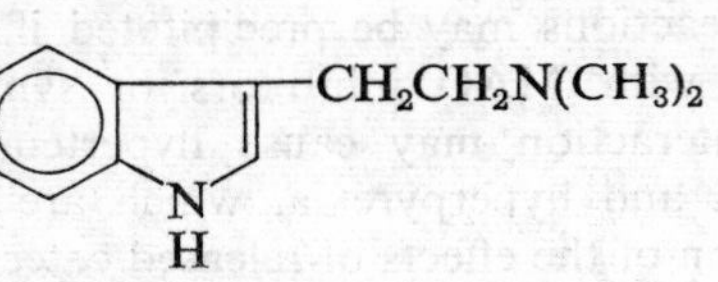

N,N, Dimethyltryptamine

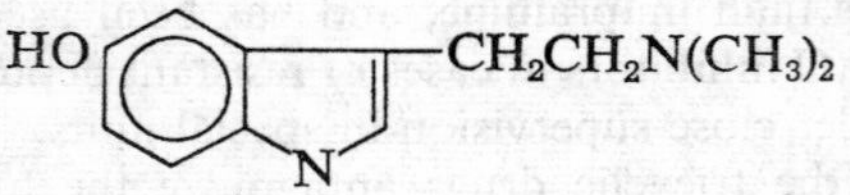

Bufotenine (5-Hydroxy *N,N*, dimethyltryptamine)

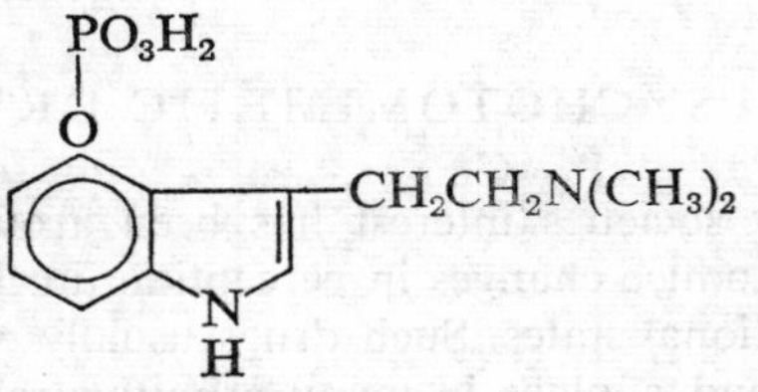

Psilocybin

COMPOUNDS RELATED TO INDOLALKYLAMINES

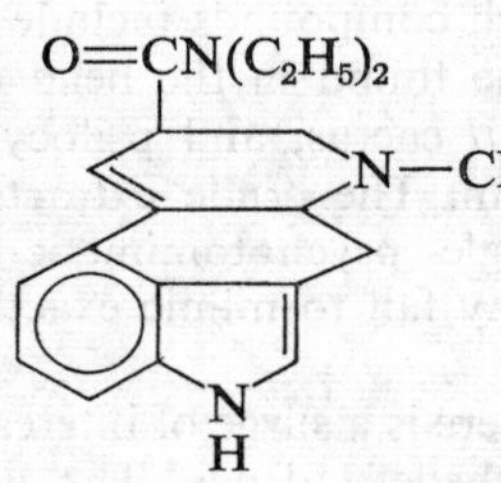

D- Lysergic acid diethylamide (LSD)

Harmala alkaloids

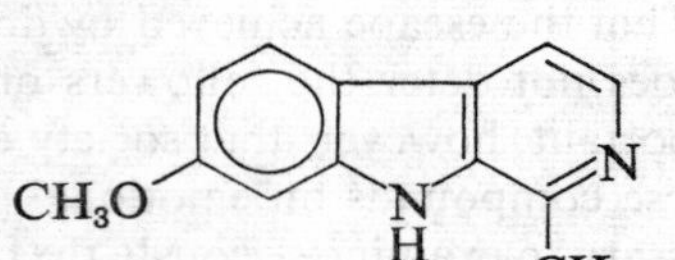

Harmine

PHENYLETHYLAMINES

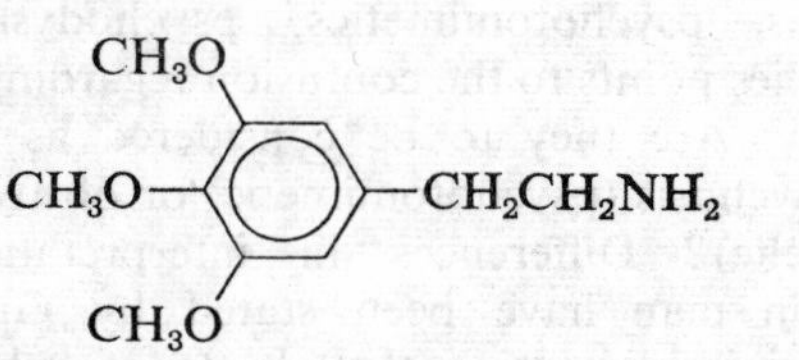

Mescaline (3, 4, 5-Trimethoxyphenylethylamine)

PIPERIDINE DERIVATIVES

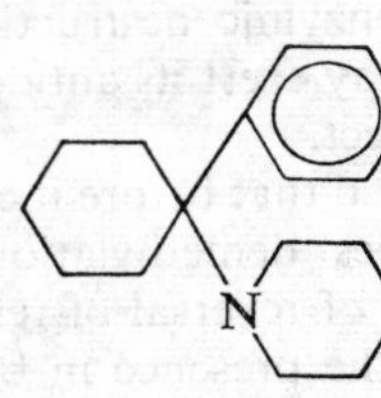

Phencyclidine (sernyl)

TETRAHYDROCANNABINOLS

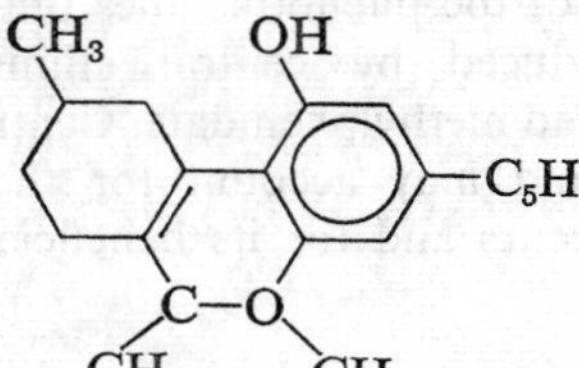

Tetrahydrocannabinol

FIG. 5.23. Some psychotomimetic drugs.

'The usual boundaries which structure thought and perception become fluid; awareness becomes vivid while control over input is markedly diminished; customary inputs and modes of thought and perception become novel, illusory and portentous; and with the loss of customary controlling anchors, dependence on the surroundings, on prior expectations or on a mystique for structure and support is enhanced. Psychiatrists recognize these primary changes as a background state out of which a number of secondary psychological states can ensue, depending on motive, capacity and circumstance. If symptoms ensue the drug is classified according to the interests of subject and observer.'

CLASSIFICATION OF THE PSYCHOTOMIMETICS
A complete classification is impracticable, but the commoner drugs grouped according to their chemical structure are given in fig. 5.23. Since it is not possible to compare fully the pharmacology of each drug, LSD is described in detail and brief comments and comparisons with other drugs are made.

D-lysergic acid diethylamide (LSD)
In most subjects a dose of 1 μg/kg produces symptoms which develop, as a rule, within 30 min and clear within 12 hours. At first there are vague feelings of apprehension and anxiety. Perceptual changes follow either in the form of heightened intensity or a change in the interpretation of perception, e.g. aspects of a situation, colours, shapes, etc., assume a prominence not usually obvious. Hallucina-

tions usually of a visual nature may occur, but sometimes these develop only with the eyes closed.

Autonomic and neuromuscular disturbances occur in some subjects and may dominate the picture. Other symptoms in a given subject depend on his expectations and interpretation of the perceptual, autonomic and affective disturbances.

In the clinical situation anxiety, irritation and hostility may predominate; whilst in the experimental or social situation gregariousness, inappropriate mood and passive acceptance of the mystical experience may occur. In doses which induce these effects LSD does not produce total confusion or disorientation.

Although psychotic symptoms disappear usually by 12 hours, prolonged mental disturbance has been recorded in the form of anxiety, depression, hallucinations or even a persistent psychosis. At the height of the effect of the drug on the mind the individual may commit a crime of violence or personal injury from disregard of reality and the normal considerations of safety.

Phenothiazine tranquillizers antagonize many of the physical and mental symptoms seen after LSD administration, and have been used to terminate its effects.

The reported effects of LSD in human subjects are confused, since many factors influence the content of the report of the symptoms. Information is available from the use of LSD in normal individuals and psychiatric patients. The verbal output is influenced by the dose, the environment and the relationship with the observer, be he a physician, author, colleague or some other person.

ANIMAL STUDIES

The ability of these drugs to affect perception and thought processes is impossible to monitor in animals. Animal studies have been confined therefore to general pharmacology and to the use of techniques to evaluate effects on behaviour.

Peripheral effects

LSD has ergot-like actions on smooth muscle, e.g. it produces contraction of the isolated rat uterus. It antagonizes the effects of 5-HT on smooth muscle preparations, an action which suggests a possible basis for its central effects.

Effects mediated via the central nervous system

LSD stimulates monosynaptic reflexes, e.g. patellar reflex, and the central sympathetic centres producing mydriasis, pyrexia, and piloerection. It increases sensitivity to sensory stimuli; large doses produce ataxia and vomiting.

LSD has been shown to exert an action on the reticular formation of the brain stem. In an *encéphale isolé* preparation, direct electrical stimulation of the reticular system or an auditory stimulus activates the cerebral cortex. LSD potentiates the response to auditory stimulation at a dose which has no effect on the response to direct stimulation. Chlorpromazine inhibits the response to auditory but not direct stimulation and antagonizes the effect of LSD. Thus LSD and chlorpromazine may act at the synapses between sensory neurones and reticular neurones, the one potentiating, the other blocking the effects of sensory stimulation. Barbiturates appear to have a direct depressant effect on the reticular neurones (p. 5.9).

Studies on animals have included various types of behavioural testing, from simple assessment of the effect on spontaneous activity to the application of conditioning methods, or the observation of changes in behavioural patterns under controlled conditions. In general it is difficult to distinguish between hallucinogens and tranquillizers by the simpler techniques.

BIOCHEMICAL EFFECTS AND MODE OF ACTION

The suggestion was originally made simultaneously by Gaddum and Woolley that the central effects of LSD might be explained on the basis of its antagonism to 5-HT. This explanation, however, does not seem probable as 2-bromolysergic acid diethylamide (Brom LSD), a more potent antagonist of 5-HT, fails to produce psychotomimetic effects, despite satisfactory penetration into brain. Other influences on cerebral amine mechanisms have been suggested, e.g. central sympathetic stimulation and increases in 5-HT in brain. LSD in high dosage (130–1500 mg/kg) in rats increases 5-HT in whole brain, the increase being mainly confined to the particulate fraction. In dogs the greatest increases occur in midbrain, medial thalamus and hypothalamus. It is postulated that LSD increases the ability of subcellular particles to bind 5-HT although the relationship of such a mechanism to the action of the drug at the behavioural level is difficult to visualize.

Mescaline, 3:4:5-Trimethoxyphenylethylamine

This substance, found in a Mexican cactus, was used by the Aztecs for the induction of mystical states. The relationship of its chemical structure to that of dopamine is obvious.

In man it produces a feeling of diffuse anxiety, intensification of colour patterns, visual hallucinations especially when the eyes are closed, coarse tremor, hyperactive tendon reflexes with ankle and patellar clonus. Autonomic disturbances include signs of sympathetic overactivity with mydriasis and tachycardia.

When given to animals, mescaline shows many of the sympathomimetic actions of the phenylethylamine series of drugs. In simple behavioural studies the drug has an excitatory effect and produces desynchronization of the EEG, an effect similar to the action of central stimulant drugs.

CH₃O

CH₃O —⟨ ⟩— CH₂CH₂NH₂

CH₃O

Mescaline

HO —⟨ ⟩— CH₂CH₂NH₂

HO

Dopamine

In tests of avoidance conditioning, using a shuttle-box with sound as the conditioning stimulus, large doses cause inhibition of the response followed by excitation, small doses producing only excitation. This profile of activity correlates well with the hallucinogenic activity of other drugs of the phenylethylamine series.

BIOCHEMICAL EFFECTS AND MODE OF ACTION

Animal studies suggest that the onset and duration of the behavioural effects are not directly related in time to the amount of mescaline in the brain; the hallucinogenic effects may depend on prior metabolism of mescaline to a more active compound which might be either the alcohol or the aldehyde, i.e. with the ethylamine side chain converted to —CH_2CH_2OH or to —CH_2CHO.

The oxygen consumption of brain slices is reduced by mescaline and this fall occurs only after a period of preincubation with the drug. This again suggests that pharmacological activity depends upon metabolic transformation.

Amines and model psychoses

Many psychotomimetic drugs have an amine structure, and resemble the naturally occurring amines of the tryptamine and catecholamine series.

Two modifications of the amine molecule are associated with an increase in hallucinogenic activity, namely O-methylation in the catechol series and N-methylation in the tryptamine series. Examples of such active compounds include mescaline and N-dimethyltryptamine. The presence of enzymes in mammalian tissues capable of catalyzing O- and N-methylation of the catechol- and indolalkylamines has led to the suggestion that such metabolites might occur in schizophrenia. Despite the attraction of such a hypothesis much experimental effort has failed to produce evidence of such an abnormality in the schizophrenic patient.

PHYSICOCHEMICAL CORRELATION WITH PSYCHOTROPIC ACTION

Although the suggestion that these drugs may release cerebral amines or mimic their actions is attractive, many facts are difficult to explain in terms of this view. BromLSD is more active as a peripheral 5-HT antagonist than LSD, but unlike LSD it has no hallucinogenic effect. Cross tolerance between LSD, mescaline and psilocybin also makes it difficult to interpret effects in terms of the metabolism of cerebral amines.

An effect common to all these compounds has recently been suggested as the basis for their action and shows a good correlation with psychotropic activity. The ability of LSD, psilocybin and the phenylethylamine series to act as electron donors correlates well with their hallucinogenic activity.

Piperidine derivatives

Hallucinatory states and delirium in poisoning with the belladonna alkaloids, atropine and hyoscine, were well known to physicians in ancient times.

Compounds with a structure based on the piperidine ring, which is present in the atropine molecule, have psychotomimetic properties. Changes in mood, delusions, auditory and visual hallucinations, occur with oral doses of 5–10 mg of phencyclidine and may last for 12–24 hours. With this group, symptoms are said not to occur in a setting of clear consciousness but are accompanied by mild delirium and loss of contact with the environment.

Phencyclidine (sernyl) was introduced as an analgesic agent, but has been found to produce psychotomimetic effects.

Morphine alkaloids

Psychotomimetic effects follow the use of various morphine derivatives, e.g. N-allylnormorphine (nalorphine) and N-allylbenzomorphine; mood changes, hallucinations and delirium occur (p. 5.53).

Cannabis sativa L or Indian hemp

Preparations of this plant have been smoked or chewed as an intoxicant or narcotic in Asia and the middle East for centuries; they are known by a variety of names, e.g. bhang, ganga, dagga, hashish, kif, marihuana. Recently they have spread to other continents. Cigarettes containing cannabis are known as reefers. One of the active principles is tetrahydrocannabinol which is present as a mixture of isomers.

The drug gives a feeling of well being and stimulates the imagination; there are often vivid auditory and visual hallucinations. A state of euphoria and detachment may predominate and accounts for the present popularity of the drug as a psychedelic. Physical changes include vertigo and tinnitus, exaggerated reflexes and increased sensitivity to stimuli. The pupils may be dilated with a diminished response to light; nausea and vomiting may occur.

Evidence suggests that the drug is nonaddicting, and its protagonists argue that it is less dangerous to the health of the individual than alcohol and nicotine although African psychiatrists have attributed prolonged psychotic episodes to its use. Arguments for control of the various preparations of cannabis in Europe and North America are based on the effect of its increasing spread in society and its use as an introduction to 'harder' drugs rather than on its ill effects on the individual.

TRANQUILLIZING DRUGS

As already indicated the search for drugs for the relief of emotional tension and excitement can be traced throughout history; opium, alcohol and more recently the bromides and barbiturates, all subserve this function. These drugs, however, exert little selectivity in their action. Thus at doses needed to control anxiety or excitement they interfere with intellectual functions and with increasing doses there is rapid and progressive clouding of consciousness and coma. Significant progress in discovering drugs which dissociate the effects on anxiety or excitement from the effects on intellectual activity and consciousness has been made only in the past two decades.

Definition and classification of drugs which possess this property has proved difficult and many names have been used to describe them, e.g. tranquillizers, neuroleptic, ataractic and anxiolytic agents. With the introduction of chlorpromazine in 1953 the term tranquillizer was coined and it remains the most widely used.

The study of the pharmacology of tranquillizers is complicated by difficulties similar to those encountered when considering the antidepressant and psychotomimetic drugs. Tranquillization and the abnormal psychic states which they influence are subjective experiences which cannot be monitored easily or reproduced in animal experiments. However, as in the case of other drugs which influence behaviour and mood, certain relationships have been established between behavioural, autonomic, neurophysiological and biochemical effects in animals and their effects in man. On this basis, tentative hypotheses may be advanced to explain their mode of action and appropriate animal tests can be used to search for new drugs.

States of excitement and anxiety constitute an important part of clinical psychiatry and are not described here. However, the neuronal systems involved in these responses include the hypothalamic centres which control autonomic and endocrine responses, the reticular activating system which has an important function in determining the degree of arousal, and the limbic system whose main function seems to be to regulate the direction and intensity of emotional response and to relate this response to both prevailing stimuli and previous experience (vol. 1, p. 24.35). The modes of action of the tranquillizing drugs may, therefore, be considered in relation to these neuronal systems, and to two other possible sites of action, the peripheral autonomic nervous system and the cerebral cortex.

From an analysis of their clinical effects tranquillizers may be divided into two categories:

(1) drugs used for the most part to ameliorate states of psychotic excitement, e.g. in mania, agitated depression, schizophrenia and organic delirium, constitute the **major tranquillizers**; discussion is confined to three groups, the **phenothiazines**, the **butyrophenenes** and the **rauwolfia alkaloids**;

(2) drugs used to treat states of emotional tension and anxiety, the so-called **minor tranquillizers**; these include **meprobamate** and the **benzodiazepine series**.

It is argued that the major tranquillizers act primarily at the level of the activating systems and central autonomic centres, whilst minor tranquillizers act primarily in relation to limbic structures, barbiturates having less selectivity in their site of action. However, none of the differences reported between the minor tranquillizers and the conventional sedatives are absolute. If large enough doses are given, the benzodiazepines, for example, induce sedation and ataxia, but in most cases small doses relieve anxiety without producing more widespread effects. The lack of specificity should, however, be emphasized and the minor tranquillizers have much in common with the barbiturates both as regards structure and activity.

Alkaloids of rauwolfia serpentina

Rauwolfia alkaloids were the first of the tranquillizing drugs to be used clinically and have been given to excited patients in India for many centuries, their use in this context being first mentioned in Europe in 1785.

In the 1930s the alkaloids were also studied for their antihypertensive properties and it was for this purpose that they were re-introduced into Western medicine in 1946. A further decade passed before the rauwolfia alkaloids were in general use in psychiatric practice following the isolation of the alkaloid **reserpine** in 1952.

The discovery of reserpine initiated a revolution in psychiatry and also played an important part in the drug therapy of hypertension. Although reserpine has now, to a large extent, been replaced by newer compounds it occupies an important place in the analysis of the action of psychotropic drugs and in the development of biochemical hypotheses of psychiatric illness. Discussion is confined to the single alkaloid reserpine, trimethoxybenzolyl reserpate.

PERIPHERAL EFFECTS OF RESERPINE

A single intravenous injection of reserpine in experimental animals produces a transient increase in blood pressure followed after 0·5–1 hour by hypotension and bradycardia which persist for several days. The effects on the blood pressure can be explained by its action on the stores of noradrenaline in the terminals of postganglionic sympathetic nerves. Reserpine depletes the granular stores by affecting the uptake or binding of noradrenaline within them. The drug first causes a sudden release

Reserpine

of large amounts of noradrenaline from storage sites. While most of the amine is removed rapidly by enzymic destruction, some acts on the receptor sites and gives an initial rise in blood pressure. After the stores have been depleted, newly synthesized noradrenaline is destroyed by intracellular MAO. Thereafter the labile stores of noradrenaline in the nerve endings, normally available for release by nerve impulses, are not replenished (p. 15.30). This results in a fall in sympathetic tone. The levels of noradrenaline in peripheral tissues innervated by the sympathetic nerves also fall rapidly, e.g. in the spleen and heart. The storage of 5-HT in peripheral tissues is also affected, in particular in blood platelets and the argentaffin cells of the gastrointestinal tract. The release of 5-HT in the gut may account for the increased motility and diarrhoea seen in many species after reserpine administration. The reduced neural release of noradrenaline is accompanied by an effect similar to that occurring after sympathectomy, i.e. increased sensitivity to the administration of exogenous noradrenaline and sympathomimetic agents that act directly on receptors (p. 15.17).

In summary, the peripheral autonomic effects of reserpine are due to a decrease in sympathetic activity and a predominance of the parasympathetic system. Pupillary constriction and ptosis occur in addition to the fall in blood pressure, bradycardia and increased gastric acid secretion.

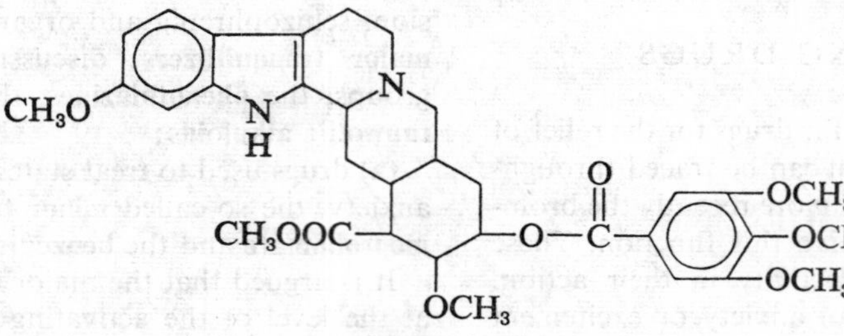

CENTRAL ACTIONS OF RESERPINE

The administration of reserpine in animals produces a sequence of behavioural changes. There is a short period of stimulation with increased activity. After 20–60 min the animal shows a general reduction in activity and may become completely immobile; it does not become unconscious and an appropriate stimulus provokes a reaction, although aggressive behaviour may be inhibited. Catatonia is also induced, i.e. the animals remain for long periods in postures in which they have been placed. Conditioned responses are suppressed.

Reserpine potentiates the effects of sedative drugs, e.g. barbiturates. It decreases the threshold to convulsant drugs and electroshock to the brain and is prone to precipitate cardiac arrest and apnoea. This appears to be due to vagal stimulation which, in the presence of sympathetic blockade, leads to cardiac arrest. The effect can be modified by atropine, but because of the dangers of a similar occurrence in man, electroconvulsive therapy is contraindicated in patients receiving reserpine.

Interesting behavioural effects are produced by the interaction between reserpine and the antidepressant drugs which are described in more detail on p. 5.22. Prior treatment of an animal with MAO inhibitors or drugs of the tricyclic series reverses the behavioural effects of reserpine inducing overactivity and excitement. The possible relationship of these effects to changes in brain amine metabolism brought about by the drugs is discussed below.

BIOCHEMICAL STUDIES IN BRAIN

After a single dose of the drug the concentrations of noradrenaline, dopamine and 5-HT in the brain fall rapidly (fig. 5.24). This is accompanied by a rise in the concentration of the acid metabolites of dopamine and 5-HT as a result of intracellular inactivation of the released amines by MAO. Under these conditions the acid metabolites of noradrenaline are difficult to detect because they undergo oxidation to glycols (p. 15.8).

The effect of a single dose of reserpine on storage of amines persists for many days and is roughly paralleled by the behavioural changes, the animals remaining tran-

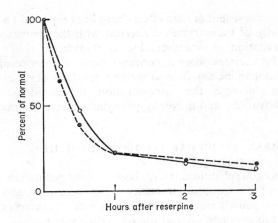

FIG. 5.24. Noradrenaline (○) and 5-HT (●) content of rabbit brain stem after intravenous injection of reserpine, 5 mg/kg. After Shore *et al.* (1957) *Psychotropic Drugs.* Amsterdam: Elsevier.

quillized during the period of amine depletion. Early studies failed to demonstrate the presence of the drug in brain after a few hours, and the prolonged behavioural response was thought to be due to an irreversible block of the storage mechanism persisting after disappearance of the drug. Studies using ^{3}H-reserpine, however, have shown that small amounts do persist in the brain throughout the period of amine depletion and may be sufficient to explain its duration of action.

Pretreatment with MAO inhibitors prevents the fall in brain amines produced by reserpine. After combined treatment, free amines within the brain cells increase and the behaviour of the animal returns to normal (p. 5.22).

The extrapyramidal effects of reserpine have also been related to the changes in cerebral amine metabolism, in this case to the fall in dopamine in extrapyramidal structures. Reserpine does not affect the concentration of acetylcholine in the brain but reduces the concentration of histamine.

CLINICAL USE OF RESERPINE
Reserpine and other rauwolfia alkaloids were used for many years in the treatment of hypertension but, to a large extent, have now been replaced by other drugs (p. 8.7). The drug has also been much used in psychiatry as a tranquillizer (2·5–10 mg/day), e.g. in the treatment of schizophrenia, but for the most part has been replaced by the phenothiazine and butyrophenone tranquillizers. Nevertheless the adverse effects are of interest from the point of view of its mode of action.

When high doses were given for the treatment of mental illness, hypotension and bradycardia were troublesome. A rare complication was the development of diffuse cardiomyopathy which was possibly related to the loss of catecholamines from the heart. This was occasionally fatal and has been produced experimentally in animals. As mentioned above, cardiac arrest can occur if patients taking reserpine are given electroconvulsive therapy.

The action of the drug on hypothalamic centres probably caused lactation, gynaecomastia and menstrual irregularities. Gastrointestinal effects included diarrhoea, increased gastric acid secretion, gastric erosions and activation of gastric and duodenal ulcers.

Central nervous system effects included vivid dreaming and a Parkinsonism-like syndrome. The most serious and common adverse effect was the precipitation of a depressive illness which occurred in up to 5 per cent of patients treated with the drug for hypertension. This complication together with the interactions between reserpine and the antidepressant drugs contributed greatly to the development of the amine hypothesis of the aetiology of depression.

Reserpine is absorbed from the gastrointestinal tract and part of it is split by an esterase in the liver into methyl reserpate which is inactive and trimethoxybenzoate. This and other metabolic products are excreted in the urine.

The phenothiazine tranquillizers
In the early years of this century phenothiazine was used as a veterinary anthelminthic but was abandoned because of its toxic effects. In 1952 Courvoisier and his colleagues in France, while investigating promethazine, a phenothiazine drug with antihistaminic properties, noticed its tranquillizing effects in experimental animals. These investigations led to the development of **chlorpromazine** (fig. 5.26) which possesses strong tranquillizing but weak antihistaminic properties. Since then the drug has been widely used to treat mentally ill patients. Other phenothiazines and newer drugs differ from chlorpromazine in their range of effects but chlorpromazine remains a valuable drug and may be taken as the prototype.

In animals large doses of chlorpromazine induce symptoms which are partly dependent on environmental temperature. At low temperatures there is somnolence and decreased activity, whilst at high temperatures there is excitation, ataxia and tremor. Further increase in dosage produces loss of muscle tone, convulsions, respiratory arrest and death.

EFFECTS OF CHLORPROMAZINE ON PERIPHERAL STRUCTURES
Chlorpromazine shows strong antagonism to adrenaline, moderate antagonism to 5-HT but weak antagonism to anticholinergic and antihistaminic activity in isolated

tissues. Its antagonism to noradrenaline produces hypotension in the intact animal and tachycardia is also seen but the metabolic effects of adrenaline, e.g. hyperglycaemia, are not affected.

CENTRAL EFFECTS OF CHLORPROMAZINE
Behaviour studies show that moderate doses of the drug (4 mg/kg) reduce spontaneous activity. The animal preserves unusual positions in which it is placed (catatonia, fig. 5.25). Lower doses potentiate the activity

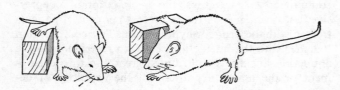

FIG. 5.25. Catatonia in rats after administration of 4 mg chlorpromazine per kg body weight. After *Triangle (En.)* (1960) 4, 245.

of other central depressants, e.g. barbiturates. In doses of 2·5 mg/kg, the drug inhibits the conditioned avoidance response without affecting the unconditioned response. In intermediate doses the drug impairs the avoidance response. In experiments designed to induce conflict, e.g. in which cats are discouraged by electric shocks from catching mice, chlorpromazine enhances their predatory activity. Operant conditioned responses for reward are also increased.

The drug has a strong anti-emetic action on the vomiting centre in the medulla and induces hypothermia by a central action on temperature regulation centres.

In animals, chlorpromazine reduces the sensitivity of the reticular system to incoming sensory stimuli, especially auditory; it inhibits the excitatory effect of circulating adrenaline on the same system.

METABOLIC EFFECTS OF CHLORPROMAZINE
In vitro, chlorpromazine can uncouple oxidative phosphorylation in brain tissue and inhibit ATPase activity. As the drug inhibits the uptake by the brain of $^{35}PO_4$ ^{22}Na and ^{42}K and also certain amino acids including methionine when injected into the ventricle, the diverse actions of the phenothiazines might be explained by their effects on biological membranes. Decrease of membrane permeability has also been demonstrated in studies on erythrocytes, e.g. inhibition of passive water movement, prevention of K^+ loss and entry of Na^+. Chlorpromazine may alter the permeability of the storage granules for the monoamines and increase the ratio of free to bound 5-HT in brain.

No consistent *in vitro* effects have been reported on the activity of the enzymes concerned with the synthesis or degradation of noradrenaline or dopamine. However, *in vivo* changes occur in concentrations of noradrenaline and dopamine and its acid metabolites. Low doses of the drug increase the concentration of noradrenaline, homovanillic and dihydroxyphenylacetic acid in brain.

COMPARATIVE PHARMACOLOGY OF OTHER PHENOTHIAZINES
Structural substitutions have been made at positions 2 and 10 in the phenothiazine nucleus. The three main groups of compounds are shown in fig. 5.26 with an example of a drug in common clinical use from each group.

The student should be familiar with the properties of one drug from each group as there are important changes of pharmacological activity with the different substitutions and these alter the clinical indications for their use. In comparison with chlorpromazine, at a dose which produces comparable efficacy in the management of states of excitement in man, the following differences are seen in the pharmacological properties of the other two groups.

The piperidine group
The blocking actions to adrenaline are similar to those of chlorpromazine but these compounds have greater antagonism to acetylcholine. They are less sedative than chlorpromazine and less liable to produce extrapyramidal effects. They have no anti-emetic activity. Clinically they are used in maintenance treatment of psychotic patients and in the management of the elderly, where the reduced incidence of extrapyramidal effects is particularly important.

The piperazine group
These drugs produce a high incidence of extrapyramidal effects; they have sedative effects comparable to those of chlorpromazine and also have strong anti-emetic properties. They are especially valuable in acutely psychotic patients.

ADVERSE EFFECTS OF PHENOTHIAZINES
Extrapyramidal and autonomic effects of these drugs have already been described; some other adverse reactions are listed as follows:

(1) agranulocytosis and photosensitivity reactions are uncommon;

(2) effects on hypothalamic structures lead to a number of endocrine disturbances, e.g. amenorrhoea, breast enlargement and lactation in females, and gynaecomastia

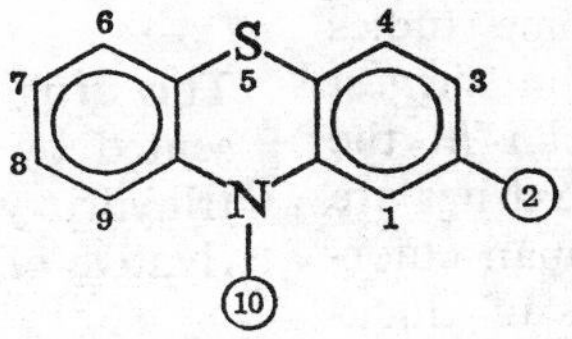

Phenothiazine nucleus

Substitution	R_2	R_{10}	Usual daily dose mg/day in man
Aliphatic group			
Chlorpromazine	—Cl	—$CH_2CH_2CH_2N(CH_3)_2$	50–500
Piperidine group			
Thioradazine	—SCH_3	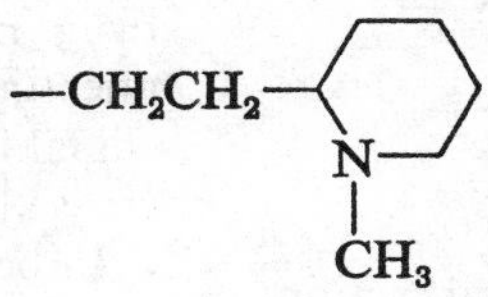 —CH_2CH_2— (piperidine with N—CH_3)	100–500
Piperazine group			
Trifluoperazine	—CF_3	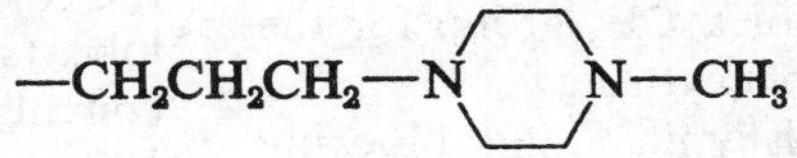 —$CH_2CH_2CH_2$—N(piperazine)N—CH_3	5–25

FIG. 5.26. The phenothiazine nucleus and commonly used phenothiazines.

and impotence in males; stimulation of the appetite and gain in weight may occur;

(3) in patients treated over long periods, myocardial lesions consisting of subendocardial deposition of muco-polysaccharides occur. These lesions lead to ECG changes, e.g. nonspecific S–T segment changes and low voltage T-waves. Similar lesions may follow treatment with reserpine;

(4) jaundice occurs with the halogenated compounds and is intrahepatic and obstructive; its occurrence is unrelated to dose or duration of treatment and is a hyper-sensitivity reaction;

(5) opacities of the lens and cornea and pigmentation of the retinae occur especially with thioradazine; and

(6) epileptic seizures are occasionally precipitated. In animals, phenothiazines lower the threshold to the action of convulsant drugs.

CLINICAL USES

Phenothiazines are used as tranquillizing agents in patients with states of excitement, e.g. mania, agitated depression, schizophrenia and delirium. Because of the absence of habituation they are also used in the treatment of anxiety, but many anxious patients gain more relief from barbiturates and the minor tranquillizers. Chlorpromazine is claimed to exert a specific antagonism to the central effects of LSD and has been used to terminate psychotic reactions in man provoked by this drug.

Because phenothiazines potentiate the effects of analgesics and anaesthetics they have been used in pre-medication for surgical operations and in the management of intractable pain.

The phenothiazines are used to inhibit vomiting, e.g. in uraemia, radiation sickness or carcinoma of the gastro-intestinal tract. They may also be valuable in the prevention of attacks of migraine and in the control of severe continuous hiccups.

Chlorpromazine and the other phenothiazines are taken by mouth or given by intramuscular injection in doses indicated in fig. 5.26. They are absorbed rapidly from the gastrointestinal tract and widely distributed throughout the tissues, including the brain. Some studies of regional distribution throughout the brain suggest greater accumulation in the brain stem than in the cerebral cortex. Numerous metabolites of the drugs are excreted in the urine as sulphoxides but in man chlorpromazine is eliminated largely as conjugates of glucuronic acid.

Butyrophenones

These drugs are chemically related to pethidine and the first to be used clinically was **haloperidol**, a halogenated derivative produced in 1958.

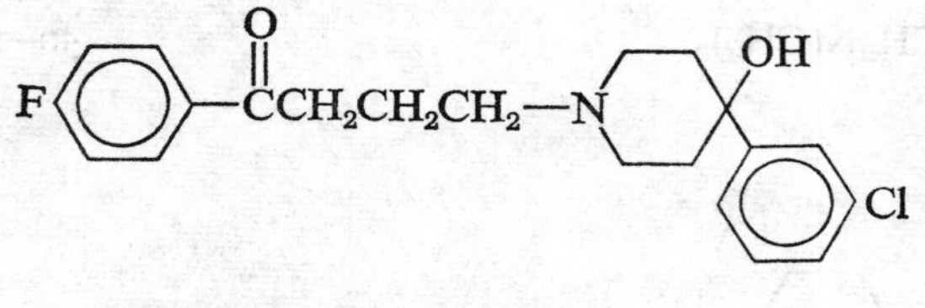

Haloperidol

Members of the series with potent central actions contain a fluorine substitute in the para-position in the benzene ring as in haloperidol. **Triperidol** differs from haloperidol by the substitution of a CF_3 group for the chlorine attached to one of the phenyl rings.

The drugs have weak antihistaminic and blocking activities to adrenaline, differing in this respect from the phenothiazines.

The effect of haloperidol on conditioned avoidance is remarkably similar to that of chlorpromazine. The butyrophenones are also anti-emetics and they potentiate the central depressants, e.g. the barbiturates; they antagonize the central effects of amphetamine.

Catatonia is produced in animals, and extrapyramidal effects are common in man. Unlike the phenothiazines, the butyrophenones have no effect on convulsive thresholds in animals.

As yet biochemical studies with these drugs are not so extensive as with the phenothiazines. Two interesting observations are (1) butyrophenones inhibit uptake of amino acids into the brain, and (2) haloperidol increases the concentration of the dopamine metabolite, homovanillic acid, in the caudate nucleus.

CLINICAL USES

Haloperidol and triperidol are used in the treatment of psychotic states, e.g. in schizophrenia and mania. Haloperidol is given by mouth in doses of 3–10 mg/day and triperidol in doses of 0·5–2·5 mg/day. Adverse reactions include extrapyramidal effects.

Meprobamate

This drug was developed from the group of drugs represented by mephenesin which is a phenyl derivative of trihydroxypropane. Meprobamate is a dicarbamyl derivative of propane.

Meprobamate

ANIMAL EXPERIMENTS

Meprobamate does not affect the activity of acetylcholine, histamine, catecholamines or 5-HT in isolated organs.

Muscle relaxant and paralysing actions are similar to those of mephenesin (p. 5.61). With high dosage the drug produces a reversible flaccid paralysis, without affecting ventilation. The drug is believed to act on spinal interneurones, because it depresses the flexor and crossed extensor reflexes.

In behavioural studies in monkeys, the drug abolishes aggressive responses and reduces fear and avoidance behaviour. It tames rats made aggressive by lesions under the corpus callosum on the medial aspect of the frontal lobes (septal nuclei). Meprobamate protects animals from convulsions induced by strychnine and electroshock. It also decreases spontaneous electrical activity of the caudate nucleus and thalamus and inhibits the after discharge seen on electrical stimulation of the amygdaloid body.

Doses which produce these effects do not appear to depress cerebral cortical activity or the reticular system.

So far biochemical studies have contributed little to knowledge of the action of the drug which itself does not change cerebral amine levels.

CLINICAL USES

The present place of this drug in clinical practice is uncertain. Soon after its introduction it reached the top of the hit parade in the USA, being prescribed more than any other drug. Controlled trials, however, indicate that it has little, if any, advantage over the barbiturates in the management of mildly anxious patients. The drug is also used in the treatment of petit mal. Meprobamate is taken by mouth in a dose of 800–1000 mg/day.

Adverse effects include drowsiness, ataxia, and skin rashes due to hypersensitivity. Anaphylactic reactions rarely occur.

The main danger of the drug is habituation or drug dependence; withdrawal reactions with exacerbation of anxiety and irritability and occasionally fits occur.

The benzodiazepines

The first drug of this series to be described was **chlordiaze-poxide** (librium), introduced in 1960 for the management of anxiety and emotional tension. Other drugs of the series have since been developed and include **diazepam** (valium), **oxazepam** (serenid) and **nitrazepam** (mogadon) (fig. 5.27).

Although these drugs are completely different in chemical structure from meprobamate they have certain features in common, e.g. they act as muscle relaxants and anti-convulsants.

In isolated organs none of them antagonize acetyl-choline, histamine, catecholamines or 5-HT and they have no specific activity on peripheral autonomic neurones.

Chlordiazepoxide has a taming effect on aggressive monkeys and also on rats made vicious by lesions of the septal nuclei. These effects are produced at doses which are not sedative.

At higher dosage, however, the drug produces ataxia and sedation and the ratio between tranquillizing and

is also used as a night sedative and induces sleep without the hangover effects attributed to the barbiturates; diazepam has recently been used in status epilepticus and tetanus for its anticonvulant properties (p. 5.58).

Although the drugs are said to relieve anxiety in doses which are not sedative this does not seem to be true for all patients. Thus some patients become drowsy and develop ataxia on small doses of the drugs. The distinction from the barbiturates in terms of selectivity of action is thus relative. The drugs are taken by mouth and their usual daily doses are given in fig. 5.27.

Adverse effects include skin rashes, muscle tenderness or weakness. Habituation is a serious problem and emphasizes again the difficulty of separating tranquillizing effects from the tendency to produce drug dependence.

The discovery of meprobamate and other minor tranquillizers, especially the benzodiazepines, has been an important advance in pharmacology, although it is

Chlordiazepoxide (5–25 mg)

Diazepam (5–25 mg)

Oxazepam (25–50 mg)

Nitrazepam (5–10 mg)

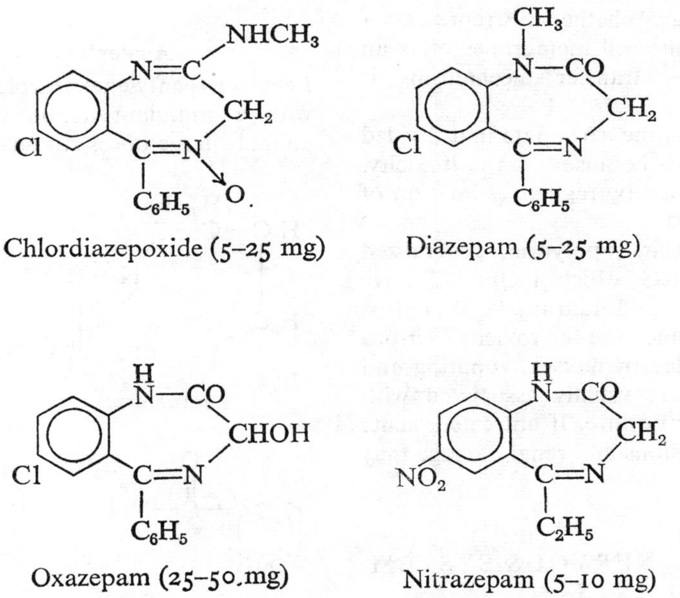

FIG. 5.27. The benzodiazepines and their usual daily doses.

general depressant effects varies between different members of the series. Thus oxazepam shows a wide margin of dosage between such effects, and sedative actions are more marked with nitrazepam.

Like meprobamate, the benzodiazepines exert a selective action on spinal neurones and on the limbic system. The drugs prevent the after discharge produced by electrical stimulation of limbic structures.

CLINICAL USES

The main use lies in the treatment of anxiety. Nitrazepam

difficult to interpret their precise mode of action. They are now fashionable but it must be some time before their role in medical practice can be assessed fully. As mentioned on p. 5.2 there are many older drugs that have been used as tranquillizing agents. It is also well to remember that satisfactory effects can be achieved with other forms of therapy. Thus Emerson, the American philosopher and essayist 'heard with admiring submission the experience of a lady who declared that the sense of being well-dressed gives a feeling of tranquillity, which religion is powerless to bestow'.

Lithium

Lithium salts were introduced into psychiatry in 1949 after Cade had observed that they caused sedation in guinea-pigs. They have been used in the treatment of acute mania and to prevent recurrent manic and depressive attacks.

Most of the pharmacological studies with lithium have little relevance to the clinical use of the drug in man. Lithium salts can replace Na^+ *in vitro* in muscle and nerve preparations and interfere with resting potentials and propagated responses. In clinical use, however, a serum $[Li^+]$ of 0·5–1 mEq/l, maintained for long periods, does not alter normal serum $[Na^+]$ and $[K^+]$.

It is difficult to provide an explanation for the effects of lithium in manic depressive illness, and further controlled clinical and pharmacological studies are needed before a unifying hypothesis is possible. However, lithium increases the uptake of noradrenaline into synaptosomal fractions of brain, an effect which might *in vivo* lead to an increased reuptake of released noradrenaline into nerve endings. Whether this represents a direct effect of lithium on the cell membranes or is an interaction with membrane transfer mechanisms is unknown.

Lithium is usually given as the carbonate in a divided dose of 250–1500 mg/day; because of the toxicity, treatment should be controlled by regular estimation of serum lithium concentrations.

Adverse effects include thirst, polyuria, generalized itching, changes in the ECG which include T-wave depression. An adequate salt and fluid intake should be maintained as low salt diets increase the toxicity. Serious adverse reactions are heralded by nausea, vomiting and coarse hand tremor, and are usually associated with serum $[Li^+]$ higher than 2 mEq/litre. If untreated, acute encephalopathy with convulsions and renal damage may occur.

GENERAL CENTRAL NERVOUS SYSTEM STIMULANTS

General stimulation and depression of the CNS by drugs follow an increase or decrease in the activity of groups of cells or whole areas of brain. They should not be equated with the terms excitation and inhibition which have an exact meaning at a cellular level. Since the CNS contains millions of nerve cells each of which receives excitatory and inhibitory inputs from a wide range of other cells, drugs might act in several ways to stimulate or depress the CNS as a whole. They might act locally by direct excitation or by removing inhibition, or at a distance by facilitating excitatory pathways or depressing inhibitory ones, and in some cases even by interfering with conduction.

Drugs that stimulate the central nervous system fall into three main groups. The **analeptic convulsants** (Greek, *analeptikos*, to restore or repair) which have a restricted clinical use, stimulating ventilation by an effect on the respiratory centre; in slightly larger doses, other levels of the brain are stimulated and convulsions occur; examples are leptazol and nikethamide. **Psychomotor stimulants** increase purposeful motor or mental activity and elevate mood. In the usual dosage, the cerebral cortex and subcortex are stimulated. In larger doses, the brain stem is affected so that these compounds may also be used to stimulate respiration; amphetamine and caffeine are examples of this group. **Miscellaneous convulsants** which have no therapeutic use, but are useful as tools in the elucidation of the physiology and pharmacology of the CNS, include strychnine and picrotoxin.

Analeptics may be tested by their ability to reduce barbiturate-induced sleep or respiratory depression. Psychomotor stimulants are measured by appropriate behavioural tests and responses.

Analeptic convulsants (fig. 5.28)

Leptazol (pentylenetetrazole) is a synthetic compound, with a stimulant action mainly on the medulla. In animals, large doses stimulate all levels of the brain and

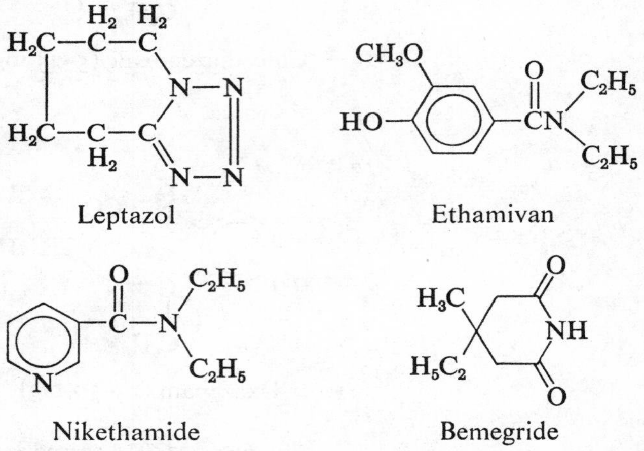

FIG. 5.28. Some analeptic convulsants.

cause convulsions. These convulsions are used to test drugs designed for the treatment of petit mal and other forms of epilepsy. In man, an overdose produces twitching at the corners of the mouth or in the fingers; these signs should be looked for when using the drug clinically.

The mode of action of leptazol is not known, though it may reduce the relative refractory period of central neurones so that repetitive firing occurs more readily. Leptazol is absorbed from the gastrointestinal tract but is never administered orally. It is distributed evenly throughout all tissues and is rapidly metabolized by the liver. The drug was formerly used in the treatment of respiratory depression associated with barbiturate overdosage (p. 5.43), but is now rarely used for this purpose because mechanical assistance of respiration is much more effective. Leptazol and other analeptic agents do not accelerate the breakdown of barbiturates nor do they exert a specific pharmacological antagonism. Today the drug is sometimes used as a first remedy in acute respiratory failure associated with chronic lung disease. The main benefit may be in raising the level of consciousness rather than in stimulating respiration. Leptazol is given in doses of up to 100 mg by slow intravenous injection every 10–20 min.

Nikethamide (coramine) is a synthetic pyridine derivative. It stimulates all levels of the nervous system, but in small doses, it affects only the medulla. Respiration is stimulated mainly by a direct action on the respiratory centre and indirectly via peripheral chemoreceptors. In high doses, it may produce convulsions. It is a less effective analeptic than leptazol but has a longer duration of action. Though capable of being absorbed orally, it is always given by intramuscular or intravenous injection to achieve a more certain effect.

Nikethamide is used occasionally as an emergency respiratory stimulant in barbiturate poisoning, while more adequate mechanical measures to support respiration are being prepared, and in CO_2 narcosis of acute respiratory failure associated with chronic lung disease. A dose of 2–8 ml of 25 per cent solution of nikethamide is given and this is repeated at intervals of 30 min to 2 hours as required (p. 9.2).

Ethamivan (vandid) is a derivative of vanillic acid and resembles nikethamide both in structure and pharmacological activity. It stimulates the respiratory centres well below a dose that causes general convulsions; there is no evidence that it is more effective than other analeptics. It is usually given by intravenous injection in doses of 50–100 mg.

Bemegride (megimide) is a synthetic analeptic which, though it has a formula resembling that of the barbiturates, is not a specific barbiturate antagonist and is of no value in barbiturate overdosage. It possesses no advantages over nikethamide. In large doses it may produce convulsions.

Psychomotor stimulants

These compounds increase alertness, affect mood and suppress appetite. They seldom induce convulsions and this distinguishes them from the analeptic convulsants.

The distinction between psychomotor stimulants and antidepressants such as MAO inhibitors is not always clear, but the psychomotor stimulants antagonize the central depressant effects of chlorpromazine in animals;

in man they have a wide range of activity in both normal and depressed patients. There are two broad classes of psychomotor stimulants:

(1) amphetamine and its derivatives, and
(2) xanthines.

AMPHETAMINE AND ITS DERIVATIVES
This substance is widely prescribed, though there are few specific indications for its use. Currently, it is favoured by young people looking for 'kicks' and addiction to it (psychic dependence) occurs. Its chemical name is β-phenylisopropylamine and it is thus related to the catecholamines.

Amphetamine

Methylamphetamine

Two stereoisomers exist; the (+) isomer is four times as potent as the (−) in its central effects, but it is slightly less potent than the (−) isomer in some peripheral sympathetic effects, e.g. on the heart.

In man, amphetamine acts both on the CNS and peripherally. The central effects predominate and constitute the basis for which amphetamine is used.

Central effects
Although all levels of the central nervous system are stimulated, the actions at the cortical level are most evident. With continued intake, tolerance occurs. There may be marked changes in mood, and feelings of confidence or anxiety. While stimulation of behaviour predominates in adults, children may be sedated. In normal subjects, the onset of fatigue is delayed and tasks are more readily completed, but there is loss of judgement and accuracy. Hence, amphetamine is not recommended for swotting before examinations; indeed when amphetamine has been taken for this purpose, candidates may leave the examinations with a feeling of success, when in fact they have written nonsense. The improvement in fatigued subjects after amphetamine has been taken is followed by feelings of depression.

In mentally or physically exhausted individuals, amphetamine has remarkable effects in removing the sense of fatigue. Some athletic performances may be improved by amphetamine, but it impairs the judgement, so often necessary for success. Amphetamine is also dangerous for athletes as its use may lead to a severe or fatal hypertension and hyperpyrexia.

Since amphetamine reduces appetite it has been used widely in the treatment of obesity. However, many studies have shown that permanent weight loss is no more likely to follow the use of amphetamine than dietary restrictions alone. As patients become habituated to the drug, it should not be prescribed for this purpose.

In man, the alerting effects of amphetamine may be of use in narcolepsy, but the subsequent insomnia is sometimes a disadvantage. In animals, amphetamine also causes EEG arousal, an effect which is also seen with hallucinogens, e.g. LSD and mescaline. This may be due to an action on the reticular formation.

In animals, amphetamine produces interesting behavioural changes; conditioned reflexes may be either augmented or depressed, depending on the reinforcement schedule used. Environmental factors influence these effects, e.g. a dose of amphetamine which is lethal to mice kept in groups does not kill litter-mates kept in isolation. In experimental animals, amphetamine facilitates both monosynaptic and polysynaptic reflexes in the spinal cord.

Peripheral effects
In therapeutic doses, amphetamine produces mild sympathetic stimulation by release of endogenous noradrenaline from postganglionic nerve endings. The blood pressure may rise but, because of reflex slowing of the heart rate, there is usually little change in cardiac output. The pupils are dilated and urinary retention may occur especially in elderly men with prostatic hypertrophy.

Poisoning
Acute effects are an exaggeration of those which occur with a therapeutic dose, i.e. excitement, anxiety, restlessness, tremors and confusion. A state resembling acute schizophrenia may occur. Cardiac arrhythmias, hypertension, palpitations, headache, nausea and vomiting may develop. In severe poisoning, hyperpyrexia, cerebral haemorrhage and coma may prove fatal.

Chronic effects include anorexia, insomnia, restlessness and physical and psychic dependence. As the patient becomes dependent on the drug, mental changes resembling schizophrenia may arise. Daily doses of up to 500 mg may be taken by dependent persons.

Mode of action of amphetamine in the CNS
Although the excitatory effects of amphetamine on behaviour are associated with changes in the metabolism and intracellular distribution of the catecholamines, the mode of action is unclear. Amphetamine does not affect the concentrations of catecholamines in the brain, except in high doses. Its action is probably comparable to that on the peripheral adrenergic neurone (p. 15.18). Thus, amphetamine may have one or both of the following actions on the brain;

(1) to release catecholamines from intracellular stores into the cytoplasm and thence to the receptor; cytoplasmic catecholamines may be protected from MAO by a weak inhibitory action of amphetamine on the enzyme (p. 5.19), and

(2) to prevent neuronal re-uptake of catecholamines after release from neuronal endings.

The effect of amphetamine is still seen in animals after treatment with reserpine, which depletes the stores but does not interfere with the formation of catecholamines. Nevertheless, the effect is abolished by treatment with inhibitors of tyrosine hydroxylase, which prevent the synthesis of catecholamines (p. 15.28).

Absorption, metabolism and fate
Amphetamine is absorbed from the gastrointestinal tract and though a small proportion is metabolized in the liver, the bulk is excreted unchanged in the urine; its excretion is increased in an acid urine. In poisoning, the administration of NH_4Cl is of value in promoting elimination.

Clinical uses
As indicated previously, amphetamine has a very restricted place in clinical practice. Although widely used to relieve mental and physical fatigue and to improve performance, it is not recommended for this purpose nor for the treatment of depression. It is occasionally of value in the treatment of narcolepsy, postencephalitic Parkinsonism and petit mal. The usual dose is 10–20 mg/day.

Amphetamine is contraindicated in the psychologically unstable (addictive risk), in hypertension, in hyperthyroidism and in patients taking MAO inhibitors.

Dexamphetamine (dexedrine), the (+) isomer, is to be preferred to (±) amphetamine (benzedrine) as it is twice as potent in the CNS and has fewer peripheral sympathomimetic effects. The usual daily dose is 2·5–5 mg.

Derivatives of amphetamine
Methylamphetamine (2·5 mg) may be used as an alternative to amphetamine to produce CNS stimulation. In acute respiratory failure, methylamphetamine (10 mg) may be given by intravenous injection. In larger doses (10–20 mg) the peripheral effects are more prominent and a sustained rise in blood pressure occurs largely due to an increase in cardiac output. It may be used to maintain the blood pressure during anaesthesia. It is interesting that some trimethoxylated amphetamines are hallucinogenic in man; 2-4-5-trimethoxyamphetamine is about seventeen times as potent as mescaline in conditioned behavioural tests in rats.

Other drugs with central amphetamine-like actions
Drugs with central effects similar to those of amphetamine and which bear some chemical resemblance to it

have been developed in the hope that they might be less liable to induce habituation and dependence. Appetite suppressant drugs include **phenmetrazine** (preludin), **chlorphentermine** and **diethylpropion** (tenuate). Their value in this respect is limited and emotional dependence has been reported.

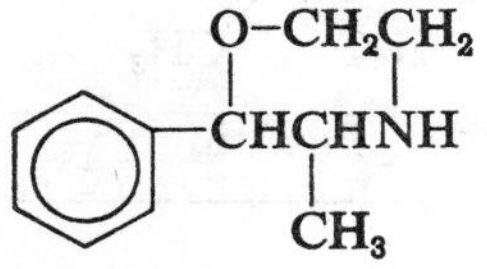

Phenmetrazine 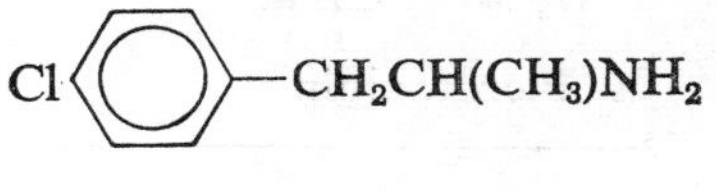   Chlorphentermine

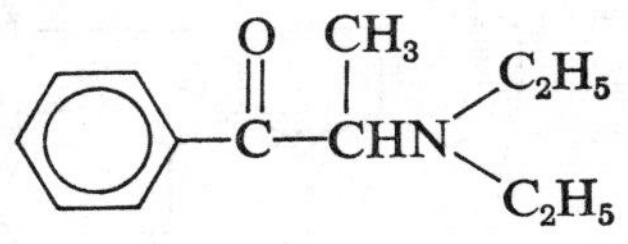

Diethylpropion

CAFFEINE, THEOPHYLLINE AND THEOBROMINE (THE XANTHINES) fig. 5.29
These alkaloids, found in a variety of seeds and leaves, are consumed habitually by millions of people in the form of coffee, tea and cocoa.

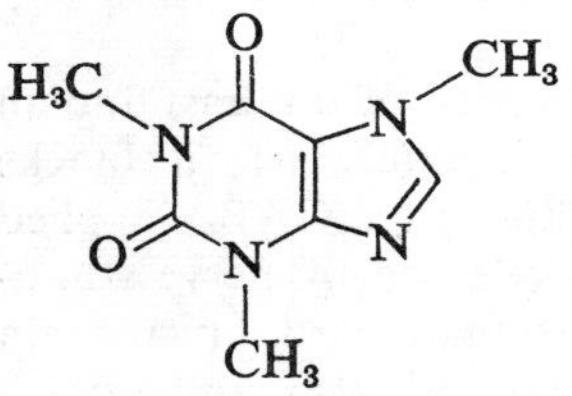

Caffeine 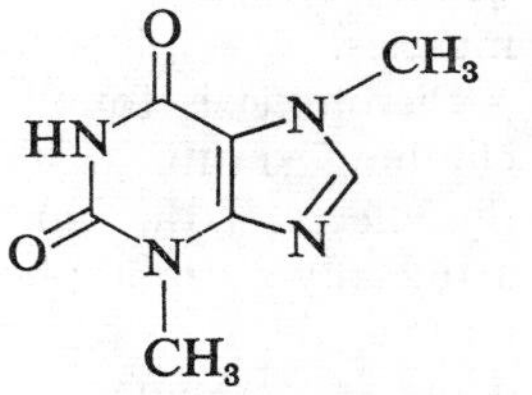   Theobromine

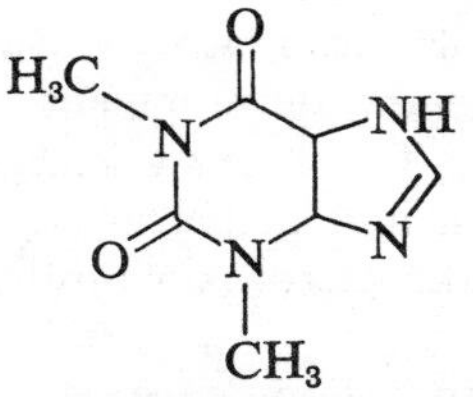

Theophylline

FIG. 5.29. The xanthines.

Caffeine is 1-3-7 trimethylxanthine and is related to theophylline (1,3 dimethylxanthine) and theobromine (3-7 dimethylxanthine). Caffeine resembles theophylline and theobromine in many of its actions on different organ systems, but there are quantitative differences; however, caffeine has more marked central effects than theophylline and theobromine, which are more active peripherally. Theophylline is more active than theobromine.

Central actions of caffeine
Caffeine is a CNS stimulant. It causes wakefulness and an increased capacity for intellectual work, and allays drowsiness and fatigue. The reaction time to visual and auditory stimuli is diminished and the rate of performing motor tasks increased. These effects may be seen with doses between 50 and 200 mg of caffeine, the amount that might be found in two cups of ground coffee or four cups of instant coffee.

With larger doses, hand tremor may impair delicate motor co-ordination. Increased excitability and insomnia occur and there may be hyperaesthesia. After large doses of caffeine, stimulation is followed by a rebound depression, such as is seen with amphetamine. Marked tolerance to the central effects of caffeine does not occur though this may develop to its peripheral effects.

Respiration is stimulated when 200 mg of caffeine is given parenterally. This is probably due to increased sensitivity of the respiratory centre to CO_2 and is the basis for its occasional use in acute respiratory depression. Certainly, caffeine would appear to be safer than amphetamine as, in man, convulsions due to caffeine are virtually unknown. In experimental animals, however, large doses of caffeine increase the reflex excitability of the cord giving rise to clonic convulsions. The EEG arousal seen in cats after large doses of caffeine differs from that seen after amphetamine in that it is not abolished by section of the midbrain and so is presumably due to an action at a higher level. The mode of action of caffeine in the CNS is unknown.

Peripheral effects of caffeine
In man these are minimal when compared with those of theophylline. The heart is stimulated directly; the force of contraction and cardiac output increase and extrasystoles may occur; indeed some coffee drinkers experience palpitations. Usually, caffeine causes little change in heart rate or blood pressure probably because of homeostatic circulatory reflexes. The coronary, pulmonary and systemic blood vessels are dilated by caffeine, but this action is slight and has no therapeutic value. Curiously, cerebral blood vessels are constricted and the cerebral blood flow and Po_2 fall. This may explain the beneficial effect in migrainous headache, and why it is often included in popular remedies. Gastric secretion is increased in man and gross overconsumption of caffeine-containing beverages leads to gastritis, nausea and vomiting. Patients with peptic ulcers should take coffee and tea in moderation, since caffeine can induce gastritis and peptic ulceration in experimental animals. The diuretic effect of caffeine may be marked but it is much less than that of theophylline.

The force of contraction of isolated skeletal muscle, stimulated both directly and indirectly, is increased by caffeine. The extent to which this contributes to improved motor performance in man is not known, and it is believed that the central actions of caffeine are mainly responsible.

Metabolic effects

Xanthines inhibit phosphodiesterase and reduce the rate of breakdown of 3'-5' cyclic AMP (p. 15.13); its accumulation in the tissues promotes glycogenolysis in the liver and other effects which are discussed in vol. 1, p. 9.9.

Absorption, metabolism and fate

Like most other alkaloids, caffeine is poorly soluble in water and is often compounded as a double salt, e.g. sodium benzoate, to increase solubility.

Caffeine is absorbed in the stomach, though if it is to be used as an analeptic, parenteral injection is required. Only a small proportion of caffeine is bound to plasma proteins. Caffeine is both demethylated and oxidized and its metabolism does not involve xanthine oxidase or increase uric acid excretion.

Clinical uses

Coffee is drunk by many as a pleasant stimulant. Caffeine is only occasionally used as a remedy for headache particularly of migraine usually in combination with ergotamine or salicylate.

Theophylline and theobromines

These have more powerful effects than caffeine on the cardiovascular system, smooth muscle and the kidneys and are described on pp. 8.7, 9.2 and 11.2.

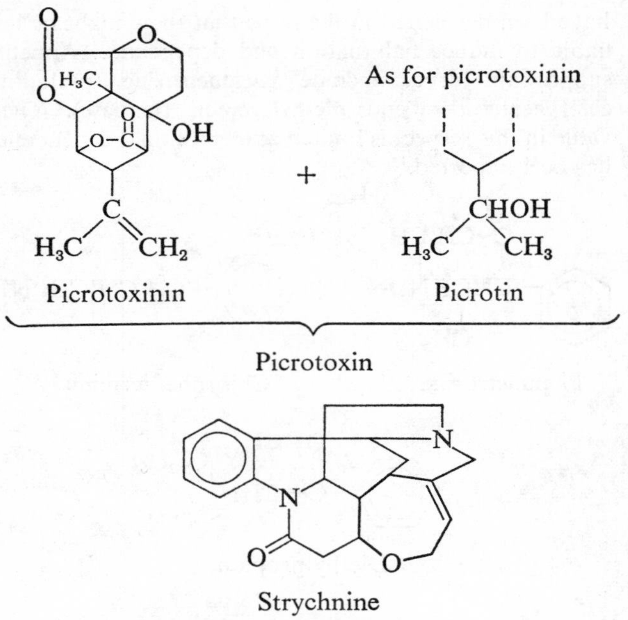

Miscellaneous convulsants (fig. 5.30)

Strychnine is the principal alkaloid present in the seeds of the Indian tree, *Strychnos nux vomica*.

Its mode of action is not completely understood. In the spinal cord it depresses inhibitory postsynaptic potentials (IPSP's vol. 1, p. 14.27) and prevents the effects of glycine, the presumed inhibitory transmitter. It does not directly excite spinal neurones; since inhibition is widespread in the spinal cord, its removal by strychnine results in 'release' excitation. Strychnine also stimulates the cerebral cortex but its mode of action here is far from clear. It does not appear to block the effects of the presumed cortical inhibitory transmitter (GABA).

Although once used widely in tonic mixtures, strychnine has no therapeutic value. However, it is still used in rat poison and this may give rise to accidental strychnine poisoning in man, in whom synchronized painful tonic convulsions occur, similar to those seen in tetanus. The convulsions are most marked in antigravity muscles so

FIG. 5.30. Experimental convulsants.

that the back becomes arched and the body supported by the feet and head. This characteristic posture is known as opisthotonus. Initially consciousness is retained. When death occurs it is due to respiratory failure as the consequence of maintained activity (spasm) in the respiratory muscles.

Picrotoxin is found in the berries of an East Indian climbing shrub, *Anamirta*. In invertebrates, it blocks the effects of the inhibitory transmitter GABA applied artificially by iontophoresis or released by nerve stimulation. In the mammalian spinal cord, picrotoxin depresses presynaptic inhibition and also antagonizes the inhibitory effects of glycine. An active component, **picrotoxinin** has been isolated, which is a powerful stimulant of the CNS. Respiratory and vasomotor centre stimulation precede the development of incoordinated clonic convulsions. The narrow margin between respiratory stimulation and convulsions, and the delayed onset of effects make picrotoxin unsuitable for clinical use.

Semicarbazide and **thiosemicarbazide** ($NH_2NHCS-NH_2$) block reactions dependent on pyridoxal such as amino acid decarboxylations. Hence GABA formation in the cortex is depressed and this might be expected to lead to the uncontrolled spread of activity, i.e. epileptic seizures by impairment of inhibitory mechanisms. This convulsant action may be prevented by the injection of pyridoxal. However, it has now been shown that convulsions induced by thiosemicarbazide do not necessarily depend on lowered GABA levels in the cortex.

α-Chloralose and **γ-hydroxybutyrate** are convulsants

which are also anaesthetics; they are used experimentally in animals to induce prolonged anaesthesia without the neurological depression associated with depressant general anaesthetics.

Fluorethyl (hexafluoryldiethylether) is a convulsant anaesthetic vapour which produces brief convulsions following a single exposure. Proposed as a convulsant agent for the treatment of endogenous depression, it has no advantages over electroconvulsive therapy. It illustrates that unconsciousness can result from uncontrolled and irregular stimulation as well as from depression of the nervous system.

GENERAL CNS DEPRESSANTS

General depressants of the CNS are capable of inducing sedation, sleep or general anaesthesia, depending mainly on the dose given. In therapeutic doses in man, hypnotics induce or predispose towards a state resembling normal sleep, in which the patient is unconscious but easily aroused; the eyes are closed and movements are reduced but the postural reflexes are intact. In larger doses, hypnotics may induce general anaesthesia. However, the nonvolatile CNS depressants used specifically as anaesthetics have a very short duration of action which makes them unsuitable as sedatives or hypnotics. Anaesthesia differs from sleep in that the immediate arousability by sensory stimuli is impaired, postural reflexes are lost and sensory reflexes and muscle tone are diminished. In smaller doses, sedation occurs, and anxiety and aggressive response are reduced. As already discussed, it is difficult to distinguish precisely between sedatives and the minor tranquillizers (p. 5.29). Occasionally, the general CNS depressants induce a state of excitement with euphoria. This is due to depression of normal behavioural restraints.

In animal tests, general depression of the CNS may be detected by reduced movements, changes in posture and prolongation of sleep. In man, drug-induced sleep should be estimated objectively by unbiased observers ideally with EEG control, and also subjectively by getting the subject to complete an appropriate check list. If this was carried out more commonly in trials of hypnotic drugs, the efficacy of many hypnotics would be known with a greater degree of certainty. In sedative doses in man depression of intellectual performance, reaction time and co-ordination in motor tasks occurs. Scales for rating anxiety are also a useful way of assessing changes of mood in response to these agents.

TYPES OF CNS DEPRESSANTS
CNS depressants fall into several classes:
   (1) barbiturates,
   (2) chloral hydrate and its derivatives,
   (3) paraldehyde,
   (4) piperidines like glutethimide, and
   (5) miscellaneous types.
This list excludes ethyl alcohol, gases and vapours used for general anaesthesia and obstetric analgesia, which are described on pp. 5.68 & 72.

Hypnotics are valuable drugs in the control of insomnia but are often prescribed unnecessarily. For most patients, barbiturates are the most acceptable form of hypnotic. Current search for new remedies arises from the dangers of overdosage and dependence with barbiturates. These disadvantages, however, occur with most of the nonbarbiturate hypnotics available and at present there is no absolutely safe hypnotic.

The barbiturates
These are derivatives of malonylurea or barbituric acid. Barbituric acid itself is not hypnotic and has acid properties because the keto form is in equilibrium with the enol form. Water-soluble salts are readily formed by reacting alkalis with the enol form. The relation of the commonly used barbiturates to this parent substance are seen in table 5.5.

STRUCTURE AND ACTIVITY
Alkyl side chains at C-5 confer hypnotic activity which is abolished by a polar group in either side chain. Increasing the length of one or both chains produces compounds which are more soluble in lipids and have a faster action and more rapid breakdown. Increase in the length of the side chain to over seven carbon atoms may decrease hypnotic activity and lead to convulsive activity. Methylation of one nitrogen atom increases lipid solubility and thus shortens the duration of action. Substituting alkyl groups in both nitrogens gives convulsive properties. The depressant and anticonvulsant properties are to some extent separable, e.g. a phenyl group at C-5 (phenobarbitone) confers anti-epileptic properties even in nonsedative doses. The substitution of a sulphur atom for the carbonyl oxygen at C-2 yields the thiobarbiturates which are very soluble in fat, act rapidly and are used exclusively for general anaesthesia.

ACTIONS OF BARBITURATES
The main action is to depress the CNS; the effects of this depression may be those of sedation, sleep or anaesthesia. Sedative doses of barbiturates impair reasoning and judgement, increase reaction time and distractability and impair motor co-ordination. Hence their use increases the likelihood of a road accident. The fact that alcohol is also a CNS depressant is easily overlooked, and the combination of barbiturates with alcohol is potent and may be lethal, either by depression of respiration or a failure to apply the brake.

As indicated in table 5.5, the duration of action of the

TABLE 5.5.

Properties, doses, uses and the chemical structure of some barbiturates.

	Compound	R_1	R_2	X		Properties, doses and uses
	Barbituric acid	H	H	=O		Not hypnotic
Group I	Thiopentone (pentothal)	Ethyl	1-Methylbutyl	=S	⎫	Used as intravenous anaesthetics on account of
	Methohexitone	Allyl	1-Methylpentynyl	=S	⎬	ultrashort activity. Very high fat solubility and
	Thialbarbitone	Allyl	Cyclohexenyl	=O	⎭	protein binding (p. 5.68).
Group II	Pentobarbitone (nembutal)	Ethyl	1-Methylbutyl	ONa	⎫	Hypnotics in current use; the usual dose of 100
	Quinalbarbitone (seconal)	Allyl	1-Methylbutyl	ONa		mg giving about 6 hours sleep. At this dosage, the
	Cyclobarbitone (phanodorm)	Ethyl	Cyclohexenyl	ONa	⎬	duration of effects is similar; thus there is no clinical basis for further subclassification. Fat
	Amylobarbitone (amytal)	Ethyl	Iso Amyl	ONa		solubility and protein binding are intermediate.
	Butobarbitone (soneryl)	Ethyl	Sec Butyl	ONa	⎭	
Group III	Barbitone	Ethyl	Ethyl	=O	0·3–0·5 g	⎧ Slow in onset; they enter the brain slowly. Not generally used as hypnotics; phenobarbitone is mainly used as an anti-epileptic. Protein binding and fat solubility are minimal.
	Diallylbarbituric acid	Allyl	Allyl	=O	0·1–0·3 g	
	Phenobarbitone	Ethyl	Phenyl	=O	0·1–0·2 g	

group II and III barbiturates makes them unsuitable for general anaesthesia except in experimental animals, since precise control over the depth of anaesthesia is not possible and the effects of an overdose cannot be reversed rapidly. In sedative or hypnotic doses, there is slight depression of the medullary centres leading to diminished respiration and slight hypotension and bradycardia. These changes are not easily distinguished from those which occur in normal sleep. With increasing dosage, however, depression of the respiratory centre by barbiturates becomes dangerous and is probably the main cause of death in poisoning; the resulting hypoxia is also a major factor in the development of hypotension and circulatory failure in these cases. With normal doses of barbiturate, hypothermia is slight but with large doses, temperatures may fall to 30°C or below.

Sedative and hypnotic doses of barbiturates induce little analgesia, and the effect is accompanied by intellectual impairment. Barbiturates may decrease the relief of pain obtained from specific analgesics. Indeed if pain is at all severe, their administration often results in a restless confused state.

In a high proportion of ambulant patients, hangover occurs after hypnotic doses. This may be detected by deterioration of tests in intellectual performance, for up to 10 hours after waking. It is more likely to occur after the group III compounds which act for a very long time.

Tolerance occurs with barbiturates as with other general CNS depressants. It is not so marked with the narcotic analgesics and only ten or fifteen times the hypnotic dose may be taken. While tolerance appears to be due partly to cellular adaptation as with the narcotic analgesics, there is induction of enzymes in the liver which metabolize barbiturates (p. 10.9). More rapid disposal of the drug, however, is not a feature of the tolerance to narcotic analgesics (p. 5.49).

Addiction is a grave problem. Both psychic and physical dependence occur and the impairment of mood, behaviour and intellectual functions cause social deterioration. When barbiturates are withdrawn from addicts, symptoms may be seen within one day and persist for two weeks. Common features are anxiety, nausea and vomiting, weakness, hypotension, tremors and disturbance of vision. Convulsions may also occur.

MODE AND SITE OF ACTION

Barbiturates are not selectively concentrated in the brain. Moreover, while they depress energy yielding reactions and oxygen consumption in the brain, this is likely to be the result and not the cause of the depressed neuronal function, though this point needs further clarification. While the barbiturates induce sleep, perhaps by action on polysynaptic pathways in the reticular formation, this is not a selective action since even small doses depress monosynaptic reflexes in the spinal cord. Barbiturate-induced sleep differs from that seen normally in one important respect; paradoxical sleep, part of the normal sleep pattern (vol. I, p. 24.91), is depressed by barbiturates, though the consequences of this effect are unknown.

It is always hard to distinguish between cause and effect, and this is evident in studying the relationship of possible transmitter substances in the brain and barbiturates. During barbiturate anaesthesia, the release of acetylcholine into cortical cups is depressed, while cerebral concentrations of acetylcholine are increased. Both effects, however, could be the consequence of diminished activity in the ascending reticular system. Barbiturate and other anaesthetic substances depress the excitatory responses of single neurones in the brain to acetylcholine 5-HT, noradrenaline and glutamate.

Peripheral effects
In contrast to the small effects seen with hypnotic doses, large or anaesthetic doses of barbiturates cause a marked fall in blood pressure. When barbiturates are given intravenously so that the plasma level rises sharply, the blood pressure falls probably because of depressant effects at several sites, e.g. the vasomotor centre, sympathetic ganglia, the heart muscle and the blood vessels.

In normal doses, the effects of barbiturates on the kidneys are small. In large doses there may be oliguria, probably due to the circulatory failure.

Adverse effects
With usual hypnotic or sedative doses, adverse effects are uncommon. Hypersensitivity reactions, especially of the skin, may occur.

Acute poisoning may occur accidentally or deliberately. In severe cases, coma with respiratory and circulatory failure occur and erythema and blisters are seen in a small number of patients. These are acute medical emergencies. Some aspects of treatment are not in dispute and include the provision of a good, clear airway, ventilatory assistance and maintenance of water and electrolyte balance. However, other aspects of treatment are less certain and in particular, the value of analeptics is disputed. It is stated that in many hands, they may do more harm than good. The converse situation, that in skilled hands they may be of benefit, remains to be proved. Where coma is not too deep and there are no renal or cardiac complications, some advantage may be gained by

inducing an alkaline diuresis. Such a treatment is of benefit only with those in group III which are excreted in the urine. The ionization of phenobarbitone (pK_a 7·2) is favoured in alkaline urine and so tubular reabsorption is reduced. The forced osmotic diuresis also reduces passive reabsorption of all the long-acting barbiturates. However, it is possible that such cases might recover just as well without the alkaline diuresis.

The indications for peritoneal or haemodialysis as a means of eliminating the drug are the subject of controversy.

Chronic poisoning occurs principally in the addict, although rarely it is iatrogenic. Apathy, intellectual impairment and ataxia, contribute to the social deterioration of the addict and are in contrast to the apparent well-being of the satisfied morphine addict.

ABSORPTION, METABOLISM AND FATE
The Group I barbiturates are given intravenously and, because of their high fat solubility and the high cerebral blood flow, reach peak concentration in the brain and cause anaesthesia within one minute after administration. Thereafter, their plasma concentrations fall, as they are taken up by muscle and fat. As this occurs, the brain gives up e.g., its thiopentone, so that within half an hour, brain levels may be only 10 per cent of their initial peak value and the peripheral stores may be saturated. This rapid redistribution of thiopentone, rather than its metabolism, accounts for the short duration of its action, and consciousness may be regained within 10 min of the induction of anaesthesia. Because of the high degree of protein binding, little thiopentone is excreted and less than 1 per cent appears in the urine. Thiopentone is metabolized at a rate of about 10 or 15 per cent/hour, mainly in the liver but also in the kidney and brain. The metabolites have not been identified (p. 5.68).

After oral administration, the hypnotic barbiturates (group II) are readily absorbed from the stomach and small intestine. The sodium salts may be absorbed more rapidly than the free acid, though possibly with an increased incidence of local gastric irritation. When given parenterally, they penetrate the brain rapidly but less readily than the group I barbiturates because of their lesser fat solubility. Thus, the depth of sleep increases for several minutes after an intravenous injection of sodium pentobarbitone. There is a significant degree of protein binding and little renal excretion of unaltered barbiturate occurs. The tissues are therefore more evenly exposed to the barbiturate, and metabolism rather than redistribution is the principal means of ending the effects. Quinal, pento- and cyclobarbitone are more rapidly metabolized (about 15 per cent/hour) than amylo- and butobarbitone (about 6 per cent/hour).

The group III compounds have a very low fat solubility and, after intravenous injection, may take up to 15 min to produce sleep which increases in depth for another 15 min. They are widely distributed throughout the body tissues and fluids. The depressant effect is terminated slowly, principally by renal excretion in the case of barbitone, where almost all the dose appears in the urine. Both metabolism and renal excretion are important for phenobarbitone since only 15–30 per cent of the oral dose is excreted in the urine. However, phenobarbitone is metabolized very slowly, about 1 per cent/hour; hence it readily accumulates. For this reason its habitual use as a hypnotic is not recommended.

CLINICAL USES OF BARBITURATES
The short-acting barbiturates are used to induce anaesthesia for short procedures, e.g. dental extractions. The group II compounds are principally used as sedatives or hypnotics. They have some use as antidotes in amphetamine or mescaline poisoning. Phenobarbitone is valuable in the treatment of epilepsy and this is considered on p. 5.58.

There are many contraindications to the use of barbiturates. In persons with an unstable personality, their habitual use may lead to addiction. Alcohol and barbiturates form a particularly potent depressant mixture and should never be taken together. Barbiturates are not recommended in the very young or very old, or where an analgesic effect is needed. While depression of the respiratory centre with normal doses is minimal, hypnotics should be used with the utmost care in patients with asthma or with respiratory insufficiency, associated with chronic lung disease. Barbiturates may cause severe reactions in some patients with porphyria (p. 31.3). Though the popular barbiturates are mainly metabolized in the liver, only severe liver disease is a contraindication to their use.

ADMINISTRATION
The group I barbiturates are given by slow intravenous injection as a 2·5–5·0 per cent solution, to reduce the risk of venous thrombosis, and to avoid respiratory and circulatory collapse from temporarily high plasma concentrations. To keep thiopentone as a sodium salt, the solution is made alkaline. Extravascular injections are damaging to tissues, and intra-arterial injections cause vasospasm and the resulting arterial insufficiency may cause gangrene.

The group II and III barbiturates are given by mouth as tablets or capsules of the sodium salt. Intramuscular injection of the hypnotic barbiturates is recommended only if oral intake is impracticable.

Nonbarbiturate hypnotics
It is evident from the preceding sections that the barbiturates have their disadvantages, particularly in their potentiality for abuse. The ideal hypnotic would be non-addictive and have a wide margin of safety making lethal overdose impossible. Despite the large number of non-barbiturate hypnotics available, these may be considered only as alternatives to the barbiturates, as they have no special advantages with respect to these hazards. Research into the new sedative and hypnotic drugs continues.

Chloral hydrate
This is a crystalline halogenated aliphatic alcohol. Its principal action is to depress the CNS. Like the barbiturates, it causes sedation, sleep and even anaesthesia. In the usual hypnotic dosage of 1–2 g for an adult,

$$CCl_3—CH(OH)_2$$

Chloral hydrate

sleep occurs within 30 min–1 hour and lasts for about 6 hours. There is usually little hangover though precise comparisons with equihypnotic doses of the group II barbiturates have not been made. Tolerance to the hypnotic effects of chloral hydrate occurs occasionally. Depression of respiration and blood pressure occurs with hypnotic doses to the same extent as in normal sleep. Chloral hydrate has no analgesic or anticonvulsant activity. The features of acute poisoning resemble those of barbiturates. Addiction can occur though it is uncommon.

Chloral hydrate is absorbed rapidly from the stomach and small intestine, and also from the rectum. It is metabolized rapidly in the liver and kidney mainly to trichlorethanol, which is also hypnotic and accounts for part of the action of chloral hydrate. Trichlorethanol is conjugated with glucuronic acid and excreted in the urine.

Chloral hydrate is a popular hypnotic in the very young and very old, and the only contraindications are active peptic ulcer or serious liver or kidney disease. It has never found favour as a sedative probably because of its unpleasant taste and smell and its irritant effect on the stomach. It is too hygroscopic to be prepared in tablet form and it is usually given in a flavoured diluted mixture. Owing to the long duration of its action, it is not used as an anaesthetic.

Various salt complexes of chloral hydrate or its active metabolite, trichlorethanol, are widely used since they can be made in tablet form, have a more acceptable taste and cause less gastric irritation. These include **dichloralphenazone** (welldorm), and **triclofos** (tricloryl). This latter is the monosodium salt of trichlorethylphosphate which is hydrolysed to trichlorethanol in the gut. Other preparations include **penthrichloral** (clorased) and **chloral betaine** (somilan).

Paraldehyde

This is a volatile liquid with disagreeable taste and smell which makes its use unpleasant for both the patient and his attendants. Chemically, it is a cyclic polyether and has no reactive aldehyde groups, though derived by the condensation or polymerization of three molecules of acetaldehyde.

Paraldehyde

In the presence of air and light, paraldehyde decomposes to acetic acid which contributes to its toxicity. It is advisable to use only recently prepared paraldehyde from an unopened light-proof container which has been stored in complete darkness.

Paraldehyde is rapidly absorbed from the stomach and small intestine or from the rectum, and sleep follows an oral hypnotic dose in about 15 min. The main action is on the CNS. Paraldehyde is more anticonvulsant than chloral hydrate though it is less depressant, and for this reason is sometimes used in the treatment of status epilepticus.

In acute overdosage, the usual triad of coma, depressed respiration and hypotension is seen. However, respiratory difficulties are more marked than with other CNS depressants, possibly because of pulmonary oedema. Liver and kidney necrosis may occur.

With chronic use, tolerance and addiction develops as with the other CNS depressants, and severe metabolic acidosis may arise in addicts. On stopping the drug, clinical features sometimes develop which resemble those which may follow the withdrawal of alcohol from the chronic alcoholic (delirium tremens).

A variable proportion, perhaps up to one-quarter of the dose, is excreted via the lungs. The remainder is metabolized to CO_2 and water, very little being excreted as such in the urine.

Paraldehyde can be used in the treatment of mania, delirium tremens and status epilepticus. Like chloral hydrate, it is a useful hypnotic in the elderly, but it is also safe in the presence of severe renal failure. Oral use is contraindicated in the presence of peptic ulcer and it should not be given rectally when anorectal pathology is present. Care should be shown in using paraldehyde in alcoholics under treatment with disulfiram (antabuse) since this delays its metabolism (p. 5.72).

Paraldehyde is popular in hospital practice and is usually given by intramuscular injection. This is not without hazard as sterile abscess and sciatic nerve lesions may occur. The intravenous injection of undiluted paraldehyde may be lethal. Right heart failure, pulmonary oedema and haemorrhage may be seen. Ideally therefore, paraldehyde should be diluted to 10 per cent of its strength in isotonic saline before injection. Alternatively, the amount of undiluted paraldehyde given at a single intramuscular injection should be limited to 5 ml. Though dilute paraldehyde has been given safely by intravenous injection, it is wiser to avoid this route.

Piperidinedione derivatives

Two of these, **glutethimide** and **methyprylone**, are now used clinically, as alternatives to barbiturates but have no special advantages. The closely related compound **thalidomide** appeared to have a high safety margin so that even with enormous doses, severe depression of medullary centres and death did not occur. As is well known, its teratogenic properties and its ability to induce neuropathy led to its withdrawal (p. 12.17).

GLUTETHIMIDE (DORIDEN)

This is a solid which is highly soluble in lipid but poorly soluble in water. Chemically, it is α-ethyl-α-phenylglutarimide. Glutethimide resembles the barbiturates in causing CNS depression. There is, however, some stimulation of the CNS, not seen with the barbiturates; with hypnotic doses, the EEG shows spike-like waves and with overdosage brisk reflexes, muscle twitching and spasticity are seen. Absorption from the gastrointestinal tract is irregular. The half-life is short and glutethimide is completely metabolized in the body. Conjugates with glucuronic acid may circulate for several days in the enterohepatic circulation.

Glutethimide

The usual hypnotic dose of 0·5 g produces a sleep which lasts for about 6 hours and resembles that seen with quinalbarbitone (0·1 g). Glutethimide is effective against motion sickness but is not commonly used for this. The analgesic and anticonvulsant properties are too weak to justify its use for these purposes.

Adverse effects

Addiction occurs and withdrawal symptoms are much more frequent than with the barbiturates. Glutethimide has atropine-like effects and dry mouth and mydriasis are commonly produced. In toxic doses, these anticholinergic effects are even more marked, and fixed dilated pupils, urinary retention and even paralytic ileus may arise.

Although hypersensitivity skin reactions, blood dyscrasias and peripheral neuropathy may occur, adverse effects are not common. It is not teratogenic and may be safely used in the first trimester of pregnancy.

The margin of safety is lower than for the barbiturates. Some studies suggest that half the patients who consume 10 g of glutethimide die. The features of overdosage differ in several ways from those of barbiturate overdosage. In particular, hyperthermia occurs and there is relatively little respiratory but marked circulatory depression. The signs of CNS stimulation referred to earlier may also be seen. Glutethimide coma has an unusual fluctuating character for reasons unknown and death may occur suddenly. Hence glutethimide overdosage is an acute medical emergency and haemodialysis is of value. If hypotension is severe, forced diuresis is hazardous, because of the risk of cerebral and pulmonary oedema.

METHYPRYLONE (NOLUDAR)

This resembles glutethimide in many respects, though it is more potent; a 250 mg dose having the same hypnotic effect as a 100 mg dose of a group II barbiturate. It occasionally gives rise to pruritus and skin rashes.

Methyprylone

NITRAZEPAM

This is a benzodiazepine (p. 5.35). It is a popular hypnotic and has several advantages over the barbiturates; it has a wider safety margin in case of overdose and a reduced incidence of morning hangover. Physical and psychic dependance are less common than with barbiturates and meprobamate. Neurophysiological studies show that, unlike the barbiturates, nitrazepam has little direct depressant effect on the reticular formation and only slight effects on arousal. This could be the basis of the clinical observation that patients are readily awakened from sleep induced by nitrazepam. The usual dose is 5–10 mg.

METHAQUALONE

This drug is used widely as an alternative to the barbiturates. The bulk of an orally administered dose of 250 mg is rapidly absorbed from the gut, concentrated in fat, metabolized in the liver and excreted in the urine. About one-third of the dose is excreted in the faeces. While in animals the margin between hypnotic and lethal doses is wide, acute poisoning in man is not uncommon. Methaqualone is antitussive, potentiates analgesics although

it is not itself analgesic, is a local anaesthetic and a weak antihistaminic. Its effects are potentiated by alcohol. Like the barbiturates, it depresses polysynaptic reflexes

Methaqualone

and probably also the rapid eye movement (REM) sleep. The advantages of methaqualone over the barbiturates are not clear, though hangover is probably less. Dependence occurs and many heroin addicts favour methaqualone and diphenhydramine (mandrax) as a hypnotic. In moderately severe poisoning the reflexes are hyperactive and muscle tone is increased. Some studies suggest that circulatory disturbances are more marked in acute methaqualone than in acute barbiturate poisoning; cardiac arrhythmias and acute heart failure may occur. In poisoning, pulmonary and tissue oedema may be due to acute cardiac failure, though it has been suggested that methaqualone has a direct toxic effect on blood vessels increasing their permeability.

The usual hypnotic dose is 100–200 mg; a dangerous degree of poisoning occurs when about ten times this amount is taken.

ANALGESICS

Pain is commonly experienced from childbirth throughout life to death and its relief by giving pain killing drugs or analgesics is commonplace in clinical practice. Knowledge of the pharmacology of these drugs contributes to their proper use and provides the understanding needed in the search for new analgesics.

PHYSIOLOGY OF PAIN (see also vol. 1, p. 24.68)

A bewildering variety of experimental and pathological stimuli give rise to painful sensations. These may act directly on the free unencapsulated nerve endings, though many of them affect the endings indirectly through the release of active pain substances, possibly 5-HT, histamine or polypeptides. Sensations of pain differ in quality and timing with the type of stimulus evoking them and also the area which is affected. Stimulation of skin receptors, e.g. with a pinprick, induces superficial pain which is well localized, has little autonomic accompaniment and causes little or no real suffering. Pain from deep somatic or visceral structures is less well localized, is characteristically more unpleasant and is often associated with profound changes in mood and sometimes intense suffering. Such pain is associated with autonomic effects such as sweating, bradycardia, hypotension and nausea. Several qualities of visceral pain may be recognized, e.g. the dull gripping pain of ischaemic heart muscle or the spasmodic colicky pain of inflamed or obstructed tubes of smooth muscle. Pain sensations reach the central nervous system via somatic and visceral (autonomic) pathways. The exact site where pain is appreciated is unknown. The cortex is not directly involved, and it is likely that the medial or possibly lateral thalamic nuclei are responsible. Lesions in the thalamus give rise to characteristically unpleasant sensations and spontaneous pain, or to severe pain in response to mild stimuli.

Analgesic drugs relieve the symptoms of pain without removing their cause, impairing conduction in peripheral nerves or causing severe CNS depression. Traditionally, these drugs are divided into two main classes, narcotic and non-narcotic or antipyretic drugs.

Narcotic analgesics are effective against visceral pain and against severe pain from any source. They have many structural features in common and are neither antipyretic nor anti-inflammatory. They tend to induce drowsiness or sleep, hence the name 'narcotic' (Greek, *narcosis*, numbness) and with the single exception of pentazocine have a remarkable capacity to induce physical and psychic dependence, i.e. addiction. Physical dependence means that the body becomes so used to the action of the drug that various abnormal reactions (withdrawal symptoms) develop when the drug is withdrawn. Psychic dependence involves an intense craving for the drug and possible pleasure from its use. Chemically different narcotic analgesics can be substituted for each other in addicts. A common additional feature is that tolerance to certain of their effects develops with regular use and larger doses are required to produce an analgesic effect; addicts, for example, can take doses which are lethal to healthy individuals.

Non-narcotic analgesics or **antipyretic analgesics** are not effective against severe pain from any source or against visceral pain. They are effective against pain of mild to moderate severity, especially when it has an inflammatory component or arises from joints or muscles. They do not induce addiction.

Narcotic analgesics

Many different chemical compounds possess the characteristic features of this group of drugs. These include,

(1) natural phenanthrene alkaloids from opium, e.g. morphine and codeine,

(2) derivatives of the opium alkaloids, e.g. diacetylmorphine (heroin), dihydrocodeine (DF 118), levorphanol and certain tetrahydro-oripavines, and

(3) synthetic analgesics:
(a) phenylpiperidines, e.g. pethidine,
(b) diphenylheptane derivatives, e.g. L-methadone and D-propoxyphene,
(c) benzimidazoles, e.g. etonitazine,
(d) benzomorphans, e.g. phenazocine and pentazocine.

Certain general chemical characteristics are common to many analgesics. The compounds are usually weak bases (e.g. morphine pK_a 9·85) and partially un-ionized at the pH of body fluids. Where two optical isomers exist, the active compound is invariably L-rotatory indicating that analgesic activity depends specifically on molecular geometry. The presence of a tertiary nitrogen atom appears to be critical and the substituent hydrocarbons on this nitrogen must not be too large or so sterically rigid that they block the reactivity of the basic component with the receptor sites which are presumably anionic. Otherwise, the molecules usually have a flat aromatic structure and the nitrogen atom centre is fairly rigid sterically. Many strong narcotic analgesics possess a γ-phenyl-N-methylpiperidine nucleus.

ASSESSMENT OF ANALGESIA

Research to discover compounds which retain the most desirable features of the narcotic analgesics but which do not possess their disadvantages continues. Though it is commonly held that a high degree of analgesic potency cannot be separated from the capacity to induce tolerance, dependence and respiratory depression, there is no *a priori* reason why this should be so, and the recent discovery of pentazocine (p. 5.53) indicates that powerful analgesics which do not cause addiction can be developed.

New analgesic drugs are tested in animals before being given to man. Possible analgesic activity may have been suggested in the preliminary screening (see below). The value of inducing pain experimentally in animals and man in order to test new drugs has been questioned, since it is impossible to reproduce the suffering caused by disease. In addition, in the case of animal testing, the experimenter is deprived of the subjective impressions of the recipient. However, the relative potency of many narcotic analgesics in animal tests compares well with their known efficacy when used clinically. The relief of pain induced in experimental animals by physical pressure to tail or limb is probably the most selective test available. Other methods, which may be used in man, include the exposure of a sensitive point to radiant heat, the induction of blisters, electrical stimulation of the tooth pulp or the inflation of a sphygmomanometer cuff on the arm to induce the pain of muscle ischaemia. Other tests are needed to differentiate drugs with true analgesic properties from general CNS depressants.

These methods depend on recording a response to the noxious stimulus. The minimal stimulus producing the response is measured before and after giving the drug, and the difference between the threshold intensities is taken as a measure of analgesia. In tests on man and larger laboratory species, the measured effect can be related to log dose, so that the dose response curves for two or more analgesics can be compared. When many compounds are screened for analgesic activity, it is more convenient to use small animals and quantal methods of assay (p. 3.6). Log dose is then related to the percentage of positive effects in groups of animals that receive a stimulus of fixed intensity. For example, when a clip is placed on the base of the mouse's tail for 10 sec, the median dose 50 is derived from the proportion of mice not attempting to bite the clip (BD-50).

The effects of analgesic drugs in man are also assessed in double blind trials to avoid observer and subject bias (vol. 1, p. 3.5). The suggestion to a patient that a drug will alleviate his suffering is in itself an analgesic, as shown by the observation that 30 per cent of patients obtain relief from moderately severe postoperative pain when given a placebo alone. In such tests the subject's own impressions of the degrees of relief from pain are noted by trained observers and this can be reinforced by objective estimates of motor activity or autonomic responses. In comparing different analgesics in man, the effects on pain threshold should be distinguished from those on the reaction to pain. Other effects, pleasant or unpleasant, should be noted and also the time of onset and duration of activity. It is important to test new analgesics for their liability to produce addiction. Such tests can be carried out on primates.

Morphine (fig. 5.31)

This is the most widely used narcotic analgesic and is the standard against which others are compared. For this reason and because it illustrates the general features of all narcotic analgesics, it is dealt with at some length.

Morphine is a natural alkaloid extracted from opium which is the dried juice of the incised, unripe seed capsule of the poppy, *Papaver somniferum*. There are two main groups of alkaloids in opium, the **phenanthrenes** which include morphine (about 10 per cent), codeine (about 1 per cent), thebaine (about 0.5 per cent) and the **benzylisoquinolines** which include papaverine (about 1 per cent) and noscapine (narcotine) (about 2–8 per cent). Papaverine has no analgesic activity and is a powerful smooth muscle relaxant. However, it has been claimed that the effectiveness of 10 mg morphine is significantly potentiated by the prior administration of papaverine. This observation needs to be carefully reassessed since it is widely believed that there is no therapeutic advantage

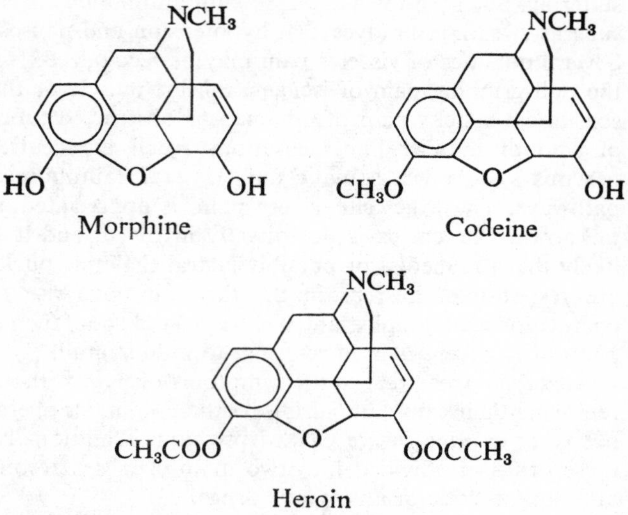

FIG. 5.31. Chemical structures of morphine, codeine and heroin. The two OH groups and the CH_3 group attached to the tertiary N atom are essential for the actions of morphine. Codeine is methyl morphine and heroin is diacetyl morphine. In apomorphine (p. 5.49) the O bridge and the internal N link are removed.

in using mixed alkaloid preparations from opium, such as **papaveretum** (omnopon).

CENTRAL ACTIONS

Homer records that, 'Helen presently cast a drug into the wine, whereof they drank, a drug to lull all pain and anger, and bring forgetfulness of every sorrow.' This concise statement of the action of morphia can be elaborated under seven headings. **Analgesia** is a constant feature in a variety of different species. It occurs without marked impairment of consciousness, sensitivity to touch, hearing or vision or of motor or intellectual function, which barbiturates and gaseous anaesthetics cause in equianalgesic doses. Morphine has only a modest effect on raising the pain threshold and is most effective when fear or anxiety accompanies natural or experimentally contrived pain; the mental distress caused by pain arises partly in memory and is aggravated by fear of its recurrence; morphine diminishes distress and thus acts principally on the affective component of pain.

Sedation and **drowsiness** or **sleep** occur even in healthy pain-free volunteers.

Euphoria and **relief from anxiety** occur readily and make morphine particularly attractive to unstable persons with a tendency to addiction. The combination of euphoric and sedative effects is of particular value in premedication before operations, in the treatment of very severe pain and in the dying. Rarely unpleasant feelings or dysphoria occur. In the case of the morphine antagonist nalorphine, dysphoric effects are sufficiently marked to prevent clinical use being made of its considerable analgesic potency (p. 5.52).

Tolerance to the analgesic, euphoric and respiratory depressant effects of morphine develop quite rapidly. In a few days larger doses may be required to produce the initial analgesic effect. This fact is often overlooked, and unnecessary suffering is caused by failure to recognize the requirements for increased doses in those with persisting severe pain. In addicts, the phenomenon of tolerance is seen on a grand scale so that large doses, e.g. sixty times the usual therapeutic dose, may be taken regularly. The mechanism of tolerance is unknown. It is thought to reside at a cellular level since the absorption, metabolism and excretion of morphine appear normal in tolerant subjects. There is, however, a marked reduction in the ability to *N*-demethylate morphine in the liver of addicted rats and this might conceivably occur also in the brain.

Addiction is the feature of narcotic analgesic drugs which gains them notoriety. Morphine and the other narcotic analgesic drugs are capable of inducing a state of physical and psychic dependence within a few days.

Respiratory centre depression occurs even with therapeutic doses of morphine, and the ventilatory response to CO_2 is reduced so that the alveolar P_{CO_2} rises and the respiratory minute volume falls. This depressant effect precedes the appearance of analgesia. In larger doses, morphine causes marked depression of respiratory rate, and ventilatory failure is the cause of death in acute morphine poisoning.

The **cough centre** is depressed. This antitussive effect is not due to the same part of the molecule as that responsible for analgesia, and it is possible to separate analgesic from antitussive activity. Dextromethorphan, which is the D-isomer of levorphan, is a useful antitussive but does not have the analgesic or addictive properties of levorphan (p. 9.4).

Other effects include constriction of the pupil (miosis) which is a characteristic action of morphine in man; but in species in which the excitant effects of morphine are more marked, e.g. the cat, dilation (mydriasis) occurs. Since tolerance does not develop to this effect, the pinpoint pupil is a useful diagnostic sign in the addict as it is in morphine overdosage in other subjects. The effect on the eye may be due to stimulation of the third cranial nerve nucleus as local application of morphine to the eye has no effect.

Nausea and perhaps vomiting may occur. However, this is more common in ambulant patients than in those confined to bed and suggests that stimulation of the vestibular apparatus or orthostatic hypotension are contributory causes. On the other hand, morphine may also stimulate the area postrema or chemoceptive trigger zone (CTZ) for vomiting. The observation that the morphine derivative, **apomorphine**, is a powerful stimulant of the CTZ in experimental animals supports this view. Morphine alters the equilibrium point of the heat regulating centre in the hypothalamus and lowers body temperature in some species, e.g. the dog, and to a slight extent in man. It stimulates the secretion of ADH by a direct effect on the supraoptic nucleus and inhibits the release of ACTH and pituitary gonadotrophic hormones. Hyperglycaemia from increased secretion of adrenaline also occurs occasionally from what is believed to be a central action.

The mechanism by which morphine produces its widespread CNS effects is unknown. There are, however, many interesting observations, the full significance of which will perhaps emerge when the roles of acetylcholine, 5-HT and noradrenaline as possible transmitter substances in the brain have been clarified. For instance, in some animals reserpine and α-methyltyrosine antagonize the analgesic effects of morphine. Morphine also reduces the release of noradrenaline from peripheral autonomic nerve endings, and antagonizes the effects of 5-HT on peripheral receptors, e.g. guinea-pig ileum, and in certain molluscan neurones. In some species where the excitant effects of morphine are marked, surprisingly it produces an elevation of brain homovanillic acid, a metabolite of dopamine. Morphine also reduces acetylcholine release from peripheral autonomic nerve endings and the cerebral cortex.

PERIPHERAL ACTIONS

In therapeutic doses, morphine causes constriction of smooth muscle tubes, thereby increasing the tone and decreasing the propulsive activity of hollow viscera. The consequences of this action are as follows:

(1) constipation (central disregard of defaecatory stimulation may also play a part),
(2) a rise in intrabiliary duct pressure,
(3) bronchospasm, and
(4) urinary retention.

Morphine is used extensively in the treatment of gastrointestinal, biliary and ureteric colic to relieve the pain; however, if a mechanical obstruction is present, e.g. calculus, morphine is likely to reduce the chances of it being passed naturally. Tolerance to the constricting effects of morphine on smooth muscle does not occur.

Morphine causes orthostatic hypotension, which may contribute to nausea and dizziness in the ambulant patient. The hypotension is mainly due to a peripheral action, possibly histamine release. Direct depression of the vasomotor centre plays little part.

The release of histamine by morphine is apparent with subcutaneous injections which may cause erythema and itching at the site of the injection. Occasionally the reaction is more general and the face becomes flushed.

MORPHINE POISONING

Accidental overdosage may occur in novices or in addicts

who have lost their tolerance. The person becomes comatose, develops severe respiratory depression and pinpoint pupils; hypodermic needle marks may help to suggest the diagnosis. These features are not specific for narcotic analgesics since pethidine overdosage does not cause pinpoint pupils. The importance however, in recognizing acute morphine overdosage is that a specific antidote, **nalorphine**, exists. A very small intravenous dose of nalorphine should be given initially to see if it reduces the respiratory depression. This guarded use of nalorphine is recommended for two reasons:

(1) in overdosage with narcotics, a large dose of nalorphine may precipitate a withdrawal state which is difficult to control, and

(2) when the respiratory depression is due to some other agent, e.g. a barbiturate, it may be aggravated by nalorphine (p. 5.53).

Chronic morphine intoxication occurs in the addict and is considered in vol. 3. Until recently in the United Kingdom, many young addicts obtained their initial supplies because of over-prescribing by practitioners to their existing addict patients. This has now been stopped by restricting the treatment of addicts to selected centres.

ABSORPTION, METABOLISM AND FATE
Morphine is absorbed irregularly from the small gut and is not given orally except to control diarrhoea (p. 10.6). When given by intramuscular injection it acts within a few minutes. It is not concentrated selectively in the CNS; it readily passes the placental barrier and is metabolized mainly by the liver, principally by conjugation with glucuronide. In man, the main route of excretion is via the kidney and though the clinical effects of morphine persist only for some 4–6 hours after the usual therapeutic dose (10 mg), excretion takes much longer; 90 per cent of the dose is usually excreted in the urine in the first 24 hours.

CLINICAL USE
Morphine is widely used as an analgesic on a short term basis in many conditions. It is standard treatment for the severe pain of a myocardial infarction and for the distressing breathlessness of acute left ventricular failure.

The usual analgesic dose of morphine sulphate is 10 mg given subcutaneously, intramuscularly or intravenously. This may be repeated in 4–6 hours, but the hazards of inducing tolerance and dependence should be remembered.

Given by mouth in small doses morphine is used in the treatment of diarrhoea in the form of a kaolin and morphine mixture, each dose containing about 1 mg morphine. Tolerance does not occur to the constipating effect. For chronic diarrhoea, codeine rather than morphine is frequently used (p. 10.6).

Morphine is a traditional premedication before anaesthesia (p. 5.69).

Morphine is a popular cough suppressant (antitussive), about 1 mg being given in the form of a linctus. Other narcotic analgesics, e.g. codeine, pholcodine and methadone, are also used as cough suppressants but synthetic nonanalgesic nonaddicting cough suppressants, e.g. dextromethorphan, are now available (p. 9.4).

CONTRAINDICATIONS
(1) Morphine and other narcotic analgesics should be used cautiously in those with chronic pain and whose life expectancy exceeds 6 months. In these circumstances, e.g. rheumatoid or osteoarthritis, there is real risk of addiction and/or tolerance.

(2) There is no advantage to be gained by giving morphine for severe recurrent pain, e.g. that of a peptic ulcer or angina, when other simpler measures are available.

(3) In general, the hasty administration of narcotic analgesics to allay pain before accurate diagnosis has been made is best avoided. Further, the repeated use of morphine subcutaneously to the shocked patient whose absorption from this site is poor might unwittingly give rise to overdose. Also, the use of morphine in patients with head injuries by altering the state of consciousness, the pupil size and by depressing respiration, may confuse the clinical picture from which the presence or extent of intracranial injury may be assessed.

(4) Morphine should be avoided in patients where bronchospasm is the primary feature, e.g. bronchial asthma. A combination of histamine release and morphine-induced bronchospasm may be fatal in an asthmatic patient. The respiratory depression induced by morphine is dangerous in patients with chronic respiratory insufficiency.

(5) Morphine is best avoided in biliary colic as it may precipitate acute pancreatitis, and it should not be used to control the pain of acute pancreatitis.

(6) Morphine should be avoided when certain brain, eye or abdominal operations are contemplated in which postoperative vomiting is likely.

(7) Because morphine readily passes the placental barrier it is best avoided as an analgesic in childbirth.

(8) Morphine and pethidine should be used with care in patients receiving MAO inhibitors (p. 5.22).

Codeine

Codeine is a naturally occurring phenanthrene alkaloid found in opium. Chemically, it is the 3-methylether of morphine (fig. 5.31). The range of activity of codeine resembles that of morphine. However, on a weight-for-weight basis, it is less potent and this has given rise to confusion over its advantages and disadvantages with respect to analgesia, addictive hazard, respiratory depression and constipation. Codeine is one-twelfth as potent an analgesic as morphine; 120 mg codeine is equianalgesic with 10 mg of morphine. At this dose, respiratory depression, constipation and tolerance occur. Codeine can partially suppress morphine withdrawal symptoms and cross-tolerance between codeine and other narcotic analgesics occurs. Psychic dependence on codeine can be demonstrated in monkeys. With frequent use of large doses in man, physical dependence can be produced and withdrawal symptoms are similar to, though less intense than those produced by morphine. Thus, like morphine, codeine is potentially a drug of addiction and the precise reasons why few become addicts are not known. It is possible, however, that its reputation for low potency plays a part, and it appears to be less euphoriant than morphine.

Codeine is traditionally used in lower doses that are not equianalgesic with 10 mg morphine. Thus a dose of 60 mg is effective against moderately severe pain. It is often prescribed in fixed dose analgesic mixtures, e.g. containing codeine (8 mg) acetylsalycylic acid (250 mg) and phenacetin (250 mg). Codeine is also used as an antitussive agent but effective nonnarcotic antitussives exist and should be used in preference. It is popular as a symptomatic remedy in acute diarrhoea and colic (p.10.6). Codeine has less sedative effect than morphine, and in large doses it may produce behavioural excitement due to central stimulation.

Codeine is given by mouth in doses of 30–60 mg. It is about one-third as effective when given orally as when given parenterally, whereas morphine is only about one-tenth as effective orally.

Derivatives of the opium alkaloids

Heroin or diacetylmorphine (diamorphine) is synthesized from morphine by acetylation of both the phenolic and alcoholic OH groups (fig. 5.31). On a weight-for-weight basis, it is more potent than morphine but in equianalgesic doses, trials have failed to show that it has significantly different effects in terms of respiratory depression, euphoria or sedation. It is possible that heroin posesses fewer adverse effects, e.g. nausea and vomiting, than morphine, and it has a smaller effect in depressing the blood pressure when used in the management of myocardial infarction, but these advantages have not yet been clearly established. There is no compelling reason why heroin should be used in clinical practice and indeed, it has been prohibited by law from medical use in the USA. The World Health Organization has advocated a total ban on the manufacture of heroin and many countries are following this advice. Objections to this policy are based on subjective clinical impressions that it is superior to morphine or other narcotics.

Though heroin is used extensively by addicts and

5

accorded journalistic pride of place as a drug of addiction, addicts are often unable to distinguish between heroin and morphine when both are given by subcutaneous injection though they may do so when given intravenously, probably on account of heroin's more rapid action which is perhaps related to its higher lipid solubility. In many trials, however, addicts have not expressed a preference for heroin over morphine, even when given intravenously, though some claim that heroin produces a unique orgiastic sensation. One can only assume that the addictive popularity of heroin is a reflection of its potency on a weight basis and extensive 'advertising'.

The usual dose of heroin hydrochloride is 5–10 mg by subcutaneous or intravenous injection.

Levorphanol (dromoran) is the 3-hydroxy derivative of *N*-methylmorphinan. It is more potent than morphine with a similar range of activity and is readily absorbed by mouth. Its D-isomer (**dextromethorphan**) is neither analgesic nor addictive, but is a useful antitussive (p. 9.4).

Levorphanol

Oxymorphone (dihydroxymorphinone) is a semisynthetic derivative of morphine. The equianalgesic dose is five times less than that of morphine. It is less constipating but respiratory depression may be more marked.

Dihydrocodeine (DF118) possesses about one-third of the analgesic activity of morphine but has more serious adverse effects when the dose is elevated. Other semisynthetic compounds include **dihydromorphinone** (dilaudid), **methyl dihydromorphinone** (metapon) and **pholcodine** or β-morphinylethyl morphine (p. 9.4).

Of particular interest because of their extraordinary potency are a series of experimental narcotic analgesics e.g. M 99 or **etorphine** and M 183. These substances have a very similar structure to that of **thebaine**, the third major phenanthrene alkaloid of opium (fig. 5.32). In mice, M 183 is about 1500 times more potent an analgesic than morphine, while M 99 is about 1300 times more potent.

Synthetic analgesics (fig. 5.33)

Pethidine (meperidine) is a phenylpiperidine and was developed during a study of synthetic atropine-like antispasmodic compounds. In general, its actions resemble those of morphine and it causes analgesia presumably by

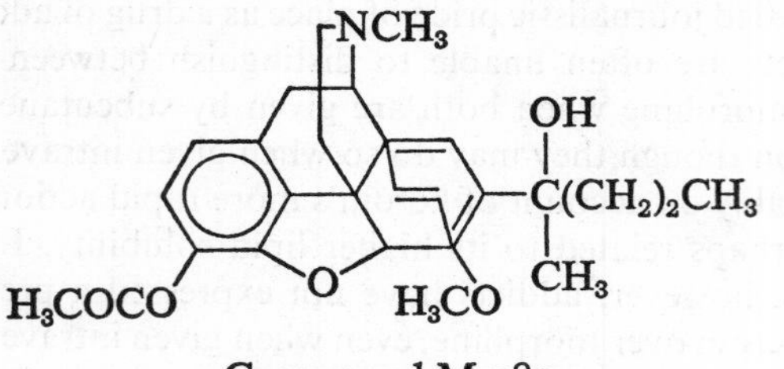

Compound M 183

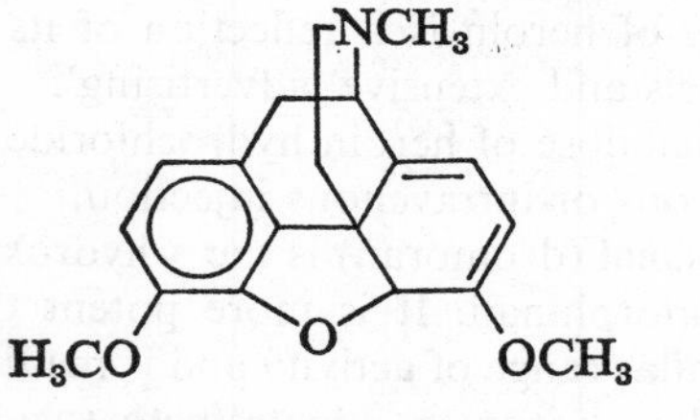

Thebaine

FIG. 5.32. Thebaine and compound M183.

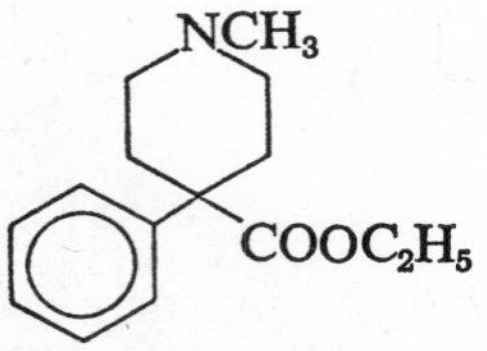

Pethidine

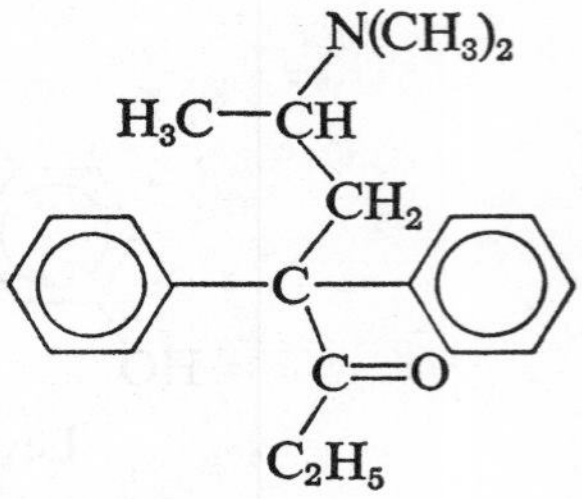

Methadone

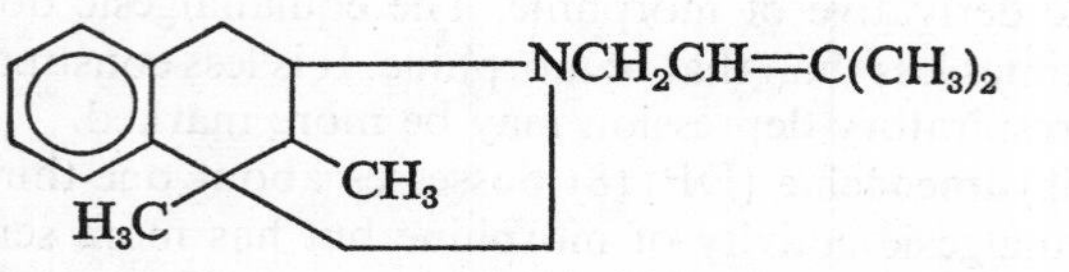

Pentazocine

FIG. 5.33. Some synthetic morphine-like analgesics.

the same mechanism. It is less potent on a weight basis than morphine but in equianalgesic doses (100 mg) it causes a similar degree of sedation, euphoria and respiratory depression. Nevertheless it is not a complete substitute for morphine in addicts and tolerance develops more slowly, but addiction may occur and constitute a social problem. Unlike morphine pethidine does not constrict the pupils; in fact, mydriasis may be seen. In therapeutic doses, pethidine is less antitussive than comparable doses of morphine.

In equianalgesic doses, smooth muscle is less affected by pethidine than by morphine and constipation and bronchospasm are uncommon. This may be due merely

to a shorter duration of action. Pethidine also increases intrabiliary pressure and causes orthostatic hypotension, probably due to histamine release. Pethidine is well absorbed from the gut, metabolized in the liver and the products of metabolism excreted in the urine. The excretion is increased in acid urine.

Its short action makes it preferable to morphine in obstetrics or for diagnostic procedures. Given as the hydrochloride either orally or intramuscularly in doses of 50–100 mg, its effects last 3–4 hours.

Methadone (physeptone) is similar to morphine in its effects but is about three times more potent as an analgesic. It has less sedative activity than morphine and is effective when given by mouth in doses of 5–10 mg. Addiction to methadone also occurs but is less severe.

D-**Propoxyphene** (doloxene) is related to methadone and is of the same order of potency as codeine but is less constipating and has fewer central effects. It is given orally in doses of 50–100 mg; addictive liability is small.

Phenazocine is five times as potent as morphine and more prolonged in its action. It has no advantage over morphine in its addictive or other effects.

Etonitazone, a benzimidazole, is of particular interest as it is much more potent an analgesic than morphine. Indeed, in mice, it may be several thousand times as potent though the ratio is smaller in man.

Pentazocine is described on p. 5.53.

Narcotic antagonists

These are substances which specifically counteract the main actions of the narcotic analgesics. They include nalorphine, levallorphan, pentazocine and cyclazocine.

NALORPHINE (*N*-allylnormorphine)

When given to nonaddicts and in the absence of other narcotic drugs, the effects of nalorphine resemble those of morphine. Ten to 15 mg of nalorphine given subcutaneously produce the same degree of analgesia as 10

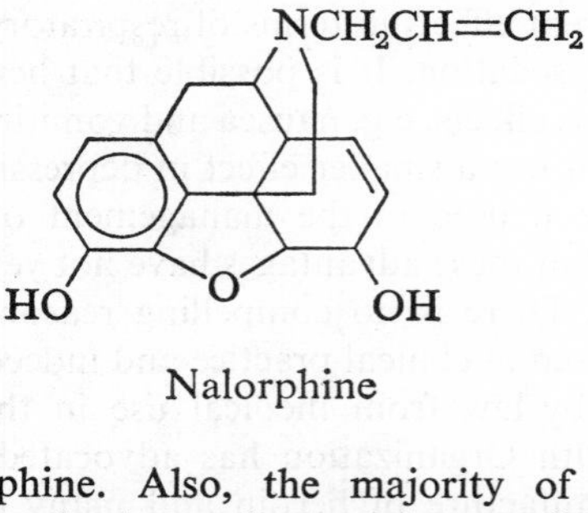

Nalorphine

mg of morphine. Also, the majority of nonaddicts experience euphoria and drowsiness with analgesic doses of nalorphine. However, a small number of people show dysphoria and complain of malaise, anxiety, nausea and visual hallucinations. Because of these effects nalorphine does not find favour as an analgesic for therapeutic use.

Nalorphine is a rapid and highly specific antagonist of morphine and other narcotics, being effective in antagonizing the respiratory depression. It also antagonizes the euphoriant, sedative and miotic effects of morphine. While nalorphine itself is an analgesic, when given with morphine, it reverses the analgesia to a variable extent. Nalorphine is not an analeptic, and as it may cause mild respiratory depression in some circumstances it is not used in the treatment of barbiturate overdosage.

Nalorphine is poorly absorbed by mouth and is administered parenterally. Its action lasts between 1 and 3 hours; it is conjugated in the liver, and excretion by the kidney may be complete within 4 hours.

Nalorphine is given intravenously to relieve narcotic-induced respiratory depression. Five to 10 mg may be given to the nonaddict suffering from the depressant effects of morphine and this can be repeated up to a total of 40 mg. In addicts, the initial dose of nalorphine should not exceed one tenth of this amount to avoid provoking a withdrawal reaction. It is useful in the treatment of respiratory depression in the newborn, arising as a result of administration of a narcotic analgesic to the mother.

Nalorphine is a useful laboratory tool. If its administration to an animal receiving a new analgesic causes withdrawal symptoms, it is likely that the new drug is an addictive hazard.

LEVALLORPHAN

This is the *N*-allyl derivative of levorphanol and is related structurally to it as nalorphine is to morphine. It is similar to nalorphine in its actions but is more active, the dose being 1–2 mg.

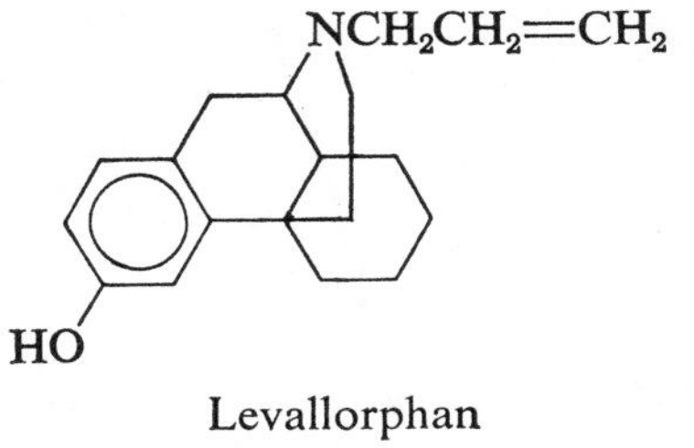

$NCH_2CH_2{=}CH_2$

HO

Levallorphan

PENTAZOCINE (fig. 5.33)

Pentazocine (fortral) is a benzmorphan derivative and is a narcotic antagonist. Its importance, however, lies in the fact that it is as effective as morphine in controlling severe pain and is believed to be without addictive properties. One-third of patients show sedation with pentazocine though it is less marked than with equianalgesic doses of morphine. Respiratory depression, nausea and vomiting are also less marked. Euphoria and tolerance do not occur. Pentazocine is probably safer than morphine for other reasons since the margin between therapeutic and lethal dose is greater. Though the sphincter of Oddi is stimulated, smooth muscle elsewhere is little affected as judged by the absence of constipation and urinary retention in clinical trials. The usual dose is 30 mg given intramuscularly; analgesia occurs between 15 and 30 mins and lasts 3–4 hours. As a narcotic antagonist, pentazocine has only 1/50th potency of nalorphine, so care should be taken in administering it to addicts. Pentazocine may well replace morphine in many of its applications.

Non-narcotic analgesics and analgesic antipyretics

These may be divided into three groups:

(1) salicylates including acetylsalicylic acid (aspirin),

(2) paraminophenol derivatives including phenacetin and paracetamol, and

(3) pyrazolone derivatives including phenylbutazone and oxyphenylbutazone.

The chemical structures of these compounds are shown in fig. 5.34.

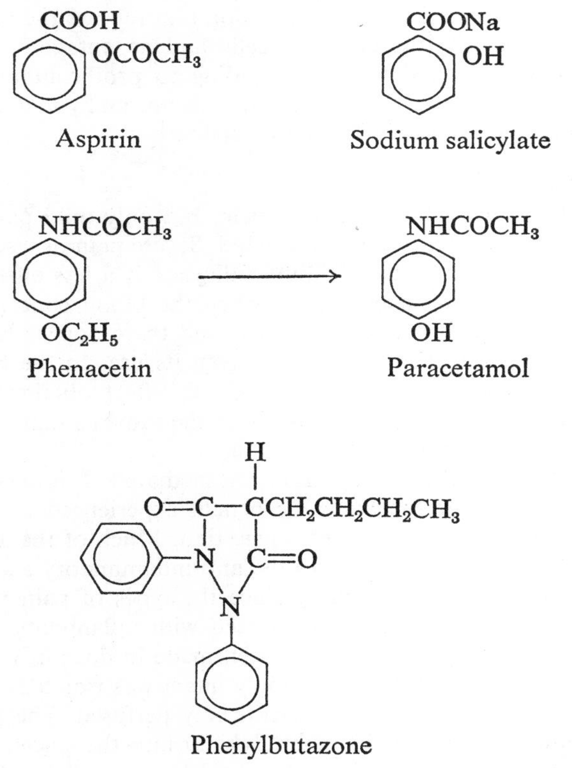

COOH $OCOCH_3$

Aspirin

COONa   OH

Sodium salicylate

$NHCOCH_3$ OC_2H_5

Phenacetin

$\longrightarrow$

$NHCOCH_3$ OH

Paracetamol

Phenylbutazone

FIG. 5.34. Chemical structure of non-narcotic analgesics and antipyretics.

SALICYLATES

The willow bark (*Salix alba*) was a traditional remedy for fevers but unlike the Peruvian bark, which contains quinine, it was not specific for malaria. The active principle was the glycoside, **salicin**, which on hydrolysis yields glucose and salicyl alcohol. In 1838, salicylic acid (*O*-hydroxybenzoic acid) was first prepared from the alcohol but later, after the discovery of phenol in 1860, it was made synthetically. It was not until 1875 that sodium salicylate came to be used as an antipyretic and, shortly after, as an effective remedy in the symptomatic treatment of acute rheumatic fever, where reduction of pain and swelling in joints represents the anti-inflammatory action of the drug. In 1879, sodium salicylate was found to increase the urinary excretion of uric acid and so began its use in the treatment of gout. In 1899, the acetyl ester of salicylic acid was introduced as the first solid preparation of the drug. It came at a time when machines were being invented for dispensing drugs as tablets. The new drug was named 'aspirin' from *spirsäure* (German, salicylic acid), which is also found in the free state in the buds of *Spiraea ulmaria*. Today, aspirin is a household word and the world annual consumption of the drug is measured in thousands of tons. Salicylates act on the CNS as antipyretics and analgesics, on cellular metabolism by uncoupling oxidation from phosphorylation and in other ways, as inhibitors of the reaction that follows the union of antigen with sensitized cells and as antagonists of vitamin K in the liver so leading to prothrombin deficiency and bleeding. Their actions are many and complex and even now poorly understood.

Analgesic activity (fig. 5.35)

This is a useful effect of aspirin, but only mild pain in superficial structures is alleviated. Severe pain or visceral pain is not affected. Sodium salicylate is a less effective analgesic than aspirin even when the blood concentrations of salicylate are identical and there appear to be few advantages to be gained from its use. In the relief of postoperative pain the analgesic effect obtained by 600 mg of aspirin orally is about the same as that given by 30 or even 60 mg of codeine.

How are these analgesic effects mediated? It is possible that some of the analgesic benefit experienced in self-medication is due to autosuggestion. Much of the analgesic effect may be due to the anti-inflammatory actions of salicylates, particularly since the types of pain most effectively relieved are associated with inflammation or oedema. Experiments have been made in dogs in which the spleen with its nerve supply intact was isolated from the main circulation and artificially perfused. The pain induced by injections of bradykinin into the spleen was prevented by injection of salicylates into the splenic circulation, but not if it was injected systemically, though by this route it could reach the brain. Using experi-

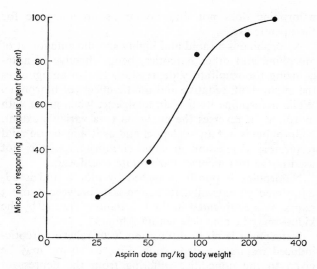

FIG. 5.35. Analgesic effect of aspirin in different doses to the subcutaneous injection of a noxious chemical. After Collier H.O.J. (1963) *Sci. Amer.* Offprint 169.

mental pain in man in which there is very little inflammatory component, various studies show little or no elevation of pain threshold by aspirin. Similarly, in animals, the best procedures for assessing the potency of non-narcotic analgesics are those which have a substantial component of inflammation.

Antipyretic activity

In therapeutic doses, salicylates have no effect on normal body temperature, but they rapidly reduce body temperature raised in disease, i.e. salicylates are antipyretic (fig. 5.36). Where the temperature is raised physiologically

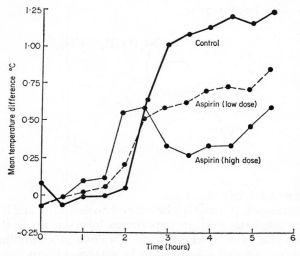

FIG. 5.36. Antipyretic effect of aspirin. Rise in temperature of rabbits treated with pyrogen and aspirin. Low dose 22 mg aspirin/kg; high dose 67 mg aspirin/kg. After Collier H.O.J. (1963) *Sci. Amer.* Offprint 169.

e.g. by working in hot environments, salicylates are without effect. The temperature regulating centres lie in the hypothalamus and it seems likely that salicylates act on this site. Local intracerebral applications of salicylates may provoke heat loss by inducing vasodilation and sweating, and hypothalamic lesions have been shown to prevent the antipyretic effect of salicylates. In toxic doses, salicylates cause pyrexia in normal subjects, a consequence of metabolic stimulation and increased heat production.

Anti-inflammatory activity

The most successful uses of salicylates are in the treatment of inflammatory processes. One of the most important actions of salicylates is to reduce the increased capillary permeability that occurs in inflammation. Salicylates inhibit paw oedema in rats following injection of 5-HT, histamine, dextran or foreign protein. The increased vascular permeability produced by bradykinin is not blocked, though the pain response which it evokes is. Dye leakage experiments show that the increased capillary and venular permeability induced by histamine injection or local antigen–antibody reactions is blocked by salicylates. Salicylates are also effective against a variety of experimental immunological phenomena and when given in large doses, suppress antibody production and interfere with antigen–antibody aggregation. Salicylates are widely used in the treatment of acute rheumatic fever; and some of the symptoms of this disease, malaise, fever and some of the signs, polyarthritis, visceral effusions and a raised ESR, are suppressed. Unfortunately, the worst aspects of acute rheumatic fever, i.e. the development and progression of carditis, are unaffected. The role of salicylates and other drugs in influencing the inflammatory response is discussed further on p. 24.7.

Gastrointestinal effects

With repeated administration of aspirin, epigastric discomfort and exacerbation of ulcer symptoms may occur. Blood loss from the gastrointestinal tract occurs in about 70 per cent of patients but is rarely severe (1.5–3 g Hb/day) and is usually unnoticed by patients. However, a high proportion of ulcer patients who develop major gastrointestinal haemorrhage give a history of recent aspirin ingestion. The cause of aspirin lesions in the stomach is not known. Local irritation by insoluble particles is likely and crystals may be seen in the mucosal folds of the stomach in the region of the lesion with areas of haemorrhage surrounding them. Even the application of buffered aspirin tablets to the buccal mucosa may cause local tissue damage, but local irritation is not the complete explanation since in dogs and rats, gastric mucosal lesions may follow the parenteral administration. The concentration of acetylsalicylate anion in the gastric mucosal cells and capillary endothelial cells may be the damaging factor. Gastric irritation can be reduced by lowering the concentration of non-ionized aspirin, by reducing particle formation or by enhancing the rate of passage of drug from the stomach to the intestine. The ingestion of aspirin in an alkaline fluid to raise the gastric pH generally meets these aims. At the normal pH of gastric juice, aspirin is poorly soluble and may be slow to dissolve, but the fraction in solution is poorly ionized and is quickly absorbed.

Respiratory stimulation

Therapeutic doses of salicylates i.e. 8–10 g/day which yield blood concentrations of approximately 35 mg/100 ml are usually associated with hyperventilation in man. At first, there is an increase in the depth rather than in the rate of respiration. The factors responsible for this and other disturbances in acid base composition of the body fluids are described on p. 9.3.

Metabolic effects

Salicylates act on the mitochondria to prevent the formation of ATP and to quicken the rate of its destruction. On the one hand, they uncouple oxidative phosphorylation, possibly by competing with NAD; on the other, they stimulate adenosine triphosphatase activity. As a result, many ATP dependent reactions in the body are inhibited and energy of oxidation which would normally be transferred to phosphate bonds in ATP is instead dissipated as heat. Thus, in the presence of high concentration of salicylates, mitochondrial oxidation proceeds at a faster rate, oxygen consumption and CO_2 production are increased; these effects may explain the rise in body temperature which occurs in man or animals after large doses.

In large doses, salicylates have other important effects. The daily loss of amino acids in the urine increases 10–100 fold and the nitrogen balance becomes negative. Increased protein catabolism, reduced incorporation of amino acids into proteins and failure in the renal transport of amino acids contribute to the amino aciduria.

In man and animals large doses of salicylates cause hyperglycaemia, glycosuria and depletion of muscle and liver glycogen. In certain diabetic patients, toxic doses of salicylates may lower blood sugar and reduce glycosuria. Full therapeutic doses of salicylates also inhibit fatty acid synthesis and lower both plasma phospholipid and cholesterol levels. Salicylates in large doses reduce the plasma prothrombin level. Animals on diets low in vitamin K are more susceptible to this action and it is possible that salicylates compete with vitamin K for a receptor site on enzymes in the liver responsible for the synthesis of prothrombin and other coagulation factors. Care should be exercised in the use of salicylates in those with abnormal liver function. The uricosuric effect of salicylates is only seen with doses in excess of 5 g/day.

It is mainly due to the inhibition of renal tubular absorption of uric acid. In smaller doses, however, salicylates may actually raise the serum uric acid due to the selective inhibition of tubular secretion. For this reason aspirin is not used therapeutically to reduce the serum uric acid in gout and even in small doses may offset the benefit of potent uricosuric agents, like probenecid.

In the treatment of rheumatic disorders salicylates are usually employed in doses that are limited by the appearance of adverse effects. The high concentration attained in body fluid is maintained for days or weeks. Since the salicylates are as effective as corticosteroids in the control of rheumatic symptoms, it might be supposed that they act centrally, through the release of ACTH, to increase the output of adrenocortical hormones. There is, however, no clear evidence that they act in this way, and it is probable that their metabolic effects are due mainly to a direct action on cells.

Adverse effects
Mild symptoms of toxicity or salicylism frequently occur when salicylates are given in high doses, e.g. in the treatment of acute rheumatic fever. Typically, salicylism includes headache, dizziness, tinnitus or ringing in the ears, high tone deafness, visual disturbances, mental confusion and drowsiness. Hyperventilation, nausea and vomiting due to the central effects may be seen. Salicylism in itself does not represent a major hazard except in children in whom serious toxicity occurs.

Severe salicylate intoxication is an acute medical emergency which may be lethal. This may occur in self poisoning or accidentally. Very young children are particularly prone to aspirin poisoning from fond and unsuspecting parents administering overlarge fractions of adult tablets to them. The clinical picture is more severe than salicylism. Vomiting, hyperventilation, confusion, delirium, hyperpyrexia or severe prostration occur. Respiratory alkalosis and metabolic acidosis also develop (p. 9.3). In young children, metabolic acidosis is particularly severe. Hyperglycaemia and ketonuria are also seen.

In the management of severe salicylate poisoning, intravenous infusion of isotonic $NaHCO_3$ and mannitol are useful in increasing the rate of elimination of salicylate in the urine and in some cases haemodialysis is needed.

The incidence of hypersensitivity to salicylate in the general population may be as high as 0·2 per cent which is important in view of the vast consumption of aspirin. It is much more common in asthmatic subjects in whom small doses may cause urticaria, bronchospasm, angioneurotic oedema or anaphylactic shock.

Absorption, distribution and fate
Salicylates are absorbed from the stomach and small intestine. Appreciable blood concentrations may be found 30 min after the oral ingestion of a single 600 mg dose but the peak plasma levels may not occur for 2 hours. Aspirin is rapidly hydrolysed to salicylic acid in plasma and in the tissues. Salicylates are evenly distributed throughout body water, and as with the majority of drugs, selective distribution is not the basis for its therapeutic effects. Brain concentrations of salicylate are low and it does not accumulate in inflammatory effusions. The bulk of the salicylate in plasma is combined with plasma albumin, and salicylates compete with thyroxine and triiodothyronine for binding sites. Thus, plasma bound iodine (PBI) falls, serum thyroxine rises and ^{131}I uptake by the thyroid is actually depressed. Only a proportion of the salicylate administered is metabolized. This occurs in many tissues but particularly in the liver. The main metabolites are salicylic acid, phenolic and acyl glucuronides and a small proportion as di- and tri-hydroxybenzoic acid. The metabolites constitute only a small fraction of the total plasma salicylates. Excretion is mainly via the kidney but the process is so slow that only half of a given dose is excreted in 24 hours. The proportion of free salicylic acid excreted in the urine varies greatly depending on the amount of nonionic renal tubular reabsorption (p. 2.15). About 10 per cent of the oral dose may be excreted in acid urines, while in alkaline urines, some 80 per cent of the dose may appear.

Clinical uses
Aspirin is widely used as an analgesic for headache and other minor aches and pains, a single dose of 600 mg often being sufficient. In colds and 'flu, where there is also fever, its analgesic and antipyretic properties are valuable. Aspirin is one of the most valuable drugs in the treatment of acute rheumatic fever, where it is given for several weeks.

Aspirin administration should be avoided in asthmatics, in patients with known or suspected peptic ulcer and in patients receiving anticoagulants.

Aspirin is available in pure form or as soluble calcium aspirin (disprin), which may reduce the incidence of gastric erosions. Aspirin is also available in various fixed dose drug mixtures, e.g. aspirin and phenacetin, or aspirin and codeine; all aspirin-containing tablets should be kept dry in storage to avoid decomposition.

Other antipyretic analgesics
PHENACETIN AND PARACETAMOL (fig. 5.34)
These are the only two aminophenol derivatives in current use, all other derivatives, e.g. acetanalid and amidopyrine having been discontinued because of toxicity.

In therapeutic doses (about 600 mg) phenacetin and paracetamol appear equally effective in relieving mild pain for 3–4 hours. The analgesic effect is similar to that of aspirin. Some studies show that the pain threshold is raised, but severe somatic or visceral pain is not affected. Like the salicylates, aminophenol derivatives are potent anti-inflammatory and analgesic agents. However, in comparison with salicylates they have little effect on antigen-antibody reactions (p. 5.55).

In a few individuals, phenacetin may induce feelings of euphoria and relaxation or feelings of drowsiness. These effects encourage mild psychic dependence and habit formation but not physical dependence.

In contrast to the salicylates, therapeutic doses of phenacetin and paracetamol do not affect the respiratory centre, change acid base balance or cause gastrointestinal irritation. However, they lower adrenal ascorbic acid in laboratory animals like the salicylates and the pyrazolones.

Adverse effects
Adverse effects are more severe with phenacetin than with paracetamol. This may be partly due to the presence of a contaminant, 4-chloroacetanalide. Cyanosis may develop due to the formation of methaemoglobin and sulphaemoglobin.

Haemolytic anaemia may occur with long continued ingestion of both drugs. The lowered concentrations of NAD and reduced glutathione make the red cells susceptible to injury by drugs or substances produced in normal metabolic processes, and thereby shorten red cell survival. A haemolytic anaemia also occurs due to hypersensitivity and in individuals with genetically determined deficiency of glucose-6-phosphate dehydrogenase (p. 31.10).

Chronic renal failure may occur in individuals consuming large doses of analgesics containing phenacetin and salicylates over long periods of time. All the constituents of the popular analgesic mixtures including salicylates and caffeine can cause renal lesions in experimental animals and it is not certain which constituent is responsible for the renal disease in man. Skin reactions may occur with long continued ingestion. Poisoning with large doses of paracetamol may lead to hepatic necrosis.

Absorption, metabolism and fate
The absorption of both compounds from the gastrointestinal tract is rapid and nearly complete. About 25 per cent of the compound in the blood is combined with plasma protein. After a single dose of paracetamol peak plasma levels are achieved in 0·5–1 hour, earlier than with phenacetin. Seven hours after an oral dose, these compounds are virtually undetectable in the circulation. Phenacetin is de-ethylated largely in the liver to form paracetamol, though it possesses analgesic properties of its own. Paracetamol is conjugated in the liver, a small proportion is deacetylated to oxidizing substances like

p-aminophenol which may then cause methaemoglobinaemia.

Paracetamol is preferred to phenacetin; it acts more quickly and has fewer unwanted effects. It is a useful alternative analgesic to aspirin when hypersensitivity or gastritis are troublesome. Paracetamol is inferior to aspirin when inflammation is present.

PYRAZOLONE DERIVATIVES
Phenylbutazone (butazolidin) and oxyphenbutazone (tanderil) are too dangerous to be used as routine analgesics or antipyretics. Their use is confined almost solely to conditions where joints are painful and/or inflamed.

Phenylbutazone has little pure analgesic effect; however, where pain is associated with inflammation, it is more effective than the salicylates, and approaches the efficacy of the corticosteroids. The basis of its anti-inflammatory action is probably similar to that of the salicylates, i.e. it counteracts increases in vascular permeability (p. 24.7). Though phenylbutazone displaces the glucocorticoids from their plasma protein binding sites and might act via the potentiation of adrenal steroids, its anti-inflammatory effects are seen in adrenalectomized animals.

As with the salicylates, small doses of phenylbutazone may raise the serum uric acid due to an initial inhibition of uric acid renal tubular secretion, while larger doses depress the serum uric acid by preventing tubular reabsorption. A derivative of phenylbutazone, **sulphinpyrazone,** is a potent uricosuric agent used in the treatment of chronic gout; though it lacks the anti-inflammatory and analgesic properties of phenylbutazone, it is less toxic and does not cause salt and water retention.

In therapeutic doses, phenylbutazone causes salt and water retention, the mechanism for which is unknown. Peripheral oedema occurs and increased plasma volume may give rise to a dilution anaemia. Acute pulmonary oedema or congestive heart failure may be precipitated.

Like the salicylates, phenylbutazone is strongly bound to the plasma proteins, and consequently displaces thyroxine. Oxidative phosphorylation is also uncoupled by phenylbutazone though metabolism is stimulated less than by salicylates. Several active transport mechanisms in the kidney are competitively inhibited so that renal tubular transport of PAH and PAS is diminished.

Phenylbutazone is rapidly and completely absorbed after an oral dose from the gastrointestinal tract so that peak blood concentrations occur in 2 hours. Curiously, however, the absorption of phenylbutazone after an intramuscular injection is slower than with oral administration. The transformation of phenylbutazone is very slow, about 20 per cent/day, so that the half-life of a single dose is about 3 days in man. Very little phenylbutazone appears unchanged in the urine and most of the metabolites are unknown. About 4 per cent of phenylbutazone is converted to oxyphenbutazone and this compound is used sometimes as an alternative to phenylbutazone though if anything, it appears to be more toxic.

Clinical uses of phenylbutazone

Phenylbutazone is used in painful chronic joint diseases after other less toxic remedies have been tried, but should not be used in patients with peptic ulcer or ischaemic heart disease in view of the adverse effects. These are seen in one form or another in about 20 per cent of patients and may be dangerous. The most common are salt and water retention, and gastric irritation. Blood dyscrasias, thrombocytopenia and purpura are less common, but unfortunately occur sometimes even with low doses and after short exposure to the drug. Gastric irritation is diminished by dividing the oral dose which should seldom exceed 400 mg/day.

ANTICONVULSANT DRUGS

Epilepsy is a disease characterized by paroxysmal electrical disturbances in the brain. These recur at intervals and are often accompanied by loss of consciousness, disturbance of sensation or behaviour and sometimes by involuntary movements or convulsions. High frequency electrical discharges begin in a small area or seizure focus; these may then spread to normal tissue to involve the entire brain. A disturbance in the EEG is usually seen. Epilepsy occurs in about 0·5 per cent of the population and several main varieties exist. **Grand mal epilepsy** characterized by major convulsions, alone or in association with petit mal or psychomotor epilepsy, accounts for nearly 75 per cent of all cases. Of the remainder, **psychomotor epilepsy**, characterized by attacks of confused behaviour, accounts for about 15 per cent of cases, and **petit mal**, in which brief periods of loss of consciousness occur, for about 10 per cent. **Focal epilepsy** is used to describe the condition in which the abnormality is confined to localized sensory disturbances or convulsions which involve only limbs or some muscle groups. The clinical features of these and other types of epilepsy are described in vol. 3. *Status epilepticus* consists of persisting or recurring generalized convulsions. However, the different varieties of epilepsy respond to different drugs and these are now described (table 5.6).

Drugs capable of controlling the tonic phase of grand mal may be assessed by estimating the power to control convulsions induced with high frequency stimulation in rodents. Drugs used in petit mal and psychomotor epilepsy may be assessed against the clonic convulsions induced by leptazol or against the temporary behavioural arrest induced by low frequency stimulation

of the rat brain. Specially bred strains of mice in which convulsions are induced by sound (audiogenic seizures) may also be employed; alternatively the local application of a variety of chemical substances, e.g. penicillin or cobalt can be used to induce cortical or subcortical lesions and seizures in animals. At present, however, seizure-prone animals have not been widely used in the investigation of anticonvulsant drugs.

The investigation of anticonvulsants in man poses difficult ethical and technical problems; the decision to withdraw satisfactory therapy from a patient who is leading a full and useful social life and subject him to an unknown drug is not easily taken. It may also be misleading to assess new anticonvulsant drugs by giving them to chronic epileptic patients who are often resistant to therapy.

PHENOBARBITONE

This is a widely used, potent and cheap anticonvulsant which is effective in grand mal and focal epilepsy. However, psychomotor epilepsy and petit mal occurring with grand mal epilepsy are unaffected or may even be aggravated. In therapeutic doses it is a more specific anticonvulsant than other barbiturates.

Phenobarbitone

The administration of phenobarbitone for the treatment of epilepsy may continue for years and systemic toxicity is small. Skin rashes occur in about 2 per cent of patients. Although phenobarbitone is often the first drug given to children with 'fits', this is probably unwise. Children often become irritable with this drug and petit mal, which is more common at this age, may be made worse.

In the treatment of epilepsy in the adult the correct dose

TABLE 5.6. Main drugs used in the treatment of epilepsy

Type of epilepsy	Drug treatment
Grand mal Psychomotor	Phenobarbitone, phenytoin, primidone
epilepsy	Primidone, phenytoin, ethosuximide
Petit mal	Ethosuximide, tridione
Status epilepticus	Phenobarbitone or amylobarbitone IV, paraldehyde IM, phenytoin sodium IV, or general anaesthetics, either volatile or thiobarbiturates

is that which controls the fits with minimum side effects. This is usually from 100–200 mg/day.

Alternatives include **methylphenobarbitone** and **methbarbitone,** which are converted to phenobarbitone in the body.

PRIMIDONE (MYSOLINE)

This is a congener of phenobarbitone in which the oxygen in the urea group is replaced by two atoms of hydrogen. It is mainly used for the treatment of grand mal but is also effective against petit mal. Drowsiness, nausea, ataxia and dizziness are common initially but decline with continued treatment. Other unwanted effects are oedema, skin rashes, psychosis, impotence, leukopenia

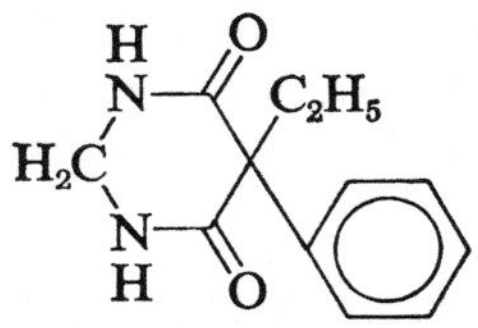

Primidone

and megaloblastic anaemia which responds to folic acid. About 20 per cent of primidone is converted to phenobarbitone, the remainder is degraded via other pathways. Primidone is seldom given alone; it is best used as an alternative to phenobarbitone since severe drowsiness results if the two drugs are given together. The dose of primidone is between 0·5 g and 2·0 g/day.

PHENYTOIN (EPANUTIN)

This is diphenylhydantoin and has a five membered ring structure which closely resembles the six membered broad ring structure of phenobarbitone. It is highly fat soluble.

In contrast to phenobarbitone, it has little sedative or depressant effect when given in full anticonvulsant doses and large doses are not hypnotic. Grand mal and psychomotor epilepsy are controlled, but petit mal is unaffected and the frequency of attacks may be increased.

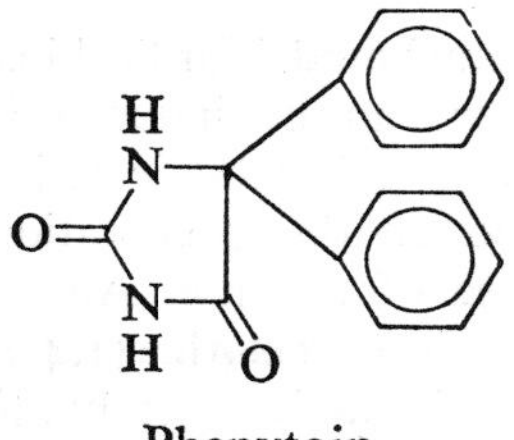

Phenytoin

Unfortunately therapeutic effects are often achieved only with doses near to the upper limit of tolerance; thus adverse effects are common, and include ataxia, tremor, slurred speech, nystagmus and diplopia; they may be accompanied by irritability or infrequently by apathy and drowsiness. Peripheral effects include hyperplasia of the gums which is especially common in children. Hirsutes also occurs and may be troublesome in female patients. Macrocytosis with or without a megaloblastic marrow picture is uncommon but responds promptly to folic acid. Sodium phenytoin is alkaline and may cause gastric irritation with pain, nausea and vomiting. In some cases, enlargement of the liver, spleen and lymph nodes occurs with fever. These features subside rapidly when the drug is stopped. Nevertheless there is a wide safety margin between anticonvulsant and lethal doses.

The principal action of phenytoin seems to be stabilization of the neuronal membrane. This limits facilitation of synaptic transmission which occurs during rapid repetitive stimulation. In peripheral nerve fibres, phenytoin prevents repetitive firing without affecting the threshold of excitability for single impulses. It is believed that this effect is brought about by an enhancement of the Na^+ pump with a consequent reduction in intracellular sodium. In electroshock convulsions in animals, the intracellular $[Na^+]$ increases; phenytoin reduces the seizures, limits their spread and also prevents the increase in intracellular sodium. It is more active than phenobarbitone while troxidone is ineffective in this respect. When the EEG is diffusely abnormal in grand mal, phenytoin may abolish the epileptic phenomena, so that only localized foci of seizure activity remain.

Phenytoin is slowly absorbed and after a single dose the antiepileptic effect may last for many hours; by 24 hours, half the dose is excreted in the urine and no free drug is detectable in the plasma.

Other hydantoins have been prepared, e.g. **ethotoin** and **methoin** (mesontoin); these have no advantages over phenytoin. Indeed, methoin on demethylation gives a much more toxic product. The usual dose of phenytoin is 0·3 g/day. Gastric irritation can be minimized by taking these capsules after meals in divided doses.

ETHOSUXIMIDE (ZARONTIN)

Chemically this is a water-soluble solid, α-ethyl-α-methyl succinimide.

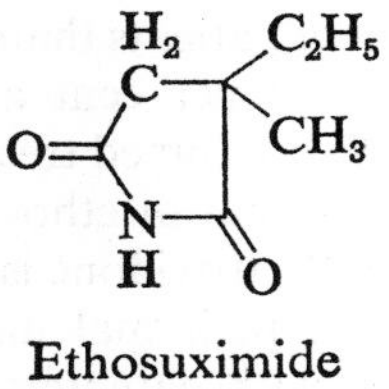

Ethosuximide

It is the drug of choice in the treatment of petit mal, giving complete control in 40–50 per cent of patients and a substantial reduction in the number of attacks in another 40 per cent. It is suitable for long term therapy since its effectiveness increases with use while that of troxidone declines. It is slightly more active than troxidone and has fewer adverse effects. Grand mal, if it occurs with petit mal, may be exacerbated with ethosuximide. The mode of action is unknown.

Adverse effects may occur initially but decline with continued treatment. These include drowsiness, depression, mild euphoria, headache and ataxia or dizziness and psychotic symptoms. Gastric irritation may occur with nausea and vomiting. Very rarely marrow depression develops.

The initial daily dosage is 0·5 g and this is increased up to a maximum of 2·0 g until control is achieved.

The congeners, **methsuximide** (celontin) and **phensuximide** (milontin), are of less value in petit mal as their initial effectiveness declines with continued treatment so that after a few years only half as many patients are controlled with these two compounds as with ethosuximide.

TROXIDONE (TRIDIONE)
This produces a striking and selective reduction in the incidence of petit mal seizures especially in children.

Troxidone

Grand mal seizures are not improved and, when they occur together with petit mal, may be exacerbated. In patients undergoing electroconvulsion treatment the seizure patterns are not modified by troxidone as they are by phenobarbitone and phenytoin. Troxidone does not induce sleep, although slight sedation and analgesia may be seen. In adults, blurring of vision in bright light may develop. In very large doses, ataxia and respiratory depression occur. Uncommonly, blood dyscrasias, skin reactions, and proteinuria are found.

Troxidone initially gives complete control of petit mal in a higher proportion of patients than does ethosuximide, and at 6 months, 30–40 per cent are controlled completely. However, with continued treatment over 2 years, the effect declines while that of ethosuximide increases.

When given by mouth, troxidone is slowly absorbed so that maximal effect on petit mal may not be seen for several days and even with parenteral injections, control takes several hours. The drug is evenly distributed throughout the body water and shows no preference for nervous tissue. It is metabolized in the liver and slowly excreted in the urine.

Troxidone is given in divided doses, the initial daily dose of 0·6 g being increased to a total of 1·8 g if necessary.

Paramethadione may be preferable to troxidone, to which it is closely related. Dosage, adverse effects and toxicity are similar, but the incidence of serious complications including the precipitation of grand mal is less. Patients who develop adverse effects with troxidone do not necessarily suffer similar effects with paramethadione.

Miscellaneous drugs used in epilepsy include **acetazolamide**, occasionally used in petit mal. **Sulthiame** (ospolot), a sulphonamide congener with weak carbonic anhydrase inhibitory properties, is useful in psychomotor epilepsy but causes serious liver and marrow toxicity and may precipitate psychotic behaviour; the usual dose is 100–500 mg/day. **Pheneturide** is a phenylacetyl urea compound which like sulthiame is most useful in psychomotor epilepsy. The usual dose is 200–1000 mg/day. Others include meprobamate (p. 5.45) and diazepam (p. 5.35).

ANTIPARKINSONISM DRUGS AND CENTRALLY ACTING MUSCLE RELAXANTS

ANTIPARKINSONISM DRUGS
Parkinsonism is a common neurological disease, characterized by slowness and poverty of movement, tremor and muscle rigidity. It is associated with degeneration of neurones in the basal nuclei, particularly the globus pallidus and the substantia nigra and their interconnecting and extrapyramidal pathways. This may be due to atherosclerosis, viral infection or drugs, notably reserpine, phenothiazines and methyldopa. The disturbed nervous activity in Parkinsonism may be relayed through the cholinergic synapses, which would explain how many anticholinergic drugs alleviate the condition. Dopamine, noradrenaline and 5-HT in the caudate and lentiform nuclei are abnormally low in patients with Parkinsonism and it is possible that this permits cholinergic activity to predominate. The drugs which induce a Parkinson-like syndrome deplete the brain of these amines.

A satisfactory animal model for Parkinsonism does not exist though tremor can be induced in monkeys by stereotactically placed subthalamic lesions. Antitremor drugs can be tested on this preparation but it is not widely used because of expense. Another method involves the use of the drug **tremorine** (1.4 dipyrolidinobut-2-yne) (fig. 5.37), or its active metabolite oxotremorine which induce tremor, rigidity, akinesia, analgesia and signs of peripheral cholinergic stimulation in many animal species. These features are reduced by drugs effective in Parkinsonism or by pretreatment with 5-hydroxytryptophan or an MAO inhibitor, both of which elevate brain 5-HT.

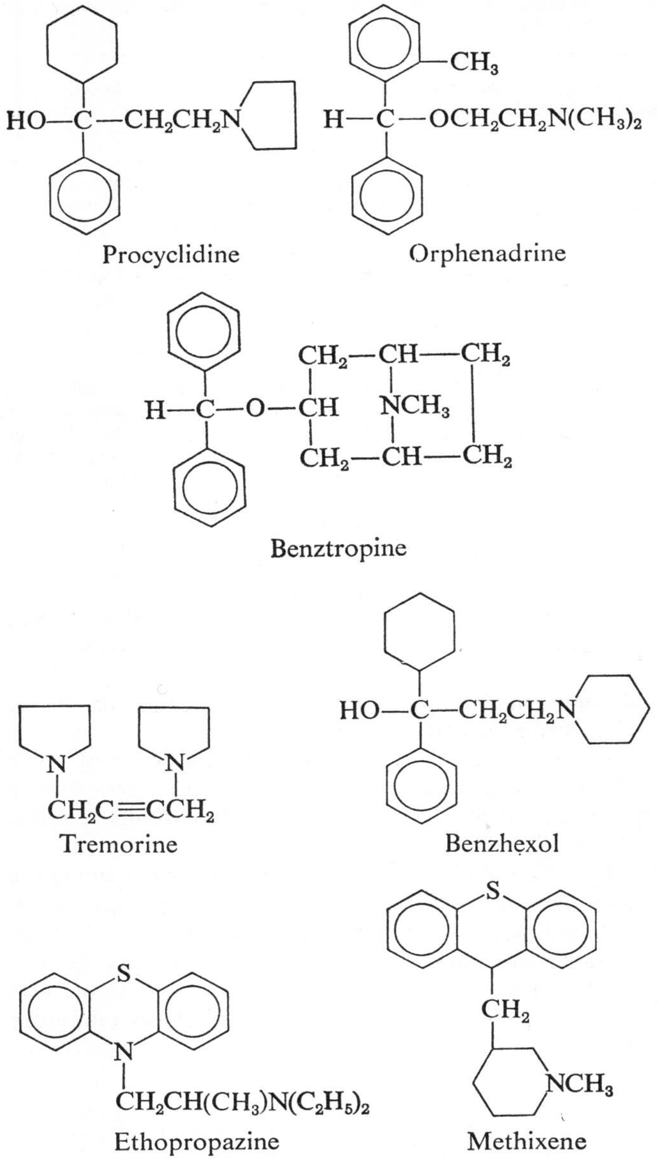

benztropine; orphenadrine which structurally resembles diphenhydramine has also a mild antidepressive effect.

Table 5.7 shows that the bulk of prescriptions for anti-Parkinsonism drugs in the United Kingdom are for either benzhexol or orphenadrine. However, it is by no means certain that their clinical popularity is justified; although they are especially indicated for akinesia and depression, they are probably inferior to benztropine or ethopropazine in the control of rigidity. When tremor is a major problem, **hyoscine, ethopropazine** or **methixene** are most useful.

The dose of the drug chosen is increased gradually until the symptoms are controlled or adverse effects become severe. If one drug fails or adverse effects occur, another drug should be tried and the first drug withdrawn gradually. Current clinical practice favours combinations of drugs rather than single drugs, but knowledge of the value of different combinations is incomplete, though suitable combinations may be deduced from the information in table 5.7. AntiParkinsonism treatment is of long duration and tolerance to drugs occurs.

Other drugs with limited value in the treatment of Parkinsonism are amphetamine (p. 5.37) and diphenhydramine (p. 14.18). It is likely that the antihistamine drugs act by virtue of their cholinergic blocking properties. Diphenhydramine is especially useful in severe tremor and amphetamine when akinesia is troublesome. Reports of the beneficial effects of DOPA also lends support to the dopamine–acetylcholine balance hypothesis. DOPA is given by mouth in doses up to 16 g/day of the racemic mixture or up to 8 g of L-DOPA. DOPA readily crosses the blood–brain barrier while dopamine does not do so. A number of adverse reactions occur which include hypertension, anorexia and vomiting, and psychiatric disturbances.

CENTRALLY ACTING MUSCLE RELAXANTS

Mephenesin (3 o-tololyl 1, 2 propanediol) was discovered in 1946 and found in animals to produce flaccid paralysis of skeletal muscle as a result of selective action on the CNS without loss of consciousness. In smaller doses it reduces spontaneous activity. Mephenesin has no influence on the neuromuscular junction, neuronal conduction or muscle excitability. It acts within the spinal cord where it depresses polysynaptic more than monosynaptic reflexes. The action, however, is not limited to the spinal cord but extends to the reticular system. Arousal, however, is little affected and the drug shares some of the sedative properties of meprobamate to which it is chemically related. Given by oral or intravenous routes it is distributed throughout the tissues and metabolized rapidly in the liver. The drug is used as a muscle relaxant in the treatment of the convulsions of tetanus in which it is given by continuous intravenous infusion. Adverse effects include nystagmus,

FIG. 5.37. Chemical structure of some antiParkinsonism drugs and also tremorine.

At the end of the last century in Paris, Charcot introduced atropine and hyoscine, alkaloids of solanaceous plants, in the control of Parkinsonism. Although hyoscine is still used in patients in whom tremor is severe, the alkaloids have been largely replaced by synthetic compounds with atropine-like activity. The chemical structure of some of these are shown in fig. 5.37 and their comparative effects and adverse reactions in table 5.7. Like the alkaloids they probably act by blocking muscarinic receptor sites on central neurones. Some possess antihistamine activity notably **benzhexol, orphenadrine** and

TABLE 5.7. Effectiveness of antiParkinsonism drugs on the different elements of Parkinson's disease and the proportion of patients showing improvement. Derived mainly from Nodine & Siegler, Doshay & Constable and Strang.

Drug and daily dose	Prescribing frequency in UK	Rigidity	Tremor	Akinesia	Depression	Excessive salivation	Oculogyric crises	Adverse effects	Special indications for use
Benzhexol (trihexiphenidyl, artane) 2·5–10 mg oral	+++	++(+)	+(+) (occasionally) exacerbated)	++++(+)	++	++	++	Dry mouth, blurred vision, giddiness, confusion, agitation, delirium, hallucinations	Rigidity, akinesia, depression
Orphenadrine (disipal) 200–400 mg oral	++++	++	+	++++	++++	O	++	Drowsiness; mild euphoria	Akinesia, contractures, depression, rigidity
Methixene (tremonil) 15–60 mg oral	+								
Procyclidine (kemadrin) 7·5–30 mg oral	+	++(+)	+(+)	+++	+		+	Similar to but less severe than benzhexol	Particularly good in the elderly and for drug-induced extra-pyramidal syndrome
Ethopropazine (lysivane) 50–500 mg oral	+	++	+++ (occasionally exacerbated)		++	(O+)	+	Constipation drowsiness, tingling extremities, vertigo	Major tremor
Benztropine (cogentin) 0·5–6 mg oral	+	++(+)	+(+)	+(+)	++	+++	+	Constipation, sedation and depression, numb fingers	Rigidity, contractures, depression
Hyoscine 0·3–0·9 mg IM	+	+	++++	++	—	++	+	Dizziness, drowsiness	Major tremor

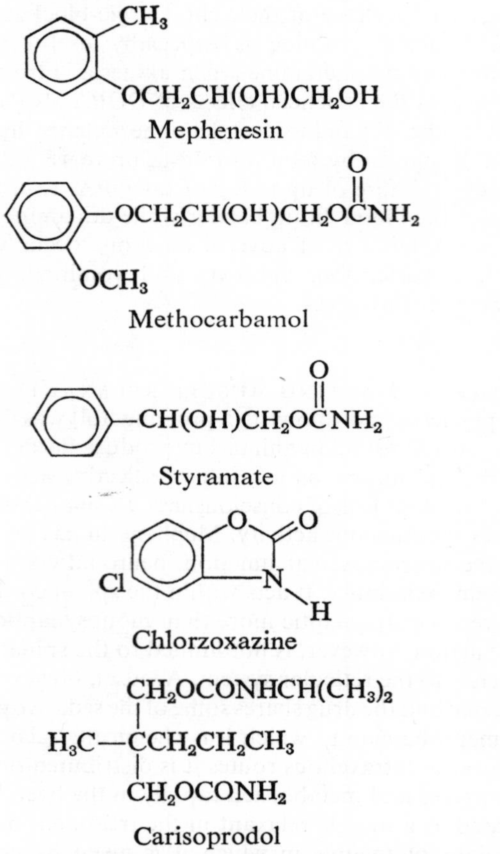

FIG. 5.38. Chemical structures of some centrally acting muscle relaxants.

diplopia, nausea and vomiting. Overdosage results in death from respiratory failure.

The structure of mephenesin and a number of other related and unrelated compounds which possess similar properties to mephenesin but which have limited clinical use are given in fig. 5.38.

The effect of nicotine on sympathetic ganglia and in the neuromuscular junction are described on pp. 4.1 and 7. Although not used in clinical medicine it is the most important constituent of tobacco and a cigarette may contain as much as 7 mg. It is a weak muscle relaxant. This may be exerted by its stimulating effect on inhibitory Renshaw neurones.

GENERAL AND LOCAL ANAESTHETICS

The term 'anaesthesia' was used in its modern sense by Oliver Wendell Holmes in the latter part of the nineteenth century, though it had been employed by the Greeks as a description of philosophical detachment many centuries earlier. The definition 'loss of sensation' implies loss of consciousness and general anaesthetics produce a reversible state of unconsciousness during which surgical operations can be carried out. Though the soporific effects of alcohol, mandragora and opium had been used for this purpose for hundreds of years a controllable loss of consciousness did not become possible until specific gases, e.g. nitrous oxide and ether, and other agents, had been identified. In the case of nitrous oxide Sir Humphry

Davy had pointed out its anaesthetic possibilities half a century before it was used for this purpose. Early accounts of anaesthesia are studded with bizarre events occurring during the inhalation of anaesthetic agents, the behaviour of the participants ranged from powerful oratory to antics matched only in the Victorian music hall.

Most general anaesthetics are gases or volatile liquids and are given by inhalation but some are nonvolatile and given by intravenous injection. A variety of hypnotics and analgesics are used to sedate the patient and allay anxiety prior to the operation and to induce a clinical state where general anaesthesia is more easily achieved. This is called premedication.

Signs and stages of anaesthesia

An attempt was made by early anaesthetists to correlate the depth of anaesthesia and the amount of agent administered. John Snow, in 1858, was the first to improve upon the open administration of ether, which was for many years merely dropped over a pad of cotton held over the mouth and nose, by inventing an inhaler which produced a concentration of vapour that could be assessed approximately and controlled. He added to this advance by designing a chloroform inhaler and described the four stages of anaesthesia. A few years later Joseph Clover carried out similar observations, especially with air–chloroform mixtures, and both anaesthetists assessed the level of anaesthesia by observing the frequency and depth of respiration and by monitoring the pulse, a practice still of great importance.

However, it was not until 1937 that the clinical signs and the various depths of ether anaesthesia, which apply to other volatile agents, were defined and accepted as a clinical guide. The four stages are as follows:

(1) the **stage of analgesia** which lasts until consciousness is lost; the patient is able to talk and obey commands but sensation to pain is reduced;

(2) the **excitement stage** follows when involuntary movement and respiratory irregularity may be marked and muscular tone increased;

(3) the **stage of surgical anaesthesia** sets in when respiration becomes regular, muscle tone diminishes and tendon and other reflexes (e.g. conjunctival) disappear;

(4) **overdosage** is characterized by shallow respiration and fall in blood pressure.

The stage of surgical anaesthesia is further divided into four planes on the basis of the movement of the eye, the character of respiration, the presence or absence of certain reflexes and the state of the pupils.

The limitations of such a classification should be stressed. The depth of anaesthesia is determined by the concentration of the anaesthetic in the brain and the rate at which anaesthesia occurs is related to the rate of rise of its concentrations. Furthermore, the use of muscle relaxants and other drugs makes it possible to carry out surgical operations without achieving the depths of anaesthesia needed in former days. Thus, the three components of modern anaesthesia are (1) narcosis, (2) suppression of reflexes and (3) muscle relaxation. These may be varied independently by the use of appropriate drugs. Sleep or narcosis and reflex suppression may be ensured by the anaesthetic gases and volatile agents supplemented with hypnotics or tranquillizers given preoperatively or by the use of nonvolatile anaesthetics, whilst relaxation is produced by drugs which induce muscle paralysis.

The art of anaesthesia consists in assessing the clinical state of the patient who is unconscious and partially paralysed. Clinical experience with the monitoring of pulse and blood pressure remains the most important method of assessing depth of anaesthesia, despite attempts to correlate it with electrical activity of the brain as indicated by the EEG. The size of pupil and its reaction to light are influenced by many factors and are not an accurate guide. Nevertheless, hypoxia is an important cause of dilation of the pupil.

Inhalational anaesthesia

The sequence of events on inhaling any gas or vapour is dependent upon the physical characteristics of the particular gas and the laws which govern its passage across the barriers between the body tissues. The inhalational agents are not metabolized within the cells and are not known to play a direct part in any enzymic reaction. They act indirectly by altering the lipids in the membranes of cells (p. 1.4). Thus, the solubilities of the gases in water and lipid are important in determining their concentration in the blood and in the various tissues.

The process of anaesthesia may be conveniently divided into three steps, (1) induction, (2) maintenance, and (3) recovery.

During these three steps the objects are to establish, maintain and then reduce the partial pressure of anaesthetic in the brain. All three steps are influenced by changes in the frequency and depth of ventilation.

The amount of anaesthetic gas passing from the upper airway to the alveolus depends upon the partial pressure at which it is inspired and upon the respiratory rate and tidal volume.

Initially the inspired mixture is diluted in the anatomical dead space. If the patient inspires inadequately as a result of nervousness, excitement, or the irritant nature of the vapour, e.g. ether, alveolar ventilation may be insufficient and anaesthesia will not proceed.

Provided pulmonary ventilation is satisfactory, however, the partial pressure of anaesthetic in the alveoli rises rapidly and this is followed by rapid diffusion across the alveolar wall into the blood. Equilibrium between the inspired and alveolar pressure is never complete, however, because there is a continued passage of gas into the pulmonary capillaries and the tissues. This uptake is extremely important and the rate of diffusion across the barrier is closely related to the solubility of the agent in the blood.

The ratio of the concentration on two sides of any membrane, in this case pulmonary capillary blood and alveolar content, is termed the partition coefficient and this is a function of solubility. The higher the solubility the larger the coefficient (table 5.8).

TABLE 5.8. Approximate blood–gas partition coefficients for common anaesthetics.

Anaesthetic	Blood–gas partition coefficient
Cyclopropane	0·46
Nitrous oxide	0·47
Ethylchloride	2·0
Ethylene	2·8
Halothane	3·6
Chloroform	7·3
Trichlorethylene	9·0
Methoxyflurane	13·0
Diethyl ether	13·0

The more soluble the anaesthetic is in blood the more of it must be dissolved to elevate its partial pressure and so its pressure rises more slowly. Fig. 5.39 illustrates the rise in arterial partial pressure with time for a variety of anaesthetic gases and should be compared with their solubilities. The rate of rise of partial pressure is rapid for insoluble gases and slower for soluble agents. The curves are constructed on the basis that the inhaled gas concentration, cardiac output and pulmonary ventilation remain constant.

Initially the pulmonary venous blood does not contain the agent but as circulation throughout the body occurs the blood returning to the lungs contains an ever increasing amount. If inhalation anaesthesia were allowed to continue at a constant concentration of inspired anaesthetic, saturation of the body would occur and the partial pressure in the pulmonary, arterial and venous blood would be the same and would be in equilibrium with the alveolar pressure. Equilibration seldom if ever occurs in practice since the action of the anaesthetic agents upon the brain is sufficiently selective to establish anaesthesia before this happens.

The extent to which the agent is carried throughout the body depends upon cardiac output and regional blood flows and the brain receives about 15 per cent of cardiac output.

Most general anaesthetics have a tissue–blood partition

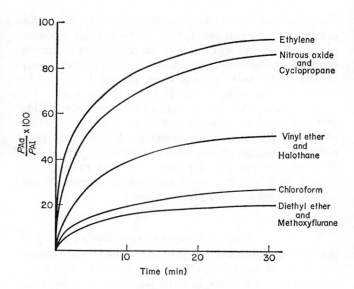

FIG. 5.39. Partial pressure (P) of anaesthetics (A) in arterial blood (a) expressed as a percentage of the inspired air (I).

coefficient of nearly one, i.e. they are equally soluble in both. Fat is an exception and has a higher affinity for these agents. In spite of the fact that brain has a high lipid content, the brain–blood coefficient for inhalational anaesthetics, except for halothane and methoxyflurane is near unity; anaesthetic properties therefore cannot be attributed to this factor alone.

The fat–blood coefficient is also relevant to the potency of an anaesthetic agent and the rapidity with which the patient loses consciousness as observed clinically is directly correlated with this coefficient. Table 5.9 shows the fat–blood coefficient for selected anaesthetics.

During maintenance of anaesthesia unconsciousness is maintained by providing in the inspired mixture sufficient anaesthetic to sustain the partial pressure in the brain which establishes the desired clinical effect. As anaesthesia proceeds, the tissues acquire a higher content and if the concentration of anaesthesia being administered were not reduced, progressively deeper anaesthesia would develop.

TABLE 5.9.
Fat–blood partition coefficients for common anaesthetics.

Anaesthetic	Fat–blood partition coefficient
Nitrous oxide	3
Diethyl ether	5
Cyclopropane	21
Halothane	60
Methoxyflurane	63

The skill in giving of anaesthetics consists in the adjustment of the concentration of anaesthetic to maintain the necessary level of anaesthesia for the particular surgical procedure.

Recovery rapidly follows the stopping of the anaesthetic. Since these anaesthetics are not metabolized and only small amounts are lost in the urine, the main route of excretion must be the lungs. The excretion rate is usually rapid and about half the amount absorbed is usually eliminated in 30 min. The process is the reverse of induction.

Different areas of the brain are not affected by anaesthetics simultaneously or in a uniform manner. It appears that the newer areas phylogenetically are affected first. Thus the higher centres, e.g. the cerebral cortex, are those that are initially depressed, the process spreading down towards the medulla and spinal cord.

It may be that the reticular system which is extremely rich in synaptic junctions is particularly sensitive to depression. This is true of the action of the barbiturates,

and there is evidence that gaseous anaesthetics have a similar propensity for blocking transmission at this site.

The difficulties of measurement and insufficient knowledge of the basis of consciousness and of mechanism of transmission in the CNS have made it impossible to define the mechanism of action of anaesthetic agents. Reference is made to the possible physical basis of the action on p. 1.4.

Anaesthetic gases and volatile agents

Table 5.10 gives the chemical structure, boiling point, and the range of concentrations in the inspired air and in the arterial blood for the common anaesthetic gases and volatile agents.

NITROUS OXIDE

Nitrous oxide is the only inorganic gas used to produce anaesthesia and was the first general anaesthetic to be employed in man. Although nonexplosive it supports

TABLE 5.10. Some physical values for anaesthetic gases and the commoner volatile agents.

	Structure	Boiling point °C	Range of inspired concentrations for anaesthesia (V/V per cent)	Arterial blood concentration associated with anaesthesia (mg/100 ml)
Oxygen	O_2	−182	—	—
Nitrous oxide	N_2O	−89	50–80	45–55
Cyclopropane	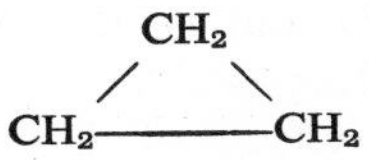 CH_2 / CH_2——CH_2	−33	10–20	5–20
Diethyl ether	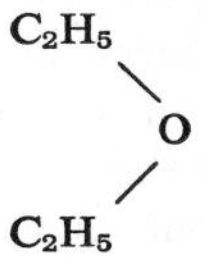 C_2H_5 \ O / C_2H_5	36	3–4	10–20
Methoxyflurane	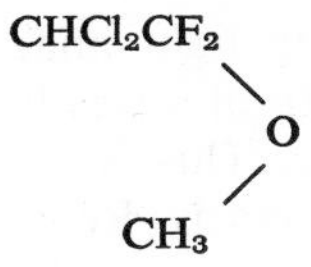 $CHCl_2CF_2$ \ O / CH_3	105	0·25–3	0·3–2
Chloroform	$CHCl_3$	61	0·5–2	5–20
Trichlorethylene	$CHCl=CCl_2$	87	1–2	5–10
Halothane	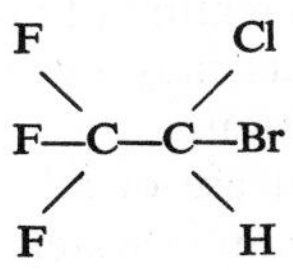 F—C—C—Br with F, F, Cl, H	50	0·5–4	5–20

combustion. N_2O is a weak anaesthetic but has substantial analgesic activity. When given with 20 per cent O_2 it causes unconsciousness which is not sufficiently deep to allow major surgical procedures. Surgical anaesthesia is produced only when it is given in higher concentration, i.e. with concentrations of O_2 which cause hypoxia. The gas has been used alone for induction or very short procedures as, for example, in dentistry. Anaesthesia develops in 60 sec but can be maintained thereafter using a 50 per cent mixture of N_2O and oxygen. Cyanosis, irregular respirations and dilated pupils indicate the lack of O_2. N_2O is still widely used and provided hypoxia is avoided it is free from significant danger. For these reasons it is often combined with other anaesthetics which allows the proportion of O_2 to be increased without loss of the depth of anaesthesia.

CYCLOPROPANE

Cyclopropane is a colourless gas with a sweet smell, which liquefies under 5 atmospheres of pressure and is stored in liquid form. It is almost insoluble in water but very soluble in fat.

During cyclopropane anaesthesia, the production of endogenous catecholamine is increased and whilst blood pressure is usually well maintained, the depressant effects of the gas upon respiration may lead to the retention of CO_2. These two factors partially account for the cardiac arrhythmias which may occur during its use. Adrenaline should not be used with cyclopropane because of the liability to produce ventricular arrhythmias.

The main disadvantage of cyclopropane is its liability to detonate in low concentrations in air and when mixed with oxygen. Nevertheless, this property which cyclopropane shares with diethyl ether has not displaced it entirely from anaesthetic practice.

Like halothane, high concentrations of oxygen may be given with little loss of anaesthetic power. This and its nonirritating characteristics make cyclopropane an attractive agent for rapid induction or descent in level of anaesthesia.

For induction several breaths of cyclopropane alone or with oxygen may be inspired; for maintenance a concentration of 20 per cent cyclopropane and 80 per cent oxygen is usually adequate. Its high cost and explosive nature make it necessary to use a closed rebreathing circuit in which CO_2 is removed by soda lime.

ETHYL CHLORIDE

This agent was popular at the beginning of the century. Ethyl chloride is the most volatile anaesthetic used, having a low boiling point and it must, therefore, be stored in containers at slightly above atmospheric pressure. It is nonexplosive. The high volatility may easily lead to an overdosage if care is not used in administration. Though

respiration is initially stimulated, apnoea may readily occur as the blood concentration rises rapidly.

The heart rate is commonly slowed during this period and blood pressure falls by a direct action upon the heart and medullary centres. For this reason it has been largely superseded. Ethyl chloride is still occasionally used as a local or surface anaesthetic by virtue of its cooling effect on the skin.

DIETHYL ETHER

The use of ether as a general anaesthetic started with the dramatic demonstration given by William Morton whilst still a medical student at Massachusetts General Hospital in 1846. Synthesized by Valerius Cordus in 1540, it was used on at least two separate occasions as an anaesthetic agent in the 10 years that preceded its public appearance, but this particular event was responsible for its introduction. It is a drug that has radically altered the history of medicine.

Diethyl ether is manufactured by the fractionation of the product of sulphuric acid and ethyl alcohol. Ether, is a colourless liquid, and its pungent odour is easily recognizable. The stored agent commonly contains small amounts of impurities which are the result of decomposition and this process is accelerated by air, heat and light. Storage should be, where possible, in a cool, dark place.

Diethyl ether stimulates respiration by its irritant effects upon the bronchial mucosa. Both the rate and depth of respiration are increased during its inhalation and an increased flow of salivary and bronchial secretions may be troublesome in practice. Ether, however, dilates the bronchi and is, therefore, a suitable anaesthetic when bronchospasm is present.

The effects of diethyl ether upon the cardiovascular system depend on the depth of anaesthesia and state of the peripheral circulation. The myocardium is least affected and vagal action upon the heart is partially blocked. Ether induces release of endogenous catecholamines, but does not sensitize the heart to their effects.

During light anaesthesia vasodilation occurs but as the depth of anaesthesia increases vasoconstriction takes its place. This is visible in the skin but also occurs in deeper vessels. Renal vasoconstriction occurs. The compensatory powers of the circulation to counteract haemorrhage and shock may therefore be lost.

Relaxation of skeletal muscle by a block at the neuromuscular junction similar to that produced by tubocurarine is a feature of diethyl ether anaesthesia so that additive effects may occur when the two drugs are used in combination.

The release of adrenaline produced by stimulation of the autonomic system leads to hyperglycaemia but this is usually without serious effects.

The wide margin of safety in inexperienced hands and the low cost have made ether a popular anaesthetic. The amounts needed, however, limit portability to a certain extent. Used with air or N_2O and O_2 for induction, patience and skill are required. The irritating vapour readily provokes coughing or breathholding, particularly when the inspired concentration is increased too rapidly. These characteristics make induction by thiopentone or halothane preferable whenever possible. Postoperative nausea and vomiting occur in up to 50 per cent of patients.

Diethyl ether is inflammable in air in a concentration of up to 36 per cent. The mixture is heavier than air, sinking to floor level and burns if ignited slowly as a 'cold' flame which may become the source of ignition for a more serious fire.

With oxygen, a readily explosive mixture is formed and a number of accidents have occurred even with strict precautions. Violent detonation throughout the circuit, including the patient's respiratory tract, may occur with fatal results.

DIVINYL ETHER (VINESTHENE)

This agent shares characteristics with ethyl chloride and diethyl ether. It is of high volatility, having a boiling point between the two of 28°C. The vapour is nonirritating but is explosive over a range comparable with ether. It is much more unstable and is rapidly oxidized *in vitro*.

Divinyl ether is at least four times more potent than the diethyl ether; being less soluble in blood, induction and recovery are more rapid. It has similar effects upon the cardiovascular and respiratory systems but has a smaller margin of safety and is reserved for short procedures; it causes liver damage when used for longer periods.

METHOXYFLURANE (PENTHRANE)

Methoxyflurane is methyl ether with substituted chlorine and fluorine. It is a noninflammable gas with a high boiling point and is of low volatility. Induction is slow since it is as soluble in blood as diethyl ether and although the vapour is less irritating, coughing may disturb the patient before complete loss of consciousness ensues.

Methoxyflurane is a powerful depressant of the respiratory system so its use is generally confined to conditions where ventilation can be controlled. Depression of the cardiovascular system also occurs and bradycardia and hypotension may develop during light planes of anaesthesia. These effects may be reversed by the administration of atropine or a lowering of the inspired concentration. Methoxyflurane may be used as an alternative to halothane or diethyl ether.

CHLOROFORM

Sir James Young Simpson and his colleagues, Duncan and Keith in Edinburgh, introduced chloroform in 1847, just twelve months after Morton's use of ether in America. The use of chloroform followed a suggestion of its potentialities by Waldie, a Liverpool chemist.

Chloroform is a clear liquid of boiling point 61°C which is not unpleasant to inhale.

Direct depression of the myocardium and conducting tissues produces cardiac irregularities predominantly of ventricular origin. A progressive fall in blood pressure is due to these effects and to a loss of tone in the peripheral vessels. Hypoxia and CO_2 retention subsequent upon respiratory depression may aggravate the circulatory changes.

Hepatic necrosis was an occasional cause of death, when large doses were used for long periods.

Convenient to carry, noninflammable and of relatively low volatility, chloroform fulfils some of the requirements for anaesthesia in remote underdeveloped areas, but owing to its toxic effects it is regarded with caution by most anaesthetists. Though many thousands of 'successful' anaesthetics have been given using chloroform, it is now retained only by those skilled in its use who regard it with trust and particular affection.

TRICHLORETHYLENE (TRILENE)

Like chloroform trichlorethylene is of low volatility and is noninflammable in the clinical range of concentrations. Coloured blue for identification, the liquid is stabilized by the addition of thymol. Though tachycardia or bradycardia may occur, few adverse cardiovascular effects develop if anaesthesia is maintained at a light level.

Trichlorethylene has strong analgesic properties, which weighs in its favour as an alternative to halothane as a supplement to nitrous oxide anaesthesia.

During spontaneous respiration it almost invariably produces tachypnoea, thought to be due to reflex stimulation from the lung. This may be controlled by the injection of small amounts of pethidine.

Trichlorethylene is unsuitable when muscular relaxation is needed because this effect occurs only in deep anaesthesia.

The use of trichlorethylene with soda lime (calcium and sodium hydroxide) should be avoided. Interaction with soda lime produces powerful neurotoxins; dichloracetylene is the most important, and its formation is accelerated by the heat that accompanies the absorption of CO_2. Modern types of soda lime, whilst lessening the risk, do not ensure freedom from these toxic products.

HALOTHANE (FLUOTHANE)

Halothane is a colourless, nonirritating liquid with a sweet odour. It is stabilized by thymol. Since its introduction over 10 years ago, it has become the most widely used volatile agent in spite of its high cost. It is noninflammable.

Halothane tends to lower the blood pressure to an extent that is directly related to the inspired concentration. This effect is attributable to depression of the myocardium, vasomotor centre, sympathetic nervous system and the vessel wall itself. The blood pressure may fall rapidly if drugs such as tubocurarine have also been given. In addition halothane enhances the action of the vagus upon the heart. The resultant bradycardia may be avoided or reduced by the administration of atropine.

When the inspired concentration of halothane is increased, respiration is also directly depressed. This is most marked when the patient has been heavily premedicated. For this reason hypoventilation should always be looked for during and after halothane anaesthesia.

Halothane lacks the analgesic properties of anaesthetics such as trichlorethylene, and postoperative sedation is needed at an earlier stage than with these agents. In a number of patients shivering occurs during the period of recovery from anaesthesia, and the fall in temperature is attributed to loss of reactive vasoconstriction.

A bronchodilator, like ether, it is suitable for patients with chronic lung disease, and the ease with which ventilation may be controlled has led to its use in thoracic and paediatric surgery. Like ether it has a direct relaxant effect on skeletal muscle.

Reports of liver damage have caused anxiety, but the incidence is low in relation to the number of anaesthetics given and the risk is small.

Nonvolatile general anaesthetics

Certain of the barbiturates are commonly used to induce anaesthesia which may then be continued with other agents, or alone to produce general anaesthesia for minor operative or diagnostic procedures. Thiopentone, methohexitone and thialbarbitone are all employed for this purpose. Their chemical composition and general properties are described on p. 5.41 and in table 5.5. The effect of these agents depends not only on the dose given but on the rate of administration. A rapid injection induces unconsciousness followed by rapid recovery while the same injection given slowly induces sleepiness. The difference in effect is due to the extent to which the drug is distributed to other tissues than the brain. The chief danger of barbiturates is their depression of respiration and laryngospasm particularly with high dosage.

In anaesthetic doses the barbiturates depress the action of all muscular tissue including the myocardium, but arrhythmias are uncommon. They also, like curare, impair transmission at the neuromuscular junction. These effects, with some depression of the autonomic ganglia, may contribute to the hypotension which follows their use.

PROPANIDID (EPONTOL)

$$OCH_2CON(C_2H_5)_2$$
$$OCH_3$$
$$CH_2COOCH_2CH_2CH_3$$

Propanidid

This nonbarbiturate short-acting intravenous anaesthetic agent is propyl 4-(*N*, *N*-diethylcarbamayl methoxy)-3 methoxy phenylacetate. It is insoluble in water but is solubilized with polyoxyethylated castor oil to give a 5 per cent aqueous solution which is extremely stable. Given intravenously (100–750 mg) it induces anaesthesia smoothly; this is associated with hyperventilation lasting about 1 min. The anaesthesia lasts 3–6 min after which recovery is rapid, due to its rapid metabolism by liver and plasma esterases. There are few adverse effects; laryngospasm and bronchospasm do not occur and respiratory and circulatory depression is less marked than that with thiopentone. Propanidid is also a potent local anaesthetic which probably accounts for its antiarrhythmic properties.

It is probably safer than thiobarbiturates when short duration anaesthesia is required. The rapid and complete recovery make it particularly suitable for out-patient use.

HYDROXYDIONE (21-HYDROXYPREGNANEDIONE)
This was the first steroid to be used to produce anaesthesia. Given intravenously (1–1.5 g) it has no hormonal activity. It induces drowsiness in 15 min which is followed by sleep and anaesthesia and its effects last up to two hours. Depression of the cardiovascular and respiratory system is unpredictable. Its chief disadvantage is a tendency to produce thrombophlebitis.

γ-HYDROXYBUTYRIC ACID (GHBA)
GHBA is chemically related to GABA (vol. 1, p. 24.88). In the brain, GABA is deaminated to succinic semialdehyde which then undergoes oxidation to succinic acid. Some have claimed that the semialdehyde may also be reduced to form GHBA and the cyclic form, butyrolactone. The identification of these substances as normal metabolites in brain remains uncertain.

Intravenous injection of a single dose (5 g) of GHBA acts within 15 min to produce deep sleep and sedation, but not total anaesthesia. Unlike barbiturates, GHBA is effective in doses which do not depress respiration. Rapid destruction of the drug by oxidation to CO_2 and water ensures prompt recovery of consciousness; about 2 per cent of the dose appears in the urine. GHBA is used as a basal anaesthetic.

Neuromuscular blocking agents

Before the discovery of neuromuscular blocking agents the only means of providing muscular relaxation during surgery was by the establishment of a deep plane anaesthesia. The curare-like effects of ether and halothane assist the surgeon in gaining access to deep abdominal or thoracic regions. The use of specific peripheral muscular relaxants, however, allows still greater muscular relaxation so that even safer amounts of general anaesthetics can be used.

The mode of action of postjunctional blocking agents is given on p. 4.6. The **depolarizing drugs** act in the same way as acetylcholine at the motor end plate. They produce prolonged depolarization and after intravenous administration fasciculations of the muscles are seen. Suxamethonium (p. 4.7) is the drug most used in clinical practice. An intravenous injection of 50 mg **suxamethonium chloride** ensures relaxation for 5 min and is thus useful for rapid intubation or short procedures, though repeated doses may be given. Suxamethonium chloride is rapidly destroyed by pseudocholinesterase first to succinylmonocholine, a weaker relaxant, and then to succinic acid and choline. A genetically determined defect of inactivation, in which prolonged apnoea develops, is described on p. 31.10. Artificial respiration must be maintained for as long as inadequate ventilation persists and transfusion of enzyme-rich fresh blood accelerates disappearance of the block. Suxamethonium causes transient bradycardia and a fall in blood pressure followed by tachycardia and hypertension. Cardiac arrhythmias may also occur. Muscular discomfort is a common complaint for 24 hours after operation.

Nondepolarizing relaxants act by blocking the access of acetylcholine to the receptors of the motor end plate. D-tubocurarine is a pure crystalline alkaloid (p. 4.7). Like acetylcholine and the depolarizing relaxants, its molecule contains quaternary ammonium groups which account for its affinity for receptors in the postjunctional membrane.

It is active only when given by intramuscular or intravenous injection. An injection of 30 mg causes muscular paralysis which lasts for up to 30 min. The short action of the drug is due to dilution in the ECF rather than to rapid metabolism. Degradation in the liver takes several hours, and the free drug and its metabolic products are excreted in the urine.

Both classes of relaxants produce progressive paralysis of the eye and face muscles, the musculature of the head and neck, the limbs and the diaphragm in that order. D-tubocurarine also produces a sympathetic blockade followed by a fall in blood pressure. This effect is enhanced by drugs with a similar action, e.g. halothane.

Bronchospasm due to release of histamine may occur in asthmatics.

Dimethyltubocurarine in which the two OH groups are replaced by two methoxy groups is more potent, but it acts for a shorter time. Toxiferines are curare alkaloids and one of these, **Toxiferine I**, is sometimes used as an alternative to tubocurarine.

Gallamine triethiodide (flaxedil) is a synthetic compound with one-third of the potency of D-tubocurarine; the paralysing action lasts for up to 20 min. The molecule is a trisquaternary structure but unlike the curare alkaloids the drug is wholly excreted unchanged in the urine.

Gallamine shows more affinity for parasympathetic ganglia than curare and this block causes tachycardia. Bronchoconstriction is less evident than with D-tubocurarine; gallamine more readily crosses the placental barrier and tubocurarine is preferable in obstetrical procedures. The dose is 80–120 mg intravenously.

The anticholinesterases and neuromuscular blocking agents

Neostigmine inhibits cholinesterase and leads to the accumulation of acetylcholine. The competitive block produced by the nondepolarizing relaxants is thus overcome and the muscular paralysis reversed.

Muscarinic effects of the anticholinesterases such as bradycardia and excessive secretions should be prevented by the intravenous administration of atropine.

Up to 2·5 mg of neostigmine intravenously are usually preceded by 1·0 mg of atropine intravenously though some anaesthetists inject these drugs together. Neostigmine and atropine may cause sudden cardiac arrhythmias.

Certain antibiotics also impair transmission at the neuromuscular junction. These are **neomycin, kanamycin** and **streptomycin**, sometimes used to treat infections in the peritoneal or pleural cavity. Thus at operation solutions instilled into these cavities may be absorbed into the blood stream; respiratory depression usually appears within 5–15 min. Since these drugs produce a nondepolarizing block, they act synergistically with D-tubocurarine, gallamine or ether. The block, however, is not identical with that of curare since its reversal by neostigmine is incomplete. Ca^{++} reverse the block rapidly and completely.

Premedication

This term describes the use of drugs to ensure sedation, diminish anxiety and reduce the quantity of secretions before general anaesthesia and operation. Their use facilitates induction and reduces the amount of volatile anaesthetic required. A number of hypnotics, tranquillizers and analgesics are used and their selection is commonly dictated by personal choice and by the extent to which pain or anxiety are likely to be most troublesome. Morphine (10 mg) and atropine (0·6 mg) are traditional and still employed commonly. Hyoscine (0·6 mg) has a similar effect to atropine but occasionally causes excitement in the elderly. Pethidine is an alternative to morphine. In the absence of pain quinalbarbitone and pentobarbitone (100–200 mg) are useful. In young children a simple hypnotic, e.g. chloral hydrate or one of the phenothiazines may be adequate.

Local anaesthetics

When applied directly to peripheral nerves or spinal roots local anaesthetics prevent the conduction of nerve impulses. Motor and sensory nerves are equally susceptible but small fibres are more vulnerable than are large fibres; the smallest unmyelinated fibres, are blocked more easily than the myelinated fibres. Differential fibre sensitivity appears to be the main reason why there is a definite order in which different sensations are affected. Pain is first to disappear, followed by temperature discrimination, touch and deep pressure.

Local anaesthetics are used to induce limited zones of anaesthesia by direct application to mucous membranes (surface anaesthesia), by injection around nerve endings (infiltration anaesthesia), by injection near nerves (conduction anaesthesia), by injection into the subarachnoid space in the lumbar region (spinal anaesthesia) and by injection into the extradural space (extra or epidural anaesthesia). Surface anaesthesia is used to abolish sensation in areas covered by mucus membranes, e.g. larynx or urethra. Infiltration anaesthesia is used for minor operative procedures, e.g. lumbar puncture or dental extraction. Surgical operations can be carried out in limbs with conduction anaesthesia; spinal and extradural anaesthesia which induce anaesthesia up to the thoracic regions can be used for major procedures in the abdomen or pelvis. Ideally these agents should interrupt nerve transmission completely and reversibly, and without causing tissue damage; systemic toxicity should be low. The onset of action should be rapid and the duration should conform to the limits required for surgery.

Most local anaesthetic drugs are esters of aromatic acids and amino alcohols. A lipophilic aromatic residue is joined by an ester link to a hydrophilic amino group, the latter being a secondary or tertiary amine. The basic structure is thus,

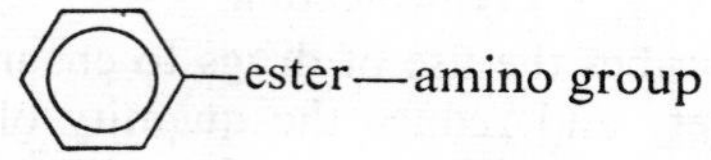

ester—amino group

Changes of the molecular structure alter potency, toxicity and stability. The structures of some of the more important local anaesthetics are shown in fig. 5.40.

These drugs are weak bases and those in common use have pK_a values between 8·0 and 9·0. They are administered as the water-soluble salt, usually hydrochloride, and only a small part exists in the nonionized

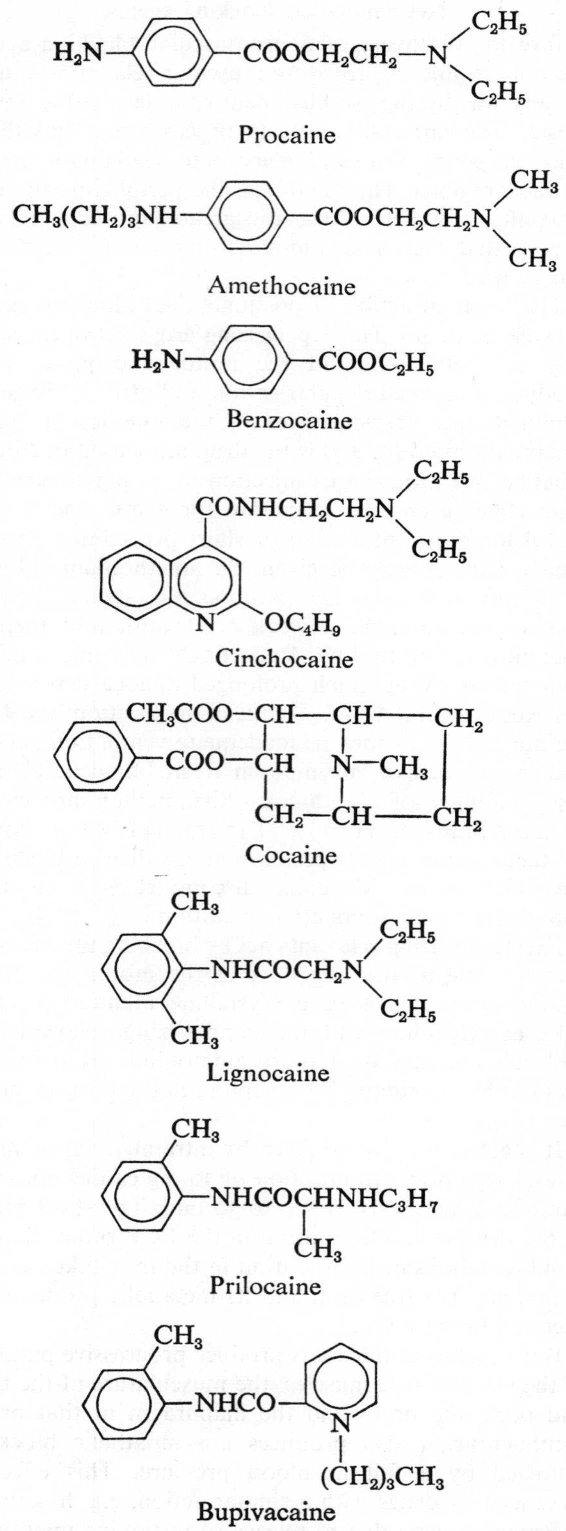

FIG. 5.40. Chemical structure of some local anaesthetics.

form at the pH of body tissues. This component easily penetrates the lipid membrane of the cell, while the cationic or charged form of the drug does not do so. Once the agent has penetrated the axonal membrane it acts in the charged cationic form. This is demonstrated by the fact that in nonmyelinated nerves, conduction can be inhibited merely by adjusting the pH of the medium bathing the nerve to 9·0. Thus the uncharged amine is important in penetrating the nerve while the charged cationic form appears important for activity. Local anaesthetics interfere with the generation of the nerve action potential by preventing the large increase in permeability to Na^+ normally associated with depolarization. Block in conduction is not associated with significant changes in resting potential, but alteration in the permeability to K^+ also occurs. The means by which the agents alter cell membrane permeability are unknown. As might be expected from their actions, local anaesthetic drugs influence the function of all excitable tissues. After absorption they first stimulate and then depress the CNS. Restlessness, tremor and convulsions occur and are toxic effects of these drugs. Cocaine also induces euphoria and this may contribute to its addictive properties.

These drugs also act on the cardiovascular system. Rarely their administration is followed by cardiac arrest and death due either to block of the sinuatrial node or ventricular fibrillation. Procaine in particular possesses quinidine-like actions on the myocardium, i.e. it increases the refractory period, diminishes the force of contraction, and raises the threshold for excitation. These actions led to the development and therapeutic use of procainamide (p. 8.6). Local anaesthetics also depress smooth muscle contraction, neuromuscular and ganglionic transmission.

The action of the drugs upon blood vessels is important since this determines their clearance from the site of application and therefore the blood concentration. Since most local anaesthetics are vasodilators, they are commonly employed in conjunction with adrenaline. This delays absorption into the blood stream and the maximum safe local dose can be increased.

Cocaine, however, is a vasoconstrictor because it inhibits the reuptake of noradrenaline at the sympathetic nerve ending (p. 15.20).

Local anaesthetics are metabolized in the plasma or liver by hydrolysis. In man cocaine and lignocaine are hydrolysed chiefly in the liver, whereas procaine is hydrolysed by esterase in the plasma.

SPECIFIC LOCAL ANAESTHETIC DRUGS

Cocaine is an alkaloid extracted from the leaves of the tree *Erythroxylon coca*. Although a potent anaesthetic it has actions peculiar to itself. The most striking effect is marked central nervous stimulation with a feeling of well being, alertness and loss of fatigue. This has led to

its use as a drug of addiction enshrined in Conan Doyle's famous novels about Sherlock Holmes.

Stimulation of the medullary and sympathetic centres leads to an increase in respiratory and cardiac rate. This is followed by depression in higher dosage. The sympathomimetic actions of cocaine have already been referred to and include dilation of the pupil. Although originally attributed to inhibition of monoamine oxidase, cocaine appears to sensitize the tissue to adrenaline by reducing or preventing the uptake of the transmitter into the nerve terminals and is the only local anaesthetic known to have this action (p. 15.20).

Cocaine is rapidly absorbed from mucous membranes of the body and as absorption greatly exceeds the rate of destruction in the liver, toxic effects may be rapid and severe. This drug is now used solely as a topical anaesthetic. Cocaine may be applied to the nose in solution or spray and to the throat in a 1–5 per cent solution. It should never be given by injection.

Cocaine poisoning is characterized by excitement, restlessness and mental confusion. Headache and a rise in temperature occur. The pupils are dilated, the pulse rapid and breathing irregular. Convulsions, collapse and unconsciousness rapidly follow. Death has occurred after injection of only 20 mg.

Procaine is one of the weakest local anaesthetics and is readily hydrolysed. Hydrolysis produces the parent acid para-aminobenzoic acid which may inhibit the action of the sulphonamides and para-aminosalicyclic acid derivatives.

Procaine is unsuitable for topical use because it is poorly absorbed from mucous membranes and to be effective it must be injected near nerve fibres. However, it has been replaced in most of its applications by more stable drugs. When given intravenously it may produce general anaesthesia.

Solutions containing 0·5–2·0 per cent (with adrenaline) are suitable for infiltration or nerve block. Maximum adult dosage given with adrenaline is in the region of 1·0 g.

Lignocaine (xylocaine) is a synthetic anilide with potent local anaesthetic properties. It is an extremely stable compound in solution and is rapidly absorbed from mucous membranes. It is more than twice as potent as procaine and since it has vasodilator activity, adrenaline is usually given when it is used. Though toxic effects have been reported, used in correct dosage and with appropriate technique, lignocaine is a safe local anaesthetic. It is destroyed only in the liver. Drowsiness may occur when larger doses are absorbed.

Local anaesthesia is achieved more rapidly, i.e. in minutes and lasts longer (up to 3 hours) than with procaine. Solutions of 0·5–2 per cent are used for nerve infiltration or nerve block. The maximum dosage of lignocaine (with adrenaline) in the adult is 500 mg.

Prilocaine is a synthetic local anaesthetic which is similar in structure and action to lignocaine. An adverse effect is the production of methaemoglobinaemia. With dosages under 1 g the risks, however, are small.

Bupivacaine is chemically related to lignocaine and prilocaine but is more potent and has a more prolonged action. It is used as a 0·25–0·5 per cent solution.

Cinchocaine (dibucaine) is a synthetic amine with potent local anaesthetic properties. It is more toxic than cocaine and is mainly used as a topical agent in jelly, cream or suppository form.

Amethocaine (tetracaine) is one of the most potent and rapidly absorbed local anaesthetics. As with cinchocaine its use is limited to application of the jelly or ointment to areas of mucous membrane. Other local anaesthetics used in this way are butacaine, benzocaine and orthocaine.

ETHYL ALCOHOL

The absorption, metabolism and excretion of ethyl alcohol, the alcoholic content of various beverages and its value as a source of energy are given in vol. 1, pp. 30.37, 31.7, 4.4 & 4.6. Although originally considered to be of use in the treatment of many diseases and in the form of whisky called 'the water of life' in the Gaelic language, its clinical value is limited. It exerts its most important influence on the CNS on which it acts as a general depressant like the general anaesthetics. Behavioural tests show deterioration of all types of performance requiring skill or patience. Logical thought and purposeful activity are progressively disorganized. Self-restraint, discrimination and sobriety are lost and the personality becomes vivacious and expansive. At high blood concentrations unconsciousness ensues and this level is very close to the lethal concentration which depresses the respiratory centre (500 mg/100 ml).

Although it is used widely by the laity as a mild analgesic and regarded as a general stimulant and cure for a variety of ills, it probably owes its effects in these directions to its power to alter the patient's attitude to pain or distress to one of detachment.

The metabolic basis of these events is unknown but they are greatly enhanced in individuals who have taken simultaneously barbiturates, chlorpromazine, meprobamate and other agents. Fig. 5.41 neatly summarizes the general effects of alcohol and the legal limits of the blood concentration in relation to driving. The considerable variation in response to a given dose of alcohol is also shown. Repeated use of alcohol induces tolerance but not to the same extent as does morphine. The basis of the tolerance is unknown and is not due to an increased rate of oxidation. There is no doubt that the mental and physical consequences of small amounts of alcohol on behaviour

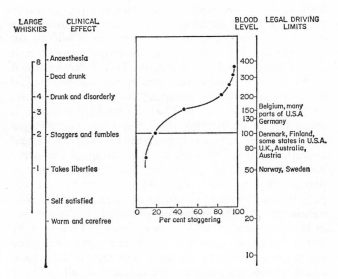

FIG. 5.41. Average effects produced by different concentration of alcohol in the blood. After Gaddum (1956) *Lectures on the Scientific Basis of Medicine*, vol. 4. London: Athlone Press.

can be consciously resisted and it is possible that the habitual drinker has learned to compensate for these. Addiction to alcohol occurs in some individuals who drink excessively and this may lead to disintegration of the personality. This constitutes a serious medical and social problem which is discussed in vol. 3. Other pharmacological effects of alcohol include peripheral vasodilation which leads to a feeling of warmth and a fall in body temperature. Reflex stimulation of the salivary and gastric secretions have led to its use as an appetizer, and its diuretic effect is due partly to inhibition of secretion of ADH. It also inhibits the release of oxytocin (p. 12.16). Alcohol by injection is irritant to tissues but is occasionally used to inject nerves or ganglia to relieve pain, e.g. trigeminal neuralgia. In a concentration of 70 per cent it is a moderately effective antiseptic.

TETRAETHYLTHIURAM DISULPHIDE (DISULFIRAM ANTABUSE)

$$C_2H_5 \quad\quad\quad\quad\quad C_2H_5$$
$$\text{N—C—S—S—C—N}$$
$$C_2H_5 \quad \| \quad\quad \| \quad C_2H_5$$
$$\text{S} \quad\quad \text{S}$$

Disulfarim

The sensitizing action of thiuram disulfide to alcohol was known as an industrial hazard, particularly in the rubber industry, where the tetraethyl derivative is used as an antioxidant. The full significance of this observation did not become apparent until the drug was tested as a potential cure for worms. In the course of these investigations, two Danish physicians took the drug and, to their astonishment, became ill after a few beers some hours later.

The drug is now used as an adjunct in the treatment of chronic alcoholism. By itself it has few metabolic effects but it influences the metabolism of alcohol by reducing the rate of oxidation of acetaldehyde in the liver and thus allows the concentration of this substance in the blood to rise. Acetaldehyde dehydrogenase is a copper-containing enzyme with which disulfiram combines. The rise in blood acetaldehyde is accompanied by unpleasant sensations which include flushing, headache, nausea and vomiting and which may last for several hours after alcohol is taken. The daily dose is 0·25–0·5 g and should be taken in the morning when the resolve to abstain is often greatest. Circulatory collapse may follow a large consumption of alcohol if the patient is taking disulfiram. Hypersensitivity reactions which include blood dyscrasias, skin reactions and gastrointestinal disturbances occasionally occur. In the treatment of alcoholism it is not a substitute for psychiatric care.

FURTHER READING

ADAMS E. (1958) *Barbiturate*. Scientific American Offprint No. 1081.

BARRON F., JARVIK M.E. & BUNNELL S. (1964) The hallucinogenic drugs. *Sci. Amer.* **210**, 29.

DIXON A.St. *et al.* (1963) *Salicylates*. London: Churchill.

DOMENJOZ R. (1966) Synthetic anti-inflammatory drugs: concepts of their mode of action. *Adv. Pharmac.* **4**, 143.

EDSTROM R. (1964) Recent developments in the blood–brain barrier concept. *International Review of Neurobiology*, vol. 7, p. 19.

GATES M. (1966) *Analgesic Drugs*. Scientific American Offprint No. 304.

GLOWINSKI J. & BALDESSARINI R.J. (1966) Metabolism of norepinephrine in the central nervous system. *Pharmacol. Rev.* **18**, 1201.

GOTH A. (1966) Antidepressant and psychotomimetic drugs, in *Medical Pharmacology*, 3rd Edition. St. Louis: Mosby.

GREEN J.P. (1964) Histamine and the nervous system. *Fed. Proc.* **23**, 1095.

HIMWICH H.E. & HIMWICH W.A. eds. (1964) Biogenic amines, in *Progress in Brain Research*, vol. 8. Amsterdam: Elsevier.

HORNYKIEWICZ O. (1966) Dopamine (3-hydroxytryptamine) and brain function. *Pharmacol. Rev.* **19**, 925.

KETY S.S. (1951) The theory and applications of the exchange of inert gas at the lungs and tissues. *Pharmacol. Rev.* **3**, 1.

KEYS T.E. (1963) *The History of Surgical Anesthesia*. New York: Dover.

LASAGNA L. (1964) The clinical evaluation of morphine and its substitutes as analgesics. *Pharmacol. Rev.* **16**, 47.

MILLICHAP J.G. (1965) Anticonvulsant drugs, in *Physiological Pharmacology*, vol. 2. ed. Root W.S. & Hofmann F.G., New York: Academic Press.

PATON W.D.M. & SPEDEN R.N. eds. (1965) Anaesthetics and the central nervous system. *Brit. Med. Bull.* **21**, 1.

PSCHEIDT G.R. (1964) Monoamine oxidase inhibitors, in *International Review of Neurobiology*, vol. 7, p. 191.

RITCHIE J.M. & GREENGARD P. (1966) on the mode of action of local anaesthetics. *Ann. Rev. Pharmacol.* **6**, 405.

WINTER C.A. (1965) Physiology and pharmacology of pain and its relief, in *Analgetics*, ed. de Stevens G. New York: Academic Press.

Chapter 6
Hormones and drugs that act on the endocrine glands

HORMONES OF THE PITUITARY GLAND

Six hormones have been isolated from the anterior lobe of the pituitary gland and two from the posterior lobe. The former six comprise growth hormone, corticotrophin, thyrotrophin, follicle stimulating hormone, luteinizing hormone and prolactin; the last three are known collectively as the gonadotrophins and are discussed in chap. 12. Growth hormone is species-specific, so that only material from primates is active in man. By contrast, corticotrophin of animal origin is satisfactory for pharmacological and clinical use in man.

Human growth hormone (HGH)

This is also known as somatotrophin (STH). Potent material is obtained from extracts of acetone-dried powdered preparations of cadaver glands and has been used extensively for clinical and laboratory investigations. HGH contains 188 amino acids and its mol. wt. is about 21,500. For purposes of assay, extracts are standardized in terms of the international reference preparation provided by WHO, 1 i.u. being equivalent in biological activity to 1 mg of this material. Preparations of HGH are assayed by their capacity to increase the rate of growth of normal or hypophysectomized rats or to increase the width of the proximal tibial cartilage of immature hypophysectomized rats.

Immunoassay procedures are sufficiently sensitive to follow the changes in concentration of the hormone in normal human plasma (vol. 1, p. 25.12).

Given intramuscularly, a single dose of HGH in man is followed by a series of metabolic changes which indicate that the mobilization of lipid as a source of fuel for energy requirements is a major function of the hormone. Although the half-life of the hormone in the blood is only about 25 min, some of the metabolic effects of a single dose persist for several days. The changes which may be observed include a rise in the plasma concentration of free fatty acids, together with a fall in the respiratory quotient. The plasma urea and amino acid concentrations both fall and increased protein synthesis is reflected in a reduction of the urinary excretion of nitrogen (fig. 6.1). Urinary calcium excretion is raised and, with prolonged administration, absorption of calcium from the gastrointestinal tract increases. When HGH is given to diabetic patients, the blood glucose concentration rises and the excretion of glucose and ketone bodies increases sharply.

Repeated injections of 5 mg of HGH at intervals of two or three days for periods of months accelerate the

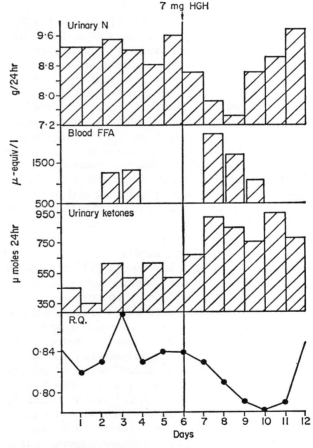

FIG. 6.1. Effects of human growth hormone on a woman with hypopituitarism. Changes in basal R.Q., in the urinary excretion of ketones and nitrogen and in the level of free fatty acids in the blood (FFA) following an injection of HGH. From Basu A., Passmore R. & Strong J. A. (1959) *J. Physiol.* **148**, 39P.

rate of growth of dwarfed children who are deficient in HGH. Some develop HGH antibodies and cease to grow with continuing treatment, but others maintain their growth despite the presence of antibodies.

Thyrotrophin

This is also known as thyroid stimulating hormone (TSH) and is obtained from extracts of the pituitary gland as a glycoprotein with a mol. wt. of between 25,000 and 30,000. The hormone is available as freeze dried material which is given by intramuscular injection, usually in doses of 10 i.u. These units refer to an international standard of bovine TSH, which differs antigenically from TSH of human origin. Many methods of bioassay have been described. The most satisfactory at present available depends on the discharge of ^{131}I from the thyroid gland of the mouse following administration of the test preparation.

The thyroid gland is almost completely dependent upon TSH for its continued function and the hormone acts on the thyroid gland at several points in the iodine cycle. When given by injection, the normal gland responds with an increased uptake of ^{131}I, an acceleration of the rate of thyroid hormone synthesis, and an increased output of thyroid hormones (vol. 1, p. 25.14). Using ^{131}I or ^{132}I uptake as an index of response, TSH, in doses of 10 i.u. intramuscularly daily for 3 days, distinguishes primary failure of the thyroid gland from the secondary hypothyroidism occurring as a sequel to pituitary failure; only in the latter form does increased uptake of iodine occur. A refractory state develops with repeated intramuscular injections of the commercial preparations of bovine TSH at present available, so that the use of thyrotrophin for clinical purposes is virtually restricted to this diagnostic test (fig. 6.2).

Corticotrophin

The adrenocorticotrophic hormone (ACTH) is much the most fully studied of the pituitary hormones and is widely used in clinical medicine. Preparations of ACTH from several species have been shown to contain thirty-nine amino acids, and to have a mol. wt. of 4500. Several fractions of the molecule have been prepared which retain biological activity, and active synthetic forms with as few as twenty-four amino acids have been used successfully for several years past (vol. 1, p. 25.8). One fraction of the molecule of ACTH with melanocyte stimulating hormone (MSH) activity has been prepared and found to contain thirteen amino acids (αMSH), and another, (βMSH) varies in composition between species but in man contains twenty-two amino acids.

Commercial preparations of ACTH are obtained from extracts of the pituitary glands of such species as sheep, pig, ox and whale and are standardized in units of an international standard. The official British reference

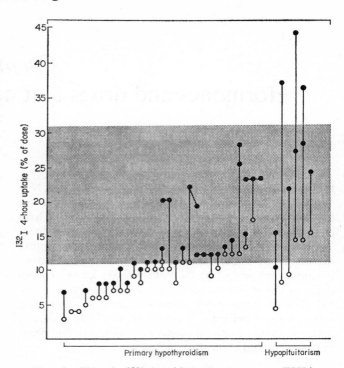

FIG. 6.2. The 4 hr ^{132}I thyroid uptake response to TSH in patients with primary hypothyroidism, and with hypothyroidism due to hypopituitarism. $\bigcirc$, Before TSH; $\bullet$, 18–24 hours after TSH intramuscularly. The shaded area shows the normal range of uptake. Redrawn from Bayliss (1967) Symposium on the Thyroid Gland, *J. Clin. Path.* (suppl.) **20**, 360.

preparation contains 1 i.u./mg, and the bioassay used depends upon the depletion of ascorbic acid in the adrenal glands of hypophysectomized rats. Changes in the output of steroid hormones by the adrenal cortex provide a useful alternative method. In addition, however, methods employing immunoassays have been developed and shown to be sufficiently sensitive to detect the hormone in the blood of man under a variety of circumstances.

Since the response elicited by ACTH varies with the route of administration, for purposes of standardization it must be given by intravenous or intramuscular injection. With the increasing use of synthetic analogues, it is likely that the dose of this material will soon be prescribed by weight, rather than in arbitrary units.

Administration of corticotrophin by intravenous, intramuscular or subcutaneous injection is followed by an increased output of steroids from the adrenal cortex. Repeated doses lead to an increase in the weight and in the secretory capacity of the adrenals. The output of steroids by the adrenal gland is dependent on the stimulus provided by ACTH, with the exception of aldosterone secretion by the zona glomerulosa of the cortex which is more closely dependent on angiotensin, activated by renin produced in the kidney (vol. 1, p. 33.17).

Numerous metabolic effects of ACTH on tissues other than the adrenal glands have been described, but most of these follow very large doses and are probably of little physiological importance. Pigmentation in animals and man after ACTH has been attributed to melanocyte stimulating hormone-like activity of ACTH. The main pharmacological activities of ACTH in man can, however, be ascribed largely to the increase in the production of cortisol.

Following a single intravenous dose of ACTH, the hormone disappears very rapidly from the circulation, so that continuous infusion is required if more than a transitory response from the adrenal is required. Absorption and inactivation of the hormone after intramuscular injection are also rapid and levels of corticosteroids in the blood are elevated for only a few hours. Prolongation of the effect is achieved by suspending the ACTH in gelatine, or conjugating it with zinc or zinc hydroxide. A single intramuscular injection of **ACTH-gel** or **ACTH-Zn hydroxide** acts for 24–48 hours. The 24-amino acid synthetic analogue, **tetracosactrin** (β^{1-24} corticotrophin) adsorbed on to a zinc–phosphate complex has been shown to have an action similar to that of corticotrophin-gel, and is used when it is necessary to obtain a therapeutic effect by a sustained increase in output of adrenal steroids. Long-acting ACTH preparations may be used clinically in diseases which respond to corticosteroids (p. 6.12). They are of greatest value in stimulating the adrenal cortex after a course of corticosteroid therapy which induces hypofunction. About 1 mg of synthetic tetracosactrin Zn phosphate is equivalent to 100 i.u. of ACTH-gel (fig. 6.3). As a test of responsiveness of the adrenal cortex, 0·25 mg of β^{1-24} corticotrophin given intravenously as a single injection should be followed by a rise of 50 per cent or more above the preinjection level of the plasma concentration of cortisol.

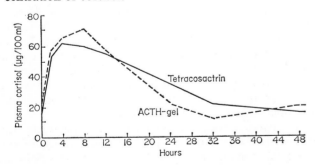

FIG. 6.3. Mean plasma cortisol concentrations after 80 units of ACTH-gel and 1 mg tetracosactrin Zn phosphate given by IMI. After Besser, Butler & Plumpton (1967) *Brit. med. J.* **4**, 391.

Vasopressin

The earliest active preparation of vasopressin was an aqueous extract of the mammalian neurohypophysis. Such extracts contained oxytocin as well as vaso-

pressin and their biological activity, therefore, resembled that of the physiological secretion. Subsequently, the two hormones were isolated in pure form and their structures were elucidated by du Vigneaud and his colleagues who, in 1953, synthesized both octapeptides. Such synthetic preparations have been widely employed in the investigation of the fundamental properties of the posterior pituitary hormones and have introduced a new degree of specificity in therapy.

Only the pharmacology of vasopressin is discussed here, oxytocin being described on p. 12.13.

CHEMICAL STRUCTURE

Study of the comparative chemistry of vasopressin has shown that the octapeptide structure of the hormone (vol. 1, p. 25.16) is common to man and all other mammals with the exception of the pig and the hippopotamus. In the vasopressin of the latter species, lysine replaces arginine as the penultimate amino acid residue of the straight chain part of the molecule (lysine-8-vasopressin).

The finding that this modified molecule exhibits in man some 60 per cent of the antidiuretic activity of arginine-8-vasopressin led to the synthesis of other cyclic octapeptides, each varying slightly from the natural hormones in amino acid sequence, in the hope of discovering yet more powerful antidiuretic principles. That it proved impossible to prepare a synthetic analogue of greater potency than arginine-8-vasopressin provides a fascinating commentary upon the effectiveness of the biological evolution of peptide structures.

BIOASSAY AND STANDARDIZATION

In common with many other polypeptides in therapeutic use, doses of vasopressin are expressed in terms of units of activity, the assay system being based, in this case, upon the effect of the intravenously administered hormone in raising the blood pressure of anaesthetized animals. This assay allows an unknown preparation of vasopressin to be standardized in terms of the activity of an internationally accepted posterior pituitary reference standard, 0·5 mg of which contains, by definition, 1 unit of pressor activity and 1 unit of antidiuretic activity.

Assayed in this way, synthetic arginine-8-vasopressin has an activity of some 500 units/mg. Since the relationship between antidiuretic and pressor activities is constant, the potency of a preparation expressed in pressor units provides an adequate indication of its antidiuretic activity.

ABSORPTION, FATE AND EXCRETION

Vasopressin cannot be given by mouth as it is inactivated by trypsin in the gut and must, therefore, be administered parenterally. The half-life of the hormone in the blood is about 5 min after an intravenous dose, 10 per cent being excreted in the urine and the remainder destroyed by peptidases, mainly in the liver and kidneys. As a result of rapid inactivation, the effect of an aqueous solution of the hormone, given intravenously, is transitory while, even by the subcutaneous and intramuscular routes, its duration of action is only some 1–2 hours.

Two preparations have been devised to overcome the need for frequently repeated injection. The first of these is the insoluble tannate of purified vasopressin suspended in an inert oil (pitressin tannate in oil, 5 units/ml), from which the active principle is released slowly, providing a sustained antidiuretic effect of about 48-hour duration following a single dose given intramuscularly. An alternative preparation takes the form of a nasal spray of synthetic lysine-8-vasopressin in aqueous solution and is absorbed in an active form from the mucosa of the upper respiratory tract. Its effect when given by this route, however, lasts for only 2–3 hours.

CLINICAL USE
In diabetes insipidus (vol. 1, p. 25.16), treatment requires the replacement of defective vasopressin secretion by an exogenous source capable of maintaining a sustained level of circulating hormone sufficient to restore renal water handling to normal. The precise plasma concentration of vasopressin required to exert such an effect is not known, but in normally hydrated subjects levels of 1–3 microunits/ml appear to be characteristic; this level rises some fivefold in response to water deprivation over a period of 24 hours.

In individual cases of diabetes insipidus, the appropriate dose of vasopressin is determined indirectly in terms of the clinical response, satisfactory control usually being achieved by the administration, on every second or third day, of 2·5–5·0 units of the hormone in the form of vasopressin tannate in oil by deep intramuscular injection. This can be supplemented, if necessary, by the use of the nasal spray of lysine-8-vasopressin when recourse to injection is inconvenient.

While replacement therapy is the most important application of vasopressin in medicine, the hormone is occasionally employed in two other situations, in which its pharmacological rather than physiological properties are exploited. In these cases, 10–20 units of aqueous vasopressin are given intravenously over periods of 15–30 min, these doses being many times greater than those required to effect maximum antidiuresis.

(1) Large doses of the hormone exert a direct stimulatory effect upon the contractile elements of the walls of blood vessels (vol. 1, p. 25.16). In the conscious animal, the impact of the resultant vasoconstriction upon blood pressure is normally minimized by the moderating influence of the vascular reflexes. Whatever the blood pressure response, however, reduced tissue blood flow inevitably results. This effect is employed therapeutically in the control of bleeding from the distended veins of the

oesophageal wall secondary to portal venous obstruction (p. 10.14).

(2) Unphysiologically large doses of lysine-8-vasopressin given intravenously may be used as a test of anterior pituitary function. This procedure depends upon the fact that the hormone exerts an effect upon the anterior pituitary similar to that of the corticotrophin releasing factor of the hypothalamus. Thus, in a healthy subject, the pituitary responds to an infusion of vasopressin by releasing ACTH in greater than normal amounts. This response can be detected either by the immunological estimation of the trophic hormone in plasma or indirectly in terms of an increase in the activity of the target gland. Failure of response implies a defect of anterior pituitary function. For the reasons set out below, however, the test is dangerous and is seldom employed clinically.

ADVERSE EFFECTS
Vasopressin replacement therapy in diabetes insipidus should be unattended by adverse effects which are seen only when the hormone is employed in unphysiologically large doses. The toxicity of vasopressin is due to its stimulating effects on smooth muscle and include nausea, eructation, intestinal colic and diarrhoea. Overshadowing all of these is the effect on the heart that results from a reduction in blood flow to the myocardium due to coronary arterial constriction together with a direct depressive effect exerted upon the heart muscle. This combination leads commonly to transient abnormalities in cardiac function and in the electrocardiogram; permanent ischaemic damage to the heart may be sustained in persons with coronary insufficiency.

THE THYROID GLAND

The physiological role of the thyroid gland depends mainly upon two amino acids formed and secreted by it, L-**thyroxine** (T_4) and L-**tri-iodothyronine** (T_3, or **liothyronine**). In addition, a further and separate function of the gland is performed by **calcitonin**, a hormone produced in its cells. The parafollicular (C) structure, synthesis, transport, metabolic fate and function of these hormones are described in vol. 1, p. 25.17.

The two hormones T_4 and T_3, as well as the related but physiologically inactive amino acids mono- and di-iodotyrosine, contain iodine. This element, therefore, is essential for the function of the thyroid gland. As it has no other known role in the body than to serve as a component of the thyroid hormones, iodine metabolism within the gland and elsewhere provides a valuable indication of the function of this organ and the metabolism of its secretions.

Radioiodine (p. 6.8) is used for the investigation of iodine metabolism in the thyroid gland, and for the treatment of increased thyroid function; in suitable doses the ionization it provokes leads to a reduction of function or even to destruction of the cells of the gland. Numerous organic compounds capable of interfering reversibly with the synthesis of T_4 and T_3 are also available, and are used as antithyroid drugs for the treatment of disorders of function of the gland.

The long acting thyroid stimulator (LATS), an immunoglobulin, is of great importance in the aetiology of hyperthyroidism and its origin and effects are described on p. 23.3.

The thyroid hormones

L-Thyroxine is the main physiologically active member of the four iodinated amino acids formed; it is stored as thyroglobulin in the colloid of the thyroid gland. When released into the circulation, the hormone is carried in two forms, a small free portion (<0·1 per cent) and the remainder which is bound to the thyroxine-binding globulin (TBG) of the plasma. Only the free form of the hormone is active. L-Tri-iodothyronine is similarly carried but has a lesser affinity for protein and is bound to a considerably less extent than T_4. The binding of T_4 to protein can be affected by a number of drugs which displace it from the protein. These include sulphonamides, chlorpromazine, salicylates, diphenylhydantoin and bishydroxydicoumarin. After their administration the total T_4 content of the blood is reduced but thyroid function is not disturbed. The increased binding of T_4 which occurs in pregnancy (vol. 1, p. 25.21) can be reproduced by giving oestrogens and is occasionally seen in the course of liver disease and rarely as a genetically determined variant. Androgens lower the level of TBG. In molar terms, T_3 is approximately five times more active that T_4.

These differences in binding and potency are largely responsible for the difference in the onset and duration of action of the two hormones. After giving T_3 by subcutaneous injection to a hypothyroid subject a metabolic response can be detected within 6 hours, in contrast to the interval of approximately 48 hours that elapses before the effect of a dose of T_4 five times larger begins to be apparent. The pharmacological effects of T_3 are short-lived in contrast to those of T_4, the former persisting for a few days whereas the response to T_4 may last for several weeks, depending in both instances on the dose used. In both cases, however, the metabolic effect outlasts the presence of the hormones in the blood.

ACTIONS OF THYROID HORMONES
The qualitative effects of T_3 and T_4 are identical. The methods of study include observation of the naturally occurring states of hyperthyroidism and hypothyroidism and the responses to effective treatment.

Shortly after extracts of the thyroid gland had first been used in 1891 by Murray to treat thyroid insuffi-

ciency, it was shown that the response to treatment was associated with an increased oxygen consumption. Ever since then changes in the resting or basal metabolic rate (BMR) have been used as an indication of the state of thyroid function, of the need for treatment and of the response to any treatment that may have been given. The development of many other measurable indices of thyroid function has reduced greatly the use of the BMR, but it remains a useful guide (vol. 1, p. 4.8).

The increase in oxygen consumption promoted by thyroid hormones should not be regarded as their primary action, but rather as a change accompanying the stimulation of a variety of metabolic processes. These include the following.

Increased heat production accompanies the increased oxygen consumption and the patient becomes more sensitive to warm environments.

Lipid catabolism is usually increased and hence the amount of body fat reduced when the concentration of thyroid hormone in the circulation increases; this response may not occur if the patient's appetite increases. The serum cholesterol concentration falls with increasing levels of T_4 or T_3, and it may rise to very high levels in hypothyroidism. These changes appear to be related mainly to redistribution rather than formation or degradation of cholesterol.

Carbohydrate metabolism changes with increased T_4 concentrations and carbohydrate tolerance may be impaired and resemble a mildly diabetic state; diabetes, if present, is aggravated. This effect is associated with depletion of glycogen stores, particularly in the liver.

Protein synthesis is stimulated by the thyroid hormones, but large doses also promote its breakdown and lead to muscle wasting. Urea nitrogen, creatine and creatinine excretion are all increased by abnormally high concentrations of the thyroid hormones.

Growth and development are both promoted by normal amounts of thyroid hormones. Hormone deficiency in man, on the other hand, is associated with profound delay of both, as exemplified in the cretin. Most of the features can be corrected by hormone administration, except for mental development which may be permanently defective unless hormone treatment is started soon after birth. Minor acceleration of growth and physical development above normal rates may occur with raised levels of circulating T_4 and T_3, e.g. in dental development. Increased rate of growth of thyroidectomized rats and metamorphosis of tadpoles are used as specific methods of assessment of thyroxine-like compounds.

Reproductive capacity may be impaired, but the mechanism of this failure is complex and indirect. Some derangement of menstrual function in the female is common with increased or reduced thyroid function, and is generally corrected when this is rectified.

The cardiovascular system, particularly the heart, responds vigorously to changes in T_4 and T_3 concentration. Administration of T_4 in hypothyroidism usually increases the heart rate modestly, but cardioacceleration is very marked with the excessive concentrations of hormone found in hyperthyroidism. High concentrations are associated with marked vasodilation, tachycardia and disorders of cardiac rhythm such as extrasystoles and atrial fibrillation, especially in older patients. The effects of thyroid hormones on the heart may be mediated in part at least by alterations in the responsiveness of the organ to catecholamines. These considerations are particularly important in patients with ischaemic heart disease; small doses of T_4 may be sufficient to aggravate angina pectoris or to precipitate myocardial infarction in such a patient. Propranolol (p. 15.23) may be used to reduce or prevent these effects.

The central nervous system shows marked responses to changes in T_4 concentration. Mental development is arrested in the cretinous infant or child. Development progresses in response to treatment, but is seldom complete unless the hormone has been given continuously from an early stage of life. Thyroid insufficiency at any stage of life is associated with depression and slowing of cerebral cortical function; psychoses may appear, but these effects are all potentially reversible by treatment with T_4. Excess of thyroid hormone in the circulation, as in hyperthyroidism, may be associated with excitement or maniacal behaviour. All these changes are reflected in EEG abnormalities and respond to appropriate adjustments of the circulating level of thyroid hormone.

Administration of T_3 and T_4 inhibits the release of TSH by the anterior pituitary, by the feedback mechanism described in vol. 1, p. 25.7. If T_3 and T_4 secretion is inhibited by antithyroid drugs, the secretion of TSH rises and the thyroid gland undergoes hyperplasia and enlargement. Such a preparation may be used experimentally to test the effectiveness of thyroxine-like preparations which are given along with the antithyroid drug.

The time-course of muscular relaxation after a stretch reflex is also susceptible to alterations in the level of T_4. Delay in the relaxation phase of, e.g., the ankle jerk, is found in hypothyroidism; it may be detected clinically and is reversible with treatment.

Water and electrolyte metabolism are affected by altered thyroid function. Retention of water in severe hypothyroidism (myxoedema) is corrected by treatment, and the excess of water lost by sweating and evaporation in hyperthyroid states is usually balanced by an increased intake of fluids and restriction of losses in the urine. Sodium is retained in excess along with water in hypothyroidism, and both are excreted in response to treatment. Potassium metabolism reflects the changes in the muscle mass that may occur. Calcium metabolism is also sensitive to major alterations in thyroid function. A long standing excess of T_4 may be associated with a negative calcium balance sufficiently severe to lead to the radiological changes of osteoporosis.

Haemopoiesis may be depressed in hypothyroidism and responds to treatment with T_4.

CLINICAL USE
T_3 and T_4 may both be used in the treatment of hypothyroidism in doses of about 20–100 μg and 0·1–0·3 mg/day respectively. T_4 is preferred for general use because its effect is slower in onset and more prolonged than T_3. T_3 may be given intravenously in the treatment of severe hypothyroidism (myxoedema coma) in which cortisol should also be given to overcome the functional adrenocortical insufficiency which accompanies this condition. Formerly a dried extract of thyroid was used in the treatment of hypothyroidism. This was standardized chemically to contain 0·1 per cent iodine as thyroxine. The use of such a preparation has been abandoned because there was little correlation between its biological activity and iodine content.

Overdosing with T_3 or T_4 reproduces the features of hyperthyroidism and induces tachycardia, nervousness, insomnia, sweating, weight loss, vomiting and diarrhoea.

THYROID HORMONE ANALOGUES
Since it has been realized that only the laevorotatory isomers of T_4 and T_3 are physiologically active and that the dextrorotatory forms have only a small effect on oxygen consumption, but may lower the serum concentration of cholesterol, many analogues of T_4 and T_3 have been synthesized and tested for thyroxine-like activity. These investigations have been directed mainly towards finding an analogue that would selectively reduce the serum concentration of cholesterol without producing signs of overdosage, as with T_4. It has not proved possible to segregate these two effects. In any case it is far from clear that even were this possible, lowering of the serum cholesterol concentration has any real advantage for the patient with hypercholesterolaemia and potential or established atherosclerosis (p. 8.11).

Antithyroid Drugs
Reduction of the effects of the thyroid hormones on the tissues can be accomplished in several ways, apart from surgical removal of a large part of the thyroid gland. Three separate methods exist which reduce the rate of formation of the thyroid hormone and which are em-

ployed in the treatment of hyperthyroidism. First, a temporary effect is obtained by administering iodine; second, a reversible inhibition of hormone formation can be established by the thiocarbamide group of drugs and related compounds, and third, complete and permanent, or incomplete but progressive, destruction of the gland by irradiation can be produced with radioactive iodine.

IODINE

It is paradoxical that iodine, the element on which the formation of the thyroid hormones depends, should be used as an antithyroid drug. However, if it is recalled that the total body store of iodine is about 50 mg, and that this element forms about 65 per cent by weight of T_4, the amount of iodine required to provide for the normal daily output of about 0·2–0·3 mg of T_4 is seen in proper perspective. Furthermore, since most of this iodine is reutilized by the thyroid gland, the total daily intake of iodine normally required is of the order of 100–200 μg.

It has been realized for more than 40 years that giving iodine before and after thyroidectomy performed for hyperthyroidism reduces rapidly the severity of the illness and the thyrotoxic manifestations, but the quantity of iodine needed to achieve this effect is usually 100 mg daily and often more is given. This suppressive effect is transient, but the clinical signs and the histological appearances in the thyroid gland all revert towards the normal state under this treatment. The maximal effect is reached in about 2 weeks and, after a variable period of time the effect gradually wears off. Iodine does not inhibit the formation of thyroglobulin but rather promotes its storage; hence the effect may be due to a block in the release of thyroid hormones from these stores into the circulation. This suggests that the amount of iodine in the gland may influence the rate of secretion of thyroid hormones, and suppressive activity by iodine can be demonstrated also in animals given TSH.

Iodides have been shown to be goitrogenic and when taken for prolonged periods in large doses, e.g. in proprietary asthma remedies, reduce the concentration of thyroid hormones; with this treatment the thyroid gland becomes hyperplastic and depleted of iodine. About 10 per cent only of those who take iodides in this way develop a goitre, and a few may also become hypothyroid. It has been shown experimentally that iodide transiently inhibits iodine binding to protein in the gland.

Iodine deficiency on the other hand has long been recognized as a cause of simple or endemic goitre. Since the amount of iodine in a normal diet in most parts of the world approximates to the minimal requirement of about 100 μg daily, the condition is relatively common. In many instances other factors besides absolute iodine deficiency probably contribute to the incidence of goitre, but these can also be overcome by an adequate intake of the element.

Iodide when taken in excessive doses may produce characteristic features resembling those accompanying a common cold (iodism), and a papular or vesicular rash may develop.

THE THIOCARBAMIDE COMPOUNDS (fig. 6.4)

The discovery of the antithyroid thiocarbamides arose from a chance observation at Johns Hopkins Hospital made in 1928; rabbits raised in the laboratory for the study of syphilis and fed largely on cabbage developed

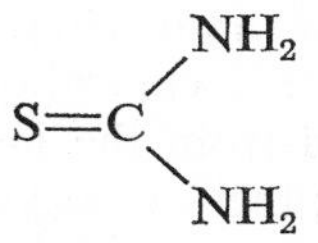

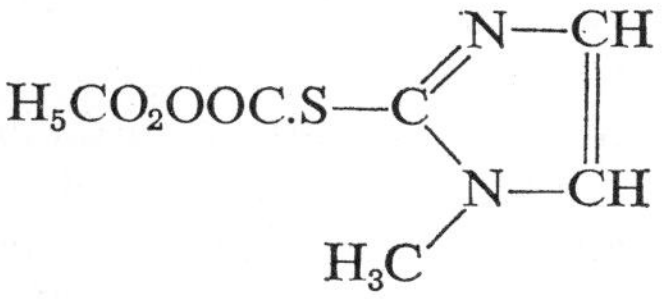

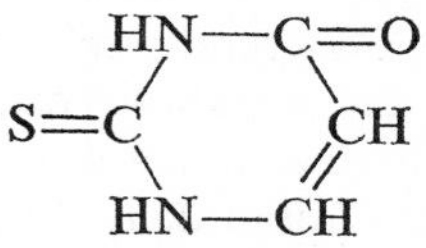

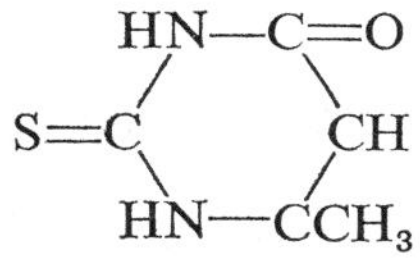

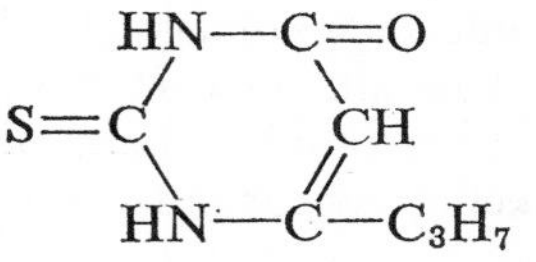

FIG. 6.4. Goitrin and antithyroid compounds of the thiocarbamide group. The doses represent usual daily maintenance requirements for the treatment of hyperthyroidism in the adult.

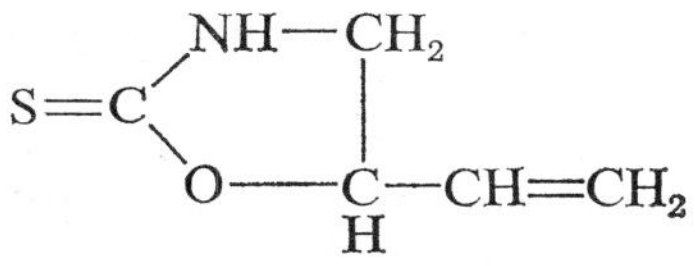

goitre. New Zealand workers then showed that many vegetables, e.g. cabbage, turnip, mustard and rape seeds had goitrogenic properties. The thyroid enlargement appeared to be a compensatory hypertrophy consequent upon interference with synthesis of T_4; TSH secretion was increased but hypothyroidism developed. The substance responsible was shown to be goitrin or related substances which are released from the food by gastrointestinal micro-organisms (fig. 6.4). This chance discovery of a natural inhibitor of thyroid function pointed the way to the development of modern antithyroid drugs which were first used in 1943 by Astwood at Harvard. This group of compounds inhibit hormone formation in the gland. Among them **carbimazole** is as satisfactory as any; the comments which follow apply generally to the group though the effective doses vary.

The action of these drugs probably involves more than one of the steps in thyroid hormone synthesis, including the iodination of tyrosine, the coupling of the iodinated tyrosines to form T_3 and T_4 and possibly their de-iodination as well. Studies in animals and man have shown that the dose can be adjusted not only to block all hormone synthesis, but also to allow normal thyroid hormone synthesis to proceed, but at less than full capacity. That the compounds probably interfere with the peripheral action of the thyroid hormones as well as with their formation is shown by the observation that thiouracil-treated rats respond less well to thyroxine than animals subjected to thyroidectomy. While these effects may contribute to the goitrogenic activity of antithyroid drugs they are probably of little importance in clinical dosage.

These drugs are readily absorbed from the intestine and are widely distributed in tissues; they are excreted in the urine and also in milk, so that breast feeding may inhibit thyroid function in an infant. Thiourea labelled with ^{35}S is oxidized to sulphate in the thyroid gland and liver. In the treatment of hyperthyroidism these drugs are given in high doses for a period of several weeks during which there is a slow fall in the metabolic rate to normal. Thereafter the drug is maintained at a lower dose for a minimum of 1 year. The usual initial daily dose of **methyl** and **propylthiouracil** is 300 mg and that of carbimazole 40–60 mg. They are liable to produce a wide range of untoward effects, including nausea and vomiting, diarrhoea, skin rashes, lymph node and salivary gland enlargement, and most important of all, bone marrow depression which may progress to agranulocytosis, or aplasia. These effects are most likely to occur in the first few weeks of treatment.

Reduction in the output of thyroid hormones by thiocarbamides promotes TSH secretion which in turn increases the vascularity of the thyroid gland and causes hypertrophy of the acinar cells. In excessive doses marked enlargement of the thyroid gland occurs.

THIOCYANATE AND PERCHLORATE

Sodium or potassium salts of either of these ions are potent inhibitors of the iodine concentrating mechanism in the thyroid gland. Potassium perchlorate is occasionally employed as a substitute for the thiocarbamides in treating hyperthyroidism, but it produces most of the adverse effects of this group of drugs, and so enjoys no special advantage. Since both salts inhibit thyroid hormone synthesis at the earliest or trapping stage of the iodine cycle in the thyroid gland, they are used occasionally in the investigation of disordered thyroid function to show that ^{131}I is discharged from the gland when hormone synthesis is blocked at the next stage by a peroxidase deficiency. Such a disorder is a cause of one rare form of congenital goitre.

ANILINE AND HETEROCYLIC COMPOUNDS

A number of drugs which are employed for a variety of clinical purposes, e.g. para-aminosalicylic acid, sulphonamides and the sulphonylureas, when given over long periods and in large doses, may cause hypothyroidism and thyroid gland enlargement.

RADIOACTIVE IODINE

This term is used to describe a series of nineteen radioactive isotopes (radionuclides) of the stable isotope of iodine, ^{127}I. Only a few of these are suitable and available for use in biology and medicine, depending on their physical and other characteristics. Since radioisotopes of iodine are metabolized in precisely the same way as stable iodine, they can be used not only as tracer indicators of the metabolism of iodine and of the thyroid hormones, but also in order to irradiate the thyroid gland for therapeutic purposes.

Radioiodine is also used extensively in chemistry, biology and medicine as a label for a large variety of substances which either contain iodine, or can be made to react with iodine in such a way that they acquire this radioactive label.

The isotope of radioiodine most widely used at present is ^{131}I. This has a half-life of 8 days, and decays with the emission of β-particles and relatively high energy γ-rays. ^{132}I has a shorter half-life of 2·3 hours, and is particularly valuable for repeated tests in adults or when radioiodine studies are required in children, since the dose of radiation delivered is so much smaller than with ^{131}I. A third isotope, ^{125}I, with a half-life of 60 days, is widely used to label compounds required for biochemical and similar purposes, but at present it is seldom used *in vivo* in animals or man.

Radioiodine is readily available commercially as a pure solution of sodium iodide (Na ^{131}I), or alternatively as Na ^{132}I or Na ^{125}I. Since the specific activity of these preparations is very high, and because of the extremely small quantities of iodine present, it is common practice to add a small quantity of stable 'carrier' iodide to solutions of radioactive iodine, so as to reduce losses in handling, on glassware and in syringes.

When used for diagnostic purposes, radioiodine is usually given by mouth in a dose of 5–15 microcuries and is very rapidly absorbed from the stomach. If necessary it can be sterilized and given by intravenous injection. Provided there is not already an excess of iodine in the circulation, the isotope is concentrated rapidly in the thyroid. The rapidity of uptake and the speed with which the plasma is cleared of radioiodine provide measures of the activity of the thyroid gland. At this stage if a biopsy is taken of the gland and autoradiographs prepared, the radioiodine is found within the thyroid parenchymal cells and in the colloid of the follicles. Chemical analysis shows that the isotope has been incorporated into the thyroid hormones which have been labelled in this way, and the rate and extent of labelling of the serum protein bound iodine (PB ^{131}I) provides a further measure of the activity of the thyroid gland. Ultimately the hormone is degraded and the iodine is either recovered by the thyroid gland or excreted in the urine. Since about 99 per cent of inorganic iodide present in the circulation at any time, whether stable or radioactive, is normally either taken up by the thyroid gland or excreted in the urine, the ratio between these two fractions provides a further useful measure of thyroid function.

When ^{131}I decays, it emits γ-rays and β-particles, both of which, especially the latter, create a state of ionization in surrounding tissues. The average range of β-particles in tissue is about 0·5 mm, whereas the γ-rays are absorbed by the tissue of the thyroid to a small extent only, and most escape into the surrounding air where they can be detected by suitable apparatus and their source and quantity determined.

Irradiation of the thyroid gland with interference in cell function is readily achieved by the administration of radioiodine, and the treatment of hyperthyroidism is frequently undertaken in this way. The dose is determined by the size of the thyroid gland and its activity as judged by the rapidity of uptake of a tracer dose of ^{131}I. Amounts of 5–15 millicuries are commonly used. Because of the theoretical but remote danger of inducing thyroid carcinoma this method of treatment is usually limited to patients over 40 years of age. The effect of the radioactivity on the gland is slowly progressive and the incidence of hypothyroidism some years after treatment is high. Cancer of the thyroid gland is also occasionally amenable to treatment with radioiodine, but only a few of these tumours have much affinity for iodine.

Like other radioactive isotopes, radioiodine must be handled with care and used with discretion, since it is not only potentially destructive in the intended recipient, but is also a danger to the handler or to any other person who might be accidentally contaminated. The biological effects of ionizing radiation are cumulative, so that repeated relatively small doses may in time lead to an accumulated potentially toxic dose of radiation.

Calcitonin
This polypeptide is secreted by the parafollicular or C cells of the thyroid gland and assists in maintaining calcium homeostasis. Like the parathyroid hormone, it acts on bone as well as on the kidney. It suppresses bone resorption, and lowers the serum concentration of calcium as well as of phosphorus. These effects on bone are the reverse of these of parathyroid hormone. Calcitonin enhances the excretion of phosphate by the kidney and in this respect resembles parathyroid hormone. It does not appear to affect the absorption of calcium (vol. 1, p. 25.26).

6

Limited studies in man suggest that the hormone might be of value in the management of hypercalcaemia, and when it becomes available in sufficient quantities, it will certainly merit a trial in the treatment of osteoporosis and Paget's disease.

THE PARATHYROID HORMONE

Potent aqueous extracts of bovine parathyroid glands, assayed by their ability to elevate serum calcium, have been available commercially for many years, and are given by intramuscular or intravenous injection. A single dose exerts an effect on serum calcium which lasts up to 36 hours. These preparations have been of limited clinical value for two reasons; firstly, the patient readily becomes tolerant to them, and secondly, therapy with calciferol and calcium salts is more effective in the treatment of hypocalcaemia associated with hypoparathyroidism.

Much more pure and potent extracts of the parathyroid glands have now been prepared, and it is likely that a relatively pure preparation of the active polypeptide will be available commercially in the near future. Immunoassay procedures have also been developed which are suitable for studying the hormone in plasma (vol. 1, p. 25.25).

Excessive doses of parathyroid hormone reproduce the biochemical features of hyperparathyroidism, namely an increase in the serum concentration of calcium, and a fall in the serum concentration of phosphorus. Grossly excessive doses lead to nausea, vomiting, thirst, polyuria stupor, coma and even death. These features occur when the serum concentration of calcium rises to 17 mg/100 ml or more.

THE ADRENAL CORTEX

The corticosteroids
In 1931 Swingle and Pfiffner prepared an extract of adrenocortical tissue which was capable of maintaining life in the adrenalectomized animal. The administration of such extracts to patients suffering from Addison's disease represented the first form of hormone replacement therapy in this otherwise fatal condition. During the next twenty years, the work of Kendall, Reichstein and others led to the isolation and synthesis of a number of corticosteroids including the most important of the naturally occurring hormones, cortisol. These preparations supplanted the use of gland extracts in replacement therapy.

In the late 1940s, a second therapeutic role was defined for the corticosteroids. It had been known for some years that striking remission of the signs and symptoms of rheumatoid arthritis often occurred in pregnancy and the recognition that this physiological state was associated with increased synthesis of steroid hormones led Hench and his colleagues in 1948 to investigate the effect of the newly synthesized steroid, cortisone, in patients suffering from rheumatoid arthritis. The success of this therapy led to the recognition that glucocorticoid hormones were able to control many inflammatory and allergic conditions. Similarly, large doses of glucocorticoids have been found therapeutically useful in modifying the abnormal haemopoiesis in some forms of leukaemia (p. 7.8) and in the treatment of bacterigenic shock (p. 18.30). In all these conditions, the amount of steroid required to exert a therapeutic effect is much greater than that necessary for replacement therapy. This is explained by the fact that in patients with normal hypothalamo-pituitary–adrenal function, doses of a glucocorticoid equal to or less than the replacement dose simply suppress adrenocortical function to an extent which maintains the pretreatment concentration of circulating steroid.

Suppression of hypothalamic and pituitary function in this way is invoked in a further clinical application of steroid hormones. In some genetically determined adrenal disorders, the contribution of sex hormones by the adrenal glands is undesirable. In such cases, the administration of replacement doses of a glucocorticoid suppresses the liberation of ACTH from the pituitary and with it the undesirable secretions of adrenocortical sex hormones. The normal physiological situation is, however, otherwise maintained, as aldosterone secretion, being largely independent of ACTH, remains at a normal level while the exogenous glucocorticoid replaces the resulting cortisol deficiency.

MECHANISM OF ACTION
The efficacy of corticosteroid therapy in the replacement and suppression of adrenal function is readily understood in the light of what is known of the physiology of the adrenal cortex (vol. 1, p. 25.33). Despite extensive investigation, however, little is known of the mechanism by which large doses of glucocorticoids suppress inflammation, influence allergy or exert their other effects. The hormones cause a reduction in fibroblastic activity and in collagen formation, and decrease capillary permeability, phagocytic activity and the deposition of fibrin. In addition, the *in vitro* enzymic conversion of kininogens to vasoactive kinins is inhibited by cortisol, a fact which may in part account for the ability of the glucocorticoids to reduce the intensity of the allergic response in which kinins are known to play an important part (p. 24.6).

Glucocorticoids have no curative property in inflammation or allergy but merely minimize the local and systemic effect of the underlying disorder. It is important to recognize that both inflammatory and hypersensitivity reactions represent normal tissue responses to injurious stimuli and that the former fulfil an important defensive

and reparative function. It is only in those cases where the response is clearly excessive or inappropriate, therefore, that its suppression is desirable; examples are provided by such diseases as bronchial asthma, idiopathic ulcerative colitis, rheumatoid arthritis, acute rheumatic fever and other connective tissue disorders, some forms of glomerulonephritis and hypersensitivity manifestations occurring in the skin (p. 23.7).

Glucocorticoids have been shown to be effective in protecting experimental animals from the effects of endotoxin given intravenously and are now widely used in the treatment of circulatory collapse in man especially when due to septicaemia (bacteraemic shock syndrome). In these circumstances hypotension and shock are not due to absolute adrenocortical insufficiency, as the rate of secretion of cortisol and its concentration in the blood are many times higher than the basal levels. In spite of this, cortisol in doses of the order of 500–1000 mg/day are valuable in the treatment of shock which fails to respond to more conventional methods. The mechanism of action is uncertain but in man the cardiac output and blood pressure rise and the peripheral resistance falls (p. 8.7).

Another interesting effect concerns the influence of high concentrations of glucocorticoids on the integrity of lysosomes (vol. 1, p. 25.34). Lysosomes are believed to be disrupted by hypoxia and endotoxins, and the hydrolases and proteases which are released may contribute to the genesis of the circulatory failure. Glucocorticoids are known to stabilize lysosomal membranes and thereby prevent their disruption, suppressing the release of the enzymes into the tissues. The relationship of this effect to the action of the steroids in shock and to their anti-inflammatory effect is unknown.

STRUCTURE–ACTIVITY RELATIONSHIPS
In the early years of the use of the corticosteroids in the control of hypersensitivity and inflammatory conditions, only the naturally occurring hormones were available. Large doses of these agents were required and their use was attended by the occurrence of serious adverse and unwanted effects. For example, the prototype glucocorticoid, cortisol, a potent anti-inflammatory steroid, also exerts powerful undesirable effects upon water, mineral, carbohydrate, protein and fat metabolism. It soon became clear that the successful application of corticosteroids to the suppression of allergic and inflammatory disorders was dependent upon the development of agents modified in such a way as to minimize the undesirable effects associated with their use.

Consideration of the two hormones, cortisol and aldosterone, provided the key to the solution of the problem since, despite their close structural similarity, their actions are entirely different (vol. 1, p. 25.33). This observation led to the finding that relatively minor changes in the structure of the steroid molecule may lead

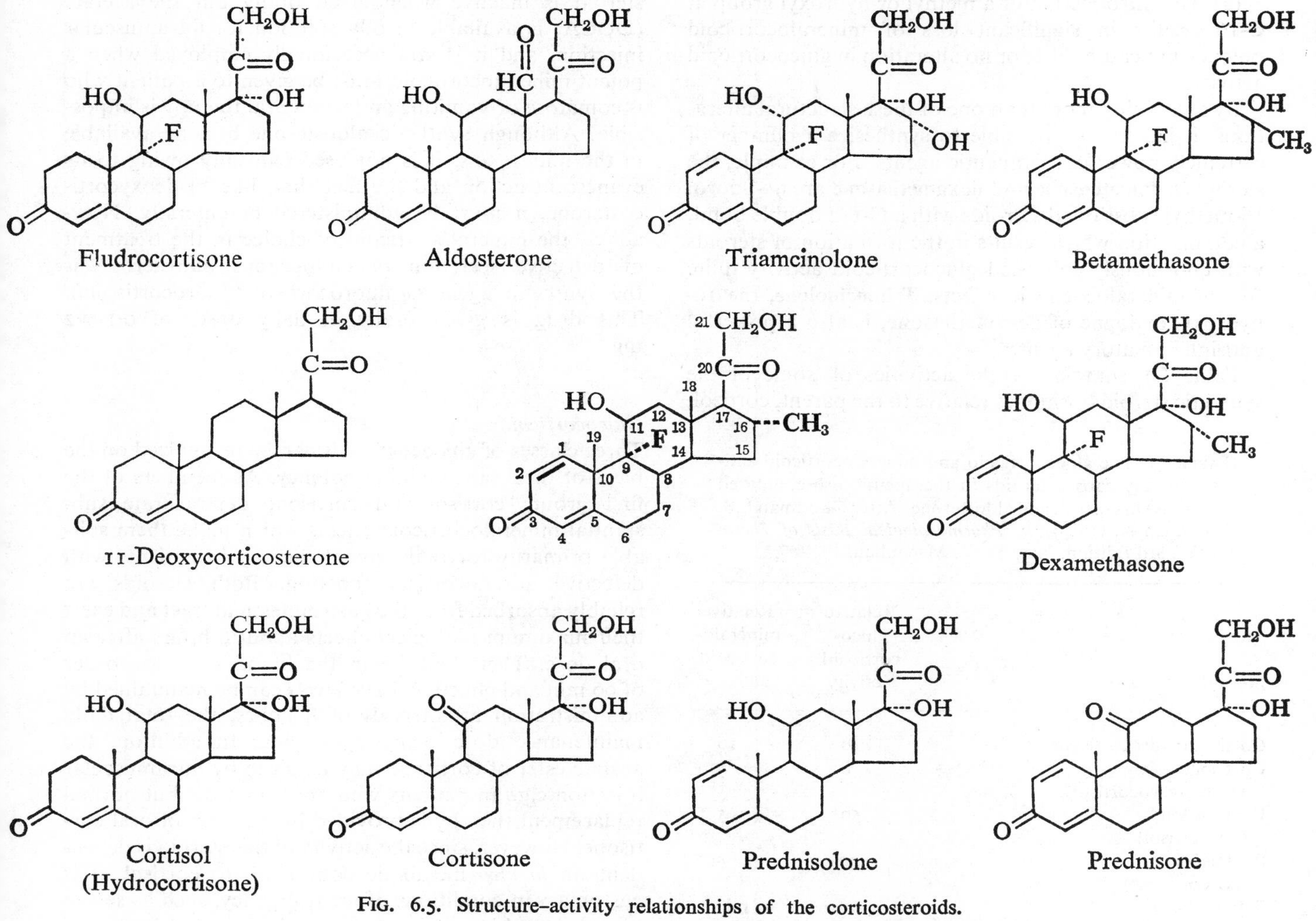

FIG. 6.5. Structure–activity relationships of the corticosteroids.

to major modifications in biological activity. These modifications are at least to some extent predictable and it has proved possible to synthesize steroid analogues with specified desirable features.

Fig. 6.5 represents a guide to the structure–activity relationship of the corticosteroids together with the structural formulae of the more important synthetic derivatives. The bold type in the central formula indicates four structural alterations which are employed in the preparation of those steroids in therapeutic use. These alterations are as follows.

(1) The molecular configuration at C-11 of the steroid nucleus is of fundamental importance in determining activity. Thus, an oxygen radical in this position is an essential characteristic of all glucocorticoids although its absence is not inconsistent with sodium retaining activity. An example of this phenomenon is provided by **11-deoxycorticosterone** (DOC) which is a powerful mineralo-corticoid free from glucocorticoid activity. Moreover,

the form in which the oxygen function occurs may be of importance. For example, cortisone, which differs from cortisol only by its possession of an 11-keto instead of an 11-hydroxyl group, is devoid of corticosteroid activity, its effectiveness *in vivo* being dependent upon enzymic reduction to cortisol in the liver.

(2) The introduction of a double bond between carbon atoms 1 and 2 of the steroid nucleus increases glucocorticoid at the expense of mineralocorticoid activity. In addition, it delays the *in vivo* inactivation of the steroid, so potentiating its biological effect. Modification of cortisol and cortisone in this way results in the production of **prednisolone** and **prednisone** respectively.

(3) Introduction of a fluorine atom in the 9α position leads to a significant increase in all of the activities of the corticosteroids. In the particular case of cortisol, this modification results in the formation of **9α-fluorocortisol (fludrocortisone)** which possesses greatly enhanced mineralocorticoid activity.

(4) The introduction of a methyl or hydroxyl group at C-16 results in significant loss of mineralocorticoid potency but causes little or no alteration in glucocorticoid activity.

By combining more than one of these structural alterations, it has proved possible to synthesize a number of extremely powerful therapeutic agents. For example, the steroids **betamethasone** and **dexamethasone** are 9α-fluoro, 16-methyl substituted steroids with a C-1–2 double bond, a combination which results in the formation of steroids with enormously enhanced glucocorticoid activity quite free of mineralocorticoid effects. **Triamcinolone**, the 16-hydroxy analogue of dexamethasone, is also a powerful anti-inflammatory agent.

Table 6.1 summarizes the activities of some of the synthetic steroid hormones relative to the parent, cortisol,

TABLE 6.1. The glucocorticoid and mineralocorticoid activities of the corticosteroids in therapeutic use compared with those of cortisol and aldosterone. After Goodman L.S. & Gilman A. (1965) *The Pharmacological Basis of Therapeutics*, 3rd Edition. New York: Macmillan.

Steroid	Relative gluco-corticoid activity	Relative mineralo-corticoid activity
Cortisol (hydrocortisone)	10	10
Cortisone (11-dehydrocortisol)	8	8
Prednisolone (Δ1-cortisol)	50	5
Prednisone (Δ1-cortisone)	40	5
Betamethasone (9α-fluoro-16β-methylprednisolone)	300	nil
Dexamethasone (9α-fluoro-16α-methylprednisolone)	300	nil
Triamcinolone (9α-fluoro-16α-hydroxyprednisolone)	100	nil
Aldosterone	?	4000
11-Deoxycorticosterone	nil	300
Fludrocortisone (9α-fluorocortisol)	150	1500

in terms of glucocorticoid activity, which parallels their anti-inflammatory effect, and mineralocorticoid potency. While many other steroid analogues exist, in general they have no distinct advantage over those listed in the table.

CLINICAL USE, ABSORPTION, FATE AND EXCRETION
Mineralocorticoids
For many years, 11-deoxycorticosterone (DOC) was employed in the treatment of mineralocorticoid deficiency that might arise, e.g. in Addison's disease. This steroid is inactive when given orally but the acetate (DOCA) is available in oily solution for intramuscular injection, and it is still occasionally employed when a potent mineralocorticoid must be given to a patient who is comatose or vomiting and when oral therapy is impossible. Although synthetic aldosterone became available in the mid 1950's, it is not used clinically owing to its evanescent action and the fact that, like 11-deoxycorticosterone, it must be administered parenterally. Nowadays, the mineralocorticoid of choice in the treatment of defective secretion of endogenous aldosterone is the synthetic agent 9α-fluorocortisol (fludrocortisone). This drug is given orally in daily doses of 0·1–0·2 mg.

Glucocorticoids
Three classes of glucocorticoids can be recognized on the basis of their salt retaining potency. As members of the first group, cortisol and cortisone demonstrate substantial mineralocorticoid effects which make them suitable primarily for replacement therapy in patients with defective adrenocortical function. Both steroids are reliably absorbed from the gastrointestinal tract and exert their maximum biological effects about 6 hours after an oral dose. Their half-life in the blood is of the order of 90 min and effective tissue levels can be maintained by administration at intervals of 8 hours, the total daily maintenance dose being 25–50 mg. In addition, the acetate ester of cortisone may be given by intramuscular injection e.g., in patients who are comatose, but normal replacement therapy is provided in the form of oral cortisone. However, since the activity of this steroid is dependent on *in vivo* metabolic conversion to cortisol, it is customary in conditions of great urgency, such as severe acute adrenal insufficiency, to employ cortisol itself and to hasten the attainment of adequate tissue levels of the hormone by the intravenous administration of its soluble salt, **cortisol sodium succinate.** In these circumstances much larger doses than those used for maintenance therapy are needed, 10–40 mg being given hourly for several hours followed by 100 mg/day for several days. Thereafter, once the crisis has subsided cortisone in usual replacement doses should be given by mouth.

The second group of glucocorticoids is represented by prednisolone and prednisone which have, weight for weight, anti-inflammatory potency about four times that of cortisol but which are slightly less active than cortisol in the regulation of mineral metabolism. Both are well absorbed after oral administration and have a slightly longer duration of action than cortisol. They are not used in replacement therapy but are the most widely employed anti-inflammatory steroids. They are given in daily doses of up to 100 mg/day for some days or weeks and thereafter in doses of 5–20 mg/day (p. 24.6).

In the future, however, it seems likely that members of the third group, represented by betamethasone and dexamethasone (0·5–5 mg/day), will enjoy greater popularity in the suppression of allergy and inflammation as a result of their freedom from unwanted mineralocorticoid effects. These steroids are normally given by mouth but the sodium phosphate salt of dexamethasone is also available for intramuscular or intravenous injection. Triamcinolone is almost as powerful as dexamethasone or betamethasone but is more toxic and is particularly liable to induce muscle damage with wasting and weakness. For this reason it should probably never be used clinically.

Specialized preparations of cortisol, cortisone, prednisolone and dexamethasone as creams or ointments are available for local application to the skin, mucosal surfaces and the conjunctiva.

The mechanisms of metabolic inactivation and excretion of the synthetic corticosteroid derivatives do not differ significantly from those described for the naturally occurring steroids cortisol, corticosterone and aldosterone (vol. 1, p. 31.11).

ADVERSE EFFECTS
The use of fludrocortisone and of 11-deoxycorticosterone is, in general, restricted to the replacement of defective endogenous secretion of aldosterone and is, therefore, usually unattended by significant adverse effects. If unusually large doses are administered, however, undue retention of sodium and water with alkalosis and loss of potassium, together with arterial hypertension, may result. The same untoward effects follow unphysiologically large doses of glucocorticoids with significant electrolyte regulating activity. These effects have precluded the use of cortisone as an anti-inflammatory agent but even with prednisolone, which has greatly attenuated mineralocorticoid activity, supplements of potassium chloride must often be given with the steroid in order to forestall the potassium depletion which might otherwise follow prolonged administration. Similarly, the accumulation of oedema in a patient treated with prednisolone may require the concurrent use of diuretic therapy together with a diet restricted in its sodium. These complications can be avoided by the use of beta- or dexamethasone in cases in which only the anti-inflammatory action of the steroid is required.

That the rather false physiological distinction between mineralo- and glucocorticoid activities has been realized pharmacologically represents a triumph of molecular engineering and allows agents such as betamethasone to be used without attendant mineralocorticoid effects. Unfortunately, however, the application of structure–activity relationships is subject to considerable limitation and it has so far proved impossible to enhance selectively one glucocorticoid activity at the expense of others by molecular modification. Thus, for example, the use of betamethasone in doses sufficiently large to exert a powerful anti-inflammatory effect is necessarily accompanied by untoward side effects attributable to glucocorticoid activity. These undesirable effects are seen usually after prolonged administration of the hormones in doses in excess of the replacement dose of cortisol or its equivalent and are, to some extent, predictable from knowledge of the physiological actions of the glucocorticoids (vol. 1, p. 25.33). Thus, prolonged administration results in negative nitrogen balance leading in adults to muscle wasting, and in children to retardation of growth. Long continued use of glucocorticoids also leads to negative calcium balance and osteoporosis. Calcium absorption from the gastrointestinal tract is reduced and there may be arrest in linear growth of bone as a consequence of failure of growth of epiphyseal cartilage. In addition, impaired tissue integrity marked, for example, by recurrent peptic ulceration and by bleeding into the subcutaneous tissues occurs. There is also a reduction in the resistance to and in the signs and symptoms of systemic infections, of which tuberculosis is perhaps the best known instance. Another important effect of the glucocorticoids is impairment of carbohydrate tolerance leading to increase in the insulin requirements of those patients already suffering from diabetes mellitus and the not infrequent appearance of glycosuria in those patients not hitherto regarded as diabetics. Other effects include psychological abnormalities such as euphoria, depression or psychotic reactions, together with the development of the external features of Cushing's syndrome such as mooning of the face and increasing obesity mainly affecting the trunk. In this context, it is worthy of note that the more potent glucocorticoids, when applied to the skin in large quantities or over a wide area, may be absorbed in sufficient amounts to result in systemic effects of the types outlined above.

Perhaps the most important unwanted effect of the glucocorticoids, however, is their impact upon the feedback control of the hypothalamo–pituitary axis. The resultant suppression of adrenal function is not rapidly reversible and may persist for prolonged periods extending to months or even years, so that withdrawal of the supply of exogenous steroid must be gradual if adrenal insufficiency is to be avoided. In addition, intercurrent stress or illness occurring in a patient treated with steroids increases the patient's corticosteroid requirements often to as much as three times the normal replacement dose and, since endogenous production of the hormones is in abeyance, supplementary therapy must be given.

For these reasons, all patients on steroid therapy must be aware of possible dangers and must carry at all times a printed card giving details of their treatment. Such information may be of life-saving importance in situations where the patient is admitted to a hospital where he is not known, for example, unconscious after a motor accident. These considerations apply equally to patients suffering from chronic adrenal insufficiency receiving replacement therapy.

Steroids are, in a real sense, dangerous drugs and their use places a heavy burden of responsibility on doctor and patient alike, if therapeutic disasters are to be avoided.

In all cases, the risks attending the use of glucocorticoid hormones in the unphysiologically large doses required to modify haemopoiesis, hypersensitivity and inflammation must be weighed against the gravity of the underlying disease and the beneficial effects which may be expected, before this form of therapy is undertaken.

Adrenocortical inhibitors

Apart from the glucocorticoids, the application of which to the selective suppression of the secretion of adrenal sex hormones was discussed on p. 6.10, a number of agents which modify cortical function are recognized.

For example, during investigation of the animal toxicity of *p,p'*-dichloro-diphenyl-trichloroethane (dicophane, DDT), it was found that several analogues of the insecticide interfere with adrenal steroidogenesis. Two of these derivatives, **metyrapone** and *o,p'***-dichlorodiphenyldichloroethane** (*o,p'*-DDD), are employed clinically and their structures, together with that of DDT, are illustrated in fig. 6.6.

METYRAPONE (metopirone)

Metyrapone is a selective inhibitor of the enzyme,

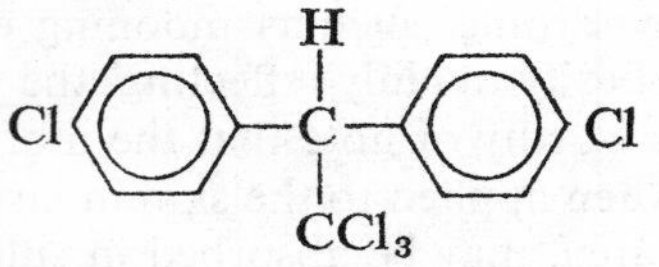

p,p'-Dichlorodiphenyltrichloroethane
(DDT)

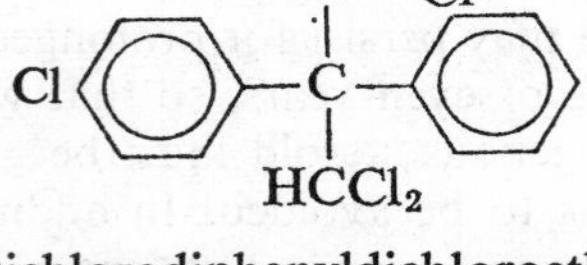

o,p'-Dichlorodiphenyldichloroethane
(*o,p'*-DDD)

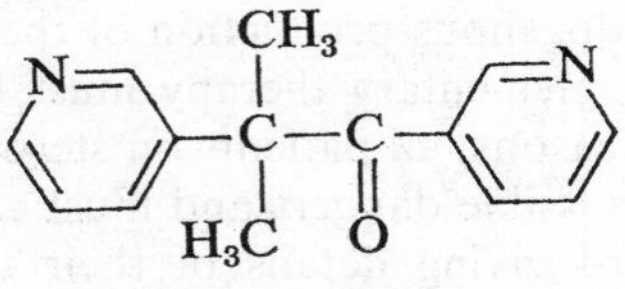

Metyrapone

FIG. 6.6. The insecticide DDT and its derivatives *o,p'*-DDD and metyrapone.

11-β-hydroxylase, which catalyses the *in vivo* synthesis of cortisol and aldosterone from their respective precursors, 11-deoxycortisol and 11-deoxycorticosterone (vol. 1, p. 25.32). The drug is active after oral or intravenous administration but its biological half-life is short so that optimum enzyme inhibition requires its administration either by constant intravenous infusion, or by mouth, at intervals not longer than 2 hours. The usual total daily dose is 3 g.

In the past, the use of metyrapone has been advocated in disorders of adrenocortical function associated with excessive secretion of aldosterone or cortisol. The suppression of aldosterone secretion by this drug, however, has never been of convincing therapeutic value since the 11-deoxysteroids, whose secretion is increased by the drug, are themselves powerful mineralocorticoids. With the introduction of the spironolactones (p. 11.9), the use of metyrapone in cases of inappropriate aldosterone secretion was therefore abandoned. In patients suffering from Cushing's syndrome metyrapone is still occasionally employed to suppress the excessive secretion of cortisol either as a preliminary to surgical treatment or when, for some reason, this is impossible.

The most important clinical application of metyrapone, however, is in the assessment of hypothalamo–pituitary function. The metyrapone test depends upon the fact that the feedback control mechanism between the adrenal cortex and the hypothalamo–pituitary axis is mediated by the circulating concentration of unbound cortisol, the 11-deoxysteroids being ineffective in the suppression of ACTH secretion. By blocking cortisol synthesis, metyrapone frees the hypothalamo–pituitary axis from its normal constraints and this results in the secretion of ACTH at a rate determined only by the functional capacity of the axis system.

The test involves the oral administration of ten doses of metyrapone, each of 250 mg, at intervals of 2 hours. In the normal subject, this regime results in an increase in the plasma concentration of ACTH which stimulates the adrenal cortex to secrete increased amounts of 11-deoxysteroids, the metabolites of which are detected in the laboratory as urinary 17-hydroxycorticosteroids (17-OH-CS). Failure to detect the expected increase in urinary 17-OH-CS excretion implies either that the hypothalamo–pituitary axis is unable to respond normally to the metyrapone-induced reduction in the concentration of circulating cortisol or that the adrenals are incapable of response to the increased plasma concentration of endogenous ACTH. This ambiguity in interpretation can be avoided by demonstrating the responsiveness of the adrenals to exogenous ACTH before metyrapone is given. This preliminary allows unequivocal interpretation of 'metyrapone unresponsiveness' in terms of hypothalamo–pituitary failure and has the additional advantage that it obviates the need to use metyrapone in patients with primary adrenal disease, in whom it is liable to induce acute adrenal insufficiency.

The metyrapone test has been used clinically for several years but its indirect approach is likely to be replaced, in the near future, by methods based upon the radio-immunoassay of ACTH which will allow the direct assessment of hypothalamo–pituitary function in terms of plasma concentration of the trophic hormone.

Adverse effects are commonly encountered with metyrapone and include rashes and gastrointestinal disturbances such as nausea, vomiting and diarrhoea. The hazard of acute adrenal insufficiency occurring during administration of the drug requires particular emphasis.

o,p′-DDD

This highly toxic derivative of DDT causes profound anorexia, nausea and skin eruptions. The fact that it exhibits selectively enhanced toxicity towards cells of adrenocortical origin, whether normal or neoplastic, has led to its use in the management of malignant tumours of the adrenal cortex for which surgical treatment is precluded. For example, in the recent past the drug has been employed in oral doses of up to 10 g/day, as a palliative agent in cases of adrenal carcinoma with extensive metastatic deposits. In favourable cases shrinkage of the tumour mass due to cellular necrosis has resulted, together with significant reduction in associated hormone production by the tumour cells, which may be so great as to provoke a state of adrenal insufficiency. For this reason, maintenance therapy with oral cortisone, supplemented if necessary by fludrocortisone, is often administered concurrently.

AMINOGLUTETHIMIDE

Originally employed as an anticonvulsant, aminoglutethimide, in oral doses of 1–2 g/day, inhibits steroid biosynthesis at the stage of the conversion of cholesterol to pregnenolone (vol. 1, p. 25.32). As may be anticipated from the site of the resulting metabolic block, the drug suppresses the production of all steroid hormones but, unlike o,p′-DDD, it does not result in structural damage to the cortex. Aminoglutethimide can be used, therefore, to suppress both adrenal and gonadal steroid production but it is not free from toxic effects which include anorexia, ataxia and somnolence, and the precise place of this agent in therapy has not yet been established.

INSULIN AND HYPOGLYCAEMIC DRUGS

Insulin

The British Pharmacopoeia defines insulin as a 'sterile solution of the specific antidiabetic principle of the mammalian pancreas'. It is used in the treatment of diabetic patients who are deficient in endogenous insulin. Given by mouth it is ineffective because to retain its potency insulin must also retain its integrity as a protein. Thus, it is generally injected subcutaneously. Intramuscular and intravenous injection of the short-acting insulins (see below) can also be used in certain circumstances. The chemistry, physiological actions, mechanism of action and degradation of this hormone are discussed in vol. 1, p. 25.39.

For clinical use insulin is prepared from the fresh or frozen pancreas of either cattle or pigs, usually by extraction with acid. It is then purified by repeated crystallization in the presence of zinc. The zinc is probably incorporated into the crystal lattice and pure insulin, crystallized as the sulphate or the phosphate, contains from 0.3 to 0.6 per cent zinc.

ASSAY OF INSULIN

Insulin in serum is essentially a trace protein, a single molecule occurring among 2 million other protein molecules. This makes its detection and still more its estimation extremely difficult. Moreover, there are substances in the blood which may influence the activity of insulin, e.g. proteins, other hormones, nonhormonal antagonists of various kinds, and antibodies. Thus, any test must be not only extremely sensitive but also either highly specific or involve some preliminary extraction procedure.

Chemical methods for the estimation of insulin are not available and their development in the immediate future is unlikely. Several bioassay procedures are available, each measuring insulin-like effects, but there is no assurance that the effects are due to insulin alone. Three types of assay are employed.

In vivo methods are based on the blood sugar response of suitably sensitive animals to injected extracts of biological material. These are used mainly for testing and standardizing therapeutic insulin preparations.

In vitro methods are based on a metabolic response of an isolated tissue to added serum or plasma containing insulin, e.g. measurements of,

(1) glucose consumption and glycogen deposition by the isolated diaphragm of the rat,

(2) glucose consumption and CO_2 production by the epididymal fat pad of the rat,

(3) CO_2 production by slices of lactating mammary gland of the rat and

(4) glucose uptake of the perfused isolated heart. All these methods measure effective insulin-like activity.

In *immunoassay methods* antisera to beef insulin are prepared in guinea-pigs. Beef insulin labelled with ^{131}I is added and this combines with antibody to form complexes. The reaction is reversible and after a time equilibrium is reached and the ratio of insulin bound in complexes to free insulin is constant (bound:free ratio). The addition of human insulin for assay competes for binding and displaces labelled insulin, causing an increased amount of free labelled insulin and a fall in the bound:free ratio. The ratios obtained with the test and standard preparations are then compared. Immunoassay methods are extremely sensitive and precise. However, since they give no information about the biological activity of the insulin estimated, it is unlikely they will replace completely the older bioassay procedures.

STANDARDIZATION OF INSULIN PREPARATIONS
The treatment of diabetes mellitus with insulin became possible only because of the development of accurate methods of standardization. The dose is measured in units, each unit representing a degree of hypoglycaemic activity. This was first defined in 1922 by Banting and Best and was based on the ability of samples of insulin to lower the blood glucose level in rabbits. In 1925, the unit of insulin was defined by reference to a standard preparation with an activity of approximately 24 units/mg. Today, insulin is assayed by comparing it with the fourth International Standard Insulin Preparation (1958) in its effect on lowering the blood glucose concentration of mice to a lethal level. Therapeutic preparations of insulin usually contain 20, 40 or 80 units/ml.

PREPARATIONS OF INSULIN (table 6.2)
There are two main types of insulin in clinical use, those with a rapid onset and short duration of action, and those whose action is slow in onset and lasts longer, the depot insulins.

Short-acting insulins
Insulin injection, commonly termed **soluble insulin** (sometimes known as unmodified or regular insulin) is a clear aqueous solution of insulin extracted from the pancreas of cattle or pigs, purified by crystallization and prepared at a pH of between 3.0 and 3.5, a trace of preservative being added. When injected subcutaneously, it produces an effect in 30–60 min which lasts about 6–8 hours.

Neutral insulin injection (insulin novo actrapid; nuso neutral insulin) is a clear solution of insulin extracted from pig pancreas and buffered with acetate at pH 7. Its effect lasts for approximately the same time as soluble insulin but the onset is faster.

Depot insulins
A number of preparations have been made which prolong the action of subcutaneous doses and reduce the need for frequent injections.

TABLE 6.2. Summary of insulin preparations.

Type of activity	Preparation and units/ml	Appearance	pH	Animal source	Protein modifier	Buffer	Miscible with
Rapid onset and short duration	Soluble insulin injection (20, 40, 80)	Clear solution	3–3.5	Pig, cattle, pig/cattle mixed	None	None	Globin, isophane
	Neutral insulin injection (40, 80) actrapid	Clear solution	7.2	Pig	None	Acetate	Crystal II
Intermediate	Globin zinc insulin injection (40, 80)	Clear solution	4.0	Pig, cattle, pig/cattle mixed	Globin	None	Soluble insulin
	Insulin zinc suspension (amorphous) (40, 80) semi-lente	Cloudy suspension	7.2	Cattle	None	Acetate	Other insulin zinc suspensions
	Isophane insulin injection (40, 80)	Cloudy suspension	7.2	Pig, cattle, pig/cattle mixed	Protamine	Phosphate	Soluble insulin
Slow onset and long duration	Protamine zinc insulin injection (40, 80) PZI	Cloudy suspension	7.2	Pig, cattle, pig/cattle mixed	Protamine	Phosphate	None
	Insulin zinc suspension (crystalline) (40, 80) ultra-lente	Cloudy suspension	7.2	Cattle	None	Acetate	Other insulin zinc suspensions
	Crystal II insulin injection (40, 80)	Cloudy suspension	7.2	Cattle	None	Acetate	Actrapid

Protamine zinc insulin injection (PZI) is prepared by adsorbing insulin on to a foreign protein molecule, protamine, in the presence of zinc; the protein–zinc–insulin complex, when injected subcutaneously, breaks up slowly in the tissues, and gradually releases the bound insulin over a period of 24 hours.

Globin zinc insulin injection is prepared with globin, obtained by removing haem from haemoglobin, and then combined with insulin. The mixture forms a clear solution at pH 4 but, when injected, the higher pH of the subcutaneous tissue causes precipitation. The precipitate breaks up slowly, releasing the insulin. The duration of the action of globin zinc insulin is intermediate between that of soluble and protamine zinc insulin, i.e. about 12 hours.

Insulin zinc suspensions do not contain foreign protein. The duration of their action depends on the size and form of the insulin crystals as well as on the rate at which these crystals are dissolved and are absorbed. The former is achieved by carefully controlling the conditions of precipitation; the latter is delayed by buffering with acetate (rather than phosphate, as with most insulins) and by adding small quantities of zinc. Because they do not contain a foreign protein they are less likely than other depot insulins to cause sensitization. Three forms are available.

(1) **Insulin zinc suspension (crystalline)**, commonly known as ultra-lente, contains comparatively large crystals which dissolve slowly, so that the effect does not begin for over 4 hours and lasts for 24 hours or longer.

(2) **Insulin zinc suspension (amorphous,** semi-lente), has smaller crystals and the maximal effect is apparent within 6–7 hours and persists for about 12 hours.

(3) **Insulin zinc suspension** (lente), is a mixture of three volumes of semi-lente with seven volumes of ultra-lente.

Isophane insulin injection (NPH, neutral–protamine–Hagedorn) is similar to protamine zinc insulin but has a much smaller percentage of protamine so that it contains some soluble insulin which is not complexed. The onset of action is therefore quicker than with insulin zinc suspensions, although the duration of action is similar.

Crystal II insulin injection has the same chemical composition and pH as actrapid but is prepared by crystallizing beef insulin. These crystals, unlike those of pig insulin remain undissolved at pH 7. They are absorbed slowly after subcutaneous injection and have an intermediate onset of action, the duration of which depends on the physical properties of the crystals and not on the presence of added zinc or protein.

Biphasic insulin injection (insulin novo rapitard) is a mixture of actrapid and crystal II insulins.

Table 6.2 summarizes important facts about the different kinds of insulin. A combination of protamine zinc and soluble insulin is commonly prescribed, but these should not be mixed together prior to injection, since the excess protamine simply converts the soluble insulin to protamine insulinate. Soluble insulin should not be mixed with the lente insulin since the critical pH of the zinc suspension is liable to be disturbed. However, globin and isophane insulin can be mixed with soluble insulin to provide preparations with intermediate characteristics.

Fig. 6.7 shows the duration of action of some common

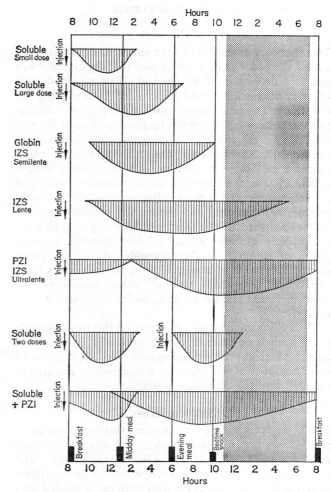

FIG. 6.7. Duration of action of insulins in common use.

insulin preparations. The degree and duration of hypoglycaemic effect depends on the size of the dose as well as on the type of preparation; generally the larger the dose the more profound the depression of blood glucose and the longer the effect.

ADVERSE EFFECTS

Overdosage with insulin leads to hypoglycaemia with its characteristic symptoms. Eventually loss of consciousness, sometimes with convulsions, may occur. These effects are reversible provided the degree and particularly the duration of hypoglycaemia have not been so great as to cause permanent neurological damage.

Nonspecific local reactions at the site of injection, and allergic reactions such as skin rashes and urticaria occasionally occur. Insulin preparations derived from pig pancreas and those which do not contain other protein material are less likely to give rise to allergic responses.

Subcutaneous atrophy of fat sometimes occurs at the site of injection, particularly in women.

Oral hypoglycaemic agents

The discovery of insulin in 1922 appeared at first to have solved the problem of diabetes mellitus; the disorder was due to a deficiency of insulin and all its metabolic and other consequences could be avoided by replacing the deficiency. The continuous search since then for alternative methods of treatment has had two sources of inspiration, firstly, the inconvenience caused by the need to inject insulin and secondly, the growing realization that diabetes mellitus may not be due to primary insulin deficiency. For these reasons the introduction in 1954 of the **sulphonylureas** for the treatment of diabetes mellitus was of both practical and theoretical interest; they are now established in the treatment of many middle aged and elderly diabetic patients. More recently, another group of compounds, the **biguanides**, have been introduced. The mode of action of these compounds is completely different from that of either insulin or the sulphonylureas and the indications for their use are also different.

Today, approximately one-third of the total diabetic population is being treated with an oral hypoglycaemic agent. Moreover, the development and application of these compounds has provided a tremendous impetus to research into the aetiology of diabetes.

Sulphonylureas

The hypoglycaemic effect of several sulphonamide compounds was first reported in 1930, but was not systematically studied until 1942. Grave, sometimes fatal neurological disturbances were observed in patients suffering from typhoid fever who were being treated with a thiadiazole derivative of sulphanilamide; these were found to be due to hypoglycaemia. The mechanism of the hypoglycaemic action of this compound was then studied experimentally and it was found to have no hypoglycaemic effect in depancreatectomized animals. It was not, however, until 1954, when Franke and Fuchs accidentally recognized the hypoglycaemic property of an antibacterial sulphonamide, **carbutamide**, that the therapeutic usefulness of these compounds as hypoglycaemic agents was demonstrated. Since then many related sulphonyl compounds have been synthesized and tested for their effect on the blood sugar. The most commonly used today are **tolbutamide** (artosin, rastinon, orinase) and

chlorpropamide (diabinese); **acetohexamide** and **tolazamide** are also sometimes used. Because it has toxic effects on the bone marrow, carbutamide has been largely abandoned. Similarly, metahexamide, one of the most potent hypoglycaemic agents in this group, is no longer used clinically because of the high incidence of liver damage and blood dyscrasias.

The arylsulphonylurea molecule may be considered as a urea derivative, with an arylsulphonyl group at one

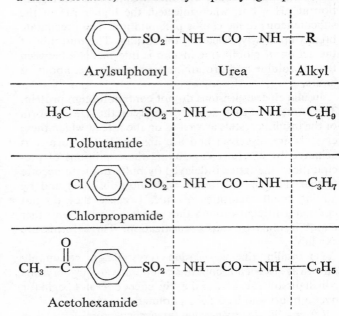

FIG. 6.8. Sulphonylurea derivatives.

end, and another group 'R', usually an aliphatic side chain, at the other end (fig. 6.8). The various modifications of the molecule affect not only its action on the blood sugar, but also the toxicity and the persistence of the drug in its active form in the body.

MECHANISM OF ACTION

Animal experiments and clinical studies have established the following three facts concerning the mechanism of the hypoglycaemic action of the arylsulphonylureas.

(1) The presence of functioning β-cells in the pancreatic islets is essential for the hypoglycaemic effect. This was first demonstrated by Loubatières in 1944 and has since been amply confirmed (fig. 6.9). Sulphonylureas do not lower the blood glucose concentration significantly in experimental animals in which the β-cells are ablated, e.g. by alloxan or in depancreatized or eviscerated animals. By contrast, hypoglycaemia occurs when the β-cells are intact, even after hepatectomy. These compounds are ineffective therefore in treating diabetic patients who are insulin deficient, but they are of value in treating patients in whom the pancreas retains some capacity to produce insulin.

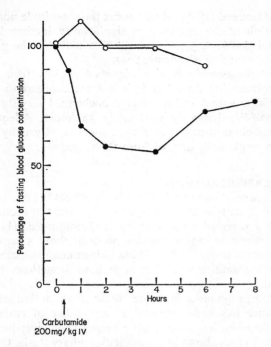

FIG. 6.9. Action of carbutamide on the blood glucose concentration of eight normal (●) and four depancreatectomized dogs (○). The points are the mean figures for each group plotted as a percentage of the fasting blood glucose level. Note the lack of effect in the depancreatized animals. Redrawn from data of Houssay B.A., *et al.* (1957) *Ann. N.Y. Acad. Sci.* **71**, 12.

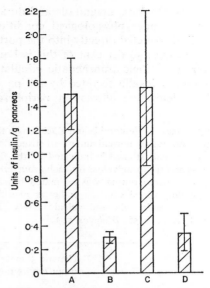

FIG. 6.10. The effect of 14 days' treatment with carbutamide on the amount of insulin extractable from the pancreas of dogs. The columns represent the mean values ± SEM.

A, three control dogs; B, three dogs given carbutamide 2·4 g daily by mouth; C, three dogs given 2 units of depot insulin subcutaneously twice daily; D, two dogs given both carbutamide and insulin twice daily. Note the fall in the amount of insulin extractable from the pancreas in the animals treated with carbutamide. Redrawn from data of Root M.A. *Diabetes* (1957) **6**, 12.

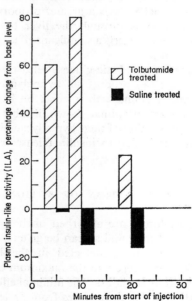

FIG. 6.11. Changes in plasma insulin (measured by the rat diaphragm bioassay) in the pancreatic venous blood of four dogs given 1·0 g sodium tolbutamide intravenously and four dogs given isotonic saline. Experimental animals showed a rise in ILA which was maximum at 10 min after injection. Control animals exhibited a slight fall in ILA. From Colwell A.R. Jr. & Metz R. (1962) *Diabetes* **11**, 504.

(2) They stimulate, at least initially, the release of insulin from the pancreas. The evidence in support of this has been derived from perfusion experiments in which a vascular anastomosis has been made between the pancreaticoduodenal vein of a normal donor dog and the jugular vein of an alloxan diabetic recipient. Following the administration of carbutamide to the intact animal, hypoglycaemia occurs in the diabetic recipient. In addition, a fall in the amount of insulin extractable from the pancreas (fig. 6.10), and a rise in the insulin-like activity of pancreatic venous blood follows the acute administration of sulphonylureas (fig. 6.11). Although doses of carbutamide producing therapeutic blood levels may decrease the insulin content of the pancreas when the drug is first started, longer treatment does not maintain this and after 8 weeks' treatment the pancreas recovers its normal concentration of insulin.

The view that the sulphonylureas act by increasing endogenous insulin release is difficult to reconcile with the failure to demonstrate consistently either an increase in peripheral glucose utilization or an increase in peripheral blood insulin following their administration. However, the failure of the sulphonylureas to reproduce the peripheral actions of exogenous insulin is probably due to the fact that the metabolic effects of insulin are influenced by the site, rate, magnitude and duration of its administration. Under physiological conditions, endogenous insulin is secreted directly into the portal circulation and more than 50 per cent of this is bound in the human liver in a single transhepatic circulation. Thus small amounts of insulin secreted by the pancreas may not produce detectable effects on peripheral glucose

TABLE 6.3. Effect of tolbutamide and glucagon on the hepatic glucose output of normal unanaesthetized dogs. The number of animals studied is indicated by the figures in parentheses and the mean values for each group are shown. The hepatic glucose output was estimated by simultaneously sampling blood through catheters placed in the portal vein, hepatic vein and splenic artery. Data of Ashmore J., *et al.* (1958) *Diabetes*, **7**, 1.

	Hepatic glucose output mg/kg/min
Controls, no injection (6)	6
60 minutes after tolbutamide, 0·5 g/kg (3)	0
15 minutes after glucagon, 1.0 mg IV (3)	19

utilization. Only when hepatic insulin binding sites are saturated or blocked does a greater proportion of endogenous insulin pass through the liver to the systemic circulation where it exerts a significant effect on peripheral glucose utilization.

(3) They reduce hepatic glucose release. Although the sulphonylureas can produce an hypoglycaemic effect in hepatectomized animals, their effect on hepatic glucose release in the intact animal shown in table 6.3 accounts for a large proportion of their hypoglycaemic action; it is likely that this is due to insulin release from the pancreas.

ABSORPTION, DURATION OF ACTION, FATE AND EXCRETION
The sulphonylureas are absorbed unchanged from the gastrointestinal tract and so can be given orally.

Tolbutamide can be detected in the blood within 30 min of an oral dose and the maximum concentration is reached within 3–5 hours. The minimal effective plasma concentration of the drug varies from patient to patient but is about 6–10 mg/100 ml. These levels follow a single dose ranging from 0·5 to 1·5 g. Since tolbutamide is oxidized rapidly in the body to its inactive carboxy derivative (biological half-life 4–8 hours), two or even three doses are required to maintain an adequate hypoglycaemic effect throughout the 24 hours. No single dose

should exceed 1·5–2 g, since neither the magnitude nor the duration of the response is significantly increased by greater doses. A 5 per cent solution may also be given intravenously in diagnostic tests.

Chlorpropamide is also absorbed rapidly from the gastrointestinal tract but it is not metabolized to any significant extent and is excreted unchanged very slowly, its half-life being approximately 36 hours. Adequate plasma concentrations of 2·5–5·0 mg/100 ml usually follow a single daily dose of from 100 to 500 mg.

ADVERSE REACTIONS
Adverse reactions to tolbutamide are infrequent and mild. Blood dyscrasias are occasionally observed but these are quickly reversed when therapy is discontinued. Hypersensitivity reactions in the skin occur in about 5 per cent of patients treated with tolbutamide or chlorpropamide; nausea, vomiting and diarrhoea have sometimes been noted.

Chlorpropamide is more toxic than tolbutamide. Jaundice has been reported in a number of patients, usually when large doses have been given. Liver biopsy in these cases shows intracanalicular biliary stasis. Other unwanted effects include intolerance to alcohol, and symptoms of lethargy, muscular weakness, ataxia and dizziness which seem to be due to the direct action of the drug on the CNS.

Hypoglycaemia with symptoms is a relatively uncommon complication of sulphonylurea therapy, as compared with insulin, and when it occurs it tends to be less severe and abrupt in onset. It is usually easily relieved by carbohydrate, but more profound hypoglycaemia, accompanied by loss of consciousness, may be very refractory to treatment. Severe and sometimes fatal hypoglycaemic coma may occur in patients treated with chlorpropamide, and less frequently with tolbutamide.

Patients who have an allergic response with one drug, do not necessarily have one with the others.

Biguanides
In 1918, guanidine was shown to have a hypoglycaemic effect, but the neurotoxic properties of this compound precluded its clinical use. In 1926, two diguanides, synthalin A and B were introduced as an oral treatment for diabetic patients. The belief that these compounds caused liver damage in man led to their being abandoned in the early 1930s.

In 1929, various biguanides were synthesized and their hypoglycaemic effect tested in animals, but it was not until 30 years later in 1957 that Ungar and his colleagues reported on the hypoglycaemic activity of a newly synthesized biguanide, phenformin, and since then over 200 related biguanides have been tested in animals. At the present time, two are used in the treatment of diabetic

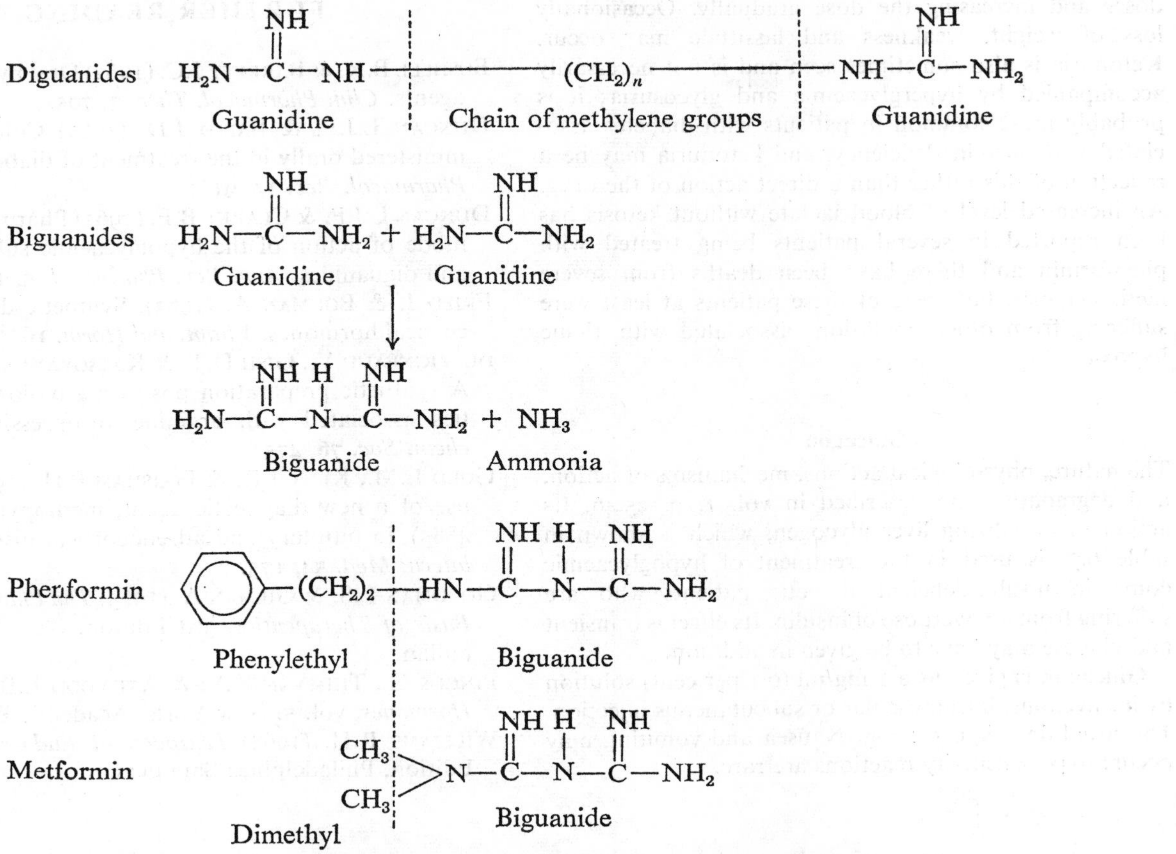

Diguanides

$$H_2N-\overset{\overset{\text{NH}}{\|}}{C}-NH \underbrace{\hspace{3cm}(CH_2)_n\hspace{3cm}} NH-\overset{\overset{\text{NH}}{\|}}{C}-NH_2$$

Guanidine   Chain of methylene groups   Guanidine

Biguanides

$$H_2N-\overset{\overset{\text{NH}}{\|}}{C}-NH_2 + H_2N-\overset{\overset{\text{NH}}{\|}}{C}-NH_2$$

Guanidine   Guanidine

$$\downarrow$$

$$H_2N-\overset{\overset{\text{NH}}{\|}}{C}-\overset{\overset{\text{H}}{|}}{N}-\overset{\overset{\text{NH}}{\|}}{C}-NH_2 + NH_3$$

Biguanide   Ammonia

Phenformin

$$\bigcirc-(CH_2)_2-HN-\overset{\overset{\text{NH}}{\|}}{C}-\overset{\overset{\text{H}}{|}}{N}-\overset{\overset{\text{NH}}{\|}}{C}-NH_2$$

Phenylethyl   Biguanide

Metformin

$$\overset{CH_3}{\underset{CH_3}{>}}N-\overset{\overset{\text{NH}}{\|}}{C}-\overset{\overset{\text{H}}{|}}{N}-\overset{\overset{\text{NH}}{\|}}{C}-NH_2$$

Dimethyl   Biguanide

FIG. 6.12. Chemical derivation of biguanides from two molecules of guanidine with the elimination of one molecule of ammonia.

patients, **phenformin** (dibotin) and **metformin** (glucophage). Although the biguanides can probably be used in a wider range of patients than the sulphonylureas, their main use is in the noninsulin-dependent diabetic whose pancreas is still secreting some insulin.

Chemically the biguanides may be considered to be derived from two molecules of guanidine with the elimination of one molecule of ammonia (fig. 6.12). Thus, each molecule of biguanide contains five nitrogen atoms in contrast to the six nitrogen atoms of the diguanide molecule.

MECHANISM OF ACTION

The mode of action of these compounds is not clearly defined. An early theory that anaerobic glycolysis was stimulated and tissue respiration inhibited is no longer valid. The presence of some insulin is necessary for their action. On the other hand, they do not lower the blood glucose level of normal individuals and, unlike the sulphonylureas, they do not stimulate the secretion of insulin. Again, they have no effect on insulin degradation, although studies in both diabetic animals and patients show that insulin is utilized to better effect in a diabetic

under the influence of the biguanides. Thus, the biguanides seem to act as antidiabetic agents in correcting some disturbance of the normal regulating mechanism which occurs in the diabetic with regard to the secretion, release and activity of insulin. There is some evidence that the antidiabetic hypoglycaemic effect of biguanides and the sulphonylureas is synergistic.

ABSORPTION, FATE, EXCRETION AND DURATION OF ACTION

Both metformin and phenformin are rapidly absorbed from the gastrointestinal tract and are quickly excreted by the kidney in an unchanged form. The hypoglycaemic effect of each lasts for 4–5 hours and they are, therefore, given in two or three daily doses of 25 mg and 50 mg respectively.

Either drug may be used alone or in conjunction with a sulphonylurea.

ADVERSE REACTIONS

Anorexia, nausea, vomiting and diarrhoea are common, but can often be avoided by starting treatment with small doses and increasing the dose gradually. Occasionally loss of weight, weakness and lassitude may occur. Ketonuria is also sometimes seen and is not necessarily accompanied by hyperglycaemia and glycosuria; it is probably most common in patients with diabetes associated with insulin deficiency, and ketonuria may be a reflection of this rather than a direct action of the drug. An increased level of blood lactate without ketosis has been reported in several patients being treated with phenformin and there have been deaths from severe lactic acidosis, but some of these patients at least were suffering from other conditions associated with tissue hypoxia.

Glucagon

The nature, physiological actions, mechanisms of action, and degradation are described in vol. 1, p. 25.46. Its action in mobilizing liver glycogen, which is shown in table 6.3, is used in the treatment of hypoglycaemic coma in insulin-deficient diabetic patients who are suffering from an overdose of insulin. Its effect is transient and glucose may have to be given in addition.

Glucagon is given as a 1 mg/ml (0·1 per cent) solution by intravenous, intramuscular or subcutaneous injection. The usual dose is 0·5–1 mg. Nausea and vomiting may occur; hypersensitivity reactions are rare.

FURTHER READING

BOSHELL B.R. & BARRETT J.C. (1962) Oral hypoglycaemic agents. *Clin. Pharmacol. Ther.* **3**, 705.

DUNCAN L.J.P. & BAIRD J.D. (1960) Compounds administered orally in the treatment of diabetes mellitus. *Pharmacol. Rev.* **12**, 91.

DUNCAN L.J.P. & CLARKE B.F. (1965) Pharmacology and mode of action of the hypoglycaemic sulphonylureas and diguanides. *Ann. Rev. Pharmacol.* **5**, 151.

FRIED J. & BOUMAN A. (1963). Synthetic derivatives of cortical hormones. *Vitam. and Horm.* **16**, 303.

DU VIGNEAUD V., GISH D.T. & KATSOYANNIS P.G. (1954) A synthetic preparation possessing biological properties associated with arginine vasopressin. *J. Amer. chem. Soc.* **76**, 4751.

GOLD E.M., KENT J.R. & FORSHAM P.H. (1961) Clinical use of a new diagnostic agent, methopyrapone (SU-4885), in pituitary and adrenocortical disorders. *Ann. intern. Med.* **54**, 175.

GOODMAN L.S. & GILMAN A. (1965) *The Pharmacological Basis of Therapeutics*, 3rd Edition. New York: Macmillan.

PINCUS G., THIMANN K.V. & ASTWOOD E.B. (1964) *The Hormones*, vol. 5. New York: Academic Press.

WILLIAMS R.H. (1968) *Textbook of Endocrinology*, 4th Edition. Philadelphia: Saunders.

Chapter 7
Drugs that influence the formation and coagulation of blood

DRUGS THAT INFLUENCE THE HAEMOPOIETIC SYSTEM

Agents that influence the haemopoietic system may be classified as follows.

(1) Some drugs, vitamins and hormones cure anaemia by correcting deficiencies in substances necessary for normal haemopoiesis; these are iron, vitamin B_{12}, folic acid, pyridoxine and thyroxine.

(2) Other substances stimulate haemopoiesis nonspecifically; these are corticotrophin, adrenocorticosteroids and cobalt.

(3) Some drugs inhibit mitosis and suppress normal and abnormal haemopoiesis; these include drugs used in the chemotherapy of tumours (p. 29.2). In addition, numerous drugs may damage the haemopoietic elements in the bone marrow or suppress the production of red cells, white cells or platelets; although adrenocorticosteroids and their analogues stimulate the bone marrow, paradoxically they suppress lymphopoiesis.

(4) Drugs may produce haemolysis either through direct damage to the red cell or because of hypersensitivity or genetic defect (p. 23.2).

(5) Other drugs and chemicals may convert haemoglobin into the nonfunctional pigments, met- and sulph-aemoglobin, e.g. phenacetin and nitrites.

Iron

Iron has been known from the earliest times, and its therapeutic use is far older than the explanation for its effects. Hippocrates used iron salts for a variety of ills probably because it was believed to give strength, imbued with a magical force by Mars, the god of war. The same belief underlies accounts in the Middle Ages of the sufferer hoping to acquire something of its strength by drinking water in which a sword had rusted.

Sydenham introduced iron into clinical medicine for the treatment of anaemia in the seventeenth century. He described the management of 'chlorosis', a severe iron-deficiency anaemia in young girls, by bleeding and purging followed by the administration of iron or steel filings steeped in cold Rhenish wine. The reason for Sydenham's good results was not discovered until the early eighteenth century when iron was found in the ash of blood; when the iron content of blood was shown to be increased by feeding iron-containing foods. The modern use of iron in medicine dates from 1831 when the Frenchman, Pierre Blaud, introduced his famous antichlorotique pills. He was the first to use iron salts in adequate doses for a sufficiently long time in the treatment of iron-deficiency anaemia.

ABSORPTION, FATE AND EXCRETION

The metabolism of iron is discussed in vol. 1, pp. 5.8 & 26.8. The body conserves ingested iron and only about 1 mg is lost each day. This is not excreted in the usual sense but is lost in cells which are shed from the skin and mucosal surfaces and in sweat. In health it is necessary for men and nonmenstruating women to absorb only 10 per cent of their daily dietary iron of about 10–15 mg to remain in iron balance. Women in the child-bearing period, growing children and those who give regular blood donations need to absorb an additional 1–2 mg/day and their iron nutrition is more precarious.

When iron is given by mouth in larger than physiological amounts a wide range in the percentage absorbed is found. For example, fasting subjects who are not anaemic absorb 10–70 per cent (mean 30 per cent) of a dose of 5 mg of iron given as a ferrous salt, and iron-deficient subjects absorb 15–95 per cent (mean 55 per cent). When ^{59}Fe haemoglobin is given by mouth in an amount which contains 5 mg of iron, healthy subjects absorb 1–30 per cent (mean 15 per cent) and iron deficient patients 1–70 per cent (mean 25 per cent). These observations show that under experimental circumstances healthy subjects may absorb more than their theoretical requirements, and that iron-deficient people on average absorb more; many individuals who need iron may absorb only a small amount of either medicinal iron or of the organic iron in food.

Medicinal iron is used in the correction of iron-deficiency anaemia and increasingly in its prevention. Prophylactic use of iron is especially valuable in the premature infant, born with poor iron stores, in the woman with heavy menstrual bleeding, in pregnancy, in the patient with intestinal malabsorption of iron or with a chronic bleeding disorder which cannot be cured, and in the habitual blood donor. For most purposes, iron is given as an iron salt in tablets by mouth; therapeutic trials show that in iron deficiency, various salts containing equivalent amounts of elemental iron raise the haemoglobin level at approximately the same rate and give a similar incidence of adverse effects. Liquid preparations are used when there is difficulty in swallowing pills; they have their greatest value in children and in the very young for whom they may be added to the feeding bottle. Common iron salts given orally are shown in table 7.1.

TABLE 7.1. Common iron salts given orally.

	Content of iron in recommended dose usually given three times a day
Ferrous sulphate	60 mg in 200 mg tablet
Ferrous gluconate	36 mg in 300 mg tablet
Ferrous succinate	35 mg in 150 mg tablet
Ferrous fumarate	65 mg in 200 mg tablet
Ferric ammonium citrate mixture	400 mg in 15 ml
Elixir of ferrous gluconate	36 mg in 4 ml
Elixir of ferrous succinate	35 mg in 4 ml
Syrup of ferrous fumarate	32.5 mg in 4 ml
Elixir of sodium iron edetate	27.5 mg in 4 ml

EFFECTS OF ORAL IRON THERAPY IN IRON-DEFICIENCY

When a patient with iron-deficiency anaemia receives adequate amounts of medicinal iron, and there is no other nutritional deficiency or complicating disorder such as infection, renal failure, endocrine insufficiency or malignant disease, the iron deficiency is promptly corrected. There is first an increase in reticulocytes in the blood which begins about the third or fourth day, is maximal about the fifth to seventh day and subsides about the tenth day. The lower the initial haemoglobin level, the higher is the reticulocyte response. Seven to ten days after starting treatment, the haemoglobin level begins to rise and thereafter increases at the rate of 1–2 per cent/day or 1 g/100 ml/week. The new cells appearing in the circulating blood contain their full complement of Hb, and therefore the MCHC returns gradually to normal as the hypochromic red cells of iron deficiency disappear (fig. 7.1). The reduced concentration of serum iron is corrected and the body stores of iron are then repleted.

Over the next few weeks the associated clinical features of chronic severe iron deficiency, i.e. atrophy of the tongue papillae and brittleness and flattening of the nails,

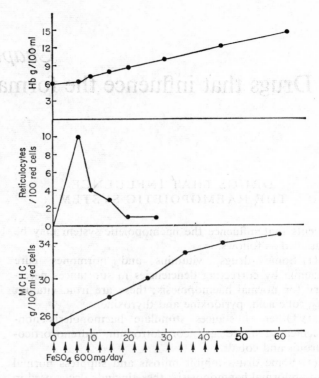

FIG. 7.1. The response of iron-deficiency anaemia to oral iron therapy. The time scale in the abscissa is in days.

disappear. In most patients, the impairment of gastric acid secretion improves also.

ADVERSE EFFECTS OF ORAL IRON PREPARATIONS

About 15–20 per cent of patients have epigastric discomfort, heartburn, colicky lower abdominal pain, constipation or diarrhoea, when taking iron-containing tablets in common use. Ferrous fumarate, however, has been found to produce the lowest incidence of complaints which occurred in less than 3 per cent in two studies. Usually these untoward effects are no more than an inconvenience and are allayed by reassurance and by asking the patient to take the tablet or mixture after meals. If the effects are particularly unpleasant with one preparation, another preparation is nearly always found to be acceptable.

Psychological factors appear to play a part in the development of adverse effects. In one study, patients had gastrointestinal symptoms when given green ferrous sulphate tablets but none when white tablets, identical in every other way, were given. Even more surprisingly, a group of nurses taking part in a trial of different iron pills showed the same incidence of side effects (20 per cent) from a lactose-containing pill which they believed contained iron as with iron-containing tablets, but no symptoms from an identical lactose-containing pill which they knew was given.

Ferric ammonium citrate mixture may blacken the teeth and oral iron preparations cause the stools to appear greyish-black; this latter effect is useful in ascertaining that a patient is actually taking iron that has been prescribed.

PARENTERAL IRON PREPARATIONS

Iron–dextran is a colloidal solution containing a complex of ferric hydroxide with dextrans of mol. wt. 5000–7500 and buffered at pH 5·2–6·5. It contains 50 mg iron/ml. It is best given by deep intramuscular injection but can also be given intravenously.

Iron–sorbitol is an isotonic solution containing a complex of iron–sorbitol and citric acid stabilized with dextrin at pH about 7·5. The average mol. wt. of the complex is less than 5000. It also contains 50 mg iron/ml and is best given by deep intramuscular injection.

Iron–dextrin is a complex of ferric hydroxide and dextrin in colloidal solution; it contains 20 mg iron/ml and is given only by intravenous injection. It has replaced another intravenous preparation, saccharated iron oxide, which is no longer used.

Indications for parenteral iron therapy

Parenteral iron preparations in any form may have unpleasant effects, and they are therefore given only in the following special circumstances.

(1) Malabsorption of iron is rare but may follow disease of the small intestine, e.g. idiopathic steatorrhoea and after partial gastrectomy. Even in these cases a satisfactory clinical response is usually seen following oral iron therapy.

(2) When the patient is completely intolerant of all oral preparations. This is very rare.

(3) When the patient suffers from chronic irremediable bleeding, and when it is impossible to keep pace with iron losses using oral iron preparations.

(4) In patients who do not co-operate in taking oral preparations.

When parenteral therapy is used it is customary to begin with small doses of 25 mg and 50 mg of iron and then to continue with 100–250 mg daily or at convenient intervals. Twenty-five mg of injected iron can be expected to raise the haemoglobin level in the blood by 1 per cent and this estimate is used in the calculation of dosage. In practice the total dose is estimated from the amount required to raise the haemoglobin level to 100 per cent, 1–1·5 g being added for the body stores which are always depleted before iron deficiency anaemia develops. About 25 per cent more of iron–dextran and iron–sorbitol than the expected amount is required, because in the case of iron–dextran about one-quarter of that injected remains at the injection site, while in the case of iron–sorbitol about one-quarter of each injection is excreted in the urine.

Iron–dextran may be given in a 'whole-dose' intravenous infusion. The patient's requirement for iron is calculated and the appropriate amount of iron–dextran is added to 500 ml of isotonic saline which is given intravenously over 6–8 hours (table 7.2).

TABLE 7.2. Iron preparations given parenterally.

Preparation	Fe in mg/ml	Route of administration	Recommended daily dose in ml
Iron-dextran	50	IM and IV	2
Iron-sorbitol	50	IM	2
Iron-dextrin	20	IV	5

Adverse effects of parenteral iron therapy

Iron–dextran causes aching at the site of intramuscular injection and permanent staining of the skin if the injection is not made deeply. Its administration may be followed by headache, dizziness, flushing, nausea, vomiting and sometimes by a metallic taste in the mouth. Anaphylactic and other hypersensitivity reactions have also been observed; the first include dyspnoea, angioneurotic oedema and circulatory collapse; the others, fever, skin rash, generalized pains, arthralgia and enlargement of lymph nodes. These reactions may be associated with the transient discharge of primitive blood cells from the marrow into the circulation, a condition sometimes termed a leuko-erythroblastic or leukaemoid reaction. The main additional disadvantage of the whole-dose intravenous infusion of iron-dextran is thrombophlebitis.

In rats and rabbits large doses of iron–dextran given intramuscularly regularly produce sarcomata at the site of injection. The amount of iron–dextran required is about 300–400 times greater than is used in man for therapeutic purposes and so far there is no proof of a causal relationship between iron–dextran injections and malignant disease in man.

Iron–sorbitol also causes aching at the site of intramuscular injection but staining of the skin is transitory. It has not been shown to be carcinogenic in animals. Adverse effects are rare and include nausea, vomiting, metallic taste in the mouth, dizziness and urticaria. The high urinary excretion of injected iron-sorbitol is often associated with blackening of the urine, believed to be due to iron sulphide.

Iron–dextrin has similar adverse systemic effects to the intramuscular preparations but it causes circulatory collapse slightly more frequently. For this reason it is important to begin therapy with small doses given slowly.

IRON POISONING

When iron is given over years to a patient who does not suffer from iron deficiency but in whom the rate of erythropoiesis is increased, e.g. in haemolytic anaemia, it may be absorbed in excess of requirements and leads to iron deposition in the tissues, i.e. siderosis. The iron accumulates mainly in the parenchymal and reticuloendothelial cells of liver and also in the spleen and bone marrow. Siderosis induced in this way has been reported only rarely as being harmful. In the African Bantu a more severe siderosis accompanied by cirrhosis of the liver is seen; it results from excessive absorption of high dietary intakes from native beers and from the use of iron cooking pots. There is also evidence that siderosis of the liver may be an aetiological factor in the genesis of primary liver carcinoma. Forty per cent of patients with Bantu siderosis and cirrhosis have liver carcinomata at autopsy, and this tumour accounts for about 50 per cent of all cancers in these people. In one American series, carcinoma of the liver was seen in 15 per cent of patients dying of haemochromatosis, a condition which in the liver resembles Bantu siderosis, while the incidence in patients with portal cirrhosis was 8 per cent.

All parenteral iron preparations cause siderosis when given in excessive amounts and there are reports of two patients who developed a clinical picture resembling primary haemochromatosis after receiving 85 g of iron in the course of 17 years in one case, and 130 g during 13 years in another.

Acute poisoning from overdosage with iron salts is not uncommon, particularly in young children who may ingest large amounts of medicinal iron tablets, mistaking them for sweets. In the first hour after ingestion there is nausea, vomiting, diarrhoea and gastrointestinal bleeding. In severe poisoning large amounts of iron enter the circulation and hyperventilation, circulatory collapse and death occur in 4–6 hours. In less severe poisoning there may be transient recovery from the alimentary symptoms due to uptake of the iron by the reticuloendothelial cells; after 12–24 hours, iron is released from these cells and causes progressive collapse, coma and convulsions. There is a high mortality from liver cell necrosis. For those who recover, gastrointestinal scarring may be a late result, with pyloric stenosis the main complication.

Vitamin B_{12} (cyanocobalamin)

The story of the introduction of liver therapy for pernicious anaemia and of Castle's theory of a dietary extrinsic factor combining with a gastric factor to form the anti-anaemic principle in liver is well known (vol. 1, pp. 5.15 and 26.9). These developments were followed in the 1930s by the therapeutic use of proteolysed liver and desiccated hog's stomach given by mouth; then crude liver extracts and later refined liver extracts by parenteral injection were used. In 1948 Rickes in the United States and simultaneously Lester Smith in England isolated from liver red needle-shaped crystals containing cobalt and a cyano group which was named vitamin B_{12} or cyanocobalamin. All subsequent experience indicates

that vitamin B_{12} is identical with Castle's extrinsic factor and is the active principle in liver which is deficient in pernicious anaemia.

Vitamin B_{12} is synthesized only by micro-organisms and the most intensive natural synthesis is by rumen bacteria. Foods in our diet that contain vitamin B_{12} are for all practical purposes of animal origin. The antibiotic-producing moulds, *Streptomyces griseus* (streptomycin) and *Str. aureofaciens* (aureomycin) synthesize large amounts and provide inexpensive commercial sources. A number of organisms, e.g. *Euglena gracilis* and *Lactobacillus leichmanii*, cannot synthesize the vitamin and, because they depend on exogenous sources for growth, are suitable for assay purposes.

The chemical structure of vitamin B_{12} was elucidated by Hodgkin and her colleagues in 1955. The molecule was found to have two portions, a planar moiety bearing some resemblance to a porphyrin ring and a nucleotide moiety. A number of natural and semisynthetic analogues of cyanocobalamin have now been discovered. Many of these, even without the CN group, have physiological activity similar to vitamin B_{12} itself. For example in **aquocobalamin** (vitamin B_{12b}) H_2O replaces the CN group while **hydroxocobalamin** (vitamin B_{12a}) is the anhydrous form of vitamin B_{12b}. In **nitritocobalamin** (vitamin B_{12c}) NO_2 replaces CN. The most important of these and of several other analogues used in replacement therapy is hydroxocobalamin. The chemical structure of vitamin B_{12} and its analogues and their spatial configuration are illustrated in fig. 7.2.

The term **cobalamin** is frequently used to describe the analogues of vitamin B_{12} which do not contain the cyano group. In 1959, to avoid confusion, a systematic nomenclature was introduced by international agreement. The planar group or macro ring is now termed the **corrin nucleus** and derivatives **corrinoid compounds**. It seems likely from major advances in recent years that many of the metabolic activities of vitamin B_{12} depend upon corrinoid compounds known as **cobamides** acting as coenzymes. While, strictly, the term vitamin B_{12} means cyanocobalamin, by general usage it has come to embrace all the cobamides active in man.

Many fundamental questions regarding vitamin B_{12} metabolism remain unresolved. The most significant activities of vitamin B_{12} in man are summarized as follows:

(1) deoxyriboside synthesis in the course of DNA synthesis (vol. 1, p. 12.18),

(2) the isomerization of methylmalonyl CoA to succinyl CoA and hence propionate catabolism (vol. 1, p. 11.22),

(3) the synthesis of methionine methyl groups (vol. 1, p. 11.28).

ABSORPTION, FATE AND EXCRETION

Intrinsic factor is concerned with the intestinal absorption

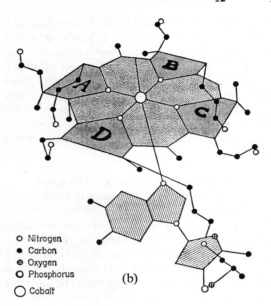

FIG. 7.2. (a) Chemical structure of vitamin B$_{12}$ and its analogues. (b) Semidiagrammatic representation of three-dimensional structure showing relations of planar and nucleotide moieties. Hydrogen atoms and a number of oxygen atoms are omitted.

Cyanocobalamin, Vitamin B$_{12}$	X = CN$^-$
Hydroxocobalamin, Vitamin B$_{12a}$	X = OH$^-$
Aquocobalamin, Vitamin B$_{12b}$	X = H$_2$O
Nitritocobalamin, Vitamin B$_{12c}$	X = NO$_2$$^-$

From *Drill's Pharmacology in Medicine*, 3rd Edition. ed. Joseph D. DiPalma. New York: McGraw.

of about 1 μg/day of vitamin B$_{12}$ ingested either in protein or peptide bound form in food or as the purified vitamin. Intrinsic factor has not yet been identified, but it appears to be a mucoprotein, mol. wt. 5000–15,000, secreted by the mucosal glands in the body and fundus of the stomach. It binds vitamin B$_{12}$ and modifies it to facilitate absorption in the ileum. It is not yet known whether the complex between intrinsic factor and vitamin B$_{12}$ or vitamin B$_{12}$ alone enters the mucosal cell; in the former case the cell could assimilate such a large molecule only by pinocytosis. In studies with ^{58}Co vitamin B$_{12}$ it has been found that physiological amounts of vitamin B$_{12}$ using the intrinsic factor pathway enter the bloodstream and the liver 2–4 hours after ingestion. Large oral doses of purified vitamin B$_{12}$ appear in the bloodstream almost at once and are thought to enter the body by simple diffusion. Sorbitol, food and some cholinergic drugs, e.g. carbachol, and adrenocorticosteroids enhance the absorption of vitamin B$_{12}$ perhaps by stimulating intrinsic factor secretion. Phytate and other calcium chelating agents have an inhibitory effect. The dietary intake of vitamin B$_{12}$ is about 15 μg/day and of this 1–4 μg is absorbed through the mediation of intrinsic factor; when 0·4–1 μg doses of radioisotope-labelled pure vitamin B$_{12}$ are ingested, between 5 and 50 per

cent is excreted unabsorbed in the faeces. Vitamin B$_{12}$ is carried in the plasma, bound to an α-globulin believed to be a specific B$_{12}$ binding protein; the binding capacity of this protein is in the region of 1000 pg/ml, and the normal serum vitamin B$_{12}$ level is in the range 170–1000 pg/ml. When the serum vitamin B$_{12}$ level is raised above this level, the vitamin is bound to other proteins. Small injected doses of vitamin B$_{12}$ are retained in the body, but when the dose exceeds 50 μg, increasing amounts are excreted in the urine. When serum levels reach 10–25 μg/ml the rate of urinary excretion approximates that of the glomerular filtration rate.

In the adult, the body content of vitamin B$_{12}$ is believed to be in the region of 4 mg. The largest amount, about 1 mg, is in the liver, mainly in the form of cobamide coenzyme; otherwise the highest concentrations are found in the kidney and adrenal gland. The body stores are depleted at the rate of about 0·2 per cent/day by faecal loss; studies using ^{58}Co indicate that the biological half-life of vitamin B$_{12}$ in the liver is about 1 year.

CLINICAL USE OF VITAMIN B$_{12}$

Cyanocobalamin and hydroxocobalamin both correct vitamin B$_{12}$ deficiency. However, during the first few days of treatment, the urinary excretion is lower and the serum level of vitamin B_{12} higher with hydroxocobalamin. The difference is due to the fact that it is bound to protein to a greater extent than cyanocobalamin. In one study in which four injections of 1000 μg of one or other preparation were given to untreated patients with pernicious anaemia over 5 days, the serum vitamin B_{12} level had fallen to less than 150 pg/ml at 31 weeks in all patients receiving cyanocobalamin, while in all those receiving hydroxocobalamin the level remained above 200 pg/ml at this time.

INDICATIONS FOR VITAMIN B_{12} THERAPY

Although large oral doses of vitamin B_{12} are absorbed to some extent even in the absence of intrinsic factor, parenteral injections of vitamin B_{12} are recommended for vitamin B_{12} deficiency. This is because vitamin B_{12} given by mouth may not maintain the serum vitamin B_{12} level and the body stores of the vitamin. Hence, although vitamin B_{12} deficiency anaemia may be corrected or improved, the patient may not be protected from neuropathy which is a serious complication of vitamin B_{12} deficiency (vol. 1, p. 26.10).

When vitamin B_{12} therapy is indicated, it should be given for life, except in nutritional deficiency and some disorders of the small intestine which are amenable to surgery. It should be given in all vitamin B_{12} deficiency states, the commonest in Europe being Addisonian pernicious anaemia.

It is administered initially in doses of 250–1000 μg weekly or twice weekly by intramuscular injection till the effects of B_{12} deficiency are corrected and the body stores are repleted. Thereafter it is usually given in 250–1000 μg amounts every 1–2 months. These high doses exceed the patients' theoretical requirements with a large safety margin.

In view of the better retention of hydroxocobalamin in the body this is now the preparation of choice.

EFFECTS OF VITAMIN B_{12} IN VITAMIN B_{12} DEFICIENCY

The main results of vitamin B_{12} deficiency are atrophy of the tongue papillae, macrocytic anaemia due to megaloblastic erythropoiesis, hypersegmentation of the blood neutrophil polymorphs, leukopenia, thrombocytopenia and, rarely, peripheral neuropathy and degenerative changes in the posterior and lateral columns of the spinal cord.

When a deficient subject is given the vitamin in the dosage recommended above there is usually an improvement in well being; the temperature, which is commonly slightly elevated, becomes normal and the erythrocyte sedimentation rate falls to normal before there is any significant effect on the haemoglobin level.

After 3–4 days, reticulocytes appear in increased numbers in the blood, reaching a peak usually after 5–7 days and returning to normal values after 10 days. The reticulo-

cyte response varies with the initial degree of anaemia and may reach 30–40 per cent of the erythrocyte count. Seven to 10 days after giving vitamin B_{12}, the haemoglobin level begins to rise, and abnormalities in the white cells and platelets disappear; the haemoglobin rises at the rate of 1–2 per cent per day (fig. 7.3). The anaemia is fully

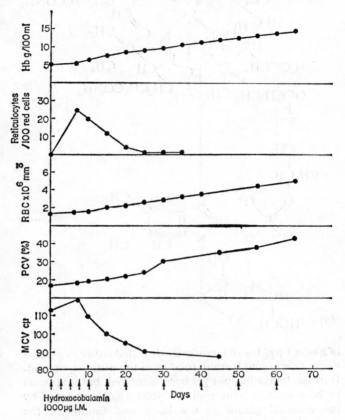

FIG. 7.3. Response of pernicious anaemia to specific therapy with vitamin B_{12}.

corrected provided there is no concomitant iron or folic acid deficiency or coexistent infection, inflammation or other generalized disease. Megaloblasts disappear gradually from the bone marrow in 3–4 days.

The tongue atrophy recovers in a few weeks and the features of peripheral neuropathy may remit completely in a similar length of time. However, long standing peripheral neuropathy and spinal cord damage tend to be partially irreversible.

The gastric mucosal atrophy and the histamine-insensitive achlorhydria which are features of the classical case of Addisonian pernicious anaemia are permanent and uninfluenced by therapy.

ADVERSE EFFECTS OF VITAMIN B_{12} THERAPY

Vitamin B_{12} is virtually free of any adverse effects. One example of anaphylactic shock has been reported in a patient aged 29 years. This contrasts with liver extracts formerly in use which sometimes caused troublesome hypersensitivity reactions.

Folic acid

Folic acid in therapeutics means **synthetic pteroylmonoglutamic acid**, but the term is sometimes used to embrace all naturally occurring substances with folic acid activity. This is confusing and it is preferable to refer to the many folic acid analogues collectively as **folates** (fig. 7.4). All the folates support the growth of *Lactobacillus casei*, which is a most useful organism for microbiological assay.

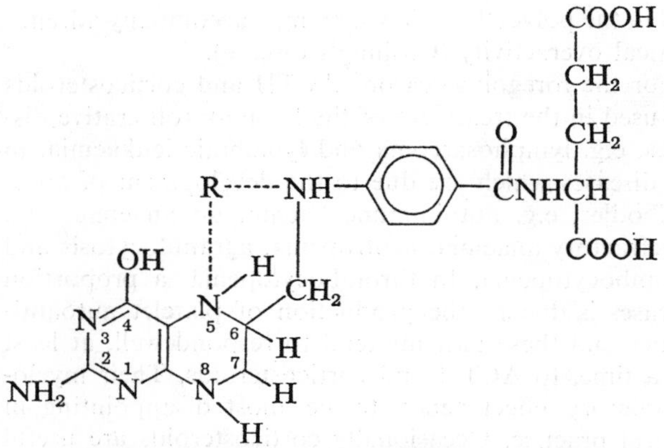

Tetrahydrofolic acid (THF) (R = —H)

	R
N^5 formyl THF (folinic acid)	—CHO
N^{10} formyl THF	—CHO
N^5 formimino THF	—CH=NH
$N^{5.10}$ methenyl THF	CH
$N^{5.10}$ methylene THF	CH₂
N^5 methyl THF	—CH₃

FIG. 7.4. Structures and nomenclature of folates. The names of the folates may be given without the 'N', e.g. N^5 formimino THF = 5 formimino THF. From Goodman L.S. & Gilman A. (1965) *The Pharmacological Basis of Therapeutics*, 3rd Edition. New York: Macmillan.

In foods, folates are found free and in conjugated forms, the latter being polyglutamates such as pteroyltriglutamate and pteroylheptaglutamate. The daily dietary requirement is uncertain, but in the adult is believed to be 50–100 μg; in pregnancy the mother's requirement is increased and is in the region 200–350 μg. Because of heat lability, a large amount of the folates in foods is destroyed by cooking.

ABSORPTION, FATE AND EXCRETION

When 5 mg of folic acid is taken by mouth by a healthy person, 50–75 per cent is absorbed and, if there is no folate deficiency, most of this is excreted in the urine in the next 6 hours, excretion being complete in 24 hours. Folic acid is assimilated throughout the small intestine and in experimental animals active transport has been demonstrated for amounts of the order of micrograms; larger amounts are believed to enter the body by simple diffusion, particularly in the jejunum. The conjugates in the diet require preliminary hydrolysis by conjugases to monoglutamates to facilitate absorption. The adult body contains 5–10 mg of folates and about half of this is in the liver. The form in which folic acid is found in highest concentration in the liver and blood is N^5-methyltetrahydrofolic acid (5 methyl THF).

When folic acid is given intravenously in a dose of 1 mg/kg body weight, about 65 per cent is cleared from the blood in one circulation. This is taken to indicate active uptake in cells. The renal tubules also reabsorb folic acid filtered by the glomerulus. After a 5 mg dose intravenously or intramuscularly the amount appearing in the urine in the next 6 hours is very nearly the same as after an oral dose, i.e. 2–3 mg.

METABOLIC FUNCTIONS

The complex interrelationships of vitamin B_{12} and folic acid have not been fully elucidated. The therapeutic administration of either may reverse, at least for a time, the megaloblastic erythropoiesis induced by deficiency of the other. However, folic acid does not correct and may aggravate the neuropathy sometimes associated with deficiency of vitamin B_{12}.

Absorbed folic acid, pteroylmonoglutamic acid, is reduced in the body to tetrahydrofolic acid (THF) which can accept various one carbon units in the N^5 or N^{10} position or balanced between the two. The various folate coenzymes with metabolic functions and their formulae are shown in fig. 7.4. The main reactions involving the transfer of one carbon units which utilize these folate coenzymes are:

(1) purine synthesis ($N^{5.10}$ methenyl THF and N^{10} formyl THF),

(2) pyrimidine nucleotide synthesis ($N^{5.10}$ methylene THF),

(3) interconversion of serine and glycine ($N^{5.10}$ methylene THF),

(4) conversion of histidine to glutamic acid (N^5 formimino THF),

(5) conversion of homocysteine to methionine (N^5 methyl THF), and

(6) production of formate (N^5 formyl THF and N^{10} formyl THF) (vol. 1, pp. 11.29, 12.18 & 23).

The interconversion of glycine and serine is dependent on pyridoxine. Vitamin B_{12} is concerned in the interconversion of methionine and homocysteine and probably also interrelates with folate coenzymes in pyrimidine nucleotide synthesis.

CLINICAL USES
Folic acid tablets (5 mg) are suitable for almost all conditions requiring folic acid therapy. Only on rare occasions when there is marked intestinal malabsorption is parenteral therapy necessary and for this purpose a folic acid solution containing 15 mg/ml is available for injection.

Folic acid is given for the treatment of macrocytic and megaloblastic anaemia due to folic acid deficiency. This occurs in malnutrition, pregnancy, malabsorption from the small intestine and rarely after the prolonged use of certain anticonvulsant drugs, e.g. the hydantoins. Its use is justified also in the prevention of folic acid deficiency in pregnancy. A number of preparations combining iron and folic acid are available. Their use is recommended in the last trimester of pregnancy and the first few weeks of the puerperium provided that they contain at least 100 mg of iron and 350 μg of folic acid per day.

Folic acid is of no value in counteracting overdosage with folic acid analogues which act by competitive inhibition of the enzyme folate reductase. This enzyme system is concerned with the formation of THF from precursor folates and interference with its function prevents the production of the metabolically active forms of folate. Analogues in this category include the antimetabolites aminopterin and amethopterin (methotrexate) used in the leukemias and other malignant diseases and the antimalarial drug pyrimethamine; pyrimethamine intoxication is unlikely to occur in the management of malaria (p. 20.20).

THF is too unstable to be therapeutically useful but its derivative N^5 formyl THF (folinic acid) may be given by intramuscular injection in a dose of about 20 mg/day. Treatment of overdosage with the antimetabolites must be undertaken within hours; the effect of methotrexate for example is not only severe but also protracted because the enzyme inhibition is slow to disappear (p. 29.7).

EFFECTS OF FOLIC ACID IN FOLIC ACID DEFICIENCY
The response in well being, correction of anaemia and improvement in tongue atrophy consequent on the giving of folic acid is similar to that described for vitamin B_{12} deficiency (p. 7.6), provided there is no concomitant deficiency of iron or other nutrients and no coexisting disease.

ADVERSE EFFECTS
When folic acid is given in uncomplicated folic acid deficiency there are no known adverse effects. When it is given alone to a patient with vitamin B_{12} deficiency, it may cause the vitamin B_{12} neuropathy to worsen or appear for the first time, for reasons unknown.

Adrenocorticotrophic hormone (ACTH) and adrenocorticosteroids

The pharmacological effects of ACTH and corticosteroids are discussed on p. 6.9. Their actions which are relevant to the haemopoietic system are:
(1) dissolution of lymphocytes in lymphoid tissue,
(2) suppression of immune responses (p. 24.6), and
(3) stimulation of the marrow, which is best seen in the neutrophil leucocytosis and reticulocytosis that often accompanies the clinical use of ACTH and corticosteroids, and in the polycythaemia which may accompany adrenocortical overactivity (Cushing's disease).

For the foregoing reasons ACTH and corticosteroids are used in the treatment of the lymphoproliferative diseases, e.g. lymphosarcoma and lymphatic leukaemia, in the diseases which are due to the development of autoantibodies, e.g. autoimmune haemolytic anaemia, and in refractory anaemia, neutropenia, agranulocytosis and thrombocytopenia. In thrombocytopenia, a proportion of cases is due to the production of platelet autoantibodies and these patients tend to respond well, at least for a time, to ACTH and corticosteroids. Their myelostimulatory effect tends to be most disappointing in clinical practice. Occasionally corticosteroids are useful in disorders of the blood when there is no rational explanation; this is seen in the acute leukaemias other than lymphocytic leukaemia when temporary remission may be obtained, and in thrombocytopenic purpura when bleeding may improve dramatically although the platelet count in the blood may remain unchanged. A direct action on the permeability of the capillaries has been suggested to explain this effect.

The absorption, fate and excretion, the mode of administration of ACTH and the various corticosteroids and their adverse effects are described on p. 6.13. In general, when dealing with disorders of the blood, ACTH is little used because it has to be given parenterally. Of the oral corticosteroids, prednisone and prednisolone are preferred because they cause less electrolyte disturbance; they are, however, just as prone to give rise to serious adverse effects, e.g. osteoporosis, when given over long periods.

Substances which are used occasionally in blood disorders
ASCORBIC ACID
The clearest indication for the clinical use of ascorbic acid is in scurvy. Although anaemia is common in this condition it is usually due to bleeding and to concomitant nutritional deficiencies of iron and folic acid rather than to lack of ascorbic acid. Ascorbic acid as a reducing agent improves iron absorption both in healthy and iron defi-

cient subjects, presumably by converting ferric to ferrous iron. This action of ascorbic acid is seldom used clinically except when a patient with iron deficiency anaemia responds poorly to adequate iron therapy; this may occur in malnourished people particularly if achlorhydria is present.

PYRIDOXINE

Pyridoxine is involved in haem synthesis at the porphobilinogen stage (vol. 1, 26.10). A rare disorder inherited as a sex-linked recessive characteristic and presenting as a refractory hypochromic anaemia is responsive to pyridoxine; it is believed that this is an inborn enzyme defect.

In later life, a similar haematological picture may be seen in relation to many chronic diseases and also after the taking of certain drugs, e.g. isoniazid, pyrazinamide and cycloserine. These anaemias may also respond to pyridoxine, suggesting that in them there is interference with haem synthesis at the point of action of the coenzyme, pyridoxal phosphate. Pyridoxine is given in doses of 20–200 mg/day.

COBALTOUS CHLORIDE

This has been shown to cause a rise in reticulocyte count and later in haemoglobin and packed cell volume in occasional patients with refractory anaemia, notably that associated with renal failure The mode of action is unknown but it may be relevant that in animals cobalt has been shown to increase the secretion of erythropoietin. Its clinical effect in anaemia is irregular and it gives rise to reactions which include skin rashes, precordial pain, temporary nerve injury and thyroid enlargement.

ANDROGENS

Remission in aplastic anaemia at puberty and occasional improvement in anaemia in patients receiving androgens for carcinoma of the breast has led to the use of androgens in aplastic anaemia and in the anaemia associated with myelofibrosis with limited success. The most frequently used preparations are testosterone propionate and oxymetholone (p. 12.12).

PHYTOHAEMAGGLUTININ

This substance obtained from the seeds of *Phaseolus vulgaris* stimulates mitosis in lymphocytes. Its value as a therapeutic agent has still to be assessed but occasional remissions from its use in various refractory anaemias have been reported.

DESFERRIOXAMINE MESYLATE

Ferrioxamine B is a naturally occurring substance isolated as a metabolite from *Streptomyces pilosus*. It belongs to the sideramines and contains trivalent iron as

a chelate. The corresponding iron-free compound desferrioxamine B is an iron-chelating agent which facilitates the elimination of iron from the body. The preparation in clinical use is the methane sulphonate, desferrioxamine mesylate (desferal). It is a trihydroxamic acid derivative which reacts with iron to form the octahedral iron complex ferrioxamine B.

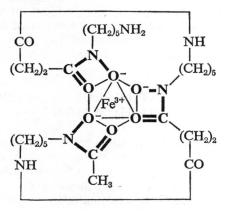

Ferrioxamine B

Ferrioxamine B has a basic amino group which renders it readily soluble in water. It is not absorbed to a significant extent from the alimentary tract but being of low molecular weight it is excreted readily by the kidneys. *In vitro* and *in vivo* desferrioxamine is virtually a specific chelating agent for iron, the effect on other elements being negligible.

When iron is removed from the tissues following the parenteral injection of desferrioxamine mesylate, the serum iron rises due to the presence of ferrioxamine B. Sixty to 70 per cent of the mobilized iron is excreted in the urine in 24 hours causing it to have a reddish-brown appearance; the rest appears over the next 2 days. Desferrioxamine does not chelate haemoglobin iron and has no adverse effects on erythropoiesis or on the kidneys.

Orally administered desferrioxamine blocks the absorption of inorganic iron from the intestine; the degree to which it can chelate organic iron in food is still uncertain.

No significant adverse effects have been reported from the therapeutic use of desferrioxamine in man. In animals acute poisoning has led to ataxia and acute respiratory failure, while chronic toxicity tests have caused minor inhibition of growth and leucopenia.

There are several clinical applications of desferrioxamine.

(1) In diseases of iron overload it has been used mainly in the prevention and treatment of transfusion-induced siderosis. The usual dose is 500–1000 mg/day given intramuscularly. The daily output of iron in the urine is of the order of 10–15 mg.

(2) In acute iron poisoning, gastric lavage is carried out with a solution of desferrioxamine; 5000 mg of

desferrioxamine is then left in the stomach to prevent absorption of iron still in the intestine and 2000 mg is injected intramuscularly and repeated if necessary 12 hourly. In severe cases an infusion of desferrioxamine in saline is started, initially at a rate of 15 mg/kg body wt./hr, the maximum dose being 80 mg/kg in 24 hrs.

(3) It is used as a test to measure the body stores of iron. This is still at the research stage, but it appears likely that the output of iron in the urine in a fixed time after a standard dose of desferrioxamine may prove useful in assessing the body content of iron.

DRUGS THAT INFLUENCE BLOOD COAGULATION

The haemostatic mechanism depends on a dynamic balance between the clotting mechanism on the one hand and the fibrinolytic system on the other (vol. 1, p. 26.14). An imbalance can result in a bleeding diathesis or a thrombotic state. These arise in a variety of pathological conditions. They are also induced by drugs which cause haemostatic disturbances either as an unwanted effect or when given clinically for their effect on the haemostatic mechanism. Most drugs in the latter class affect the clotting or fibrinolytic systems and are considered in detail in this chapter; however, much research is now being devoted to drugs that influence platelets, particularly to reduce platelet 'stickiness', excess of which may be a major factor in the pathogenesis of thrombosis (p. 26.2).

Drugs that damage vascular endothelium and platelets
Because vascular endothelium and platelets are closely linked in haemostasis, it is probable that drugs which alter or damage vascular endothelium exert an action also on platelets. A drug may act as a hapten by combining with the vascular endothelium or with the platelets to form an antigen which stimulates the production of antibody. This antibody then damages those cells forming part of the hapten complex and results in the development of either vascular or thrombocytopenic purpura (p. 23.3). Other drugs exert a toxic action on the bone marrow, either selectively on the megakaryocytes or as part of an action on all blood-forming elements; in the former case thrombocytopenia, and in the latter pancytopenia, i.e. depression of all the blood cells in the peripheral blood and of the appropriate blood forming cells in the marrow, follow (p. 32.4). In other instances it is possible that the offending drug may inhibit or impair platelet stickiness or adhesiveness; this, for instance, is one effect of clofibrate (p. 8.11).

Drugs that inhibit the coagulation mechanism
These drugs which are commonly called the **anticoagulants** fall into two main classes, heparin and the oral anticoagulants; the latter are either coumarins or indanediones.

HEPARIN
In 1916, McLean, a medical student at Johns Hopkins, first demonstrated anticoagulant activity in extracts of liver. The active principle was named heparin and immediately it became a practical aid to mammalian physiologists, who speculated that it might have a role in the prevention of intravascular clotting. Whether it does or not is still uncertain, but now other possible physiological roles have been discovered. Since purified samples became available, they have been widely used in clinical practice to reduce the coagulability of the blood.

Heparin is prepared commercially from mammalian lung, liver or intestinal mucosa, organs which are rich in mast cells, and it is usually dispensed as a sterile solution of the sodium salt in strengths varying from 1000–25,000 units/ml. The drug is standardized biologically, a unit being defined in terms of the ability of the preparation to delay blood clotting *in vitro* in relation to a standard preparation. The product must contain not less than 110 units/mg if manufactured from lung and not less than 130 units/mg if manufactured from intestinal mucosa. The drug is administered parenterally, usually intravenously. Purified preparations on partial hydrolysis yield sulphuric acid derivatives of D-glucosamine and D-glucuronic acid in approximately equimolar amounts. The molecule was shown to be formed from repeating units each consisting of two substituted hexoses joined by a glycosidic link (fig. 7.5); it is chemically related to the mucopolysaccharides hyaluronic acid and chondroitin sulphuric acid (vol. 1, p. 16.7). Preparations from different

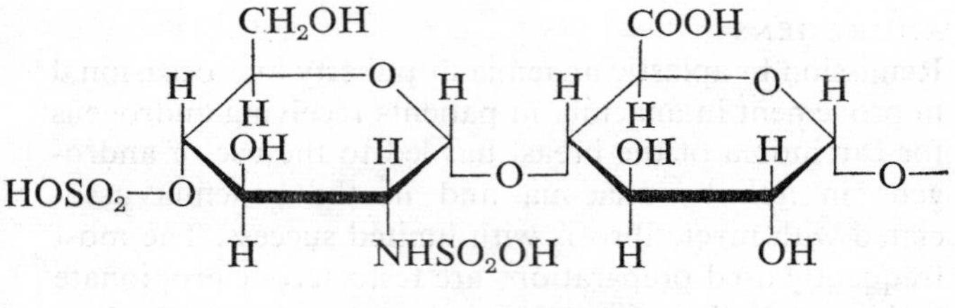

FIG. 7.5. The probable structure of the repeating unit of heparin.

species and tissues differ in sulphate content, anticoagulant potency and molecular weight (8000–17,000).

The anticoagulant action is due to the strong anionic activity created by its sulphuric acid content and is lost if this group is removed by hydrolysis or neutralized by compounds with cationic groups, e.g. protamine.

The fate of injected heparin is uncertain; its rate of disappearance from the plasma is exponential and after normal doses it is not excreted in the urine. It does not cross the placental barrier nor is it excreted in the milk.

Actions of heparin

The physiological function of heparin is unknown. Its pharmacological effect is to inhibit blood coagulation both *in vitro* and *in vivo* and to produce a 'clearing action' on lipaemic plasma *in vivo* but not directly *in vitro* (vol. 1, p. 10.12).

Its principal effect on the blood clotting mechanism is to inhibit the action of thrombin on fibrinogen and thus to prevent the formation of fibrin (fig. 7.6).

$$\text{Fibrinogen} \xrightarrow[\text{Ca}^{++}]{\text{Thrombin}} \text{Fibrin monomer}$$

$$\text{Fibrin monomer} \longrightarrow \text{Fibrin polymer}$$

$$\text{Fibrin polymer} \xrightarrow[\text{(Factor XIII)}]{\text{Fibrin stabilizing factor}} \text{Physiological fibrin}$$

FIG. 7.6. Stages in the formation of fibrin from fibrinogen.

This action requires the presence of a heparin cofactor from the α-globulin fraction of plasma and it can be shown *in vitro* that heparin does not inhibit this reaction significantly in its absence.

Heparin also inhibits the formation of plasma thromboplastin and its subsequent action on prothrombin. The effect of the drug therefore is to increase markedly the whole blood clotting time and this is its principal use *in vitro* and *in vivo*.

Other than haemorrhage, adverse effects of heparin are few and rare. The commonest are hypersensitivity reactions such as urticaria, asthma, rhinitis, lacrimation and fever. Patients who have a history of hypersensitivity or of previous reaction to the drug should be given a small test dose before receiving it again. Alopecia and thrombocytopenia have been occasionally reported.

Heparin is usually given by intermittent intravenous injection. After a loading dose of 10,000–15,000 units a maintenance dose varying between 5000 and 15,000 units is given every 4–8 hours. It may also be given by intramuscular or subcutaneous injection but absorption is unreliable.

COUMARINS AND INDANEDIONES

In 1920 a severe bleeding disease in American cattle was found to be due to feeding the animals with inadequately cured sweet clover hay. It was subsequently shown that this effect was caused by the presence in the fodder of a substance known as dicoumarol. Many allied coumarins have now been synthesized for medicinal use from the basic 4-hydroxycoumarin nucleus. Indanediones, derived from indane-1:3-dione, also have an anticoagulant effect, similar to that of the coumarins.

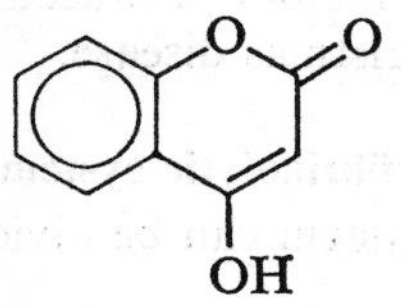

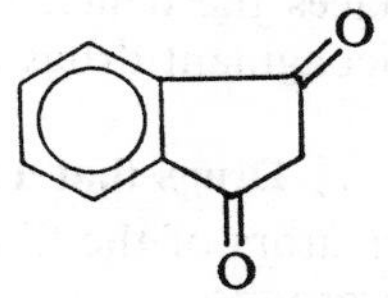

Action on blood clotting mechanism

The only important pharmacological effect of the coumarin drugs is to inhibit blood coagulation and, in contrast to heparin, they are active only *in vivo*. They are fairly well absorbed from the alimentary tract and are distributed in plasma and thence to tissues. The drugs interfere with the synthesis in the liver of Factors II (prothrombin), VII, IX and X possibly by competing with the action of vitamin K as a prosthetic group in an enzyme system which synthesizes these Factors. The drugs act only after a latent period of 12–24 hours, determined by the rate of absorption and handling of the drug by the liver, and by the half-life of the clotting Factors. The time of the peak effect and duration of action depends upon the drug used (table 7.3).

TABLE 7.3. Speed of action and duration of effect of some of the commonly used oral anticoagulant drugs.

Type of drug	Name	Peak effect (hours)	Duration of action (days)	Initial dose/day mg
Coumarin	Warfarin	36–72	5–6	30–50
	Phenprocoumon	48–72	6–7	15–20
	Nicoumalone	36–48	2–3	20–30
	Dicoumarol	36–48	5–6	300
	Ethyl biscoumacetate	24	2–3	1000–1200
Indanedione	Phenindione	24–48	3–4	200–300

The drugs depress rapidly the blood levels of Factors VII and IX, which have half-lives of 12 hours and reach low levels within 48 hours. The level of Factor X, with a half-life of nearly 3 days, falls more slowly. The summation of these effects on Factors VII and X can be detected simply *in vitro* by a one-stage prothrombin time test (vol. 1, p. 26.16), which is also used to control the dosage. These drugs also lower the blood level of Factor II (prothrombin) in the same way, but this is less easily detected by the usual one-stage prothrombin time techniques, which are also insensitive to changes in Factor IX. 'Thrombotest', a more recently introduced variation of the classical one stage prothrombin test, is sensitive to changes in Factor IX levels.

Of the oral anticoagulant drugs, only warfarin can be given parenterally. The dosage varies widely between different drugs but involves the administration of a large loading dose followed by a maintenance dose which is

4-Hydroxycoumarin   Indane-1:3-dione

adjusted on the basis of the one-stage prothrombin time or similar test.

Adverse effects, other than haemorrhage, are rare with the coumarins and consist mostly of mild gastrointestinal disturbances. Alopecia and allergic reactions, mainly urticaria, have been reported. More serious adverse effects such as leucopenia, agranulocytosis, jaundice, skin rashes and nephropathy have occurred, though infrequently, with the indanediones. As all these drugs pass the placental barrier, they are potentially dangerous in pregnancy.

The actions of the drugs can be modified in many ways. A decrease in the vitamin K supply, as a result of malabsorption or the action of antibiotics on intestinal bacteria which synthesize the vitamin or impaired liver function, either through disease or immaturity in the newborn, enhance their action. Renal insufficiency, infection and certain drugs, particularly salicylates, clofibrate and phenylbutazone, produce the same effect. Phenylbutazone potentiates the coumarin anticoagulants by a special mechanism of particular interest. Both drugs compete for the same binding site on the serum albumin molecule. Phenylbutazone has a high affinity constant and displaces the protein-bound coumarin. The concentration of coumarin free in the plasma water rises and the effect on prothrombin synthesis is enhanced. Debilitated and cachectic patients are more sensitive to the drugs. Diarrhoea may impair absorption and increase the dosage requirement of the drug.

GENERAL CONTRAINDICATIONS TO THE USE OF ANTICOAGULANT DRUGS

The use of anticoagulant drugs is contraindicated either absolutely or relatively in a patient who has a haemostatic defect or a blood dyscrasia, an ulcerative lesion of the gastrointestinal tract, liver or renal disease, and in pregnancy, in severe hypertension, in subacute bacterial endocarditis, in diseases associated with haemorrhage in the retina and in the early stages after injury or operation. The administration of other drugs, e.g. long-term salicylate therapy, may preclude their use and they should not be prescribed for unintelligent or non-cooperative patients.

ANTAGONISTS TO HEPARIN

Three drugs, **toluidine blue, protamine sulphate** and **hexadimethrine bromide,** have all been used clinically as antagonists to heparin, but protamine sulphate is now the drug of choice.

The protamines are strongly cationic proteins obtained from the sperm of certain fish, which combine rapidly with the heparin anion and thereby neutralize its anticoagulant effect. The protamine–heparin complex does not readily dissociate in solution. The drug, as protamine sulphate, in a 1 per cent sterile aqueous solution, is given intravenously at the rate of not more than 50 mg every 10 min. If given too rapidly hypotension, bradycardia, warmth and flushing may occur. Extravascular leakage of the drug causes tissue irritation.

Protamine can act as an anticoagulant. In high doses it blocks the action of thrombin on fibrinogen and, in a lower concentration, it inhibits thromboplastin generation. For this reason not more than 100 mg of protamine SO_4 should be given to a patient as a single dose or over a short period of time, in the absence of laboratory control of the clotting mechanism.

ANTAGONISTS TO THE COUMARINS

Vitamin K is the pharmacological antagonist to the coumarins and indanediones. Vitamins K_1 and K_2 are derived from 2-methyl-1:4-naphthaquinone (vol. 1, p. 10.9), are lipid soluble and are absorbed orally only in the presence of bile salts, but the water soluble, synthetic analogues are absorbed unaided.

The coumarins and indanediones depress the production of clotting factors by interfering with the synthetic activity of vitamin K. If a patient receives too large a dose of anticoagulant, vitamin K increases the production of clotting factors but 6–8 hours may elapse before bleeding is controlled though an *in vitro* effect in the blood can be detected sooner. The maximum effect is obtained in about 24 hours. Vitamin K_1 (**phytomenadione**) is the most effective form of the drug, and it should always be used. Active derivatives of vitamin K include **menaphthone** (menadione) and **acetomenaphthone.** Vitamin K_1 is available in oral and parenteral forms and a single dose by either route is up to 20 mg. Acetomenaphthone is available also in oral and parenteral forms and the usual dose by either route is up to 100 mg. Repeated doses are usually given if the patient's prothrombin time remains prolonged. A form of the drug used intravenously, **menaphthone sodium bisulphite,** should be given slowly, otherwise it produces chest tightness, paraesthesiae and sweating; the oily forms should be diluted with sterile water for injection immediately before use.

Adverse effects from the drug are rare but chest pain, cramp, convulsions and cardiac arrhythmias have been reported. The drug can cause haemolysis in individuals whose red cells lack glucose-6-phosphate dehydrogenase (p. 31.10). A fraction prepared from human plasma containing Factors II, VII, IX and X is becoming available, and when given in appropriate amounts intravenously replaces the deficit in clotting factors produced by oral anticoagulant drugs and in Christmas disease.

Drugs that activate the fibrinolytic system

Activators of the fibrinolytic system can be divided into two groups,

(1) those used prophylactically to enhance endogenous fibrinolytic activity,

(2) those used therapeutically to produce massive enhancement of fibrinolytic activity.

PROPHYLACTIC USE
An imbalance between coagulation and fibrinolysis (vol. 1, p. 26.16) in favour of the former may be an important cause of degenerative and thromboembolic vascular disease. If this is so, a rational approach to the prophylaxis of such diseases would be by regular use of a drug enhancing endogenous fibrinolytic activity. Unfortunately, at present, knowledge in this field is fragmentary, and no satisfactory therapy is available. About 20 years ago adrenaline, when given by injection, was found to increase fibrinolytic activity transitorily and it appears to do so in part by causing the release of plasminogen activator. Attempts to exploit this finding by using oral sympathomimetic amines have so far been unsuccessful. Many drugs, e.g. the sulphonylureas, nicotinic acid, insulin and the male sex hormones, produce some increase in fibrinolytic activity which is of no practical value due either to fleeting action or to development of resistance to the drug. Clofibrate (p. 8.11) was reported to be effective but this has not been confirmed.

However, phenformin (p. 6.20) is the most promising drug at present available. When given orally it produces, in the majority of patients, a significant and sustained increase in fibrinolytic activity and resistance to it has not been reported. In many patients it causes gastric disturbances which preclude an effective dose being given.

THERAPEUTIC USE
Filtrates from cultures of certain strains of haemolytic streptococci lyse human fibrin *in vitro*. However, they are inactive against fibrin prepared from highly purified fibrinogen unless a small amount of human serum is added. It has therefore been postulated that the filtrate contains an enzyme, **streptokinase**, which converts inactive plasma plasminogen into plasmin. However, streptokinase does not activate bovine plasminogen unless a small amount of human serum is added and hence human blood is presumed to contain a substance, named proactivator, which bovine blood lacks and which is necessary for the action of streptokinase. A possible mechanism is as follows:

Streptokinase + proactivator → activator
Plasminogen + activator → plasmin
Plasmin + fibrin → soluble fibrin degradation products

There is, however, no proof that proactivator exists and some workers believe that the action of streptokinase could be explained equally well by a direct action on human plasminogen.

Streptokinase has been purified and is a protein with a mol. wt. of 50,000. It is active *in vivo* only when given parenterally, and it is antigenic, stimulating the production of antistreptokinase. Since most people have had haemolytic streptococcal infections on one or more occasions in their lives their plasma already contains this antibody; the more recent the infection, the higher its titre.

Streptokinase is usually supplied commercially as a sterile lyophilized powder containing 100,000, 250,000 or 600,000 international units for intravenous use. An international unit is defined in terms of the least quantity of streptokinase which lyses a standard blood clot completely in 10 min.

An activator obtained from culture filtrates of certain strains of staphylococci, **staphylokinase**, has an action similar to streptokinase but has been much less used.

Most tissues and body fluids contain plasminogen activators in variable amounts. The urine contains an activator, **urokinase**, which may have been present in the blood and excreted or produced in the urinary tract. It may have a function in maintaining the patency of the tract. Urokinase has been isolated in a form suitable for clinical use but most preparations contain a small amount of undesirable thromboplastic, or clot promoting, activity. It is a protein, nonantigenic in the human, and is active only when injected; it converts plasminogen to plasmin, by a first order reaction.

Urokinase is expensive. It is supplied in ampoules containing either 5000 or 25,000 ploug units. The ploug unit is expressed in terms of the fibrinolytic activity brought about by the interaction of plasminogen and urokinase under carefully defined conditions.

Thrombolytic therapy
The discovery of streptokinase and urokinase suggested the possibility that they might be used to lyse freshly formed thrombi and thus restore the patency of an occluded vessel. Such therapy could be useful in patients with venous thrombosis and in those with pulmonary embolism and multiple emboli in small arteries. It would be especially useful when the vitality of organs peripheral to the obstruction was threatened because of inadequate collateral circulation and when surgical removal of an embolus was impractical. Thrombolytic therapy has now been extensively and successfully used to treat such conditions.

Before describing the therapeutic use of activators, a brief account of the nature of thrombolysis is given. When whole blood clots *in vitro*, the clot is a uniform mixture of fibrin and the formed elements of the blood; when a thrombus is formed in flowing blood at the site of intimal damage, it is a heterogeneous structure (p. 26.2). A thrombus consists of a white head of platelets and other formed elements anchored to the damaged surface, from which a red tail, composed mainly of fibrin and red cells, grows by accretion and oscillates in the flowing blood. Although the platelet head may sometimes be large enough to occlude the lumen of a vessel, it is usually the fibrin tail that is responsible for this and also for the formation of emboli (p. 26.2).

Fibrin has a strong affinity for plasminogen (vol. 1, p. 26.16) and, in consequence, free plasmin is formed rapidly when activator diffuses into a fibrin clot and in amounts which exceed the capacity of the antiplasmin to neutralize it; as a result the fibrin undergoes lysis. In whole blood, plasminogen is present in much smaller concentrations and plasmin is formed so slowly by activator that the blood antiplasmin can neutralize it (fig. 7.7).

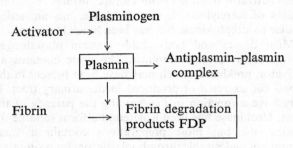

FIG. 7.7. Mode of action of fibrinolytic mechanism.

If, however, activator is released suddenly into the intact circulation (see below) or is injected therapeutically, the plasma plasminogen may be converted into plasmin so rapidly as to exceed the neutralizing power of the antiplasmin present in the blood. Free plasmin then appears in the blood and the condition is known as hyperplasminaemia. In the absence of fibrin which is its substrate of choice, plasmin attacks other blood proteins, particularly Factors V and VIII. In this way it produces a hypocoagulable state. Plasmin may also attack fibrinogen, reducing its concentration and, more importantly, forming fibrinogen degradation products. These have a half-life of about 9 hours and by blocking the polymerization of fibrin monomer (vol. 1, fig. 26.6) interfere with the formation of physiological fibrin, which alone can safely occlude damaged blood vessels. This is of no consequence in an intact blood vessel but results in pathological bleeding at sites of injury because of interference with normal fibrin deposition. Hyperplasminaemia is thus responsible for a state of pathological proteolysis.

The principle of treatment is to maintain an increase of plasma fibrinolytic activity, if possible only locally, of such an order that clot lysis is expedited without producing systemic proteolysis. This is achieved by infusing an exogenous activator, such as streptokinase or urokinase, either locally by arterial cannulation of a limb proximal to the obstruction or systemically by the intravenous route. Of the two preparations streptokinase

is at present most used. It is the cheaper, but has the disadvantage that a loading dose sufficient to neutralize the patient's own antistreptokinase titre has to be given; theoretically a preliminary laboratory titration is needed to calculate the initial dose. There is no naturally occurring plasma antibody to urokinase. After the loading dose the thrombolytic state is maintained by infusing the activator in isotonic saline. Control of the dose is at present difficult.

All assays which measure blood activator are too complex and protracted to be useful in a rapidly changing dynamic system. Empiricism, based on experience, seems to give satisfactory results. A recommended scheme for streptokinase is an initial dose of 1,250,000 units given into either a vein or an artery over a period of 15–30 min and thereafter 100,000 units/hour for up to 3 days. With this procedure clinical results are usually satisfactory; it does, however, produce systemic hyperplasminaemia which continues until the plasminogen content of the blood has been virtually exhausted. It is therefore unsuitable for a patient with a potential bleeding lesion or who may require urgent surgery. There is also the potential danger of inducing a secondary hypercoagulable state. This can occur if the blood plasminogen becomes totally exhausted by excessive and prolonged therapy so that plasmin production ceases and clot accretion and thrombus formation are no longer controlled. Such patients require a prophylactic heparin cover while the plasminogen level is being naturally restored.

Streptokinase infusions stimulate the production of antistreptokinase and subsequent therapy may be less successful because of the high titre produced. Urokinase is not antigenic. Streptokinase may occasionally cause minor adverse effects such as headache, nausea, vomiting and fever which are usually controlled by concomitant corticosteroid therapy.

Inhibitors of fibrinolysis

How activator suddenly released into the circulation in large amounts can produce hyperplasminaemia (pathological proteolysis) has already been described. It occurs most commonly when tissues rich in activator such as lung, prostate, brain, uterus and thyroid are handled roughly during operations but it can occur also in complications of pregnancy such as amniotic fluid embolus, abruptio placentae, a retained dead foetus and eclampsia. It has been reported in patients with cirrhosis of the liver, leukaemia, shock and haemorrhage and is not uncommon in operations using extracorporeal circulation. It can be produced also by overdosage with thrombolytic drugs.

There are many endogenous and exogenous substances that act as antiactivators and antiplasmins. The only two important drugs used for this purpose at present are ε-aminocaproic acid (EACA) and aprotinin.

ε-AMINOCAPROIC ACID (EACA)

This synthetic amino acid has the following structure,

$$H_2NCH_2CH_2CH_2CH_2CH_2COOH$$

It resembles lysine and ornithine in having an NH_2 group attached to the end of the C chain. Plasminogen is converted to plasmin by the removal of the lysine and ornithine molecules by activator. EACA competes with plasminogen for activator. This it does effectively at a concentration of 10^{-4} M; at concentrations of 5×10^{-2} M or higher, it is a noncompetitive inhibitor of plasmin, i.e. it is an antiplasmin. It is used therefore in the treatment of hyperplasminaemic states whether spontaneous or iatrogenic in origin. It is equally effective by the intravenous and oral routes and the dose required to inhibit plasminogen activator in an adult is 5–7 g initially, followed by 1 g hourly. When used intravenously, it is given slowly in a 5–10 per cent solution in saline. EACA is rapidly excreted in the urine, about half the ingested dose being so lost in 12 hours. It is supplied in ampoules for parenteral use and as an effervescent powder and syrup for oral use.

EACA is of low toxicity, but may sometimes cause nausea, diarrhoea and urticaria or, when infused too rapidly, hypotension. It does, however, carry the risk of causing thrombosis by blockading fibrinolytic activity completely and thereby inducing a hypercoagulable state. It is also particularly liable to produce obstruction by clot retention in ducts in which bleeding is occurring, e.g. in the ureter in haematuria. As normal lysis is inhibited, such clots become organized and in inadequately drained or closed body cavities this can be dangerous, e.g. in the pericardium.

APROTININ (TRASYLOL)

Aprotinin is a basic, water-soluble polypeptide with a mol. wt. of about 6500 and is prepared commercially from bovine lung. It is a potent protease inhibitor and is effective against plasmin and possibly against plasminogen activator. It blocks formation of thromboplastin. Theoretically it can be used therefore to control either hyperplasminaemic or hypercoagulable states; unlike EACA its use in the former condition is not attended by the risk of inducing intractable thrombosis. Its action in hyperplasminaemia can, if necessary, be augmented by simultaneous therapy with EACA which appears to be a more effective antagonist to plasminogen activation.

Aprotinin is biologically standardized in terms of its ability to inactivate kallikrein (p. 17.1) or trypsin. It can be given only parenterally and is very expensive. In the treatment of disordered haemostasis or hyperplasminaemia, the recommended dosage is 50,000–100,000 kallikrein inhibitor units initially by slow intravenous infusion and thereafter a similar dose hourly until haemostasis is satisfactory. Similar doses may be used prophylactically in procedures known to be associated with a high risk of hyperplasminaemia.

Aprotinin is virtually nontoxic in man. Rarely, when injected too rapidly, it may produce nausea. As hypersensitivity to it may develop after repeated use, it is advisable to test the sensitivity of a patient who has been previously treated with the drug, by the intradermal injection of 1000 units before therapy is started.

OTHER FIBRINOLYTIC INHIBITORS

Adrenocorticotrophin and corticosteroids enhance physiological fibrinolysis but reduce excessive or pathological proteolysis and are therefore useful adjuncts in the treatment of hyperplasminaemic states.

Alicyclic amino compounds such as aminomethyl cyclohexane carboxylic acid (AMCHA) and para-aminomethyl benzoic acid (PAMBA) are both more potent than EACA weight for weight. AMCHA is a mixture of two stereoisomers, one of which possesses all the fibrinolytic activity of the mixture. The active isomer

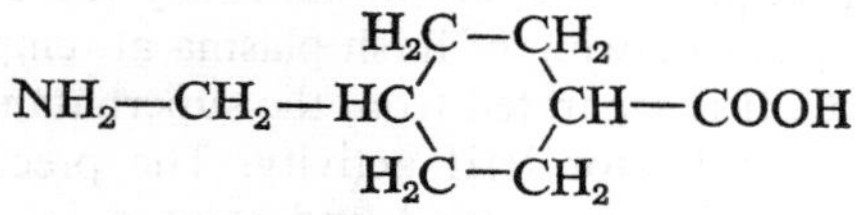

$$NH_2-CH_2-HC \overset{H_2C-CH_2}{\underset{H_2C-CH_2}{\diagup}} CH-COOH$$

Tranexamic acid

is called **tranexamic acid** and is available for therapeutic use. It is about 7–10 times more potent than EACA as a fibrinolytic inhibitor, possibly because of its more rigid chemical structure. It is less toxic even than EACA in animals. This compound probably heralds the introduction into therapeutics of newer and more potent antifibrinolytic drugs.

Blood products used in the treatment of deficiency of coagulation factors

Reference is made to the use of a plasma concentrate containing Factors II, VII, IX, and X for the treatment of overdosage of anticoagulant drugs and of Christmas disease on page 7.12. It is also given to patients with advanced liver disease who are bleeding severely or before surgery, in whom these factors are often deficient.

Dried plasma is used chiefly as a blood volume expander and also in double or triple strength as a source of fibrinogen. It is prepared by freeze drying out of date plasma from blood donor banks. Bottles made from ten or twelve donors can be stored at room temperature for several hours and reconstituted in distilled water when required. When made up to its original strength the $[K^+]$ is in the region of 15 mEq/l due to leakage from the ageing red cells.

Fresh frozen plasma is used as a source of Factor VIII

for patients with haemophilia. It contains also Factor IX, useful in the treatment of Christmas disease, and Factors V and VII. It is prepared from fresh blood from two donors from which the plasma is separated and frozen immediately. Stored at −30°C it is effective for at least three months. When required it is thawed in a water bath and administered to the patient with the minimum of delay. In a mild case of haemophilia, fresh frozen plasma from two donors usually raises the patient's circulating Factor VIII to a safe level for several hours. Fresh plasma with the same properties may be prepared by freeze drying. Both preparations are also employed as sources of pseudocholinesterase for the treatment of the apnoea caused by depolarizing relaxants (p. 5.69).

A **freeze dried preparation** obtained from the blood of three to six donors and stored under refrigeration containing more Factor VIII concentrate is used in the treatment of severe haemophilia in patients bleeding from injury or who require surgery. In contrast to fresh frozen plasma, and fresh freeze dried plasma, this concentrate does not contain Factor IX and so is unsuitable for the treatment of Christmas disease.

A **cryoprecipitate** is easily obtained by rapid freezing and subsequent thawing of fresh plasma at temperatures from 4–6°C. It is separated from the supernatant plasma and is rich in Factor VIII activity. The precipitate is stored frozen or freeze dried and is used in the same way as fresh frozen and freeze dried plasma.

A **fibrinogen** concentrate is made by freeze drying plasma, usually from eight to ten donors, in which over half the protein is coagulable. This is valuable in the treatment of fibrinogenopenia which may occur after obstetric haemorrhage, thoracic and prostate surgery, major vascular surgery and extensive injuries where there has been much tissue trauma.

All these products carry the risk of transmitting serum hepatitis (p. 18.117). The incidence of this disease varies in different parts of the world but in Edinburgh, for example, the risk is about 1 in 400 blood donations. It is obvious that the blood products that are prepared from pooled blood donations from a number of donors carry a correspondingly higher risk of transmitting infection.

FURTHER READING

BIGGS R. & MACFARLANE R.G. (1966) *Human Blood Coagulation*, 3rd Edition. Oxford: Blackwell Scientific Publications.

DE GRUCHY G.C. (1964) *Clinical Haematology in Medical Practice*, 2nd Edition. Oxford: Blackwell Scientific Publications.

DI PALMA J.R., ed. (1965) *Drill's Pharmacology in Medicine*, 3rd Edition. New York: McGraw-Hill.

DOUGLAS A.S. (1962) *Anticoagulant Therapy*. Oxford: Blackwell Scientific Publications.

FEARNLEY G.R. (1965) *Fibrinolysis*. London: Arnold.

GOODMAN L.S. & GILMAN, A., eds. (1965) Drugs acting on the blood and blood-forming organs, in *The Pharmacological Basis of Therapeutics*, 3rd Edition. New York: Macmillan.

HARDAWAY R.M. (1966) *Syndromes of Disseminated Intravascular Coagulation*. Springfield, Ill.: Thomas.

MCNICOL G.P. & DOUGLAS A.S. (1966) Aminocaproic acid and other inhibitors of fibrinolysis. *Practitioner*, **197**, 102.

VERSTRAETE M., VERMYLEN J., AMERY A. & VERMYLEN C. (1966) Thrombolytic therapy with streptokinase using a standard dosage scheme. *Brit. med. J.* **i**, 454.

Chapter 8
Drugs that act on the cardiovascular system

Many of the most effective drugs employed in the treatment of cardiovascular disease do not act directly on the cardiovascular system. For example, heart failure results in retention of water and sodium (p. 26.10) which can be ameliorated by diuretics (p. 11.1); bacterial endocarditis calls for the use of antibiotics, infarction and embolism for anticoagulants (p. 7.10), while rheumatic fever with carditis is treated with anti-inflammatory drugs such as salicylates and corticosteroids.

Here we are concerned with drugs whose principal site of action is the heart and blood vessels. These alter the response of the heart muscle itself or of vascular smooth muscle, either directly or indirectly, through neural or humoral pathways.

There are various sites at which such drugs may act on muscle. In the heart itself the variables which may be altered are the frequency of the heart beat and the strength of contraction of the heart muscle. In addition, drugs may influence the rate of blood flow through the coronary arteries, thus affecting indirectly the myocardial efficiency. In the case of the blood vessels the smooth muscle which extends throughout the vascular system except the capillaries, may be constricted or relaxed by direct action or indirectly through neural control.

Digitalis glycosides

The use of extracts of the foxglove (*Digitalis purpurea* or *Digitalis lanata*) as a treatment for dropsy, the oedema of heart failure, is of great antiquity and is described in medieval texts. The related substance squill was mentioned in the Ebers Papyrus (*c.* 1500 B.C.) and was also used in Roman times. The first scientific account was given by William Withering of Stafford who in 1785 (*An Account of the Foxglove and Some of its Medical Uses*) drew attention to the beneficial effect of the plant in cases of dropsy. He believed it to act on the kidney. Since then digitalis, or its purified components, have been universally used in the treatment of heart failure. The active principles are called **digitalis glycosides** which characteristically have:

(1) a steroid structure,
(2) a five- or six-membered lactone ring, and

(3) a carbohydrate compound of up to four sugar residues.

Molecules consisting of (1) and (2) are responsible for the action on the heart and are known as **aglycones**. All cardioactive aglycones have hydroxyl groups attached to C-3, C-14, methyl groups to C-10 and C-13, and an unsaturated lactone group at C-17. Different sugar residues affect potency and duration of action; glucose, rhamnose and fucose are most commonly found.

Digitalis itself consists of powdered leaf or a hydroalcoholic extract and contains a mixture of glycosides. Because of this it has to be standardized biologically against an international standard. The standard preparation is a powder made from dried digitalis leaves, and a unit of digitalis activity corresponds to 80 mg of this preparation. Two biological methods are employed, based on the amounts needed to arrest the heart of either a frog or a decerebrate cat. The results obtained by these and other bioassays do not always agree and attempts were made to assay digitalis by its effects in man using the T wave of the ECG as the index of response. Because the digitalis glycosides are variable in their onset and duration of action they are rarely used in this form nowadays and the difficulties of standardizing such mixtures have been overcome by the introduction of chemically pure glycosides which possess all the actions of the crude drug. Such glycosides are **digoxin, digitoxin, gitalin, lanatoside C, ouabain** and **strophanthin**. The last two, though obtained from different botanical sources, are identical chemically.

Of these cardiac glycosides only digoxin is widely used today.

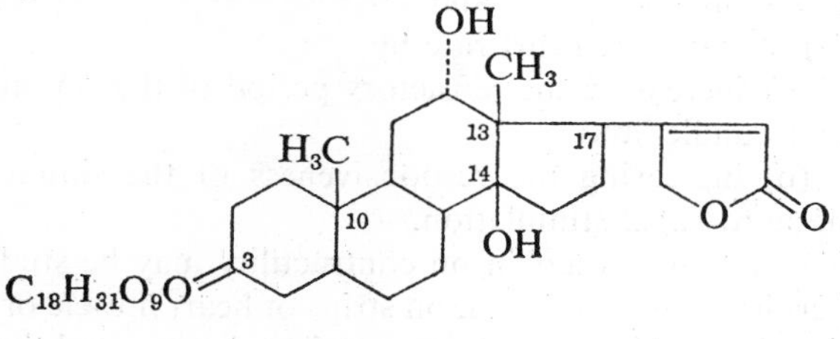

Sugar   Steroid   Lactone

Digoxin

Digoxin is a white crystalline powder and is given usually by mouth though it can be injected in solution, intramuscularly or intravenously. It is absorbed rapidly from the gastrointestinal tract. Its effects are maximal in 2–5 hours and are prolonged for several days. It is inactivated in the liver and is also excreted unchanged in the urine.

Occasionally for rapid digitalization ouabain is used. It comes from the woody bark of the *Acokanthera ouabaio* or *Schimperi*. It is chemically identical with strophanthin. This substance, obtained from a different botanical source, was introduced into clinical medicine originally as a result of the work of Sir Thomas Fraser in 1890.

ACTIONS OF DIGITALIS GLYCOSIDES

All digitalis glycosides have the same actions in the body. They differ, however, in potency and in rate of excretion which determine how frequently and how much of each glycoside must be given. Because of their slow excretion the glycosides are cumulative and excessive cumulation is detected by clinical effects and not by chemical determination of the concentration in body fluids. Fortunately the therapeutic effects are usually obtained at concentrations below those at which the adverse effects become troublesome and the dosage of glycoside must be adjusted to maintain concentration in the body within this range. The patient is then said to be fully **digitalized**. Before this stage is reached a larger **digitalizing dose** must be given initially over a short period of time in order to bring the concentration of drug in the body to an effective level. Thereafter, digitalization is sustained by the **maintenance dose** (p. 2.18).

Digoxin disappears rapidly from the blood stream and is distributed throughout the organs of the body. Blood concentration is, therefore, no guide to the state of digitalization. There is no selective uptake of digoxin by cardiac muscle. Approximately 70 per cent of an administered dose is excreted via the urine and 20 per cent via the faeces. In each case about 10 per cent is recoverable as unchanged digoxin.

Of its many actions in the body those on the heart are by far the most important and they result in:

(1) increased myocardial contractility known as positive inotropic action, and

(2) slowing the heart rate by

    (a) increasing the refractory period of the AV node and bundle, and

    (b) increasing the responsiveness of the sinuatrial node to vagal stimulation.

The action of digoxin on contractility may be studied experimentally in animals, on strips of heart muscle or on isolated amphibian and mammalian hearts and heart lung preparations. In man, the improvement in contractility is demonstrable as an increased rate of rise of pres-

sure in the ventricle (dp/dt), a shortened ejection period, more nearly complete ventricular systolic emptying and increased ventricular stroke work for a given end-diastolic pressure. The ventricular function curve (vol. 1, p. 28.34) is moved towards the left (fig. 8.1). The drug increases

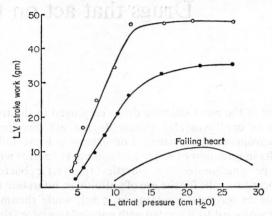

FIG. 8.1. Effect of ouabain on myocardial function. Left ventricular function curves were obtained in a normal dog, before (●) and after (○) administration of ouabain, 0·05 mg/kg. Left atrial pressure was increased by infusion of blood into the atrium at appropriate rates. The normal and ouabain curves were obtained experimentally. For comparison, a hypothetical curve for a failing heart has been added. Note that a reduction of atrial pressure from 30 to 20 cm H_2O would increase the work output of the failing heart. Ouabain, by increasing contractility, shifts the heart to a new function curve, permitting greater work output at any given atrial pressure. Adapted from Cotten & Stopp (1958), *Amer. J. Physiol.* **192**, 114.

cardiac output where this is lowered by cardiac failure but not in normal individuals. There is some evidence that the increase in output is achieved without a proportional increase in oxygen consumption or coronary blood flow, i.e. by improved utilization of energy rather than increased energy production. However, careful studies on the non-failing dog heart indicate that the increased contractility in response to digoxin is accompanied by increased O_2 consumption. The explanation of this discrepancy may lie in the fact that in the failing heart, digoxin reduces ventricular volume. Hence, for a given systolic pressure less tension is developed in the ventricular wall (vol. 1, p. 28.14) and the consequent saving of O_2 offsets the increase required by enhanced contractility.

Clinically the drug shows its most dramatic effects where both contractility and heart rate are affected, e.g. in cases of heart failure with atrial fibrillation and a rapid ventricular rate. In atrial fibrillation, atrial contraction is uncoordinated and the fibres contract asynchronously. The ventricular response is irregular and rapid (150–200/min). By prolonging the refractory period of the AV bundle and node, digoxin slows the ventricular response and improves output by allowing time for adequate diastolic filling. Apart from this, however, when rhythm and rate are normal the drug can relieve severe left ventricular failure due, e.g., to high blood pressure in a matter of hours (fig. 8.2). It has no direct effect on the coronary flow but this increases with the rise in cardiac output. Because of its action on the AV node and bundle it is clearly an unsuitable drug in patients with heart block.

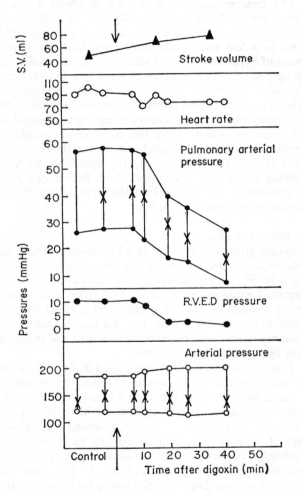

FIG. 8.2. Effect of digoxin given at arrow in a patient with hypertensive heart failure affecting left and right ventricles.

In addition to systemic hypertension the patient had a reduced cardiac output and pulmonary hypertension. After intravenous digoxin (1·5 mg), cardiac output and stroke volume increased to normal, pulmonary arterial and right ventricular end-diastolic (RVED) pressure decreased to normal, and the heart rate decreased to normal. Note the stroke work of the left ventricle was increased as the cardiac output was restored; the work load imposed on the right ventricle was sharply reduced by the reduction of pulmonary arterial pressure. Adapted from Harvey, Ferrer, Cathcart & Alexander (1951), *Circulation.*

In addition to its myocardial action digitalis has other effects. In healthy subjects it has a direct constrictive action on peripheral arterioles and veins, i.e. it **increases** the peripheral resistance. In patients with heart failure, however, who already maintain a high peripheral resistance to conserve the arterial blood pressure in the face of a low cardiac output, the myocardial effects of the drug are of greatest benefit and the peripheral resistance usually falls.

The central venous pressure decreases after administration of digoxin to patients with heart failure. This is due to improved cardiac contraction and emptying. There is a prompt increase in excretion of sodium and water largely due to increased glomerular filtration and renal plasma flow, but also to a small extent to a direct inhibition of tubular reabsorption of sodium. The increased circulating blood volume which is characteristic of heart failure is diminished by the renal effects of the drug.

MECHANISM OF THE CARDIAC ACTION
Some facts are known about the way in which digoxin exerts its effect on the myocardium, but these do not provide a clear picture of how digitalis glycosides exert their inotropic effect. Digoxin enters the myocardial cells and there yields the active aglycone, i.e. the molecule without the sugar fraction. It is mainly located in the cytoplasmic portion of the cell which contains the contractile protein and the transport system. It has been claimed that the drug is specifically localized in the tubular system of the sarcoplasmic reticulum (vol. 1, p. 15.6), the site of excitation–contraction coupling, and that its effect may be mediated through this coupling rather than through any direct action on the contractile muscle filaments. There is, however, evidence of binding of the aglycone to actomyosin and this has given rise to the idea that the action may be concerned with the myocardial contractile protein. Inactive glycosides, however, also show this binding.

Digoxin also inhibits movement of Na^+ and K^+ across the cell membrane. Thus it tends to deplete the cell of potassium and increase the sodium content. Since the source of energy for the sodium pump is ATP, it is suggested that digoxin may inhibit ATPase (vol. 1, p. 14.15). High extracellular levels of potassium inhibit and low levels enhance the effect of digoxin on membrane transport.

The inhibitory effect of cardioactive glycosides has been studied on the ATPase activity of the red blood cell membrane but similar observations have also been made on myocardial membranes. A good correlation has been found between the inotropic activity and the power to influence sodium and potassium transport. However, it is doubtful if the concentration of digitalis attained in therapeutic doses is sufficient to inhibit the influence of ATPase *in vivo*, and in low doses it has even been shown to have a stimulating effect on ATPase in microsomal fractions.

An important relationship has also been discovered between extracellular [Ca^{++}] and digitalis. Digoxin produces an increase in the uptake of cell Ca^{++} and it is possible that this facilitates the association between actin and myosin and the contractile process (vol. 1, p. 15.12). Depolarization of the cell membrane is followed by release of Ca^{++} from the sarcoplasmic reticulum which initiates the ATPase activity of myosin, with resultant actin-myosin contraction. Relaxation is accompanied by withdrawal of Ca^{++} from the cytoplasm into the sarcoplasmic reticulum. Inhibition of this Ca^{++} flux results in poor contractility. Ouabain and other cardiac glycosides have been shown to increase the binding of Ca^{++} by the sarcoplasmic reticulum, increase its turnover and augment the calcium-stimulated ATPase (fig. 8.3).

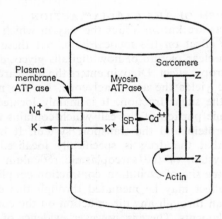

Fig. 8.3. Proposed cellular action of digitalis. Digitalis glycosides reduce the activity of plasma membrane ATPase. Na^+ enters cell and tubules of the sarcoplasmic reticulum (SR) where it releases Ca^{++} which initiates contraction by contractile proteins. After Sonnenblick, Sponitz & Spiro (1964), *Circulat. Res.*

The electrical phenomena associated with cell depolarization are affected by digoxin, resulting in ECG changes. In the individual cell, the action potential shows a smaller spike and a more rapid repolarization. The lowered membrane potential due to the ionic changes makes the cell more excitable and one of the toxic effects of digoxin when given in excessive amounts is the production of ventricular extrasystoles. On the other hand, its beneficial effect on tachycardia is due to depression of the junctional conduction tissues in the region of the AV node, thus slowing AV conduction. In toxic doses this effect leads to varying degrees of AV block. There is also evidence of sinuatrial slowing through vagal stimu-

lation by the drug. This effect can be shown in experimental animals by the fact that it can be inhibited by atropine but it is probably of little importance in man.

The toxic effects of digoxin thus include vagal stimulation with nausea and vomiting and sinuatrial slowing, AV block, ST segment and T wave changes in the ECG, ventricular ectopic beats, paroxysmal tachycardia and myocardial potassium depletion. The border line between a therapeutic and a dangerously toxic dose is fairly narrow.

The concentration of potassium in blood and cells affects the cardiac response to digoxin. The clinical setting in which digoxin is used is frequently one in which there is a low body potassium; potassium is lost as a result of hypoxia associated with heart failure itself, while many diuretics induce a further renal loss of potassium. Potassium depletion alone is known to predispose to atrial tachycardia and sensitizes the myocardium to the excitatory effects of digoxin while leaving unchanged the AV blocking effect. Thus the most characteristic arrhythmia induced by digitalis is an atrial tachycardia with AV block. This is generally reversible by withholding digitalis and giving potassium. Reference is made to the effect of propranolol on the arrhythmias of overdosage with digitalis on p. 8.6.

CLINICAL USES

Digitalis glycosides are used in all conditions of low output cardiac failure, with few exceptions. Its effects are seen most clearly in myocardial failure when there is a rapid ventricular rate as a result of an atrial arrhythmia, usually atrial fibrillation. Such a patient has a rapid irregular pulse (120–180 beats/min), low cardiac output, raised pulmonary and systemic venous pressures and is breathless, cyanosed and oedematous.

Digoxin is the most commonly used digitalis glycoside. In such a patient it is commonly given by mouth. A usual digitalizing dose is 0·5 mg 6 hourly. Little effect is noted until two to four such doses have been given. The pulse rate then starts to fall, reaching a ventricular rate of 70–80/min after a further 12–24 hours. Atrial fibrillation persists, but the ventricular rate is now slow and ventricular filling is improved. At the same time the pulse volume improves, the blood pressure may rise, and because of improved contractility the cardiac output increases and pulmonary and systemic venous pressure falls towards normal. This stage is marked by relief of breathlessness and by diuresis with loss of the accumulated water and salt. The patient's colour improves. At this stage of digitalization the high rate of dosage must be reduced to a maintenance level, sufficient only to replace digoxin excreted or detoxicated by the body. This is usually 0·25–0·5 mg/day.

If a high dosage is continued, however, further changes take place. The patient first loses his appetite, then becomes nauseated and vomits; this is believed to be due to medullary chemoreceptor stimulation. He may complain of headache and drowsiness and more rarely develop diarrhoea or visual disturbances. The ventricular rate slows further to 40 beats/min or below. If he is in sinus rhythm, AV block may appear. Ventricular extrasystoles, either singly or coupled may occur or paroxysmal atrial tachycardia with AV block. These arrhythmias, which may be lethal, are much more prone to occur when the body is depleted of potassium.

Should the patient develop any of the manifestations of digitalis overdosage the drug should be stopped for 24–28 hours, and then resumed in a maintenance dose and, when appropriate, supplementary potassium should be administered. In patients whose renal or hepatic function is impaired, or in the elderly, digitalis is more likely to cumulate, and smaller maintenance doses of the drug should be given.

Apart from arrhythmias induced by overdosage, patients receiving digitalis in therapeutic doses have characteristic alterations in the electrocardiogram which may complicate interpretation. These changes consist of T wave flattening or asymmetrical T wave inversion, often associated with ST depression. The QT interval may be shortened.

OTHER GLYCOSIDES

Although digoxin is by far the most commonly used glycoside, others are sometimes employed in clinical practice. Lanatoside C (cedilanid) is frequently used in the USA. Ouabain is used sometimes in acute emergencies, e.g. arrhythmias complicating myocardial infarction, because of its extremely rapid action and rapid excretion. In general the maintenance dose of these drugs is inversely proportional to the half life of the drug in the body. The main features of some of these drugs is shown in table 8.1.

Myocardial depressant (antiarrhythmic) drugs

A large group of drugs is employed to reduce the irritability, i.e. to raise the threshold stimulation, of myocardial cells in tachycardias where the normal sinuatrial pacemaker is usurped by abnormal irritable foci in atria or ventricles. These arrhythmias include paroxysmal atrial or nodal tachycardia, atrial flutter, frequent ventricular extrasystoles, ventricular tachycardia and flutter. Most of these drugs have the disadvantage that they depress contractility in addition to excitability and are therefore prone to induce heart failure. While **quinidine** is historically the best known of these drugs it has largely been superseded.

The use of these drugs in general has been much less frequent with the development of electrical methods of treating arrhythmias.

Pharmacologically the activity of antiarrhythmic drugs may be examined by measuring the threshold of electrical stimulation required to cause contraction of rabbit atria. In this and other myocardial tissues the effective refractory period can also be shown to be prolonged. The form of the action potential recorded from myocardial cells shows a decreased speed of depolarization.

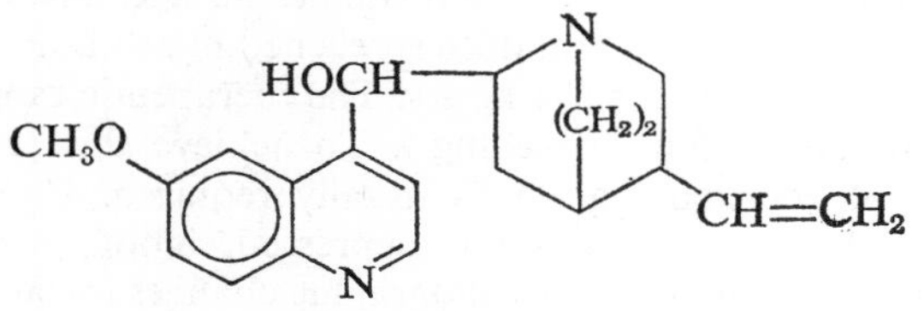

Quinidine

In 1914 Wenckebach observed that a patient who suffered from atrial fibrillation taking quinine for malaria reverted to sinus rhythm. This led to its use, and subsequently its more effective optical isomer quinidine, in arrhythmias. These substances are alkaloids which were originally derived from the bark of various species of Cinchona and Remijia trees native to the high Andes but now grown in India and Java. By a direct action on cardiac muscle quinidine decreases the velocity of conduction in atria, AV node and ventricles and reduces their excitability. It prolongs the functional refractory period of

TABLE 8.1 Pharmacological properties of cardiac glycosides.

Glycoside	Source	Effect of single IV dose				Maintenance dose mg/day	Remarks
		Dose mg	Start min	Maximal hours	Finished days		
Ouabain	*Acokanthera ouabaio*	0·5	5	1–2	1–3	—	Used for rapid IV digitalization only
Lanatoside C	*Digitalis lanata*	1·5	15	1–2	3–6	0·5–2·0	Cedilanid, name used in USA
Digoxin	*Digitalis lanata*	1·0	20	2–5	2–6	0·25–0·5	Lanoxin, name used in UK
Digitoxin	*Digitalis purpurea*	1·25	60	4–12	15–30	0·50–0·15	Slow digitalization sometimes avoids toxic effects

myocardial cells by slowing depolarization without affecting the half-time for repolarization which determines the absolute refractory period. Quinidine also exerts an anticholinergic action which enhances its direct effect on atrial conduction and refractory period. In addition it reduces the activity of the pacemaker, diminishes myocardial contractility and relaxes arteriolar smooth muscle.

The cellular mechanisms for these electrophysiological effects are unknown. The chemical structure that appears important for the antiarrhythmic properties of quinidine and procainamide (see below) is that of a ring joined to a tertiary amine nitrogen via an oxygen or hydroxyl containing bridge. Since quinidine chelates Ca^{++}, it has been suggested that the negative inotropic actions are mediated through this action. There is also evidence that it inhibits ATPase activity. The depolarization phase of the action potential is due to an increase in the permeability of the cell membrane to sodium (vol. 1, p. 14.25) and there is evidence that this is decreased by quinidine.

Absorption from the gastrointestinal tract is erratic and blood levels are poorly related to dosage. The maximum effect after an oral dose is reached in 2–4 hours and its effects persist for 6–8 hours. The therapeutic range in the blood stream is 3–6 mg/l. To achieve this level a dose of 200–400 mg/day is usually required. Contractility of the myocardium is depressed, blood pressure tends to fall and electrocardiographic changes (prolonged PR interval, ST depression and T inversion) are produced. Adverse manifestations of excessive dosage are vertigo, tinnitus, deafness, blurred vision, gastrointestinal disturbances, thrombocytopenia and ventricular fibrillation or asystole. About 50 per cent of quinidine is bound to plasma proteins and the drug is taken up quickly by cardiac muscle where radioautographic studies show it bound to cell membranes and mitochondria. Quinidine is metabolized in the liver but up to 50 per cent is excreted unchanged in the urine.

Many drugs have antiarrhythmic properties similar to those of quinidine. These include propranolol, lignocaine and procainamide, and phenytoin. All of these drugs, with the important exception of lignocaine, depress myocardial contractility, apparently by inhibiting the Ca^{++} flux into and out of the sarcoplasmic reticulum. **Lignocaine** (p. 5.70) is therefore the safest drug in the treatment of acute ventricular arrhythmias even though it is toxic in high dosage, and it must be given parenterally. Lignocaine is given slowly intravenously in doses of 50 mg. For long term use **procainamide** is the drug of choice. Adverse effects include gastrointestinal symptoms and

Procainamide

rarely agranulocytosis. Procainamide is readily absorbed from the gastrointestinal tract. Given in a dose of 500–750 mg three or four times per day, therapeutic blood levels of 10–20 mg/l are reached.

Phenytoin, long used as an antiepileptic drug, has also valuable antiarrhythmic properties of the quinidine type (p. 5.59). Given intravenously in a dose of 250 mg it is especially useful in the treatment of digitalis-induced supraventricular or ventricular arrhythmias.

Propranolol (p. 15.27) has separate quinidine-like and β-receptor blocking activities. It is useful in the treatment of supraventricular and ventricular arrhythmias, especially in those which are digitalis-induced. It slows the ventricular rate in sinus tachycardia and atrial fibrillation. It has however the unwanted effect of reducing myocardial contractility and lowering the cardiac output. Left heart failure, bradycardia, hypotension and cardiac arrest can be caused by incautious dosage in the presence of heart disease, and other adverse effects are reduced ventilation and bronchospasm. Because it reduces left ventricular work it is useful in angina pectoris. In the treatment of arrhythmias the initial intravenous dose should not exceed 0·5 mg or the oral dose 5 mg.

Recently the D-isomer of propranolol has been introduced. This possesses the quinidine-like effect with minimal β-blocking activity and is likely to be of great value in the treatment of arrhythmias.

The treatment of cardiac arrhythmia is a difficult branch of clinical cardiology and the place of these drugs in therapeutics is discussed in vol. 3.

Nitrites

Narrowing or occlusion of the coronary arteries impairing the blood supply of the heart muscle is the commonest cause of death in Great Britain and America. Restriction of coronary blood flow results in cardiac pain (angina), arrhythmias and heart failure (p. 25.5). The consequences of myocardial hypoxia are also seen in the ECG where changes in the T waves are seen. Drugs which improve the blood supply to the myocardium are therefore of great importance. Only one group of drugs, nitrites and the organic nitrates which possibly owe their action to being reduced to nitrite in the body, has been convincingly shown to do this. The discovery of the dramatic effect of one of these, amyl nitrite in relieving angina, we owe to Lauder Brunton, an Edinburgh physician, whose account appeared in 1867.

In animals the effect of drugs on the coronary circulation may be studied by flowmeters or by radioisotope clearance techniques. However, the effect in humans with diseased coronary arteries is more difficult to study. Cardiac pain is a notoriously variable symptom and placebo effects are common. Rigorously controlled standardized exercise tests using as end points the onset of pain or the time sequence of ECG changes offer the most reliable assessment of therapeutic effect.

The three nitrites which are commonly used in this respect are **amyl nitrite**, a volatile liquid which is inhaled after breaking a capsule of the substance wrapped in cloth (0·2 ml), **glyceryl trinitrate** which is sucked in tablet form (0·4 mg) and absorbed through the oral mucosa, and **sorbide nitrate** (10 mg) which is taken orally and has a rather weaker but longer acting effect. **Penta-erythritol tetranitrate** is also a long acting compound but is weak and its clinical usefulness disappointing.

Amyl nitrite acts in seconds and glyceryl trinitrate in minutes. Their effects are over in 5 and 30 min respectively.

CH₃
  \
   CHCH₂CH₂ONO
  /
CH₃
    Amyl nitrite

CH₂—O—NO₂
|
CH—O—NO₂
|
CH₂—O—NO₂
Glyceryl trinitrate
(nitroglycerine)

MODE OF ACTION
Although often classified as drugs which act on the heart, the nitrites relax smooth muscle everywhere in the body. In normal individuals these drugs cause generalized vasodilation with flushing, throbbing headache, palpitations and tachycardia; they lower the blood pressure, increase cardiac output and decrease coronary resistance causing a rise in coronary blood flow of up to 100 per cent. In patients with a structurally diseased coronary arterial system, however, the mode of action is much less certainly due to increased myocardial blood flow. In many cases it is probably at least as much due to the sudden unloading of the left ventricle by reduction in blood pressure and venous filling pressure. Observations in man show that glyceryl trinitrate dilates the capacitance vessels at least in the limbs while simultaneously diminishing peripheral vascular resistance. Pooling of the blood then explains the fall in cardiac output and the fainting episodes which are occasionally seen. The pressure load on the ventricle is the main factor in determining oxygen requirement and reduction of the requirement may allow its blood supply to catch up. Slowing the heart rate also lowers oxygen requirement and angina can regularly be stopped by carotid sinus pressure. No doubt in many cases both factors, decreased oxygen requirement and decreased coronary vascular resistance, are operative.

Nitrites relax smooth muscle probably by inhibiting ATPase activity. They cause oxidation of haemoglobin to methaemoglobin and in large doses may cause cyanosis for this reason. This is the basis of the dangerous nitrate poisoning which can occur in children who swallow **glyceryl trinitrate** tablets.

Reference is made to the effect of propranolol on angina pectoris on p. 15.27.

The xanthines
The xanthine alkaloids are described on p. 5.39. Theophylline and theobromine have more powerful effects than caffeine on the cardiovascular system, smooth muscle and the kidneys and these are of clinical value. Theophylline, and to a lesser extent theobromine, stimulate the myocardium directly, increasing the force of contraction and the cardiac output, achieving more efficient emptying of the ventricles during systole. These effects are particularly marked in acute left ventricular failure due, for example, to hypertension where the intravenous injection of theophylline is clinically valuable, although comparatively short-lived. Theophylline also relaxes smooth muscles of the coronary arteries and of the bronchi especially when constricted by histamine or in asthma. Clinically theophylline is used in its water-soluble form, **theophylline ethylenediamine** or **aminophylline**. It is usually given intravenously in doses of 250–500 mg; it may be also given as a suppository. The diuretic effects of theophylline are described on p. 11.2.

Drugs and the regulation of blood pressure
Like other biological variables blood pressure has a fairly wide distribution in the population and there are no sharp dividing lines between normal values and high or low blood pressure (vol. 1, p. 28.32). Nevertheless very high or very low values both carry serious consequences to health.

In western societies life insurance statistics show
(1) that blood pressure tends to rise with age, and
(2) that cardiovascular disease and premature death occur more frequently in those in whom the level is disproportionately higher for their age group.

Hypertension may be induced experimentally by renal artery constriction and the role of the renin angiotensin system and of salt in this experimental model is discussed in vol. 1, p. 33.20. It may also be induced or aggravated in man or animals by large doses of corticosteroids especially those with powerful salt retaining effects (p. 6.11). It may be produced in rats by section of the afferent nerves from the carotid sinus and aortic arch and by repeated exposure to stressful stimuli, e.g. a cacophony of noise or hot air blasts in certain strains of rats. It occurs in man in Cushing's syndrome, in aldosterone secreting tumours and in phaeochromocytoma (p. 15.3) and more commonly in a variety of renal diseases in which the role of the angiotensin–renin mechanism is uncertain. In the majority of patients, however, no underlying cause can be detected and in these individuals it is uncertain whether it is a disease entity or a polygenetically inherited characteristic (p. 31.13). Whatever its origin a major part of the management of the patient with elevated blood pressure consists of the use of drugs which modify the physiological factors which are concerned in the control of the circulation.

With the exception of reserpine, almost all antihypertensive drugs have been discovered by studies on normal animals. These may be tested for their vasoactive effects in a variety of pharmacological models. The majority of effective drugs are those possessing adrenergic blocking activity (p. 4.15) and can be tested by their effect in the nictitating membrane of the cat. The disadvantage of this preparation is that it provides little or no information of the suitability of the drug in man who spends much of his life in the upright position and in whom a number of homeostatic influences operate to maintain the blood pressure within limits. More recently hypertensive animals have been employed to assess potentially useful agents but their clinical acceptability still depend on trials in man.

In basic haemodynamic terms the systemic blood pressure is the product of the cardiac output and the peripheral resistance. With the possible exception of early labile hypertension, chronically elevated blood pressure is due to increased peripheral resistance, the cardiac output being normal. Possible causes of increased resistance are structural changes in arterioles (increased wall/lumen ratio), increased reflex vasoconstrictor activity, increased blood viscosity as in polycythaemia, and the presence of a circulating vasoconstrictor humoral agent such as noradrenaline. When the blood pressure is elevated in disease, the baroreceptor reflex is reduced in sensitivity and set at a higher level. All drugs used to control blood pressure do so by reducing vascular tone though they have different sites of action. These can be classified as follows:

(1) those that reduce sympathetic vasomotor tone,

TABLE 8.2. Antihypertensive drugs which reduce sympathetic activity

Decreased release of nor-adrenaline	Decreased vasomotor centre activity	Decreased transmission at sympa-thetic ganglia	Decreased action of catecholamines
Bethanidine		Pentolinium	α-Receptor block-ing drugs
Debriso-quine			
Guan-ethidine	Hydrallazine	Mecamyl-amine	Sodium de-pleting drugs
Bretylium	Sedatives and tranquillizers	Pempidine	Cardiac β-receptor blocking drugs
Rauwolfia	Veratrum alkaloids	Trimethaphan	
Methyldopa			
MAO inhibitors			

(2) those that induce direct vasodilation, and
(3) those that reduce blood volume or cause sodium depletion.

Drugs which reduce sympathetic vasomotor activity are by far the most important and may be subdivided into the groups shown in table 8.2. The ideal antihypertensive drug would lower the blood pressure without interfering with the control mechanisms which are responsible for the adaptations to posture or exercise. No drug has yet been discovered which comes near this ideal.

PREJUNCTIONAL ADRENERGIC BLOCKING DRUGS
The basis of the action of prejunctional blocking drugs is discussed on p. 15.29 and the chemical structures of bretylium, guanethedine, bethanidine and debrisoquine are given in table 4.8, p. 4.15. These drugs block circulatory reflexes and inhibit the response to sympathetic nerve stimulation. While they all do so by reducing the release of noradrenaline at the receptor site, they have different relative effects on the neuronal stores of noradrenaline. In addition, guanethidine appears to have a greater effect in blocking low rates of sympathetic discharges while bretylium has more effect interfering with the consequences of higher rates, bethanidine and debrisoquine occupying an intermediate position. Some difference in the antihypertensive effect in the upright and supine position might be anticipated from these observations but this does not appear to be borne out in practice. In hypertensive patients blood pressure is reduced in the standing position. The cardiac output shows either a small fall or no change in the recumbent position but decreases significantly on standing. Renal blood flow is also maintained in recumbency but tends to fall on standing upright, GFR showing similar changes but to a lesser degree. These changes are due to interference in circulatory control in which peripheral vasoconstriction fails to compensate the falling cardiac output. In addition they reduce venoconstriction in the legs in the upright position which further reduces cardiac output.

Guanethidine, a guanidine derivative, is a powerful antihypertensive drug which is partially but reliably absorbed from the gastrointestinal tract and has a prolonged action which lasts for several days. The usual oral daily dose ranges from 50–150 mg and tolerance to the drug is uncommon. When guanethidine is injected intravenously in man or animals, a transient rise in blood pressure occurs and is probably due to a release of noradrenaline from the stores in the nerve. Apart from orthostatic hypotension which is due to failure of the vasoconstrictor responses normally associated with standing, other troublesome effects include diarrhoea and impotence. A small number of patients retain water and salt for reasons that are unknown.

Bethanidine is a benzylguanidine with a more rapid and

shorter action of 8–12 hours. Like guanethidine the fall in blood pressure achieved is greater in the upright than that in the supine position and a further fall with exercise also occurs. The main disadvantage to bethanidine is the tendency for tolerance to develop which in some patients gives rise to the need for increasing doses of the drug. The usual daily oral dose is 50–150 mg.

Debrisoquine is the most recent compound of this type and closely resembles bethanidine in its duration and mode of action. Its effective dose usually lies between 30 and 100 mg/day; tolerance not infrequently develops but it is notably free from other adverse effects.

Bretylium, a quaternary ammonium compound, was among the first adrenergic neurone blocking drugs to be discovered. Its action is also shorter than that of guanethidine, being complete in 24 hours after a single dose. Although widely used in the treatment of hypertension for some years, its absorption from the gastrointestinal tract is unreliable, and it is no longer generally available. It occasionally induces pain in the parotid glands.

RAUWOLFIA ALKALOIDS
The chemical structure of reserpine and its pharmacological properties are described on p. 5.30 and its influence on the stores of catecholamines in adrenergic neurones is given on p. 15.30. Depletion of noradrenaline at adrenergic nerve endings is the most important cause of the hypotensive effect but other mechanisms may be involved. Intra-arterial injection of reserpine produces vasodilation in sympathectomized vessels in man. Reserpine may also induce cardiac failure perhaps due to increased sensitivity to circulatory catecholamines in conditions of hypoxia or under general anaesthesia.

As an antihypertensive agent, reserpine has not proved satisfactory, being of use only in mild cases. Only relatively low doses (0·25–0·5 mg/day) can be given by mouth in order to keep central effects to a minimum and even this dose produces lethargy, apathy and sometimes severe mental depression. With such doses the hypotensive action is slow to develop and persistence of the effect for a long time after stopping the drug is an additional drawback. Increasing the dose increases the central actions at a faster rate than the hypotensive action. Adverse effects commonly produced are diarrhoea which in part may be related to the action of 5-HT released from the intestinal tract, increased salivation possibly due to central parasympathetic stimulation, flushing and nasal congestion due to decreased sympathetic tone. Gastric secretion is stimulated and dormant peptic ulcers may be activated. Fluid retention with oedema has been noted in the absence of cardiac failure. The patients sometimes develop a Parkinsonian-like syndrome. In some patients with severe hypertensive crisis a single intramuscular injection of 1–5 mg may be of value and lower the blood pressure within a few hours.

METHYLDOPA (α-methyl dihydroxyphenylalanine, α-methyldopa)
Methyldopa is an optically active compound, the synthetic preparation containing equal amounts of D and L forms. Pharmacological activity resides in the L isomer and this is used clinically. The chemical formula of methyldopa is given on p. 4.15 and a discussion of its mode of action in reducing the blood pressure is given on p. 15.32. Although originally believed to act by diminishing the synthesis of noradrenaline by competitively inhibiting dopa decarboxylase, it more probably owes its hypotensive action to the formation of α-methylnoradrenaline which acts as a false transmitter. Unlike other sympathetic blocking drugs, it does not inhibit the nictitating membrane of the cat following stimulation of its adrenergic nerves.

Methyldopa is well absorbed from the gastrointestinal tract and given by mouth in doses of 0·5–3·0 g/day. It is also rapidly excreted in the urine, about 90 per cent of a single dose being found there in 12 hours. It exerts some hypotensive effect in the supine as well as the erect position, the blood pressure fall being greatest in the hypertensive individual. Although postural hypotension occurs, it is less severe and less common than with adrenergic neurone blocking agents. This observation is consistent with the false transmitter theory of its mechanism of action. Methyldopa often produces drowsiness and tranquillity. This sedative effect is limited to the first few days of treatment, but is liable to reappear if the dose is increased. Mental depression and a Parkinsonian-like condition may then develop. These effects on the CNS may possibly be due to the depletion of catecholamines and 5-HT in the brain. Tolerance to the drug is uncommon. Water and salt retention is common and may lead to oedema and the development of cardiac failure. Nasal stuffiness is an annoying effect and presumably results from decreased sympathetic tone to the blood vessels of the mucosa. Dry mouth, nausea and vomiting and diarrhoea also occur. A haemolytic anaemia due to the presence of an auto-immune antibody to the patient's own red blood cells occasionally occurs, but responds to the withdrawal of the drug (p. 23.3).

DRUGS THAT DEPRESS THE VASOMOTOR CENTRE
Antihypertensive drugs which act wholly or partly by reducing the output from the vasomotor centre include sedatives and tranquillizers (p. 5.29), hydrallazine and alkaloids of *Veratrum viride* and *album*. Barbiturates (p. 5.41), chlorpromazine (p. 5.32), anaesthetics (p. 5.62), alcohol (p. 5.72), morphine (p. 5.48) and other central depressants when given in large doses all reduce the blood pressure but are rarely used for this purpose because of their other effects. The tranquillizing effect of chlorpromazine, however, reduces the excitation

of the vasomotor centre which arises from external stresses and stimuli. There is also evidence that it impairs to some extent release of noradrenaline from the adrenergic neurones and it possesses slight ganglion blocking activity. It is particularly valuable in the treatment of hypertensive crises induced by MAO inhibitors when these are taken in conjunction with sympathomimetic amines (p. 5.22).

Hydrallazine (apresoline) is a derivative of phthalazine. Although classified here as a centrally acting agent its precise mode of action is uncertain. The drug possesses weak antiadrenaline and noradrenaline activity and it

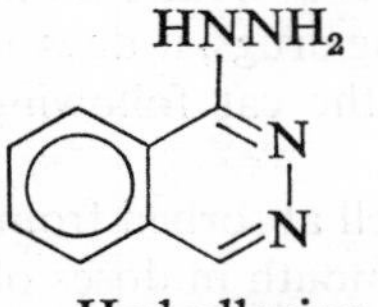

HNNH$_2$

Hydrallazine

reduces the response to sympathetic nerve stimulation. It also induces vasodilation in denervated extremities. Peripheral resistance is reduced and there is an increase in cardiac rate and stroke volume. Postural hypotension is less prominent than with prejunctional blocking drugs. Hydrallazine is readily absorbed from the gastrointestinal tract, acts within a few hours of ingestion and a single dose lasts for about 12 hours. Little is known about its metabolism and only a small fraction of a given dose is excreted in the urine. The usual dose is 100–400 mg/day. Although widely employed in the United States, its use in Britain is limited. Adverse effects are common and may be serious. These include headache, diarrhoea, dizziness, tremors, fever, urticaria, polyneuritis and blood dyscrasias. It has been implicated in the production of myocardial infarction in patients with angina pectoris. Higher dosage or long continued administration leads to a condition resembling rheumatoid arthritis and systemic lupus erythematosus (p. 30.12).

The **veratrum alkaloids** are obtained from *Veratrum viride* and *album*. A large number of alkaloids exist but the most adequately studied and important clinically are ester alkaloids which include protoveratine A and B, veratridine and geomerine. When given to man or intact animals the most striking effect is bradycardia and a fall in blood pressure. The depression of the vasomotor centre is induced reflexly by stimulation of excitatory nerves in the heart, lungs and carotid sinus baroreceptors. The cardiovascular effects of protoveratine are reduced or abolished by atropine, vagotomy and section of the carotid sinus nerves. At a cellular level, the alkaloids induce repetitive responses in excitable cells to single stimuli and the pharmacological effects of the alkaloids are due to selective effects on pressure receptors giving

rise to depressor reflexes in the cardiovascular and respiratory systems. The increased traffic from these sites is interpreted as representing high blood pressure and this leads to reduction in sympathetic tone and increased vagal activity on the heart. Because the alkaloids have the effect of resetting the level of the baroreceptor postural hypotension does not occur as the circulatory reflexes remain intact.

Although theoretically desirable agents, protoveratrine A and B are only occasionally used nowadays and on a short term basis to deal with severe hypertensive crisis

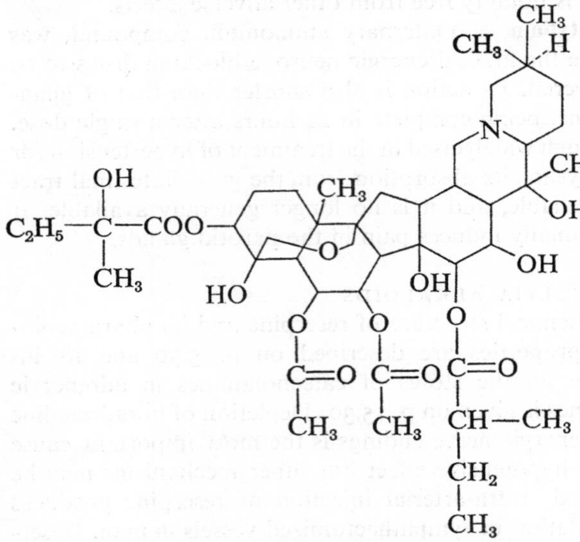

Protoveratrine A

resistant to other measures; it is given intramuscularly in doses of 0·1–0·2 mg. The objection to more widespread use lies in the difficulty in obtaining therapeutic benefit without inducing nausea, vomiting, salivation and a feeling of substernal oppression.

MAO INHIBITORS

The effect of MAO inhibitors on the level of blood pressure is discussed on p. 5.22. **Pargyline**, a nonhydrazine compound, possesses modest antihypertensive potency and its effect begins several days after the drug is given and continues for 2–3 weeks after treatment is stopped. The occurrence of orthostatic hypotension suggests impairment of sympathetic function but the mode of action is unknown. As discussed more fully on p. 15.32, one possibility is that by inhibiting noradrenaline synthesis, other less potent amines, e.g. octopamine, compete for the storage sites in the adrenergic neurone. Stimulation of the sympathetic nerve then results in their release as false transmitter. The usual dose of pargyline is 10–50 mg/day. Adverse effects of MAO inhibitors are described on p. 5.22. Nausea, elevation of mood and serious psychiatric reactions occur with pargyline which should be reserved for those very few patients who do not respond to more conventional drugs.

GANGLION BLOCKING DRUGS

The action of more important ganglion blocking drugs and their structural formulae are given on p. 4.8. The quaternary ammonium compounds **hexamethonium** and **pentolinium** are poorly and irregularly absorbed from the gut and are now given only parenterally for short periods to control hypertensive crises. Pentolinium (0·5 mg) given intravenously usually reduces the blood pressure within minutes.

The discovery of nonquaternary ganglion blocking drugs, **mecamylamine, pempidine** and **trimethaphan** represented a major advance in the drug treatment of hypertension, but all ganglion blocking drugs suffer the serious disadvantage that they impair transmission at parasympathetic as well as sympathetic ganglia. The consequent widespread adverse effects, e.g. blurring of vision, ileus, retention of urine, dry mouth and impotence have led to their almost complete abandonment in clinical practice.

SALT DEPLETING DRUGS AND DIAZOXIDE

The benefits of salt depletion and restricted intake of salt in the treatment of hypertension have been known for over 50 years and salt depleting diuretic drugs (p. 11.1) all exert a mild hypotensive effect. When used to supplement more potent antihypertensive drugs, smoother control of blood pressure can be obtained. However, there is dispute over the mechanism of this effect. Several studies

Chlorothiazide   Diazoxide

show that although mild degrees of salt depletion are induced initially the hypotensive effect of diuretic drugs persists after this has been replenished, and a direct action on smooth muscles has been postulated. Support for this theory has come from the discovery of **diazoxide**, a thiazide derivative which closely resembles chlorothiazide but which causes water and salt retention while retaining its hypotensive activity. Because of a high incidence of toxic effects diazoxide is not recommended but it may be the forerunner of safer drugs possessing similar activity.

POSTJUNCTIONAL ADRENERGIC BLOCKING DRUGS

α- and β-Receptor blocking drugs are described on p. 15.22. α-Blocking drugs are not useful in the treatment of hypertension, because in the absence of β-blocking activity, reflex tachycardia occurs. The use of

phentolamine in the diagnosis of hypertension due to phaeochromocytoma is given on p. 15.3. Propranolol, a β-blocking drug (p. 4.6 and p. 15.27), also reduces blood pressure in hypertensive patients. This is believed to be due to reduction in cardiac output due to blockade of sympathetic activity in the heart. Peripheral resistance remains unaltered or rises. Although theoretically this carries the advantage that postural hypotension will not occur, the place of propranolol in the drug treatment of hypertension is uncertain.

The pharmacological effects and clinical uses of adrenaline, noradrenaline and isoprenaline and of other sympathomimetic amines and of adrenergic blocking drugs on the cardiovascular system are discussed on p. 15.24. The structure and actions of angiotension are given on p. 17.4.

Drugs that decrease serum cholesterol

One group of drugs is used in vascular disease, not because of a vasoactive or haemodynamic effect, but because of a presumptive but as yet unproved effect in limiting or reversing the pathological process of atherosclerosis of blood vessels. These agents all have the effect of lowering the concentration of serum cholesterol. They include clofibrate, oestrogens, thyroxine and triiodothyronine, nicotinic acid, β-sitosterol, neomycin, triparanol and cholestyramine (p. 10.12).

Atherosclerosis (p. 25.12 and p. 26.3) is a pathological process resulting in the deposition of quantities of a porridge-like material containing cholesterol esters, lipoproteins and mucopolysaccharides within the intima. The process reduces the lumen and may obstruct flow of blood and lead to thrombus formation; it also alters compliance, elasticity and volume of the arterial system. Its occurrence is strongly correlated with prevailing levels of serum cholesterol, reflecting certainly dietary and possibly genetic factors. Some forms of hypercholesterolaemia occur early in life and are genetically determined. Other secondary forms are associated with myxoedema, diabetes, biliary obstruction, alcoholism, some forms of glomerulonephritis and with corticosteroid therapy. The common factor in all forms is a disorder of lipid transport in which the concentration of one or more of the lipoproteins fractions of the blood (vol. 1, p. 10.11) are raised. Hypercholesterolaemia occurs in five different phenotypes characterized by their electrophoretic pattern.

CLOFIBRATE (Atromid-S)

This drug is the principal cholesterol reducing agent and is particularly effective in reducing raised serum concentrations of triglyceride and cholesterol associated with lipoproteins of low and very low density. It is least effective in patients with familial hyper β-lipoproteinaemia. Skin manifestations of hypercholesterolaemia, e.g. xanthomata, arcus senilis, and other features regress over periods of 1–2 years during administration of the drug which produces on average a 20 per cent reduction in

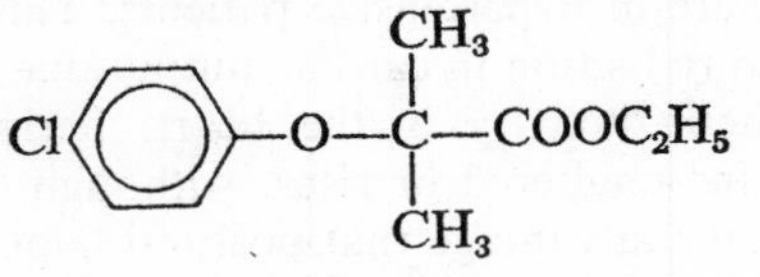

$$Cl—\langle\bigcirc\rangle—O—\overset{\displaystyle CH_3}{\underset{\displaystyle CH_3}{\overset{|}{\underset{|}{C}}}}—COOC_2H_5$$

Clofibrate

serum cholesterol concentration. Evidence of a similar effect on the more important vascular lesions of human atheroma in the coronary cerebral and skeletal circulations is awaited, and is probable.

Clofibrate is ethyl-2-p-chlorophenoxy-2-methyl propionate. It is given in a dose of 1–2 g/day, and is well absorbed after oral administration. It is believed to displace L-thyroxine and L-triiodothyronine from the thyroid binding fraction of the serum globulin. Cholesterol is metabolized in the liver, and the rate of metabolism is increased by thyroxine. Hence in thyroid deficiency the cholesterol lowering action of clofibrate is small. In terms of metabolism, clofibrate produces a relative hyperthyroid condition in the liver and a relative hypothyroid activity at the periphery. In contrast to the effect of exogenous thyroxine there is a diminished release of FFA from adipose tissue. Serum uric acid is reduced, prothrombin time increased, platelet adhesiveness and agglutination decreased.

After discontinuance of clofibrate, serum lipid concentrations rise within a few weeks to pretreatment levels.

The drug is excreted to the extent of 85 per cent in the urine as a glucuronate.

Adverse effects are uncommon apart from slight gain in weight and an elevation of the serum transaminases, but nausea, weakness and giddiness, skin rash, drowsiness and diarrhoea may occur.

Large clinical trials are in progress in Britain and the USA to evaluate the drug in healthy men as a prophylactic agent against morbidity and mortality from atherosclerotic disease. Other lipid-reducing drugs, nicotinic acid, oestrogens and D-thyroxine, are also under study. **Sitosterols** are plant sterols which reduce cholesterol absorption but a plasma lowering effect is not sustained. **Heparin** which activates lipoprotein lipase *in vivo* (vol. 1, p. 10.12) does not influence the concentration of cholesterol.

FURTHER READING

BRAUNWALD E. & POOL P.E. (1968) Mechanism of action of digitalis glycosides. *Mod. Conc. cardiov. Dis.* **37,** 129.

LEVY R.I. & FREDRICKSON D.S. (1968) Diagnoses and management of hyperlipoproteinaemia. *Amer. J. Cardiol.* **22,** 576.

SCHLITTER E. (1967) *Antihypertensive Agents.* Medicinal Chemistry Monographs. New York: Academic Press.

Symposium on Beta-adrenergic receptor blockade (1966) *Amer. J. Cardiol.* **18,** 303.

TANZ R.D., KAVALER F. & ROBERTS J. eds. (1967) *Factors influencing Myocardial Contractility.* New York: Academic Press.

Chapter 9
Drugs that act on the respiratory system

Many drugs affect respiration and their effects may be exerted in the following ways:

(1) on the respiratory centre in the brain stem, e.g. narcotics, analeptics, xanthines, acidifying and alkalinizing substances, salicylate, and CO_2, and secondarily via alterations in medullary blood flow;

(2) on the chemoreceptors in the carotid and aortic bodies, e.g. oxygen, cyanide, lobeline and nicotine, nikethamide, and secondarily via alterations in systemic blood pressure;

(3) on the central pathways serving the cough reflex, e.g. morphine and codeine, and secondarily in drug-induced coma;

(4) on sensory nerve endings in larynx, trachea and bronchi, e.g. ether, local anaesthetics and dusts, and secondarily via alterations in bronchomotor tone or pulmonary compliance;

(5) on the smooth muscle and glands of the bronchi, e.g. sympathomimetic or parasympathomimetic drugs and adrenergic blocking agents, histamine and histamine releasing drugs and ether;

(6) on the epithelium of the respiratory tract, e.g. oxygen;

(7) on the striated muscle serving ventilation, e.g. neuromuscular blocking drugs.

Drugs acting on the respiratory centre

The central mechanisms concerned in the control of breathing are described in vol. 1, p. 29.22, where the integration of the effects of $P\text{CO}_2$, $P\text{O}_2$ and pH of the body fluid is discussed. The effects of drugs on the control of respiration are best described in terms of changes they induce in the responses to physiological stimuli, particularly CO_2 and hypoxia, the response to CO_2 having received by far the greater attention.

The ventilatory response to CO_2 (vol. 1, p. 29.24) is described graphically by a straight line relating ventilation to alveolar or arterial $P\text{CO}_2$. The slope of this line, i.e. the rise in ventilation per unit rise in $P\text{CO}_2$, is termed the CO_2 **sensitivity**. The intercept of the line on the $P\text{CO}_2$ axis is the imaginary **threshold** below which ventilation is zero.

RESPIRATORY DEPRESSANTS

Most **general anaesthetics** (p. 5.66) depress ventilation in proportion to the depth of anaesthesia induced and prior treatment with opium alkaloids enhances this. **Ethyl ether**, which acts as a central depressant, also stimulates breathing reflexly; the afferent impulses may arise from irritation of the bronchial tree and bronchial secretions are increased. Even in ordinary anaesthetic doses ether has a curare-like effect on neuromuscular junctions. **Halothane** strongly inhibits laryngospasm, bronchospasm and cough; it directly relaxes bronchial smooth muscle and for this reason is probably the best choice of anaesthetic for asthmatic patients.

Hypnotics and **sedatives** (p. 5.41) similarly cause respiratory depression appropriate to the depth of sleep they induce. The CO_2 threshold is slightly raised and the CO_2 sensitivity may be markedly diminished. These changes are similar to those found in natural sleep. When sleep is prevented after giving hypnotics the response to CO_2 is normal; this is true, for instance, after a dose of cyclobarbitone three times greater than that usually used for sedation (fig. 9.1). However, barbiturates may depress the response to moderate hypoxia even in the waking state, although the response to severe hypoxia is preserved. It is widely stated that the ventilatory response to severe hypoxia is the last to be affected by an overdose of drugs. Barbiturates, when injected intravenously, are liable to induce laryngospasm, possibly by disrupting the normal coordination by which the larynx relaxes during inspiration. Respiratory depression by **ethanol** is preceded by a phase of augmentation. **Methanol** is metabolized to formic acid and results in acidotic stimulation of breathing (p. 25.16). **Paraldehyde** depresses cholinergic transmission, a possible advantage in status asthmaticus in which it is widely used as a sedative, but paraldehyde is no exception to the general rule regarding respiratory depression.

The majority of **tranquillizing** and **antidepressive drugs** (p. 5.29) depress respiration when taken in large doses as in self-poisoning. An interesting exception is **diazepam** (p. 5.35), a benzodiazepine, which in large doses produces a sleep-like state in which pharyngeal reflexes are retained and respiration is unaffected. Its property of relaxing muscle spasm by a central action, without depression of breathing, promises to be of some benefit in the treatment of tetanus. The **phenothiazines**, as well as causing central respiratory depression in high doses, block the actions of histamine and 5-HT to some extent, but these properties have not found much application in status asthmaticus.

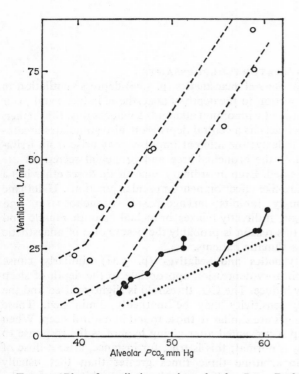

FIG. 9.1. Plot of ventilation against alveolar P_{CO_2}. Both variables have been standardized so that normal waking limits (shown by the parallel broken lines) and data from two subjects can be displayed in the same figure. The dotted line is for deep sleep, from Bülow (1963). ●, one set for each of two subjects given 500 mg and 600 mg cyclobarbitone respectively show the sleeping response. Waking responses after the drug (○) lie mostly within the normal waking range. From Harris E.A. & Slawson K.B. (1965) *Brit. J. Pharmacol.* **24**, 214.

Morphine and its derivatives, **codeine**, **pethidine** and **methadone**, all depress the ventilatory response to CO_2, even in doses too small to cause sleep. After giving codeine, the response to moderate hypoxia in wakeful subjects is depressed but the response to severe hypoxia is unaffected.

Nalorphine in small doses depresses the CO_2 response as morphine does, but the depression does not increase with the dose. Small doses of nalorphine abolish the respiratory depression caused by large doses of morphine,

pethidine and methadone, replacing this by the much smaller effect of the nalorphine itself (p. 5.52).

Neomycin, **kanamycin** and **streptomycin** depress respiration during anaesthesia by a neuromuscular blocking action (pp. 20.30 & 32 and p. 5.69).

RESPIRATORY STIMULANTS

Analeptic drugs, experimental convulsants and the psychomotor stimulants (p. 5.36) all stimulate medullary and other functions of both the normal and the depressed nervous system. They are all more or less potent convulsants, but vary widely in the margin between the dose producing respiratory stimulation and that causing convulsions. Fits, if they occur, are followed by respiratory depression.

Respiratory stimulation by all analeptics is due to a medullary action; the alkylamides, e.g. **nikethamide** and **ethamivan**, in addition, stimulate the carotid and aortic chemoreceptors in some, but not all, species. When given to a subject whose respiration is moderately depressed by hypnotic or narcotic drugs, the analeptics decrease the CO_2 threshold and increase the CO_2 sensitivity. When given to a subject already awake, a stimulant effect on respiration is observed only when air or low concentrations of CO_2 are breathed; at higher CO_2 concentrations the drug produces no additional stimulation. This suggests that respiratory stimulation by analeptics is part of a general arousal, as a fully alert subject is not affected. The study of analeptics in waking subjects is complicated, however, by side effects, e.g. itching, flushing, restlessness, pain at injection site etc. which themselves cause hyperventilation as a secondary effect.

The **xanthines** (p. 5.39) (caffeine, theophylline and aminophylline or theophylline-ethylenediamine) have other respiratory actions. Their main effect is to relax the smooth muscle of the bronchi, and aminophylline is used in the treatment of asthma. They also stimulate the myocardium, dilate the coronary and peripheral arteries and increase cardiac output; the abolition of Cheyne–Stokes breathing by aminophylline is due to improvement in medullary blood flow resulting from these actions.

CARBON DIOXIDE

Carbon dioxide is the most powerful respiratory stimulant, the inhalation of up to 10 per cent CO_2 increasing ventilation up to 70 l/min in an adult (vol. 1, p. 29.25). These concentrations, however, depress the cerebral cortex and protect against convulsions induced by analeptic drugs or electroshock. Greater concentrations do not increase ventilation further and, above an alveolar P_{CO_2} of about 80 mm Hg, actually begin to depress it. At an alveolar P_{CO_2} of 150–200 mm Hg convulsions may occur. Still higher concentrations of CO_2 (50 per cent) cause cerebral depression and anaesthesia.

DRUGS WHICH AFFECT ACID-BASE BALANCE

Drugs which cause a change in acid-base composition of the body fluids, especially acidifying substances, affect ventilation. The effects of ammonium chloride are discussed in vol. I, p. 25.26, where it is shown that the ventilatory threshold to CO_2 is reduced but the sensitivity to CO_2 is unaltered. **Carbonic anhydrase inhibitors** such as **acetazolamide** and **dichlorphenamide** induce acidosis by their action on the renal tubular cells (p. 11.6). Their stimulation of respiration may, however, be greater than can be accounted for by the degree of extracellular acidosis produced. It is known that large doses of these drugs cause retention of CO_2 by inhibiting carbonic anhydrase in red blood cells, and an increased cellular P_{CO_2} in the brain may be one factor in the ventilatory stimulation. It is also possible that even therapeutic doses of carbonic anhydrase inhibitors interfere with the escape of hydrogen ions formed by the metabolism of brain cells; thus the change in acidity of the cells controlling respiration might be greater than the pH change in the blood indicates.

The respiratory effects of **salicylate** are also complex. Two types of acid-base abnormality occur.

(1) By direct stimulation of the respiratory centre, ventilation is increased, arterial P_{CO_2} falls and respiratory alkalosis results. Salicylate acts in this way when applied directly to the floor of the fourth ventricle in animal experiments.

(2) Metabolic acidosis results from an excess of metabolic acids in the blood, i.e. (a) acetylsalicylic acid when salicylate has been taken as aspirin, (b) lactic, pyruvic and acetoacetic acids due to salicylate-induced disturbance of carbohydrate metabolism, and (c) phosphoric and sulphuric acids due to renal failure secondary to hypotension which occurs when salicylates are taken in excess. Respiratory alkalosis is usually the first effect, and is often detectable in adults with plasma salicylate concentration of 35 mg/100 ml. Metabolic acidosis becomes superimposed, especially in children, and the blood pH, elevated by the increased ventilation, falls to normal values or below.

Tris-hydroxymethyl aminomethane (THAM) is a basic organic buffer which has been advocated in the treatment of acidosis. It reacts with H^+ and CO_2 as follows:

$$(CH_2OH)_3CNH_2 + H^+ \rightleftharpoons (CH_2OH)_3CNH_3^+ \quad (1)$$
$$(CH_2OH)_3CNH_2 + CO_2 + H_2O$$
$$\rightleftharpoons (CH_2OH)_3CNH_3^+ + HCO_3^- \quad (2)$$

Transforming equation (1) we have,

$$R.NH_2 + H^+ \rightleftharpoons R.NH_3^+$$

By the Law of Mass Action

$$[H^+] = K. \frac{[R.NH_3^+]}{[R.NH_2]}$$

$$pH = pK + \log \frac{[\text{Nonionized THAM}]}{[\text{Ionized THAM}]} \quad (3)$$

Since pK for THAM is 7·82 at 37°C, the degree of ionization of the base for any given value of pH can be calculated from equation (3). Fig. 9.2 shows the effect of pH on ionization.

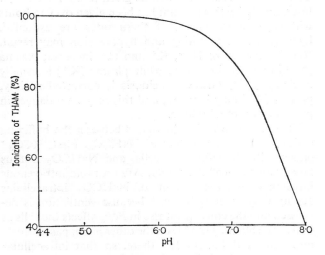

FIG. 9.2. pH and the ionization of THAM.

After injection of THAM into nephrectomized animals, the volume of distribution is approximately that of total body water. In its nonionized form, THAM readily penetrates cell membranes; inside the cell its ionization is governed by intracellular pH. The pH inside cells is sufficiently close to that of extracellular fluid to ensure almost uniform distribution of total THAM throughout the body water, but there is a delay in achieving this which varies from one tissue to another. Ionized THAM is not reabsorbed by the renal tubules; in severe acidosis (save that due to renal failure), when urinary pH may be as low as 4·4, excretion of THAM is thus more rapid than when the urine is neutral or alkaline (fig. 9.2). Entry into cells is limited if the drug is very rapidly excreted. In normal volunteers, 20 per cent of a dose of THAM was excreted in 1 hour and 80 per cent in 3 days.

The sequence of events after administration of THAM is not fully understood but the following seems likely. Equations (1) and (2) take place both inside and outside cells, pH rises and P_{CO_2} falls. The rise in pH diminishes the ventilatory stimulus, ventilation falls and there is a secondary rise in P_{CO_2}, on both sides of the cell membrane, to levels higher than before the drug was given. Since $[HCO_3^-]$ rises relatively more than P_{CO_2}, the change towards alkalinity persists. Ionized THAM carrying H^+, together with HCO_3^- formed by equation (2), are excreted by the kidneys. Because more CO_2 is excreted in the urine as HCO_3^-, less is excreted by the lungs.

THAM is poorly absorbed when given by mouth because it is largely ionized at the pH of the gut. Given intraveneously, as a 0·3 molar solution in 5 per cent glucose or isotonic saline, its alkalinity tends to cause spasm or thrombosis of the vein at the site of infusion. One litre of this solution can be given to an adult over 1 hour, and twice this amount has been given over 12 hours without adverse effects. If these rates are exceeded, hypoglycaemia, vomiting and hypotension may result. Renal excretion of Na^+, K^+ and Cl^- increase; plasma $[Na^+]$ and $[Cl^-]$ decrease while plasma $[K^+]$ is usually unchanged. If, however, acidosis is corrected rapidly, plasma $[K^+]$ may increase, and this may be a danger in patients with renal failure.

There are two main differences between the buffering action of THAM and that of $NaHCO_3$. First, HCO_3^- passes with difficulty into cells, and $NaHCO_3$ is thus largely an extracellular buffer. After a rapid intravenous infusion of a large amount of $NaHCO_3$, intracellular acidity may actually increase because ventilation is depressed and the consequent rise in $P\text{co}_2$ affects the cells as well as the blood. THAM, on the other hand, passes freely into cells and buffers H^+ there, so that intracellular acidosis is avoided. Secondly, while THAM disposes of CO_2 as shown in equation (2), generating HCO_3^- in the process, $NaHCO_3$ obviously cannot do this.

In spite of these apparent advantages over $NaHCO_3$ in the treatment of acidosis, THAM has not found a secure place in clinical practice. Its action in depressing ventilation makes it useless in respiratory acidosis unless the patient is artificially ventilated at the same time, and artificial ventilation is fully effective by itself. Its virtues in metabolic acidosis, i.e. the avoidance of a sodium load in patients with cardiac failure and the intracellular buffering, do not outweigh the ease of administration and lack of toxicity of $NaHCO_3$.

Drugs acting on the carotid and aortic chemoreceptors

Cyanide blocks oxidative processes in the cells of the carotid and aortic bodies, allowing anaerobic products, e.g. lactic acid, to accumulate in them and stimulate respiration. The only use to which this action has been put is in the measurement of circulation time; 0·1 mg of NaCN/kg body weight is injected rapidly intravenously and the time of onset of hyperventilation noted. **Nicotine and lobeline**, alkaloids of tobacco and lobelia, increase ventilation in small doses by exciting the chemoreflex; large doses cause respiratory failure by medullary depression. Parasympathomimetic drugs and nitrites also stimulate the chemoreflex.

Blood flow through, and O_2 consumption by, the carotid and aortic bodies are very high in relation to their size, but their cellular $P\text{o}_2$ is almost equal to arterial $P\text{o}_2$ so long as blood flow is maintained. Hypotension, by reducing perfusion through them, stimulates the chemoreceptors and hypotensive drugs may have this effect.

Drugs affecting the cough reflex

Measurement of cough may be made either by counting the frequency of paroxysms or by recording airflow during the inspiratory and/or expiratory phase of the reflex. In man, a satisfactory test stimulus is the inhalation of citric acid aerosol. A concentration is chosen which, when inhaled a specified number of times, produces a given number of coughs in a given subject; this 'titration' is necessary because of marked individual variations in susceptibility. The test drug is then given and the response to citric acid inhalations is observed at intervals for several hours. In this way **codeine** (15 mg), **noscapine** (narcotine) (15 mg), **dextromethorphan** (10 mg), **pholcodine** (10 mg) and **methadone** (2·5 mg), have been shown to be approximately equipotent in suppressing cough.

In cats, antitussive drugs may suppress the two types of cough reflex (vol. 1, p. 29.23) rather selectively. Morphine is most potent in both types, but pholcodine is more potent than codeine when the cough is caused by mechanical stimulation, whereas the reverse is true of the chemically induced type. Pentobarbitone suppresses both types of reflex only in doses which are fatal.

In coma induced by drugs, cough may be abolished. Ventilation in these patients must be sustained artificially and the return of cough when a suction catheter is passed down the trachea may herald the return of adequate spontaneous ventilation.

When cough suppressants are assessed in conscious patients in whom cough is a symptom, relief is often claimed even though the frequency of coughing is unaltered. It is likely that the intensity of and effort associated with coughing are as important subjectively as its frequency; studies such as those described above have shown that antitussive drugs may reduce expiratory or inspiratory flow without affecting cough frequency.

Codeine's effect on the ventilatory response to CO_2 and hypoxia has been mentioned. Noscapine has no effect on either response in doses up to 100 mg.

MECHANISM OF COUGH SUPPRESSION

The known central actions of morphine, codeine and other antitussives suggests that suppression of cough is due to a central mechanism. The central pathways serving the cough reflex are not well understood but lie mainly in the medulla. On the other hand, the selective effect of some drugs on the two types of cough reflex suggests an action on the afferent side of the reflex. A purely afferent effect also explains the abolition of the cough reflex which follows the spraying of solutions of local anaesthetics down the trachea.

Drugs acting on afferent nerve endings in the airway

Many substances, when inhaled as aerosols, cause constriction or dilation of the air passages. Some of them act by stimulating or depressing afferent nerve endings in the bronchial tree, starting a vagal reflex, but other factors may be concerned. Substances which stimulate afferent endings and cause bronchoconstriction include **irritating substances**, whether gaseous, liquid or solid, e.g. ether, chloroform, phosgene and some antihistamines, and any fine, inert, particulate matter. Constrictor responses can be prevented or abolished by inhalation of sympathomimetic dilators. **Surface anaesthetics** such as cocaine or procaine depress afferent endings and result in reflex dilation. Constrictor responses to inhaled substances may involve alveolar ducts and atria as well as bronchi, to judge from the large volume changes which can occur. In some species the release in the bronchial wall of histamine or 5-HT is involved in pneumoconstriction caused by 'inert' dusts. Other processes may be involved; in cats, for instance, aluminium dust has been shown to reduce alveolar surface tension while moderately constricting smooth muscle. Organic dusts, e.g. cotton, jute and flax, may contain histamine or other unidentified substances which directly cause bronchoconstriction; extracts of such dusts are active, *in vitro*, on human bronchial muscle.

Drugs acting on smooth muscle and bronchial glands

MUSCLE

Knowledge of the function of the autonomic nervous supply to the lungs is derived largely from pharmacological evidence. Thus **sympathomimetic drugs** relax and **parasympathomimetic drugs** constrict the bronchial smooth muscle; bronchial glands are inhibited and stimulated respectively. Isoprenaline and ephedrine (p. 15.18), which have relatively strong β-receptor stimulating effects, are more active in relaxing bronchial muscle than is noradrenaline. Drugs which block β-receptors, such as **propranolol**, constrict the bronchi and are thus potentially dangerous in asthmatic patients. Sympathomimetic effects predominate over parasympathomimetic; thus, after isoprenaline has been given vagal stimulation does not constrict the bronchi. **Atropine**, by blocking the muscarinic effects of acetylcholine, has a slight bronchodilatory effect. Bronchial constriction is a marked feature of poisoning by **organophosphorus insecticides**, and may be blocked by atropine; these insecticides also cause respiratory paralysis due to depolarizing neuromuscular blockade, which may be reversed by cholinesterase reactivators such as **pralidoxime** (2-pyridine aldoxime methochloride, p. 32.2).

Histamine, when inhaled as an aerosol in low concentrations, dilates the air passages in man, but in higher concentrations, and in most species, it has a powerful, direct constrictor effect. Patients with asthma are particularly susceptible to its constrictor action. Drugs which liberate histamine, e.g. morphine, D-tubocurarine

and diamidines must be used with caution, or not at all, in asthmatic patients. Intravenous injection of **5-HT** causes constriction of the bronchi, mainly due to a direct action on bronchial muscle; it also stimulates the carotid body in dogs and man, increasing ventilation, but in other species it may inhibit respiration.

Theophylline and **aminophylline** by injection, inhalation or rectal suppository, dilate the bronchi directly. Intravenous aminophylline is of value in status asthmaticus.

BRONCHIAL GLANDS AND SECRETIONS

Several drugs increase the secretions of bronchial glands. Parasympathomimetic drugs have been mentioned; secretions may also be increased reflexly from gastric irritation as by ipecacuanha and squill, or during excretion of a drug through the bronchial glands, as by iodides and volatile oils. These and other substances have been used as expectorants for a very long time and still have their devotees. Iodides are the most commonly used today, but it is doubtful if they are of any clinical value.

Recently *N*-acetylcysteine has been recommended for liquefying or reducing the viscosity of bronchial mucus. Its molecule has a sulphydryl group which is thought to reduce disulphide bonds in mucus and so bring about a change in its molecular shape. *In vitro*, acetylcysteine reduces mucus viscosity more quickly and extensively than detergent solutions, and its effect is more prolonged, *in vivo*, than that of trypsin. It is given by inhalation as an aerosol. It may irritate the airway and is still under trial.

THE PHARMACOLOGY OF ASTHMA

The bronchoconstrictor effect of administered histamine is prevented by antihistamines (p. 14.16). In bronchoconstriction occurring as part of the anaphylactic state (p. 24.4), the protection given by antihistamines varies with the species of animal, and in man it is weak; in asthma, too, patients are as a rule poorly protected by antihistamines. Three explanations can be advanced to account for these findings.

(1) When histamine is released very near to, or within, the smooth muscle cell, antihistamines are less effective than when histamine reaches the cell by diffusion through the extracellular fluid.

(2) Histamine is not the only substance responsible for anaphylactic responses. In some species, 5-HT is involved. In others, perhaps including man, slow-reacting substance (SRS-A), which causes intense constriction in human bronchioles, and which is not antagonized by antihistamines, may be released in hypersensitivity reactions, and the kinins may also play a part.

(3) While hypersensitivity is undoubtedly important in asthma, other mechanisms may predominate in some patients.

Many of the substances most useful in asthma, e.g.

sympathomimetic drugs, such as adrenaline, isoprenaline and ephedrine, and aminophylline, act not as specific agents but by producing an opposing, and often over-riding, effect on the bronchi. Adrenaline given by sub-cutaneous injection as 1 ml of a 1 in 1000 dilution of ad-renaline HCl usually produces an effect within a few minutes in an asthmatic attack. Adrenaline may be given also in oil and then has a more prolonged effect. Iso-prenaline may also be effective when taken by inhalation as an aerosol (1 in 100 solution) or as a tablet (5 mg) sucked under the tongue. Salbutamol (10 mg), a derivi-tive, may be used similarly and has a lesser cardiac effect. Ephedrine is equally effective but acts more slowly in 1–2 hours. It is taken by mouth in a dose of 15–60 mg. The use of corticosteroids (p. 24.6) may be life-saving in severe asthma, but evidence does not allow the firm assumption of an anti-allergic mechanism; nonspecific suppresion of inflammatory response (bronchial oedema, mucus-secretion) may account for some of the benefits observed when these drugs are given. The use of **disodium cromoglycate** is discussed on p. 24.4.

Aerosol therapy

Most drugs which act on the bronchial muscle may be inhaled as an aerosol in doses which, while active in the respiratory tract, have little systemic effect. An aerosol is a suspension of solid or liquid particles in a gas, and is most stable when the particles are about 0·5 μm in dia-meter. A given volume of gas contains much more liquid as an aerosol than it could carry in the vapour phase, e.g. a water aerosol with a mean particle size of 1·0 μm and 1 million particles/ml contains some 520 mg of water/l. On the other hand, air saturated with water vapour at 37°C contains 44 mg water/l.

Deposition occurs in the respiratory tract in three ways;

(1) large, and therefore heavy, particles that travel in an airstream possess momentum; when the stream changes direction these particles tend to continue in a straight line, hitting the wall of the airway;

(2) deposition in the larger bronchi occurs mainly by gravitational sedimentation, and

(3) very small particles are subject to Brownian move-ment, and are deposited in the alveolar ducts, atria and alveoli, largely due to the projection of particles against their walls by molecular collisions.

The retention in the respiratory tract of particles big-ger than 5 μm is almost complete, but practically all are deposited in the nose, larynx, trachea and larger bronchi. As the size of particles is reduced, their retention becomes less and less complete, but their penetration becomes deeper. At 0·2–0·4 μm, penetration is complete, but be-cause such particles are too light to acquire much momen-tum or to sediment, and too heavy to acquire much Brown-ian movement, their deposition in both upper and lower respiratory tract is minimal. Particles smaller than this have appreciable Brownian movement with resulting increase in deposition. If the diameter is less than 0·01 μm, intense Brownian movement causes deposition high in the respiratory tract.

There is difficulty in determining the optimal size of particle for aerosol therapy. Particles between 1 and 5 μm in diameter probably lead to maximum deposition in the bronchioles. However, claims have been made for better clinical responses from particles of the order of 0·1 μm and results are conflicting. Present understanding of the behaviour of the inhaled particles is insufficient to resolve this problem.

Many drugs have been shown to be absorbed into the circulation if inhalation is sufficiently prolonged, that is, if the dose of aerosol is big enough. Catecholamines, digitalis glycosides, various diuretics, ergotamine, vaso-pressin and insulin are all absorbed. Partly because the dose is hard to regulate, the method is not yet practicable.

Substances acting on the respiratory epithelium

This group includes all irritant and corrosive materials accidently inhaled, as well as the carcinogenic factor in tobacco smoke (p. 28.16). Changes in the respiratory epithelium are observed also in oxygen poisoning, an account of which is given in vol. 1, p. 43.6.

Drugs acting on the striated respiratory muscles

Competitive neuromuscular blocking drugs, e.g. D-tubo-curarine and gallamine, and depolarizing agents, e.g. succinylcholine, paralyse the respiratory muscles; the march of paralysis and recovery is the same for all. The intercostal muscles are affected after the accessory muscles, and the diaphragm last of all; the order is reversed during recovery. Potassium depletion and the administration of streptomycin, neomycin, kanamycin or polymyxin tend to prolong respiratory paralysis. Com-petitive blockers release histamine and cause bronchocon-striction; depolarizing drugs do not, and are perhaps to be preferred when a relaxant is needed in asthmatic patients.

The effects of competitive blockers are antagonized by acetylcholine and anticholinesterase drugs, which reverse the paralysis caused by curare. Respiratory and other paralysis occurring in myasthenia gravis is likewise reversible. Paralysis induced by depolarizing blockade is enhanced by anticholinesterases (p. 4.5).

FURTHER READING

GOODMAN L.S. & GILMAN A. (1965) *The Pharmacological Basis of Therapeutics*, 3rd Edition. New York: Mac-millan.

Chapter 10
Drugs that act on the gastrointestinal tract and the liver

Indigestion is one of the most common of human complaints and it arises more frequently from disturbances of function than from organic disease of the alimentary tract. As the functions of the tract are controlled mainly by the autonomic nervous system, they are susceptible to the influence of the emotions; psychosomatic factors therefore are important in the development of many gastrointestinal disorders and in the response to therapy. The general public consumes vast quantities of drugs for indigestion, and the majority of those used in alimentary disorders are given to relieve symptoms.

Much the most common organic disease of the gut is ulceration of those parts of the mucosa exposed to the acid secretion of the stomach. About 10 per cent of the population in prosperous urban societies suffer at some time in their life from peptic ulceration. Unfortunately the factors responsible for this disorder are not clear, nor do we know accurately what factors influence the tendency of peptic ulcers to heal spontaneously. A great number of drugs and dietary regimes have been used for treatment, but their scientific evaluation is difficult and it is uncertain if any of them alter significantly the course of the disease. Nevertheless, there are drugs which can modify the actions of the alimentary canal for the benefit of the patient, although their prescription should be accompanied by appropriate dietary advice and in some patients by rest. These drugs may be classified as follows:

(1) drugs that stimulate or inhibit secretion; secretogogues are particularly useful for diagnostic tests of function;

(2) enzymic and other preparations that replace deficiencies in secretion;

(3) drugs that modify the motility of the gut wall and the function of the various sphincters; these act either on parasympathetic or sympathetic nerves or directly on smooth muscle;

(4) drugs that modify the contents of the gut; these may neutralize excess acid (antacids), alter the pattern of the bacterial flora (antibiotics), or remove specific substances (chelating and binding agents);

(5) drugs that alter the cellular structure of the gut wall and so modify inflammatory reactions, e.g. corticosteroids used in ulcerative colitis;

(6) drugs that influence blood flow, e.g. vasopressin;

(7) radio-opaque and radioactive substances used to visualize or scan organs, or the lumen of the intestines, ducts or blood vessels.

DRUGS THAT ACT ON THE STOMACH AND INTESTINES

Drugs which increase gastric secretion

Stimulants of gastric secretion include ethyl alcohol and many bitter substances which form the basis of appetizers or aperitifs. In addition, many amino acids and meat extracts initiate acid secretion. All these substances act through the release of gastrin which stimulates the stomach to produce acid.

HISTAMINE, ITS ANALOGUES AND INHIBITORS
Although there is no proof that histamine is a physiological stimulus for the secretion of gastric acid, it is a potent secretagogue and has a direct action on oxyntic cells of isolated gastric mucosal preparations from animals. Furthermore, in the rat, histidine decarboxylase inhibitors which deplete the gastric mucosa of histamine reduce the resting secretion of acid and the response to a variety of secretagogues, while the response to histamine itself is unaffected.

Histamine is formed by the decarboxylation of histidine (p. 14.2). This reaction is catalysed by the histidine decarboxylases, a co-factor being pyridoxal phosphate. In the rat, the effect of the potent decarboxylase inhibitor, **4-bromo-3-hydroxybenzyloxyamine**, can be reduced by an excess of pyridoxal phosphate and enhanced by reagents which react with pyridoxal such as

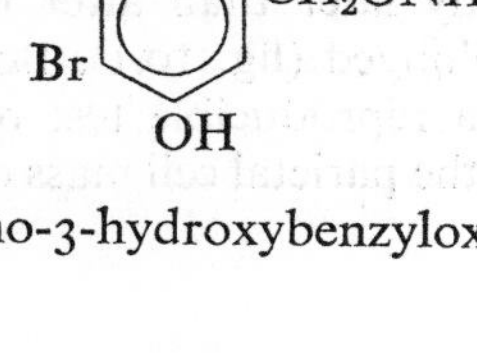

$$Br-C_6H_3(OH)-CH_2ONH_2$$

4-Bromo-3-hydroxybenzyloxyamine

semicarbazide. In addition, acid secretion in the rat is diminished in pyridoxine deficiency. While histidine decarboxylase can be assayed in rat gastric mucosa, this has not yet been done in other species or in man.

Betazole is an isomer of histamine and has a similar action on the gastric mucosa, the groupings $=N-C$ or $-N=C$ being important in evoking gastric secretion which antihistamine drugs fail to oppose. The main

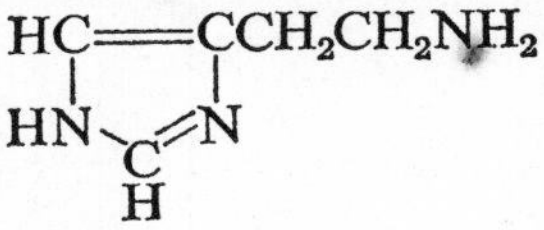

HC===CCH₂CH₂NH₂

HN   N

C
H

Histamine

HC——CCH₂CH₂NH₂

HC   N

N
H

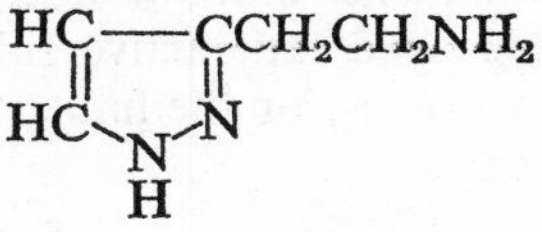

Betazole

difference between the two agents is that while histamine has a marked effect on smooth muscle and on blood pressure, betazole has only a feeble action in these respects.

In general, however, histamine is a gastric secretagogue in doses below those which influence blood pressure. When given to man in a single dose (0·04 mg/kg by subcutaneous injection) it causes the secretion of a reproducible amount of gastric acid, but antihistamine drugs need to be given beforehand to reduce facial flushing and headache, wheal and flare at the site of injection and in some patients a fall in blood pressure. Betazole (2 mg/kg SCI) produces the same effect on the stomach as hista-

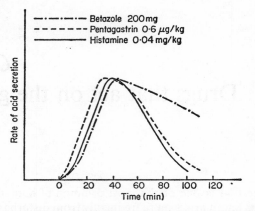

FIG. 10.1. Effect of histamine, pentagastrin and betazole on secretion of gastric acid.

GASTRIN

Several animal gastrins have been prepared and their actions on the human stomach evaluated. The active part of the gastrin molecule has been synthesized and is a gastric stimulant (vol. 1, p. 30.17).

Naturally occurring gastrins are polypeptides of similar composition (fig. 10.2). They occur in sulphated and unsulphated forms, gastrin I and gastrin II, the significance of which is unknown. The differences between the peptide chains of the various species are small and involve the amino acids near the glutamyl residues, but they do not appear to be responsible for physiological differences. All the physiological activities of gastrin are exhibited by the C-terminal tetrapeptide. This fact led to the synthesis of a pentapeptide, **pentagastrin**, for use as a

Hog I—Pyro·Gly·Pro·Try·**Met**·(**Glu**)₅·Ala·Tyr·Gly·Try·Met·Asp·Phe·NH₂

II   ↑
                                          (SO₄)

Human I—Pyro·Gly·Pro·Tyr·**Leu**·(**Glu**)₅·Ala·Tyr·Gly·Try·Met·Asp·Phe·NH₂

II   ↑
                                          (SO₄)

Dog I—Pyro·Gly·Pro·Try·**Met**·(**Ala, Glu₄**)·Ala·Tyr·Gly·Try·Met·Asp·Phe·NH₂

II   ↑
                                          (SO₄)

Sheep I—Pyro·Gly·Pro·Try·**Val**·(**Ala, Glu₄**)·Ala·Tyr·Gly·Try·Met·Asp·Phe·NH₂

II   ↑
                                          (SO₄)

FIG. 10.2. Naturally occurring gastrins.

mine and has a much smaller effect on blood pressure; other adverse effects are also unusual, so antihistamines need not be given. The output of acid after betazole reaches a peak slightly later than after histamine and secretion is more prolonged (fig. 10.1). Both substances are used to provide a reproducible test of acid output which correlates with the parietal cell mass of the stomach (vol. 1, p. 30.15).

gastric secretagogue. Its structure is t-butyl-oxycarbonyl Ala. Tyr. Met. Asp₂. Phe (NH)₂.

This substance displays the important actions of pure gastrin in stimulating the output of acid, pepsin and intrinsic factor by the gastric mucosa. It also stimulates the pancreas and colonic motility and affects the rate of movement of ions across the mucosa of the small intestine. In humans, gastrin II is thirty times more potent than the pentapeptide on a molar basis, but in appropriate doses (gastrin 2 μg/kg, pentagastrin 6 μg/kg SCI) the resultant secretory activity of the stomach is the same. Gastrin II is about 250 times more potent than histamine on a molar basis. For gastric function studies, pentagastrin has the important advantage over histamine in having no circulatory effects and there is therefore no need to give a prior injection of an antihistamine. In a small proportion of patients it causes nausea and headache.

Because gastrin is probably the most important physiological gastric secretagogue, knowledge of its chemical structure is important in the search for antagonists. In animal studies, one such compound, **2-phenyl-2-(2 pyridyl) thiocetamide**, inhibits the secretory response to gastrin II and pentagastrin. While it bears some resemblance to the terminal amino acid phenylalanine, it has yet to be shown that it acts by inhibiting this substance. While this drug is too toxic for clinical use it may be the forerunner of other compounds which will inhibit gastrin.

2-Phenyl-2-(2 pyridyl) thiocetamide

INSULIN

Insulin stimulates gastric secretion via the vagus nerves by producing hypoglycaemia. Thus it is often given to patients who have undergone vagotomy for peptic ulcer to confirm that the vagi have been divided. Although hypoglycaemia is the stimulus to the vagal centres, gastric secretion of acid may continue at an increased rate for some hours after the correction of hypoglycaemia by parenteral glucose. The usual dose is 20 units soluble insulin intravenously.

Similar effects can be produced by the drug **2-deoxy-D-glucose** (50 mg/kg) when given parenterally. This forms 2-deoxy-D-glucose-6-phosphate which cannot be metabolized and so deprives the vagal centres of glucose as a source of energy without lowering the concentration of blood glucose. Other parts of the vagal centre are not affected so that heart and respiratory rates remain unchanged. In contrast to the action of insulin, where there is a 30 min delay, stimulation with 2-deoxy-D-glucose is immediate and the output of acid and pepsin is greater. Results obtained by using insulin are difficult to interpret as there may be a late response which is not always mediated by the vagus and, furthermore, it is difficult to select the dose of insulin that produces hypoglycaemia. For this reason 2-deoxy-D-glucose may replace insulin

in the assessment of vagally mediated gastric secretion. Other drugs such as **tolbutamide** (p. 6.18) can also be used to stimulate gastric secretion by producing hypoglycaemia.

CAFFEINE AND DILUTE ETHANOL

These drugs are both gastric secretagogues. Caffeine probably acts directly on the oxyntic cells and dilute ethanol promotes gastric secretion by increasing gastrin secretion. Cholinergic drugs, such as **pilocarpine** (p. 4.9) stimulate the gastric glands and produce a copious flow of saliva.

AZURE-A CATION EXCHANGE RESIN

This can be used together with a gastric stimulant such as caffeine to determine whether the stomach can produce acid. When gastric juice with a pH of below 3·0 acts on this compound, the azure-A dye is released, absorbed from the small intestine and excreted in the urine, where it is easily detected by its colour. Since the resin may be taken by mouth, no intubation of the stomach is needed.

Drugs which reduce or neutralize stomach secretions

ANTACIDS

Large amounts of antacids are consumed by the lay public for the relief of dyspepsia and other real and imagined disorders of gastric function. Although there is doubt whether a greater than normal amount of acid secretion is the cause of duodenal ulceration, symptoms arise when acid and pepsin come in contact with the ulcer and are relieved when the acid is neutralized.

Antacids are used clinically to raise the pH of the stomach contents. In addition, if the pH is maintained at or above 5, the proteolytic activity of pepsin is abolished. Some antacids, for example aluminium hydroxide, may have further action in that they adsorb pepsin.

Antacids are commonly classified as systemic and nonsystemic. A **systemic antacid** alters the extracellular pH because it is readily absorbed. **Sodium bicarbonate** taken by mouth neutralizes HCl in the stomach and so spares an equivalent amount of HCO_3^- in the duodenum and small intestine. The net effect is similar to the infusion of an equivalent amount of $NaHCO_3$ into the blood. Provided renal function is normal, the ingested bicarbonate is excreted in the urine. When taken in large doses over long periods of time, however, the blood $[HCO_3^-]$ rises and metabolic alkalosis develops. Under these circumstances calcium phosphate tends to be precipitated in the renal tissue (nephrocalcinosis).

A **nonsystemic antacid** remains in the stomach and intestine because it forms an insoluble compound. Neutralization of HCl occurs as in the case of systemic antacid but the alkali is reformed in the small intestine. Thus **calcium carbonate** reacts with gastric HCl to form H_2O, CO_2 and $CaCl_2$. The latter passes into the intestine and reforms $CaCO_3$ with the alkaline secretions and is ultimately excreted in the faeces. Alkalosis is therefore not produced. **Magnesium oxide, trisilicate** and **carbonate**, and **aluminium hydroxide** are other examples of nonsystemic antacids. When given in large doses a rise in serum magnesium or calcium may occur, but aluminium is not absorbed. In general, the drugs which are of greatest value because of their rapid action and high neutralizing capacity may cause serious systemic effects when their anions or cations are absorbed.

The amount of antacid required to neutralize a given amount of acid *in vitro* can be easily calculated. Table 10.1 gives some commonly used antacids and their

TABLE 10.1. Neutralizing capacity of antacids measured in ml N/10HCl; time after mixing in minutes. After Piper and Fenton (1964) *Gut.*

		Time (min.)				
		0	5	10	30	120
$NaHCO_3$	1 g	115	115	115	115	117
$CaCO_3$	1 g	50	72	110	137	162
MgO	1 g	15	30	87	187	305
Mg trisilicate	1 g	5	7	10	12	15
$MgCO_3$	1 g	5	5	7	7	7
$Al(OH)_3$ (suspension) 4%	10 ml	10	10	12	12	17

relative neutralizing capacity. It is difficult to relate these results to their effect *in vivo* because increasing the dose of antacid does not increase the degree or duration of neutralization. This is mainly because of the rapid rate of gastric emptying. For example, 4 g $CaCO_3$ neutralizes 80 mEq of hydrochloric acid *in vitro*, and on the basis of a resting acid secretion of 3 mEq/hour this should neutralize all the acid produced in 27 hours. In fact the pH of the stomach contents remains above 3 for only 40 min. An additional problem is that any observations which involve the sampling of the gastric contents after the administration of antacids may be invalidated by incomplete mixing within the stomach.

With these points in mind, table 10.1 shows that $CaCO_3$, $NaHCO_3$ and MgO are the most potent antacids, but all may have adverse effects when given in therapeutic dosage. $CaCO_3$ tends to cause hypercalcaemia and, when taken for long periods, calcification of the kidney; in one study one-fifth of patients receiving 40–60 g/day of $CaCO_3$ developed hypercalcaemia. Sodium bicarbonate causes alkalosis and should not be given to patients with oedema. MgO may cause magnesium intoxication especially in patients with impaired renal function. Since $CaCO_3$ may cause constipation and Mg

salts diarrhoea, these two substances are often given together. MgO is a much more potent preparation than the trisilicate. $Al(OH)_3$ is a weak antacid but it adsorbs pepsin. On the other hand, it should not be given when other oral preparations, such as antibiotics, are being taken, because it tends to adsorb these as well.

ANTICHOLINERGIC DRUGS

Anticholinergic drugs are widely used for their effects on the motility and secretion of the stomach in peptic ulcer. These drugs are also antispasmodics or antimuscarinics because they competitively inhibit the actions of acetylcholine on structures innervated by postganglionic cholinergic nerves, including smooth muscles which normally respond to acetylcholine.

A large dose of atropine is required to reduce significantly the gastric secretion of acid. Such a dose usually causes a reduction in the secretion of saliva, dilation of the pupil and inhibition of accommodation, and it may also cause retention of urine. A number of synthetic anticholinergics have been produced in an attempt to alter the balance of effect in favour of gastric secretory depression. However, the only essential difference in action from atropine is that those with a quaternary ammonium structure exert, in addition, a ganglion blocking effect which is thought to have a greater influence on the gastrointestinal tract. These compounds include **methantheline, propantheline, poldine methylsulphate** and **glycopyrrolate**. They are poorly and variably absorbed from the alimentary tract. Once absorbed they act for a longer time than atropine and, in addition, have no effect on the central nervous system since they do not penetrate the blood–brain barrier. Because of the variability of absorption and the different individual responses, the doses are difficult to define. Usual daily doses are as follows, methantheline 50–100 mg, propantheline 30–60 mg, poldine methylsulphate 4–12 mg, and glycopyrrolate 1–3 mg.

Methantheline

Propantheline

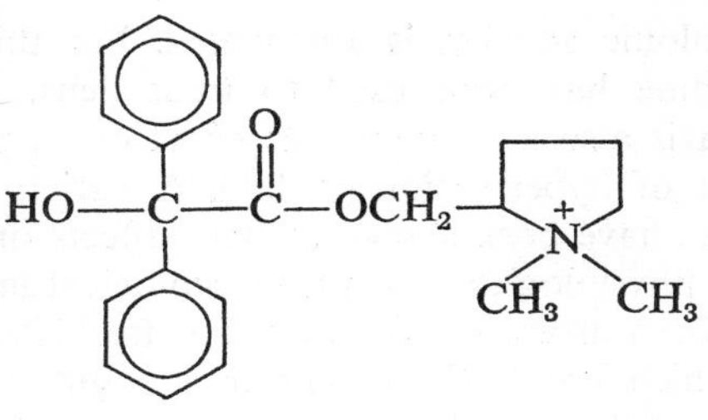

Poldine methylsulphate

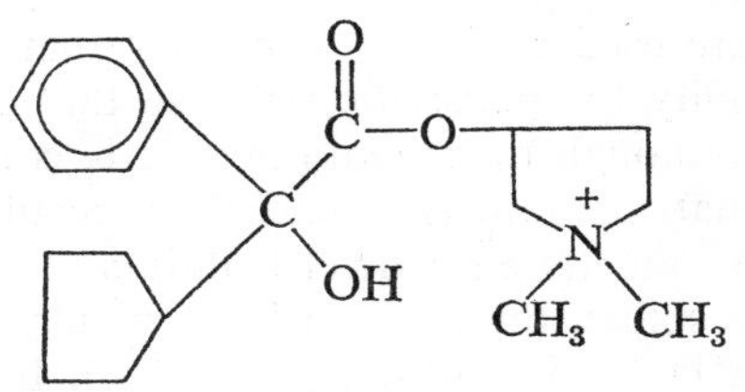

Glycopyrrolate

In full therapeutic doses these drugs partially inhibit the motility of the stomach and gastric emptying is slowed. They also reduce the volume of gastric secretion and the concentration of acid. Since the output of pepsin and mucus remain almost unaltered, their concentration may actually rise. Thus the basic action of these drugs is to facilitate neutralization of gastric juice by food and antacids. An important action is a reduction of the resting secretion of acid, but there is evidence that the pH of the stomach contents after food is not altered by their administration.

The extent to which their pharmacological activity is the basis for their clinical effect is uncertain. They may give symptomatic relief by reducing gastric hypermotility which can be associated with pain, and perhaps also by reducing the frequent swings in duodenal pH which are characteristic of duodenal ulcer. This may be accomplished by delaying gastric emptying and by reducing the resting secretion of acid. The main disadvantage of these drugs lies in the great individual variability of response to any one drug and in particular in the fact that in any one individual different anticholinergic drugs affect the function of various organs to a different degree.

ANTIPEPSINS

Much of the therapy of duodenal ulceration is aimed at increasing the pH of the gastric juice in order to inactivate pepsin, and so substances which directly inhibit peptic activity may have some importance. The mucus of gastric juice contains mucopolysaccharides (vol. I, p. 30.16). Naturally occurring sulphated polysaccharides, such as heparin and chondroitin sulphate, inhibit the proteolytic action of pepsin *in vitro*, while the antipeptic and anticoagulant activity of synthetic sulphated polysaccharides rises with an increase of molecular weight and sulphate

content. However, the sodium salt of **sulphated potato amylopectin** which is a high molecular weight substance, inhibits pepsin without being an anticoagulant. In man it reduces the pepsin content of gastric juice and clinical trials indicate that it may be of value in the treatment of duodenal ulceration, but its place in therapy has not been finally determined.

Drugs which act on the gastric mucosa

CARBENOXOLONE

Liquorice is an ingredient in many traditional indigestion remedies. Glycyrrhizic acid can be extracted from liquorice root, and **glycyrrhetinic acid** is prepared from this. Carbenoxolone is the disodium salt of glycyrrhetinic acid hemisuccinate. Its structure is somewhat similar to that of the corticosteroids. On the basis of several favourable clinical trials carbenoxolone is now used widely in the treatment of chronic gastric ulceration.

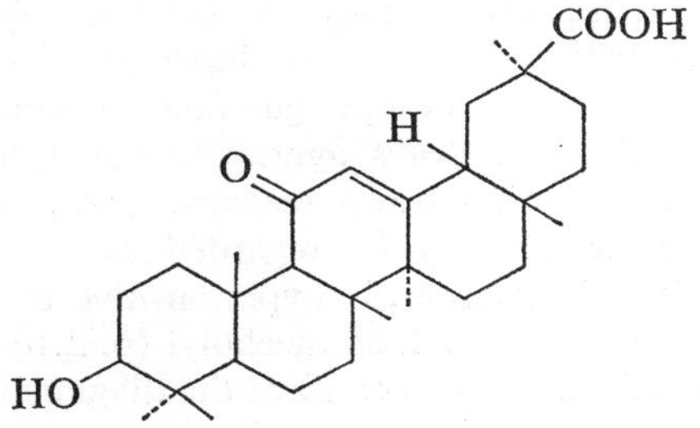

Glycyrrhetinic acid

It has been shown to have an anti-inflammatory action and to promote wound healing in some animals (p. 24.7). In man it causes retention of sodium and water, urinary loss of potassium, weight gain and hypertension. It may also cause muscle weakness and wasting. Heartburn occurs soon after its administration in some patients.

On oral administration the drug is absorbed within 30 min mainly from the stomach and is excreted in the bile and urine. It is absent from the duodenal aspirate of both rat and man and this may be the reason for its failure to act in duodenal ulceration. Two mechanisms of action have been suggested, first, an increase in gastric mucus production, which probably has a protective effect, and second, stimulation of cellular proliferation at the base of the ulcer. If the main action of the drug is to increase mucus production, then it would be expected to benefit cases of duodenal as well as of gastric ulceration. The drug has no effect on gastric acid secretion or motility. It is given after meals in doses of 50–100 mg.

CORTICOSTEROIDS

The action of corticosteroids on gastric secretion is discussed on p. 10.13.

The effects of drugs on intestinal motility

Abnormal gastrointestinal motility occurs in many gastrointestinal disorders either primarily as in achalasia and irritable colon, or secondarily as in the carcinoid syndrome (p. 16.5) or in paralytic ileus. There is a notable absence of information on the physiological and pharmacological aspects of gut motility in man. Most studies relate to animals and many are performed on isolated muscle strips and the results of these experiments cannot always be applied to man.

THE OESOPHAGUS AND THE GASTRO-OESOPHAGEAL JUNCTION

At the lower end of the oesophagus the high resting tone of the smooth muscle prevents the reflux of gastric contents. The gastro-oesophageal junction is contracted by both acetylcholine and adrenaline. Anticholinergic drugs decrease this resting tone and may permit a reflux of gastric contents. They also decrease secondary peristaltic waves in the oesophagus. In **achalasia**, in which postganglionic innervation is deficient, the lower end of the oesophagus fails to relax; despite this, anticholinergic drugs aggravate the dysphagia in this condition for unknown reasons. The body of the oesophagus, which may be regarded as a denervated structure in this disorder, is hypersensitive to parasympathomimetic drugs such as mecholyl (p. 4.10) and this fact is sometimes used to confirm the diagnosis.

STOMACH AND INTESTINES

Throughout the intestinal tract there are marked regional differences in the ability to react to drugs and in the effect they produce. A drug may act on more than one site, for example, on the extrinsic or intrinsic nerve supply, or on the smooth muscle fibre itself.

The motor activity of the alimentary tract is controlled through the parasympathetic nervous system. In general terms the stomach and proximal duodenum possess little intrinsic nervous activity, whereas intrinsic nervous control predominates in the distal duodenum and jejunum. The colon occupies an intermediate position. Thus vagotomy has a much greater effect on the motility of the stomach than it has on the small intestine and colon.

The sympathetic nervous system inhibits motor activity through both α- and β- receptors. Colonic inhibitory activity in particular is mediated through β-receptors. In contrast, α-receptors may predominate in the small intestine.

With these points in mind, the effects of various drugs on gastric and intestinal motility are considered. The effects of some drugs on the stomach, particularly the anticholinergics, are described on p. 10.41. These drugs have little effect on small intestinal or colonic activity. When adrenergic neurone blockade is produced, e.g. by guanethidine (p. 4.14), small intestinal and to a lesser degree colonic activity, is augmented. For this reason, guanethidine has been used to treat ileus. Explosive diarrhoea is also an undesirable effect of its use in the treatment of hypertension (p. 8.8). A variety of other substances have been shown to have effects on motility but their physiological and pharmacological importance has not been assessed. Among these are histamine and 5-HT, which are both present in the gut and which both act on the smooth muscle cell, and gastrin, which may act by the release of acetylcholine.

Morphine (p. 5.48) and some related drugs, particularly **codeine**, are used clinically to control diarrhoea. These drugs modify the peristaltic reflex so that propulsion is reduced, although the smooth muscle is contracted and intraluminal pressure is increased, especially within the colon. In patients with diverticulitis and perhaps also ulcerative colitis, the rise can be particularly great and may be a factor in causing perforation. In contrast to the drugs mentioned below, morphine and codeine carry some danger of addiction and tend to cause nausea.

Diphenoxylate hydrochloride is structurally related to pethidine (p. 5.52). Lengthening of either the ethyl or

Diphenoxylate

Pethidine

the CH_3—N grouping of pethidine-like drugs reduces their analgesic activity whereas their constipating activity is retained. In diphenoxylate, the pethidine-like structure is linked to an atropine-like compound. The resultant effects are that diphenoxylate acts on intestinal muscle in the same way as morphine, but it is devoid of analgesic and atropine-like activity and it is not a drug of addiction. It is used for the symptomatic treatment of diarrhoea and is given in a dose of 5 mg three or four times per day.

Metoclopramide hydrochloride is an antiemetic which acts both on the vomiting centre and on the stomach. For example, in the dog it opposes the emetic action of copper sulphate on the stomach and the action

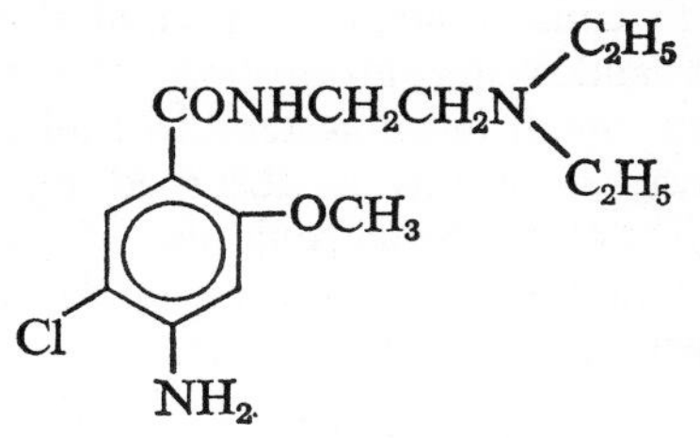

Metoclopramide

of apomorphine on the vomiting centre. In contrast to the phenothiazines (p. 5.31), which are also used as anti-emetics, no significant effects have been detected on the cardiovascular system and it is not a sedative. It is useful in controlling nausea and vomiting particularly due to upper gastrointestinal disorders, malignancy and radiotherapy. On the other hand it does not prevent vomiting secondary to labyrinthine dysfunction.

In several animal species metoclopramide increases gastric tone and peristalsis and gastric emptying is enhanced. In contrast to other drugs such as cholinergics, which have these actions, metoclopramide does not increase acid secretion by the stomach. In the dog the gastric motor stimulation produced by the drug is antagonized by anticholinergic drugs but is not blocked by vagotomy; thus it appears to act on the intramural cholinergic neurones. For its action in increasing gastric peristalsis and dilating the pylorus it is sometimes useful in the barium meal examination and it facilitates intubation of the duodenum. It may also promote peristalsis in the atonic stomach such as may occur in diabetes and other conditions.

It is given orally or parenterally in a dose of 10 mg, but may cause constipation and slight drowsiness. It should not be given with a phenothiazine since both drugs can affect the extrapyramidal system.

NONSPECIFIC MUSCLE RELAXANTS
These drugs act directly on the intestinal smooth muscle and are used for functional disorders of the bowel, e.g. irritable bowel syndrome.

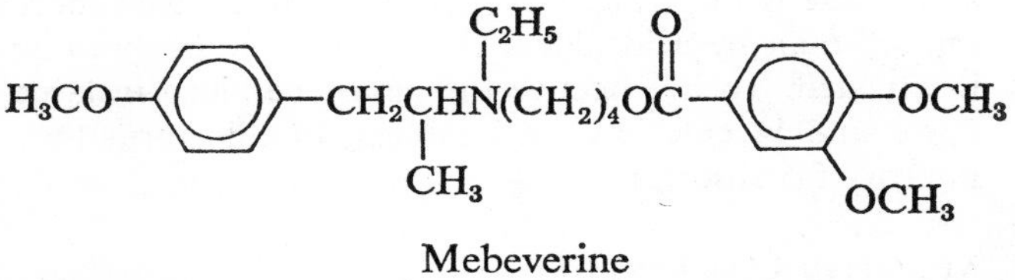

Mebeverine

Mebeverine is a phenylethylamine derivative of reserpine which has little or none of the central nervous effect of the parent compound. In man it appears to have no atropine-like effects. It acts directly on smooth muscle to inhibit peristaltic reflexes. It is given in a dose of 50–100 mg three times each day.

Dicyclomine has a direct relaxant action on smooth

muscle and it has very little atropine-like effect. It is given in a dosage of 10–20 mg three times per day.

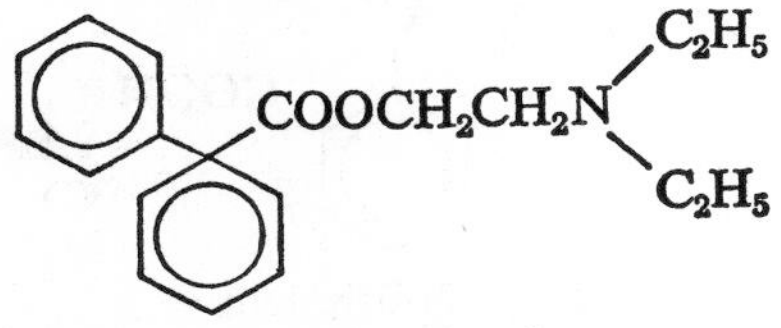

Dicyclomine

LAXATIVES
Laxatives are useful in keeping the stool soft in painful conditions of the anal region, such as haemorrhoids or fissure, and in preventing straining at defaecation in postoperative patients and following myocardial infarction. Their use is also often indicated in the elderly bedridden patient. Laxatives have been much abused by the public as a result of widespread ignorance of what constitutes normal bowel action, and dependence on them is not uncommon. They are prescribed much less frequently than formerly.

Laxatives are usually classified as **stimulant laxatives** which increase the motor activity of the bowel and **bulk laxatives** which increase peristalsis secondary to an increase of bulk within the bowel lumen. In addition, certain salts retain water within the bowel lumen by osmosis, and mineral oil and some other agents act as **lubricants.**

Stimulant laxatives
Anthraquinones include senna and cascara sagrada. Senna is a glycoside derivative of anthraquinone. The glycoside is slowly hydrolysed in the small intestine, absorbed, and broken down to form **emodin** which stimulates the muscle

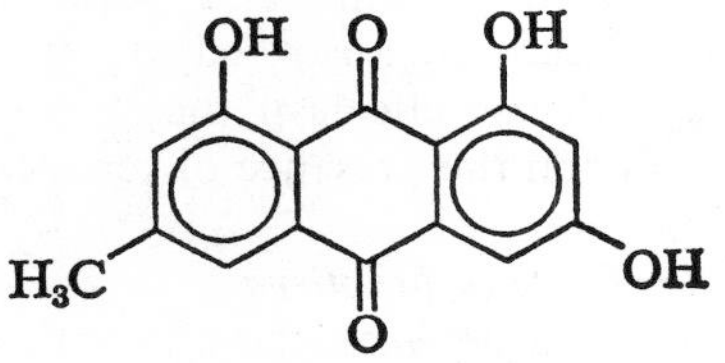

Emodin

of the large intestine. This effect occurs 6–12 hours after an oral dose; it persists in experimental animals after the continuity of the intestine has been interrupted. Emodin appears in the milk during lactation and can also colour the urine.

Phenolphthalein and **bisacodyl** are derived from diphenylmethane and act 6–8 hours after oral administration on both colon and small intestine. Phenolphthalein colours alkaline urine pink and may cause hypersensitivity and skin reactions. Bisacodyl has the advantage

Phenolphthalein

Bisacodyl

that it acts mainly on the colon, is not absorbed and can be given rectally.

Bulk-forming laxatives

These are natural and semisynthetic polysaccharides or cellulose derivatives. They increase the residue within the bowel and so stimulate peristalsis. Some also have the property of swelling in water. They are devoid of systemic side effects but have been known to cause intestinal and even oesophageal obstruction when taken dry. Examples are **methylcellulose, carboxymethylcellulose** and **bran**. A diet which is rich in vegetable roughage provides the same effect as any of these preparations.

Saline laxatives

Salts which are slowly absorbed retain fluid in the gastrointestinal tract by their osmotic action and so stimulate peristalsis. Magnesium and sodium sulphate are examples. Because they are absorbed to some degree, the ions may cause adverse effects if they are taken in excessive amounts or in the presence of renal failure.

General adverse effects of laxatives

There are similarities between the alimentary tract and the kidney in the control of electrolytes. As in the kidney, sodium is conserved in the intestine both proximally and distally, and is associated with the secretion of potassium in the colon. The effect of laxatives on the gut tends to be similar to that of diuretics on the kidney. The analogy may be taken further in that sodium absorption in the colon is increased in disease states characterized by oedema formation. This is probably due to aldosterone, which increases sodium, chloride and water absorption from the intact healthy human colon. Diuretics act also on the intestine but the effect is not sufficiently powerful to upset water or electrolyte balance. The action of laxatives is to cause colonic hurry and this interferes with sodium and water absorption. Laxatives which act also on the small intestine tend to lead to excessive potassium loss, since this is absorbed mainly in the distal small intestine. The chronic use of laxatives may lead to signs and symptoms attributable to excessive loss of potassium, sodium and water.

ACTION OF DRUGS ON THE PANCREAS

PANCREATIC SECRETION

Pancreatic secretion can be stimulated by injection of **secretin** and **pancreozymin**. These hormones are prepared commercially from hog intestine, and because they have a variable activity there is as yet no maximal function test comparable to that which exists for the assessment of gastric function. As well as stimulating the pancreas, secretin inhibits gastric secretion probably by blocking the action of gastrin, since it does not inhibit acid secretion stimulated by histamine. Sensitivity of the pancreas to secretin may be decreased by giving atropine or ganglion blocking drugs and, as would be expected, acute or chronic vagal interruption also reduces the response. A synthetic secretin has now been produced which is based upon the amino acid sequence of porcine secretin, and while it is not as potent as natural secretin it has the same actions. Secretin also increases bile flow.

In the dog, histamine causes a transient increase in the volume of pancreatic secretion and its HCO_3^- content. Gastrin also stimulates the production of pancreatic juice but the volume and HCO_3^- content is less than after stimulation by secretin, although the protein output is greater.

PANCREATIC EXTRACTS (PANCREATIN)

Preparations of hog pancreas containing trypsin, amylase and lipase are given orally to patients with inadequate pancreatic secretion. Since purified trypsin is inactivated by peptic digestion in gastric juice at a pH of less than 3·5 and lipase is inactivated by pepsin mixtures even more rapidly than by acid alone, the extracts are likely to be inactivated. To be effective they must be given in large doses and in enteric coated tablets; in this form they improve fat absorption.

APROTININ (TRASYLOL)

In acute pancreatitis, enzymes are released into the surrounding tissues and their actions may cause profound shock, e.g. trypsin activates kininogen to form bradykinin, a powerful vasodilator, causing shock (p. 17.3). Aprotinin is a kallikrein inhibitor obtained from bovine parotid gland and lung. In addition, it is an inhibitor of trypsin and has antifibrinolytic activity (p. 7.15). The extract may be given intraperitoneally or intravenously. In experimental preparations it prevents the actions of bradykinin but its benefit in acute pancreatitis in man is not yet proven; in clinical trials it has been given by continuous intravenous infusion in doses ranging from 30,000 to 300,000 units/day.

ACTIONS OF DRUGS ON THE LIVER

The liver is the principal organ in the body for the metabolism of drugs and chemicals. While some drugs pass through the liver unchanged, e.g. hexamethonium, and some are concentrated in its tissues and stored for long periods, e.g. vitamins and some antimalarial drugs, many drugs undergo chemical change, being converted into inactive metabolites or sometimes into the active form of the drug (p. 2.11). Hence the duration and intensity of action of drugs frequently depend, among other factors, on the rate at which the drugs are metabolized in the liver. When liver cells are homogenized and the fragments separated by centrifugation, the enzymes which metabolize drugs are found in the microsomal particles, which are derived from the smooth endoplasmic reticulum (p. 2.13). In the cell, these enzymes are continuously broken down and resynthesized so that the amount of each microsomal enzyme depends on the balance between these processes. Drugs may inhibit, or induce formation of these enzymes or interfere with their breakdown; when two or more drugs are given either simultaneously or in sequence, their effects may interact in a complicated way.

ANIMAL EXPERIMENTS

As discussed on p. 2.14, SKF 525-A inhibits certain microsomal enzymes and consequently potentiates the actions of a variety of drugs. Similarly drugs that inhibit the mitochondrial enzyme, monoamine oxidase, also inhibit microsomal enzymes and so interact with the effects of other drugs.

More than 200 drugs, insecticides, carcinogens and other chemicals, are now known to affect the activity of microsomal liver enzymes (table 10.2). Although diverse in structure, most of these substances are lipid soluble at physiological pH.

Phenobarbitone was among the first to be studied; it was discovered that tolerance which developed on repeated dosage was due to increased metabolism of the drug in the liver. Previous treatment with phenobarbitone was found to modify also the effects of other drugs; for example it increases the hydroxylase activity for zoxazolamine, a centrally acting muscle relaxant, and in this way reduces its paralytic effect in rats. In animals, phenobarbitone induces the formation of many microsomal enzymes and so modifies the metabolism of many drugs.

TABLE 10.2. Effect of drugs on liver microsomal enzymes. Adapted from Bowman W.C., Rand M.J. and West G.B. (1968) *Textbook of Pharmacology.* Oxford: Blackwell Scientific Publications.

Type of drug	Stimulates activity	Depresses activity
Anaesthetic	Ether, chloroform, nitrous oxide, halothane	
Hypnotics and sedatives	Barbiturates, glutethimide, urethane, chlorobutanol, carbromal, methyprylone	
Tranquillizers	Phenaglycodol, meprobamate, chlorpromazine, triflupromazine, chlordiazepoxide	
Anticonvulsants	Primidone, phenytoin, trimethadione, methoin paramethadione	
Muscle relaxants	Orphenadrine, mephenesin	
Analeptics and psychomotor stimulants	Nikethamide, bemegride, imipramine	Hydrazine and hydrazide MAO inhibitors
Analgesics	Phenylbutazone, amidopyrine, pethidine, levorphan	Morphine and congeners
Antihistamine	Diphenhydramine, chlorcyclizine	
Sulphonamides	Tolbutamide, carbutamide	
Antibiotics		Chloramphenicol
Steroids	Androgens, adrenocorticoids	Oestrogens, progestagens
Polycyclic hydrocarbons	3,4-Benzpyrene, 3-methylcholanthrene, 1,2,5,6-dibenzanthracene	
Insecticides	Chlorinated hydrocarbons DDT, dieldrin, aldrin, etc.	

This action of phenobarbitone is typical of various hypnotics, anticonvulsants, tranquillizers, insecticides and steroid hormones (table 10.2). By contrast, the effect of polycyclic hydrocarbons, such as 3-methylcholanthrene, is more selective and more potent; these drugs stimulate only *N*-demethylases and hydroxylases.

Enzyme induction may not only cause tolerance but also reduces toxicity. Strychnine, warfarin and bishydroxy-coumarin are all less toxic for rats after treatment with a polycyclic hydrocarbon or with the insecticide DDT. Indeed, it was the spraying of animal rooms with this insecticide which led accidentally to the discovery that it was possible to modify the action of drugs by stimulating drug metabolizing enzymes. Hence, enzyme induction can affect tests of drug metabolism or of chronic toxicity (p. 32.9).

As drug-induced increases in microsomal enzyme activity involves synthesis of more enzyme protein, inhibitors of protein synthesis or DNA-dependent RNA should prevent the effect. This was confirmed when ethionine, puromycin or actinomycin D was found to block the induction of drug-metabolizing activity by phenobarbitone or 3-methylcholanthrene. Ethionine probably acts by reducing the concentration of ATP in liver, puromycin by blocking the transfer of soluble RNA-bound amino acid into microsomal protein, and actinomycin D by blocking the DNA-directed synthesis of nuclear RNA required for protein synthesis. These findings suggest:

(1) that *S*-adenosylmethionine may be important for the synthesis of microsomal enzymes,

(2) that the enzyme-inducers accelerate the DNA-directed synthesis of RNA molecules which are the templates for the formation of enzymes on ribosomes.

Among the various enzymes that are induced, $NADPH_2$-cytochrome c reductase has been chosen for special study because it can be purified. *In vivo*, the turnover of the enzyme can be measured after incorporation of ^3H-L-leucine. The enzyme catalyses hydroxylation in such a way that one of the oxygen atoms goes into the substrate and the other is reduced to H_2O. This enzymatic reaction has been called a 'mixed function oxidation', since the substrate and $NADPH_2$ are both oxidized (fig. 10.3). The system for hydroxylation contains not only the flavoprotein but a haemoprotein cytochrome P-450.

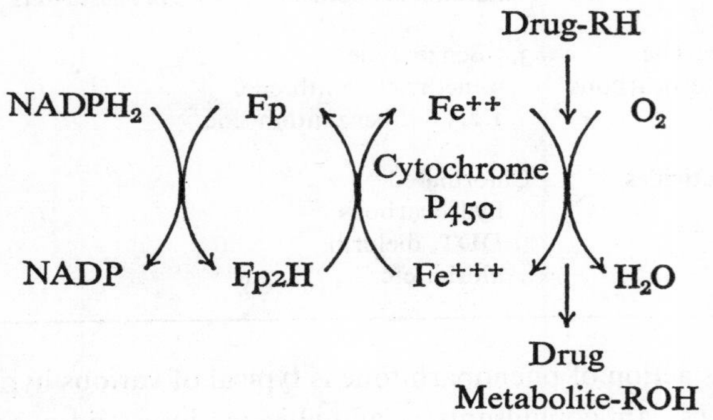

Apart from the mechanisms discussed, the induction of microsomal enzyme activity might occur in other ways. The substrate could react with repressors made by a regulator gene or with other regulators of gene function. Inducers may interact with endoplasmic reticulum so as to enhance the translation of messenger RNA on ribosomes. Again, the inducer could act directly on the enzyme to interfere with its breakdown, or with the feedback for inhibition of enzyme synthesis.

Many drug inducers of microsomal liver enzymes stimulate the growth of normal or regenerating liver. The polycyclic hydrocarbons differ from phenobarbitone in that they increase liver protein proportionately more than they increase microsomal protein. These anabolic effects have been confirmed by studying the incorporation of amino acids into liver microsomal protein, after treatment with inducers. Thus, phenobarbitone stimulates incorporation of ^{14}C-leucine and other amino acids into microsomal protein *in vivo*, but has no effect on their incorporation in other subcellular fractions. The anabolic effects of inducers, whether on the microsomes or the entire hepatic cell, are difficult to interpret at the present time.

The metabolism of drugs by the liver and the modification of this by drugs depend on the age and species of animal. The liver microsomes of newborn animals have little ability to metabolize drugs such as hexobarbitone, amphetamine and chlorpromazine; further the genetic make-up of members of a population within a given species may be important in determining the occurrence or magnitude of enzyme induction. Thus newborn mice treated with 10 mg/kg hexobarbitone sleep for at least 6 hours, whereas adult mice with 10 times this dose regain righting reflexes in less than 1 hour. The development of drug-metabolizing enzymes as the animal matures parallels drug metabolism *in vivo*, and drugs tend to act for a shorter time. Various hormones may also influence microsomal activity in the growing animal. The steroid sex hormones, thyroid hormones and insulin stimulate activity whereas noradrenaline depresses it. After adrenalectomy, the microsomal enzyme action falls but can be restored by treatment with cortisol.

The many similarities between hepatic hydroxylation of drugs and steroidal hormones prompted detailed studies of the effects of liver microsomal enzyme inducers on the metabolism of steroids. Treatment of animals with phenobarbitone increases the hydroxylation of testosterone, oestradiol, oestrone, progesterone, and various corticosteroids. The increased rate of hydroxylation of steroid hormones by microsomal enzymes diminishes their physiological actions. For example, pretreatment with phenobarbitone greatly reduced the effect of oestrogens on the uterine weight of immature mice.

FIG. 10.3. System for hydroxylation of drugs.

ENZYME INDUCTION IN MAN

Information obtained in animal experiments provides some indication of the potential hazards in man. Many of the substances which increase the activity of microsomal drug-metabolizing enzymes in animals are also drugs in therapeutic use. For example, phenobarbitone diminishes the anticoagulant action of bishydroxycoumarin by lowering the plasma concentration of this drug. If the dose of anticoagulant is increased, it should be reduced when the phenobarbitone is stopped to avoid the danger of bleeding. Phenobarbitone also stimulates the metabolism of phenytoin and so reduces the plasma concentration of the drug in patients with epilepsy. Phenylbutazone, like the barbiturates, stimulates its own metabolism, thereby limiting the rise of concentration in the plasma when the dose of this drug is increased; it also increases the rate of disappearance of aminopyrine.

Enzyme induction may also affect the concentrations of normal body substrates. Phenobarbitone stimulates bilirubin metabolism in children and increases the urinary excretion of D-glucaric acid in adults, suggesting an induced alteration in the glucuronic acid pathway. The role of sex hormones and related compounds used as oral contraceptives in regulating the metabolism of drugs, and the effect of drugs on the metabolism of sex hormones and other steroids, have yet to be fully investigated in man.

Disease in man may arise from specific derangement in the synthesis or activity of enzymes that are important for metabolism. Inherited enzymic defects are the cause of galactosaemia, phenylketonuria, glycogen storage disease and congenital nonhaemolytic jaundice. Drugs that induce enzyme formation might therefore have value in the treatment of these conditions. When infants with congenital nonhaemolytic jaundice are treated with phenobarbitone, the bilirubin concentration falls and the jaundice disappears. Parallel tests with salicylamide, which is normally conjugated with glucuronic acid, reveal a failure in conjugation which is corrected by treatment with phenobarbitone. When the treatment is stopped, the concentration of bilirubin rises to its previous level.

Man, animals and plants are being exposed more than ever to new drugs and chemicals in the form of herbicides, pesticides, food additives and hydrocarbons. Many of these compounds have been shown experimentally to modify their own metabolism or the metabolism of other drugs and of naturally occurring substances in the body. The presence of certain microsomal enzymes in the liver and in other organs raises the question of how they evolved and of their protective role against foreign molecules that might be lethal. Today, the actions of drugs on the microsomal enzymes have assumed a new importance in the understanding of genetic defects, and in forecasting the combined effects of drugs whether in laboratory toxicity tests or in the treatment of patients.

CHOLERETICS

Bile salt secretion is the most important stimulant for the production of bile. A secondary mechanism probably involves the secretion of inorganic ions by the biliary ducts which are under the control of secretin and perhaps other hormones. The choleretic effect of bile salts is partly due to their osmotic activity. Taurocholate and glycocholate have a much smaller effect than dehydrocholate because they form micelles, and this reduces their osmotic activity. Secretin characteristically produces a rise in the pH of the bile and the $[HCO_3^-]$ and $[Cl^-]$ increase. Gastrin produces an effect similar to that of secretin, though smaller.

A variety of substances are actively secreted into the bile and are choleretics because of their osmotic activity, e.g. phenol red, fluorescein and phloridzin. Some antibiotics are also actively secreted into the bile. Some of those listed under high biliary excretion in table 10.3

TABLE 10.3. Antibiotics classified according to their biliary excretion.

HIGH	Some synthetic penicillins, erythromycin, oleandomycin, rifamycin, novobiocin.
MODERATE	Benzyl penicillin, tetracyclines, polymyxin.
LOW	Streptomycin, chloramphenicol, neomycin, bacitracin, viomycin.

may be especially useful in the treatment of cholecystitis when the cystic duct is not obstructed.

Bile salts

In the liver, cholesterol is oxidized to cholic acid and to chenodesoxycholic acid. These are conjugated with either taurine or glycine to be secreted in the bile as bile salts. The conjugates resist hydrolysis by proteolytic enzymes and are reabsorbed from the lower ileum. Any that pass into the colon are metabolized by bacteria to a variety of metabolites. One of these, desoxycholic acid, is absorbed, transported to the liver, conjugated and re-excreted in the bile (vol. 1, p. 31.7). In the absence of bile, about 50 per cent of the dietary fat can be absorbed, but cholesterol and vitamins A, D and K are almost completely dependent on bile for their absorption. About 30 g of bile salts are secreted each day and this large amount is estimated to be about six times the total pool size. The amount secreted each day is also much greater than can be synthesized and the enterohepatic circulation can thus be regarded as a conserving mechanism.

Bile salts stimulate the flow of bile when given by intravenous or oral routes. Intravenous administration causes a fall in blood pressure and bradycardia, and both these features can accompany obstructive jaundice when bile salts accumulate in the body. Under normal conditions, less than 1 g of endogenous bile salt reaches the colon each day. Larger amounts cause diarrhoea, probably by inhibiting water absorption and affecting large intestinal motility. The normal enterohepatic circulation of bile salts may be interrupted by biliary obstruction, by the oral administration of substances which bind bile salts, e.g. cholestyramine, or by disease of the terminal ileum. In any of these circumstances, steatorrhoea may result from lack of bile salts in the intestine. Treatment of this steatorrhoea with oral bile salt preparations is not always desirable, since in biliary obstruction these are absorbed and increase pruritus, and in disease of the terminal ileum they pass into the colon and may cause diarrhoea.

CHOLESTYRAMINE

This is an anion exchange resin which contains quaternary ammonium groups attached to a polymer. When given by mouth it adsorbs bile salts so that they are excreted in the stool, thus interrupting the enterohepatic circulation. The drug is sometimes used for the relief of pruritus due to the retention of bile salts in obstructive jaundice where the obstruction is not complete. However, because of its adverse effects it is indicated only when the patient suffers from an irremediable disease. When given in a dose of 3–4 g with each meal the unwanted effects of the drug are steatorrhoea and malabsorption of vitamins A, D and K. It also causes nausea, diarrhoea and constipation. The excessive loss of bile salts increases their resynthesis from cholesterol and the free serum cholesterol falls. There is also a fall in other lipid fractions. However, the serum cholesterol rises again during long term treatment. Calcium absorption may also be impaired and the chloride released from the drug in the intestine may be absorbed and increase plasma chloride levels. Safer compounds employing the same principle may be discovered in the future.

Other drugs used to relieve pruritus in obstructive

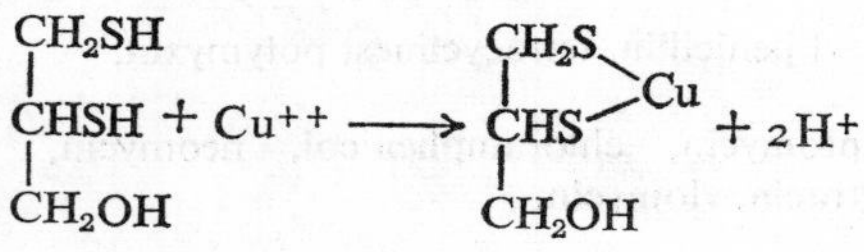

Dimercaprol

2.3. dimercaptopropanol (BAL)

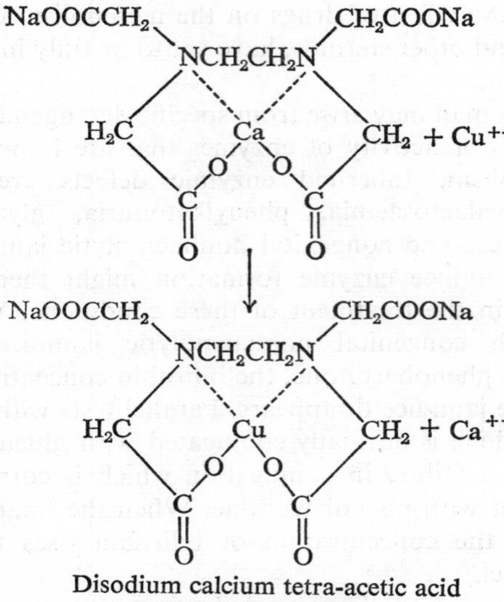

Disodium calcium tetra-acetic acid
(sodium edetate, EDTA)

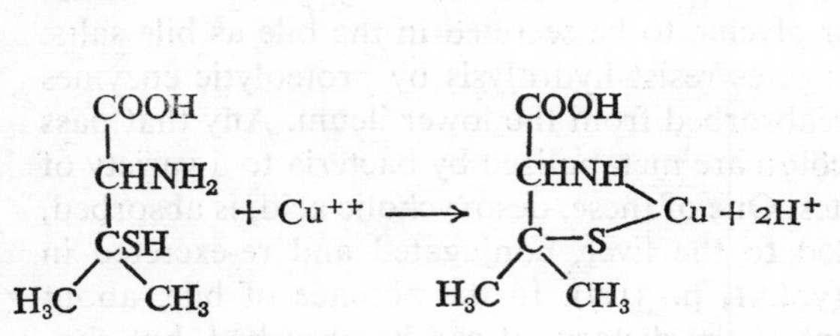

D-Penicillamine

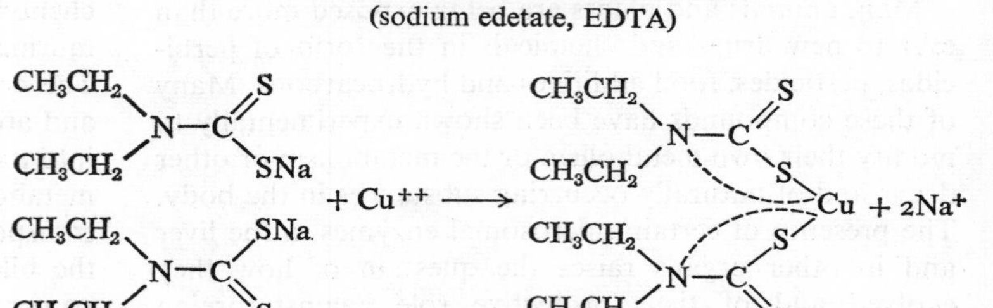

Sodium diethyldithiocarbamate

FIG. 10.4. Chemical reactions involved in chelation.

jaundice are methyltestosterone and norethandrolone (p. 12.11). Their mechanism of action is unknown, for they actually increase the level of jaundice and can cause intrahepatic cholestasis in some patients. For these reasons they are given only in severe cases.

DRUGS USED IN THE TREATMENT OF WILSON'S DISEASE

Wilson's disease or hepatolenticular degeneration is an uncommon disorder of copper metabolism in which excessive amounts of copper are deposited in the liver and other tissues (p. 25.38).

The drugs shown in fig. 10.4 are used in its treatment because they chelate copper. The most important of these are D-penicillamine and sodium diethyldithiocarbamate.

D-Penicillamine

This drug is an amino acid derived from penicillin and has no antibiotic activity. It is a chelating agent used particularly to increase the urinary excretion of copper in Wilson's disease. Part of its action on copper excretion may be due to its ability to supply sulphydryl groups to replace those blocked by copper. However, its general effect is to reduce body stores of copper when present in excess, and it does not have much effect upon normal stores. The effect of a single oral dose lasts for about 6 hours during which there is a great increase in the urinary copper excretion. Daily requirements of the drug are between 1 and 2 g; the correct dose for any patient is adjusted in accordance with the levels of urinary copper and is continued indefinitely

The drug is used also in the treatment of cystinuria. Here it acts by combining with the poorly soluble cystine to form a cysteine–penicillamine compound which is much more soluble. A further action is that it increases the solubility of collagen and increases the ratio of soluble to insoluble collagen in the skin and other organs. For this reason it is being tried in the treatment of connective tissue disorders such as systemic sclerosis (p. 30.11).

It should be noted that there may be cross hypersensitivity to penicillin. The most important adverse effects are leucopenia and thrombocytopenia and it may cause skin rashes, fever and occasionally proteinuria. When given over long periods it may also have an antipyridoxine effect in man.

Sodium diethyldithiocarbamate

When this drug is given by mouth it does not increase urinary excretion of copper. On the other hand, there is an increase in faecal excretion and a negative copper balance is produced. Paradoxically the drug seems to be effective also when given intravenously and in these circumstances it does not induce a negative copper balance.

Its beneficial role may be partly due to its ability to supply sulphydryl groups.

CORTICOSTEROIDS AND THE GASTROINTESTINAL TRACT

The corticosteroids are useful in the treatment of many gastrointestinal disorders by virtue of their anti-inflammatory and immunosuppressive actions (p. 24.6).

When corticosteroids are given to man or to animals, no effect on gastric acid secretion is apparent for 24 hours and there is much controversy as to whether or not acid secretion is then increased. Nevertheless, patients receiving corticosteroids are probably at increased risk of peptic ulceration. This may be due to changes in the composition of gastric mucus. Observations in dogs show that cortisone reduces the concentration of sialic acid in mucus, as does ACTH. The effect of other drugs which induce mucosal erosion or influence the healing of peptic ulceration may be via such mucosal defence mechanisms. For example, pregnancy has a beneficial effect on the healing of duodenal ulcer and oestrogens may have a favourable effect on healing by increasing the production of mucus. Other anti-inflammatory drugs such as phenylbutazone, indomethacin and perhaps aspirin may induce or aggravate peptic ulcers by decreasing or altering mucus production.

Although corticosteroids have little or no effect on acid or pepsin secretion by the normal human stomach, they have a slight effect on abnormal mucosa. For example, in pernicious anaemia, where there is an almost total absence of oxyntic and chief cells, corticosteroids may cause their reappearance in small numbers and the secretion of acid and intrinsic factor increases in some patients. The mechanism of this action is not known, but it may be due to inhibition of abnormal immunological factors which cause cell destruction in the mucosa. (p. 23.9). It has no therapeutic application at the present time.

Corticosteroids are used particularly in the treatment of some cases of malabsorption and ulcerative colitis. In ulcerative colitis abnormal immunological mechanisms may be at work, and in some cases of steatorrhoea an abnormal sensitivity to wheat gluten can be demonstrated. Corticosteroids may suppress these responses.

Corticosteroid therapy produces an improvement in appetite and lessens the jaundice in patients with some acute hepatic disorders, yet the long term benefits and mechanisms of action are open to dispute. In patients with jaundice due to hepatic cell necrosis, the drugs cause a sudden fall in the serum bilirubin level. This is not due to increased excretion of bile into the intestine, increased renal clearance of bilirubin or to a decrease in production, and its mechanism is unknown. Corticosteroids also have a beneficial effect in chronic active hepatitis where there is evidence of abnormal immunological mechanisms (p. 23.5).

Sulphasalazine

This drug is of value in the treatment of ulcerative colitis and is given orally in divided doses of 4–16 g/day. It is a diazo compound of salicylic acid and sulphapyridine.

Sulphasalazine

Its action is not antibacterial but on the connective tissues of the colon. In the mouse it has been shown that, after injection, the drug is split in the tissues at the N=N linkage to give sulphapyridine and 5-aminosalicylic acid. Both the 5-aminosalicylic acid and the unsplit sulphasalazine have an affinity for connective tissues. In addition, the unsplit drug is secreted through the intestinal wall. Its affinity for these tissues has been attributed to the acid-azo structure. Adverse effects are nausea, vomiting and headache, and also skin rashes, febrile reactions and joint pain. It may also cause agranulocytosis.

DRUGS AND INTESTINAL BLOOD FLOW

While adrenaline and noradrenaline constrict both the arterial and the venous sides of the mesenteric circulation, vasopressin and 5-HT constrict only the arterioles. Histamine and acetylcholine dilate the arterioles. With regard to the stomach, the relationship between gastric secretion and mucosal blood flow is still disputed, but a redistribution of blood flow to the mucosal tissue appears to take place during secretion and vice versa. Clearly the application of drugs which influence gastrointestinal blood flow might prove to be of value in the control of bleeding from superficial erosions and in other disorders. So far the only drug of proven therapeutic value is vasopressin.

VASOPRESSIN (p. 6.3)

This drug is used to reduce bleeding from oesophageal varices. Fig. 10.5 shows that intravenous injection lowers portal venous pressure and the hepatic blood flow. Splanchnic resistance increases and the mean arterial pressure also rises. The effect on the splanchnic circulation lasts for only one hour after a single injection of 20 units. Reduction in hepatic blood flow is undesirable because regenerating nodules of liver cells derive most of

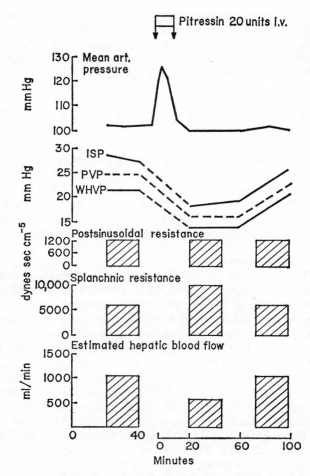

FIG. 10.5. The effect of 20 units of pitressin on the splanchnic haemodynamics in a patient with portal venous hypertension. The portal pressure was reduced by 36 per cent and the estimated hepatic blood flow fell by 34 per cent, while the splanchnic resistance increased by 68 per cent. The postsinusoidal resistance was not affected. ISP, intrasplenic pressure; PVP, calculated portal venous pressure; WHVP, wedged hepatic venous pressure. After Sherlock S. *et al.* (1961). *Circulation*, **94**, 801.

their blood supply from the hepatic artery. On the other hand, hepatic oxygen consumption does not seem to be reduced during vasopressin administration. It should be remembered that the drug is a coronary artery constrictor. It causes abdominal cramps, defaecation and often marked facial pallor.

PHENOXYBENZAMINE

Splanchnic vasoconstriction is an inherent part of endotoxic shock (p. 18.30). Vasoconstrictor drugs such as noradrenaline or angiotensin amide, given to raise the systemic blood pressure, probably increase the degree of splanchnic ischaemia. Phenoxybenzamine blocks α-adrenergic receptors and its use in experimental endotoxic shock prevents many of the haemodynamic alterations of endotoxaemia. Its use in the treatment of bacteriogenic shock is not established (p. 15.26).

SCANNING AGENTS AND CONTRAST MEDIA

Various substances which can be labelled radioactively are taken up by the liver or pancreas and are used to localize abnormalities in these organs by means of external scanning. Pathological lesions are defined because they do not take up the substance. Rose Bengal

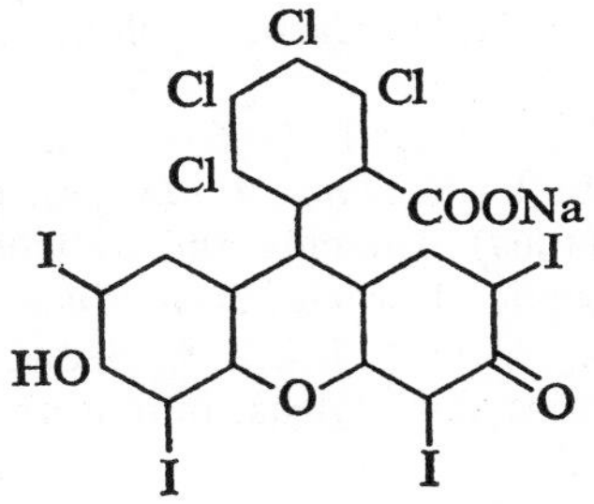

Rose Bengal sodium ^{131}I

labelled with radioactive iodine is taken up by the liver cells. Colloidal gold and technetium sulphur colloid accumulate in the reticuloendothelial system, an action which does not depend on hepatocellular function.

Radioactive selenomethionine, $CH_3SeCH_2CH_2CH(NH_2)COOH$, which behaves in the same way as methionine, is localized in hepatocytes and pancreas and is used for pancreatic scanning.

This is possible because the pancreas concentrates amino acids from the blood and utilizes them for the synthesis of digestive enzymes. However, uptake of selenomethionine by the liver often interferes with visualization.

Radio-opaque materials are used to visualize the alimentary and the biliary tracts, and to define the blood vessels of certain organs. Substances which outline the biliary tract are excreted into the bile and may be administered orally or intravenously, or they may be injected directly into the intrahepatic bile canaliculi percutaneously or at operation. For cholecystography, halogenated phenolphthalein derivatives are used, e.g. iopanoic acid and sodium ipodate; sodium iodipamide can be used intravenously.

All cholecystographic materials must be absorbed from the gastrointestinal tract, excreted by the liver, and concentrated in the gall bladder. There is a maximum rate at which the liver is able to excrete iodipamide and there is no advantage in increasing the dose further. The use of two contrast media at the same time simply results in competition for the available secretory mechanism. This

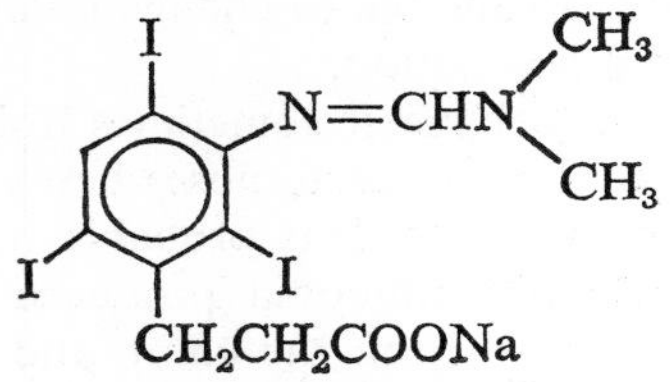

Sodium ipodate

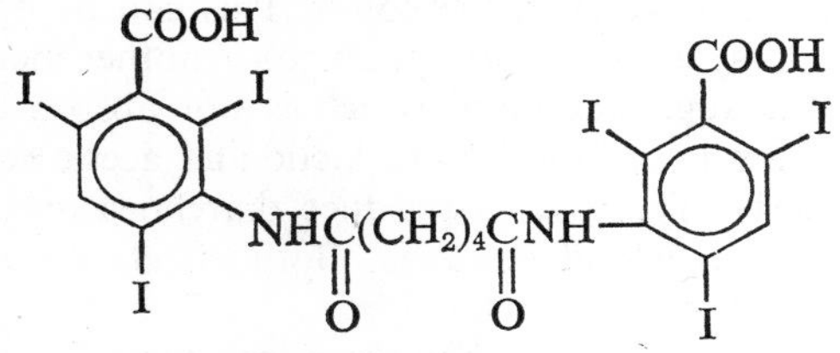

Sodium iodipamide

is also the explanation for the transient elevation of serum bilirubin which may follow cholecystography. Adequate visualization depends on a normally functioning liver. The main adverse effects of these drugs are hypotension and rarely acute renal failure, both of which are more likely to occur in the patient with hepatic impairment. They also remain bound to plasma protein for months after their use and this interferes with the estimation of protein bound iodine as a measure of thyroid function.

Halogenated substances can also be used to visualize the alimentary tract, for example meglumine diatrizoate (gastrografin), the radioactive component of which is diatrizic acid.

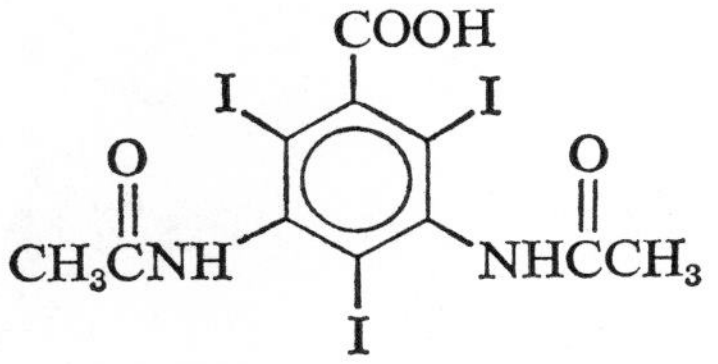

Diatrizic acid

Barium sulphate is the mainstay of alimentary roentgenography because of its insolubility in body fluids and its opacity to X-rays.

DRUGS USED TO ALTER THE BACTERIAL FLORA OF THE BOWEL

Most micro-organisms harboured in the intestines in health can exert pathological effects under certain conditions. Conversely many bacteria which are classified as pathogens can persist *in vivo* without causing overt disease. The effects of antibiotics on such pathogens are described in chap. 20. However, under certain clinical circumstances it is valuable to change quantitatively the normal bacterial population.

Psychiatric disturbances sometimes follow the development of abnormal anastomoses between the portal and systemic circulations. It is probable that toxic substances, in particular ammonia produced by bacterial ureases, are absorbed from the colon and pass directly into the systemic veins without passing through the liver. Clinical improvement can be achieved by reducing the numbers of bacteria in the colon. This can be done by giving neomycin by mouth (p. 20.30). Another method is to use the sugar lactulose which is not absorbed, and in the colon is metabolized to lactic and acetic acids by the bacteria. These acids produce diarrhoea and lower pH of the intestinal contents. Both effects reduce the number of bacteria in the colon.

Proliferation of bacteria in the upper part of the intestine, e.g. in diverticula or blind loops, affects the metabolism of bile salts and causes steatorrhoea; the bacteria also bind and utilize vitamin B_{12} so that it is not absorbed. Under certain circumstances it can be shown that oral tetracycline improves fat and vitamin B_{12} absorption and reduces the number of bacteria present. Neo-mycin also reduces the number of bacteria but induces a mild degree of malabsorption of fat and other nutrients. Neomycin, being a polybasic substance, binds bile salts in the same manner as cholestyramine (p. 10.12).

FURTHER READING

CONNEY A.H. (1967) Pharmacological implications of microsomal enzyme induction. *Pharm. Rev.*, **19**, 317.

HAVERBACK B.J. & DYCE B.J. (1967) Vasoactive substances and the gastrointestinal tract. *Gastroenterology*, **53**, 326.

HOLZ S. (1968) Drug action on the digestive system. *Ann. Rev. Pharmacol.* **8**, 171.

LANGMAN M.J.S. (1968) Carbenoxolone sodium. *Gut*, **9**, 5.

MOORE J.G. & ENGLERT E. (1967) Some pitfalls in anti-secretory drug trials. *Amer. J. dig. Dis.* **12**, 973.

PIPER, D.W. (1967) Antacids and anticholinergic drug therapy of peptic ulcer. *Gastroenterology*, **52**, 1009.

TURNER M.D., MILLES L.L., & SEGAL H.L. (1967) Gastric protease and protease inhibitors. *Gastroenterology*, **53**, 967.

Chapter 11
Drugs that influence renal function

The relation of the kidney to the action of drugs is important from two different points of view. The kidney is the major excretory organ for a large number of drugs and their derivatives. Changes in renal function therefore have a profound effect upon the rate of excretion of the drug in the urine and upon the duration of drug action. The mechanisms by which the normal kidney excretes drugs are described on p. 2.15. In addition, a number of drugs act directly on the kidney and are capable of altering renal function. Many of these are useful in correcting abnormalities of kidney function which arise in the course of disease. Drugs influence renal function either by altering renal tubular activity or by changing the rate of glomerular filtration or renal blood flow. Drugs which influence tubular transport mechanisms are pharmacologically and clinically by far the most important.

DIURETIC AGENTS

Diuretics are loosely defined as agents which increase the flow of urine. In this sense water and alcohol are diuretics, for it is common knowledge that consumption of either gives rise to an increase in the rate of urine flow. The ingestion and absorption of water dilutes the body fluids and this inhibits the release of ADH by the posterior pituitary. The ensuing water diuresis is sufficient to eliminate a volume of water equal to the amount ingested and, unless very large volumes of water are taken, there is little change in the excretion of electrolytes. Alcohol is customarily taken with large volumes of fluid as a beverage. Alcohol itself, however, induces a water diuresis by a direct action on the supraopticohypophyseal system, inhibiting the secretion of ADH. Taken orally by itself or injected directly into the carotid artery of experimental animals, alcohol produces a temporary diabetes insipidus with a marked water diuresis leading to water depletion, again with only slight electrolyte loss.

The clinical need for diuretics which significantly increase electrolyte as well as water excretion arises from the fact that in oedema, which commonly accompanies many diseases, salt accumulates in the body as well as water. Thus, agents which increase the urinary elimination of both components of oedema fluid are much more effective than those which increase the rate of water

excretion alone. Prior to the discovery of the modern diuretics, excessive retention of water and salt within the body was commonly fatal.

The history of the discovery of diuretic drugs has followed a consistent pattern. It has usually begun with the accidental discovery of the diuretic property of a drug used for an entirely different clinical purpose. This has led to pharmacological investigations to modify the molecular structure and increase the potency of the compound. At present the number of powerful and clinically effective diuretic drugs is almost embarrassingly large, and the details of their clinical use are given in vol. 3.

A satisfactory classification of diuretics is difficult to achieve. The following is based upon the main mechanism of action of the diuretics (table 11.1). It is imperfect

TABLE 11.1. Classification of diuretics.

Drugs which act primarily on the renal circulation
  Digitalis glycosides
  Colloidal substances
  Xanthine derivatives*

Osmotic diuretics
  Mannitol, urea, sodium sulphate

Acidifying agents
  Ammonium chloride

Drugs which specifically inhibit Na^+ transport, interfere with Na^+/H^+ exchange or alter tubular cell permeability to ions
  Organic mercurial diuretics
  Carbonic anhydrase inhibitors
  Benzothiadiazides, frusemide and other sulphonamyl diuretics
  Ethacrynic acid
  Aldosterone antagonists
  Triamterene

---

* Some xanthine derivatives act predominantly by inhibiting Na^+ transport.

because several diuretics act in more than one way. With the exception of the use of digitalis glycosides in cardiac failure, diuretics which improve the renal circulation or act as acidifying or osmotic agents are weak compared with more recently discovered compounds and are usually employed in a supporting role. The modern chemical diuretics specifically inhibit the transport of sodium ions by the renal tubules or alter the cell permeability to ions; some interfere with Na^+/H^+ exchange. They are generally employed as the first choice in the treatment of oedema.

Drugs that act primarily on the renal circulation

The rate of glomerular filtration is raised by agents which increase renal blood flow, cardiac output or blood volume.

CARDIAC GLYCOSIDES

The classic description of William Withering (p. 8.1) of the effect of digitalis in ameliorating dropsy did not link its diuretic properties with its action on the heart. Indeed, it was not until a few years afterwards that the primary cardiac effect was recognized and the renal activity relegated to a secondary place. Thus digitalis glycosides increase the cardiac output of the failing heart and cause a secondary rise in renal blood flow and filtration, with increased elimination of water and salt and the relief of oedema. The dependence of the diuretic properties of digitalis glycosides upon improvement in cardiac function is confirmed by the fact that they have little diuretic effect in healthy individuals or in patients with oedema of noncardiac origin. In recent years digitalis glycosides have been shown to have a small but definite inhibitory effect on sodium reabsorption by the renal tubules and on active sodium transport in other cells. Whether this effect is related to the steroid configuration of the glycosides and to the superficial resemblance they bear to aldosterone or cortisol is unknown. In any case it appears to be of minor importance compared with their action on the heart (p. 8.3).

COLLOIDAL SUBSTANCES

When the blood volume is reduced because of blood loss or because of a fall in the concentration of plasma proteins, renal blood flow (RBF) and glomerular filtration rate (GFR) fall. As a result the rate of urine flow is reduced. If colloidal substances are then given intravenously, plasma volume may be restored, RBF and GFR rise and urine flow increases. Colloidal substances are occasionally used as diuretics in oedema due to loss of plasma proteins (p. 26.11). The best preparation in these circumstances is salt-poor albumin. This is prepared by fractionating human blood plasma and is given slowly by intravenous injection in amounts of 20 g dissolved in sterile water. In view of its expense, attempts have been made to discover other substances which might act as plasma expanders. Of these the most successful is dextran.

Dextran

Dextran is a naturally occurring branched polysaccharide with a molecular weight of about 40 million. The glucose units are joined by glucoside linkages. By controlled hydrolysis, dextrans of a wide range of molecular weight may be produced. When used as a plasma expander, the average molecular weight is 70,000–80,000. Given as a 10 per cent solution it causes an increase in blood volume, cardiac output and renal blood flow. Small molecular weight fractions of dextran are excreted in the urine while the larger particles remain in the body for days or weeks and are slowly oxidized. The greatest disadvantage of the large molecular weight fractions of dextran is that they are antigenic and allergic reactions occasionally occur.

In recent years dextrans of lower molecular weight (20,000–40,000) have become available. While this mixture does not act as a plasma expander it may have a desirable effect on the microcirculation in shock in which it is claimed to reduce the stasis and the aggregation of red blood cells and platelets (p. 26.5).

XANTHINES AND AMINOURACILS

The diuretic action of coffee and to a lesser extent of tea is well known to most of us. It is due to the xanthines (p. 5.39) which they contain and which have been used as diuretics for over 100 years. In comparison with modern diuretic drugs they are weak and nowadays their use is limited to a supporting role. Xanthines have widespread pharmacological effects but promote a mild transient diuresis which was originally shown in isolated perfused kidney preparations. In intact animals, however, a large part of their diuretic action is due to an increase in RBF. The GFR may also be increased either as a result of a rise in cardiac output or by a direct effect on the renal afferent arteriole. However, the xanthines also depress renal tubular reabsorption of NaCl in man, and this effect contributes to their diuretic action.

Theophylline is the most powerful of all the xanthine diuretics and it is most commonly employed as aminophylline (theophylline ethylenediamine, p. 5.39). Its cellular mode of action as a diuretic is unknown but theophylline increases the permeability of the amphibian bladder in a way similar to vasopressin. This effect and other cellular metabolic effects of theophylline appears to depend upon the fact that methylxanthines, particularly theophylline, are competitive inhibitors of phosphodiesterase, an enzyme which inactivates cyclic 3'5'-AMP (15.13). The relation of this action to the diuretic effect of the drug is unknown.

The diuretic activity of the xanthines has led to the synthesis of a large number of related heterocyclic nitrogenous compounds in a search for improved diuretic activity. **Aminometradine** is representative of this group. It has an effect similar to that of theophylline on the renal tubules causing an increased excretion of water and NaCl. Neither compound influences urinary pH or HCO_3^- excretion. Unlike aminophylline, however, aminometradine has no effect on RBF or GFR. No information is available on its site of action within the nephron.

Aminophylline is particularly useful in increasing the effectiveness of more powerful diuretics in acute cardiac failure. For this purpose it should be given intravenously (0·25–0·5 g) 1 hour after the main diuretic has been given, when a significant potentiation of the diuretic response occurs. Aminometradine is given orally but is of limited value in view of its weak diuretic potency.

Osmotic diuretics

Any substance filtered by the glomerulus and subsequently excreted largely in the urine acts as an osmotic diuretic. In health the urinary volume depends in part on the quantity of urea to be excreted and urea is a natural diuretic. The diuresis occurs because osmotically active molecules within the tubular lumen reduce the passive reabsorption in various parts of the nephron. Similarly the diuresis of diabetes mellitus is due to the osmotic action in the tubules of the excess glucose which cannot be absorbed. An ideal osmotic diuretic is a substance of small molecular weight and high osmotic activity which, when introduced into the blood stream, is completely filtered by the glomerulus and not reabsorbed at all by the renal tubules. As water is reabsorbed by the tubules in response to active sodium transport, the concentration of an osmotic diuretic in the tubular fluid increases, so that it contributes significantly to the osmolal concentration. Tubular water reabsorption is thus reduced to an extent which depends on the osmotic concentration of the diuretic, and renal excretion of water is increased. However, osmotic diuretics increase not only the rate of water excretion but also that of NaCl. Sodium reabsorption itself is limited by a concentration gradient across the tubular lumen (vol. 1, p. 33.14). Thus, when a nonreabsorbable osmotically active substance retains water within the tubular fluid, sodium is reabsorbed only up to its limiting concentration. The presence of excess water within the renal tubule thus reduces the amount of sodium which can be reabsorbed and this is excreted in the urine. **Mannitol,** an inert sugar, meets many of the criteria of an ideal osmotic diuretic. Its renal clearance is nearly as high as that of inulin. It is, however, a much smaller molecule having the same molecular weight as glucose. However, in contrast, almost none is absorbed by the renal tubules. A suitable dose is 10 ml/kg of a 10 per cent solution in water given intravenously. Urea given by mouth also leads to an osmotic diuresis, but it is less effective than mannitol, because about 50 per cent is reabsorbed by the tubules. Glucose is an unsatisfactory osmotic diuretic since it is entirely reabsorbed by the tubules at normal blood concentrations.

The clinical indications for the use of osmotic diuretics are limited; they are employed usually to supplement the activity of diuretics which block tubular sodium transport chemically. Mannitol has also been recommended in the treatment of oliguria in acute renal failure but its value and mechanism of action in this disease are controversial.

Electrolytes may act as osmotic diuretics. Sodium sulphate introduced into the circulation is capable of inducing an osmotic diuresis because the sulphate ion is largely unreabsorbed. When given to oedematous subjects, however, its activity is slight and it has now fallen into disuse.

Acidifying drugs

AMMONIUM CHLORIDE

The diuretic properties of acidifying drugs were described over 50 years ago. Only ammonium chloride remains in use. It induces a mild temporary diuresis and increases the acidity of the urine. The NH_4^+ is converted in the liver to urea and H^+ is released. The hydrochloric acid thus formed is buffered and Cl^- is excreted in the urine initially as its sodium and potassium salts and a slight negative balance of these cations occurs. In the course of a few days, however, filtered Na^+ is conserved in exchange for H^+, some of which are combined with ammonia generated in the renal tubular cells. The amount of ammonium chloride then excreted in the urine equals the amount of ammonium chloride originally ingested and the sodium excretion falls. Nowadays ammonium chloride is used clinically only to test the acidifying power of the kidney and occasionally to potentiate the action of mercurial diuretics (p. 11.4). It is best given by mouth in doses of 2–4 g/day but tends to cause nausea.

Drugs that interfere with Na⁺ transport

These drugs reversibly inhibit tubular cell mechanisms concerned with sodium transport. They do so either by interfering with the reabsorption of sodium chloride or with Na^+/H^+ exchange which reduces the reabsorption of sodium bicarbonate. Some exert both effects though not usually to the same degree. Important pharmacological problems concern their cellular mode of action and the site of action within the nephron. Little is known of the cellular mechanisms involved. Some, notably the mercurial diuretics and ethacrynic acid, combine reversibly with SH groups in the renal tubules. Their diuretic activity may be due to interference with enzymes which are dependent for their activity on these groups. Others interfere with Na^+/H^+ exchange by reversible inhibition of carbonic anhydrase.

Knowledge of the site of action of diuretics within the nephron is imperfect and has been obtained largely from three types of study:

(1) stop–flow experiments in animals,

(2) studies of relationships between solute and water excretion in animals and in man, and

(3) micropuncture studies.

In stop–flow experiments an osmotic diuresis is first established by the infusion of mannitol. The ureter is then clamped for 5–10 min, when a stationary column of fluid is held in contact with the tubular cells. These cells then act on this static column of tubular fluid at different levels within the nephron and perform in an exaggerated way their normal operations. The ureteric clamp is then released and the urine is collected in twenty to forty small serial samples. The composition of the samples of urine collected first reflects distal tubular activity, while those collected last indicate the influence of the proximal tubules. One shortcoming of this method is that urine collected from the proximal tubules has to pass the distal system before it is excreted and its composition may be modified at this site.

Analysis of solute–water relationships is based on the knowledge that concentration or dilution of urine occurs in the distal tubules or loop of Henle. Diuretics which interfere with the concentrating or diluting ability of the kidneys must act in regions of the nephron beyond the end of the proximal convoluted tubule.

Micropuncture studies are likely to provide the most direct information on the site of action. The results of these studies, however, are difficult to interpret; this is due to the fact that reduction in the tubular reabsorption of salt and water induced by diuretics in one part of the nephron, alters the hydrostatic pressure and rate of flow of fluid throughout the nephron and causes secondary changes in reabsorptive activity.

Important comparisons between the chemical diuretics concern their relative potency and the pattern of electrolytes eliminated in response to them. The activity of diuretics can be tested in normal or salt loaded animals or in patients with oedema in a stable state. It must be remembered, however, that diuretics may not be equally active in oedema due to different causes. Fig. 11.1 gives a summary of the relative potency and pattern of electrolyte excretion of the more important chemical diuretics discussed here.

MERCURIAL DIURETICS

The diuretic properties of organic mercurial compounds were discovered as a result of a chance observation in 1920 upon a patient receiving an organic mercurial compound for the treatment of syphilis. These drugs were the first powerful inhibitors of sodium transport to be discovered. While their importance in clinical medicine has fallen in recent years, the description of their pharmacological properties is given in detail as they remain the arbitrary standard against which the potency and usefulness of other newer diuretics are compared. They also

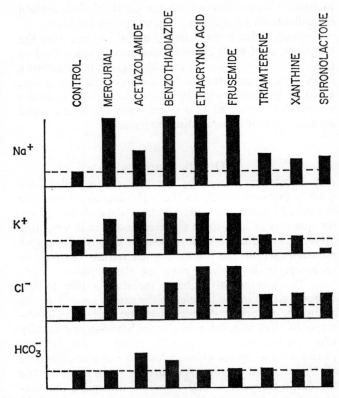

FIG. 11.1. Relative potency and pattern of electrolyte excretion in common diuretics given as a single therapeutic dose.

illustrate some of the classical methods used in the investigation of diuretics. The injection of a small dose of an organic mercurial diuretic into one renal artery results in an increased urinary excretion mainly of NaCl and water which is confined initially to the injected kidney. The diuresis occurs in the absence of a measurable increase in GFR and is therefore due to interference with tubular reabsorption. The negative potential which exists in the lumen of the proximal tubule of the Necturus is greatly reduced by mercurial diuretics. This is consistent with a primary effect of the drug on active Na^+ transport, Cl^- transport being reduced secondarily. The tubules then reabsorb less water because they reabsorb less sodium chloride.

Stop–flow studies in dogs have suggested that the proximal tubule is a major site of action, the reabsorption of sodium in the proximal portion of the nephron being strikingly depressed (fig. 11.2). Other evidence points to a more distal site of action. The maximum capacity to reabsorb solute-free water (Tc_{H_2O}) under the influence of vasopressin is reduced by mercurial diuretics. Furthermore, when mercurial diuretics are given to dogs excreting moderate amounts of potassium, a fall in urinary K^+ occurs which is probably due to an inhibition of distal

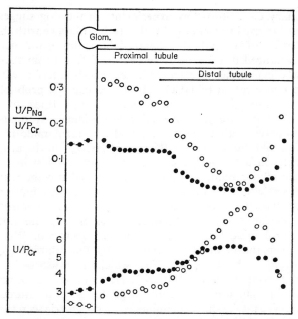

FIG. 11.2. Stop–flow experiment in dog, ●, control samples; ○, after mercurial diuretic. Reduction in Na⁺ reabsorption in the proximal tubule is shown. Reduction in U/P creatinine is due to the increased amount of water in the tubular lumen. After Kessler R.H. *et al.* (1958) *Amer. J. Physiol.* **194**, 540.

tubular K^+ secretion. The secretion of H^+ is not affected by mercurial diuretics. Micropuncture studies confirm a distal site of action of mercurial diuretics but, for reasons discussed on p. 11.4, have so far failed to show that they act proximally.

At a cellular level, mercurial diuretics may react with the SH groups of enzymes providing energy for sodium transport. Their diuretic effect can be prevented or reversed by dimercaprol (p. 10.12) which has a greater affinity for mercury than do the SH groups in renal enzymes. However, the diuretic effect of mercurial compounds cannot be explained solely by this mechanism. The compound, *p*-chloromercuribenzoate, also reacts with SH groups and is concentrated in the tissues of the kidney and yet is devoid of diuretic activity. Another theory is that the capacity for slow release of free divalent mercuric ions determines the diuretic properties of a particular compound. A divalent mercuric ion could block two adjacent sites of a receptor by attaching itself to a sulphydryl group and an amino or carboxyl group as follows:

$$\underset{Hg-O}{\overset{S\ \ \ \ \ \ \ \ C=O}{|\ \ \ \ \ \ \ \ \ \ |}} \qquad \underset{Hg-O}{\overset{S\ \ \ \ \ \ \ \ N-H}{|\ \ \ \ \ \ \ \ \ \ |}}$$

The potentiation of the activity of certain mercurials by ammonium chloride or other acidifying agents may be due to the increase in the number of divalent mercurial ions capable of making a two-point attachment with receptor sites, possibly on the cell membrane or enzyme. One important observation, however, cannot be reconciled by this otherwise attractive theory. The inhalation of 10 per cent CO_2 in dogs, which ought to be an effective means of lowering cell pH, fails to potentiate the diuretic activity of mercurials. Nevertheless, the dependence of mercurial diuretic activity upon acid base balance is reflected by the diminution in the response which occurs in metabolic alkalosis.

Most mercurial diuretics are essentially derivatives of mercuripropanol and have the general formula:

$$\overset{OR_1}{\underset{\beta\ \ \ \ \ \ \ \ \alpha}{R_2-CH_2-\overset{|}{C}H-CH_2-Hg-X}}$$

When the β-carbon is unsubstituted, the compound is non-diuretic. However, it is substituted (R_1) usually by a hydroxy, methoxy or ethoxy group and R_2 is a complex organic moiety of aromatic or heterocyclic rings or an aliphatic chain. It has been argued that the diuretic properties of organic mercurials depend not upon the ability to yield a divalent mercuric ion but upon configuration of the molecule as a whole. Many of these have the terminal univalent mercury atom separated by three carbon atoms, or their steric equivalent, from a terminal hydrophilic group R:

$$\overset{Hg^+ \qquad\qquad R}{\underset{C-C-C}{\frown\qquad\frown}}$$

However, there appear to be exceptions to this rule.

The most important mercurial diuretics are **mersalyl, meralluride** and **mercaptomerin**. Mersalyl and meralluride both contain equimolar amounts of theophylline attached at the X position, which encourages more rapid absorption from the site of injection. These compounds are not effective by mouth and need to be given by intramuscular injection. The diuresis starts within an hour and usually lasts for several hours. In general the diuresis is associated with an almost equivalent loss of Na^+ and Cl^- and there is initially no loss of HCO_3^- or K^+. Repeated doses thus deplete the body of Na^+ and Cl^- and a progressive rise in plasma HCO_3^- occurs as the volume of extracellular fluid shrinks. This contraction alkalosis is an acid base disturbance which might be expected to be adjusted spontaneously by the renal excretion of HCO_3^- during intervals between injections. While this may occur, alkalosis often persists, especially if the diet is low in NaCl. In these circumstances Cl^- deficiency may promote the tubular reabsorption of HCO_3^- and raise the threshold level of plasma HCO_3^- (vol. 1, p. 33.26), thus helping to perpetuate the alkalosis. Excessive urinary loss of K^+ may develop if the diuretics are administered for long periods of time and combined with low salt diets. In these circumstances more of the Na^+ which escapes reabsorption in the proximal parts of the nephron appears to be reabsorbed distally in exchange for K^+ and H^+ ions so that the final urine contains Cl^- with balancing amounts of K^+ and NH_4^+ and relatively little Na^+. Resistance to the action of mercurial diuretics may develop as a result of metabolic alkalosis or if the rate of glomerular filtration is greatly reduced.

Immediate and fatal reactions have been reported with the intravenous use of these drugs. Death is then due to ventricular fibrillation and is the result of a hypersensitivity reaction. Less severe reactions include flushing, pruritus, urticaria, dermatitis, fever, nausea and vomiting. Most of the mercury of a single dose is excreted in the urine within 24 hours. If mercurial diuretics are given too frequently or to individuals with reduced renal function, systemic mercury poisoning may develop with gingivitis, stomatitis and colitis. A direct nephrotoxic effect is also seen; this includes tubular necrosis, massive proteinuria and finally oliguria or anuria and acute renal failure. Mersalyl, meralluride and mercaptomerin are given by intramuscular injection to adults in doses of 1–2 ml. Each ml contains 39–40 mg Hg.

INHIBITORS OF CARBONIC ANHYDRASE

During the last 10 years a number of drugs have been discovered which cause diuresis when given by mouth. Many belong to the sulphonamyl group which contains an unsubstituted sulphonamyl radicle, $—SO_2NH_2$, or give rise to metabolites which contain this group. These substances are potent inhibitors of carbonic anhydrase and the first to be discovered, **acetazolamide**, owes its diuretic properties solely to its ability to inhibit the enzyme (vol. 1, p. 33.22).

When sulphanilamide was first introduced (p. 20.2) it was observed that it led occasionally to the development of acidosis, a rise in urinary pH and an increase in the excretion of Na^+, K^+, HCO_3^- and water. A large number of sulphonamides were synthesized and ultimately acetazolamide (diamox) was discovered.

Acetazolamide   Sulphanilamide

Studies of the enzyme kinetics in purified systems suggest that acetazolamide is a non-competitive inhibitor of carbonic anhydrase. It is rapidly absorbed from the gastrointestinal tract and causes an increase in the urinary excretion of Na^+, K^+, HCO_3^- and water within 30 min. The urinary pH rises and there is little or no increase in urinary Cl^-. Stop–flow experiments in the dog suggest that the rise in urinary pH is due to interference with the secretion of H^+ in the distal part of the nephron, and there is enhanced distal tubular secretion of K^+. From these and other studies, acetazolamide appears to interfere with the reabsorption of HCO_3^- by H^+ exchange, probably throughout the entire nephron, and this leads to a marked increase in the excretion of sodium bicarbonate. Compared with organic mercurials, acetazolamide is a weak diuretic. Moreover the loss of HCO_3^- in the urine results in a fall in the concentration of this ion in the extracellular fluid, so that with continued use the drug loses its efficacy. The resulting acidosis may also interfere with its action. Hydrogen and potassium ions compete for exchange with Na^+, which probably explains how acetazolamide leads to increased K^+ secretion. When the generation of H^+ is blocked by the inhibition of carbonic anhydrase, any Na^+ which is reabsorbed requires to be exchanged for K^+. Doses of acetazolamide that in man are sufficiently large to have a diuretic effect (10 mg/kg) have no influence on the gastric secretion of hydrochloric acid or upon the transport of carbon dioxide in the red blood cells, in both of which carbonic anhydrase is involved. The drug, however, may cause paraesthesia, drowsiness and disorientation, possibly due to its effect on carbonic anhydrase in the brain. It may also inhibit carbonic anhydrase present in the ciliary processes of the eye. This results in a fall in the intra-ocular tension and, for this reason, the drug is sometimes used in the treatment of glaucoma. None of these adverse effects is serious. Hypersensitivity is rare but may result in depression of the bone marrow, skin reactions and fever. Renal calculi have been produced in experimental animals.

Newer carbonic anhydrase inhibitors include **ethoxyzolamide** and **dichlorphenamide**, which is a disulphonamide and is ten times more potent than acetazolamide. These drugs and the parent compound have essentially similar actions.

Ethoxyzolamide   Dichlorphenamide

Oral doses of 0·5–1 g are rapidly absorbed and diuresis may persist for over 24 hours.

BENZOTHIADIAZIDES

In attempts to find carbonic anhydrase inhibitors more potent than acetazolamide, benzenedisulphonamides were

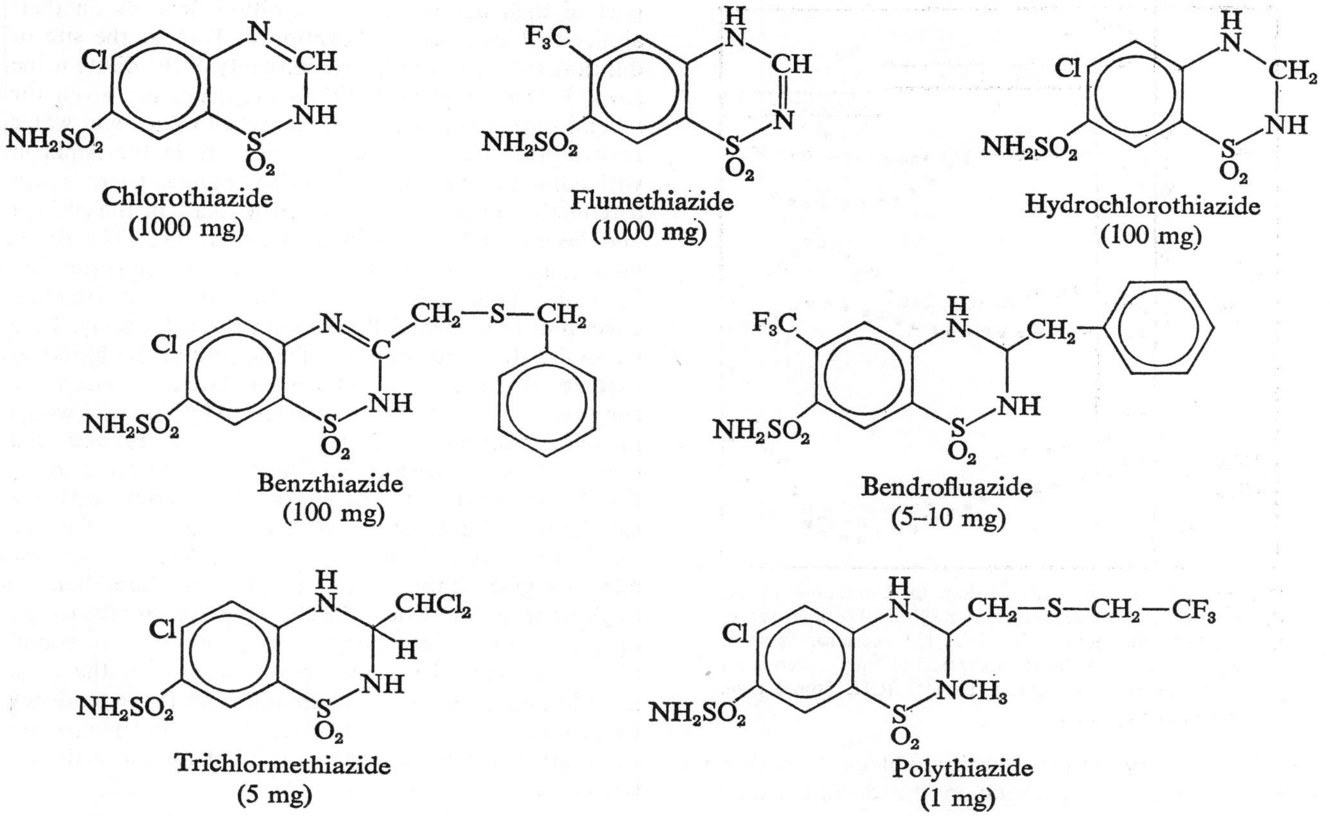

FIG. 11.3. Some benzothiadiazide drugs. The usual adult dose for each compound is indicated to show their relative potency.

examined. During synthesis a two-ring compound was formed which caused a marked increase in the urinary excretion of sodium and chloride, a response very different from that of the older carbonic acid inhibitors. This substance was called chlorothiazide. The basic molecule has since been modified in various ways and a number of these are now available (fig. 11.3). **Chlorothiazide** and **flumethiazide** are poorly absorbed from the gastrointestinal tract and over 80 per cent can be recovered from the faeces. After absorption they are distributed in the extracellular fluid and do not penetrate cell membranes readily. Other benzothiadiazine compounds are better absorbed from the gut and because of a greater lipid solubility can enter the cells as well as the extracellular fluid. This increases the activity of the drug per unit weight.

Chlorothiazide and other benzothiadiazines either by mouth or by intravenous injection cause a diuresis of Na^+, K^+, Cl^-, HCO_3^- and water. With low doses the increased excretion of Na^+ and Cl^- is most prominent, while at higher doses the secretion of H^+ is also depressed and HCO_3^- excretion increased. The drugs therefore combine the properties of carbonic anhydrase inhibitors with the ability to induce a marked diuresis of Na^+ and

Cl^-, and it is to this latter effect that they owe their powerful diuretic properties. Stop–flow studies have been carried out in dogs in order to try to determine the sites of action of chlorothiazide. Fig. 11.4 compares the pattern seen after the administration of a relatively large dose (10 mg/kg body weight/hr) with that seen in the preceding control period. Because of the size of the dose, the effects of carbonic anhydrase inhibition are particularly well marked. They are shown by the depression of distal tubular secretion of H^+ and the enhanced secretion of K^+ in this region. Proximal tubular reabsorption of Na^+ and Cl^- is also seen to be depressed. The experiment also showed that chlorothiazide is secreted into the proximal tubules, the U/P ratio for chlorothiazide exceeding that for creatinine. However, there is other independent evidence which suggests that Na^+ and Cl^- reabsorption is diminished also in the distal nephron. The renal capacity to form a dilute urine, i.e. to excrete water free of solute, depends primarily upon the absorption of sodium from the tubular fluid in a portion of the distal nephron which, in the absence of vasopressin, is relatively impermeable to water (vol. 1, p. 33.14). Chlorothiazide and its derivatives reduce the capacity of the kidney to excrete solute-free water in man, and they

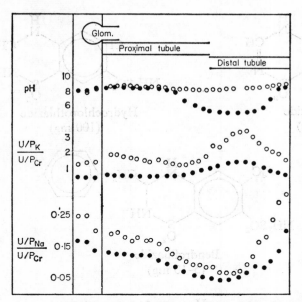

FIG. 11.4. Stop–flow study in dog. ●, Control samples; ○, after chlorothiazide. Depression of distal tubular secretion of H^+ and increase in distal K^+ secretion is seen. Some decrease in tubular reabsorption of Na^+ is seen in all parts of the nephron. After Kessler R.H. (1962) *Clin. Pharmacol. Ther.* **3**, 109.

owe this property to their capacity to block the reabsorption of sodium and chloride in the distal convoluted tubule.

Their activity is not blocked by dimercaprol and is uninfluenced by metabolic alkalosis or acidosis. When chlorothiazide is given to an animal under the influence of a mercurial diuretic, a further brisk diuresis of NaCl and water occurs. This does not depend upon its ability to inhibit carbonic anhydrase, and there is little correlation between the ability of the different drugs to inhibit this enzyme *in vitro* and their capacity to induce a sodium chloride diuresis in the living animal. A free $—SO_2NH_2$ group is necessary for carbonic anhydrase inhibitory activity, and stable substitutions of this group destroy activity. If this is done, the capacity to eliminate NaCl is reduced, but is not abolished. The increased loss of K^+ which occurs is due both to the delivery of large amounts of Na^+ to the distal part of the nephron, where K^+ is secreted in exchange for Na^+, and to the inhibition of the Na^+/H^+ exchange at this site.

Benzothiadiazine drugs have a number of other effects. Paradoxically, they reduce urinary output in experimental animals with diabetes insipidus induced by damage to the hypophyseal–posterior pituitary system and in many patients with diabetes insipidus. The mechanism by which this is brought about is obscure but the drugs do not possess vasopressin-like properties, nor do they increase the capacity of the patient with diabetes insipidus to form a urine more concentrated than plasma. It is likely that part of their action in this condition depends on their ability to block the reabsorption of Na^+ at the site of dilution, thereby raising the osmolality of the dilute urine towards that of plasma. When the drugs are given for several days a compensatory increase in Na^+ and water reabsorption occurs at some other site in the nephron with consequent reduction in urine volume. There is also a reduction in the concentration of Na^+ in the plasma and because of this the patient drinks less. The drugs also cause a fall in blood pressure in hypertension in man. This may be due to their salt-depleting effect and to a slight fall in blood volume (p. 8.11). They also raise the concentration of uric acid in the blood so that attacks of gout may be precipitated in susceptible subjects. Uric acid is normally secreted by a process which involves glomerular filtration, proximal tubular cell reabsorption and secretion. Chlorothiazide secreted by the proximal tubular cells appears to interfere with the tubular secretion of uric acid, as a consequence of which its clearance is reduced. These drugs have an adverse effect on glucose tolerance and may precipitate diabetes mellitus in prediabetic subjects. Hypersensitivity to the drug is rare but thrombocytopenia, agranulocytosis and aplastic anaemia have been reported. One of the most troublesome effects of benzothiadiazines is the tendency to produce K^+ depletion. Potassium supplements are necessary when the diuretics are used for more than a few days.

CHLORTHALIDONE

Although this sulphonamyl drug is not a benzothiadiazide, it possesses similar properties and combines a slight degree of carbonic anhydrase inhibiting power with the power to increase the excretion of NaCl. In a dose of 100–200 mg/day its diuretic action lasts over 24 hours.

Chlorthalidone

CLOPAMIDE

Clopamide is another nonthiazide substituted sulphonamyl halogen benzene derivative which contains a bridge N—N group similar to some hydrazine compounds and has the formula shown opposite.

The hydrazine group here does not inhibit monoamine oxidases. The compound is about 200 times more potent than chlorothiazide in terms of its effect on NaCl excretion and about ten times less active as a carbonic anhydrase

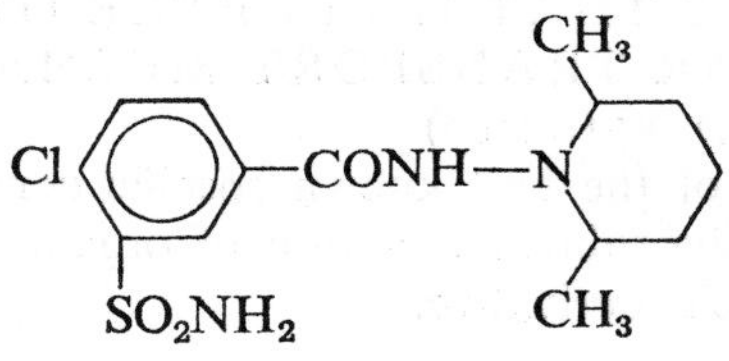

Clopamide

inhibitor. Early results suggest that in man it increases the urinary excretion of equivalent amounts of Na^+ and Cl^- and has little effect on K^+ or H^+ secretion.

FRUSEMIDE (FUROSEMIDE)

With the success of the benzothiadiazine drugs, a large number of sulphonamyl analogues have been studied. Frusemide is an important and extremely powerful compound in which the thiadiazine ring, common to the thiazide drugs, has been replaced by a furfuryl group substituted in the amino nitrogen of the anthranilic acid.

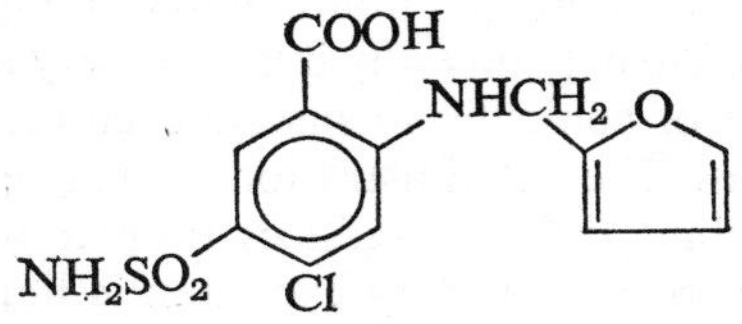

Frusemide

When this substance is given orally or intravenously to man, diuresis starts at once, is extremely intense and lasts up to 6 hours.

Experimental studies show that it acts on the proximal and distal tubules. Carbonic anhydrase is not inhibited although there is often a large K^+ loss in the urine. Proximal tubular inhibition occurs at the height of the diuresis in man since Na^+ excretion may rise to 60 per cent of the filtered load, more than twice the level reached after thiazide drugs. The greater diuretic potency of frusemide is not solely due to more complete inhibition of Na^+ reabsorption at the same site of action as other diuretics with the sulphonamyl group. Under hydropenic conditions water reabsorption (Tc_{H_2O}) is almost completely inhibited in man. This may be due to inhibition of Na^+ reabsorption in the loop of Henle or to interference with the equilibration of fluid between the collecting duct and the medullary interstitial fluid. The drug has also been shown to reduce the excretion of solute-free water due to a direct action on the diluting segment in the distal tubule. These marked effects on the concentrating and diluting abilities of the kidney are shared only by ethacrynic acid to which it is structurally unrelated.

Frusemide is a drug of great clinical value and is indicated especially in the treatment of severe pulmonary oedema attended by excessive water retention and hyponatraemia. The drug appears to have no serious adverse properties although major degrees of electrolyte imbalance may quickly result from massive diuresis produced in very oedematous subjects. A suitable dose is 40–80 mg/day.

ETHACRYNIC ACID

A search for compounds which might react with renal SH groups in a way similar to organic mercurials (p. 11.5) led to the synthesis of ethacrynic acid, an unsaturated ketone derivative of ardyloxyacetic acid.

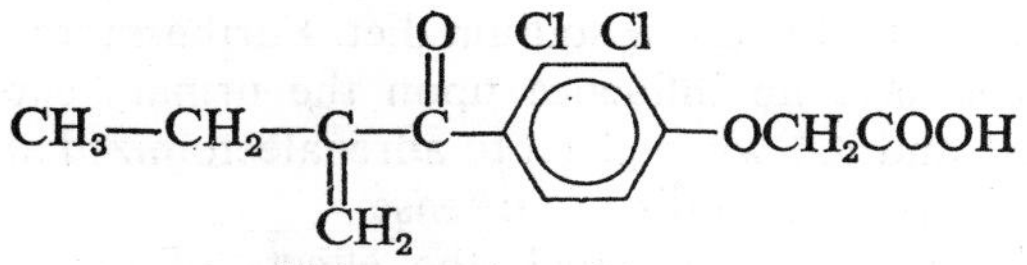

Ethacrynic acid

It causes a reduction of protein-bound SH groups in all segments of the nephron. Diuresis follows rapidly after an oral or intravenous dose and the urine contains increased amounts of Na^+, Cl^- and K^+, but not HCO_3^-. The drug does not inhibit carbonic anhydrase *in vitro*. As with frusemide, the amount of sodium excreted at the height of a diuresis indicates that the drug acts at all sites of active sodium transport within the nephron. It shares with frusemide the property of reducing the concentrating power of the kidney as well as the ability to dilute the urine, and therefore it acts on the ascending limb of the loop of Henle and possibly on the distal diluting system. For this reason its use is indicated in severe oedema when the plasma Na^+ level is low. An increase in blood uric acid and a metabolic alkalosis arising from K^+ and Cl^- deficiency may occur with its use. A suitable dose is 50–100 mg/day. Few adverse effects occur but nerve deafness has been reported.

ALDOSTERONE ANTAGONISTS

The role of aldosterone in conserving body sodium is well known. It was therefore natural to look for chemical analogues which might oppose its physiological action and so cause loss of sodium.

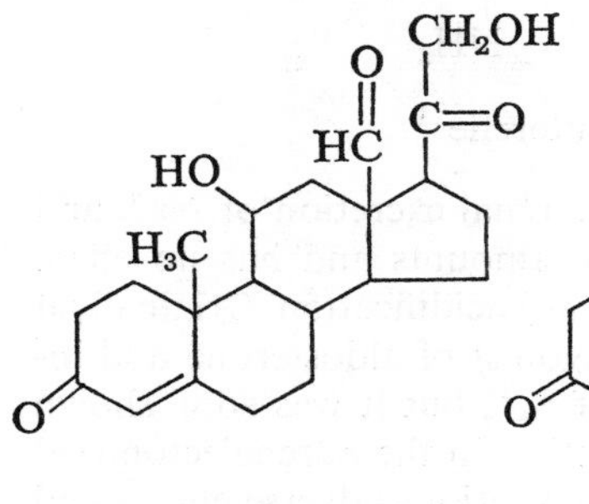

Aldosterone 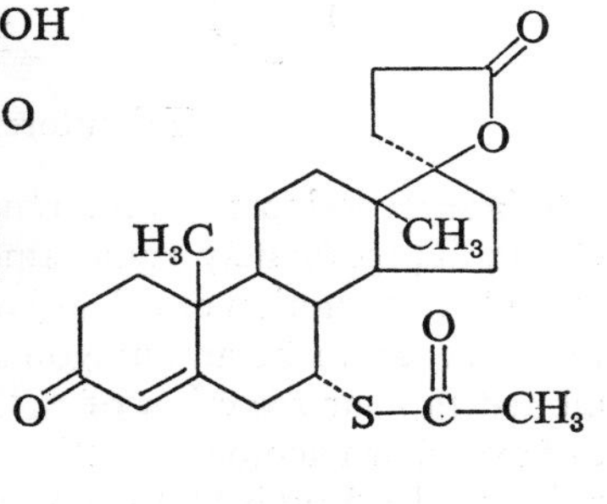   Spironolactone
                     (Aldactone A)

The most powerful spirolactone which has this effect is **spironolactone**. The main reason for believing that spirolactones are aldosterone antagonists is that they reverse all the renal effects of aldosterone. When the drug is given to a normal subject, urinary excretion of Na^+ is increased while the output of K^+ and H^+ in the urine is slightly diminished. The effect of spirolactones is, however, influenced by the intake of salt. When a normal subject receives large amounts of salt, these drugs have less effect on Na^+ and K^+ balance than when given to an individual taking a low sodium diet. Furthermore, spirolactones have no influence upon the urinary excretion of Na^+ and K^+ when given to adrenalectomized animals or patients with Addison's disease.

Spirolactones also block the effects of other corticosteroids on Na^+ and K^+ excretion but not their effects on intermediary metabolism. The site of action within the renal tubules at which the spirolactones interfere with the action of aldosterone and other adrenocorticoids is uncertain. As aldosterone increases the excretion of K^+ and H^+ in exchange for Na^+, it must act on the distal tubule ion exchange mechanism. However, in certain circumstances aldosterone produces a greater reduction of Na^+ excretion than can be accounted for by the rise in urinary K^+, and it must therefore interfere with the reabsorption of Na^+ at some other point.

Aldosterone antagonists are of limited value in clinical medicine as their diuretic powers compare unfavourably with many other diuretics. They are occasionally used in conjunction with other compounds, as they reduce K^+ loss in the urine. A suitable dose of spironolactone is 100–200 mg/day orally. Adverse effects are rare but include drowsiness and skin rashes.

TRIAMTERENE

Triamterene, a phenylpteridine, is a weak diuretic which should not be given alone but used in conjunction with other agents such as one of the thiazide drugs.

Triamterene

Triamterene increases the renal excretion of Na^+ and Cl^- in approximately equal amounts and has no effect on HCO_3^- excretion or urinary acidification. Originally it was believed to be an antagonist of aldosterone and inhibited tubular secretion of K^+, but it was soon shown to have pharmacological action in the adrenalectomized animal. The drug is free from serious adverse effects and when given by mouth is rapidly absorbed. A therapeutic dose is 150–250 mg/day.

DRUGS THAT INFLUENCE OTHER TUBULAR TRANSPORT MECHANISMS

PROBENECID (BENEMID)

This is one of the best known specific competitive inhibitors of the tubular secretion of organic acids; it is a benzoic acid derivative.

Probenecid

Historically probenecid was synthesized at a time when penicillin was scarce and it was the outcome of a planned investigation to reduce the rate of excretion of penicillin. Penicillin is excreted by the kidney, approximately 10 per cent by glomerular filtration and 90 per cent by proximal tubular secretion. The value for Tm for penicillin has been estimated to be about 3 million units (1·8 g)/hr. This high value for Tm explains why it is necessary to give very large amounts of penicillin to sustain even modest blood concentrations. The administration of probenecid to a patient receiving penicillin reduces tubular secretion of penicillin to zero and urinary excretion is limited to the small amount removed by glomerular filtration. Probenecid also inhibits the tubular secretion of other organic acids such as para-amino hippuric acid, phenolsulphonphthalein, salicylic acid and pantothenic acid. However, probenecid is most widely used in the treatment of gout in which it increases the urinary excretion of uric acid, and is one of a number of uricosuric agents. Its action in this regard appears at first sight to be paradoxical. Uric acid is a substance which the renal tubules both reabsorb and excrete. Normally a large part of the amount present in the glomerular filtrate is reabsorbed and only a small amount is secreted into the proximal tubules. Probenecid in small doses depresses proximal tubular secretion, so lowering the rate of uric acid excretion. In full therapeutic doses tubular reabsorption is impaired to an even greater extent and net loss of uric acid is increased. Probenecid is given by mouth, 1–2 g/day, and is readily absorbed.

SULPHINPYRAZONE (ANTURAN)

This drug is a derivative of phenylbutazone (p. 5.57) and was discovered among the metabolites of a phenylbutazone derivative. Like probenecid, it competitively inhibits the renal tubular secretion of organic acids such as PAH and salicylic acid. It also blocks the component of uric acid secreted by the proximal tubule. In therapeutic doses in gout (200–500 mg/day), it causes a rise in uric acid excretion in the urine by inhibition of tubular reabsorption. Sulphinpyrazone is given by mouth, is readily absorbed and largely bound to plasma proteins. Nevertheless it has a short half-life because it is itself secreted by the proximal tubules and, because of its low pK_a, little back diffusion into the blood occurs.

DRUGS THAT REDUCE RBF AND GFR

Drugs which reduce RBF and GFR are not used clinically for this purpose. These haemodynamic effects arise as an undesirable action of drugs given for other reasons. Among the most important are adrenaline and noradrenaline. They produce vasoconstriction of the renal arterioles by their action on the α-receptors. When given in small doses renal vascular resistance is increased and renal blood flow falls to about 50 per cent. Indirect evidence suggests that all segments of the renal vascular bed are affected but that the greatest increase in resistance occurs in the afferent arterioles. Glomerular filtration is usually maintained at this stage in spite of a fall in renal blood flow, presumably by an increase in the resistance of the post-glomerular efferent arteriole. Larger doses of these substances reduce RBF further and GFR then falls. Similar changes in renal function may be induced by other sympathomimetic drugs and especially metaraminol, phenylephrine and methoxamine (p. 15.19).

Various drugs which lower systemic blood pressure and which interfere with reflex vasoconstrictor pathways and peripheral resistance are capable of reducing renal blood flow in certain circumstances (p. 8.8). However, the effect of many of these agents is variable and is influenced by secondary adjustments within the kidney and by changes in the vascular resistance in other parts of the body. Thus ganglion-blocking drugs, e.g. hexamethonium, may produce only a slight fall in GFR and RBF at rest, but a more severe reduction occurs with exercise as a larger volume of blood is pooled in the muscles and limbs. Hydrallazine, which also reduces systemic blood pressure, unaccountably increases RBF in patients with high blood pressure. Little is known concerning the effects of prejunctional blocking drugs such as guanethidine and bretylium on renal function in man, but marked reductions in RBF and GFR occur if systemic hypotension is produced. There is some evidence that RBF is better maintained in both normotensive and hypertensive subjects following the use of methyldopa (p. 8.9).

DRUGS THAT INFLUENCE BLADDER FUNCTION

Although not strictly related to renal function, it is appropriate to consider here the few drugs which influence the bladder. The parasympathomimetic agents, carbachol (p. 4.10) and the closely related compound bethanechol (carbamylmethylcholine), are the most important. Both are virtually totally resistant to the action of acetylcholinesterase and have more powerful effects on the detrusor muscle of the bladder and smooth muscle of the gut than mecholyl, while at the same time producing little cardiovascular effect. For this reason they are used to treat urinary retention when organic obstruction to the outflow tract of the bladder is absent. This may arise postoperatively, in the elderly or after spinal injuries (neurogenic bladder). Bethanechol is best given by subcutaneous injection in a dose of 5 mg (or 20 mg orally), carbachol in a dose of 0·5 mg subcutaneously (1 mg orally).

FURTHER READING

LANT A.F. & WILSON G.M. (1967) Diuretics, in *Renal Disease*, 2nd Edition, ed. D. Black. Oxford: Blackwell Scientific Publications.

SELDIN D. ed. (1966) Physiology of diuretic agents. *Ann. N.Y. Acad. Sci.* **139**, 273.

Chapter 12
Sex hormones and drugs that act on the reproductive system

This chapter is concerned with the pharmacology of gonadotrophins, sex steroids and other drugs which act on the reproductive tract.

Gonadotrophins

The physiology of pituitary and chorionic gonadotrophins has already been discussed (vol. 1, p. 37.16 and 44). Two types of trophic stimulus are involved in the cyclical control of ovarian functions, a follicle stimulating hormone (FSH) and a luteinizing hormone (LH). The latter might better be called an 'ovulatory hormone' as it triggers ovulation in an FSH-primed follicle. If this trophic control of ovarian function is lost, a doctor is confronted with the problem of its replacement and for this purpose preparations of both FSH and LH are required.

PREPARATIONS WITH FSH ACTIVITY

Gonadotrophin of pregnant mare's serum (PMS) is produced by specialized structures of the endometrium (endometrial cups) during pregnancy in the mare. It reaches a high blood concentration in early pregnancy, but its physiological role is unknown. It is not excreted by the kidneys and so cannot be recovered from urine. A highly potent gonadotrophin preparation that has predominantly FSH-like activity can be extracted readily from the serum of pregnant mares. This substance was used for clinical trials in the 1940s, but its therapeutic value was limited by the fact that, as a heterologous protein, it rapidly induced neutralizing antibodies in the recipient. Consequently its effectiveness was limited to the first few administrations. This preparation has been largely superseded by homologous human extracts, but it still has an occasional use, e.g. in the selection of patients suitable for induction of ovulation.

Human pituitary FSH (HPFSH) is extracted from human pituitaries, but a large number of glands is required to produce useful quantities, and this difficulty has so far limited its availability. Nevertheless, in the future it should be practicable to prepare an adequate quantity of FSH from autopsies. It is only over the last ten years that HPFSH has been available for clinical trials. The extracts are not highly purified and contain small amounts of other trophic hormones, in particular, a significant percentage of LH.

Gonadotrophin from urine of postmenopausal women (HMG) is commercially available for limited use in several countries. Following the menopause, gonadotrophin, principally FSH, is released continuously by the pituitary (vol. 1, p. 37.21), and some of this escapes in the urine, from which it can be extracted. The quantity excreted is small and large volumes of urine are required to provide useful quantities. Like HPFSH, HMG is not a highly purified extract and contains a variable amount of LH activity.

PREPARATIONS WITH LH ACTIVITY

Chorionic gonadotrophin (CG) is produced by the human trophoblast in large quantities especially in early pregnancy (vol. 1, p. 37.44). It has potent LH-like activity and can be extracted readily from the urine of pregnant women. It has been available for clinical purposes for thirty years and has proved to be effective.

Pituitary LH has proved to be more difficult to extract and purify than FSH, and preparations are not yet available for clinical purposes. Fortunately CG is a satisfactory substitute for LH.

ESTIMATION AND STANDARDIZATION OF GONADOTROPHINS

The estimation of gonadotrophins depends on biological and immunological methods, none of which are reliably specific. Results are difficult to interpret since the responses of test animals to a gonadotrophin stimulus vary between strains of the same species and depend on a variety of environmental factors that are difficult to control; consequently results from different laboratories vary widely. The main difficulty of immunoassay is the lack of a pure preparation of gonadotrophin that is required to raise specific antibodies.

The lack of an acceptable scale for expressing assay results has made it difficult to compare data from different laboratories. Until recently results were expressed in terms of the amount of the test substance required to produce a given physiological response; e.g. the amount of gonadotrophin required to double the weight of a mouse uterus has been used as a 'mouse uterine unit'. This type of standardization is open to serious error, and has been replaced by reference to international reference preparations. Standard preparations of HMG, FSH and LH are now readily available, and results of gonadotrophin estimations are best expressed in terms of these standards.

The following methods are those in widest use.

Test for FSH

The **ovarian augmentation test** is based on the increase in ovarian weight in intact immature animals. Tests may be invalidated by the variable effects of endogenous pituitary gonadotrophins, but this can be overcome by the use of hypophysectomized animals, a laborious procedure which is impracticable on a large scale. Furthermore, even slight contamination with LH acts synergistically with FSH and adds to ovarian size. This difficulty is avoided by treating rats simultaneously with CG to induce an LH response, and by measuring the extent to which this LH effect is augmented by FSH in the unknown test preparation.

Tests for LH

The **ovarian ascorbic acid depletion test** relies on the depletion of ascorbic acid in the ovaries of immature rats pretreated with PMS and CG. Several days after the completion of this preliminary treatment, the test substance is injected intravenously, and 3 hours later one ovary is removed and analysed for its content of ascorbic acid.

The **ventral prostate enlargement test** depends on the specific action of LH on the prostate gland in hypophysectomized immature rats. The precision of this method is improved if the ventral lobe, rather than the whole gland, is weighed.

Nonspecific tests for pituitary gonadotrophins

These tests do not distinguish between FSH and LH, and may be thought of as estimating total gonadotrophin activity. However, this is not synonymous with the sum of separate FSH and LH activities as there may be either synergism or interference between the two components. They include the **mouse uterus test** which depends on the increase in uterine weight of intact immature mice in response to subcutaneous injections of gonadotrophin, and the **ovarian weight test** in which the increase in ovarian weight of intact immature rats in response to subcutaneous injections of gonadotrophin is measured.

Tests for chorionic gonadotrophin

Highly purified preparations of CG have been available for many years, and it has been possible to use these as international standards. One international unit repre-

sents the activity contained in 0·1 mg of standard. It is, therefore, customary to express CG estimations in terms of international units (IU).

Bioassays may utilize the measurement of direct responses to CG; e.g. the production of haemorrhagic follicles and corpora lutea in intact, immature mice (Ascheim–Zondek), the induction of ovulation in rabbits (Friedman), the induction of ovulation in the South African clawed toad, *Xenopus laevis* (Hogben), or the expulsion of spermatozoa in amphibia (Galli–Mainini). Alternatively, one may quantitate the responses which are secondary to the release of sex steroids from the gonads, e.g. the increase in uterine or prostatic weight.

Immunoassays utilize the ability of CG to inhibit the agglutination reaction between stabilized CG-coated sheep erythrocytes and an antisera to CG raised in rabbits. Complement fixation tests, which require a specific antiserum to CG, have been also used. Radioimmunoassay methods are being developed.

Immunological assays have virtually replaced bioassays for routine qualitative purposes, particularly for **pregnancy diagnosis**. They have the merits of being rapid, inexpensive and reliable. However, they have not yet replaced bioassays for quantitative determinations.

ABSORPTION, METABOLISM AND EXCRETION OF GONADOTROPHINS

Gonadotrophins, being glycoproteins, are digested in the gastrointestinal tract and so cannot be administered orally but require parenteral, usually intramuscular, injection.

Due to their size (mol. wt. about 30,000) they are not freely excreted by the kidney. Chorionic gonadotrophin is the only member of this group to appear in large quantities in urine.

There is little information about the metabolism of gonadotrophins. Injected isotope-labelled FSH and LH both have a short half-life of about 1 hour, although the site and nature of their metabolism is unknown. Chorionic gonadotrophin is destroyed more slowly, having a half-life of several hours. It is excreted by the kidney but there is evidence that the CG which appears in the urine may be partly inactivated, certainly in terms of its biological activity. This may explain the difference between gonadotrophin assays based on biological and immunological methods. PMS is destroyed even more slowly and does not appear in the urine.

CLINICAL USES

The greatest experience has been gained in the treatment of female disorders, and they have had little application to male disorders. Gonadotrophins are both scarce and potentially dangerous, and consequently should be given only to carefully selected patients. They should be used when it is required to restore both gametogenic and endocrine ovarian functions; they should not be used simply to control menstrual disorders but only to restore fertility.

Gonadotrophin therapy is indicated only if the failure of ovulation is due either to lack of pituitary stimulation or possibly to reduced ovarian responsiveness to endogenous gonadotrophins. This form of therapy is of no value in the presence of intrinsic ovarian failure, as it requires responsive target organs. Furthermore, in order to achieve fertility, there should be no other barrier to conception in either male or female partner. As the object of treatment is to induce ovulation in order to achieve gestation, success can be measured only in terms of successful pregnancies.

The most serious risk is overstimulation of the ovaries, leading to multiple ovulation and to multiple pregnancy with its attendant hazards. Pregnancies with up to seven foetuses have been produced, and this constitutes one of the major obstacles to the successful outcome of induced pregnancies.

Overstimulation also causes gross enlargement and excessive hyperaemia of the ovaries. Ovarian enlargement can be detected by pelvic examination in most patients under treatment. This may produce only pain, which subsides spontaneously, but bleeding may occur from rupture of the enlarged ovaries, and a few deaths have been recorded.

The aim of therapy is to find the minimum effective dose which avoids ovarian overstimulation. It is customary to give a preliminary course of FSH, in the form of either HMG or HPFSH. This may be spread out over a period of days, either in prefixed amounts or calculated daily according to ovarian steroid production, or it may be administered as a single injection. About 10 days after the start of FSH therapy, a single injection of CG is given in the hope that ovulation will follow within 12–24 hours. Coitus is timed so that insemination precedes ovulation by a few hours.

Success depends largely on the selection of cases. In experienced hands, the ovulation rate in response to FSH and CG is over 80 per cent, and the pregnancy rate is about 50 per cent. Of these conceptions, approximately 25 per cent abort; many of these abortions are associated with multiple pregnancies, but others may be due to complex endocrine errors. The incidence of serious ovarian overstimulation is about 3 per cent. It is hoped that greater experience and better control will increase the number of pregnancies and reduce the incidence of adverse reactions

There is very limited experience in the use of gonadotrophins in the treatment of male infertility, but a few infertile males with hypopituitarism have been successfully treated. Failure of descent of the testes is a common problem, and chorionic gonadotrophin has been used to induce descent.

Oestrogens

The biochemistry and physiology of sex steroids are discussed in vol. 1, pp. 37.11 & 29. Substances with oestrogenic activity are distributed widely in animal species and are found in both sexes. The stallion has a larger daily output than any other known animal. Several plants are sources of oestrogens, and these have caused impairment of fertility in grazing animals. Equally remarkable is the wide range of chemical substances which can exhibit oestrogenic activity, e.g. stilboestrol and steroids. There is no apparent correlation between structure and function of these molecules. In this respect, oestrogens are probably unique amongst hormones.

ESTIMATION OF OESTROGENS

Well established chemical methods are available for the measurement of several natural oestrogens and most information on human sex steroid physiology is based on these techniques. However, for purposes of observing the physiological role of compounds it is necessary to use bioassays, since oestrogenic activity must be defined in biological rather than chemical terms.

The most widely applied test is the induction of vaginal cornification in the spayed mouse or rat. To increase sensitivity, the thickness or mitotic activity of vaginal epithelium may be measured. Further sensitivity may be achieved by applying the test substance locally to the vagina rather than by subcutaneous injection. Alternatively, the increase in uterine weight of oophorectomized animals may be used as an index of activity.

These methods are subject to several criticisms. All are poorly repeatable, especially between different laboratories. The measurement of 'oestrogenic activity' varies according to the test used; e.g. vaginal cornification methods show that oestrone is more active than oestriol, whereas rat uterus tests show oestriol to be the more active substance. This emphasizes the arbitrary nature of the term 'oestrogenic activity'. This expression is valid only in terms of the physiological end-point used. Finally, these tests are difficult to interpret when mixtures of substances are assayed, because of potentiation or interference between different compounds. For example, the addition of progesterone inhibits vaginal cornification induced by oestrogens, whereas it augments the increase of uterine weight produced by oestrogens.

SUBSTANCES WITH OESTROGENIC ACTIVITY

One of the first nonsteroidal oestrogens to be synthesized

$$HO\text{--}\bigcirc\text{--}C\underset{\underset{C_2H_5}{|}}{\overset{\overset{C_2H_5}{|}}{=}}C\text{--}\bigcirc\text{--}OH$$

Stilboestrol

was **diethylstilboestrol** (stilboestrol). The discovery of this substance by Dodds in 1938 was a landmark in endocrinology, and it is still one of the most potent synthetic oestrogens. The related compounds, **hexoestrol** and **dinoestrol**, are less potent and are rarely used.

Ethinyloestradiol is closely related to the natural oestrogen, oestradiol-17β, having an ethinyl group

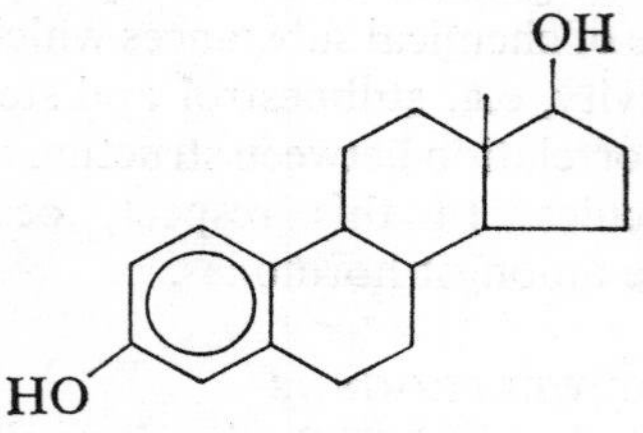

Oestradiol–17β

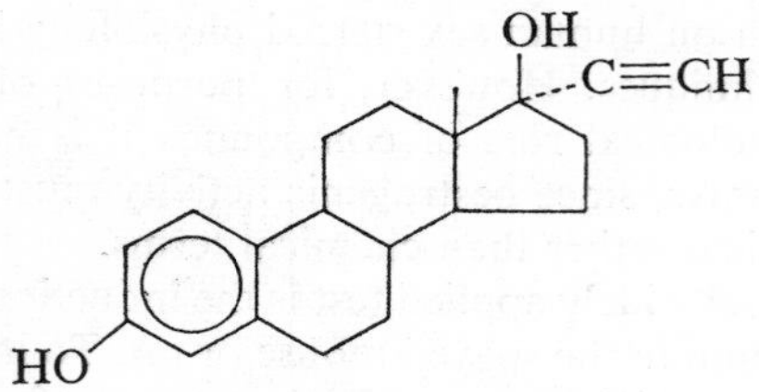

Ethinyloestradiol

attached at C-17. This substance is about twenty-five times more potent than stilboestrol.

The 3-methyl ether of ethinyloestradiol, **mestranol**, is equally potent and is widely used as a constituent of oestrogen–progestagen mixtures.

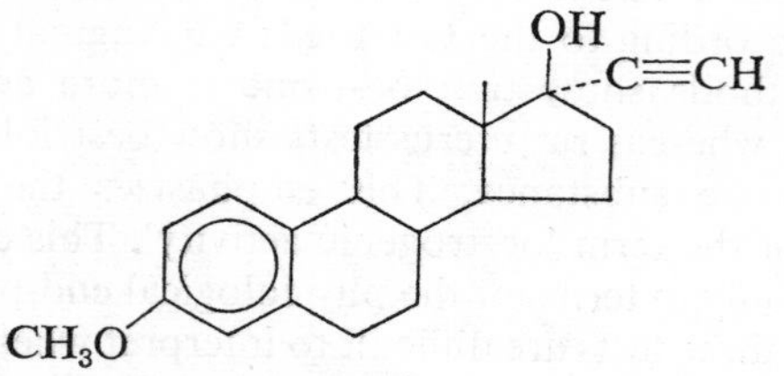

Mestranol

Conjugated equine oestrogens are derived from the urine of pregnant mares and are available as a commercial preparation, **premarin**. The detailed composition of this preparation is unknown, but it consists largely of oestrone sulphate.

Chlorotrianisene is another nonsteroidal compound. This substance is not itself actively oestrogenic, but it is converted in the body into active oestrogens. In this sense, it may be described as a pro-oestrogen.

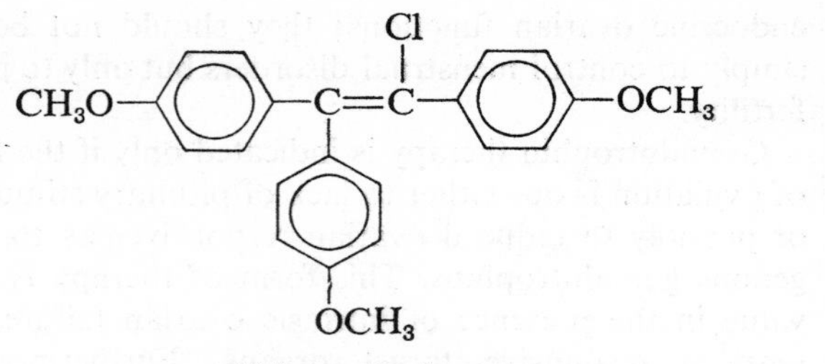

Natural oestrogens are of little clinical value. Oestradiol is available as a number of esters, benzoate, valerate and dipropionate, each having a different duration of action. All of these substances require to be administered paren-

Chlorotrianisene

terally and are rarely used. Several preparations of natural and synthetic oestrogens are available for topical application and these are of some restricted value. The compounds in widest use are ethinyloestradiol and stilboestrol, together with mestranol in steroid mixtures.

ABSORPTION, METABOLISM AND EXCRETION

Most oestrogens are absorbed rapidly from the gut and other mucous membranes and this provides a rational basis for topical application. However, natural oestrogens, after absorption from the gut into the portal circulation, are metabolized rapidly and inactivated by the liver (vol. 1, p. 31.11). Nonsteroidal compounds such as stilboestrol are equally rapidly absorbed but are degraded much more slowly in the body. Similarly, acetylation protects ethinyloestradiol from rapid degradation. The routes of metabolism and excretion of ethinyloestradiol and stilboestrol are unknown.

Sex steroid therapy usually uses mixtures of oestrogens and progestagens, and so the clinical uses of oestrogens are discussed with those of progestagens (p. 12.7).

ANTI-OESTROGENS

These are substances which inhibit or modify the action of natural oestrogens. They include androgens and progestagens, but greatest interest attaches to some weak oestrogens which may compete with more potent compounds.

In the search for synthetic oestrogens to be used as antifertility agents, compounds similar to stilboestrol were prepared. One of these, chlorotrianisene, proved to be of considerable value and consequently several analogues of this substance were prepared. One analogue, now known as **clomiphene**, was shown to have antifertility properties in mice, and this led to clinical trials of its contraceptive value. However, rather than suppress ovulation, it was found to induce ovulation in amenorrhoeic women.

The mode of action of clomiphene is still not understood and experimental findings are controversial and equivocal. Clomiphene probably causes an increase in the release of pituitary FSH, but its effects on LH are uncertain. It is likely that this pituitary stimulation is due to its anti-oestrogenic effect. Thus, clomiphene produces a low cornification index and loss of ferning of cervical mucus; it has been shown to induce regression of endometrial hyperplasia, atrophy of the vaginal epithelium of infants with precocious puberty, and regression of gynaecomastia. It can also nullify ovarian suppression by ethinyloestradiol.

Clomiphene

It is, therefore, postulated that clomiphene competes for binding sites in target organs with natural oestrogens. Such an effect on the hypothalamus may be responsible for its stimulating effect on the adenohypophysis by removing the inhibitory influence of oestrogens. This carries the implication that clomiphene acts most effectively in the presence of adequate levels of circulating oestrogens.

Clomiphene is at present the only alternative drug to human gonadotrophin for the induction of ovulation. It is effective only in the presence of an intact hypothalamic–pituitary–ovarian axis. Theoretically it should be most useful when gonadotrophin levels are either normal or subnormal and when there is an adequate level of circulating oestrogens. In practice, however, because of the vagaries of gonadotrophin estimations, it is doubtful if this is an accurate clinical screening device, and it is still uncertain what constitutes an adequate level of urinary oestrogen excretion.

Clomiphene is synthesized commercially and is readily available in many countries. While this drug should not be used indiscriminantly, it has wider uses than human gonadotrophins, e.g. for the correction of anovular menstrual disorders even when there is no desire for pregnancy.

A daily dose of 50 mg for 5 days is the usual initial course for the induction of ovulation. If this fails, it may be raised to 100 mg or 150 mg for 5–10 days. However, as the dose increases the success rate does not increase proportionately whereas the incidence of complications increases steeply. As with gonadotrophins, there is a wide variation in responsiveness to clomiphene between patients.

Success rate should be judged in terms of the incidence of ovulation, but the anti-oestrogenic properties of clomiphene make it difficult to detect ovulation accurately by the routine indirect methods; e.g. by vaginal cornification or cervical mucus ferning. However, depending on the selection of cases for treatment, ovulation may be induced in 50–90 per cent of patients. Despite this the number of pregnancies may be disappointingly low. Thus, in two recent series, fifty clomiphene cycles induced twenty-seven ovulations but only six conceptions. In general, clomiphene is less useful than are gonadotrophins in the treatment of infertility.

Clomiphene also carries the risk of overstimulation leading to ovarian enlargement and multiple pregnancies. When conception occurs the abortion rate is high. In addition, 20–30 per cent of patients experience 'hot flushes', presumably because of the anti-oestrogenic properties of the drug; other less common adverse effects include blurred vision and skin rashes.

Progestagens

Over the last 15 years there have been important developments in the synthesis of compounds with 'progestational activity'. Their application to the problem of population control has been largely responsible for this interest.

ESTIMATION OF PROGESTAGENS

There are accurate chemical methods for the measurement of progesterone and its metabolites in body fluids and tissues. However, quantitative estimates of biological activities are equally necessary to define the complex behaviour of the many new compounds which are being synthesized.

Physiological end points which have been used include the induction of 'progestational' endometrial changes in oestrogen-primed immature rabbits in response to the injection or intrauterine instillation of test compounds, the ability to induce deciduomata in rats in response to intrauterine trauma, the maintenance of pregnancy after bilateral oophorectomy in pregnant rodents, the ability to suppress ovulation in rabbits and the ability to delay the onset of menstruation in normal cyclic women. This latter test is particularly relevant to the therapeutic value of these compounds.

The same problems attach to these procedures as apply to oestrogens. None of these tests is specific; they may give some response to androgens, or alternatively oestrogens can inhibit the progestational activity of test compounds.

COMPOUNDS WITH PROGESTATIONAL ACTIVITY (Figs. 12.1, 12.2 and table 12.1)

The first useful synthetic oral progestational compound to be introduced was 17α-ethinyl testosterone, **ethisterone**. In the early 1950s it was demonstrated that testosterone derivatives which lacked the angular methyl group (C-19) attached at C-10 (19-nortestosterones) were even more effective oral progestagens. 19-Nortestosterone was itself inactive, but 17-alkyl compounds proved to be useful; of these, 17-ethinyl-19-nortestosterone (norethisterone) proved to be the most potent.

The newer compounds which have been synthesized

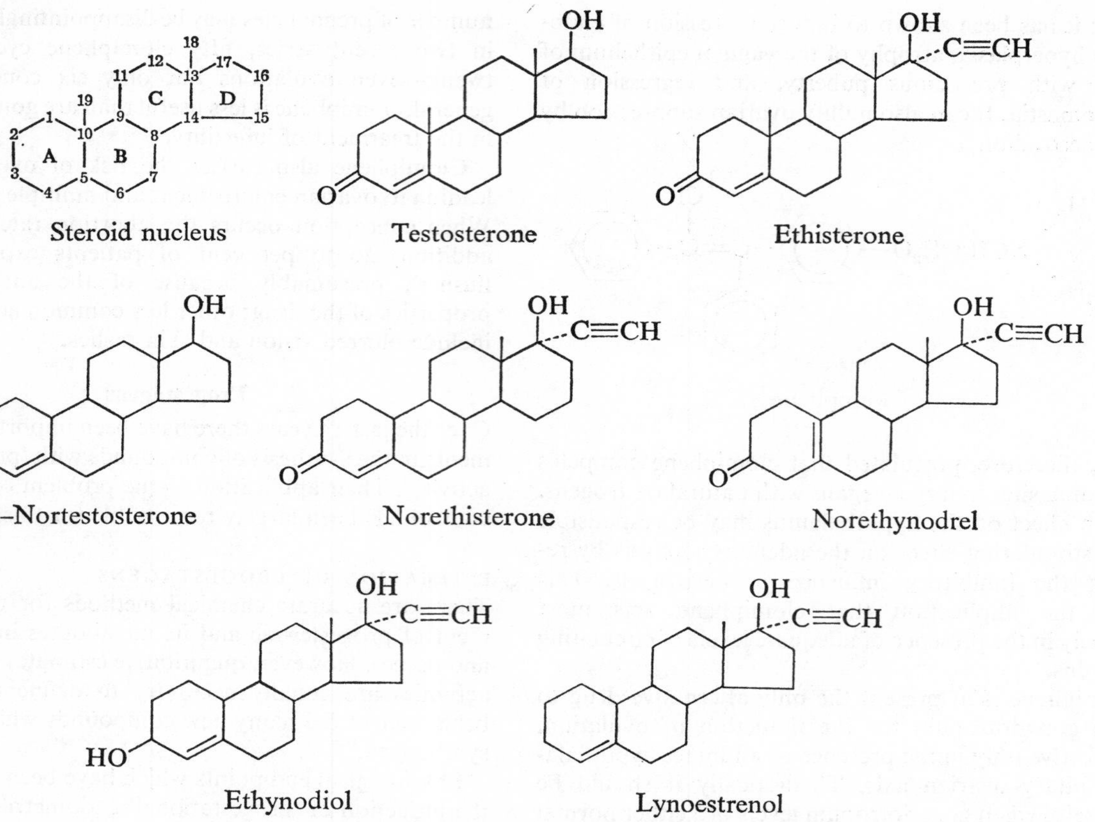

FIG. 12.1. Synthetic progestagens related to 19-nortestosterone.

TABLE 12.1. Biological activities of some progestagens. After Drill (1966).

Progestagen	Pituitary inhibition	Progestational activity	Oestrogenic activity	Androgenic activity	Anabolic effect
Norethynodrel	+	+	+	O	O
Norethisterone	+	+	O	+	+
Norethisterone acetate	+	+	O	+	+
Ethynodiol diacetate	+	+	+	+	O
Medroxyprogesterone acetate	+	+	O		
Chlormadinone acetate	+	+	O		

+, active; O, inactive.

fall into two main categories depending on their chemical nature:

(1) those similar to testosterone and 19-nortestosterone, and

(2) those related to 17α-hydroxyprogesterone.

Compounds similar to 19-nortestosterone (fig. 12.1)
Shift of the double bond in the A ring of norethisterone from the 4–5 to the 5–10 position produces the isomer, **norethynodrel**. Reduction of the 3-keto group of norethi-

sterone provides the compound **ethynodiol**, which is closely related to ethinyloestradiol. The diacetate of ethynodiol is a commonly used progestagen. Removal of the ketone group at C-3 gives rise to a series of compounds known as oestrenols. 17-Ethinyl oestrenol, **lynoestrenol**, is the most useful member of this series.

Compounds similar to 17α-hydroxyprogesterone (fig. 12.2)
17α-Hydroxyprogesterone is itself useful in the form of esters. The caproate and valerate are long-acting

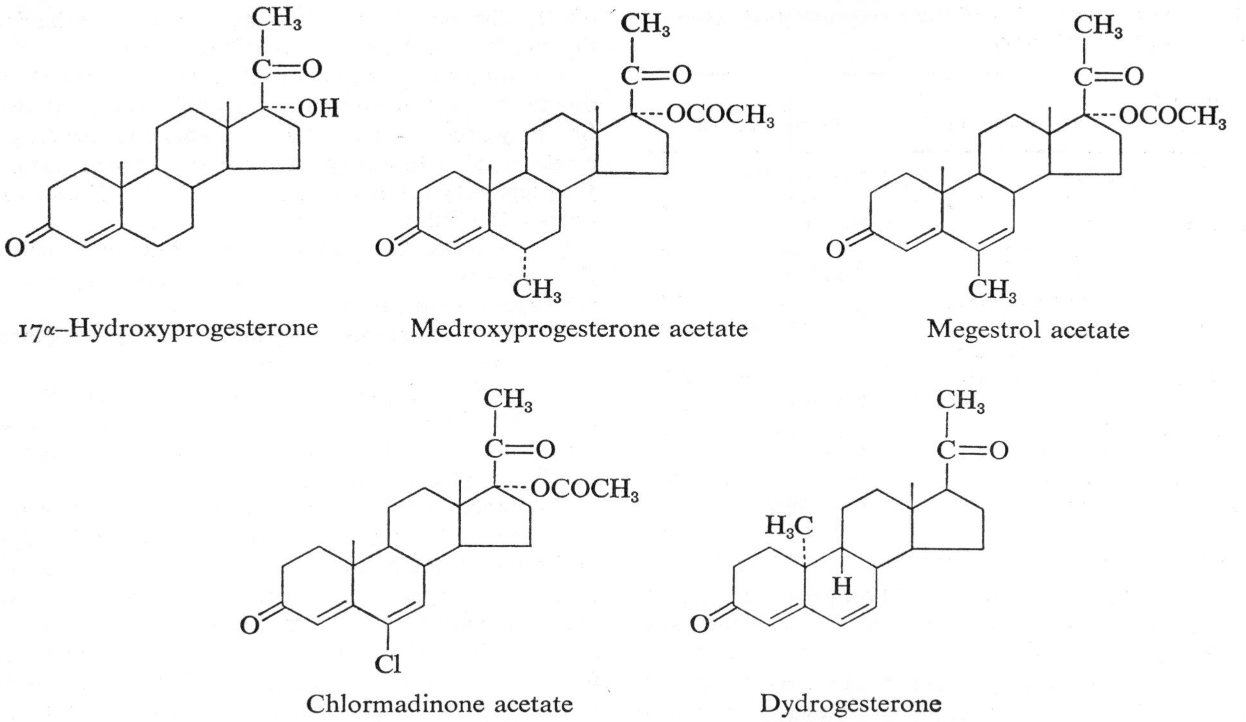

FIG. 12.2. Synthetic progestagens related to 17α-hydroxyprogesterone.

progestagens when administered intramuscularly in oil, but are virtually inactive by mouth. The acetoxyprogesterone derivatives are acetic acid esters at the C-17 position of 17 α-hydroxyprogesterone. The 6-methyl derivative, **medroxyprogesterone acetate** is effective; **megestrol acetate** has an additional double bond in the 6–7 position; in **chlormadinone acetate** the 6-methyl group is replaced by a chlorine atom. **Dydrogesterone** is a retroprogesterone, i.e. the angular methyl C-19 group is in the α-rather than the β-position (vol. 1, p. 10.6).

PHYSIOLOGICAL PROPERTIES OF PROGESTAGENS

These new synthetic compounds have been tested against the range of physiological activities of natural oestrogens, progestagens and androgens as indicated by many bio-assays (table 12.1), and it can be seen that the activities overlap. There is no 'pure' synthetic progestagen, as they all exert some oestrogenic and androgenic effects.

In general, the 17α-hydroxyprogesterone derivatives appear to be mainly progestational, and have relatively little oestrogenic activity. They are relatively poor inhibitors of ovulation. By contrast, the 19-nortestosterone compounds have marked oestrogenic properties, possibly because they are converted to oestrogens in the body.

It is clearly misleading to label any of these compounds simply as a progestagen, and there is at best only a crude correlation between physiological functions and molecular structure.

ABSORPTION, METABOLISM AND EXCRETION OF PROGESTAGENS

The fate of endogenous progestagens is described in vol. 1, p. 37.15. Progesterone is absorbed freely from the gut but is metabolized rapidly by the liver and loses its biological activity. As the half-life in the blood is very short, natural progestagens are of no clinical value.

Synthetic progestagens are protected from this rapid conversion in the liver. Thus, the half-life of megestrol acetate in therapeutic doses is about 24 hours and 70 per cent is excreted within 72 hours. This partly determines the duration of action of these compounds. They are subject to a variety of hydroxylations in the liver and are partly conjugated with glucuronic acid. They are excreted mainly in the urine, but 20 per cent is lost in the the faeces.

CLINICAL USES

The introduction of mixtures of oestrogens and progestagens was largely fortuitous and occurred during the early stages of the development of sex steroids for the suppression of ovulation. Norethynodrel contaminated with mestranol was used and found to be highly effective. Most of the sex steroid preparations which are now in clinical use are mixtures of various synthetic progestagens with either ethinyloestradiol or mestranol (table 12.2).

Sex steroids are used most effectively either to suppress normal ovarian functions (both steroid- and egg-produc-

TABLE 12.2. Composition of some combined oestrogen–progestagen preparations.

Proprietary Preparation	Oestrogen (mg)		Progestagen (mg)	
Norlestrin	Ethinyl oestradiol	0·05	Norethisterone acetate	2·5
Gynovlar	Ethinyl oestradiol	0·05	Norethisterone acetate	3·0
Anovlar	Ethinyl oestradiol	0·05	Norethisterone acetate	4·0
Volidan	Ethinyl oestradiol	0·05	Megestrol acetate	4·0
Conovid E	Mestranol	0·1	Norethynodrel	2·5
Conovid	Mestranol	0·075	Norethynodrel	5·0
Lyndiol 2·5	Mestranol	0·075	Lynoestrenol	2·5
Lyndiol	Mestranol	0·15	Lynoestrenol	5·0
Ortho-novin	Mestranol	0·1	Norethisterone	2·0
Ovulen	Mestranol	0·1	Ethynodiol diacetate	1·0

ing functions) or to mimic ovarian hormone effects in the absence of ovarian activity. In the first category sex steroids are given in order to suppress either ovulation or ovarian steroid hormone production. However, at present it is impossible to control either oogenesis or steroidogenesis independently and attempts to control one inevitably interfere with the other. Thus, inability to inhibit ovulation selectively for purposes of contraception is the cause of many of the undesirable effects of contraceptive preparations. Attempts are being made to avoid this by using small quantities of sex steroids to modify the action of ovarian steroids at the target organ without interfering with ovarian cyclical activity.

The second clinical use refers to conditions where the ovaries are either absent or inactive (prepubertal or postmenopausal). Finally there are a small number of occasional uses for sex steroids in relation to pregnancy, specific pathological conditions, or in the male.

Contraception

Oestrogen–progestagen mixtures are commonly used as a method of contraception with the aim of suppressing ovulation. Oestrogens alone are effective for this purpose and ethinyloestradiol, at a dose level of 80–100 μg/day, suppresses ovulation. However, a lower dose of 50 μg/day is effective in combination with a progestagen. The addition of a progestagen also ensures a prompt and acceptable withdrawal bleeding between monthly cycles of treatment. It is likely that ovulation is suppressed by interference with the secretion of pituitary gonadotrophin, although information on this point is confusing because of the lack of specificity of gonadotrophin assays. Both FSH and LH production may be affected, although the absence of a midcycle surge of LH is probably the most important

effect. The possibility of exogenous steroids having a direct effect on the ovaries is still unproven.

The antifertility properties of sex steroids are not solely due to their role in suppressing ovulation. Indeed, ovulation may occur occasionally in patients on these drugs, at a rate of thirty to ninety times per 100 women years, and yet pregnancy rarely occurs. Other effects of these drugs include the following:

(1) the progestagen reduces the volume and increases the viscosity of cervical mucus, and this may interfere with sperm penetration;

(2) steroid mixtures alter the timing of endometrial cyclical development, and in particular accelerate the appearance and subsequent regression of secretory changes and induce pseudodecidual appearances, and

(3) tubal motility is hormone-dependent and is modified by exogenous steroids.

Combined oestrogen–progestagen therapy can be administered by two types of regime. Using the regular oral mixture, the patient takes a 20–21 day course of an oestrogen–progestagen preparation, with a gap of 7 days between courses, during which time uterine bleeding occurs. Alternatively a sequential regime may be used with the aim of more closely mimicking the normal menstrual cycle, i.e. an oestrogen is taken for 14–16 days followed by an oestrogen–progestagen mixture for 5–7 days. Again a gap of 7 days separates courses. The sequential regime offers no appreciable advantages over the regular mixture, and it is slightly less effective in terms of contraception.

Efforts have been made to achieve an antifertility effect without suppressing ovulation. A continuous daily low dose of chlormadinone acetate, 500 μg/day, may fulfil this role. This may be achieved by its effects on cervical mucus and sperm migration, by alterations in endometrial development or by interference with the functions of the corpus luteum.

A postcoital contraceptive agent which would prevent conception following intercourse would be invaluable. Preliminary results using a large dose of oestrogen, e.g. 0·5 mg ethinyloestradiol, are encouraging but this method is not yet suitable for routine contraceptive purposes.

Finally, long-acting preparations would be useful in situations where it is impossible to ensure a regular daily intake. Long-acting oestrogens can be used either by mouth or by injection, and large doses (about 150 mg IM) of medroxyprogesterone acetate may also be effective.

All of these regimes are highly successful in preventing unplanned pregnancies. Failure rates are assessed by observing the number of unplanned pregnancies occurring during a large number of cycles in many women. The total number of cycles divided by thirteen (average number of cycles per year) gives an index of 'women years use', and failure rate is usually expressed as 'pregnancies per 100 women years'. For combined preparations this is of the order of 0·1–0·2, and for sequential regimes one to two pregnancies per 100 women years.

Dysfunctional uterine bleeding
This term refers to abnormal uterine bleeding in the absence of a demonstrable organic cause. This is assumed to be due to changes in the hypothalamic–hypophyseal–ovarian axis which controls the endometrial cycle. It can frequently be benefited by cyclical treatment with oestrogen–progestagen mixtures used in the same way as for contraception. This effectively blocks the ovarian control of the endometrium and imposes an artificial cycle of vaginal bleeding which is usually more acceptable to the patient. Alternatively, these drugs may be used in higher dosage for a short period of time simply to produce temporary haemostasis in the emergency management of excessive uterine bleeding.

Primary dysmenorrhoea and ovulation symptoms
Primary dysmenorrhoea refers to painful periods which occur with the onset of regular ovular menstruation, usually within one to two years after the menarche. It is well established that suppression of ovulation usually relieves this symptom. Midcycle pain or bleeding may occasionally be troublesome at the time of ovulation and give rise to problems of diagnosis and management. Steroids may be used to inhibit ovulation in these cases.

Replacement therapy in prepubertal, postmenopausal or castrate patients
Oestrogens have widespread effects throughout the lower reproductive tract which protect against inflammatory changes. Before puberty, after the menopause or in the castrate the genital tract epithelium is thin and susceptible to infection. A small replacement dose of ethinyloestradiol, 0·01 mg daily, is usually adequate to improve these epithelia and reverse the inflammatory changes.

In the congenital absence of ovarian tissue, oestrogens may be used at the time of puberty to induce some degree of feminization. A dose of about 0·05 mg ethinyloestradiol thrice daily is required for this purpose.

The menopause is not infrequently followed by troublesome symptoms, particularly generalized flushings. These can be relieved by as small a dose as 0·01–0·05 mg ethinyloestradiol daily.

Finally, there is an increasing interest in attempts to avoid some of the long-term undesirable sequelae of the climacteric, especially osteoporosis, a rise in blood lipids and a tendency to loss of libido. This may be achieved by regular cyclical therapy with sex steroids following the cessation of periods at the menopause.

Miscellaneous uses
Oestrogens are commonly used for the suppression of lactation. How they achieve this effect is unknown, and there is doubt about their efficacy. High doses are required over a period of 1–2 weeks.

Endometriosis describes the condition where islets of endometrium may be found outside the uterine cavity, most commonly on the peritoneal surface of pelvic viscera. This ectopic endometrium responds cyclically to ovarian hormones causing interstitial bleeding and dense adhesions. Symptoms associated with endometriosis may be relieved by long-term use of sex steroids, usually in high dosage over many months. The introduction of this regime followed the observation that endometriosis may improve during pregnancy, and this treatment was designed to produce a 'pseudopregnancy'.

Advanced inoperable endometrial carcinoma may regress in response to prolonged therapy with high doses of progestagens.

ADVERSE EFFECTS
Over one million women in the United Kingdom regularly use sex steroids for contraception. In 1966, at least 10 million women throughout the world used these drugs. It is estimated that by 1985 there may be 12 million users in the United States alone. These figures serve to emphasize the need to be aware of their possible undesirable consequences.

Immediate adverse effects
The immediate adverse effects of treatment are important because they partly determine the patient's acceptance of these drugs. The most common complaints are of nausea (usually maximal during the first course of treatment), breast discomfort, weight gain, bleeding occurring during courses of treatment (breakthrough bleeding), and failure to bleed between cycles. It is meaningless to quote any incidence for these effects, because of the enormous variability in reported incidence in various trials using the same compound (table 12.3.) Other troublesome symptoms may include abdominal fullness, depression, fatigue, hirsutism, skin pigmentation and decreased libido.

TABLE 12.3. Range of incidence of adverse effects in nine separate trials of anovlar (total of 18,568 cycles studied) From Jeffery & Klopper (1968).

	Per cent
First-cycle nausea	1·2–25
Breast discomfort	1·8–13
Weight change (over 3 lb)	1·5–54
Spotting	3·0–17
Breakthrough bleeding	2·1–5·2
Amenorrhoea	0·8–3·6

Thrombosis and embolism
The effects of sex steroids on coagulation and fibrinolytic

mechanisms are still controversial, but several contraceptive preparations cause an increase in levels of Factor VII and fibrinogen together with an increase in fibrinolytic activity. However, it is not possible to argue from these observations to conclusions about the coagulability of the blood.

A Medical Research Council Survey in 1967 reported on three studies into the relation between oral contraceptives and subsequent thromboembolism. Groups of women with venous thrombosis or thromboembolism were questioned as to their previous use of steroid contraceptives. The proportion of users was compared with well-matched control groups. These reports suggested some causal relationship between the use of oral contraceptives and deep venous thrombosis, pulmonary embolism and, to a lesser extent, cerebral thrombosis and embolism. There was no clear association with coronary thrombosis. It is difficult to estimate the magnitude of this risk. 'It would appear that in women of child-bearing age, the risk of developing any type of phlebitis may be increased three-fold to a level of about five cases per 1000 women per year—a risk which is approximately half that recorded during pregnancy and the puerperium.' 'Mortality from these conditions attributable to the use of oral contraceptives . . . is about three per 100,000 users per year.' This compares with a maternal mortality rate in this country of about 12 per 100,000 deaths during delivery and the puerperium.

Carcinogenesis
Sex steroids, especially oestrogens, have been shown to be carcinogenic in several experimental animals. However, there is no evidence so far to show any such effect in the human subject.

Recent claims have been made of an increased incidence of cervical dysplasia, or preinvasive cervical carcinoma in women taking contraceptive steroids.

However, further study is required to establish this as control observations have not so far been adequate. Although there is indirect evidence of a relation between abnormal oestrogen activity and endometrial carcinoma, there is no increased incidence of this tumour following sex steroid therapy. Indeed, synthetic progestagens may be used for the treatment of endometrial carcinoma. Breast carcinoma may be hormone-dependent, but no harmful effect of sex steroids has been demonstrated in this condition.

Despite these negative findings, these drugs may have a slow cumulative effect. Long-term observations are required and caution is needed in their use in the presence of known neoplasia.

Liver functions
Delayed excretion of bromsulphthalein and raised levels of serum bilirubin, alkaline phosphatase, serum aspartate and alanine aminotransferases (GOT and GPT) have been commonly reported in users of contraceptive steroids. The incidence of severe liver damage and jaundice is much higher in Scandinavia and Chile than in the United Kingdom and United States. Liver biopsy studies show evidence of intrahepatic biliary stasis and slight hepatic cell necrosis. However, these appearances are rapidly reversible after the drugs are stopped.

Endocrine and metabolic disturbances
Protein-bound iodine levels in the plasma are raised during use of contraceptive steroids. This effect is due to an increase in thyroxine-binding globulin, and there is no increase in free thyroxine or triiodothyronine levels and no evidence of hyperthyroidism. Similarly, plasma cortisol levels are raised secondary to an increase in the binding capacity of transcortin (vol. 1, p. 25.37), but there is no increase in cortisol secretion rates.

Glucose tolerance is impaired in some patients taking contraceptive steroids, particularly in those with a family history of diabetes. However, there is no evidence that these drugs induce diabetes. Plasma levels of triglycerides, cholesterol and low density lipoproteins are raised to levels comparable to those found in males and postmenopausal women, but it remains to be established that this has any relevance to the development of atherosclerosis (p. 25.36).

Fertility
Claims that fertility is unusually high after discontinuing contraceptive steroid therapy as a rebound phenomenon are not well founded, but there is normally a return to regular ovular cycles. However, there is frequently a slight delay in the recurrence of ovarian cyclical activity, and a small number of women experience a prolonged period of secondary amenorrhoea.

Fears that suppression of ovulation by oral contraceptives would delay the age of the menopause are unfounded. The menopause is associated with a virtual depletion of oocytes, and this occurs mainly by a gradual process of atresia rather than secondary to ovulation, and there is no reason to believe that sex steroids have any influence on the time scale of oocyte atresia.

Emotional disturbances
The immediate premenstrual phase is frequently associated with changes of mood, particularly a tendency to depression. Similar changes in mood occur in women taking contraceptive steroids, and they are more likely to occur in women who are already prone to depression.

Many animals show cyclical oestrous patterns of sexual activity, and this can be also demonstrated in subhuman primates who have a menstrual pattern. Sexual activity is increased at mid-cycle and is affected by exogenous steroids. In a minority of patients contraceptive steroids are associated with a loss of libido and reduced coital frequency.

Effects on foetal development

Contraceptive steroids may be given unwittingly to pregnant women, or these drugs may be used deliberately for therapeutic purposes in early pregnancy. Some of the nortestosterone derivatives occasionally induce masculinization of a female foetus. However, this is usually a superficial anomaly involving no more than clitoral enlargement and fusion of the labia.

Androgens

The physiology and biochemistry of gonadal androgens are discussed in vol. 1, p. 37.29. Their role as masculinizing agents has been recognized for over a century. However, there is increasing interest in their ability to promote general body and bone growth, and to stimulate protein anabolism, as evidenced by a positive nitrogen balance and an increase in the mass of muscle tissue. This has led to attempts to dissociate the masculinizing and anabolic effects in various synthetic steroids, but so far no pure anabolic steroid has been produced.

ESTIMATION OF ANDROGENS

Specific chemical methods are available for the measurement of testosterone and its metabolites in body fluids and tissues. However, biological methods must be used to assess the activities of new compounds. The classical method depends on the fact that the cock's comb involutes after castration, and this involution can be reversed by the injection of androgens. The sensitivity of this test can be increased either by local application of the test substance to the comb or by using newly hatched chicks rather than capons. Tests which measure the enlargement of the seminal vesicles or prostate in castrated rats may give a better correlation with clinical effectiveness.

For the estimation of anabolic potency, the growth of a muscle, usually the levator ani, of the castrated rat is measured. If growth of the accessory sex organs is observed in the same animal, a direct comparison between masculinizing and anabolic effects can be made, and these compared against testosterone as a control.

COMPOUNDS WITH ANDROGENIC ACTIVITY (fig. 12.3)

Given by mouth, testosterone is well absorbed but is rapidly inactivated by the liver; even after parenteral administration it is destroyed too quickly to exert any significant androgenic effect. Testerone esters are less polar and more lipid soluble and are absorbed slowly if they are injected in oil. **Testosterone propionate**, given intramuscularly in oily solution, is active over a period of 1–3 days. **Testosterone oenanthate** and **testosterone cypionate** are absorbed even more slowly and can be effective for 1–2 weeks. Pellets of testosterone implanted under the skin can act for 4–8 months.

17α-Methyltestosterone is active by oral administration; it is usually given in the form of linguets for buccal absorption. The halogenated derivative, **fluoxymesterone**, is even more active than 17α-methyltestosterone in terms of androgenicity in bioassays, but it has not been shown to be more effective as an androgen in clinical use.

COMPOUNDS WITH ANABOLIC ACTIVITY (fig. 12.4)

Norethandrolone has anabolic activity comparable to that of testosterone, but it exerts only about 5 per cent of its androgenic effects. Comparable preparations include **methandrostenolone, nandrolone, oxymetholone, stanolone, stanozolol** and **ethylestrenol**. There is little to choose between these preparations in terms of clinical efficiency. For men, it is possible to use fluoxymesterone which has powerful anabolic activity in addition to its virilizing properties.

Testosterone esters are metabolized and excreted in a similar way to that of testosterone. Structural modifications, such as methylation or halogenation, block these metabolic pathways and the mode of degradation of these compounds is unknown.

CLINICAL USES

Hypogonadism

This constitutes the most rational use of androgens. In children hypogonadism leads to delayed puberty, and it is usual to begin treatment between the ages of 15 and 17 years. If untreated, the boy develops a eunochoid stature and contours, absence of secondary sex characteristics and sexual drive. Androgens are effective in the development of secondary sex features, but they do not

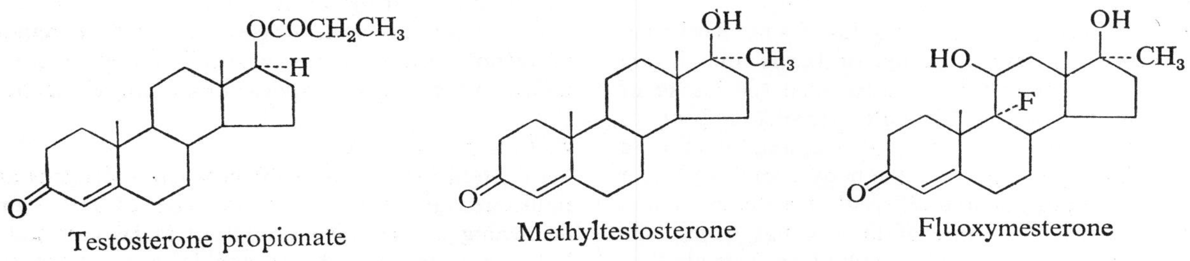

FIG. 12.3. Androgenic steroids.

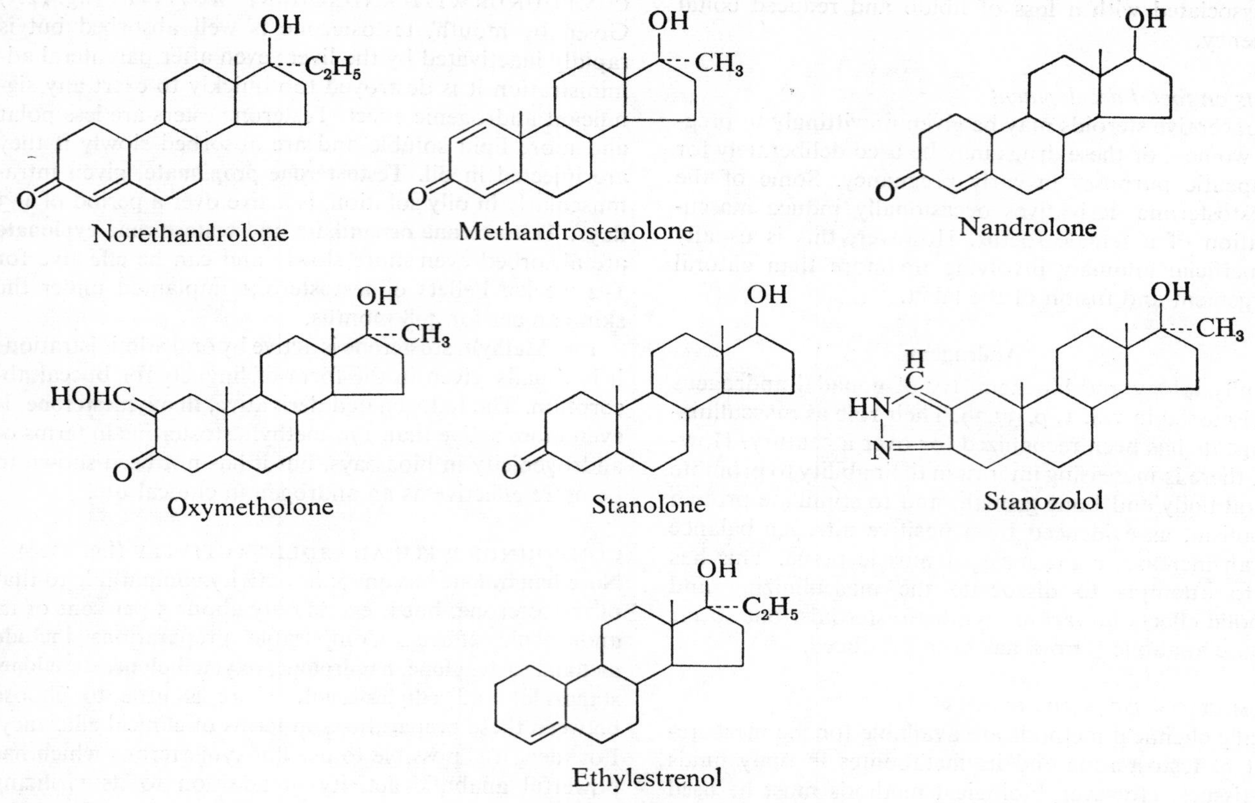

FIG. 12.4. Anabolic steroids.

stimulate spermatogenesis. In these cases, prolonged treatment with replacement therapy is required, either injections of testosterone propionate, 25–50 mg thrice weekly for 2–3 years, or, more conveniently, injections of testosterone oenanthate, 250 mg every 2 weeks for the same period. Oral methyltestosterone or fluoxymesterone (5–20 mg) are less effective for this purpose.

Hypogonadism in adult life presents a different problem, and usually constitutes partial rather than total testicular failure. The significant sequelae are loss of libido and sexual potency. Androgens may improve libido and impotence, if these are not psychosomatic; there is no evidence that they improve spermatogenesis.

Promotion of anabolism
Anabolic steroids may be used in states of general wasting, for example after severe trauma or burns and during prolonged debilitating illnesses. Provided the intake of protein and calories is adequate, steroids appear to facilitate a positive nitrogen balance and ameliorate tissue wasting. However, since the body contains protein of different composition and different turnover rates, it is difficult to assess the value of these drugs from their overall effect. Studies on healthy volunteers indicate that

these drugs may promote the formation of S-poor proteins at the expense of S-rich proteins. For these and other reasons anabolic steroids are not recommended.

Probably many athletes have taken anabolic steroids, although this contravenes athletic codes. There is no evidence that they improve performance.

Miscellaneous uses
In some hepatic diseases the degradation of oestrogens in the liver is impaired; this may cause a rise in blood oestrogen and induce feminization. This may be prevented by the use of androgens. The androgens may also relieve the generalized pruritus which is associated with jaundice, but this must be balanced against the possible damaging effects of these drugs on the liver.

Pain due to bony metastases from breast carcinoma in premenopausal women may be relieved by large doses of androgens, but at the expense of causing virilization.

ADVERSE EFFECTS
Virilization presents a problem when androgens are administered to female patients. The earliest signs are deepening of the voice, growth of facial hair and acne, but these are usually reversible after discontinuing

therapy. Later developments include a male pattern of baldness and clitoral hypertrophy, and these are likely to be irreversible. A degree of virilization may follow administration of anabolic steroids.

Several androgens are liable to cause intrahepatic obstructive jaundice. Testosterone and its esters do not cause jaundice, and it occurs most commonly in response to methyltestosterone and related compounds. The incidence of the complication is dose dependent, and it subsides when the drug is stopped.

Salt and water retention frequently accompanies administration of androgens, but this is rarely severe enough to constitute a clinical problem.

Antifertility drugs in the male

Despite the enormous clinical success of sex steroids as female contraceptives they have limitations because of their side effects and possible long term hazards. Consequently efforts are being directed in various directions to provide other means of planned parenthood. One possibility is the prevention of implantation or the rejection of the early implanted blastocyst. A number of substances are effective in this way in experimental animals, particularly oestrogens, various triphenyl ethylene derivatives and some amine oxidase inhibitors, but none of these are yet applicable to human pregnancy. It should be noted that recent legislation in Britain, which has liberalized indications for the medical termination of pregnancy and has therefore enormously increased the frequency of therapeutic abortion, makes it an urgent concern to develop drugs which will terminate pregnancy safely and effectively. Such an abortifacient drug does not yet exist.

Another possibility is the control of male fertility. A clinically useful male antifertility compound should have the following properties. It should act specifically on spermatogenesis and should not interfere with the endocrine functions of the interstitial cells of the testes; it should not impair libido or potency; it should arrest spermatogenesis totally rather than partially, since even a small number of spermatozoa might allow a degree of fertility; it must be rapidly reversible, nontoxic, nonmutagenic and effective by oral administration. Such an ideal preparation is not yet available, but some hopeful progress has been made.

Nucleotoxic substances, bisulphan and sulphonic acid esters, arrest spermatogenesis but are too toxic for clinical use. Nitrofurans, previously used for their bacteriostatic properties, and thiophenes both inhibit

Diamidine (WIN. 13099)

spermatogenesis and have no action on the interstitial cells, but they are also toxic. More recently a number of diamines, known for their amoebicidal effects, have been studied. Their only clinical disadvantage is that they have adverse effects similar to those of disulfiram (p. 5.72).

Steroids operate both directly on the testes and also via the hypothalamus and hypophysis. Oestrogens block spermatogenesis, but they also inhibit testosterone secretion and impair libido and potency. Androgens are equally effective as inhibitors of spermatogenesis and do not reduce sexual drive. Parenteral long acting androgens and intramuscular injections of large doses of medroxyprogesterone acetate are both effective. Oral androgens have proved to be less successful.

DRUGS THAT ACT ON THE MYOMETRIUM

Several problems complicate any study of the effects of drugs on the human myometrium. The interpretation of apparent drug effects on spontaneous uterine activity is hazardous because of the inherent variability and unpredictability of uterine behaviour. This is undoubtedly responsible for many divergent reports, for example, on the efficacy of drugs in suppressing premature labour. Furthermore the correlation between *in vitro* and *in vivo* activity is uncertain; the problem of defining adequate parameters to describe uterine activity is unsolved; the background of oestrogen–progestagen balance or autonomic activity may modify the action of drugs and species variations make it unwise to transfer data from one species to another; for example, the rabbit myometrium is progesterone dominated in pregnancy in a way which cannot be demonstrated in the human uterus.

Despite this a number of substances are known to be powerful stimulants of the myometrium, i.e. they show oxytocic properties. These include both naturally occurring substances, such as oxytocin and noradrenaline, and synthetic drugs. No compounds which are comparably effective as uterine relaxants are yet available.

Myometrial stimulants

OXYTOCIN
The physiological properties of this hormone and the neural control of its hypothalamic secretion and hypophysial release are described in vol. 1, p. 25.15.

The structural formula of oxytocin was elucidated and the substance was synthesized by du Vigneaud in 1953. This was the first polypeptide hormone to be synthesized and for this work he was awarded a Nobel prize for chemistry. Oxytocin proved to be a polypeptide with a pentapeptide ring and a side-chain of three amino acids (fig. 12.5).

It has been possible to synthesize a number of com-

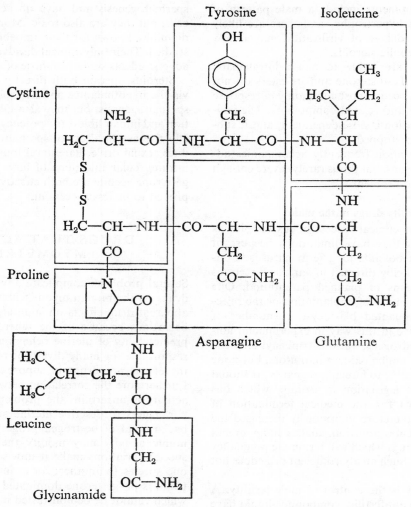

FIG. 12.5. Structural formula of oxytocin (after Berde).

pounds with varying amino acid sequences and, by so doing, to modify their pharmacological properties. Thus, if the glutaminyl or asparginyl components are replaced by other amino acids, the oxytocic property is lost. By contrast, replacement of isoleucine in the pentapeptide ring by valine increases oxytocic activity. Synthetic oxytocin (syntocinon) has virtually replaced extracts of posterior pituitary for clinical use because it does not contain any vasopressin or foreign protein. It is freely water soluble and is stable in acid solutions.

Estimation of oxytocic activity
There is no chemical method for the measurement of oxytocin and it is necessary to rely on bioassay. The most clearly identified biological effects of oxytocin are the stimulation of uterine muscle, the ejection of milk from the lactating breast and a lowering of blood pressure in fowls. Each of these effects has been employed

for bioassays of oxytocin. Unfortunately all of these assays are relatively inaccurate and nonspecific, and this has hindered physiological studies of this hormone. An international standard of powdered beef posterior lobes is used in these assays, 0·5 mg of this extract containing 1 unit of oxytocic activity.

Pharmacological effects
On the uterus. Dale demonstrated in 1906 that extracts of posterior pituitary gland stimulate the uterus, and it is now certain that this activity is a function of oxytocin. Vasopressin has some oxytocic effect but only about 5 per cent that of oxytocin. Little is known of the mode of action of oxytocin; it has no direct effect on the actomyosin-ATP system of the uterus but acts rather on the permeability of cell membranes. The effects of oxytocin on the myometrium are modified by the local oestrogen–progestagen balance; oestrogens increase oxytocin sensi-

tivity whereas progestagen dominance may block the myometrial response to oxytocin. However, the inter-relations of oxytocin, oestrogen and progestagen in controlling the myometrium, particularly in relation to the mechanisms which determine the onset of labour, are still unknown.

Despite these uncertainties, it is well established that intravenous infusions of low doses of oxytocin (1–16 mU/min) in late pregnancy increase the frequency and ampli-tude of uterine contractions without raising uterine tonus, as indicated by intra-amniotic pressures between con-tractions (vol. 1, p. 37.48). It is this property which makes it suitable for clinical use in the induction of labour. Higher doses produce greater uterine activity and a rise in tonus. The response of the uterus to oxytocin increases throughout pregnancy, but there is probably no dramatic increase in sensitivity prior to the onset of labour.

On the kidneys. Oxytocin has some antidiuretic activity, but only about 5 per cent that of vasopressin. In the dose in which it is usually used clinically it has no demon-strable antidiuretic activity in man, but at levels of 100 mU/min in the postpartum period antidiuresis may occur. In some species, especially rat and dog, higher doses of oxytocin may exert a paradoxical diuretic effect, but the underlying mechanisms are unknown.

On the cardiovascular system. The depressor effect of intravenous oxytocin in birds, which is the basis of one bioassay for oxytocin, is due to peripheral vasodilation. The circulatory effects of oxytocin in man are complex. Older reports of 'pituitary shock' following the injection of posterior pituitary extracts were due either to the vasopressin content or to anaphylaxis due to foreign proteins. In usual therapeutic doses oxytocin has little demonstrable circulatory effects, but higher doses may cause a transient fall in blood pressure. The peripheral circulatory effects of oxytocin are variable. In small doses oxytocin is vasodilator, but if the sympathetic system is blocked it shows vasoconstrictor properties. Pretreatment with oestrogens also produces a vasoconstrictor effect in response to oxytocin.

Metabolism
Intravenously administered oxytocin has a half-life of about 10–15 min in nonpregnant women or men. It is inactivated mainly by the kidneys but also by the liver. Furthermore, an oxytocinase appears in steadily increas-ing quantities in the blood throughout pregnancy and this increases the rapidity of clearance of oxytocin; the half-life of oxytocin in late pregnancy is about 1–3 min. A similar oxytocinase is present in human placentae. The physiological role of this oxytocinase is unknown, but it is unlikely to be relevant to the mechanisms controlling the onset of labour. Oxytocin is rapidly absorbed from

mucosal surfaces, especially those of the buccal and nasal cavities. It is rapidly destroyed in the gut if administered orally.

Clinical uses
Oxytocin is most commonly administered intravenously as a solution in 5 per cent dextrose in concentrations of about 1–10 units/l at infusion rates of about 1–16 mU/min. Intravenous infusion allows for precise control of oxytocic activity. However, there is some convenience in using linguets containing oxytocin. These are retained in the buccal cavity, between teeth and cheeks, and are clinically effective. An oxytocin snuff has also been em-ployed.

Oxytocin is used almost exclusively for the induction of labour or abortion. The main risk of this therapy is overstimulation of the uterus. This may cause uterine rupture, or interfere with uterine blood flow and produce foetal asphyxia. Circulatory or renal effects of oxytocin are of no clinical significance.

ERGOT ALKALOIDS
These are discussed in chap. 13. Ergometrine (or ergono-vine) is the alkaloid most widely used for its oxytocic properties. However, the type of uterine response to ergometrine differs from that to oxytocin. Ergometrine induces a prolonged tonic uterine contraction upon which rapid clonic contractions are superimposed. This means that ergometrine cannot be safely used during gestation, and its use is virtually confined to the immediate post-partum or postabortal period when the induced tonic contractions serve to arrest bleeding from the placental site.

Ergometrine maleate is water-soluble and is the pre-paration in general clinical use. It is effective both orally and parenterally, in a standard dose of 0·5 mg. Given intramuscularly it takes about 7 min to act and this may be too slow for safety. A more rapid action can be ob-tained either by intravenous administration (about 45 sec) or by combining ergometrine with oxytocin as syntome-trine which contains 0·5 mg ergometrine and 5 units syntocinon. Oxytocin acts within 1–2 min, and this rapid action is followed by the prolonged effect of ergometrine. This makes syntometrine an ideal preparation for post-partum use.

Ergometrine has a negligible vascular effect. However, in women who are already hypertensive, a transient but sometimes massive increase in blood pressure may follow intravenous injections of ergometrine. Ergotamine has little oxytocic activity.

SPARTEINE SULPHATE
Sparteine is an alkaloid extracted from the flowering broom, *Sarothamnus scoparius*. It was isolated over 100 years ago. Its structure has been determined and syn-

thesized. It has been widely used in the treatment of cardiac irregularities but has been superseded by quinidine and other compounds. It was this action of sparteine on the heart which led to the original observation that it

Sparteine

has oxytocic properties, and since 1939 it has been widely used in European and Latin American countries in clinical obstetrics. Over the last ten years several clinical trials have been conducted in the United States. Initial studies suggested that it had some advantages over oxytocin; it can be safely administered intramuscularly, does not require constant supervision of the patient and has a wide margin of safety.

However, subsequent studies suggest that the action of sparteine on the uterus resembles that of ergometrine more closely than that of oxytocin and it may cause tonic contractions. Furthermore intramuscular administration provides very poor control of the oxytocic action and both uterine rupture and foetal death from asphyxia have been reported. It is unlikely that sparteine is either as safe or effective as oxytocin.

OESTROGENS

It is generally accepted that oestrogens increase the contractile potential of the uterus. Intravenous infusions of oestradiol-17β in a colloidal suspension increase uterine activity. This is probably a direct effect on the myometrium rather than secondary to oxytocin release, as it is unaccompanied by any action on milk ejection. However, clinical studies have failed to show that oestrogens are of value either in altering myometrial responsiveness to exogenous oxytocin or in modifying usefully spontaneous uterine contractions.

Uterine relaxants

Several substances have been shown to inhibit spontaneous uterine activity in experimental animals or *in vitro*. However, all clinical studies have been bedevilled by the lack of controlled conditions, and no uterine relaxant has yet been established to be of proven clinical value. This is unfortunate since pregnancy wastage due to premature labour is a major problem, and it would be invaluable to have some preparation which could arrest labour in these circumstances.

ETHYL ALCOHOL

The diuretic effect of alcohol is well known and has been shown to be due to the inhibition of the release of vaso-

pressin. However, the release of oxytocin is also blocked by alcohol. Thus, alcohol inhibits the milk ejection reflex in lactating rabbits and postpones spontaneous delivery in parturient rabbits. It has recently been shown to inhibit milk ejection and uterine activity in the human subject. Alcohol can be given either orally or intravenously. Effective blood levels are between 90 and 160 mg/100 ml. This can be achieved by a loading dose of 15 ml/kg body weight of a ten per cent solution of ethanol over a period of 2 hours, followed by a maintenance dose of about 1·5 ml/kg body weight hourly, usually for a period of about 6 hours.

ISOXSUPRINE

Adrenergic nerves supply smooth muscle fibres in the human myometrium, and there is evidence for the presence of both α- and β-receptors in the human uterus, in so far as α- and β-adrenergic blocking agents influence the uterus both *in vivo* and *in vitro*. Adrenaline can also produce transient relaxation of the hyperactive uterus, but this is of no clinical value because of the circulatory

Isoxsuprine

effects of this drug. Isoxsuprine is a sympathomimetic drug of the β-phenylethylamine group which relaxes myometrial strips *in vitro*, probably acting via β-receptors. It is claimed that it can arrest spontaneous uterine activity in premature labour, but this has not been convincingly established by controlled trials. Furthermore adverse effects, particularly hypotension, tachycardia and nausea, limit its clinical use.

PROGESTAGENS

The effect of progestagens on the myometrium is poorly understood but it is likely that they inhibit uterine contractility, probably by hyperpolarizing myometrial cell membranes. Progesterone can delay the onset of spontaneous labour in rabbits; it inhibits spontaneous human uterine activity *in vitro*, and it sometimes reduces spontaneous activity in both the pregnant and nonpregnant human uterus *in vivo*. Despite this, controlled trials have failed to demonstrate that progestagens are of clinical value as a uterine relaxant, at least in terms of arresting premature labour.

MISCELLANEOUS AGENTS

General anaesthesia, at the level of the first or second planes of anaesthesia, inhibits uterine activity. Ether, chloroform and halothane are more effective in this role than cyclopropane. Spinal or epidural analgesia has no demonstrable effects on uterine activity.

The effect of heavy sedation, using morphine or diamorphine, on uterine activity is controversial; at most it may exert a temporary inhibition if given during the early latent phase of labour.

Several other substances in common clinical use have been tested for their effect on the myometrium, but none has been shown to alter uterine activity significantly. These include nitrous oxide and trichlorethylene, muscle relaxants, atropine and scopolamine, tranquillizing drugs and antihistamines.

EFFECTS OF DRUGS ON THE FOETUS

Until the thalidomide disaster in 1961 little attention was given to the effects of drugs on the foetus. From 1956 in West Germany and from 1958 in Britain thalidomide, a glutarimide derivative, was readily available as a sedative and hypnotic. Its principal advantage was that overdosage was not lethal. However, in 1960 and 1961 it appeared that thalidomide could cause peripheral neuritis and hypothyroidism and for this reason it was not approved for marketing in the United States. Between 1959 and 1961 an increasing number of infants with severe malformations of the limbs (phocomelia) was noted in West Germany, and careful questioning revealed that many of these women had taken thalidomide in early pregnancy. This information was widely publicized and similar observations were reported in this country in 1961, and the drug was withdrawn from West German and British markets in December, 1961. It has been estimated that thalidomide may have caused 10,000 birth deformities, the great majority in West Germany.

Drugs may exert two types of deleterious effect in the foetus, teratogenicity and toxicity.

TERATOGENETIC EFFECTS
All malformations are the result of either genetic or environmental influences, and drug teratogenicity is part of the overall problem of an unfavourable environment. However, the origin of only a small minority of malformations is purely genetic and another small minority is purely environmental. In the vast majority of instances, neonatal phenotype is the product of the interaction of genotype and maternal environment, and it is impossible to assess the relative importance of each factor.

This is well illustrated by thalidomide. Of the many British women who took this drug, fewer than 500 gave birth to a deformed child, and it is estimated that 80 per cent of mothers who took thalidomide in early pregnancy in West Germany delivered a normal infant. It is likely that there are genetic mechanisms which determine foetal susceptibility to drugs.

Two other major factors are the dosage of drug and the timing of administration. Excessive dosage is likely to be lethal to the foetus *in utero*, whereas a subthreshold dose may have no effect; thus, teratogenicity may occur only within a specific dose range. Drugs administered prior to implantation probably either kill the embryo or have no teratogenic effect. Teratogenic response is related to the stage of morphogenesis, and sensitivity is maximal during the first 6–8 weeks after implantation. Organs that are at a critical state of development at the time of foetal exposure to the drug are those which are liable to be malformed. After organogenesis is complete, organs are not malformed by drugs.

Although some drugs may induce characteristic anomalies in experimental animals or in man, for example, cortisone is associated with cleft palate and thalidomide with phocomelia, these are not specific for each drug. One teratogen may exert different effects depending on its time of administration, whereas several drugs may produce the same lesion; for example, over thirty teratogens can mimic the effects of thalidomide on limb development. While teratogens may act directly on the foetus, probably on cellular metabolic pathways, they may also act indirectly and damage the foetus by impairing the maternal environment, e.g. by reducing uteroplacental blood flow.

Despite a vast amount of drug testing since 1961, there are few proven teratogens in man. The teratogenic properties of thalidomide are established, and related compounds such as glutethamide and bemegride should be avoided in pregnancy. Progestagens are widely used in pregnancy; some of these, especially 19-nortestosterones, may induce virilization of a female foetus, although this rarely amounts to more than labial fusion and clitoral hypertrophy. Cortisone can induce cleft palate in some rodents, but there is no evidence that it is teratogenic in human pregnancy. Folic acid antagonists, especially aminopterin, may cause either abortion or foetal malformation. Other antimetabolites, such as 6-mercaptopurine and nitrogen mustard, may have a similar effect, although many pregnancies where these drugs have been used to save the mother's life have produced normal infants.

OTHER ADVERSE EFFECTS
Some drugs can exert an immediate toxic action on the foetus *in utero*. Thiouracil, used for the treatment of hyperthyroidism in pregnancy, may induce goitre and hypothyroidism in the infant. Thiouracil is also excreted in milk so that lactation is contraindicated. Iodides are also goitrogenic, while radioactive iodine causes severe damage in the foetal thyroid and is absolutely contraindicated in pregnancy.

The anticoagulants, bishydroxycoumarin and ethylbiscoumacetate, can cause severe haemorrhage in the foetus, even if the mother's prothrombin time is carefully controlled. Heparin probably does not cross the placenta and has some advantages for anticoagulant therapy during pregnancy.

Tetracyclines cause discolouration of deciduous teeth and may impair bone growth. Streptomycin is a possible cause of congenital VIIIth cranial nerve deafness.

Hypotensive drugs may be used for the treatment of pregnancy hypertension. Ganglion blocking agents such as hexamethonium may cause neonatal ileus, and reserpine can cause nasal congestion and drowsiness in the infant.

Other drugs exert an effect on the foetus which assumes significance only after parturition. For example, sulphonamides administered to the mother enter the foetus and interfere with the metabolism of bilirubin. They may compete with bilirubin for binding sites on serum albumin displacing protein-bound bilirubin and releasing free bilirubin to diffuse into tissues. This is not critical for the foetus *in utero* because the placenta excretes the excess bilirubin into the maternal circulation. However, jaundice may develop after birth. Similarly, powerful analgesics, such as morphine or pethidine, are regularly prescribed for pain relief in labour, and general anaesthesia is occasionally used for delivery. These analgesics and anaesthetics enter the foetus and depress the respiratory centre. These effects are not detectable during labour but become critical at the moment of birth when there should be a rapid conversion from placental to pulmonary respiration. Drug induced respiratory depression is an important cause of neonatal asphyxia.

The risks of drug toxicity on the foetus are maximal in the later weeks of pregnancy. All the examples quoted above refer to effects which are readily and immediately demonstrable. This should not be allowed to obscure the possibility that drugs may exert a more subtle later effect on behaviour and intelligence.

The problem of drug hazards to the foetus must be considered in perspective. Foetal malformation is now the greatest single cause of perinatal mortality, in addition to being a major cause of infant morbidity, the incidence of major anomalies being of the order of 1–2 per cent. In our current state of ignorance of the causes of human teratogenesis it is only sensible to minimize foetal exposure to drugs. The old concept of a 'placental barrier' which policed traffic between mother and foetus is discredited, and it should be appreciated that the majority of drugs readily cross the placental membrane. It was recently estimated in the United States that 92 per cent of women were given at least one drug during pregnancy, and 4 per cent received ten or more drugs. Casual administration of drugs is always to be deprecated, but when a drug is taken by a pregnant woman it is also being given to her foetus.

Steps have been taken to minimize drug hazards to the foetus. Before a new drug is marketed it is subjected to tests for teratogenicity and toxicity. This is not entirely satisfactory because of major species variation in drug effects, e.g. salicylates cause malformations in rats and mice but have never been reported to be teratogenic in man. This problem may be minimized by using several species for testing each drug, and there may be merit in making greater use of subhuman primates for this purpose. Secondly, when a new drug is released for clinical use, any possible case of foetal damage should be reported to the appropriate committee, e.g. Committee for Safety of Drugs in the United Kingdom. However, such clinical case reports are difficult to interpret, and the association between foetal malformation and a history of the use of a drug is not necessarily causal; in particular, it may be that the significant association is between foetal hazard and the disease for which the drug was prescribed. For example, early reports suggested that oral hypoglycaemic agents, used in the treatment of diabetes in pregnancy, might cause foetal malformation; these reports have not been confirmed, and it is recognized that maternal diabetes itself predisposes to congenital anomalies.

FURTHER READING

Austin C.R. & Perry J.S. (1965) *Agents Affecting Fertility.* Biological Council Symposium. London: Churchill.

Caldeyro-Barcio R. & Heller H. (1961) *Oxytocin.* Proceedings of an International Symposium in Montevideo in 1959. Oxford: Pergamon.

Jackson H. (1966) *Antifertility Compounds in the Male and Female.* Springfield: Thomas.

Chapter 13
Ergot, ergot alkaloids and ergotism

Ergotism is now a very rare disease and ergot is a drug with a strictly limited use. The account which follows is longer than the importance, in contemporary medicine, of either the drug or the disease. However, historically their study served as a gateway to nineteenth- and twentieth-century pharmacology. The present chapter provides an historical understanding of many of the contemporary investigations of drug action.

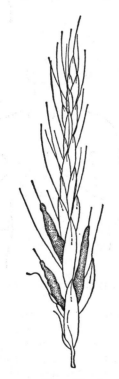

FIG. 13.1. Rye with sclerotia.

In the past ergot was known not only as a poison but also as a useful obstetrical remedy. Investigation of its constituents led to the incidental discovery of substances which, as local hormones, regulate important functions in the body. The alkaloids themselves can now be regarded as derivatives of (+)-lysergic acid. Depending on their structure, they act as antagonists of adrenaline, stimulants of uterine and smooth muscle and have complex effects on the central nervous system. The central actions of the alkaloids are poorly understood, but the discovery of D-(+)-lysergic acid diethylamide, which is psychoactive, has provided new insight into behaviour and abnormal mental states (p. 5.26).

Ergot is the fungus, *Claviceps purpurea*, which attacks edible rye, *Secale cereale*. Wind and insects carry the spores to the moist stigmata of the flower where they germinate. The mycelium eventually replaces the ovary with a soft spongy tissue that hardens to form the sclerotium. This is the resting stage of the fungus and the commercial source of the drug. The sclerotium is about 2–4 cm long, slightly curved and dark purple. Hence the resemblance to a horn or spur on the rye, and the name *Secale cornutum*, spurred rye or ergot (fig. 13.1), the latter from *argot* (old French) meaning a cock's spur. European languages and their dialects contain a multitude of names for ergot.

Rye was first cultivated in southern Europe at the beginning of the Christian era and became the chief cereal in Russia, eastern and central Europe. Rye bread was the bread of the Teutons, and for centuries it was the staple diet of the peasant. When the rye was heavily infected with fungus, whole communities were liable to be afflicted with St. Anthony's Fire, a disease which came to be known later as ergotism.

Ergotism

The history of ergotism is that of its epidemics which continued well into the nineteenth century. Soil, climate, wars and famine all contributed at different times to increase the consumption of ergot. In parts of France, such as the Sologne where ergotism was endemic, poor drainage of the soil and spells of warm, humid weather provided favourable conditions for growth of the fungus. In 1709 the rye crop from this region was reported to be as much as one-quarter ergot, and a person eating the bread might have ingested daily about 100 g of ergot. Such quantities of the fungus led to cumulative poisoning which, within days or weeks, ended in mutilation or death.

The earliest descriptions of ergotism are found in the chronicles of the Middle Ages. The disease was called Fire because of intolerable burning pain in the limbs, which became black and shrivelled and dropped off. In the thirteenth century, the Order of St. Anthony was founded in Vienne, in Dauphiné. The monks opened houses with the walls painted red, for the care of those stricken with the Holy Fire (*Ignis Sacer*) or St. Anthony's Fire, as it came to be known. The beneficial effect of a stay in hospital or of a pilgrimage to shrines might well have been due to change of diet.

The connection between eating bread containing ergot and the subsequent poisoning was recognized only gradually and many indications of the toxicity of spurred rye, both in man and farm animals, were ignored. Those who knew better avoided the infected rye; but the peasant often had no choice. In the seventeenth century a succession of severe epidemics aroused public concern and led to the first detailed descriptions of the two forms of the disease, **gangrenous** and **convulsive ergotism**. Gangrenous ergotism was seen mainly in France, whereas the

the part became dry and mummified and eventually separated. The extent of this dry gangrene varied from slight damage to the fingers and toes to the loss of whole limbs.

Severe itch, pins and needles or formication (like ants crawling all over the body) and powerful spasms which contorted the limbs or whole body, were characteristic features of convulsive ergotism (fig. 13.2). When the convulsions involved chiefly the flexor muscles 'the sick would round up their bodies like a ball'; when the extensors were affected, they became rigid 'like a statue'.

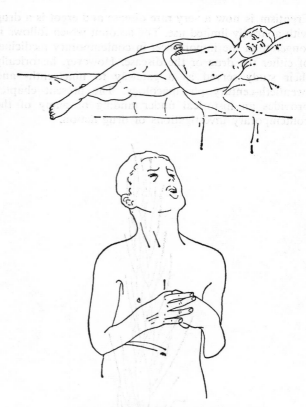

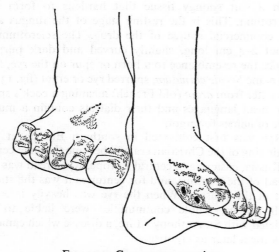

FIG. 13.2. Gangrenous ergotism.

FIG. 13.3. Convulsive ergotism.

convulsive form was more common in Germany, but mixed forms also occurred. This curious geographical distribution of the two types appears to have been related to diet. In France, the diet contained more dairy products than in Germany. Milk, eggs, butter and fats came to be regarded as foods which prevented the disease.

The onset of ergotism was often marked by a sense of lassitude and oppression, a livid colour of the skin and painful contractures. After several days or weeks, the sensation of heat in the affected part became increasingly severe and alternated with a sensation of icy cold. Gradually the limb became numbed and suddenly, all sensation might be lost. By this time gangrene had set in;

Convulsions occurred unpredictably, and in the intervals the sick felt ravenously hungry. Impairment of hearing and of sight, glaucoma, paralysis, epilepsy and dementia were complications of the convulsive form.

By the beginning of the nineteenth century, ergotism had greatly declined. Public authorities had learnt to enforce the inspection of rye crops and the removal of sclerotia by sieving and cleansing the grain. Improved methods of agriculture reduced the infection of the rye. Furthermore the consumption of rye fell after the introduction from America of the potato, which gradually spread over Europe between 1650 and 1750. With the decline of religious wars prosperity increased, and more people were able to buy wheaten bread.

Ergot as a drug

The use of ergot in midwifery was probably known to the Chinese and the Arabians. The first mention of ergot as a drug in European literature was in the sixteenth century, but it had long been a secret remedy in the hands of midwives and quacks. The recommended dose was then three sclerotia. In the eighteenth century its value in obstetrics was widely known, and ergot as a powder began to be prescribed by the physicians (*pulvis ad partum;* poudre obstètricale). At the turn of the century, John Stearns, of Saratoga County U.S.A., got to know of the powder from an old woman who had migrated from Eastern Europe. He found spurred rye in the local granaries and began to use it on his patients. In 1808 he published his *Account of the Pulvis parturiens, a Remedy for quickening childbirth*, part of which is worth quoting.

'It expedites parturition, and saves the accoucheur a considerable portion of time, without producing any bad effects on the patient. . . . Previous to its exhibition it is of the utmost consequence to ascertain the presentation . . . as the violent and almost incessant action which it induces in the uterus precludes the possibility of turning. . . . My method of administering it is either in decoction or in a powder. Boil half a drachm of the powder in half a pint of water, and give one-third every twenty minutes till the pain commences. In the powder I give five to ten grains; some patients require larger doses, though I have generally found these sufficient. If the dose is large it will produce nausea and vomiting. In most cases you will be surprised with the suddenness of its operation; it is, therefore, necessary to be completely ready before you give the medicine.'

As the use of ergot grew rapidly in popularity both in the U.S.A. and in Europe, the hazard to the foetus became apparent in the large increase in the number of still births. In 1822 Hossack wrote that as far as the child was concerned 'pulvis ad partum had become pulvis ad mortem'. The use of ergot was hereafter almost entirely restricted to aid in the expulsion of the placenta and to stop postpartum bleeding. The U.S. Pharmacopoeia of 1820 was the first official publication to include ergot. Later, in 1928, Barger wrote: 'ergot like digitalis was introduced into medicine from a popular source in Europe; it was, however, only in the New World that freedom from prejudice secured recognition of ergot; perhaps the Old World had suffered too much from its poisonous properties'.

EARLY INVESTIGATIONS

Ergot soon became an object of scientific interest and took its place among medicinal plants which were being examined for their active principles by the new chemical methods. Some of these active principles were complex organic bases which contained nitrogen in quaternary ammonium or amino form and, because they combined readily with strong acids to form water-soluble salts, these bases were called alkaloids. Since fungi are more closely related to plants than to bacteria, it was not surprising to find that ergot contained alkaloids. The first pure alkaloidal substance to be isolated from ergot was **ergotinine** in 1875, and this later turned out to be a dextroisomer of **ergotoxine** and was virtually inactive. On keeping, however, ergotinine was slowly transformed to its more potent isomeride, which for a long time gave rise to the belief that it was active. Cockerels were then commonly used to test for the activity of galenical (impure) preparations of ergot alkaloids. Within days of injecting the dose, the comb and wattles became cyanosed; gangrene then developed in the comb and the affected part was shed, leaving the comb reduced in size. This effect was later developed into a quantitative method of assay.

By the turn of the century, the extract of ergot had found its way into most of the Pharmacopoeias, but the problem of how it acted remained. The extract was presented as a liquid or a solid. The liquid extract was prepared by macerating ergot in water or in a solution of water and alcohol; if with water, alcohol was added afterwards as a preservative. The solid extract was ergot after removal of fatty substances. Obstetrical experience had shown beyond doubt that the active principle absorbed from the gut, quickly produced powerful contractions of the uterus and that the extract was remarkably free from other effects. So much was known in 1904 when Henry S. Wellcome, founder of the first laboratory for experimental pharmacology in Britain, invited the young physiologist Henry Dale to make an attempt 'to clear up the problem of ergot, the pharmacy, pharmacology and therapeutics of the drug being then in a state of obvious confusion'. The collaborative work which followed with George Barger, was to have far reaching effects on developments in physiology, pharmacology and therapeutics over the next 50 years.

Actions of ergot

Dale began by testing various impure but active preparations of ergot which were known by such cumbersome names as chrysotoxin, sphacelotoxin and cornutine, but for simplicity Dale thought of them all as ergot. Extracts were shown to raise the arterial blood pressure, and contract the uterus and the sphincter of the iris. Since the effects were still obtained after ablation of the CNS, Dale concluded that ergot must have a primary stimulating action on smooth muscle. The discovery of a second action was fortuitous and is best told in Dale's own words:

'I was finishing one of these experiments on a spinal cat, to which I had given successive doses of one of Barger's ergot preparations, when a sample of dried adrenal gland substance was delivered to me from the Burroughs

9

Wellcome factory, with a request that I would test it for the presence of a normal proportion of adrenaline. The moment seemed opportune; a boiled extract was easily prepared, and there was a cat most suitable, as it seemed, for the required test. Successive injections of the extract elicited, to my surprise, only falls of the arterial pressure, and, with the confidence of inexperience, I condemned the sample without hesitation. And then, by another and almost incredibly fortunate coincidence, the same sequence of events was repeated in detail a week later. Again I was finishing an experiment on a spinal cat, which again had been heavily dosed with an ergot preparation, when a sample of adrenal gland substance was again delivered for testing. Quite possibly it was from the same batch again, sent to control not only the quality of the material, but also the competence of the new young pharmacologist; but that was never revealed to me. The result was, of course, the same as on the earlier occasion; but reference to my notes now raised the question whether the cat's response to adrenaline might have been so altered, by the heavy doses of ergot given in both cases, that the normal pressor action had been reversed. It seemed unlikely, but control tests showed promptly that, in an animal not thus treated with ergot, both samples of the adrenal material had the usual pressor action, representing a normal content of adrenaline and then that treatment with ergot reversed the action of pure adrenaline itself' (fig. 13.4).

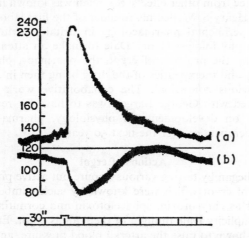

FIG. 13.4. (a) Effect on the carotid blood pressure (mm Hg) of a pithed cat of 0·025 mg of adrenaline before, and (b) 0·1 mg of adrenaline after, 10 mg of ergotoxine. From Dale H.H. (1953) *Adventures in Physiology*. Oxford: Pergamon.

This observation acquired additional significance from Elliot's suggestion that the effects of sympathetic nerve stimulation might be mediated by a substance with the actions of adrenaline. For Dale, the reversal of the pressor effect of adrenaline after ergot was the starting point of an investigation to test the effect of the drug at many other sites known to be innervated by sympathetic fibres.

Dale showed, moreover, that these effects of ergot were confined to the sympathetic part of the autonomic nervous system; ergot did not alter the responses to stimulation of parasympathetic nerves, nor did it prevent contractions produced by barium chloride or posterior pituitary extract, substances that act directly on smooth muscle. Dale concluded that ergot 'paralysed the motor elements in the structures, associated with sympathetic innervation, which adrenaline stimulates, the inhibitor elements retaining their normal function'. He left open the question why ergot failed to abolish the cardio-accelerator effect of adrenaline or to act at sites where adrenaline or the effects of sympathetic nerve stimulation were inhibitory. Thus, ergot was the first antagonist of adrenaline which in masking certain of its effects, revealed others. Today, these observations have been re-interpreted in terms of α- and β-receptors for adrenaline. The first antagonist for the β-receptors, dichloroisopropylnoradrenaline (DCI), was not discovered until 52 years later (p. 15.22).

Ergotoxine and other constituents of ergot

Barger and Dale later confirmed the effects of ergot, using ergotoxine which was the first pure alkaloidal substance with pharmacological activity to be isolated from ergot. The question arose whether ergotoxine was the principle responsible for the therapeutic action of the liquid extract. On chemical tests alone, the pharmacopoeial preparation contained only traces of the alkaloid, which might have been predicted from the low solubility of the alkaloid in water. Indeed, the alkaloid had been obtained from crude ergot by extraction with nonpolar solvents, whereas the principle of the liquid extract, whatever it might be, was water soluble. Had clinical tests to compare the oxytocic activities of ergotoxine and the liquid extract been feasible at this time, doubts about ergotoxine might have been resolved; but so, too, might the exciting discovery of other substances in ergot have been delayed, or entirely missed. Although the extract was known to possess pharmacological activity, Barger was unable to find any other active alkaloid in ergot. Hence it seemed that the oxytocic principle of the liquid extract might not be an alkaloid after all, but some other substance.

In 1907, Dale attended a physiological Congress in Heidelberg and saw for the first time a demonstration of the effect of a watery extract of ergot on an isolated horn from a cat's uterus. Kehrer, an obstetrician, was using a new method introduced by Magnus of Utrecht for studying the effect of drugs on isolated organs suspended in a bath. Dale was impressed not only by the method but also by the powerful action of the extract on the uterus, which far exceeded that previously seen with any extract of the fungus.

Now, it was well known that in the commercial manufacture of the watery extract, there was always some putrefaction, which meant that amines were probably being formed from amino acids as the result of bacterial growth. From a similar extract of ergot, Barger was soon able to obtain material which contained several pharmacologically active amines. These were separated into fractions and tested for their effects on the blood pressure of the anaesthetized or pithed cat. **Tyramine** (from tyrosine) and **isoamylamine** (from leucine) were identified as amines with pressor effects; **acetylcholine** and β-**imidazolylethylamine**, later called **histamine**, were among those bases which lowered the arterial blood pressure. Histamine isolated from ergot proved to be chemically identical with histamine which had been synthesized from β-imidazolylproprionic acid and to have the same powerful effects on the uterus, whether isolated or *in situ*. For a time, it seemed that histamine might be responsible for this effect. Both ergotoxine and histamine (also known as ergamine) were made available as chemically pure oxytocic drugs which were active when given by injection. Trials indicated not only that the uterine or oxytocic action was in each case less predictable than that of the extract, but that both produced undesirable systemic effects. It was not surprising therefore, that practitioners preferred to go on using the well tried liquid extract of ergot.

Although the problem of the identity of the oxytocic principle in pharmacopoeial preparations of ergot had not been solved, these studies led to the discovery of constitutents which differed from the alkaloids in not being specific to ergot. Apart from those already mentioned, other constituents were the amines **agmatine** (from arginine), **cadaverine** (from lysine) **putrescine** (from ornithine) and their corresponding amino acids, **ergothioneine**, the betaine of thiolhistidine and **ergosterol**.

Hence Dale's reference to ergot as a 'veritable treasure house' of substances with pharmacological interest.

LATER INVESTIGATIONS

Most of the ergot alkaloids were identified in the years between 1920 and 1940. Important among these were **ergotamine** and **ergometrine**. By 1935, studies of the degradation products of ergotinine and ergotamine had led to the isolation of lysergic acid, from which all the natural alkaloids are derived. It became possible to classify the alkaloids on a chemical basis and to make the first synthetic derivatives of lysergic acid. Further, material containing ergotoxine yielded three other related alkaloids. Hydrogenation of these alkaloids, as of ergotamine, had the remarkable effect of reducing their activity in stimulating smooth muscle, while enhancing their antagonism for adrenaline. Advances in the chemistry of the alkaloids broadened their pharmacological interest. Effects on the central nervous system were recognized for the first time and quantitative studies of the antagonism between adrenaline and the alkaloids made it possible to devise methods for their biological assay. These studies were intimately related to therapeutic applications of the alkaloids in obstetrics and in medicine.

Discovery of ergometrine

Ergotamine, first isolated from ergot by Stoll in 1920, shared all the actions then known of ergotoxine and had about the same molecular weight. But, whereas ergotoxine had not been much used in obstetric practice, ergotamine came to be widely tested on the assumption that it was the active principle of the pharmacopoeial preparations of ergot. Certain facts, however, threw doubt on this assumption. Firstly, ergotamine, like ergotoxine, was poorly soluble in water; secondly, it acted best when given by injection; thirdly, it was liable to produce undesirable effects, such as tightness in the head, vomiting about 30 min after the dose and a sense of lassitude which might persist for several hours. In all these respects it differed from the liquid extract of ergot. The claim made for ergotamine, that it possessed all the properties of a good pharmacopoeial preparation of ergot, raised the question whether it, any more than ergotoxine, was the oxytocic principle. The matter became the subject of a lively controversy between Stoll in Basel (Sandoz) and Dale in London, which was touched off in the following way. In 1930 Smith and Timmis of Burroughs Wellcome reported that in their hands Stoll's method of obtaining ergotamine from official ergot (sclerotia from rye) gave only ergotoxine, but that when they used unofficial ergot (sclerotia from New Zealand Festuca grass) the method gave an ample yield of ergotamine. Stoll pointed out that official ergots varied widely in their alkaloidal content but did not disclose the exact source and botanical description of the ergot used in Basel. He also stressed that comparisons of ergot preparations based on laboratory experiments gave no real indication of their therapeutic potency, and that in short, clinical experience had shown beyond doubt that ergotamine was as effective as any of the pharmacopoeial preparations of ergot. In this view, Stoll found support in the British Pharmacopoeial Codex (1923) which stated that although ergotoxine had been used clinically for its action on the uterus, it was disappointing and gynaecologists were now generally agreed that it was not the active constituent they wanted. Ergotamine, however, was mentioned as an alternative to the liquid extract.

The controversy served a useful purpose for it led to the first objective comparisons of the effects of the alkaloids and other constitutents of ergot on the human uterus. These were carried out in 1932 by Chassar Moir for the Medical Research Council, London. A new method of recording uterine activity was used in which on the 6th or 7th day of the puerperium a bag containing water was placed in the uterus and connected to a mercury manometer which wrote on a drum. With this method, Moir found that the effects of ergotoxine and ergotamine were indistinguishable: 0·25 mg intravenously acted in 4–10 min, 0·5 mg intramuscularly in 15–45 min and oral doses of 2–2·5 mg produced an inconstant effect in 35–60 min. Thus, the time of onset of the effect was found to vary with the route of administration. The effect lasted for less than 3 hours and was usually accompanied by a sense of depression. Histamine (1 mg) intramuscularly acted quickly but the effect was slight and there was flushing and much discomfort. Similarly, tyramine (10 mg) intravenously had a fleeting action. When histamine (2–8 mg) or tyramine (60–80 mg) was given by mouth there was no action. Finally, he gave the liquid and solid extracts of ergot. The watery extract had been prepared in strict accordance with the regulations of the British Pharmacopoeia 1914. Chassar Moir wrote:

'Judged by all previous work, the preparation ought to have been inert, for analysis showed only a trace of alkaloid. It was with the greatest surprise that I found that, far from being inert, this preparation surpassed by great measure the activity of any drug I had previously used in the same manner. An equally surprising fact was that the effect appeared in a remarkably short time. In one case, only 4 min elapsed between the swallowing of the extract and the onset of the powerful uterine contractions. The uterine contractions caused by the liquid extract were, with regard to time of onset, nature and frequency, in most striking contrast to those produced by ergotoxine and ergotamine, and it can only be supposed that they were caused by an entirely different constituent of ergot.'

Thus, Moir confirmed the precise clinical description of the effect of ergot which Stearns had given in 1808. Thus, too, was the clinician fully vindicated in his 'dogged belief in the efficiency of the old fashioned preparation'. Later Dudley and Moir isolated the water-soluble alkaloid, ergometrine. Since there was no other

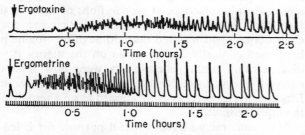

FIG. 13.5. Contractions of human uterus, 1 week after the birth of a baby, after 0·5 mg of ergometrine orally and 0·5 mg of ergotoxine intramuscularly. In spite of being given by a slow method, the ergometrine acted much more rapidly than the ergotoxine. From Chassar Moir (1935) *Proc. roy. Soc. Med.* **28**, 1660.

biological test for the presence of ergometrine than by its effect on the human puerperal uterus, the clinical method was used throughout the entire course of chemical fractionation and up to the time of discovery of the crystalline active substance. In the final tests, the action of ergometrine (0·5–1·0 mg oral) occurred within 6–8 min and was indistinguishable from that of the liquid extract. When a dose of 0·05–0·1 mg was given intravenously, the effect occurred in 65–110 sec. As with the liquid extract, ergometrine in these doses was free from other effects. The actions of ergot preparations on the human uterus are shown in fig. 13.5 and are also discussed on p. 12.15.

Discovery of lysergic acid

For many years the ergot alkaloids were known only by their molecular formulae. It had early been observed that on thermal decomposition ergotoxine yielded the amide of dimethylpyruvic acid and similarly, that ergotamine gave the amide of pyruvic acid. The discovery of new alkaloids prompted investigations into their structure which was ultimately to be proved by Hofmann's complete synthesis of ergotamine in 1963.

The first attempt to degrade an ergot alkaloid with alkali came from Smith and Timmis in 1932, who obtained from ergotinine a basic cleavage product which they named **ergine**. Jacob and Craig of the Rockefeller Institute repeated their experiments and found that ergine, on further hydrolysis, yielded ammonia and a new substance with amphoteric properties which they called **lysergic acid**. Ergine was, in fact, the amide of lysergic acid. By 1936, the structural formula for lysergic acid was proposed and contained three important features (fig. 13.6). First there is a methylated tryptamine residue which foreshadowed the antagonism of derivatives of lysergic acid for 5-HT (p. 16.4). Secondly, three of the fused rings form a rigid structure. The remaining ring, which is a piperidine residue with a double bond, contains an asymmetric carbon atom (C-8 in fig. 13.6). (+)-Lysergic acid and (+)-isolysergic acid differ only in the arrangement of the groups at this atom. In the former the carboxyl is equatorial and in the latter axial. Derivatives of isolysergic acid are pharmacologically inactive but they readily isomerize into the active forms (table 13.1), because the 9–10 double bond in the piperidine ring stabilizes the enol form of the acid. Thirdly, the carbon atom at C-5 is also asymmetric but the bonds cannot be easily rearranged to give the (−)-isomers of lysergic acid and isolysergic acid (p. 3.17).

Lysergic acid itself is not pharmacologically active but acquires activity when coupled with a basic residue. Soon after the isolation of ergometrine, it was found that the residue for this alkaloid was an amino alcohol, which explained the relatively low molecular weight of the alkaloid. The first clear indication that some ergot alkaloids contained a peptide residue was the identification

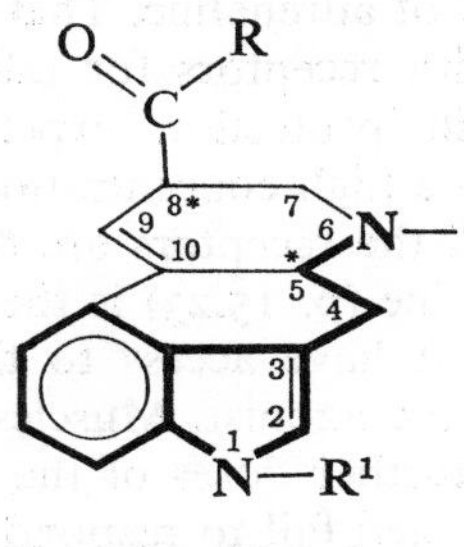

Lysergic acid nucleus

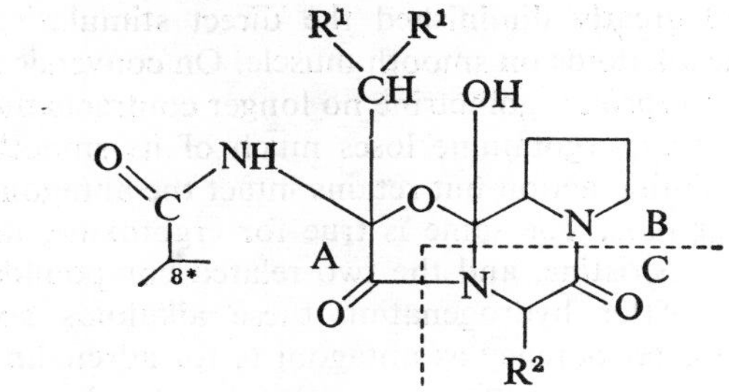

Peptide residue

R = OH,   R¹ = H,   Lysergic acid

R = N(CH₂CH₃)₂,   R¹ = H,   Lysergic acid diethylamide

R = −NHCHCH₂OH, R¹ = H,   Ergometrine
(CH₃)

R = −NHCHCH₂OH, R¹ = H,   Methylergometrine
(CH₂CH₃)

R = −NHCHCH₂OH, R¹ = CH₃, Methysergide
(CH₂CH₃)

$R^1 = H$, $R^2 = -CH_2C_6H_5$,   Ergotamine

$R^1 = CH_3$, $R^2 = -CH_2C_6H_5$,   Ergocristine

$R^1 = CH_3$, $R^2 = -CH_2CH(CH_3)_2$, Ergokryptine
$R^1 = H$, $R^2 = -CH_2CH(CH_3)_2$, Ergosine

$R^1 = CH_3$, $R^2 = -CH(CH_3)_2$, Ergocornine

---

* Asymmetric carbon.
Note: (1) methyl tryptamine structure. (2) double bond between C-9 and C-10. Saturation gives the dihydrogenated alkaloids.

A, pyruvic acid, B, proline and C, amino acid form a tricyclic structure which contains oxazoladine, piperazine and pyrrolidine ring systems.

FIG. 13.6. Ergot alkaloids.

---

of two amino acids from the alkaline cleavage of ergotoxine and ergotamine. These were identified as proline and phenylalanine and were common to the alkaloids. Later, the peptide residue as a whole was split off from nearly all the alkaloids with a peptide structure. Analysis of the structure of this fragment made it possible to classify the alkaloids on a chemical basis and to relate their structure to pharmacological action. The ergot alkaloids and their breakdown products are shown in table 13.1, and their structure in fig. 13.6. In 1943 Stoll and Hofmann together with Rothlin made the important discovery that saturation of the double bond between C-9 and C-10 of

---

TABLE 13.1. Ergot alkaloids. After Stoll A., Hofmann A. & Becker B. (1943). *Helv. chim. Acta.*, **34**, 1544.

Natural	Artificial	Breakdown products	
laevo	dextro	common to the group	specific to alkaloid
Group I			
Ergotamine	Ergotaminine	(+)-Lysergic acid NH₃ ⎫	(−)-Phenylalanine
Ergosine	Ergosinine	Pyruvic acid (+)-proline ⎭	(−)-Leucine
Group II			
Ergotoxine	Ergotinine	(+)-Lysergic acid NH₃, ⎫	(−)-Phenylalanine
Ergocristine	Ergocristinine	dimethyl pyruvic acid ⎬	(−)-Phenylalanine
Ergokryptine	Ergokryptinine	(+)-Proline ⎭	(−)-Leucine
Ergocornine	Ergocorninine		(+)-Valine
Group III			
Ergometrine	Ergometrinine	(+)-Lysergic acid	(+)-2-amino propanol

lysergic acid greatly diminished the direct stimulating action of the alkaloids on smooth muscle. On conversion to the dihydro form, ergometrine no longer contracts the uterus; similarly, ergotamine loses much of its smooth muscle stimulating action but retains intact the antagonism for adrenaline. The same is true for ergotoxine, its isomeride, ergocristine, and the two related compounds (table 13.1). After hydrogenation these alkaloids acquire even greater potency as antagonists for adrenaline and their toxicity in comparison with the natural alkaloids is reduced.

The discovery of lysergic acid made it possible to make synthetic derivatives which were closely related to ergometrine. Among these was (+)-lysergic acid diethylamide which was only slightly less active than ergometrine on the uterus. The drug did not attract attention until 1943 when Hofmann inadvertently ingested a minute amount and so discovered its hallucinogenic effects.

The alkaloids as agonists and antagonists
The pharmacology of the ergot alkaloids has been concerned mainly with their peripheral actions and much of the information has come from experiments with isolated tissues, and there are differences of opinion in their interpretation.

The amino acid alkaloids not only contract smooth muscle but also block receptors for adrenaline. The two effects, however, differ in their time relationships; whereas muscle contraction occurs soon after application of the drug, the adrenaline block is slow to develop. It has, nevertheless, been argued that this dual action is represented in a single receptor. Evidence in favour of this view is as follows. Firstly, ergotamine antagonizes its own stimulant action and that of other alkaloids; the pressor response to an initial dose of ergotamine is not repeated when subsequent doses are given. Secondly, the dihydro alkaloids which are weak agonists, block receptors for adrenaline in concentrations which do not cause contraction; they also block the stimulant action of the natural alkaloids. Thirdly, when the receptors are blocked by a different antagonist for adrenaline such as phenoxybenzamine, the stimulant action of ergotamine is reduced. Further, when adrenaline is applied in high concentration to isolated smooth muscle, the receptors are 'protected' against the blocking action of ergotamine or phenoxybenzamine. After the adrenaline has been washed out, the muscle responds once more to the action of ergotamine.

By contrast with the amino acid alkaloids, ergometrine is purely an agonist, but its action falls mainly on uterine muscle. The isolated rabbit uterus, pregnant or not, contracts strongly to adrenaline and inhibition of the response has been used to assay the potency of ergotamine and similar alkaloids. Another equally sensitive preparation is the isolated seminal vesicle of the guinea-pig. In neither of these preparations does ergometrine

oppose the motor effect of adrenaline. That ergometrine appears to combine with receptors for adrenaline can also be demonstrated in 'protection' experiments. The tissue is first exposed to a high concentration of adrenaline or ergometrine and the receptors are thereby 'protected'. Phenoxybenzamine (p. 15.23) is then applied to the muscle but does not have access to the receptors which are occupied by the agonist. Muscles that are so 'protected' respond to further doses of the agonist, but those that are not protected fail to respond because the receptors are blocked by the antagonist. Why the effect of ergometrine should fall primarily on uterine smooth muscle is not clear. Ergometrine and related derivatives of lysergic acid are much less active than the amino acid alkaloids on vascular smooth muscle, where they diminish the response to adrenaline but do not reverse it. A summary of some of their actions is presented in table 3.2. Ergot alkaloids are antagonists not only of adrenaline but also of 5-HT and, in a few instances, of histamine. The antagonism for 5-HT has been studied mainly on the rat uterus and the most potent members are ergometrine and methylergometrine. The antagonism was first discovered with (+)-lysergic acid diethylamide which is effective in concentrations of the order of 1 ug/l.

TABLE 3.2. Pharmacological actions of the ergot alkaloids.

	Pressor	Oxytocic (uterine)	Adrenaline reversal	Hyper-thermia
Natural amino acid alkaloids	+++	++ (Parenteral route)	+	+
Dihydrogenated amino acid alkaloids	+	+	++	o
Amine alkaloids	±	+++ (Oral route)	o	+

Apart from actions on smooth muscle, the ergot alkaloids interfere with certain metabolic processes that are mediated by adrenaline. For instance ergotoxine prevents the hyperglycaemia produced by adrenaline. The natural and dihydro alkaloids do not by themselves lower the blood sugar but antagonize the effect of adrenaline on glycogenolysis in the liver. Ergometrine, which elsewhere displays little or no antagonism for adrenaline, is nevertheless effective in preventing the hyperglycaemic responses.

Ergotamine and dihydroergotamine have also been reported to inhibit the lipid mobilizing effect of noradrenaline.

Central actions of the ergot alkaloids
These came to light in studies of the toxicity of the alkaloids when injected parenterally into intact animals. The

lethal dose for dogs, cats and rabbits varied from 2 to 10 mg/kg (IV) but for guinea-pigs, rats and mice, it was higher. The toxicity of the alkaloids diminished in the order ergotoxine, ergotamine and dihydro derivatives, the latter being ten to thirty times less toxic than the natural alkaloids.

The first clear description of central effects of ergotoxine (2 mg/kg) was by Githens in 1917, who injected it intravenously in rabbits. Within a minute or so, the pupils dilated and soon extreme restlessness set in and lasted for half an hour. About an hour after the injection, respiration became rapid, the body temperature rose, and the hair began to erect. There followed a period of sedation with weakness of the limbs, during which the temperature remained high and the pupils dilated. Ergotamine, ergometrine and (+)-lysergic acid diethylamide have since been shown to produce similar effects, there being a parallel between the rise of body temperature and other signs of central nervous stimulation.

In the cat, ergometrine (2 mg/kg IV) causes 'sham rage' which is best described in the words of Brown and Dale:

'Almost as soon as the injection has been completed, the onset of the effect is visible, the rapid dilation of the pupils and erection of the hairs of the tail. By the time the cat can be released, it already shows some incoordination and tendency to sprawl, and a pronounced excitability and 'sham rage', starting, snarling, spitting, baring its teeth and extending its claws in response to visual or auditory stimuli of any kind but making no purposive movement of attack or defence, so that it can be lifted without danger of bite or scratch, in spite of its apparent threatening reaction.'

After ergotoxine or ergotamine the effects were the same but the initial dilation of the pupils gave way to intense constriction, lasting many hours. During this period the animal showed muscular weakness but still responded by 'sham rage' when disturbed. The rise of body temperature in the cat is not as great as in the rabbit.

The effects seen in the whole animal suggest that the ergot alkaloids act on autonomic centres in the hypothalamus. Thus, the rise in body temperature did not occur after section of the brain stem above the superior colliculi, or when the brain was depressed by general anaesthesia.

The hypothalamus is known to contain noradrenaline and 5-HT, both of which have been implicated in the control of body temperature. In the cat, injection of noradrenaline into the cerebral ventricles causes a fall of the body temperature; injection of 5-HT has the opposite effect. It is conceivable, therefore, that the alkaloids act on central receptors for these amines. The dihydro alkaloids are less active centrally and actually produce a fall of the body temperature which may be related to their vasodilator action.

The alkaloids also act centrally to affect the arterial blood pressure. In the anaesthetized cat with central nervous system intact, ergometrine invariably lowered the pressure but after intercollicular section of the brain stem, the response became pressor. Ergotoxine and the dihydro alkaloids gave similar responses, suggesting that the alkaloids lower the pressure by acting at some point above the midbrain. The ergot alkaloids act centrally to produce bradycardia, respiratory depression and vomiting. They impair the respiratory response to CO_2 and abolish the apnoea seen after an injection of adrenaline. Both the depressor reflex (produced by central stimulation of the vagus) and the carotid sinus reflex are abolished by small doses of ergotamine in the cat and dog.

The central actions of the ergot alkaloids are complex and are liable to be obscured by peripheral effects, particularly with the amino acid alkaloids. More powerful still as a central stimulant is the synthetic derivative (+)-lysergic acid diethylamide. In the rabbit a dose of 0·5 μg/kg IV produces hyperthermia, dilation of the pupils and piloerection.

Experimental ergotism

Although it had long been known that diets rich in butter, eggs and milk protect against the onset and severity of convulsive ergotism, experimental evidence was not forthcoming until the work of Mellanby in 1932 on nutrition and degenerative changes in the nervous system. When dogs were maintained on a vitamin A deficient diet, they developed stiffness and incoordination, sometimes cramps and convulsions, and often seemed affected mentally. The addition of wheat or rye germ, or of powered ergot to the diet intensified the degenerative changes in the brain stem and spinal cord. A diet rich in vitamin A gave complete protection against these effects. Mellanby concluded that convulsive ergotism does not develop so long as the vitamin A and carotene intake are adequate. Mellanby's experiments were performed with crude ergot powder; whether the convulsive effect depends more on one alkaloid than on another, remains to be tested.

Some actions of ergot alkaloids in man

Ergometrine has already been discussed (p. 12.15). In healthy subjects ergotoxine and ergotamine in doses of 0·25–0·5 mg (IV) produce slight giddiness, frontal pressure in the head, weariness and depression lasting several hours, cyanosis of the skin, especially in the hands and feet and nausea and sometimes vomiting occur 20–30 min after the injection. Within minutes, the arterial systolic and diastolic pressures rise by 20–60 mm Hg, and remain high for one to several hours. During this period, the CSF and venous pressures rise and the pulse rate falls. Soreness and pain are felt in the muscles, particularly on walking.

Maier in 1926 introduced ergotamine for the treatment of migrainous headache for which the effective dose was 0·5 mg by subcutaneous injection or 1–2 mg by mouth. At first it was thought that the drug acted to relieve meningeal vascular spasm arising from excessive sympathetic tone. Sympathectomy, however, did not cure the condition. Later it was observed that the attacks of migraine were associated with pulsation in the distribution of the temporal artery on the affected side. The amplitude of the pulsations can be recorded with the aid of a capsule applied to the head. As the blood pressure rises after intravenous injection of the drug, so the amplitude is reduced and the headache becomes less intense.

Ergotamine is sometimes used to control itch in jaundice, but the basis for this action is not understood.

The dihydro alkaloids of the ergotoxine group lower the arterial blood pressure in doses which do not reverse the effect of adrenaline; probably they act centrally since the discharge of nerve impulses from baroreceptors is not affected. Like ergotamine or ergotoxine, the dihydro alkaloids produce vomiting, depress respiration and the response to inhaled CO_2. In these respects the actions of the alkaloids resemble morphine.

The clinical use of ergotamine reintroduced the hazard of ergotism. Should this occur because of acute overdosage, cumulative poisoning or unusual sensitivity, little can be done to avert peripheral gangrene. There is, so far, no effective antagonist of the stimulating action of the alkaloid on vascular smooth muscle.

Hardly anything is known about the fate of ergot alkaloids in the body. About 5 per cent of the dose is excreted in the urine. Excretion also occurs in the bile. Although the alkaloids act centrally, they have not so far been detected in the brain or CSF. The synthetic derivative, (+)-lysergic acid diethylamide has been detected in the brain and CSF as well as in many other tissues of the body. Less than 1 per cent of the dose disappears by excretion. *In vitro* microsomal enzymes oxidize LSD to 2-oxyLSD which does not possess LSD-like activity on the central nervous system.

Methysergide (1–6 mg orally, fig. 13.6) appears to be even more effective than ergotamine in preventing migrainous headache. Its use in this condition was suggested on the basis of its antagonism to the action of 5-HT which might play a role in inducing the vasoconstriction believed to precede the excessive vasodilation associated with the pain (p. 16.4). Its disadvantage lies in other adverse effects which include nausea and vomiting, insomnia or drowsiness, gain in weight and peripheral oedema. Another curious effect is the development of a nonspecific inflammatory reaction which leads to retroperitoneal, cardiac and pleuropulmonary fibrosis. This may extend to constrict the ureters, great vessels or lymphatic channels.

Epilogue

Sir Henry Dale was one of the really great men of science. A practical problem in the pharmacy of ergot was a trigger that fired his imagination to study the ergot alkaloids in detail and this led him to the discovery of biogenic amines and the development of the whole subject of autopharmacology. This in turn has lead to immense advances in our understanding of the homeostasis of the body, the nature of drug action and also to the discovery of new drugs which are proving of benefit to millions of patients. Even though the liquid extract of ergot has long since disappeared from the pharmacopoeia, its place in medical history is secure.

FURTHER READING

BARGER G. (1931) *Ergot and Ergotism*. London: Gurney & Jackson.
DALE H.H. (1953) *Adventures in Physiology*. Oxford: Pergamon.

Chapter 14
Histamine

Histamine is a simple natural base, formed when CO_2 is split off from histidine (vol. 1, p. 11.24). It is found in plants, notably the stinging nettle, bacterial cultures and in the tissues of many animal species including those of man. Histamine is one of the most potent drugs known and in mammals it contracts smooth muscle, dilates capillaries and small venules and stimulates glands. Its ubiquity and diversity of effects have long posed the problem of its function in the body. Although there is convincing evidence that histamine intervenes in some pathological processes, its precise physiological role remains obscure. Indeed, a famous professor of pharmacology at Sarajevo once remarked that histamine raises more problems than it solves.

Histamine or β-imidazolylethylamine was first synthesized in 1907, a year after the structure of histidine had been established. Later, and quite independently, the amine was isolated as a product of putrefaction in the watery extract of ergot and in peptone, and only then was it found to be pharmacologically active.

Histamine might have been dismissed as an interesting but unimportant drug had not Dale and Laidlaw in 1910 recognized the similarity between its toxic effects and those of the anaphylactic reaction in the guinea-pig and rabbit (p. 22.19). A few years later it was observed that trauma of soft tissues and intravenous injection of histamine both produced a dramatic and often irreversible fall of arterial blood pressure. On the strength of these analogies, Dale proposed that the effects of injury might be due to the release or formation in the damaged tissues of a substance with the actions of histamine. This theory and the contemporary work of August Krogh, the Danish physiologist, on the structure and functions of capillaries, marked the beginning of studies on the chemical control of the microcirculation. In 1924, Lewis, studying the vascular responses of the skin to local injury showed that the triple response (p. 21.3 and vol. 1, p. 28.38) was reproducible in every detail by pricking a minute quantity of histamine into the skin.

In 1927, the chemical identification of histamine as a normal constituent of mammalian tissue greatly strengthened Dale's theory and provided a firm basis for the work that followed. Thus, from 1930 onwards, bio-logical methods of assay were developed for the estimation of histamine in small samples of tissue and blood. Most tissues of the common laboratory animals were found to contain histamine and those with the highest concentration were usually the lungs, skin and gut, i.e. the organs that make contact with the external world. It was assumed that nearly all the histamine in the body was held in cells where it was pharmacologically inactive but that under certain conditions it could be released to act locally on sensitive cells or be carried by the blood to more distant sites. The first demonstration of the release of histamine from tissues was in 1932, when antigen was applied to perfused lungs from sensitized guinea-pigs. Later the alkaloidal substance curarine was shown to liberate histamine from dog's skeletal muscle *in vivo*. Out of the first experiment grew the subject of immunopharmacology; out of the second, came knowledge of the relation of chemical structure to histamine release. Of no less importance was an earlier observation by Popielski that histamine stimulated the acid gastric secretion.

The first competitive antagonists of histamine were made between 1937 and 1946. Among the most potent were mepyramine maleate and the phenothiazine derivative, promethazine (p. 14.17). In the laboratory, these compounds became valuable tools for the identification of histamine activity in extracts of tissues and body fluids and gave a fresh impetus to studies on drug antagonism. Their effectiveness in the relief of symptoms in patients with acute urticaria and other hypersensitivity states (p. 24.4) provided indirect evidence for the role of histamine in these disorders. Curiously, none of the antagonists oppose the action of histamine on the gastric secretion of hydrochloric acid.

It had long been known that histamine was virtually inactive by mouth and that a slow intravenous infusion of the drug could be maintained for hours without cumulative effects, in short, that the body disposes rapidly of histamine. Its destruction *in vitro* by tissues such as intestinal mucosa and kidney led to the discovery in 1930 of the enzyme histaminase. Because the enzyme preparation also oxidized diamines, namely, cadaverine and putrescine, it was also called diamine oxidase. In the guinea-pig, large doses of histidine by injection raised the content of histamine in the lungs and increased its excretion in the urine. *In vitro* experiments confirmed that certain tissues were able to decarboxylate histidine. These observations marked the beginning of quantitative studies on histamine metabolism.

In 1952, Schayer in the USA, was the first to apply isotopic tracer techniques to the problems of the origin and fate of histamine in the body. It was possible to distinguish between histamine that was formed in cells (endogenous histamine) from histamine that was ingested with the diet or made by bacterial decarboxylase in the gut or introduced in other ways (exogenous histamine). The identification of ^{14}C histamine metabolites in the urine made it possible to deduce pathways for its catabolism. Whereas biological methods of assay gave information on the content of histamine in cells, the new isotopic methods measured the rate of its formation and disappearance, and thus enabled the study of enzymes controlling its metabolism. Hence the older view of a static store of histamine in cells was replaced by one based on turnover; histamine was being formed and broken down continuously, some passing into stores and some being used in other ways. For example, Kahlson and his colleagues in Sweden have found that tissues which contain only a minute quantity of histamine may nevertheless be producing it at a fast rate; such are embryonic tissues, tumours and tissues undergoing regeneration or repair. The term 'nascent' was applied to histamine synthesized quickly and then immediately used in some process in the cell, possibly to do with division and growth. The functions of nascent histamine are, by definition, wholly intracellular.

In a similar way, Schayer obtained evidence in the mouse that injury, whether by heat or bacterial endotoxins, induces a faster rate of histamine formation in tissues of the body, notably the skin and lungs. Since the injection of adrenaline produces the same effect, he suggests that decarboxylase for histidine is an inducible enzyme and refers to histamine so formed as induced histamine. The latter is probably the same as nascent histamine in that it does not enter granular stores in the cell, but combines with receptors in or on the same cell and is then inactivated. On this view, histamine concerned with the control of the capillary circulation, is induced rather than preformed.

More recently techniques of differential centrifugation and electron microscopy have provided information on the intracellular location of histamine and its enzymes. Work in this field began in 1953 when Riley and West discovered that mast cells (vol. 1, p. 16.5) were rich in histamine. Although high concentrations of histamine in tissues often coincide with large numbers of mast cells, not all tissues that contain histamine possess mast cells. The histamine content of tissues therefore came to be classified as mast cell and non-mast cell histamine. In the mast cell, histamine, together with heparin, resides in large dense granules; in other cells, the granules that contain it are small and less dense. The granules, therefore, represent the intracellular stores of histamine and so protect it from destruction by cytoplasmic enzymes.

Today, the pharmacology of histamine is being pursued within the greatly enlarged framework of the cell. The cells may be of plant, bacterial or mammalian origin. In the latter they include the mast cell, the platelet, the blood basophil, the parietal cell and other cells including those in the brain. Some of these topics are now discussed in greater detail.

Properties of histamine

Histamine is 4 (or 5)-(2-aminoethyl) imidazole, $C_5H_9O_3$ (mol. wt. 111). Since the imino hydrogen (position 1) is free to move to the other nitrogen (position 3) with the formation of a double bond, the molecule is tautomeric and has two structures (I and II).

Histidine　　　　　　　　Histamine (I)

Histamine (II)

Histamine dissolves in water to give an alkaline solution. Titration of the solution with acid shows that the molecule contains two ionizable groups, the imino group (in the ring) with pK_a 5·74 and the amino group (in the side chain) with pK_a 9·80. Hence, at the pH of the body fluids, histamine behaves as a univalent cation, in which the side chain may chelate by hydrogen bonding

with the nitrogen in the ring. Since histamine is a diacidic base, it combines with one or two molecules of acid to form salts and is commonly obtained as the diphosphate or as the dihydrochloride.

Histamine forms complexes with heavy metals such as copper, zinc and cobalt which also occur in cells.

Histamine and its salts are soluble in water, ethanol and acetone but insoluble in ether. In aqueous solution, histamine withstands prolonged boiling in strong acid. This property is made use of in preparing tissue extracts for bioassay. Treatment of the extract with acid destroys other pharmacologically active substances, such as 5-HT, bradykinin, etc. which might interfere with the assay. The potencies of histamine, its derivatives and analogues are usually compared on isolated guinea-pig intestine, the arterial blood pressure of the anaesthetized cat and on the gastric acid secretion in the conscious dog.

Changes in the structure of the histamine molecule mostly diminish its pharmacological activity. Thus, acetylation of the amino group in the side chain gives *N*-acetylhistamine (p. 14.9), a conjugate formed in the body which is almost devoid of pharmacological activity. Methylation in the amino group yields *N*-mono- and dimethylhistamine both of which are more active than histamine in stimulating gastric secretion, but less active in the other two tests. By contrast, 1-methyl-4-(2-amino-ethyl) imidazole which from now on will be called methylhistamine is 300 times less active on guinea-pig intestine and inactive in the other tests. This ring-methylated compound is an important metabolite of histamine (p. 14.9).

Compounds that act like histamine are derivatives not only of imidazole, but of pyrazole and other ring structures and contain the following fragment.

Pharmacological actions

INTACT ANIMALS

Dale and Laidlaw began their study of histamine by injecting large doses into intact animals. The rabbit, after 2 mg, developed rapid breathing and cyanosis; intense constriction of the pulmonary artery caused distension and failure of the right ventricle. In the guinea-pig, 0·5 mg produced severe bronchospasm, inflation of the lungs and death from asphyxia. Similar findings had been described for the anaphylactic reaction in these two species. In the cat, 10 mg caused vomiting, purging, laboured breathing, profuse salivation and prostration, but within several hours recovery was complete. It was evident that many of the actions of histamine fell on structures that contain smooth muscle, and that the quantity, distribution and sensitivity of this muscle determine the pattern of response in different species. The dog, monkey and man are also highly sensitive, in contrast to the frog, mouse and rat which tolerate huge doses (50 mg or more) of the drug. Histamine provides a good example of how species vary in their sensitivity and responses to a drug.

PERIPHERAL CIRCULATION

Dale and Laidlaw continued their experiments on anaesthetized preparations and compared the effect of small intravenous doses (5 μg) on the arterial blood pressure.

Here again interesting differences emerged; in the guinea-pig and rabbit, the effect was always pressor, but in the cat, dog, monkey and fowl histamine produced a sharp, transient fall, which was accompanied by dilation of the peripheral vessels. The choice of anaesthetic was important to the result. For practical reasons, the herbivores were anaesthetized with urethane (ethylcarbamate) which reduced the sensitivity of smooth muscle to histamine in the pulmonary artery and bronchi but not in the arterioles. The carnivores were anaesthetized with ether which made them more sensitive to histamine. The use of different anaesthetics sharpened the contrast between the responses of the two groups of animals. On the evidence then available, the depressor action in the carnivores was difficult to explain. Experiment had shown that histamine stimulated many forms of smooth muscle including that in isolated strips of arteries and veins. If histamine was a general stimulant of smooth muscle, why did it not raise the arterial blood pressure in the cat and dog? Dale and Laidlaw argued that histamine had another and unsuspected action, namely, to dilate blood vessels at some point beyond the arterioles. The idea that arterial pressure might fall not by a lowering of the arteriolar resistance but by an increase in the capacity of the capillary bed was novel at the time. Several years later, it came to be explained in a new context, namely, that of wound or traumatic shock.

An alternative explanation of the depressor effect was that histamine reduced cardiac output by constricting the pulmonary artery or the hepatic veins or the small systemic veins. This view seemed logical and was tested in the following way. Histamine was injected into the vena cava, the portal vein and the aorta of the anaesthetized cat and the time interval between completion of the injection and onset of the effect was measured. The latency was found to be least with arterial, intermediate with caval, and longest with portal injections, and it was concluded that histamine produces its depressor effect at some point reached earliest by the blood in the arteries and that the action could not be located in the liver or the lungs. Nor was it likely to be on small systemic veins for the blood flow after small doses was actually seen to increase.

The problem of where histamine acted on the systemic vessels was studied in the cat by recording arterial blood pressure and limb volume in parallel. The nerves to one of the limbs were cut and allowed to degenerate; this procedure excluded indirect effects. In the innervated limb, a small dose of histamine always lowered the pressure but the effect on limb volume was inconstant and probably depended on the degree of arteriolar tone. In the denervated limb, the response was invariably dilation and taken to represent an effect on capillaries. Further evidence was obtained by observing the change of colour in the toe pads of cats with unpigmented feet.

Immediately after the nerves to the limb had been cut, the pads flushed. Later they became paler and warmer, indicating that capillary tone was maintained. A small dose of histamine then caused intense flushing of the pads. When capillary tone was weakened by arresting the circulation to the limb or by cooling, the vasodilator response disappeared. The dilator action on capillaries was confirmed not only by observing the effects on serosal and mucosal surfaces but by recording the responses in isolated limbs perfused with physiological solutions. In such preparations, acetylcholine always produced vasodilation whereas histamine had a reverse effect. When adrenaline and washed red cells were added to the perfusion fluid, capillary tone was restored and so was the vasodilator action of histamine. These experiments made it possible to distinguish between vasodilation produced by relaxation of arterial muscle and that by an action on the capillaries.

In summary, it was concluded that in herbivores the constrictor action of histamine on arterial smooth muscle was greater than the dilator action on the capillaries and hence the effect was pressor; that in carnivores, the action was mainly on the capillaries or minute vessels and the effect was depressor.

HISTAMINE SHOCK

During World War I, the mounting toll of deaths from battle wounds led to the recognition of traumatic shock. From 12 to 24 hours after injury, when survival seemed likely, the blood pressure might suddenly begin to fall. Intravenous infusion of saline had no more than a transient effect in restoring the blood pressure. The syndrome closely resembled that seen in the anaesthetized cat or dog after a lethal dose of histamine. The analogy suggested that the underlying cause of traumatic shock might be a chemical toxaemia. Histamine given by injection and substances formed or released in damaged tissues might thus have effects in common on the blood vessels. The experimental approach to the problem was twofold; on the one hand Dale and Richards analysed the effects of large doses of histamine on the circulation, on the other Bayliss demonstrated that mechanical trauma applied to the soft tissue produced similar effects.

The intact cat was known to withstand large doses of histamine by intravenous injection but under ether anaesthesia a dose of 1–3 mg was invariably fatal. Dale described the effects in the following terms: 'within minutes the arterial blood pressure falls to between 30 and 50 mm Hg. The respiration becomes deep and laboured, then slower and progressively weaker until it ceases altogether. Artificial respiration does not prevent the continued fall of pressure. When the chest is opened, the heart is seen to be beating strongly but the great veins are empty. An infusion of saline has no more than a fleeting effect on the pressure because the venous return

has ceased. The skin is cold, the mucous membranes are pallid, the intestines are of a dusky hue. When the tissues are cut they hardly bleed and the blood is dark and thick. Such is the picture of histamine shock'.

The clue to the missing venous blood was found in the values for the haemoglobin and the packed red cell volume. As the arterial pressure fell, so the red cells became more concentrated, indicating a progressive fall of the plasma volume. At the same time, the flow of lymph increased in the thoracic duct. Although the plasma volume fell by as much as 50 per cent, the protein concentration was virtually unchanged. Hence it was concluded that histamine not only dilated capillaries but also made them more permeable to plasma. The larger dose of histamine (1–3 mg) had not only increased the capacity of the systemic capillary network but had reduced the circulating blood volume. The venous return and the cardiac output fell and the circulation became stagnant. Hypoxia, sludging of the red cells and other effects completed a vicious circle.

In other experiments, Dale showed that the choice of anaesthetic, haemorrhage and removal of the adrenal glands all enhanced the production of shock. For example, when nitrous oxide was used instead of ether, shock did not develop. The interaction of histamine and ether and similar anaesthetics in producing shock is still not understood. Much of this older work has since been confirmed and extended. The effect of histamine on the permeability of capillaries and venules has been demonstrated by labelling the plasma proteins with dyes, such as Evans blue. Histamine increases the permeability of vessels of 20–30 nm diameter on the venous side of the capillary bed, but its mode of action is controversial. Evidence from electron microscopy suggests that the venular endothelial cells which normally overlap, are now separated thus exposing the basement membrane through which water and solutes may pass (p. 21.6).

In summary, the pharmacological effects of histamine on the systemic circulation of the cat or dog under ether anaesthesia are similar to those seen after extensive tissue injury, under the same experimental conditions. The analogy provides no more than presumptive evidence that histamine may be involved in the production of traumatic shock. There is so far no clear evidence that the plasma histamine rises during shock or that histamine antagonists minimize its effects. Nevertheless, according to Schayer, injury in some way increases the activity of decarboxylase for histidine and so increases the rate of histamine formation in tissues, possibly in the endothelial cells of capillaries.

VASCULAR RESPONSES TO HISTAMINE IN MAN

Triple response (p. 21.3 and vol. 1, p. 28.38)

When Lewis consulted Dale on what chemical of known structure was most likely to produce effects similar to the triple response, the answer he got was histamine. Lewis then measured the exact time relationships of the triple response produced by the stroke stimulus and by a minute quantity of histamine pricked into the skin, and found them to be identical. Thus, histamine is regarded as acting,

(1) to dilate capillaries,

(2) to stimulate sensory nerves and so cause dilation of arterioles through an axon reflex, and

(3) to increase capillary permeability.

Arteriolar dilation increases hydrostatic pressure in dilated capillaries and so contributes to formation of the weal.

Responses produced by the stroke stimulus or by histamine were shown to be identical in other ways. For example, arrest of the circulation to the limb delayed the fading of the flare in the triple response produced by histamine. When the blood flow was released, the flare disappeared owing to the removal of histamine by absorption. The experiment was repeated using the stroke stimulus to evoke the response, when an identical result was obtained. In another experiment, the circulation was stopped and the stroke stimulus and histamine were then applied to the skin. In each case the local red reaction appeared and was later replaced by the weal. Again, with either stimulus the flare was absent from the response in skin where the sensory nerves had degenerated. Lewis therefore advanced the hypothesis that the triple response was mediated by a diffusible substance which had been released by injury. The detection of histamine-like activity in extracts of the skin provided support for this view.

In later years, these observations were the starting point of much new work on histamine releasing drugs, urticaria and other hypersensitivity reactions, and on the actions of antihistamines. The latter were effective in controlling not only urticaria but in reducing the triple response to histamine. The antihistamines do not prevent the local release of histamine in response to injury, but antagonize its effects on sensory nerve endings and on the capillaries.

Antidromic stimulation of sensory nerves (vol. 1, p. 28.38)

Antidromic stimulation of dorsal nerve roots in the cat or dog produces peripheral vasodilation. The pads redden and the skin temperature rises, the limb increases in volume. Lewis and Marvin, in 1927, proposed that the effect was due to the release of histamine in the skin. At first the evidence seemed convincing; antidromic stimulation of a purely sensory nerve, the saphenous, not only caused vasodilation but a rise of the acid gastric secretion. On the strength of this finding, Ungar in 1935 postulated the existence of 'histaminergic' nerves. Later experiments showed, however, that the vasodilator effect of nerve stimulation was more prolonged than that pro-

duced by histamine injected intravenously and that antihistamines failed to abolish the response. Although the evidence was against the view that histamine was released in the course of antidromic nerve stimulation, the hypothesis led to the discovery of histamine in peripheral nerves and other parts of the nervous system.

The chemical mediator of this effect, like that of the axon reflex, remains to be identified.

SYSTEMIC VASCULAR EFFECTS IN MAN

Histamine (0·5 mg) injected subcutaneously produces after 0·5 to 2 min, a sensation of warmth in the face, coinciding with a flush which gradually spreads down into the neck and body. At the same time, the pulse quickens and there is a throbbing headache which frequently persists when all other effects have disappeared. These effects are greatest in 3–4 min and pass off in 20–40 min. The flush denotes the dilator action of histamine on the minute vessels and its colour may be bright red or cyanotic depending on whether the action has fallen mainly on the arteriolar or venous capillaries. The extent of the flush is related roughly to the dose, the sensitivity of the vessels tending to diminish from the head towards the feet. This difference in sensitivity can be demonstrated by injecting histamine (50 μg) into the femoral artery when the vasodilator response is greater in the upper limb than in the lower, as measured by skin temperature.

Histamine injected into the brachial artery causes pain in the fingers, throbbing and a bright red flush, the skin temperature rises and the hand swells and feels stiff.

Cerebral vessels

These are of special interest because histamine has been used both to produce headache and to cure it. The effect was first observed in patients undergoing operation for removal of a tumour of the brain. When the surface of the brain is exposed and histamine injected intravenously, the brain begins to bulge within minutes and a bright red flush appears. A large rise of pressure in the CSF coincides with the expansion of the brain, and the difference in the oxygen content of blood withdrawn from the carotid artery and from the internal jugular vein is reduced. The dose needed is so small that the effects occur without change in pulse rate, or the arterial and venous pressures. Histamine acts directly on the vessels to increase the blood flow through the brain, thereby making it larger and displacing cerebrospinal fluid. Histamine does not penetrate the blood–brain barrier.

Histamine headache

In 1936, Pickering was interested in headache and wanted a method of producing it experimentally. He tried various vasodilator drugs but none was more suitable than histamine, which enabled him to induce a 'standard' headache. A dose of 20 μg injected intravenously was followed in 50 sec by headache; this increased up to 1 min and then usually passed off in 6–10 min, but slight headache sometimes persisted for several hours. In all his experiments histamine produced a fall of the arterial blood pressure, which was maximal in 5–10 sec and lasted for 30–40 sec. This time relation is important because headache never occurred during the fall of blood pressure but only after it had returned to its previous value. The fall in systemic blood pressure is part of the vasodilator action of histamine and coincides with dilator effects on vessels of the skin and brain. Thus, as the pressure falls, the CSF pressure rises and reaches its peak in 5–20 sec and then falls to its resting level as some of the fluid disappears by reabsorption. Even before this has happened, the arterial pressure has recovered, but the increased pulsation of the brain persists. It seems, therefore, that the dilator effect of histamine on the cerebral vessels continues for some time after its effects on vessels elsewhere have disappeared.

A larger pulsation than normal appears to be a necessary condition of headache since its reduction either by raising the CSF pressure or lowering the arterial pressure, cures the headache. Thus excessive stretching of the cerebral vessels during systolic thrust might stimulate sensory nerves in the wall of the vessels. There is, however, the difficulty of explaining why histamine should appear to act longer at this site than on vessels elsewhere; in other words, why headache may occasionally persist for hours when the other effects of histamine have disappeared.

Early in his investigations, Pickering excluded the scalp as a source of the headache, but he observed that where the trigeminal ganglion had been removed, headache was abolished on the same side. This suggested that the 'stimulus responsible for headache arose in tissues innervated by the trigeminal and that impulses travel along branches of this nerve'. The dura mater, therefore, seemed a possible site of action for histamine. Other observations made in the course of arterial angiography showed that when histamine was injected into the internal carotid artery, headache is felt on the same side; when it was injected into the external carotid, headache seldom occurs. By the first route, histamine would be expected to act mainly on cerebral vessels; by the second, on the vessels of the dura mater. Hence, it might be inferred that histamine acted primarily on the cerebral vessels.

Arterial blood pressure
Doses of histamine that are large enough to cause flushing also have a slight but definite depressor effect which depends as much on the speed of the injection, when this is intravenous, as on the total amount injected. With prolonged infusion of the drug, tolerance to its vascular effects may occur. Skin vessels which were previously dilated become constricted and so the flush acquires a mottled appearance. This irregular fading of the flush may be accompanied by a rise of the arterial pressure. It seems probable that histamine stimulates a physiological antagonism, possibly through the release of adrenaline from the adrenal medulla.

Heart
During the intravenous infusion of histamine the heart rate quickens and the effect is approximately related to dose. The tachycardia may be a reflex effect in response to the depressor action of histamine and is in fact accompanied by a rise in the cardiac output. Histamine therefore quickens the circulation. This effect is difficult to interpret because histamine also stimulates metabolism. The oxygen consumption rises and although the effect increases with dose, it is maintained beyond the period of the infusion.

All these effects, like the rise of arterial pressure, might be attributable to the release of adrenaline from the adrenal medulla. In support of this view, moderate increases in the excretion of catecholamines in urine have been observed in man after subcutaneous injection of histamine.

RESPIRATION
In healthy subjects, the intravenous infusion of histamine (20–40 μg/min for 60 min) stimulates metabolism and so increases ventilation; bronchial tone is not affected. Patients with asthma or long standing bronchitis, however, are sensitive to histamine and even small doses (3–15 μg/min) reduce the vital capacity and cause dyspnoea. Sensitivity of bronchial muscle to histamine can be tested by applying the drug as an aerosol. When guinea-pigs are placed in a chamber containing a droplet cloud of histamine, they quickly develop laboured breathing, hypoxia, and collapse. The collapse time, which is measured in seconds, provides a measure of the sensitivity of the guinea-pigs to histamine. In patients, as in guinea-pigs, previous treatment with an antihistamine gives protection against the bronchoconstrictor action of histamine. In the guinea-pig this action differs from that seen in the anaphylactic reaction in that local oedema and infiltration with eosinophils are absent. The lungs not only contain histamine in mast cells but remove it from the circulating blood as they do 5-HT, bradykinin, prostaglandins and other pharmacologically active substances.

GASTRIC SECRETION
Histamine in common with pilocarpine and choline esters stimulates secretion in the salivary glands, the pancreas and the mucosal glands of the alimentary canal; by far the most sensitive glands are those of the stomach. Whereas in the dog and cat histamine acts mainly on the

parietal cells, in man it also stimulates the pepsin-producing cells. No other cell in the body is so sensitive to histamine as the parietal cell where its action in promoting secretion of hydrogen ions is not properly understood. Since histamine stimulates secretion in a transplanted fundal pouch, its action is not dependent on the extrinsic nerve supply to the glands.

Clinically, histamine given as a single subcutaneous dose is used to test for the presence or absence of functioning parietal cells although pentagastrin is rapidly replacing it in this regard (p. 10.2).

The response to histamine or pentagastrin is an important parameter of gastric secretory function since it is taken as a measure of the parietal cell mass, or the total number of functioning parietal cells in the stomach. The main evidence in support of this concept is the correlation that has been established between the maximal secretory response and parietal cell counts in a series of stomachs (vol. 1, fig. 30.14). Such tests of secretory function provide information on whether the parietal cell mass is enlarged as in duodenal ulcer or on the extent of its reduction after surgical resection or in other ways. The response to histamine, however, is contingent not only on the number of parietal cells but on the background of vagal activity, and hence on acetylcholine. Vagal stimulation or the simultaneous infusion of carbachol enhances the maximal response to histamine; conversely, vagotomy or the administration of atropine reduces the response. The dose–response relationship may be interpreted in two ways; either the dose stimulates all the parietal cells at once and the response of each cell is graded, or it stimulates only a fraction of the total population at a time when the response of each cell is all or none, or quantal (vol. 1, p. 3.15).

When histamine is given by infusion, the drug accumulates in the blood and extracellular fluids and a balance is eventually struck between the rate of infusion and the rate of its disappearance by metabolism and excretion in the urine. In man, the rate of infusion which causes a detectable and sustained rise in the acid gastric secretion is about 10 ng/kg/min. At this rate, a man weighing 65 kg would have received a total of only 39 μg at the end of 60 min and only a small fraction of this dose could have acted on receptors for histamine in the gastric glands. This extraordinary sensitivity of gastric glands and of the parietal cells in particular, long ago raised the question whether or not histamine had a physiological role in the control of gastric secretion.

In 1905, Edkins had shown that extracts of the pyloric, but not of the fundal mucosa, excited gastric secretion. He called the active substance 'gastrin' (vol. 1, p. 30.17). Later the activity came to be identified as that of histamine and because extracts of other tissues also stimulated gastric secretion the effect of pyloric mucosal extracts was regarded as unspecific. It was not until 1938 that a clear distinction was made between gastrin, then a substance of unknown structure, and histamine.

At least three substances are involved in the regulation of gastric secretion; firstly, acetylcholine as the neurochemical transmitter of vagal nerve impulses, secondly, gastrin as a hormone released from the pyloric antrum and thirdly, histamine which is present in high concentration in the gastric mucosa. In 1938, Babkin proposed that the function of acetylcholine and gastrin might be to control the release or formation of histamine in or close to the parietal cell. The evidence for this role of histamine, as the final stimulator of the parietal cells, is still indirect. Although histamine is detectable in the gastric juice, whatever the method of stimulation, an increase has not so far been demonstrated in venous effluent from the stomach during active secretion. Nevertheless, the following can be cited in support of the hypothesis. Histamine extractable from the gastric mucosa is not derived from mast cells; the profile of its concentration in the gastric glands reaches a peak in the region of the parietal cells; the gastric mucosa contains a highly active decarboxylase for histidine. According to Kahlson and his collaborators, the infusion of pure gastrin or the ingestion of a meal or vagal stimulation induced by an injection of insulin augments the histamine forming capacity of the mucosa.

The gastric mucosa, unlike that of the intestine, is devoid of the enzyme histaminase; it may, however, inactivate histamine by methylation in the ring. After a subcutaneous injection of ^{14}C-histidine, ^{14}C-histamine is formed in the stomach as well as in other parts of the gut. The intake of food increases the output of labelled histamine in the urine and at the same time reduces the stores in the stomach. Many of these experiments have been performed in the rat and the results remain to be confirmed in other species.

Histamine content in tissues

Histamine is readily extractable from tissues after precipitation of the proteins with trichloracetic acid. The supernatant or filtrate is then purified by chromatography or solvent extraction. The estimation may be performed by biological or chemical methods of assay. Of the chemical methods, the spectrophotofluorimetric is the most sensitive and specific. Histamine is made to react with O-phthaldehyde to yield a fluorescent compound which is identified by its activation spectrum.

Although chemical methods of assay are now replacing the biological, most of our information on the histamine content of tissues has been obtained using these older methods, notably the isolated guinea-pig ileum. Here the activity of the unknown is measured in comparison with a standard solution of histamine and the results are expressed as the base. The method usually detects a concentration of 1 ng/ml (10 nanomolar) of histamine. The activity is identified by repeating the assay in the presence of low concentrations of specific antagonists, such as mepyramine.

Typical values for the content of histamine in tissues and body fluids are shown in table 14.1, which illustrates

TABLE 14.1. Estimates of histamine base contained in different tissues expressed in µg/g or /ml.

	Rat	Guinea-pig	Rabbit	Cat	Dog	Man
Hypophysis	0·2	0·9	0·8	5	10	4
Hypothalamus	0·3	0·6	0·7	0·8	0·7	—
Skin	40	6	4	20	15	10
Lungs	5	30	14	40	25	15
Stomach	15	—	3	25	80	15
Liver	3	2	3	1	60	2
Blood	0·05	1	4	0·05	0·02	0·08
Urine*	60		5	10	8	30
Mast cell tumour					800	700

*Output of free histamine in µg per 24 hours.

differences in a number of species. The differences are in the main related to the number and distribution of mast cells in the various organs. For example, the rabbit differs from other species in having a high blood histamine which is contained mainly in the platelets and basophils. Elsewhere, apart from the lungs, the values for the rabbit are low and can be related to the paucity of mast cells in the tissues.

However, not all tissues that are rich in histamine contain mast cells. The gastric mucosa is devoid of mast cells yet the concentration is high. In the grey matter of brain, the concentration is low and not associated with mast cells. The precise location of histamine in tissues that are devoid of mast cells is not yet known.

Fate

Whether histamine is given by mouth or injection, the greater part of the dose is removed by the tissues and destroyed. More than 95 per cent of an oral dose is metabolized in the intestinal mucosa and only a minute fraction is absorbed as free histamine. In the lumen of the gut, bacteria inactivate histamine by acetylation and N-acetyl histamine is absorbed and excreted in the urine. After intravenous injection, histamine disappears rapidly from the plasma and only 1–2 per cent of the dose appears in the urine as free histamine (table 14.2).

Catabolic pathways for histamine are shown in fig. 14.1. Schayer injected ^{14}C-histamine into laboratory animals and recovered nearly all the radioactivity in the urine; none was detected in the expired air. All labelled metabolites were derivatives of imidazole but their relative quantities varied in the different species (table 14.2).

TABLE 14.2. Quantitative analysis for histamine and its metabolic products in urine of various species given ^{14}C histamine subcutaneously. Per cent total radioactivity in urine. After Schayer R.W. (1966) *Handbook of Experimental Pharmacology*, vol. 18. Berlin: Springer.

Species	Hist-amine	Methyl-histamine	Methyl-imidazole acetic acid	Imidazole acetic acid	N-Acetyl-histamine
Rat (Female)	12	4	6	51	3
Mouse	—	19	32	21	1
Rabbit	—	—	41	40	0·5
Guinea-pig	—	5	26	45	2
Cat	0·3	0·6	77	9	—
Dog	0	8	64	20	0
Man	1	8	60	25	—

Mammalian tissues therefore degrade histamine in at least three different ways, namely, by oxidation, methylation and conjugation. By treating animals with certain enzyme inhibitors and then analysing the urine, it is possible to study *in vivo* the enzyme systems that catalyse the reactions. Aminoguanidine, a powerful inhibitor of diamine oxidase reduces the amount of radioactivity appearing as imidazole acetic acid. Iproniazid, an inhibitor of monoamine oxidase, increases the excretion of methylhistamine which is oxidized normally to methylimidazole acetic acid.

In the rat, the principal metabolite of histamine is imidazole acetic acid indicating that metabolism depends mainly on diamine oxidase. Nevertheless after large doses of histamine or imidazole acetic acid, a conjugate of ribose and imidazole acetic acid also appears in the urine. In the cat, dog and man the principal metabolite is methylimidazole acetic acid. Since treatment with aminoguanidine does not interfere with the methylation of histamine, and methylimidazole acetic acid is not detectable in urine after the administration of imidazole acetic acid it can be concluded that histamine is first methylated in the ring and then oxidized.

The methylating enzyme (imidazole N-methyltransferase) is specific for histamine and occurs in many tissues of the body, including the nervous system. Ring methylation of histamine can be readily obtained *in vitro* by incubating a mixture containing tissue extract and S-adenosylmethionine as a source of methyl groups. Efficient inhibitors of the enzyme remain to be discovered.

Hitherto, changes in histamine metabolism were studied by estimating the daily output of free histamine in urine. Pharmacological methods made it possible to show that histamine in its free and conjugated (acetylated) form was excreted continuously in the urine, when it could not be detected in the blood plasma.

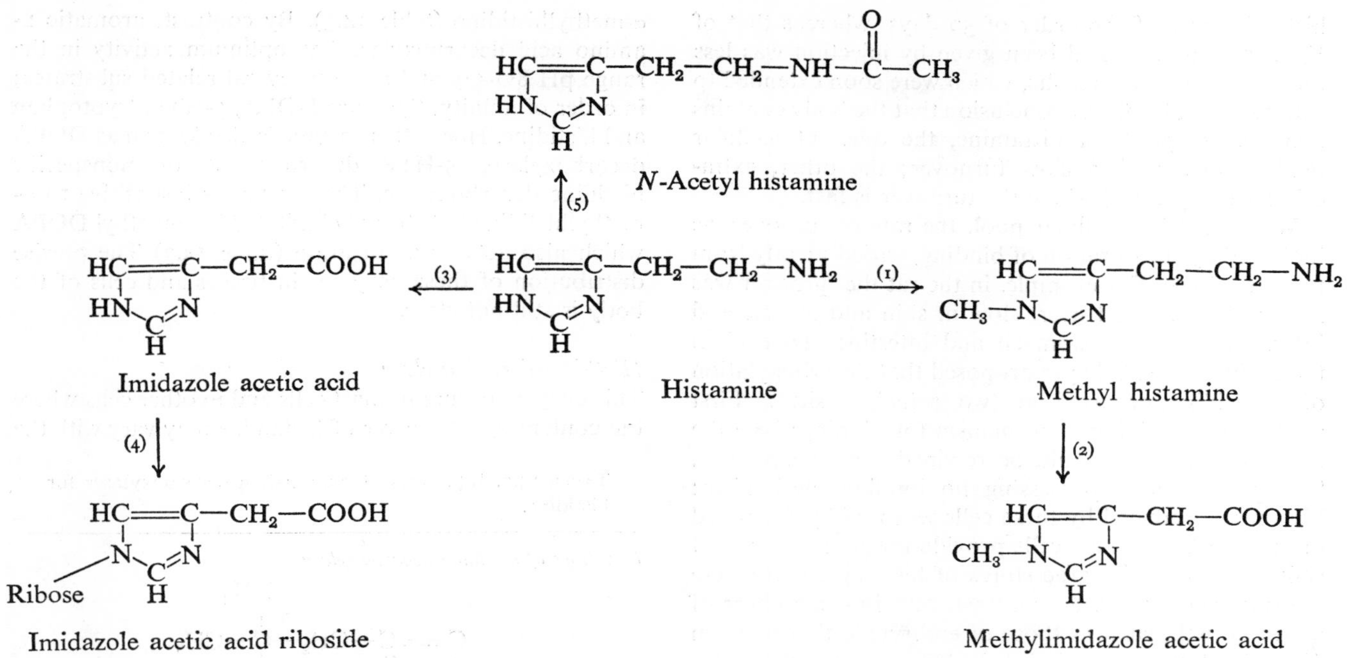

$$HC=C-CH_2-CH_2-NH-\overset{\overset{O}{\|}}{C}-CH_3$$
(imidazole ring: $HN{-}\underset{H}{C}{=}N$)

N-Acetyl histamine

(5) ↑

$$HC=C-CH_2-COOH$$ (ring $HN{-}\underset{H}{C}{=}N$)

Imidazole acetic acid

← (3)

$$HC=C-CH_2-CH_2-NH_2$$ (ring $HN{-}\underset{H}{C}{=}N$)

Histamine

(1) →

$$HC=C-CH_2-CH_2-NH_2$$ (ring $CH_3{-}N{-}\underset{H}{C}{=}N$)

Methyl histamine

(4) ↓

$$HC=C-CH_2-COOH$$ (ring Ribose${-}N{-}\underset{H}{C}{=}N$)

Imidazole acetic acid riboside

(2) ↓

$$HC=C-CH_2-COOH$$ (ring $CH_3{-}N{-}\underset{H}{C}{=}N$)

Methylimidazole acetic acid

FIG. 14.1. 1, The major pathway for the catabolism of histamine in mammalian species, including man; ring methylation by imidazole-*N*-methyl transferase; 2, oxidative deamination (via acetaldehyde) by a monoamine oxidase; 3, oxidative deamination by histaminase (diamine oxidase); 4 and 5, conjugates formed in tissues: 5, also formed by intestinal bacteria. After Schayer R.W.

Radioisotopic methods, however, are not applicable for routine use in man, and new sensitive nonisotopic methods are needed for the study of disorders of histamine metabolism; changes are most likely to be detected by measuring the urinary output not only of histamine, but of all the known metabolites, principally methylimidazole acetic acid.

Origin of histamine in tissues

Fifty years ago, the gut was regarded as the main source of histamine in the body, since it was known that the amine is present in the diet, and that many intestinal bacteria contain a powerful decarboxylase for histidine. The alternative view, that histamine is actually made in tissues that contain it, came to be tested first by pharmacological, and then by isotopic methods of assay. The pharmacological method depended on incubating extracts of tissues with histidine and then measuring the amount of newly-formed histamine by its activity on isolated guinea-pig intestine. The results first obtained by this method favoured the original theory; many tissues which contain histamine, such as the skin and lungs, fail to decarboxylate histamine under the conditions of the test. Again, there is a species difference in that decarboxylation of histidine is more easily detectable in tissues of the rat, guinea-pig and rabbit than in those of the cat and dog. The possible importance of histamine in the gut was indicated in other ways. Firstly, variations in the daily intake of histamine in the diet were reflected in the daily output of histamine in urine. Secondly, a large dose of histidine by mouth was followed by an increase in the urinary histamine; pretreatment with antibacterial drugs abolished this effect and reduced the daily output of histamine. Thirdly, although the intestinal mucosa destroyed histamine, a small fraction of an oral dose was nevertheless absorbed. Finally, histamine was readily demonstrable in contents of the colon. On these findings, histamine was likened to a vitamin.

In 1952, Schayer injected a small dose of ^{14}C L-histidine into guinea-pigs. ^{14}C-histamine was found in some tissues at the earliest interval tested, 6 hours, and was still present at the end of 56 days. ^{14}C-histamine appeared in the urine for about one week after the injection. When ^{14}C-histamine was injected into another group of guinea-pigs, none was detectable in the tissues after 4 hours. Further tests *in vitro* proved the capacity of many tissues to decarboxylate histidine. The isotopic, as compared with the pharmacological, methods were more sensitive and specific, in the sense that the results were obtained with physiological quantities of the amine and its precursor. Schayer's experiments provided the first clear demonstration that in the guinea-pig, the source of histamine in the tissues was L-histidine and not exogenous histamine. It was estimated that about 0.05 per cent of the histidine had been converted into histamine and that the half-life of the newly formed, bound ^{14}C-histamine was of the order of 50 days, whereas that of ^{14}C-histamine that had been given by injection was less than 4 hours. These results, which were soon extended to other species, led to the conclusion that the body contains two distinct pools of histamine, the one, intracellular (endogenous) with a slow turnover; the other, extracellular (exogenous) where the turnover is fast.

Within the intracellular pool, the rate of turnover, as indicated by the duration of binding, varied greatly from tissue to tissue. For example, in the rat the turnover was fast in the lung and liver, slow in skin and muscle and intermediate in the stomach and intestine. To explain these differences, Schayer proposed that decarboxylation of L-histidine occurred at two principal sites: 'First were cells containing a mechanism for binding; here the resulting histamine could be retained for long periods. Second were cells possessing no binding mechanism; histamine produced by these cells was rapidly destroyed or excreted'. The mast cells provide the best example of cells which contain large stores of histamine and where the turnover is slow. By contrast, cells in some phase of active growth, such as those of embryonic tissues, form histamine but do not bind it. In between are other cells, such as those of the gastric mucosa and brain where although the turnover may be high, some of the histamine is bound.

Histamine in germ-free rats
Evidence for the formation of histamine in tissues came from another direction. By 1955, Gustaffson had devised a simple method of rearing germ-free rats. The rat was delivered by Caesarean section into a sterile world where it grew up on a synthetic histamine-free diet. These rats did not differ from control rats maintained on the same synthetic diet, either in their daily urinary output of free histamine or in the content of histamine in the tissues. The experiment proved conclusively that the rat's own tissues synthesized histamine and suggested that the contribution by the diet or bacterial decarboxylase to the total body histamine was if any, much smaller than had been previously supposed. These findings led to a closer study of the enzymes that were responsible for the formation of histamine in tissues.

MAMMALIAN DECARBOXYLASES FOR HISTIDINE
Mammalian decarboxylase for histidine was at first thought to be a single enzyme with optimum activity at pH 8·0–9·5. Later it was found to consist of at least two enzymes, histidine decarboxylase and aromatic L-amino acid decarboxylase. The enzymes depend on pyridoxal phosphate as coenzyme. They are distinguished by their pH optima, substrates and inhibitors. Thus, histidine decarboxylase which is most active in the range pH 6–7, acts only on histidine and is inhibited by the analogue

α-methylhistidine (table 14.3). By contrast, aromatic L-amino acid decarboxylase has optimum activity in the range pH 8·0–9·5 and acts on several related substrates; in order of affinity, these are DOPA, 5-HTP, tryptophan and histidine. Hence this enzyme is also known as DOPA decarboxylase, 5-HTP decarboxylase or nonspecific histidine decarboxylase. The enzyme is insensitive to α-methylhistidine but strongly inhibited by α-methyl DOPA which also acts as a substrate (table 14.3) The precise distribution of these enzymes in tissues and cells of the body is still not clear.

Histidine decarboxylase
This enzyme occurs in mast cells and in other cells where the content and turnover of histamine may vary with the

TABLE 14.3. Inhibitors of mammalian decarboxylases for histidine.

Inhibitors of histidine decarboxylase

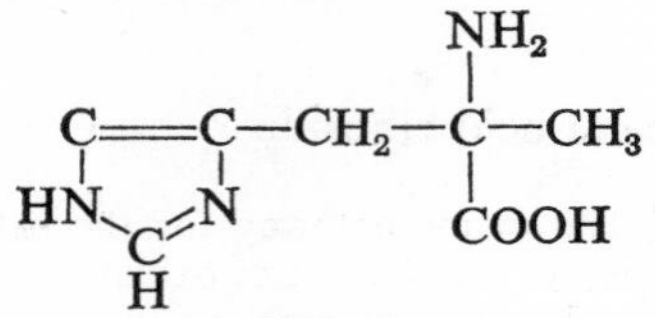

α-Methylhistidine

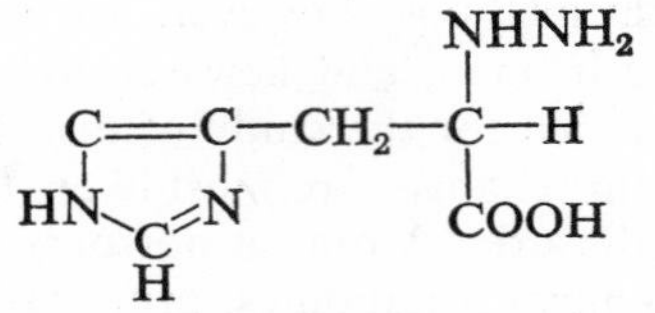

α-Hydrazinohistidine

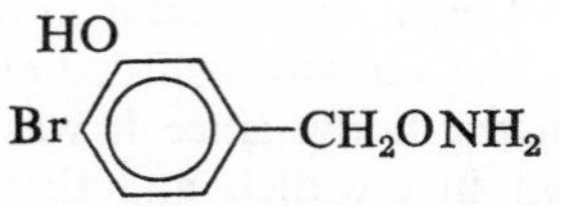

4-Bromo-3-hydroxybenzyloxyamine (NSD–1055)

Inhibitors of aromatic L-amino acid decarboxylase

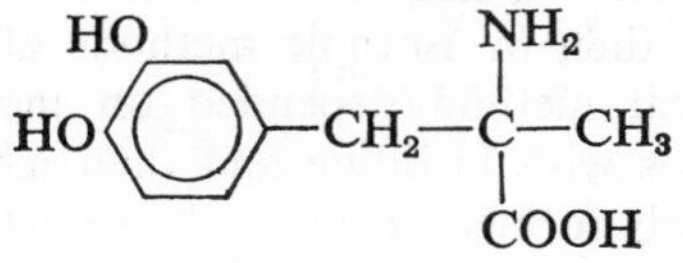

α-Methyldopa

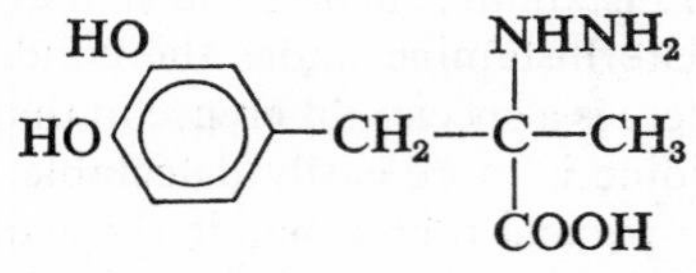

α, α-Hydrazinomethyldopa

activity and type of cell, e.g. cells in growth, cells of the gastric mucosa and probably endothelial cells of capillaries. Here the decarboxylase is seen as an adaptive or inducible enzyme which adjusts the production of histamine in the cell, whether in the process of division and growth or in response to a physiological stimulus, be it a neurotransmitter, autacoid or hormone. On this view, the importance of non-mast cell histamine is to be understood more in terms of the variable rate of its synthesis than of the stores carried in the cell. At one extreme is rat foetal liver which generates histamine at a fast rate and contains hardly any; at the other are the mast cells where the content is high but the turnover is slow. In the rat, at least, histidine decarboxylase forms the greater part of the body histamine. When rats are treated with α-methylhistidine, not only does the total body histamine fall, but the daily output in the urine is reduced. That decarboxylation is impaired can be tested by injecting ^{14}C-histidine and measuring the urinary excretion of ^{14}C-histamine and its metabolites. Treatment with α-methylhistidine does not inhibit the decarboxylation of amino acids which are substrates for aromatic-L-amino acid decarboxylase.

Aromatic-L-amino acid decarboxylase

This enzyme occurs in brain, adrenergic neurones, the adrenal medulla, chromaffin and argentaffin cells, the salivary glands, small intestine, kidney and other tissues. It has a low affinity for histidine and the contribution which it makes to the total body histamine and to the non-mast cell histamine in particular, is probably less than that of histidine decarboxylase. When rats are treated with α-methyl DOPA or the α-hydrazino analogue of α-methyl DOPA (table 14.3), which is not metabolized, the daily output of histamine is unchanged. The functional significance of the enzyme is not clearly understood; it may be to form histamine in some special relationship to acetylcholine, the catecholamines and 5-HT, as in the nervous system where histamine may act to modulate neurochemical transmission.

The search for inhibitors of the decarboxylases led, first, to the use of drugs that combine with the coenzyme and, secondly, to substituted analogues of the substrates. Compounds that interact with pyridoxal phosphate are carbonyl reagents such as semicarbazide and derivatives of hydrazine. These substances, however, were not sufficiently specific when used *in vivo* for they inhibited other pyridoxal dependent enzymes. Substituted analogues of the substrates made it possible to inhibit, either *in vitro* or *in vivo*, one or other of the decarboxylases for histidine. Thus, the α-methyl analogue of DOPA or 5-HTP inhibits aromatic-L-amino acid decarboxylase from guinea-pig kidney but not histidine decarboxylase from a transplantible rapidly growing tumour, namely rat hepatoma. The converse occurs with the α-methyl

analogue of L-histidine. Since the α-methyl analogues not only inhibit the enzyme but also act as substrates, more potent inhibitors were found in α-hydrazine analogues of the amino acids or of their α-methyl derivatives. In a different category is the compound 4-bromo-3-hydroxybenzyloxyamine (NSD 1055) (table 14.3) which acts on histidine decarboxylase and has been reported to inhibit histamine formation in man; given by mouth it reduced the daily output of histamine in the urine. Drugs which act selectively to inhibit the formation of histamine in the body and which share none of the other actions of glucocorticoids, might be of value in the treatment of disorders of histamine metabolism, e.g. urticaria pigmentosa and other conditions in which the mast cells are greatly increased in number (mastocytosis).

Histamine and endocrine glands

CATECHOLAMINES

Histamine bears an important relationship to the catecholamines. Firstly, these may be regarded as physiological antagonists of histamine; secondly, histamine acts on the adrenal medulla to release adrenaline; thirdly, catecholamines activate histidine decarboxylase to produce histamine.

The antagonism can be demonstrated on the arterial blood pressure of the anaesthetized cat, on the minute vessels and on smooth muscle particularly of the bronchioles. For example, isoprenaline (p. 15.1) is about twice as powerful as adrenaline in protecting guinea-pigs exposed to an aerosol of histamine.

In the cat, injection of histamine (1 μg) into the artery supplying the adrenal gland causes a sharp rise of the blood pressure owing to the discharge of catecholamines into the venous outflow. This effect of histamine was formerly used as a diagnostic test for phaeochromocytoma, a tumour of chromaffin tissue which produces mainly noradrenaline (p. 15.3). The release of noradrenaline provokes a pressor response which in some cases proved dangerous and for this reason the test is no longer advised. Conversely, large doses of adrenaline and sympathomimetic amines release histamine from tissues, but of greater significance from a physiological standpoint is the effect of catecholamines on the inducible form of histidine decarboxylase.

ADRENAL CORTICOSTEROIDS

After adrenalectomy, animals become more sensitive to the toxic effects of histamine and the LD50 may be reduced by five to ten-fold. Histamine tends to accumulate in the tissues possibly because more is bound in stores or less is destroyed. The disturbance in histamine metabolism is not properly understood. In the adrenalectomized rat both sodium chloride and cortisol increase the urinary output of histamine.

Treatment of normal rats with cortisol, prednisone or prednisolone reduces histidine decarboxylase activity in the lungs and skin but increases the activity of the enzyme in the stomach. This selective action so far lacks explanation. The cortical hormones do not act as antagonists of histamine but may suppress its formation or binding (storage) in cells; they do not appear to alter the pattern of its catabolism. There is some evidence that in man treatment with cortisol increases the urinary output of histamine and its metabolites.

Since cortisol and its derivatives act as immunosuppressants and histamine is released in the antigen–antibody reaction, their mode of action in affecting histamine metabolism remains important.

GONADAL STEROIDS

The effect of these hormones on histamine metabolism has been studied mainly in the rat and in man by following changes in the daily output of histamine and some of its metabolites in the urine. In rats the daily urinary output of histamine ($\sim$ 50 μg) is about the same as a human adult. The higher daily excretion of histamine in females, as compared with males, led to more detailed studies of the effects of the gonadal hormones on histamine metabolism. Castration in the male raises the output of histamine whereas treatment with testosterone reduces it by stimulating its conversion to methylhistamine (p. 14.9). The anabolic steroid, norethandrolone, is more potent than testosterone; after a single injection, the fall in output of histamine may last for several days.

In rats and mice, the output of free histamine increases steadily during pregnancy. On the day before term, however, it falls precipitously to the original value. The histamine derives mainly from foetal tissues but maternal tissues also make a contribution. In the rat foetus, histamine decarboxylase activity is greatest in the liver and in the mouse foetus in the skin. Of the maternal tissues, the kidney in the mouse and the glandular part of the stomach in the rat are the main sources of the increased endogenous histamine. When ovariectomized mice are treated with oestradiol, the urinary output of free histamine rises, largely owing to an increase in the formation of histamine in the kidney.

Oestrogens may also affect enzymes that inactivate or destroy histamine. The placenta contains histamine, histidine decarboxylase and the methylating enzyme, but principally histaminase. In women, the ratio of methylhistamine to histamine in urine tends to vary with the excretion of oestrogen. As the excretion of oestrogen increases so the output of histamine falls, because more is being destroyed by oxidation. Oestrogen is presumed to stimulate histaminase.

Histamine release

The distinction has been made between histamine that is not bound in the cell (nascent or induced) and that which is concentrated in granules, and thus protected from destructive enzymes in the cytoplasm. Little is known about how the granules are formed and the way they accumulate, store and release the substances which they contain. The granules, however, differ according to the cell. In the mast cell, for example, they are large and dense and on centrifugation they appear in the nuclear fraction. These granules contain heparin which, because of its strong anionic groups, acts as a polyanion and is bound to protein. Histamine in turn is loosely bound to the heparin protein complex. When the granules are placed in distilled water, they swell rapidly and burst, releasing their contents. In the brain, histamine is contained in smaller granules which sediment mainly with the synaptosomal and microsomal fractions.

The release of histamine normally implies the discharge of granules from the cell, as when a mast cell disrupts. Histamine and heparin are then set free to act locally, or may be carried away by the blood to more distant sites of action. Release, however, may also be intracellular as when histamine is lost from the granules to the cytoplasm, and only the metabolites leave the cell. Reserpine, which lowers the concentration of histamine in the brain probably does so by acting on the granules (p. 5.30). Release may occur in two ways:

(1) by the action of drugs on normal cells, and

(2) by the interaction of antigen with antibody fixed to cells, i.e. sensitized cells.

Substances that release histamine from tissues are roughly divisible into two groups, naturally occurring and synthetic macromolecules, and a wide range of drugs and chemicals of known structure of lower molecular weight. Complex macromolecules, such as the proteolytic enzymes in snake venoms, bacterial toxins and horse serum not only damage cells, including mast cells, but also activate enzymes in blood which catalyse the formation of kinins and other vasoactive substances. By contrast, compounds of low molecular weight, which include a number of drugs used in man, tend to act selectively on histamine stores, whether in mast cells or other cells.

METHODS OF INVESTIGATION

Histamine release can be demonstrated *in vivo* or on isolated organs and tissues, or on cells and granules that have been separated by centrifugation. In the whole animal, release is detected by measuring the rise in plasma histamine or the output of histamine and its metabolites in urine, or by recording some pharmacological effect, such as a delayed fall of blood pressure, bronchospasm, increased capillary permeability or stimulation of the gastric acid secretion. In man, the agent can be applied directly to the skin to test for the triple response. *In vitro* methods make it possible to screen large numbers of compounds and to study physical, structural and biochemical factors which influence the process of release. Thus, isolated organs such as lung or liver, or even flaps of skin, can be perfused with solutions and histamine in the perfusate may be measured before and after injection of the drug. The simplest method is to chop tissues into small blocks which are then incubated with the drug. Similar methods are applicable to suspensions of mast cells or other cells that are rich in histamine, such as rabbit platelets.

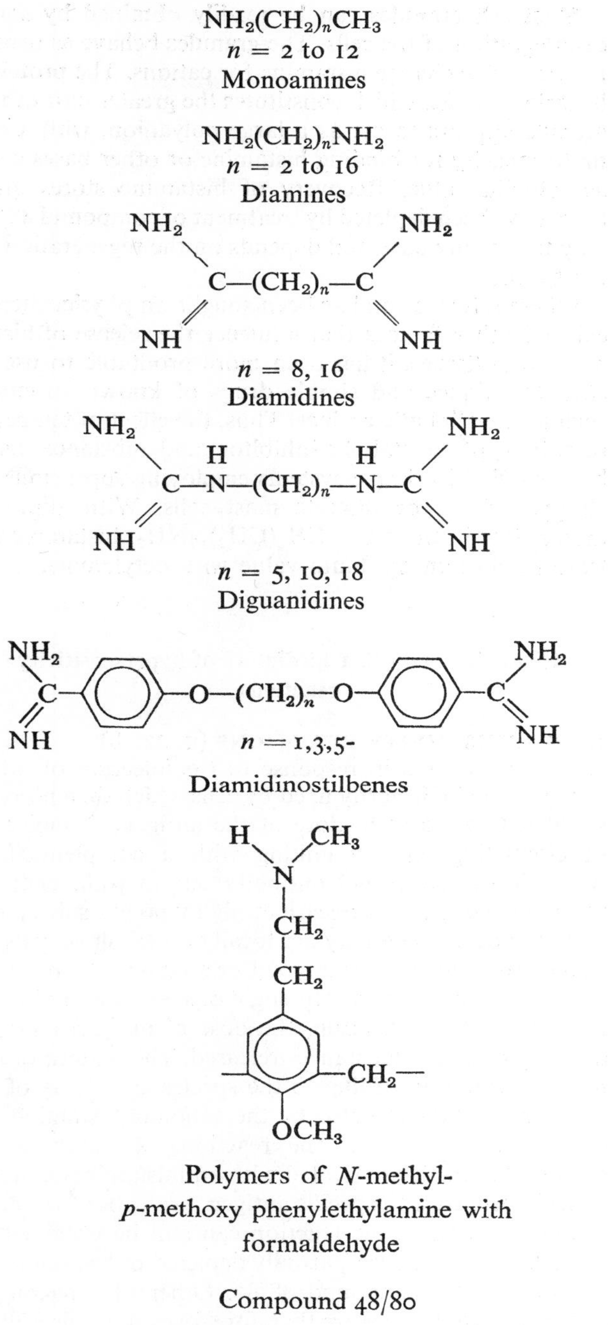

Most of the histamine releasing compounds are organic bases and include amines, amidines, ammonium substituted compounds and more complex bases (fig. 14.2). Among these are drugs which are used in man, e.g. the alkaloids D-tubocurarine, morphine and atropine and certain chemotherapeutic agents, stilbamidine, pentamidine and polymyxins. In the body, stilbamidine changes into a fluorescent compound and can be seen to accumulate in mast cells which swell and disrupt. Stilbamidine also has a strong affinity for trypanosomes, schistosomes (p. 20.19) and for cells of the tumour plasma cell myeloma (p. 28.4). In man, the intravenous injection of stilbamidine often gives rise to anaphylactoid reactions which are due to the release of histamine and the formation of other vasoactive substances. The reactions are marked by intense itching, flushing, urticarial wheals, headache and fall of blood pressure.

The potency of drugs that act as histamine releasers varies over a wide range depending on the species, the tissue and the method of investigation. In many instances the effect is unrelated to the main action of the drug; for example, the muscle relaxant action of D-tubocurarine is independent of histamine release. In tests on the whole animal or perfused organs, the most potent substance is **compound 48/80**, which is a mixture of low polymers obtained by allowing *p*-methoxyphenylethylamine to react with formaldehyde (fig. 14.2). Its potency is roughly correlated with the number and spacing of the amino groups in the polymer. In small, repeated doses it depletes tissues of histamine by disruption of mast cells. In this way, it has served to distinguish between mast cell and non-mast cell stores of histamine. For example, treatment with compound 48/80 reduces the skin histamine which is chiefly in mast cells by more than 80 per cent but hardly affects histamine stores in the gastric mucosa or intestine, where mast cells are few or absent.

Mast cells can be obtained by injecting an isotonic salt solution into the peritoneal cavity of the rat; after a short interval, the solution is withdrawn and the mast cells are separated by differential centrifugation.

Suspensions of the mast cells make it possible to study in more detail the structure of the granules, the loss of granules with drugs and the uptake of histamine and

other bases by the cells or granules. Thus, the action of compound 48/80 was found to be dependent on pH, Po_2 and temperature and could be blocked by metabolic inhibitors, such as dinitrophenol. Hence the view that compound 48/80 activates an enzyme in the membrane, possibly a lecithinase; when lecithinase A is applied to the cells, it parallels the effects of compound 48/80.

$$NH_2(CH_2)_nCH_3$$
$$n = 2 \text{ to } 12$$
Monoamines

$$NH_2(CH_2)_nNH_2$$
$$n = 2 \text{ to } 16$$
Diamines

$$n = 8, 16$$
Diamidines

$$n = 5, 10, 18$$
Diguanidines

$$n = 1,3,5\text{-}$$
Diamidinostilbenes

Polymers of *N*-methyl-
p-methoxy phenylethylamine with
formaldehyde

Compound 48/80

FIG. 14.2. Some substances able to release histamine.

Mast cell granules can be readily obtained by sonic disintegration of the cells. The granules behave as osmometers and exchange histamine for cations. The protein–heparin complex which constitutes the greater part of the granule appears to act as a large polyanion, with a definite capacity for binding histamine or other bases such as toluidine blue. Recovery of histamine stores after these have been depleted by treatment of compound 48/80 may take many days and depends on the regeneration of mast cells.

Where information has been sought on physicochemical and other factors that influence the release of histamine from tissues, it has been more profitable to use *in vitro* techniques and simple drugs of known structure such as the aliphatic amines. Thus, the effect of temperature, ions, pH, metabolic inhibitors and substances have been studied in simple systems employing supensions of chopped tissue or discrete mast cells. With aliphatic monamines in the series $CH_3(CH_2)_{12}NH_2$, histamine release reaches an optimum value with octylamine.

Histamine and other mediators of hypersensitivity reactions

HYPERSENSITIVITY REACTIONS (p. 22.18)
Antibody, formed in response to the injection of other foreign protein, is partly fixed by cells which then become sensitized to a second dose of the antigen. A molecule of circulating antigen uniting with a complementary molecule of cell bound antibody sets in train changes which may end in the release of highly potent substances from the cell. These may act locally on sensitive cells or at more distant sites. The type I or anaphylactic reaction develops rapidly and may be slight or severe depending on the extent of sensitization, the dose of antigen and the quantity of active substances released. The pattern of the reaction varies according to the species and many of its features can be paralleled by the action of histamine, an important mediator of the reaction. However, when sensitized animals are treated with antihistamines and are then challenged with specific antigen, protection is seldom complete. Further, the reaction can still be obtained in animals that have been partially depleted of histamine by treatment with compound 48/80. Other pharmacologically active substances are therefore formed or released in the anaphylactic reaction. These include heparin, 5-HT (p. 16.5), bradykinin (p. 17.3) and slow reacting substance of anaphylaxis (SRS-A). Lymph node permeability factor (LNPF) is a mediator in delayed hypersensitivity and is discussed on p. 14.16 and p. 22.20.

The classical experiments on anaphylaxis have been performed on the guinea-pig which can be readily sensitized to egg albumin. Sensitization may be demonstrated in several ways:

(1) by injecting antigen into the intact animal,
(2) by applying antigen to perfused organs, notably the lungs, and
(3) by incubating tissues or cells, such as mast cells, with antigen *in vitro*.

In (2) and (3) the tissues are washed free from blood and the reaction is therefore independent of complement or other factors in the plasma.

When isolated intestine or uterus from a sensitized guinea-pig is exposed to specific antigen, it gives a sharp contraction (the Schultz-Dale reaction); a second dose of antigen is without effect. After the first dose of antigen the reaction with antibody runs to completion; thereafter the tissue is insensitive to any further dose of antigen. This is known as desensitization. Sensitivity to specific antigen can nevertheless be restored by immersing the uterus in a solution of the same antibody. The Schultz–Dale reaction provides a useful experimental model for the study of anaphylaxis.

Other methods depend on subdividing tissues from sensitized animals, thus increasing the effective surface area of the tissue. Lungs of sensitized guinea-pig are chopped into small pieces, 0·5–1 mm in length, which are exposed to more antibody in solution so as to obtain maximum sensitization. After removal of excess antibody, antigen is added to the tissue and the amount of histamine diffusing out of the tissue in 15 min at 37°C is taken as an index of sensitization.

Mast cells, circulating basophils and, in the rabbit, platelets all fix antibody and are sensitized. On contact with the antigen, histamine is released and the mast cells and basophils lose their granules and no longer stain with toluidine blue. The anaphylactic reaction is seen only in cells that are intact. Mast cells and other cells not only fix antibody to the surface of the cell but rapidly ingest it. Intracellular granules containing histamine might then become sensitized to the antigen. So far, experiment has shown that antigen is without effect on the granules from which histamine can be released in other ways, e.g. by octylamine. The cellular basis of the anaphylactic reaction is imperfectly understood. The experimental approach is based on the view that it is a sequence of enzymic reactions which might be activated or suppressed by physical or chemical agents. Quantitative studies of the reaction have depended mainly on the estimation of histamine.

The anaphylactic reaction requires O_2 and Ca^{++}, and occurs within a narrow range of pH with an optimum at 7·8. A rise of temperature from 38°C to 43°C for 25 min inhibits it whether in the whole sensitized guinea-pig or isolated lung; the effect is usually irreversible.

The addition of antigen to particles of sensitized guinea-pig lung stimulates O_2 consumption which suggests that energy is used in the reaction. Dinitrophenol, however, does not inhibit histamine release when applied in concentrations that abolish oxidative phosphorylation; nor is the anaphylactic reaction sensitive to carbon monoxide.

Many substances ranging from general anaesthetics to selective enzyme inhibitors prevent the release of histamine from sensitized guinea-pig lung by antigen. Iodoacetate, *N*-ethylmaleimide and *p*-chloromercuribenzoate probably act by blocking SH groups; cysteine, thioglycolate, sulphite and reduced glutathione split S—S bonds in essential proteins.

Antipyretics as a group inhibit histamine release in anaphylaxis, but the effect is probably not specific since these drugs depress oxygen consumption and contractibility of smooth muscle in about the same concentrations that inhibit histamine release. Phenylbutazone is the most potent of these inhibitors.

In theory, anaphylaxis may be prevented at three stages of the reaction:

(1) union of antigen with antibody,

(2) intracellular reactions leading to the release or formation of mediators, and

(3) the action of mediators on sensitive cells, such as capillaries, glands and smooth muscle.

The Schultz–Dale reaction, histamine release and desensitization are tests which provide information on the likely sequence of reactions. Thus, a substance which inhibits the Schultz–Dale reaction and histamine release is presumed to act before stage (3); a substance which inhibits histamine release but fails to prevent desensitization is presumed to act beyond stage (1). Phenol is more generally known as the drug that denatures proteins, penetrates cell membranes and kills bacteria. Yet in low concentrations it acts to uncouple the antigen–antibody reaction from histamine release. If sensitized tissue is exposed to antigen in the presence of phenol, Schultz–Dale and histamine release reactions are inhibited, but if phenol is later removed and a second dose of antigen applied the tissue is found to have been desensitized. Phenol interferes with a mechanism, probably enzymic, which links the first to the second stage of the anaphylactic reaction. An hypothetical scheme of events is shown in fig. 14.3.

Mast cells contain proteolytic enzymes which may be activated in the anaphylaxis. Among these are chymotrypsin, aminopeptidases and cathepsins. It may be significant that di-isopropylfluorophosphate (DFP; Dyflos) which inhibits chymotrypsin also prevents anaphylaxis; SH blocking compounds act on the cathepsins. Snake and bee venoms are powerful histamine releasers *in vivo*. The venoms owe their actions mainly to the presence of highly active proteins, among which is the enzyme lecithinase-A. Sulphydryl blocking reagents and other enzyme inhibitors protect the mast cell from disruption by lecithinase A, antigen and compound 48/80. It has, therefore, been proposed that the mast cell membrane

Cell fixed antibody + antigen
↓
Enzyme precursor
Inhibition at 43°C   ↓ + Ca^{++}
Inactivated ← Active enzyme
(short lived)
Phenol inhibits →   +
Bound histamine ← Histamine
(in granules)   releaser
↓
Free histamine
↓
Receptors of effector cells
↓
Anaphylactic reaction

FIG. 14.3. Sequence of events in the immediate hypersensitivity reaction. After Mongar J.L. and Schild H.O. (1962). *Physiol. Rev.* **43**, 226.

contains a lecithinase which can be activated by antigen and compound 48/80 and inactivated by enzyme inhibitors (p. 25.16).

Lack of Ca^{++} prevents mast cell destruction by all these agents and Ca^{++} are an essential cofactor of lecithinase A *in vitro*.

So far, the term antibody has been used in a general sense; in fact, it is the fractions as defined by their physical properties that are important. For example, histamine release in sensitized tissue occurs when antigen reacts with the cell-bound IgA fraction; again, a component of this fraction specifically sensitizes mast cells (mast cell sensitizing antibody).

In the present context, the term histamine release means not only the explosive release from the granular stores in mast cells but a continuing formation and release from cells through the induction of histidine decarboxylase.

On this view, the formation of histamine would be similar to the formation of bradykinin and SRS-A which contributes to the anaphylactic reaction. Unlike histamine, neither of these substances is stored in cells. Bradykinin is formed when antigen reacts with the antibody fraction IgG which requires complement. The antigen–antibody reaction in turn activates a tissue enzyme which acts on α_2-globulin precursor in plasma (kininogen) to yield the polypeptide (p. 17.2).

Slow reacting substance-A (SRS-A) is a substance of unknown structure that shares some of the physical properties of a fatty acid. On the isolated guinea-pig ileum its potency, weight for weight, is similar to that of histamine. Whereas histamine produces a quick contraction, the response to SRS-A appears more slowly and is protracted. As an agonist the pharmacological properties of SRS-A differ from all other known agonists; antagonists for SRS-A are not yet known. Unlike histamine and bradykinin, SRS-A is not rapidly destroyed in the body. Human bronchial smooth muscle is more sensitive to the action of SRS-A than that of any other species tested so far. This fact together with the formation of SRS-A by human sensitized lung *in vitro* suggests that SRS-A may be important in the pathogenesis of asthma. The formation of SRS-A *in vitro* can be followed in tissues sensitized with antibody fraction IgG but apparently does not require complement.

As a consequence of the antigen-antibody reaction there is first the release of histamine followed by the formation of bradykinin and SRS-A. Depletion of histamine stores probably stimulates the formation of more histamine. All the mediators stimulate smooth muscle; histamine and bradykinin increase the permeability of blood vessels.

DELAYED HYPERSENSITIVITY (TYPE IV) REACTION
This type of reaction involves the interaction of sensitized mononuclear cells of the blood and tissues with specific antigen and is described on p. 22.18. Little is known about the mediators of the response. Extracts of lymph nodes from sensitized animals contain small amounts of histamine, other unidentified substances that stimulate smooth muscle and a factor which increases vascular permeability. **Lymph node permeability factor** (LNPF) can also be extracted from lymph nodes and other tissues of normal animals (p. 21.6) and is assayed by its local effect on the permeability of vessels of the skin to a blue dye. It is possibly leukotaxic but LNPF antibody does not induce leucopenia although it greatly reduces the tuberculin reaction which is a classical example of delayed hypersensitivity (p. 21.16).

Antihistamines

Up till 1937, the only substance known to oppose the actions of histamine was adrenaline. The antagonism, however, is not specific but physiological, since adrenaline occupies different receptors and acts in the opposite direction. Adrenaline brings quick relief in serum sickness and other hypersensitivity reactions in which there may be intolerable itch or danger of suffocation from laryngeal oedema (p. 24.5).

The disadvantages arising from its use were, firstly, excitation of the heart, and secondly, the short duration of its action. The discovery of specific or competitive antagonists (p. 3.12) for histamine not only met a therapeutic need but also made it possible to identify the histamine activity in extracts of tissues and body fluids and to classify histamine receptors.

The antihistamines oppose many of the actions of histamine on smooth muscle and blood vessels, but do not prevent the gastric secretory response. In guinea-pigs and other animals that are protected with antihistamines, large doses of histamine induce prolonged

secretion and eventually ulceration of the gastric mucosa.

Antihistamines also oppose weakly the actions of acetylcholine, but this action differs from their antagonism for the stimulant action of histamine on the salivary glands or on the adrenal medulla.

Antihistamines do not affect histamine metabolism nor prevent the release of histamine from cells in response to injury or drugs, or in the anaphylactic reaction. Indeed, as weak organic bases, they may act as histamine releasers. Sensitization to antihistamines may occur in patients, particularly when the drugs are applied to the skin. In this respect, the antihistamines behave as do many other drugs. Antihistamines possess important actions which appear to be unrelated to their antagonism for histamine. They act as local anaesthetics and have a quinidine-like action on the heart. In this sense, they stabilize membranes. Antihistamines act on the CNS and in usual doses frequently cause drowsiness which may be enhanced by other drugs such as alcohol or barbiturates. Some prevent vomiting in motion sickness and are also used in the treatment of Menière's disease in which the sense of balance is disturbed.

The tranquillizer, chlorpromazine, was developed from the potent antihistamine, promethazine. In pharmacological tests, antihistaminic actions are slight. Chlorpromazine is also anti-emetic but its mode of action may differ from that of the antihistamines, since it prevents vomiting induced by apomorphine, whereas the antihistamines are ineffective (p. 5.31).

RELATIONSHIP OF STRUCTURE AND ACTION
In 1937, Daniel Bovet, and his colleagues of the Institut Pasteur in Paris, re-examined the pharmacological properties of certain phenolic ethers which were designed as possible antagonists of adrenaline. In the event, tests on isolated guinea-pig intestine indicated that the drugs had a greater antagonism for histamine. This unexpected result led to the further investigation of the most active

Thymoxyethyldiethylamine (929F)

member of the series, thymoxyethyldiethylamine (929F), which had been synthesized as early as 1910 by Furneaux, an organic chemist of the Institut Pasteur.

Earlier work had shown that the drug was an antipyretic, was oxytocic and also blocked the effect of adrenaline and of sympathetic nerve stimulation. Methods were now developed which established criteria for the identification and measurement of antihistamine activity. Firstly, the antagonism of 929F for histamine was confirmed in other smooth muscle preparations; secondly, 50 mg of the drug, given intraperitoneally, protected guinea-pigs against three lethal doses of histamine, 0.5×3 mg given intravenously; thirdly, the drug gave protection against anaphylaxis; fourthly, the drug did not prevent gastric secretory response to histamine and finally clinical trial showed that the drug might be of value in the treatment of allergic disorders. The application of these and other tests in the work that followed made it possible to select the most active compounds and to increase their potency still further by changes in structure.

More active than the phenolic ethers were compounds based on the structure of phenylethylene diamine or aniline ethylamine,

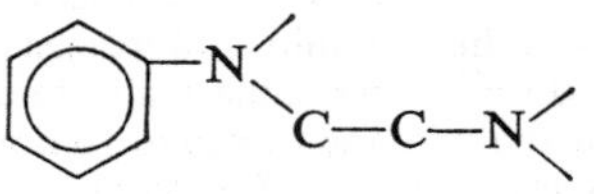

Of these, the most active was first, substance 2325 RP

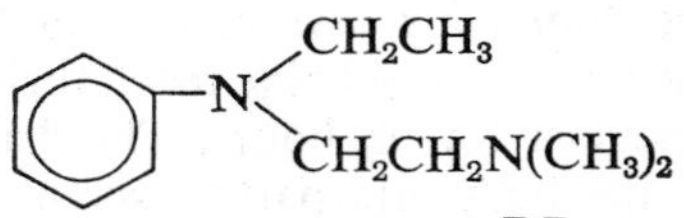

2325 RP

and then, antergan

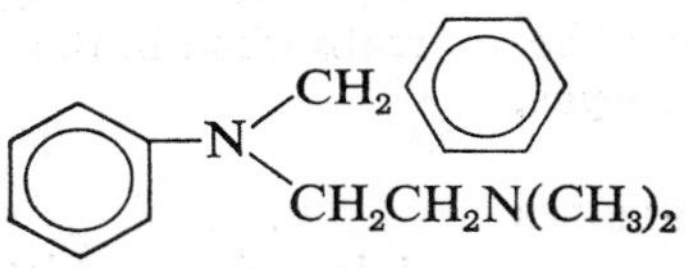

Antergan

Antergan in a dose of 5 mg/kg given subcutaneously protected guinea-pigs against forty lethal doses of histamine. Clinical trial left no doubt about its therapeutic value in the control of hay fever and urticaria (p. 24.4).

Further progress was made by replacing the benzene ring in phenylethylenediamine with other ring structures, such as pyridine. The addition of a methoxy group in the para position of the benzyl group, increased potency still further and the drug was named **neoantergan**. In the guinea-pig, 5 mg/kg subcutaneously gave protection against 300 lethal doses of histamine, and 1 mg/kg against

Neoantergan

the anaphylactic reaction. Neoantergan (mepyramine maleate) was discovered in 1944 and to this day remains one of the most potent antagonists of histamine.

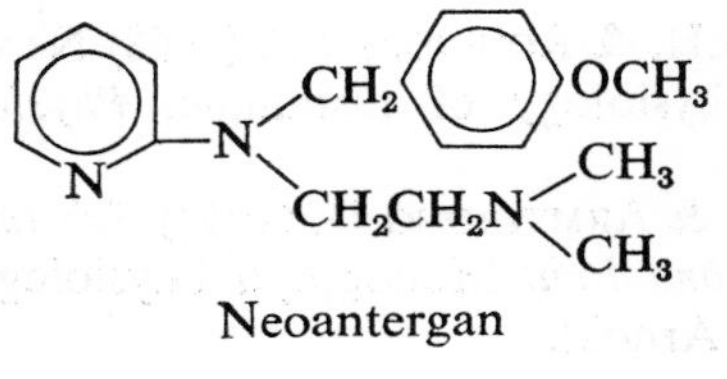

From 1945 onwards, the antihistamines were developed on a large scale in the USA and many new structural types were introduced. Most are based on an ethylamine chain which is also shared by histamine.

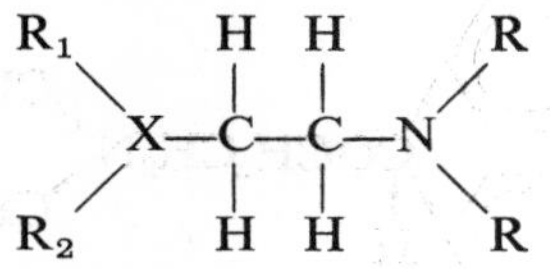

The X may stand for nitrogen, oxygen or carbon. Nitrogen gives an ethylene diamine derivative

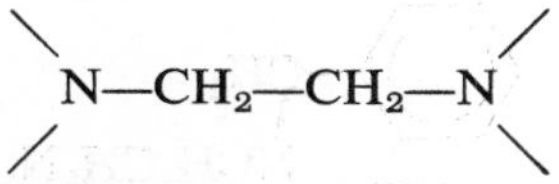

oxygen an aminoalkylether, and

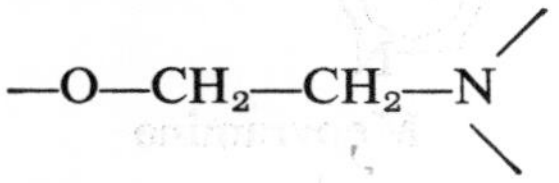

carbon an alkylamine,

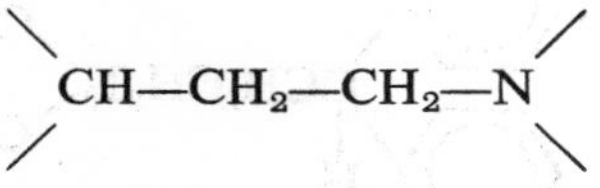

Some of the more commonly used antihistamines and their structural relation to histamine are shown in table 14.4 and fig. 14.4. Fig. 14.5 illustrates one method of assaying their activity.

TABLE 14.4. Some commonly used antihistamines and usual daily doses.

Antazoline (antistin)	50–100 mg orally
Chlorcyclizine (histantin)	50–200 mg orally
Chlorpheniramine (piriton)	5– 20 mg IM or IV,
	4– 16 mg orally
Cyclizine (marzine)	25– 50 mg orally
Cyproheptadine (periactin)	4– 20 mg orally
Dimenhydrinate (dramamine)	25– 50 mg IM,
	25–100 mg orally
Diphenhydramine (benadryl)	25– 75 mg orally,
	10– 50 mg IM or IV
Mebhydrolin napadisylate (fabahistin)	100–300 mg orally
Meclozine (ancolan)	25– 50 mg orally
Mepyramine maleate (anthisan)	25– 50 mg IM or IV,
	100–200 mg orally
Phenindamine	25– 50 mg orally
Promethazine hydrochloride (phenergan)	20– 50 mg IM,
	20– 50 mg orally
Promethazine theoclate (avomine)	25– 50 mg orally
Tripelennamine (pyribenzamine)	50–100 mg orally
Triprolidine (actidil)	5– 7.5 mg orally

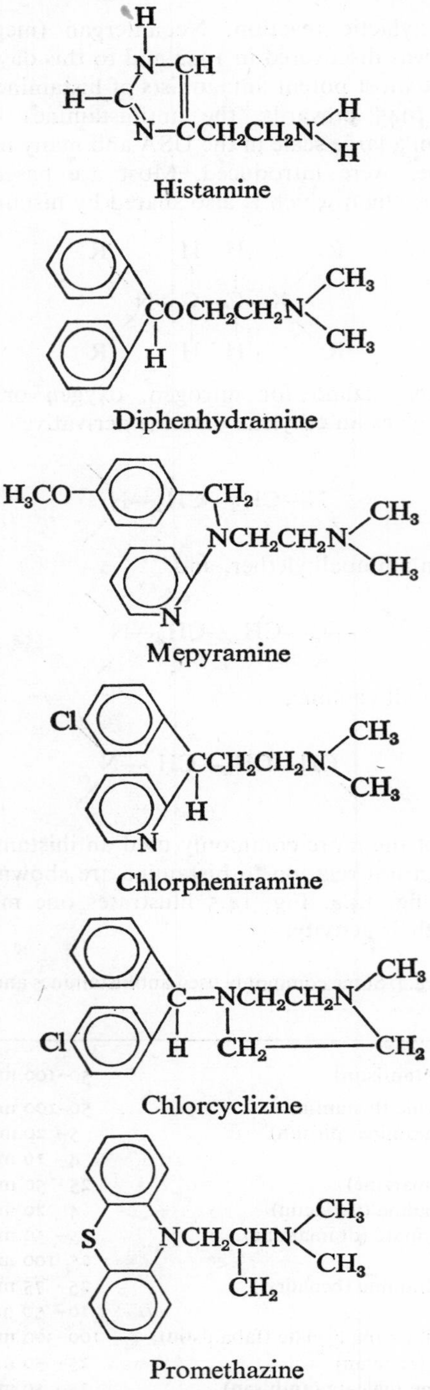

Histamine

Diphenhydramine

Mepyramine

Chlorpheniramine

Chlorcyclizine

Promethazine

FIG. 14.4. Structural relations of histamine and commonly used antihistamines.

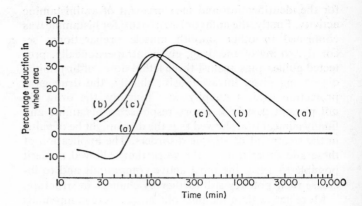

FIG. 14.5. The effect of three antihistamines given orally on the response of healthy subjects to intradermal injections of histamine. (a) 25 mg promethazine reaches a maximum effect in 200 min and persists for up to 50 hours; (b) 150 mg mepyramine malleate attains a maximum effect in 100 min and ceases in 16 hours; (c) 350 mg antazoline exerts a similar effect to 150 mg mepyramine. After Bain W.A. (1949). *Proc. roy. Soc. Med.* **42**, 615.

ABSORPTION AND FATE

The antihistamines are readily absorbed from the gut or after injection. They behave as weak bases and are widely distributed in the tissues and body fluids, including the brain. Maximum effects are obtained in 1–2 hours and the action continues for several hours; the actions of promethazine and chlorcyclizine reach their maximum in 4–5 hours and last for 24 hours. The drugs are partly destroyed in the body and partly excreted in the urine. The chief site of transformation is the liver where they may undergo hydroxylation and conjugation with glucuronic acid or be changed in other ways. Metabolites excreted in the bile are reabsorbed in the gut and finally appear in the urine.

ADVERSE EFFECTS

Apart from sedation and drowsiness which have already been mentioned, other effects are dizziness, tinnitus, incoordination, blurred vision, excitement and tremors; loss of appetite, nausea, vomiting and diarrhoea. Leukopenia and agranulocytosis are rare.

In children, the lethal dose of antihistamines is of the order of 500–1000 mg of most preparations. Fixed, dilated pupils, facial flush and raised body temperature might suggest atropine poisoning. Death is usually within 2–18 hours. There is no specific therapy for antihistamine poisoning.

FURTHER READING

DALE H.H. (1953) *Adventures in Physiology.* Oxford: Pergamon.

KAHLSON G.H. & ROSENGREN E. (1968) New approaches to the physiology of histamine. *Physiol. Rev.* **48**, 155.

KEELE C.A. & ARMSTRONG D. (1964) *Substances Producing Pain and Itch.* Monograph Physiological Society. London: Arnold.

Chapter 15
The catecholamines

The catecholamines, dopamine, noradrenaline and adrenaline are of great importance in the sympathetic nervous system and two of them, dopamine and noradrenaline, probably have major functions in the CNS. These substances have been described and discussed briefly in vol. I in relation to the adrenal medulla and neurochemical transmission (vol. I, pp. 14.23, 24.88 and 25.28).

The actions of these physiological substances are simulated closely by several drugs, and other drugs modify their release. For these reasons, a fuller account of these important substances is given here. The chemical relationship between the compounds is shown in fig. 15.1. They are derivatives of 2- or β-phenylethylamine. The group name 'catecholamine' derives from the fact that all contain a catechol group, i.e. a benzene ring with two hydroxyl groups attached at adjacent positions to the ring, and an amine group (substituted or unsubstituted) at the end of the side chain attached to the benzene ring. **Dopamine** is 2-(3-4-dihydroxyphenyl)ethylamine. **Adrenaline** differs from dopamine in having a hydroxyl group at the 2- or β-position in the side chain and a methyl group attached to the amino group. In North America it is known as epinephrine. **Noradrenaline** (USA, norepinephrine) differs from dopamine only in the presence of a hydroxyl group in the β-position in the side chain. It differs from adrenaline in lacking the methyl substituent on the amino group. To the organic chemist the prefix 'nor' indicates a compound with one methyl or methylene group less than the named substance. An alternative explanation is that it is an abbreviation of the German *N Ohne Radical* meaning nitrogen without a radical, i.e. the methyl group present in adrenaline. **Isoprenaline** (USA, isoproterenol), a contraction of *N*-isopropylnoradrenaline, is a drug which is also a catecholamine. It differs from noradrenaline in having an *iso*propyl group attached to the amino nitrogen.

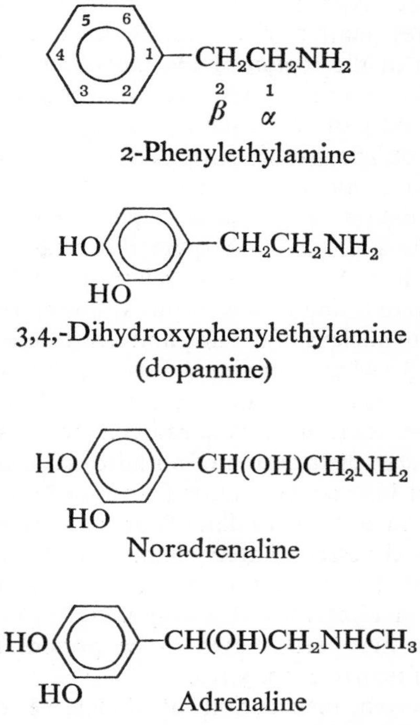

The catecholamines are weak bases because of the presence of a primary or secondary amine group. They are white crystalline solids sparingly soluble in water. They may be obtained in the form of easily water-soluble salts such as hydrochloride or hydrogen tartrate. The catecholamines are rapidly oxidized and, in neutral or alkaline solutions, they give rise to pink coloured oxidation products when exposed to air and light. The oxidation is catalysed by traces of copper or ferric ions in solution.

Adrenaline, noradrenaline and isoprenaline exist in two optically active isomeric forms because of the asymmetric carbon atom at position 2- of the side chains, which dopamine lacks. Naturally occurring adrenaline and noradrenaline are laevo- (−) rotatory, and are much more active biologically than the dextro- (+) form; this is also true of isoprenaline.

Occurrence of the catecholamines

ADRENAL GLANDS
The total amount of catecholamines in the whole gland varies from species to species in the range 0·12–14 mg/g.

FIG. 15.1. Structural formulae of catecholamines.

Human adrenal glands contain 0·3–1 mg/g, the quantity depending on the relative proportions of cortex to medulla. The proportion of noradrenaline also varies greatly. It accounts for only about 3 per cent of the total catecholamines in the rabbit, but in the whale, for almost 100 per cent. In man the proportion is about 10–20 per cent. Histochemical methods show that adrenaline and noradrenaline are contained in separate cells in the medulla and that preferential release of one or other amine into the blood can occur. Dopamine has been detected also in adrenal extracts, but accounts at most for 2 per cent of the total catecholamines.

SYMPATHETIC NERVOUS SYSTEM

In 1921, Loewi showed that on stimulating the sympathetic nerves to a perfused frog heart, the perfusate acquired the property of accelerating the rate of another frog heart, just as would adrenaline. At about the same time Cannon found that stimulation of sympathetic nerves, such as those to the liver, liberated substances with an adrenaline-like action on other tissues. These findings have often been confirmed, and for many years adrenaline was considered to be the chemical transmitter of sympathetic nerve impulses.

However, pharmacological analyses showed discrepancies between the biological actions of the liberated substances and of adrenaline and, at various times, it was suggested that noradrenaline might be involved. In 1946 von Euler showed noradrenaline to be present in peripheral organs and sympathetic nerves and that it was the predominant amine in various animals. The evidence was derived from comparisons of the biological activity of extracts of tissues with those of adrenaline and noradrenaline on pharmacological preparations, differing quantitatively in their responses to the amines. In all the extracts traces of adrenaline, amounting to 2–15 per cent of the total catecholamines, were also detected.

Direct evidence that sympathetic nerves release noradrenaline was obtained by Peart, when he stimulated the splenic nerves of the cat and collected blood from the splenic vein. Plasma from this blood was active on pharmacological preparations such as the isolated rat uterus and colon; comparisons with adrenaline and noradrenaline indicated that the main substance active in the plasma was noradrenaline. Small amounts of adrenaline, never exceeding 10 per cent of the noradrenaline concentration, were sometimes detected.

These findings have been extended to other mammalian species. It is now accepted that noradrenaline is released on stimulating mammalian sympathetic nerves, apart from a few which release acetylcholine, and that it is responsible for the physiological responses in the innervated organs. The noradrenaline is unevenly distributed in postganglionic sympathetic nerves, the lowest concentration occurring in the sympathetic ganglia (50–100 µg/g), slightly higher concentration in the mid axon part (100–500 µg/g) and highest (10 mg/g) in the terminals.

The postganglionic sympathetic nerves which release noradrenaline are referred to as **adrenergic nerves**, a term coined by Dale before the discovery of noradrenaline. This terminology is strictly accurate only in the case of amphibia such as the frog where the transmitter is indeed adrenaline.

Dopamine has also been detected in adrenergic nerves in amounts about one-tenth to one-sixth that of noradrenaline. Whether this dopamine has any functional significance other than as a precursor of noradrenaline (p. 15.4) is not known. In certain tissues of ruminants such as sheep and goats, dopamine is present in a much higher relative concentration and it is the predominant amine in some tissues such as the lung; in other species the only organ containing significant amounts is the intestine where it is present in a concentration about half that of noradrenaline. In ruminants, especially large amounts are located in some mast cells, the function of which is not known.

CATECHOLAMINES IN THE CNS

In whole brain, noradrenaline and dopamine are found in roughly the same concentration, but their distribution throughout the brain is uneven.

In studies in the cat and dog, Vogt showed that noradrenaline was confined to the grey matter and absent from white matter. The highest concentrations were present in the hypothalamus (1–2 µg/g) followed by the central grey matter of the midbrain and the reticular formation in the region of the medulla (0·35–0·4 µg/g). The corpus striatum, the cortex and the cerebellum contained only small amounts ($<$0·1 µg/g). Much smaller amounts of adrenaline were detected and it does not accumulate in any particular region (p. 5.15, fig. 5.16).

Carlsson first showed that dopamine was present in brain with a distribution quite different from that of noradrenaline. In particular, relatively high concentrations were found in the corpus striatum, e.g. 6 µg/g in the caudate nucleus of the dog and a little less in the lentiform nucleus which contains about 0·1 µg/g noradrenaline. In other areas the concentrations of dopamine were much lower than those of noradrenaline (p. 5.15).

The uneven distribution of noradrenaline suggests that in areas of high concentration ($>$0·1 µg/g) the amine has a function in addition to that of control of smooth muscle of the blood vessels. Catecholamines in tissue slices can be located by converting them to substances which fluoresce in ultraviolet (UV) light, and in this way noradrenaline has been shown to be present in complex systems of neurones (p. 5.16).

The uneven distribution of dopamine differing as it does from that of noradrenaline, especially in the corpus striatum, makes it likely that in some regions dopamine serves a function other than as a precursor of noradrenaline.

CHROMAFFIN CELLS (vol. 1, p. 25.28)

The cells of the adrenal medulla which contain the catecholamines are known as chromaffin cells; when these are treated with dichromate, a brown substance is formed from oxidation products of the catecholamines.

Tumours of chromaffin cells, which are known as **phaeochromocytoma**, may arise in the adrenal gland or from extra-adrenal chromaffin tissue. They give rise to persistent or paroxysmal high blood pressure and hyperglycaemia, because they release catecholamines into the blood stream. In adrenal medullary tumours both adrenaline and noradrenaline are present, with the latter predominating. Rarely dopamine is the predominant catecholamine. Such tumours are not innervated and the stimulus to secretion is not known. Handling of such a tumour during surgical operation for its removal may lead to secretion as can the injection of histamine (p. 14.11). Such tumours are rarely malignant and surgical removal effects a cure.

OCCURRENCE OF CATECHOLAMINE IN NATURE

Other malignant tumours secreting catecholamines arise from embryologically related sympathetic ganglia. These contain dopamine and noradrenaline, with the former in a relatively higher proportion than in phaeochromocytoma. Concentrations of the catecholamines are low compared to those in phaeochromocytoma, but there is evidence of a rapid turnover of the amines. Such tumours seldom cause a marked rise in blood pressure, probably because most of the noradrenaline found is metabolized and inactivated within the tumour tissue.

Catecholamines are found in many animals and plants. In earthworms and lugworms the ventral ganglion chain has been reported to contain about 1·5 μg noradrenaline and about 0·3 μg adrenaline/g tissue. Adrenaline in the high concentration of 50 μg/g or more is the predominant amine in the hearts of hagfish and lamprey, the noradrenaline content being 15 μg/g or less. In the frog, adrenaline also occurs in large amounts in the heart (about 1 μg/g), brain (about 2 μg/g) and other tissues; noradrenaline is present in amounts one-tenth or less. A similar ratio occurs in other amphibia.

Dopamine is the major catecholamine in insects (bees, house-flies, earwigs), with a concentration of about 10 μg/g, that of noradrenaline being about 2 μg/g; adrenaline is only just detectable (<0·3 μg/g). Dopamine is the predominant amine in the nervous tissue of sea urchins, starfish, clams and octopods. Noradrenaline is also present but adrenaline has not been detected.

Various fruits and vegetables contain catecholamines. Noradrenaline has been detected in oranges, potatoes and plums, and dopamine in avocados. The highest concentrations have been found in the banana. One report gives the concentration/g pulp as 8 μg dopamine and 2 μg noradrenaline, with the peel containing 700 μg/g dopamine and 122 μg/g noradrenaline. It is of interest that several fruits and vegetables share other biologically active amines such as 5-HT, tryptamine and tyramine with the animal world. For reasons which are given on p. 15.19, the normal person does not experience any pharmacological effect from these amines on eating such foods.

Cellular localization of catecholamines

The catecholamines in the adrenal medulla, in sympathetic nerves and in the brain must be held in the cell in a form which protects them from breakdown by amine oxidases present in the mitochondria.

Adrenal medulla

The catecholamines are held in granules, 0·1–0·5 μm in diameter, which can be separated by density gradient centrifugation. They can be released from the granules by exposure to hypotonic solutions or detergents and by freezing and thawing. This indicates that there is a membranous cover around the granules, as can be confirmed by EM. In the granules, the concentration is much in excess of that of an isotonic solution so they cannot exist in a freely soluble state, and there is a 4 to 1 ratio between the molar concentrations of the catecholamine and of ATP. Since each ATP molecule has four acidic groups and each catecholamine molecule one basic group, it has been suggested that a nondiffusible ionic complex exists between the two, stabilized by the protein present in the granules.

The granules contain soluble acidic protein which is known as chromagranin. Other proteins and probably also the lipid present in the granule are located in the membrane, which contains unusually large amounts of lysolecithin.

In phaeochromocytoma, the ratio of catecholamines to ATP may be as high as 20, indicating binding of much of the amines by processes not involving ATP.

Adrenergic nerves

Granules containing noradrenaline have been isolated from adrenergic nerves and from sympathetically innervated organs; they resemble the adrenal medullary granules but are smaller (0·05 μm diameter) and more resistant to freezing and thawing. Such granules can take up noradrenaline from the surrounding medium. How much of the noradrenaline is contained in such particles is not known. After ultracentrifugation, about 40 per cent of the noradrenaline is always found in the supernatant fraction, but this may arise from disruption of the granules during the isolation procedure. However, some noradrenaline is present in an extragranular form, possibly combined with lipid. Several different storage forms may exist, each containing limited amounts of noradrenaline; these when utilized are replaced from the main store in the granules where noradrenaline is synthesized. These minor but important stores can be depleted preferentially by certain drugs and by nerve impulses. In addition, some of the noradrenaline from the storage granules is inactivated within the axon by monoamine oxidase. The composite picture, the details of which remain controversial, is one of a complex dynamic equilibrium between synthesis, storage and utilization.

Fluorescence microscopy shows that these granules collect in groups in the terminal sympathetic axons to form thickenings, or varicosities, at points along the length of the fibre. The varicosities probably correspond to synaptic regions of the adrenergic terminals. The granules are also found in the axon of the neurone.

Neurones in the CNS
The subcellular localization of the catecholamines is probably similar to that in adrenergic nerves and at least part of the noradrenaline in brain is present in granular vesicles (p. 5.16). Although the dopamine in brain is present in neurones, its localization within vesicular storage granules similar to those containing noradrenaline is not definitely proven. In brain homogenates, part of the dopamine and noradrenaline is found in the synaptosomal fraction, but ultracentrifugation of the lysed synaptosomes shows that very little of the dopamine is in storage granules. Fig. 15.7, p. 15.16, summarizes the dynamic equilibrium between synthesis, storage and release and indicates the sites of action of certain drugs which may influence it.

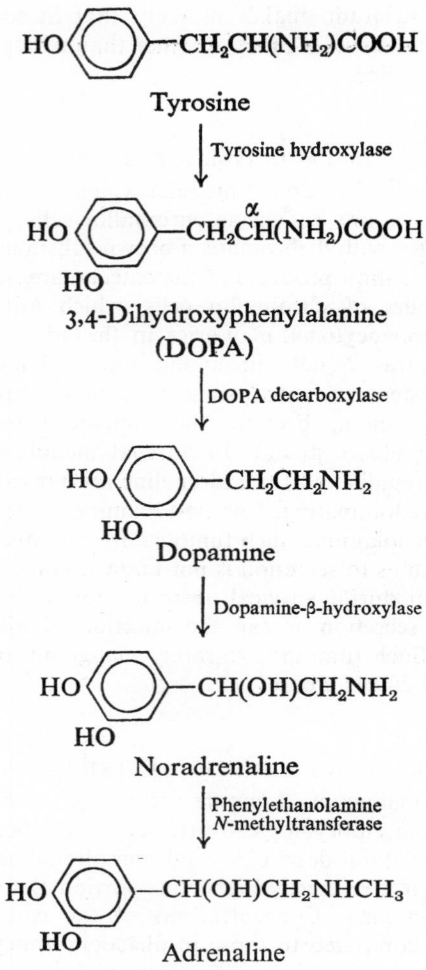

Biosynthesis of the catecholamines

The major pathway in the biosynthesis of the catecholamines, outlined in vol. 1, p. 11.25, is shown in fig. 15.2. This sequence of reactions was first postulated by Blaschko, in 1939, soon after the discovery in mammalian kidney of one of the enzymes involved, DOPA decarboxylase. ^{14}C-tyrosine, ^{14}C-DOPA and ^{14}C-dopamine give rise to ^{14}C-noradrenaline and ^{14}C-adrenaline in the adrenal medulla both *in vivo* and *in vitro*. Homogenates of sympathetic nerves and ganglia, on incubation with tyrosine or DOPA, produce dopamine and noradrenaline but, significantly, not adrenaline. Similarly rat and cat brain produce labelled dopamine and noradrenaline from ^{14}C-tyrosine. There is therefore evidence that tissues in which catecholamines are found are able to form the amines from their precursors.

FIG. 15.2. Biosynthesis of catecholamines.

DOPA DECARBOXYLASE
This enzyme is present in the adrenal medulla, sympathetic ganglia, postganglionic adrenergic neurones and in the brain where it is distributed unevenly; there is more of the enzyme in the caudate nucleus, the hypothalamus, the thalamus and midbrain than in the cortex; it is undetectable in white matter. The distribution is thus similar to that of catecholamines (p. 5.15).

DOPA decarboxylase, in common with other amino acid decarboxylases, requires pyridoxal phosphate as coenzyme. Although its action *in vitro* is specific to the L-form of DOPA, substrate specificity is only relative since the enzyme also decarboxylates L-5-hydroxytryptophan to yield 5-hydroxytryptamine. α-Methyldopa is also a substrate, a finding of significance in the action of this amino acid as an antihypertensive agent (pp. 8.9 and 15.31). *m*-Tyrosine, *o*-tyrosine and dihydroxyphenylserine (DOPA with a hydroxyl group on the β-position) are also substrates, yielding the corresponding amines. Dihydroxyphenylserine could thus give rise to noradrenaline bypassing dopamine, but there is no evidence that this amino acid is a precursor of importance in the normal biosynthesis of noradrenaline. The enzyme has a low affinity for histidine, *p*-tyrosine, tryptophan and phenylalanine. Because of its wide ranging activity towards aromatic amino acids, DOPA decarboxylase is also called 'aromatic-L-amino acid decarboxylase' (p. 14.11).

DOPAMINE-β-HYDROXYLASE

Noradrenaline is formed from dopamine by dopamine-β-hydroxylase. This enzyme has been purified from beef adrenal glands and is a copper-containing protein. Studies *in vitro* indicate that the copper at the active centre is first reduced, possibly by ascorbic acid to the cuprous form of the enzyme, which then combines with oxygen and catalyses the oxidation at the β-position, the cuprous copper of the enzyme being oxidized simultaneously. Other possible reducing agents include cysteine and the catechol group of dopamine itself.

Chelating agents, especially those with a high affinity for copper, inhibit this enzyme. Thus disulfiram is a potent inhibitor after its reduction to diethyldithiocarbamate, the actual chelating agent. In animals, disulfiram lowers noradrenaline and increases dopamine in the brain.

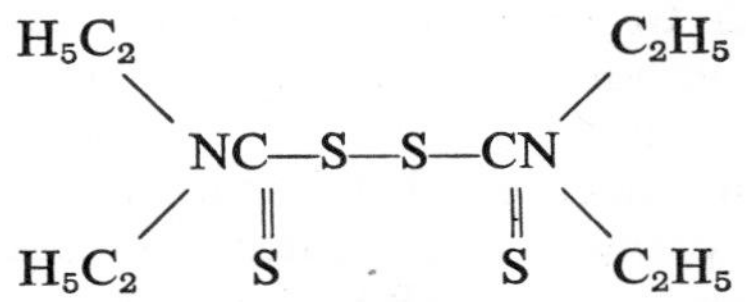

Disulfiram

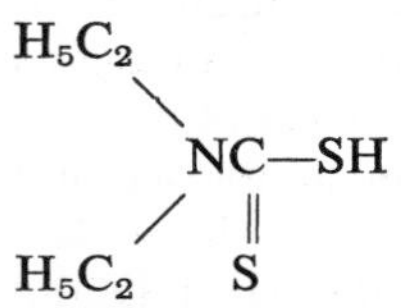

Diethyldithiocarbamate

The enzyme is not specific to dopamine, and many phenylethylamine derivatives can act as substrates. Among these are *p*-tyramine (converted to octopamine), α-methyldopamine (to α-methylnoradrenaline) and α-methyl-*m*-tyramine (to metaraminol). Isosteres of phenylethylamines in which the α-carbon atom is substituted by *O* or *N* are not substrates but have an affinity for the enzyme and inhibit its action. These compounds are also inhibitors of DOPA decarboxylase. Examples of such compounds are *N*-(3-hydroxybenzyl)-*N*-methylhydrazine and *O*-(3-hydroxybenzyl) hydroxylamine.

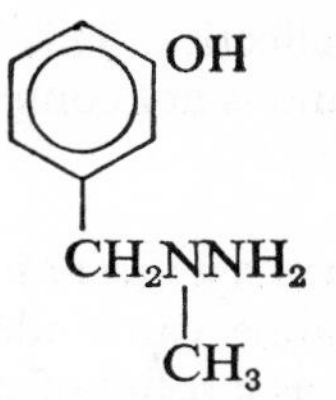

N-(3-Hydroxybenzyl)-*N*-methylhydrazine

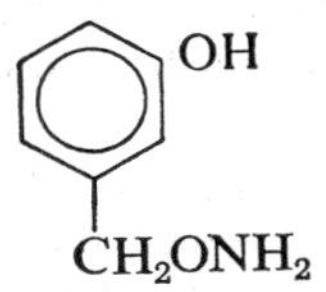

O-(3-Hydroxybenzyl) hydroxylamine

The distribution of dopamine-β-hydroxylase in brain follows a similar pattern to noradrenaline, with the exception that high enzyme activity has been detected in the corpus striatum, an area which contains high concentrations of dopamine and relatively low concentrations of noradrenaline. It would appear that the enzyme is not accessible to the major part of the dopamine produced in this region.

TYROSINE HYDROXYLASE

This enzyme is present in the adrenal gland, sympathetically innervated tissues and in the brain in mammals. It has been purified from beef adrenal medulla and requires a tetrahydropteridine as cofactor, ferrous ions and molecular oxygen. The sequential steps resemble those outlined above for dopamine-β-hydroxylase. The tetrahydropteridine reduces the enzyme; the reduced enzyme thus catalyses the aerobic oxidation of tyrosine, being itself oxidized in the process. The natural tetrahydropteridine cofactor may be the same as the reduced form of 7:8 dihydrobiopterin isolated from rat liver and shown to be a cofactor in the hydroxylating system of liver which converts phenylalanine to tyrosine. Significantly, the tyrosine hydroxylating system can also hydrolyse phenylalanine to tyrosine, although the K_m for phenylalanine is much higher than the K_m for tyrosine. On the basis of this finding, it has been suggested that the small amount of conversion of phenylalanine to tyrosine which takes place in patients with phenylketonuria, in which the phenylalanine hydroxylating system of the liver is missing, may be due to the action of the tyrosine hydroxylase in adrenergic tissues.

The enzyme is stereospecific to L-tyrosine and it does not oxidize D-tyrosine. Tyramine, *m*-tyrosine and tryptophan are not hydroxylated.

Analogues of tyrosine are competitive inhibitors of the enzyme; α-methyl-*p*-tyrosine is a potent inhibitor and *in vivo* decreases the catecholamine content of the brain, adrenal glands and peripheral tissues. Interestingly, 3-iodotyrosine and 3-5-diiodotyrosine, normal intermediates in thyroglobulin metabolism, are also potent inhibitors.

Catechol derivatives, such as noradrenaline, are also inhibitors, a substance called 3:4-dihydroxyphenylpropylacetamide being particularly effective. This inhibition involves the pteridine cofactor and is not competitive with the substrate L-tyrosine.

PHENYLETHANOLAMINE-*N*-METHYLTRANSFERASE

In the adrenal medulla, noradrenaline can undergo a further reaction to yield adrenaline, as a result of methylation of the amino group by phenylethanolamine-*N*-methyltransferase. The source of the methyl group is *S*-adenosylmethionine. Inhibition of the enzyme by *p*-chloromercuribenzoate suggests that a sulphydryl group is an active site on the enzyme surface. The enzyme is specific for phenylethanolamine derivatives. Thus dopamine or tyramine are not *N*-methylated by the enzyme, but in contrast, the substances shown in fig. 15.3 are methylated. Indeed adrenaline itself can act as

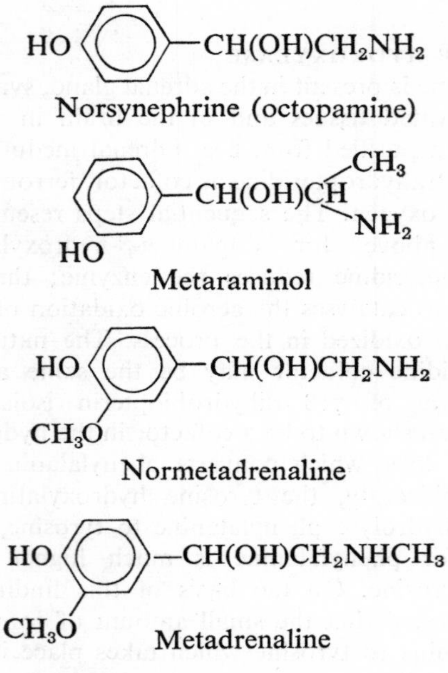

HO—⟨ ⟩—CH(OH)CH$_2$NH$_2$

Norsynephrine (octopamine)

⟨ ⟩—CH(OH)CH⟨$^{CH_3}_{NH_2}$

HO

Metaraminol

HO—⟨ ⟩—CH(OH)CH$_2$NH$_2$

CH$_3$O

Normetadrenaline

HO—⟨ ⟩—CH(OH)CH$_2$NHCH$_3$

CH$_3$O   Metadrenaline

FIG. 15.3. Various phenylethanolamines.

substrate, the product being *N*-methyladrenaline. Very small amounts of *N*-methyladrenaline have been found in the adrenal glands of various species. The physiological significance, if any, of this substance is not known.

Adrenocortical hormones modify the activity of the enzyme, and hence of adrenaline in the medullary cells. Enzyme activity falls markedly in hypophysectomized animals and is restored on giving ACTH or large doses of cortisol. The close anatomical association of the cortex to the medulla ensures that the medulla receives higher concentrations of corticoids than other parts of the body. A low ratio of cortical to medullary size is associated with a low ratio of adrenaline to noradrenaline in the medulla.

This would appear to explain the differences in the ratio of adrenaline and noradrenaline found in the glands of different species (p. 15.3).

It is doubtful if the formation of adrenaline occurs to any significant extent in peripheral nerves or in brain.

SUBCELLULAR DISTRIBUTION OF THE CATECHOLAMINE-FORMING ENZYMES

Differential centrifugation of homogenates of adrenal medulla, postganglionic sympathetic nerves and the brain shows the enzymes to be present in cells which normally contain the catecholamines. Tyrosine hydroxylase is associated with a particulate fraction, but DOPA decarboxylase is found largely in the supernatant and so may be cytoplasmic in origin. This enzyme may also be loosely associated with the noradrenaline storage granules of sympathetic nerves, and these granules may form noradrenaline from DOPA, but not from tyrosine, indicating the absence of the tyrosine hydroxylase. A similar loose association of DOPA decarboxylase with particles in brain homogenates has also been reported. Dopamine-β-hydroxylase activity is present within the catecholamine storage granules of the adrenal medulla and adrenergic nerves and probably also of noradrenaline storage granules in the CNS. The enzyme methylating noradrenaline in the adrenal medulla is found in the supernatant and is presumably in the cytoplasm of the cells. This implies that the noradrenaline formed in the granules has to be released into the cytoplasm for methylation to adrenaline, which is then taken up once more into granules.

The present evidence is that the rate-limiting step in the biosynthetic pathway of the catecholamines is the conversion of tyrosine to DOPA; the amount of enzyme is probably small and tissue concentrations of tyrosine are always sufficient to saturate it. The amounts of the decarboxylase and of dopamine-β-hydroxylase, however, are present in great excess of normal requirements. Probably for this reason inhibitors of tyrosine oxidase are more effective in lowering the content of noradrenaline in the tissues than inhibitors of DOPA decarboxylase and dopamine-β-oxidase, even when they are given in amounts which cause marked inhibition of the enzymes.

The inhibitory effect of the catecholamines on tyrosine hydroxylase activity may exert a controlling influence on their production in the tissues. Thus, it appears that noradrenaline synthesis is controlled by the rate of noradrenaline secretion and that this control takes place at the step for conversion of tyrosine to DOPA.

Fate of catecholamines

There is no enzyme analogous to acetylcholinesterase at cholinergic synapses, which can rapidly destroy catecholamine released by sympathetic nerve stimulation. The rapid termination of the biological actions of the catecholamines involves a number of processes and is not solely dependent on enzymic degradation.

UPTAKE INTO ADRENERGIC NEURONES

When ^{14}C-noradrenaline is given intravenously in small doses (0·03 mg/kg), it disappears rapidly from the blood. About 60 per cent of the dose is found unchanged in the heart, spleen, adrenal glands and other tissues. The remainder can be accounted for in the form of metabolic products, principally the *O*-methylated derivatives (see below). The unchanged catecholamine in the tissue is retained for a relatively long period of time and must be bound in a form which protects it from enzymic destruction. Adrenaline also is taken up by the tissues but not to the same extent as noradrenaline.

Uptake in the tissues is mainly in the postganglionic sympathetic neurones and is markedly reduced by postganglionic sympathetic denervation. The uptake mechanism is an active transport process which proceeds against a concentration gradient of the amines. Noradrenaline is taken up more rapidly than adrenaline but isoprenaline is not accumulated; thus uptake is dependent on chemical structure. The (−) isomers of noradrenaline and adrenaline are accumulated more rapidly than the (+) isomers. The amines are stored in the intraneuronal particles where they are protected from enzymatic inactivation. A similar uptake mechanism in the CNS system has been demonstrated by injecting labelled catecholamines into the cerebral ventricles (p. 5.18).

The return of noradrenaline into the sympathetic nerve terminals is probably the principal mechanism for ending its actions after liberation by the nerve impulse. However, some of the transmitter is inactivated by *O*-methylation in the tissue, some escapes into the blood stream to be metabolized in the liver and some appears unchanged in the urine. The uptake mechanism may also play a role in the inactivation of catecholamines from the adrenal medulla.

Inhibition of uptake mechanisms

The uptake of noradrenaline and adrenaline is inhibited by a number of drugs which include cocaine, imipramine, desimipramine, guanethidine, bretylium, chlorpromazine and phenoxybenzamine, phentolamine, sympathomimetic amines such as tyramine, amphetamine, and ephedrine and monoamine oxidase inhibitors. Under suitable conditions all these potentiate the actions of the noradrenaline and adrenaline; this action is due to the amines persisting in higher concentrations and for a longer time at the effector sites (p. 15.20).

ENZYMIC INACTIVATION

Two enzymes are principally involved, catechol-*O*-methyl transferase and monoamine oxidase. Since the products

10

of the action of one can then be metabolized further by the other there are several possible pathways of inactivation (fig. 15.4).

Catechol-*O*-methyltransferase (COMT) catalyses the introduction of a methyl group into the hydroxy group of the catechol nucleus primarily at the meta- (or 3-) position.

Thus metadrenaline, normetadrenaline (vol. 1, p. 25.30) and methoxytyramine are formed from adrenaline, noradrenaline and dopamine respectively. In rare cases depending on the constituent of R, methylation occurs primarily at the 4 position. As with other methyltransferase enzymes, e.g. phenylethanolamine-*N*-methyltransferase, the methyl group for this reaction comes from *S*-adenosylmethionine and studies with purified enzyme from rat liver show that a divalent metal such as Mg^{++} is required. Substrate specificity is low and all catechols are *O*-methylated regardless of the substituent at *R*.

The action of COMT on the catecholamines and their derivatives can be inhibited both *in vitro* and *in vivo* by pyrogallol, as well as by other catechols. These are competitive inhibitors and are themselves substrates for the enzyme. Other inhibitors are the tropolones, e.g. 4-methyltropolone, which inhibits by chelating with the divalent metallic ion essential for the activity of the enzyme.

4-Methyltropolone

COMT activity is widely distributed in the animal body with high concentrations in liver and kidney. It is fairly evenly distributed in all areas of the brain and has been found in parasympathetic and sympathetic ganglia and nerves. The enzyme has not been detected in skeletal muscle or plasma. The amount in the sympathetic nerves must be small since surgical sympathectomy with degeneration of the nerves has little or no effect on the activity in peripheral tissues. However, the presence of the enzyme in organs in which the catecholamines act suggests that it acts locally in the metabolism of these substances. The enzyme appears to be located in the cytoplasm of cells.

Monoamine oxidase (MAO), like COMT, is widely distributed and MAO activity is found in almost every

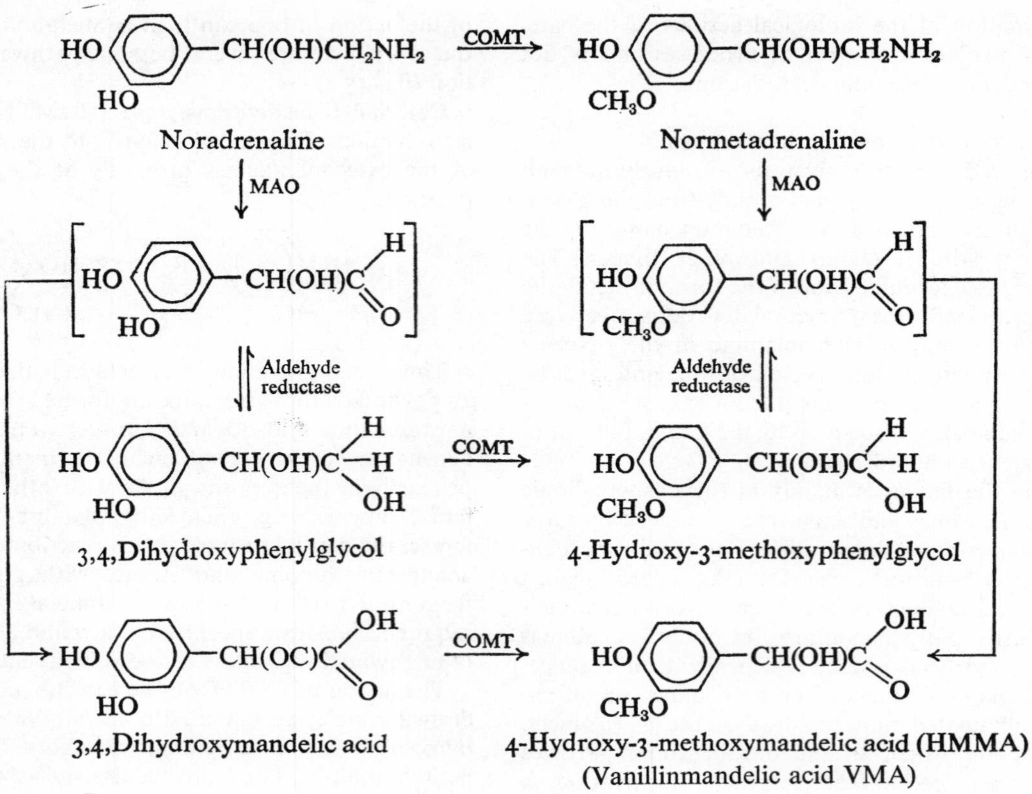

FIG. 15.4. The metabolic pathways for the degradation of noradrenaline. Adrenaline and dopamine are degraded in the same manner. The end products of adrenaline and noradrenaline are the same. The end products for dopamine are 4-hydroxy-3-methoxyphenylethanol and 4-hydroxy-3-methoxyphenylacetic acid (homovanillic acid HVA).

tissue in the body, with high concentrations in liver, kidney and intestine. It is present in all parts of the CNS and its activity is low in sympathetic nerves.

MAO catalyses the oxidative deamination of monoamines such as noradrenaline, adrenaline, dopamine and the 3-methoxy derivatives of the latter arising from the action of COMT. Other amines which also serve as substrates are 5-HT, tryptamine and tyramine. The end product of the reaction is an aldehyde.

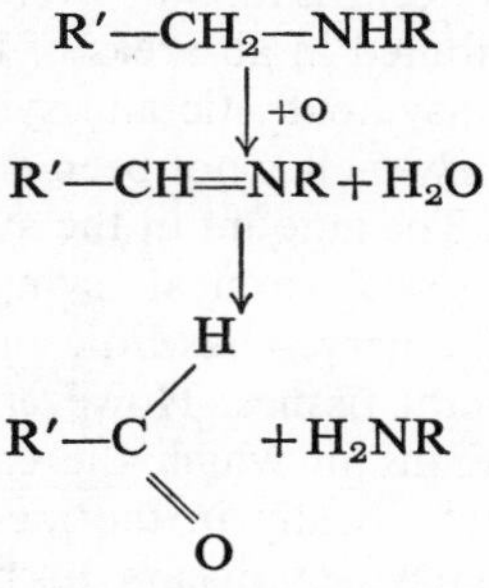

$$R'—CH_2—NHR$$
$$\downarrow +O$$
$$R'—CH{=}NR+H_2O$$
$$\downarrow$$
$$R'—C\overset{H}{\diagdown} \quad +H_2NR$$
$$\overset{\parallel}{O}$$

In tissues, the aldehyde is oxidized by dehydrogenase to the corresponding acid. In the case of adrenaline and noradrenaline and their methylated derivatives, the

aldehyde can also be reduced to the corresponding alcohol. In brain, dopamine and its methylated derivative give rise mainly to acid metabolites, and noradrenaline and its methylated derivative to alcohol metabolites.

MAO is associated mainly with the mitochondria in cells and its activity can be inhibited by a number of substances. Phenylethylamine derivatives with a methyl group in α-position in the side chain, e.g. ephedrine and

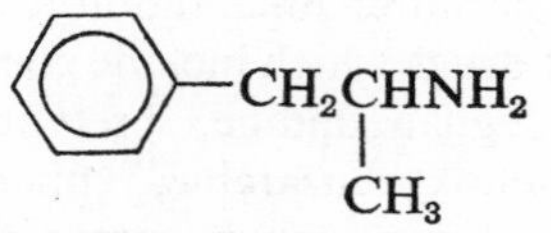

Amphetamine

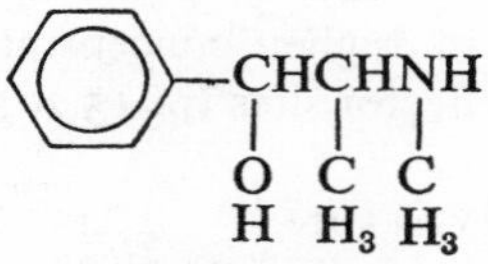

Ephedrine

amphetamine, are not substrates for MAO but act as competitive inhibitors.

More potent inhibitors have been discovered. These include various hydrazine derivatives such as iproniazid, phenelzine, pheniprazine, nialamide and isocarboxazid which produce a non-competitive inhibition of the enzyme. Tranylcypromine and pargyline produce a reversible competitive inhibition. Their formulae are shown in fig. 5.20, p. 5.21. Some of these drugs are used in the treatment of depression and of high blood pressure.

RELATIVE PHYSIOLOGICAL IMPORTANCE OF COMT AND MAO

The action of either enzyme on the catecholamines could result in the disappearance of virtually all the biological activity. For example, the *O*-methylated derivatives of adrenaline and noradrenaline possess less than 1 per cent of the pressor activity of the parent amines. The products of action of MAO are known to be biologically inactive.

Experiments with labelled catecholamines lead to the following conclusions.

The metabolism of catecholamines which are given by injection or are released into the circulation by the adrenal medulla or the peripheral sympathetic nerve endings, is carried out chiefly by *O*-methylation, inactivation by MAO playing a lesser role. From a study of the urinary excretion products after intravenous administration of adrenaline in the rat, the proportion of adrenaline methylated is found to be 70 per cent compared with 25 per cent deaminated. The remainder is excreted as unchanged or conjugated catecholamine.

The importance of *O*-methylation, as a first step in the metabolism, receives support from the fact that inhibition of COMT *in vivo* has little effect on the actions of noradrenaline but potentiates and prolongs the actions of injected adrenaline, this effect being more marked with isoprenaline. The order of potentiation is opposite to that of the uptake into sympathetic neurones in peripheral tissues. In contrast, MAO inhibition does not potentiate the effect of adrenaline or noradrenaline given intravenously or released by nerve stimulation. Inhibition of the enzymes affects the pattern of the excretion products. As might be expected after COMT inhibitors, nonmethylated derivatives increase and methylated derivatives decrease, while the converse is true after MAO inhibitors are given. For noradrenaline liberated from sympathetic nerve terminals, either by nerve stimulation or by drugs such as tyramine, that fraction which is metabolized is acted on mainly by COMT. However, when noradrenaline is liberated within the nerve, either spontaneously or by the action of drugs such as reserpine which deplete the storage granules, it is metabolized within the nerve by MAO. This enzyme within the nerve mops up noradrenaline synthesized in excess of the

storage capacity. Inhibition of this enzyme increases the concentration of noradrenaline in peripheral tissue and of catecholamines in the brain. However, for some reason not evident there is a species difference in this effect. For example, the noradrenaline in the brain of cats and dogs does not show a rise, although a marked effect is seen in rabbits and rodents (fig. 5.21, p. 5.23).

MAO is of major importance in the metabolism of other amines such as 5-HT and certain sympathomimetic amines (p. 15.28) which do not possess the catechol nucleus, e.g. tyramine, and of methyl histamine (p. 14.9).

URINARY EXCRETION

Noradrenaline, adrenaline and dopamine and their metabolites are found in the urine. Table 15.1 gives some estimates of the amounts found in normal human urine.

TABLE 15.1. Amounts of catecholamines and metabolites found in human urine (μg/24 hr excretion).

Noradrenaline	25–50
Adrenaline	2–5
Normetadrenaline	100–300
Metadrenaline	100–200
4-Hydroxy-3-methoxymandelic acid (VMA)	2000–4000
4-Hydroxy-3-methoxyphenyl glycol	2000–5000
Dopamine	100–200
Dihydroxyphenylacetic acid (dopac)	2000–4000
Homovanillic acid (HVA)	6000–10,000

These are figures culled from different sources and do not refer to the same group of individuals. They indicate the relative orders of magnitude of the different substances.

The catecholamines, the methoxy amine derivatives and the glycols are excreted partly as conjugates in man, mainly as sulphate esters. In other animals glucuronide conjugation may predominate. Such conjugations are a usual metabolic pathway for phenols.

The rate of excretion of both adrenaline and noradrenaline varies with activity, being lower during sleep or resting in bed than during normal daytime routine. Physical stress produces proportionate rises in the excretion of both adrenaline and noradrenaline. Mental stress sometimes raises only the excretion of adrenaline. However, in medical students undergoing an oral examination in anatomy, the urinary excretion of both adrenaline and noradrenaline has been found to be about twice control values. Stimulation of adrenaline secretion from the adrenal medulla is also evident in insulin-induced hypoglycaemia, in which elevated adrenaline but not noradrenaline excretion is noted. Change from the recumbent to the upright position increases the output of noradrenaline but has little effect on the adrenaline excretion; this is presumably a reflection of the increase in sympathetic tone to the blood vessels consequent on homeostatic adjustments to maintain the blood pressure. Markedly elevated levels of some or all of the endogenous catecholamines and their metabolites occur in the urine of most patients with phaeochromocytoma or other catecholamine-producing tumours and the estimation of these substances provides a useful aid to diagnosis in suspected cases.

BLOOD CONCENTRATIONS

The plasma concentrations of the catecholamines in normal human peripheral blood are extremely low and difficult to estimate. The noradrenaline concentration is less than 1 μg/l and that of adrenaline even lower. Raised levels of noradrenaline or both amines occur in patients with actively secreting phaeochromocytoma. Dopamine has not been detected in normal blood, and that found in the urine may have been formed in the kidney.

Release of catecholamines from the adrenal medulla

The chromaffin cells in the adrenal medulla are innervated by cholinergic fibres of the splanchnic nerves. Acetylcholine releases the hormones by altering the permeability of the cell membrane to ions. Experiments by Douglas showed the importance of Ca^{++} in the sequence of events leading to release of the hormones, which is called **stimulus secretion coupling**. He measured the amount of catecholamines appearing in the outflow from an isolated adrenal gland, perfused with isotonic salt solution. When acetylcholine (10 μg/ml) was added to the solution, the output of the catecholamines increased a 100-fold. The effect was still obtained in the absence of Na^+ or K^+ from the perfusing solution but not in the absence of Ca^{++}.

As $[Ca^{++}]$ was increased from zero, the secretory response to the acetylcholine also rose. Further experiments with ^{45}Ca show that acetylcholine increases the uptake of Ca^{++} by adrenal cells. Similar changes in permeability of cell membranes to ions are characteristic of the action of acetylcholine at other sites.

Histamine, 5-HT, bradykinin, angiotensin and also high concentrations of K^+ stimulate release of catecholamines and in all cases the release is dependent on the presence of Ca^{++} in the perfusing solution.

Thus the release of the hormone from the adrenal chromaffin cells by nerve stimulation is directly related to a sudden rise in $[Ca^{++}]$ at some critical point within the cell which follows the increase in permeability of the cell membrane to the ion. The Ca^{++} then enter the cell down the electrochemical gradient, the intracellular $[Ca^{++}]$ being about 1 per cent of the extracellular. Secretion of the hormone ceases when acetylcholine is removed by diffusion or hydrolysis or when Ca^{++} is bound or lost from the cell.

The release of noradrenaline on stimulation of postganglionic adrenergic nerves is usually considered to follow the change in permeability of the nerve terminals to ions, which allows the entry of Ca^{++} from the extracellular fluid. This entry of Ca^{++} then releases noradrenaline in some unknown way.

When the adrenal medulla is stimulated, catecholamines, adenine nucleotides and the soluble protein chromogranins are released in the same proportions as they occur in the chromaffin granules. Membrane protein and lipid are not released.

These findings indicate that the catecholamines are not normally released into the cytoplasm of the cell but that the first step in their secretion may be fusion of the granular membrane with the cell membrane followed by release of the soluble constituents of the granule to the exterior of the cell, by a process akin to pinocytosis but in the reverse direction.

Intracellular recording of potentials from adrenergically innervated smooth muscle cells of various organs are consistent with a quantal release of the adrenergic transmitter.

The hypothesis of a cholinergic link in adrenergic transmission

Potentiation of the effects of sympathetic nerve stimulation by cholinesterase inhibitors such as physostigmine has been observed in a number of tissue preparations. This can be interpreted as being due to prolongation of the action of acetylcholine accumulating after inhibition of cholinesterase. Burn and Rand have advanced an intriguing theory, implicating acetylcholine in the release of noradrenaline from postganglionic adrenergic neurones by nerve stimulation. Thus the primary event in adrenergic transmission, following invasion of the nerve terminals by the action potential, is the release of acetylcholine, either extra- or intra-neuronally. This is then responsible for the increased permeability of the membrane to Ca^{++}, leading to the release of the adrenergic transmitter. This postulated sequence of events has much in common with the mechanism proposed for the release of catecholamines from the adrenal medulla described above.

Some of the evidence supporting their theory is as follows. Stimulation of the splenic nerve of a cat normally causes the spleen to contract, but if the nerve is first depleted of noradrenaline by reserpine the spleen dilates. This dilation can be blocked by atropine, which inhibits the muscarinic actions of acetylcholine. Section of the sympathetic nerves to the spleen leads to a parallel loss of noradrenaline and acetylcholine from the organ, suggesting that the sympathetic fibres contain both substances. Acetylcholine was able to produce in various isolated tissues, e.g. the heart, effects similar to sympathetic nerve stimulation when its muscarinic actions were blocked by atropine. The liberation of noradrenaline by acetylcholine in the perfused heart and spleen has also been demonstrated.

The responses to postganglionic sympathetic stimulation in some preparations were prevented by hemicholium, a drug which inhibits acetylcholine synthesis, and by botulinus toxin which is known to prevent the release of acetylcholine from cholinergic nerves. Bretylium and guanethidine, two drugs which block adrenergic transmission, also block sympathomimetic actions of acetylcholine in various preparations.

In spite of this and other evidence the cholinergic link theory has not received wide acceptance. Critics point out several defects in the evidence; for example, many of the drug effects cited in support could be explained in ways which would not necessarily involve acetylcholine. The theory thus remains controversial.

PHARMACOLOGICAL ACTIONS OF THE CATECHOLAMINES

The catecholamines mimic to a greater or lesser degree responses obtained on stimulation of the sympathetic system. Other drugs, also derivatives of phenylethylamine, are **sympathomimetic agents**, but some possess additional properties, such as effects on the CNS which may be of more importance when they are used clinically. The response of the tissue depends on the interaction of the molecules of the catecholamines or sympathomimetic drugs with specific receptors.

α- and β-receptors

Reference to two distinct types of receptor for catechol amines, often called adrenoreceptors, has been made on p. 4.12. These were named the α-receptor and the β-receptor by Ahlquist in 1948. The evidence for their presence was derived mainly from his study of the relative potencies of a number of sympathomimetic amines which included adrenaline, noradrenaline and isoprenaline, in producing specific responses in a series of different pharmacological preparations. If the receptors in various tissues are of the same type, the relative potencies of the agents would be expected to be the same for all tissues tested. Such a result would suggest that the difference in potencies of the drugs resides in differences in their chemical structure. On the other hand, if each test object gives a different order for the relative potencies of the drugs then these variations must be due to differences in the receptors in the different tissues. The results of the experiments indicated that there were, broadly speaking, two orders of relative potency; in one

group of pharmacological tests noradrenaline was the most active, adrenaline was less active, while isoprenaline had only feeble activity, i.e. $NA > A \gg IsoP$. In the other group, isoprenaline was the most active, adrenaline less so, with noradrenaline showing considerably less activity, i.e. $IsoP > A \gg NA$.

Making the basic assumption that the drugs were acting on the tissues in a qualitatively similar manner, Ahlquist concluded that two types of receptors existed which he named α-receptors ($NA > A \gg IsoP$) and β-receptors ($IsoP > A \gg NA$).

The classification of these receptors into two types is further supported by the fact that tissue responses mediated by interaction of the amines with α-receptors can be blocked by one group of drugs, known as the **α-blocking agents**, which have no effect on responses mediated through the β-receptors. Another group of substances, the **β-blocking agents**, act contrariwise. Such a classification has generally been based on effects on tissues from animals but where these have been examined in man, the classification appears to hold good. α- and β-Blocking agents are discussed in more detail on p. 15.22.

In most tissues the receptors appear to be predominantly of one type or the other. In some tissues, however, receptors of both types are present in significant numbers.

In some cases, the activation of both types of receptor produces the same response in the tissue, in other cases the opposite effect. In the latter event the effect produced by a sympathomimetic agent depends on its relative potency in activating each of the two types of receptor and on the relative proportions of the two types of receptor; in the presence of an α- or β-blocking agent, the response of the tissue may well be reversed, e.g. from contraction to relaxation. In the less common situation, when activation of both types of receptor produces the same results, the response to the sympathomimetic agent persists in the presence of α- or β-blocking agents provided the drug can activate the type of receptor which has not been blocked. The distribution of some of the α- and β-receptors is summarized in table 4.6, p. 4.12. A fuller discussion is given here.

SMOOTH MUSCLE CONTAINING α-RECEPTORS
Generally, but not always, the activation of α-receptors depolarizes cell membranes leading to contraction of the muscle. Thus vasoconstriction occurs in blood vessels in skin, mucous membranes, abdominal viscera and, to a smaller degree, in kidney, lungs and brain. Contraction of the radial muscle of the iris leads to dilation of the pupil; in addition, the sphincters of the gastrointestinal tract and the smooth muscle of the spleen contract. Contraction of the pilomotor muscles leads to erection of the hair in animals and 'goose flesh' in man and that of smooth muscle of the eyelid to elevation of the lid.

SMOOTH MUSCLE CONTAINING β-RECEPTORS
The activation of β-receptors stabilizes the resting membrane potential and induces hyperpolarization; as a result in spontaneously active tissue, relaxation of the smooth muscle occurs. This leads to dilation of blood vessels in the heart, dilation of bronchi and relaxation of the detrusor muscle of the bladder.

SMOOTH MUSCLE WITH BOTH α- AND β-RECEPTORS
Stimulation of the α-receptors in arterioles in skeletal muscle causes contraction while activation of the β-receptors produces dilation. α-Receptors predominate in veins, stimulation causing constriction, β-receptor activation causing dilation.

Activation of both types of receptors in intestinal smooth muscle produces relaxation of the muscle and inhibition of spontaneous movements. In this tissue activation of α-receptors thus produces a relaxation of the smooth muscle and not contraction as in other smooth muscle.

Uterine muscle contains both α- and β-receptors but the relative responses varies with the species and may depend on whether the animal is pregnant or not.

Activation of α-receptors produce contraction, while β-receptor activation causes relaxation. Strips of human nonpregnant or pregnant uteri *in vitro* contract on exposure to adrenaline and noradrenaline. In late pregnancy or at parturition the uterus *in vivo* is relaxed by adrenaline and contracted by noradrenaline. The explanation for these different effects is unknown, and they are not clinically useful.

RECEPTORS IN THE HEART
Adrenergic receptors are of the β-type. Stimulation of these receptors leads to,

(1) an increase of heart rate by increasing the rate of depolarization of the pacemaker in the sinuatrial node (**positive chronotropic effect**),

(2) an increased force of contraction in the atria and ventricles (**positive inotropic effect**),

(3) an increase in velocity of impulse conduction throughout the heart, and possibly to

(4) the appearance of ectopi foci of contraction, ventricular arrhythmias and fibrillation.

In contrast to its weak action on β-receptors elsewhere, noradrenaline shows a strong action on the β-receptors in the isolated heart and is not very different from adrenaline. Isoprenaline, as at other sites, is the most potent activator.

EXOCRINE GLANDS
Receptors are of the α-type; stimulation of the salivary glands for example produces a sparse, thick, mucinous secretion.

Although stimulation of the sympathetic nervous system activates the sweat glands, the postganglionic fibres to the glands are in fact cholinergic. Nevertheless, adrenaline or noradrenaline injected intradermally can induce localized sweating and this response is inhibited by α-blocking agents. Apocrine glands have an adrenergic nerve supply and are stimulated during severe emotional stress, such as fear or pain and by adrenaline and noradrenaline. The type of receptor is not known.

METABOLIC EFFECTS AND RECEPTOR THEORY
The catecholamines, adrenaline, isoprenaline and, to a lesser degree, noradrenaline, alter the metabolism in many tissues. A prominant metabolic effect is the increased glycogenolysis in liver and skeletal muscle. Since liver possesses glucose-6-phosphatase, glucose is produced and the level of the blood sugar rises. In muscle which lacks this enzyme, lactic acid is produced and the concentration of this substance in the blood rises. Glycogenolysis and glycolysis occur in other tissues including the myocardium, intestinal smooth muscle and adipose tissue. The catecholamines also promote the release of fatty acid from triglycerides in adipose tissue so that the concentration of free fatty acids in the blood increases (vol. 1, p. 32.6).

It is not possible to classify the adrenergic receptors involved in these metabolic effects in all cases into either α- or β-type because much of the evidence is contradictory. Glycogenolysis in the heart and skeletal muscle appears to operate through β-receptors in all species, because the effect is blocked by β- but not α-receptor antagonists. The evidence regarding lipolysis and liver glycogenolysis however, is less clear and there are apparently species differences. For example, in man, the lipolytic effect is blocked by β- and not α-receptor antagonists while in the rat and dog both types of antagonists appear to be effective. It has been reported that neither type of antagonist blocks the hyperglycaemic response to adrenaline in man, but in the dog β- and not α-antagonists are effective inhibitors. Some believe that all the metabolic effects are initiated through activation of β-receptors, and that the effects on metabolism of α-receptor blocking agents are due to a nonspecific inhibition exerted at some later point in the sequence of reactions.

The role of adenosine-3′5′-monophosphate (3′5′ cyclic AMP)
The formation of this nucleotide from ATP in the presence of Mg^{++} is catalysed by the enzyme system adenyl cyclase bound to cell membranes; its breakdown to adenosine-5′-phosphate is brought about by the action of a phosphodiesterase (vol. 1, p. 9.9). The cellular concentration of 3′ 5′ cyclic AMP in the presence of adequate amounts of precursor ATP depends

on the balance of activities of the two enzymes; the concentration is raised by substances activating adenyl cyclase or inhibiting phosphodiesterase.

Catecholamines raise the concentration of cyclic AMP by activating adenyl cyclase, and the suggestion has been made that this enzyme system may in fact contain the β-receptor.

3'5' Cyclic AMP appears to influence many aspects of metabolic activity by acting as a cofactor in enzyme reactions. For example, it stimulates the activity of phosphorylase kinase leading to an increased conversion of inactive phosphorylase *b* to the phosphorylase *a*. The raised concentration of the active phosphorylase then speeds up the breakdown of glycogen to glucose-1-phosphate. The further conversion of the latter to glucose in liver and to lactic acid in skeletal muscle accounts for the hyperglycaemia and increased lactic acid produced by the catecholamines.

The adenyl cyclase in different tissues is activated by different hormones and shows varying degrees of specificity. Thus glucagon as well as catecholamines activate the cyclase in liver to produce glycogenolysis. In adipose tissue glucagon, ACTH, vasopressin as well as the catecholamines are effective in raising the activity of 3'5' cyclic AMP which in turn stimulates lipolysis. However, β-blocking agents competitively antagonize the response to catecholamines at doses which do not interfere with the action of the other hormones.

Attempts have been made to correlate the mechanical and electrical effects of the catecholamines with their biochemical actions. Experiments on the heart indicate that the adrenergic receptor for phosphorylase activation is the same as that responsible for augmenting the contractile force. For example the order of potency of adrenaline, noradrenaline and isoprenaline in eliciting both effects is the same and both effects are blocked by β-blocking agents but unaffected by α-blocking agents. Such evidence indicates that phosphorylase activity and the contractile force are closely associated, but not necessarily causally linked. Indeed, it appears that the muscle response is preceded by a rapid rise in 3'5' cyclic AMP but occurs prior to increased activity of the phosphorylase which suggests that phosphorylation activation is not the primary role of cyclic AMP in this response. Activation of β-receptors which produces a relaxing effect in smooth muscle also increases 3'5' AMP production. Although phosphorylase activation occurs there is evidence that it is not essential to the mechanical effect and that cyclic AMP mediates the response in some other way.

In an endeavour to produce a unifying theory, it has been postulated that, like the β-receptor, the α-receptor may be located in the adenyl cyclase system; the interaction of the catecholamines with the α-receptors may lead to a decrease in cellular cyclic AMP levels.

The methylxanthines, such as theophylline, potentiate some of the effects of catecholamines. This may be due to their inhibitory action on phosphodiesterase which catalyses the hydrolysis of 3'5' cyclic AMP. They thus raise the concentration of cyclic AMP which may then be related at least in part to some of the effect of the drugs such as cardiac stimulation, smooth muscle relaxation and lipolytic actions (fig. 15.5).

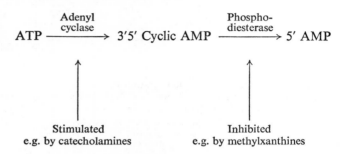

FIG. 15.5. The effect of catecholamines and methylxanthines on 3'5' cyclic AMP.

Effects of catecholamines in the intact animal

CARDIOVASCULAR ACTIONS

From knowledge of the receptors in various tissues and the relative ability of each amine to activate each type of receptor, it is possible to predict many of the effects likely to be induced in the intact animal on administration of these drugs. Before proceeding further, however, it is worth while recapitulating the following facts:

(1) adrenaline acts on both α- and β-receptors;

(2) noradrenaline produces its effects mainly on α-receptors, its ability to activate β-receptors is relatively weak with the important exception of the β-receptors of the heart, and

(3) isoprenaline exhibits marked activity on β-receptors; its capacity to activate α-receptors is very weak.

The response of the cardiovascular system to these amines is complicated by the fact that both α- and β-receptors are involved and that homeostatic reflexes play a part in the final result. It is instructive therefore to analyse observations made during intravenous infusion of low concentrations of the amines into man over a 15 min period. These are summarized in fig. 15.6. The effects of dopamine are considered separately.

The **systolic blood pressure** is increased with all three drugs, the effect being most marked with noradrenaline. The **diastolic blood pressure** shows a rise with noradrenaline, a slight fall with adrenaline and an even steeper fall with isoprenaline. The **mean pressure** thus rises with noradrenaline, shows little change with adrenaline and decreases with isoprenaline.

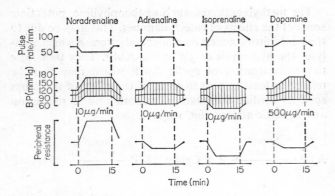

FIG. 15.6 Cardiovascular effects of infusions, made intravenously during time between broken lines, of noradrenaline, adrenaline, isoprenaline and dopamine. From Allwood M.J., Cobbold A.F. & Ginsburg J. (1963) *Brit. med. Bull.* **19**, 132.

The **heart rate** is decreased by noradrenaline, raised by adrenaline and also to a greater extent by isoprenaline.

So far as adrenaline and noradrenaline are concerned these observations are not consistent with their effect and relative potency on the isolated perfused heart preparation. In such a preparation, noradrenaline is as potent as adrenaline in increasing the heart rate and force of contraction. The decreased heart rate produced by noradrenaline *in vivo* follows the rise in mean blood pressure which stimulates baroreceptors in the aortic arch and carotid sinus and reflexly slows the heart. This reflex response overrides the direct effect of noradrenaline on the heart rate and can be prevented by atropine or, in experimental animals, by cutting the vagi. Under these conditions, noradrenaline increases the heart rate. Adrenaline and isoprenaline do not raise the mean pressure so there is no reflex stimulation of the vagus. In fact, with isoprenaline, reflex stimulation of the cardioaccelerator nerves due to the fall in mean pressure, augments the direct cardiac actions of the drug.

The **cardiac output** is unchanged or falls only slightly with noradrenaline, the decrease in frequency being offset by the increased stroke volume. With adrenaline and usually with isoprenaline the cardiac output is increased.

The total **peripheral resistance**, calculated from the cardiac output and the mean arterial blood pressure, increases with noradrenaline and decreases with adrenaline and even further with isoprenaline. Since the peripheral resistance is controlled by smooth muscle of the arterioles, it follows that these drugs act differently in certain vascular beds. These differences are best explained in terms of the concept of α- and β-receptors. Adrenaline activates the α-receptors in the blood vessels of skin, mucosae and abdominal viscera to produce a vasoconstriction. It also however, activates the β-receptors in the arterioles of skeletal muscle to produce vasodilation.

Quantitatively, the vasodilator action is more sensitive, so with a low dose of adrenaline the total peripheral resistance falls. Noradrenaline, with little or no β-activity, fails to dilate the skeletal muscle blood vessels but constricts them and those in other regions and so produces a rise in the peripheral resistance. Isoprenaline with its marked activity on the β-receptors, dilates the vessels in skeletal muscle. Consequently there is a greater fall in peripheral resistance than that observed with adrenaline.

Noradrenaline raises the systolic pressure by peripheral vasoconstriction, whereas adrenaline and isoprenaline do so only by increasing the cardiac output. Since the pressor response to adrenaline and isoprenaline is the result of two opposing actions, the systolic pressure may in fact fall if the decreased peripheral resistance more than offsets the effect of increased cardiac output. With larger doses of adrenaline, the diastolic pressure rises as well as the systolic, because the α-receptor vasoconstrictor action in skeletal muscle and elsewhere overrides the potential vasodilator action. With larger doses of isoprenaline both the systolic and diastolic pressures fall due to accentuated vasodilator actions. On stopping the infusion the various effects quickly disappear because of the rapid clearance of the drugs and the operation of homeostatic mechanisms.

In experimental animals, such as an anaesthetized rat, a large intravenous dose of adrenaline or noradrenaline produces a sharp rise in both systolic and diastolic blood pressure because of marked vasoconstriction and cardiac stimulation. The blood pressure returns quickly to normal levels over the period of a few minutes, and with adrenaline, but not noradrenaline, there is a secondary fall below the resting level. The secondary fall after adrenaline is due to vasodilator action, which is more sensitive to the small concentrations of the drugs remaining in the blood at that time than are the vasoconstrictor actions. Noradrenaline, having little vasodilator activity, does not show this secondary fall.

Prior administration of an α-blocking agent such as phenoxybenzamine converts the pressor response to adrenaline to a depressor action since the vasoconstrictor effect on the α-receptors is blocked and the vasodilator effect on the β-receptors is unmasked. This phenomenon, referred to as **adrenaline reversal**, was first reported by Dale in 1906, who noted the effect in cats that had received preparations of ergot. Because of the feeble vasodilator action of noradrenaline, an α-blocking drug abolishes the pressor response to the amine but does not cause a reversal. The depressor response to isoprenaline is little affected by the α-blocking drugs.

A drug such as propranolol, which blocks the β-receptors, usually potentiates the pressor response to adrenaline by inhibiting the β-vasodilator action more readily than the β-cardiac action, and the secondary fall in blood pressure is eliminated. The noradrenaline pressor response may decline slightly because of decreased stimulation of the myocardium, while isoprenaline may show a reversal of the depressor response as a result of the more complete block of its vasodilator actions than of its cardiac effects; the unmasking of its vasoconstrictor action, through a relatively feeble action on α-receptors, may contribute to this.

SPECIFIC HAEMODYNAMIC EFFECTS

Kidneys

Adrenaline and noradrenaline, infused in low doses (10 µg/min) in man increase renal vascular resistance and reduce the renal blood flow, adrenaline being the more active. There is an increase in the filtration fraction, but little change in the glomerular filtration rate, indicating a vasoconstrictor effect mainly on the efferent arterioles. Urine output may be increased, decreased, or unaffected. If, however, the patient's mean arterial pressure and the renal blood flow and filtration fraction are low, e.g. after administration of a ganglion blocking agent, noradrenaline increases the renal blood flow and urine formation since the rise in arterial pressure overcomes the local vasoconstrictor action in the kidney. Isoprenaline appears to have little direct action on the blood vessels of the kidney (p. 11.11).

Spleen

Infusions of adrenaline and noradrenaline cause the spleen to contract. This forces blood out of the organ into the general circulation. In some animals, but not in man, the spleen serves as a significant store of blood.

Coronary blood flow

This tends to be increased by the catecholamines and several factors seem to operate. A direct β-receptor mediated vasodilation of the arterioles occurs together with a vasodilation due to the accumulation of metabolites released during the increased cardiac work and to a relative oxygen deficiency. If the systemic blood pressure is raised this contributes to the increased flow.

Cerebral blood flow

Adrenaline and noradrenaline have little constrictor effect on the cerebral arterioles. Doses of the drugs which raise the systemic pressure therefore increase cerebral blood flow.

Pulmonary circulation

Direct pulmonary vasoconstrictor effects of adrenaline and noradrenaline can be demonstrated. However, after systemic administration, the observed rise in pulmonary pressure is due mainly to a rise in pressure in the left atrium, and to an increase of blood in the pulmonary circulation because of reduction in the systemic circulation following constriction of the great veins. Overdosage with the drugs may cause fatal pulmonary oedema due to increased capillary pressure.

ACTIONS ON THE CENTRAL NERVOUS SYSTEM

When injected into man, adrenaline produces restlessness and feelings of anxiety. Noradrenaline and isoprenaline are less active in this respect. The amines do not penetrate readily the blood–brain barrier and it is unlikely that these effects are due directly to an action on the brain.

In cats a small intravenous dose of adrenaline causes arousal from sleep, probably by an indirect effect on the reticular formation. Larger doses cause stupor, vomiting, spasticity and even convulsions. Presumably these arise from vascular or other peripheral actions.

Adrenaline or noradrenaline injected into the cerebral ventricles in order to circumvent the blood–brain barrier, produce sleepiness and a light anaesthesia, or in smaller doses into the anterior hypothalamus causes vasodilation and a fall in rectal temperature. 5-HT similarly causes shivering, vasoconstriction and a rise of rectal temperature. Similar effects are produced in the dog and monkey but opposite responses have been noted in the rabbit and goat. These observations and the fact that the hypothalamus contains relatively high concentrations of these amines have led to the suggestion that they may be concerned in temperature regulation at the hypothalamic level (p. 16.5).

RESPIRATORY EFFECTS

Adrenaline, noradrenaline and isoprenaline all stimulate respiration, increasing the depth rather than the rate of breathing. This is probably associated with the general restlessness produced by catecholamines.

Of importance clinically is the bronchodilator effect of adrenaline. This is most evident when the muscle is contracted either in asthma or by drugs such as histamine or carbachol or by vagal stimulation. The effect is due to activation of the β-receptor by adrenaline and is an example of physiological antagonism since the action is exerted independently of the nature of the agonist causing the constriction. Isoprenaline is also an effective bronchodilator but noradrenaline with its relatively feeble β-receptor action is not effective.

Adrenaline also decreases congestion in asthma. Since this is an α-receptor effect, isoprenaline does not possess this activity to any appreciable degree (p. 24.5).

Effects of dopamine

Dopamine produces similar effects to those of the other catecholamines, but its potency is 50 to 250 times less, depending on the particular response being tested. Its actions on the cardiovascular system in man during an intravenous infusion are shown in fig. 15.6. These are similar to those of adrenaline and are consistent with an action on α- and β-receptors. In its effects on metabolism, dopamine resembles noradrenaline rather than adrenaline; the concentration of blood glucose and lactate are not altered appreciably by doses producing cardiovascular changes.

THE ACTION OF DRUGS ON ADRENERGIC NERVE TERMINALS AND ASSOCIATED RECEPTORS

The reader should be aware already from vol. 1, chap. 14 and vol. 2, chap 4, that the structure and function of the nerve terminals at which impulses are transmitted to other neurones or to effector cells is complex. In adrenergic nerve terminals there are at least eight sites at which drugs may modify transmission. Understanding of how drugs may act in this way is made difficult by the fact that a drug may act at more than one site

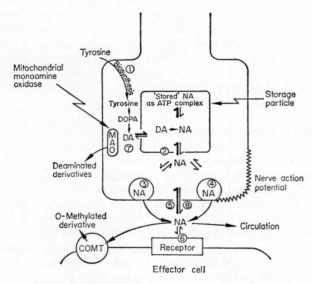

FIG. 15.7. Sites of drug action at an adrenergic nerve terminal. NA, noradrenaline; DA, dopamine; MAO, monamine oxidase; COMT, catechol-*O*-methyltransferase. For explanation, see text.

and that the actions at different sites are not necessarily complementary. Fig. 15.7 provides a map which shows the possible sites of drug action. These are,

(1) site of synthesis of the transmitter noradrenaline from the precursor tyrosine,

(2) site of active transport of the transmitter and other amines into the storage particles,

(3) site of small stores of transmitter readily released by many drugs,

(4) site of stores of transmitter released by the nerve action potential; the evidence is that sites 3 and 4 are not always identical,

(5) site of reuptake of the transmitter back into the nerve terminal by active transport,

(6) site of receptors on the effector cell,

(7) site of destruction of catecholamines within the nerve terminal by monoamine oxidase, and

(8) site of spontaneous release of transmitter.

Repeated reference to fig. 15.7 should help understanding of the following text, which is inevitably difficult. A drug may alter transmission by,

(1) mimicking the effects of catecholamines,

(2) inhibiting the uptake of noradrenaline by the neurones,

(3) blocking receptors on the effector cell,

(4) inhibiting enzymes, which synthesize catecholamines,

(5) inhibiting enzymes, which break down catecholamines,

(6) blocking the release of catecholamines from the neurones,

(7) depleting the neuronal stores of catecholamines, and

(8) forming false transmitters.

Drugs that mimic the effects of catecholamines (sympathomimetic drugs)

Many different amines can be derived from β-phenyl-ethylamine by substitution of hydrogen atoms by hydroxyl and alkyl, e.g. methyl, ethyl or propyl groups at various points in the molecule. Such derivatives are structurally related to noradrenaline and adrenaline and many of them produce biological effects similar to sympathetic nerve stimulation; in consequence, they are known as **sympathomimetic amines.**

STRUCTURE

The structural similarities and dissimilarities of a number of these substances are given in table 15.2, which shows their chemical formulae. A number of interesting structure–action relationships have been derived from studies of their comparative pharmacology, using different pharmacological preparations.

There are several other compounds, not phenyl-ethylamine derivatives, which have sympathomimetic properties to varying degrees. These include aliphatic amines, such as 2-amino heptane, which are homologues of ethylamine, and they also include imidazoline derivatives such as naphazoline.

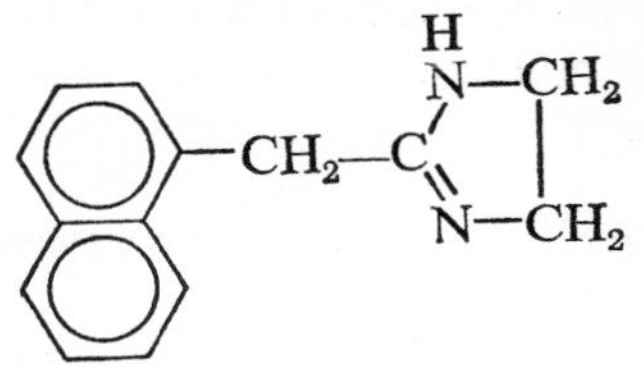

Naphazoline

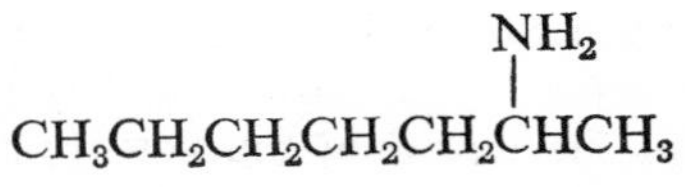

$$CH_3CH_2CH_2CH_2CH_2\overset{\overset{\displaystyle NH_2}{|}}{C}HCH_3$$

2-Amino heptane

TABLE 15.2. Chemical structures of some sympathomimetic amines, showing substitutions at five positions in the parent β-phenylethylamine molecule.

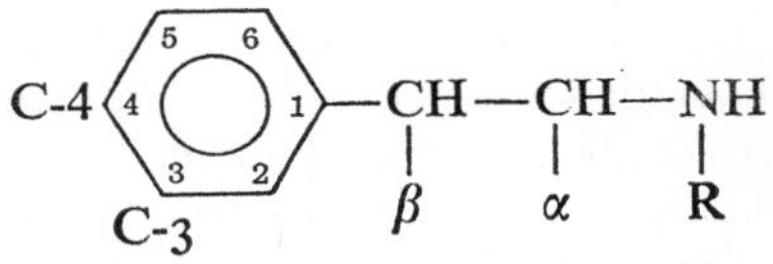

	C-4	C-3	β	α	R
β-Phenylethylamine	H	H	H	H	H
p-Tyramine	OH	H	H	H	H
Amphetamine	H	H	H	CH₃	H
N-Methylamphetamine	H	H	H	CH₃	CH₃
p-Hydroxyamphetamine	OH	H	H	CH₃	H
Phenylpropanolamine	H	H	OH	CH₃	H
Ephedrine	H	H	OH	CH₃	CH₃
Metaraminol	H	OH	OH	CH₃	H
Octopamine (norsynephrine)	OH	H	OH	H	H
Phenylephrine	H	OH	OH	H	CH₃
Dopamine	OH	OH	H	H	H
Epinine	OH	OH	H	H	CH₃
Noradrenaline	OH	OH	OH	H	H
Adrenaline	OH	OH	OH	H	CH₃
Isoprenaline	OH	OH	OH	H	CH(CH₃)₂
Methoxamine*	H	H	OH	CH₃	H

*C-2 and C-5 substituted —OCH₃

MECHANISM OF ACTION (fig. 15.7)

The sympathomimetic effects of these substances are not always explained only in terms of a direct action on α- or β- receptors (site 6). In some cases, the effects are produced mainly or partly by an indirect action through the release of noradrenaline from the nerve endings (site 3), which then produces the response in the tissues. This release of noradrenaline follows the uptake of the agent into the nerve terminals where it displaces noradrenaline from storage sites 2, 3 or 4.

Such conclusions have been drawn from comparisons of the activity of the drug when the stores of noradrenaline in the neurones are full and when they are empty. If a drug is no longer active when the stores are depleted, then it must produce its effect solely by noradrenaline release; in other words its action is wholly indirect. With some drugs, depletion of noradrenaline reduces but does not abolish activity, in which case the action is partly direct on the receptors and partly indirect through noradrenaline release. With another class of drugs, the response is not reduced in the absence of noradrenaline, indicating a wholly direct action on receptors.

In analysing the mode of action of the sympathomimetic drugs, noradrenaline is removed from the tissues by such devices as cutting the postganglionic sympathetic nerve supply and allowing the nerves to degenerate or by treating the animal with reserpine, which depletes stores of noradrenaline in nerve endings. The pharmacological preparations used include the spinal cat in which blood pressure responses are recorded, the contraction of the nictitating membrane of the cat and the mammalian isolated perfused heart in which the effects on the rate and force of contraction are observed.

In tissues depleted of noradrenaline by reserpine acting at site 2, exposure to noradrenaline partly repletes the stores of noradrenaline and restores the response to sympathomimetic amines working by noradrenaline release.

Prior treatment of the tissues with cocaine is another way of distinguishing between directly and indirectly acting sympathomimetic agents. Cocaine prevents the uptake of the amines into the nerve endings at site 5, so that they can no longer liberate the noradrenaline. Other support for an indirect action of some sympathomimetic drugs is the demonstration of the release of noradrenaline into the perfusates of isolated organs after administration of the drug.

In addition to the release of noradrenaline, the indirectly acting amines also prevent the re-uptake of the released transmitter into the nerve terminals at site 5 by competition for the uptake mechanism. This action potentiates the effect of the noradrenaline released from the nerve endings.

As with many pharmacological studies, consistent results are not always obtained for any one drug from all the tests. In some tests a drug may appear to act predominantly by an indirect action and in others predominantly by a direct one. The ratio of indirect to direct action may vary also for the same test in different species.

Nevertheless it is possible to make a rough classification of the compounds into three groups according to their mode of action.

Drugs that act indirectly at sites 3 or 5

This group includes β-phenylethylamine, tyramine, amphetamine, N-methylamphetamine and p-hydroxyamphetamine. Table 15.2 shows that these compounds lack the catechol group and the hydroxyl group on the side chain which are present in noradrenaline and adrenaline.

Drugs that act directly and indirectly at site 6 and also at sites 3 or 5

Phenylpropanolamine, octopamine, metaraminol and ephedrine are representative. These compounds differ from the members of the first group by the presence of a hydroxyl group in the side chain.

Drugs that act predominantly by direct action at site 6

This group includes adrenaline, noradrenaline, dopamine, phenylephrine and epinine. These compounds possess a phenolic hydroxyl group in the 3-position but not necessarily in the 4-position (phenylephrine). It appears that a catechol grouping is not essential for the production of direct actions if the compound possesses a hydroxyl group in the side chain; but it is essential if this hydroxyl group is missing. Furthermore, the introduction of a phenolic group in the 3-position on the benzene ring is more effective in eliciting direct actions than its introduction into the 4-position.

Compounds acting mainly indirectly produce effects predominantly on α-receptors, and relatively feeble β-effects except in the heart. Those with mixed direct and indirect actions may produce marked β-effects, if they have a relatively potent action on β-receptors in smooth muscle as a component of their direct action. Sympathomimetic amines, the action of which is predominantly direct on the receptors in the effector cells, produce effects which depend on the relative responsiveness of the α- and β-receptors to the drug.

TACHYPHYLAXIS TO SYMPATHOMIMETIC AMINES ACTING INDIRECTLY

Tachyphylaxis (p. 2.14) develops to repeated doses of the amines until eventually no response is elicited. However, noradrenaline is still found in the tissues. This probably indicates that the drugs release noradrenaline from a pool in the nerve endings (site 3), which on depletion is not refilled quickly by noradrenaline from the granular stores. It is also possible that the noradrenaline is released from particles influenced by the nerve action potential (site 4). Any noradrenaline released from particles lying deeper within the nerve terminal may be deaminated by monoamine oxidase and so is not released in active form.

PHARMACOLOGY OF SOME SYMPATHOMIMETIC AMINES

The number of these agents is too large to allow detailed discussion of all and reference is made only to those which are of interest because of their clinical applications or for other reasons.

Adrenaline and **noradrenaline** do not produce systemic effects when given by mouth. Since they are not very lipid soluble their absorption is slow and they produce vasoconstriction in the intestinal mucosa. In addition, if a small amount of drug is absorbed, it is quickly inactivated in the liver (p. 15.7). To produce a systemic effect they must be injected. Care should be taken that solutions intended for subcutaneous injection are not given intravenously. Given subcutaneously, the amines produce local vasoconstriction so that only a minute fraction of the dose reaches the circulation at any one time. The same dose of adrenaline injected intravenously may cause ventricular fibrillation or cerebral haemorrhage owing to a rise in blood pressure. In the treatment of asthma adrenaline, but of course not noradrenaline, is administered by subcutaneous injection or as an aerosol (p. 9.6). The latter route allows the drug direct access to bronchi and bronchioles. The amount absorbed into the circulation is so small that adverse effects such as tachycardia are minimal. Adrenaline solution may also be applied topically to abraded skin or mucosa, such as that of the nose, to stop bleeding. Adrenaline or noradrenaline is often added to solutions of local anaesthetics to delay absorption by their vasoconstrictor action and so prolong their action (p. 5.71).

Noradrenaline has been employed to raise the blood pressure in shock from various causes; it is given as an intravenous infusion of a very dilute solution, 4 μg/ml. The rate of infusion is adjusted to maintain the blood pressure. Since noradrenaline diminishes the blood supply to various organs to a dangerous level it is not recommended for this purpose.

Unlike adrenaline or noradrenaline, **isoprenaline is** absorbed to a variable extent from the intestine, probably because it lacks the vasoconstrictor action of the other catecholamines. Palpitation due to its marked stimulant action on the rate and force of the heart is the main adverse effect when the drug is used for its bronchodilator action in the treatment of asthma (p. 9.6). This appears most frequently when the drug is swallowed, less so when tablets of the drug are sucked and absorption takes place through the buccal mucous membrane and least of all when the drug is administered as an aerosol. Isoprenaline is also used to increase the heart rate in patients with heart block.

The effects of the catecholamines are short lived. This is because the drugs are rapidly taken up and inactivated by the tissues. Only 2–3 per cent of an intravenous dose of adrenaline or noradrenaline appears in the urine unchanged.

Absorption from the gastrointestinal tract occurs more readily with sympathomimetic amines which do not contain a catechol nucleus, but is variable in those compounds containing a phenolic group.

The clinically useful noncatechol sympathomimetic amines have a longer duration of action than the catecholamines, partly because, being less potent, they are given in higher doses and partly because they are not so readily inactivated. They are not inactivated by COMT. Those which contain a methyl group attached to α–C in the side chain are resistant to the action of MAO. Thus over 50 per cent of a dose of ephedrine or amphetamine appears in the urine unchanged, the remainder being metabolized by other enzymes in the liver.

The noncatechol sympathomimetic amines may be given by mouth, injection, or by topical application.

Tyramine is not used clinically. It is formed mainly in the gut by the bacterial decarboxylation of tyrosine and is largely and rapidly metabolized by monoamine oxidase in the mucosa. Some is present in the urine, and it has been detected in the CNS notably in the spinal cord.

Tyramine is present in high concentrations in cheeses and in some wines, strong beer and yeast extracts. Healthy persons who eat these foods are able to destroy the tyramine with MAO. However, patients under treatment with MAO inhibitors cannot do this rapidly and in them the tyramine in the blood can reach high concentrations. The pressor effects which follow are the now notorious cheese reaction (p. 5.22).

Amphetamine, the name of which is derived from the alternative chemical name, an (alpha)-methylphenylethylamine, is prescribed for its actions on the CNS which are described on p. 5.37. However, it also produces α- and weak β-effects. Vasoconstriction is produced and the blood pressure raised. The heart rate may be increased or slowed reflexly. Cardiac arrhythmias can follow administration of high doses. The weak bronchodilator effect is not clinically useful. Difficulty in passing urine may occur because of relaxation of the detrusor muscle of the bladder. Dilation of the pupil is produced.

Experiments indicate that amphetamine releases noradrenaline from and inhibits the uptake of the catecholamine into noradrenaline-containing neurones in the brain, as it does in the periphery. Thus a raised noradrenaline concentration is likely at receptor sites and the central effects of amphetamine may be in part related to this. However, amphetamine can produce central effects in animals treated with reserpine which depletes the brain of noradrenaline, but its effect depends upon continued formation of noradrenaline (p. 5.38).

Amphetamine is not a substrate for MAO as it contains an α-methyl group in the side chain. Indeed it acts as a weak inhibitor of the enzyme.

Ephedrine contains two asymmetric carbon atoms at the 1- and the 2- positions on the side chain. There are therefore, four isomeric forms known as (−) ephedrine, (+) ephedrine, (−) pseudoephedrine and (+) pseudoephedrine. The most active in the group as regards sympathomimetic activity is (−) ephedrine which is the pharmacopoieal preparation commonly used. The use of ephedrine in medicine extends back thousands of years during which it was used in China as preparations from plants of the species *Ephedra*. It was introduced into western medicine in the early 1920s, and was the first sympathomimetic agent to be employed.

Ephedrine produces both α- and β-effects. It raises blood pressure both by cardiac stimulation and by vasoconstriction. The heart rate may increase or remain unchanged, if the action of the drug is offset by reflex vagal stimulation. Like adrenaline, its vasoconstrictor action may be used to combat the vascular collapse and local vasodilation in hypersensitivity reactions. It dilates the bronchi, but it is less effective although longer acting than adrenaline or isoprenaline. However, it is useful in mild cases of asthma (p. 9.6) and also in increasing the heart rate in patients with heart block.

It dilates the pupil by stimulating the radial muscle of the iris when applied topically to the conjunctiva, an effect which incidentally is not obtained with adrenaline or noradrenaline because they fail to penetrate to the site of action. It constricts the mucous membranes of the nose and gives relief when this is congested. For this purpose it is usually applied topically.

Ephedrine stimulates the CNS, like amphetamine, but it is much less powerful. Insomnia, however, is an undesirable effect of long term medication with ephedrine in asthmatic patients.

Phenylephrine differs from adrenaline in lacking a phenolic hydroxyl group in the benzene ring at position 4. It differs also in possessing only a feeble action on β-receptors, even those in the heart, while retaining a marked stimulant action on α-receptors. The blood pressure is raised by an increase in peripheral resistance and not by cardiac stimulation. Marked slowing of the heart occurs, due to reflex vagal stimulation. It has little action on the CNS. Clinically it is used by injection to raise the blood pressure in hypotensive states but it suffers from the same disadvantage as noradrenaline. It is also used as a nasal decongestant by topical application.

Methoxamine acts like phenylephrine but has even less cardiac stimulant actions.

Metaraminol has cardiovascular effects similar to noradrenaline but is less potent. It raises the blood pressure, mainly by a vasoconstrictor action and is used occasionally for this purpose in hypotensive states. This substance is of additional interest as a possible mediator of the antihypertensive effect of α-methyl-*m*-tyrosine (p. 15.32).

INTERACTION OF SYMPATHOMIMETIC DRUGS AND PREJUNCTIONAL BLOCKING AGENTS

Sympathomimetic drugs with a major indirect action at sites 3 and 5, e.g. amphetamine and ephedrine, may displace guanethidine and related prejunctional blocking agents from their attachment at site 4 and bring to an end their hypotensive effects. Such a situation might arise when the overweight hypertensive patient is inadvisably given amphetamine to reduce the appetite in addition to the blocking agent. In similar circumstances ephedrine may be prescribed to relieve the nasal congestion which is a common annoying effect of sympathetic neuronal block; even when applied topically to the mucous membrane sufficient can be absorbed to produce a systemic effect.

As might be expected, directly acting sympathomimetic amines also antagonize the hypotensive action of the prejunctional blocking agents. During therapy with such antihypertensive drugs, the adrenergic receptors become supersensitive and respond to much lower concentrations of directly acting sympathomimetic agents.

Drugs inhibiting the uptake of noradrenaline into the neurone

The most important mechanism which restricts the intensity and duration of action of noradrenaline released on stimulation of adrenergic nerves is rapid re-uptake of the amine into the nerves. This occurs at site 5, and is to be distinguished from a second process occurring within the nerve at site 2, which involves intraneuronal redistribution of the amine already taken up, and which is then retained in specific intracellular stores. Re-uptake is carried out by active transport; the mechanism is located in the nerve membrane and it can be inhibited by a variety of drugs.

If such inhibition is the only action of the drug at the neuroeffector junction, the drug potentiates the response of the tissue to adrenergic nerve stimulation, because a higher concentration of noradrenaline than normal persists in the vicinity of the receptors. Cocaine is a good example of such a drug. It potentiates the response to nerve impulses and to noradrenaline circulating in the blood stream. The active transport mechanism at site 5 is capable of being saturated; it is not specific for noradrenaline, and other sympathomimetic agents are also substrates with varying degrees of affinity. Thus inhibitors of this active transport mechanism potentiate the action of those sympathomimetic drugs which also act on the receptors at site 6. The degree of potentiation depends on the rate of uptake since this determines to what extent the mechanism is normally responsible for reducing the concentra-

tion of agonist at the adrenergic receptors. For example, noradrenaline is taken up faster than adrenaline, while isoprenaline is not taken up at all. Thus cocaine increases the sensitivity of tissues more to noradrenaline than adrenaline and not at all to isoprenaline.

The uptake mechanism shows some stereospecificity, the naturally occurring (−) isomers of noradrenaline and adrenaline being taken up at a faster rate than the (+) isomers. Potentiation, resulting from inhibition of the uptake mechanisms, occurs irrespective of whether the tissue response is the result of α- or β-receptor activation.

Inhibition of the uptake by cocaine and other drugs can be shown experimentally by the decreased amounts of administered noradrenaline taken up by various sympathetically innervated tissues, such as the heart and spleen, both *in vivo* and in isolated perfused organs. ^{3}H- and ^{14}C-noradrenaline are used in such experiments as they are easily measured in very small amounts and are distinguishable from the noradrenaline already in the tissue. Inhibition of the uptake mechanism increases the amount of noradrenaline appearing in the venous outflow from isolated organs on stimulating the sympathetic nerve supply. This has been demonstrated in cat spleen, isolated perfused rabbit heart and other organs.

A large number of substances with a variety of chemical structures act as inhibitors of the uptake process in peripheral tissues with various degrees of efficiency. The extent to which this action is of significance in the pharmacological responses to some of these drugs and of importance in their clinical use is discussed below.

Studies of the uptake of catecholamines into brain slices, and their distribution in brain tissue following their injection into the cerebral ventricles, indicates that a similar mechanism probably operates in the CNS; inhibition of this mechanism may account for the central actions and therapeutic effects of some drugs used in the treatment of certain mental illnesses (p. 5.23).

COCAINE (p. 5.71)

Increased sensitivity of tissues to the actions of adrenaline, noradrenaline and sympathetic nerve stimulation following the administration of cocaine has been known for many years, but a satisfactory explanation was not available until its inhibitory action on the uptake mechanism was discovered. The action of cocaine on the uptake mechanism exhibits the characteristics of competitive inhibition, the degree of which is determined by the relative concentrations of cocaine, noradrenaline or other sympathomimetic agent competing for a common uptake site.

Cocaine does not appear to act in any other way at the adrenergic nerve. It is not an inhibitor of COMT and its inhibitory effect on MAO is extremely weak.

Its local anaesthetic properties are probably not related to its effect on the uptake process since other local anaesthetics, e.g. procaine, cinchocaine or lignocaine do not potentiate the action of noradrenaline, nor do they block its uptake into the nerve.

Applied topically to the eye, cocaine produces local anaesthesia of the cornea, but in addition it dilates the pupil and constricts the conjunctival vessels. The dilation of the pupil follows increased activity of the radial muscle to the iris as a result of the potentiation of the response to noradrenaline released from the adrenergic nerves. A similar explanation probably holds for the constriction of the conjunctival vessels. Vasoconstriction is also apparent if cocaine is injected into the skin. This, too, is due to an increased response of the blood vessels to the noradrenaline released by nerve stimuli. It is obviously not related to any local anaesthetic actions since this, by blocking nerve conduction, would tend to have the opposite effect on the blood vessels.

Given systemically cocaine causes a rise of blood pressure with tachycardia and peripheral vasoconstriction. This is mainly the result of central stimulant effects as shown by restlessness and excitement in man and in animals by increased motor activity, which is a prominent feature of the drug's effect.

The responses to stimulation of the cardioaccelerator and vasomotor centres are potentiated by the peripheral effect of cocaine on the re-uptake of the noradrenaline liberated from the adrenergic nerves to the heart and blood vessels.

Although it is tempting to ascribe the central excitation effects of cocaine to an inhibition of re-uptake of catecholamines released from neurones in the brain, the evidence for this is equivocal.

OTHER DRUGS WHICH INHIBIT UPTAKE OF NOR-ADRENALINE

Whereas cocaine acts only at site 5 in the nerve terminal, some drugs which have primary actions at other sites also have a cocaine-like action at site 5.

Drugs which block α- or β-receptors
Phenoxybenzamine, phentolamine, dichloroisoprenaline, and pronethalol, besides blocking either α- or β-receptors, also inhibit the uptake mechanisms. The potentiation of the response to nerve stimulation or to exogenous amines is apparent only in those tissues in which the receptor is not blocked by the drug. For example, phenoxybenzamine, an α-blocking agent, potentiates the action of adrenaline and noradrenaline on β-receptors, e.g. on isolated atria. Such a potentiation of response to the noradrenaline released from cardiac nerves may well contribute to the tachycardia which follows the hypotensive action of the drug in the intact animal.

The inhibitory effects of adrenergic receptor blocking agents on noradrenaline uptake lack the specificity of their actions on the receptors. Lack of a fundamental relationship between blocking action and inhibition of uptake is shown by the β-blocking agent, 1-(3-methyl-phenoxy)-2-hydroxy-3-isopropylamino-propane, which does not appear to inhibit uptake.

Tricyclic antidepressant drugs
Imipramine, desipramine, amitryptyline and nortryptyline are used in the treatment of mental depression (p. 5.24). They inhibit catecholamine uptake in peripheral tissues and sensitize them to the actions of adrenaline and noradrenaline. Some of the beneficial effects in mental depression may result from inhibition of the re-uptake of noradrenaline released from nerves in the brain (p. 5.24).

Chlorpromazine
This phenothiazine derivative bears a chemical resemblance to the antidepressant drugs referred to above. It too inhibits the noradrenaline uptake mechanism. However, in doses used in man, it has a marked receptor blocking action, which masks any potentiating action by the drug of the responses to adrenaline and noradrenaline. It thus seems doubtful if inhibition of the uptake mechanism plays any significant part in its complex pharmacology (p. 5.31).

Sympathomimetic amines
Many sympathomimetic amines produce their effects in part indirectly by liberating noradrenaline at site 3. A necessary preliminary is uptake of the amine into the nerve at site 5 and it appears that the uptake mechanism for noradrenaline is utilized for this purpose. Hence these amines act as competitive inhibitors of the uptake of noradrenaline.

This action would explain the potentiating effect of such substances as tyramine and ephedrine on tissue responses to exogenous noradrenaline and the marked effect produced by the very small amounts of noradrenaline released by the indirectly acting sympathomimetic amines.

The sympathomimetic agents show different degrees of affinity for the uptake site and the relationship between structure and inhibitory potency of the phenylethylamine group on the uptake mechanism has been studied by Iverson using the isolated rat heart. In summary his results are as follows.

Introduction of phenolic groups increased potency, β-hydroxylation decreased potency with the (−) isomer being more effective than the (+) compound. Substitution of the *N*-atom decreased potency, the bulkier the substitute the more the decrease. Thus the rate of uptake of adrenaline with a methyl substituent is less than that of noradrenaline. Isoprenaline with a large isopropyl group on the nitrogen atom shows little or no affinity for the uptake site.

Prejunctional blocking agents

Amongst these substances (pp. 4.14 and 15.29) bretylium and guanethidine have been found to inhibit noradrenaline uptake, the latter being the more effective. This action may explain the rapid sensitization of tissue to adrenaline and noradrenaline which develops after repeated administration of these drugs. It could also explain the tolerance which develops to their action in lowering sympathetic tone by blocking adrenergic neurones, as seen by a gradual reduction of their hypotensive effect in man. The receptors become extremely sensitive to the very much reduced amounts of noradrenaline which may be released on nerve stimulation and also to any circulating catecholamines from the adrenal medulla, the release from which is not interrupted by the prejunctional neurone blocking drugs.

The effect of such blocking agents on the uptake mechanism could also explain the observations that in low concentrations they potentiate the action of indirectly acting sympathomimetic amines, while in large doses they depress their effect by action at site 5. In low doses, the inhibitory effect on uptake is synergistic with that of the amines in decreasing the re-uptake of liberated noradrenaline. In higher doses, inhibition of uptake of the amine with consequent decreased release of noradrenaline could lead to a reduced tissue response to the amines. This occurs in spite of the potentiating action due to inhibition of the re-uptake of noradrenaline. Guanethidine more easily exerts a depressant effect than bretylium, which is in keeping with its greater effect on the uptake mechanism. It is not impossible, however, that the depressant actions on amine effects may be due to a suppression of the release of noradrenaline exerted at the level of the noradrenaline stores within the nerve. In the case of guanethidine, the lowering of catecholamine stores could also contribute to the depression of the response to indirectly acting sympathomimetic amines, although it has been shown that the responses to tyramine and amphetamine can be inhibited at a time when there is no significant reduction of the catecholamine levels.

INTERACTIONS OF INHIBITORS OF NORADRENALINE UPTAKE WITH OTHER DRUGS

Adverse effects may result from the increased sensitivity of the tissue receptors to sympathomimetic amines. A few examples will serve as illustrations. Thus, combination of imipramine with MAO inhibitors or with sympatho-

mimetic amines may result in hypertensive reactions, excitement and pyrexia. Cocaine applied to mucous membranes as a local anaesthetic may be absorbed to a sufficient degree to precipitate excessive sympathomimetic actions in patients taking a sympathomimetic amine such as amphetamine. Attempts to treat the hypertension found in patients with phaeochromocytoma by lowering sympathetic tone with prejunctional blocking agents is irrational since these drugs sensitize the tissues to the actions of adrenaline and noradrenaline liberated from the tumour and make the situation worse. It is, therefore, important that the presence of a catecholamine-secreting tumour is excluded as a cause of hypertension before embarking on treatment of the patient with a prejunctional blocking agent. Fortunately such tumours are rare.

UPTAKE OF CATECHOLAMINES INTO CELLS OTHER THAN ADRENERGIC NEURONES

This uptake becomes evident only at high concentrations of noradrenaline, but isoprenaline and adrenaline are more readily taken up. The amines may then be acted on by cytoplasmic COMT and mitochondrial MAO. Unreacted amine remains free and readily diffuses out probably because of the absence of storage mechanisms. This uptake is inhibited by drugs which may or may not inhibit neuronal uptake. Thus the 3-*O*-methylated derivatives of adrenaline and noradrenaline, which do not block neuronal uptake, are potent inhibitors. Phenoxybenzamine inhibits both whereas cocaine is more effective against the neuronal system. Phenylethylamine derivatives also inhibit both but the order of potency is different from that for neurones. Iversen has shown that, in the rat heart, *N*-substitution, or β-hydroxylation increases potency but phenolic hydroxylation or α-methylation decreases it.

It seems likely that non-neuronal uptake is of minor importance compared with neuronal re-uptake in determining the duration of action of noradrenaline released under physiological conditions; however, it may become important when, for example, neuronal uptake is blocked.

Drugs which block receptors on the effector cell

As discussed on p. 4.14 the effects of sympathetic nerve stimulation can be reduced by prejunctional blocking drugs that interfere with the release of noradrenaline from nerve endings; the decrease in response does not involve the reduction in sensitivity of the tissue to the transmitter; indeed, the responses to noradrenaline and adrenaline may be markedly increased. Furthermore, they decrease the responses of smooth and cardiac muscle to sympathetic stimulation irrespective of whether α- or β-receptors are involved.

On the other hand, the **postjunctional blocking agents** inhibit the response of the tissues to adrenergic nerve stimulation. They also inhibit responses to catecholamines, either released in the body or administered, and to other directly acting sympathomimetic amines. Unlike the prejunctional blocking agents, they do not interfere with the release of noradrenaline on nerve stimulation, but they may inhibit its re-uptake (p. 15.21).

The individual members of this group of substances are specific with regard to the type of adrenergic receptor involved so that they may be divided into **α-receptor blocking agents** and **β-receptor blocking agents**. Some of these are listed in table 15.3 and the formulae for several

TABLE 15.3. α- and β-Receptor blocking agents.

Class of compound	Examples
α-Receptor blocking agents	
Lysergic acid derivatives (ergot alkaloids)	Ergotamine, dihydroergotamine, hydergine
Imidazoline derivatives	Tolazoline, phentolamine
Haloalkylamines	Dibenamine, phenoxybenzamine
β-Receptor blocking agents	
Analogues of isoprenaline	Dichloroisoprenaline, pronethalol, propranolol, MJ 1999

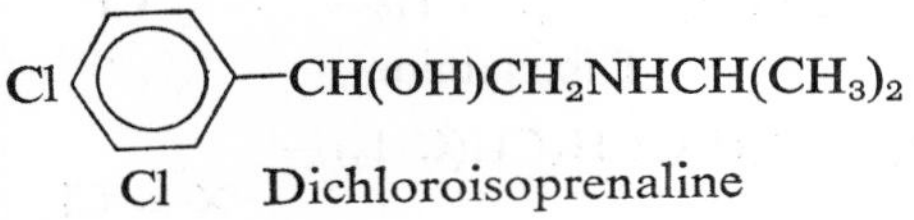

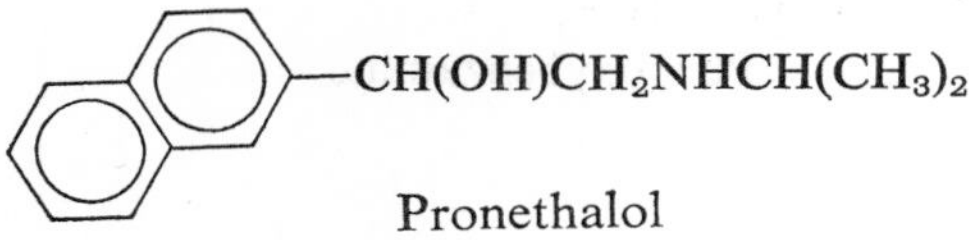

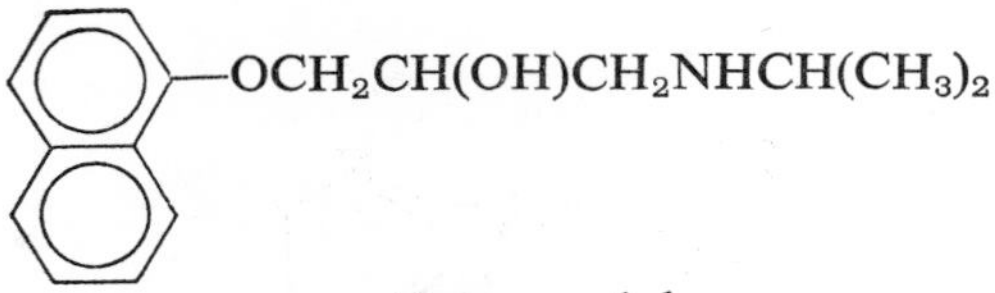

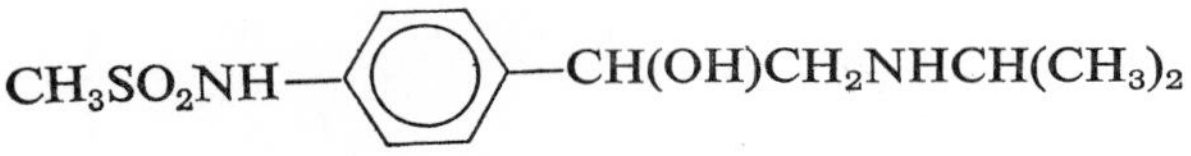

of them are shown in figs. 15.8 & 9. Reference has already been made to the adrenergic blocking agents in the discussion of the classification of adrenergic receptors (p. 15.11) and to their effects on the blood pressure responses to noradrenaline, adrenaline and isoprenaline (p. 15.14).

While α-receptor blocking activity is shown by compounds of diverse chemical structures, β-receptor blocking activity is found only in compounds resembling isoprenaline, which is a potent activator of β-receptors. Apparently the ring structure determines whether the substance stimulates or blocks the receptors. As with isoprenaline the L-isomers of these substances are much more active than the D-isomers.

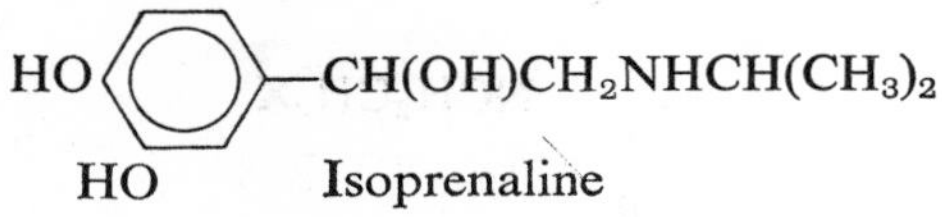

MODE OF ACTION OF POSTJUNCTIONAL BLOCKING AGENTS

The postjunctional blocking agents prevent the actions of noradrenaline and allied drugs by occupying the receptors in the tissues to the exclusion of the agonist drug. With the majority, the antagonism is of the competitive equilibrium type and is therefore reversible by high doses of the agonist. However, the α-receptor blocking agents which chemically belong to the β-halo-

β-Receptor agonist

β-Receptor antagonists

FIG 15.8. Formulae of some β-receptor blocking agents.

alkylamine group exert a non-equilibrium type of antagonism which, once developed, is not reversible even by high doses of the agonist.

The α-receptor blocking agents inhibit the vasoconstrictor actions and other excitatory responses of smooth muscle to the catecholamines and other sympathomimetic amines. The β-receptor blocking agents prevent the cardiac stimulant effects, the inhibitory effect on smooth muscle, e.g. the vasodilator and bronchodilator actions and some of the metabolic effects of noradrenaline, adrenaline and isoprenaline.

The administration of an α-blocking agent unmasks the actions of an agonist drug on β-receptors, while the administration of a β-blocking drug unmasks the actions on α-receptors. This is illustrated in the effects of these blocking agents on the blood pressure response of an anaesthetized animal to adrenaline, noradrenaline and isoprenaline (p. 15.14).

Other tests, which may be used to show α-blocking activity, are inhibition of the contraction of the cat

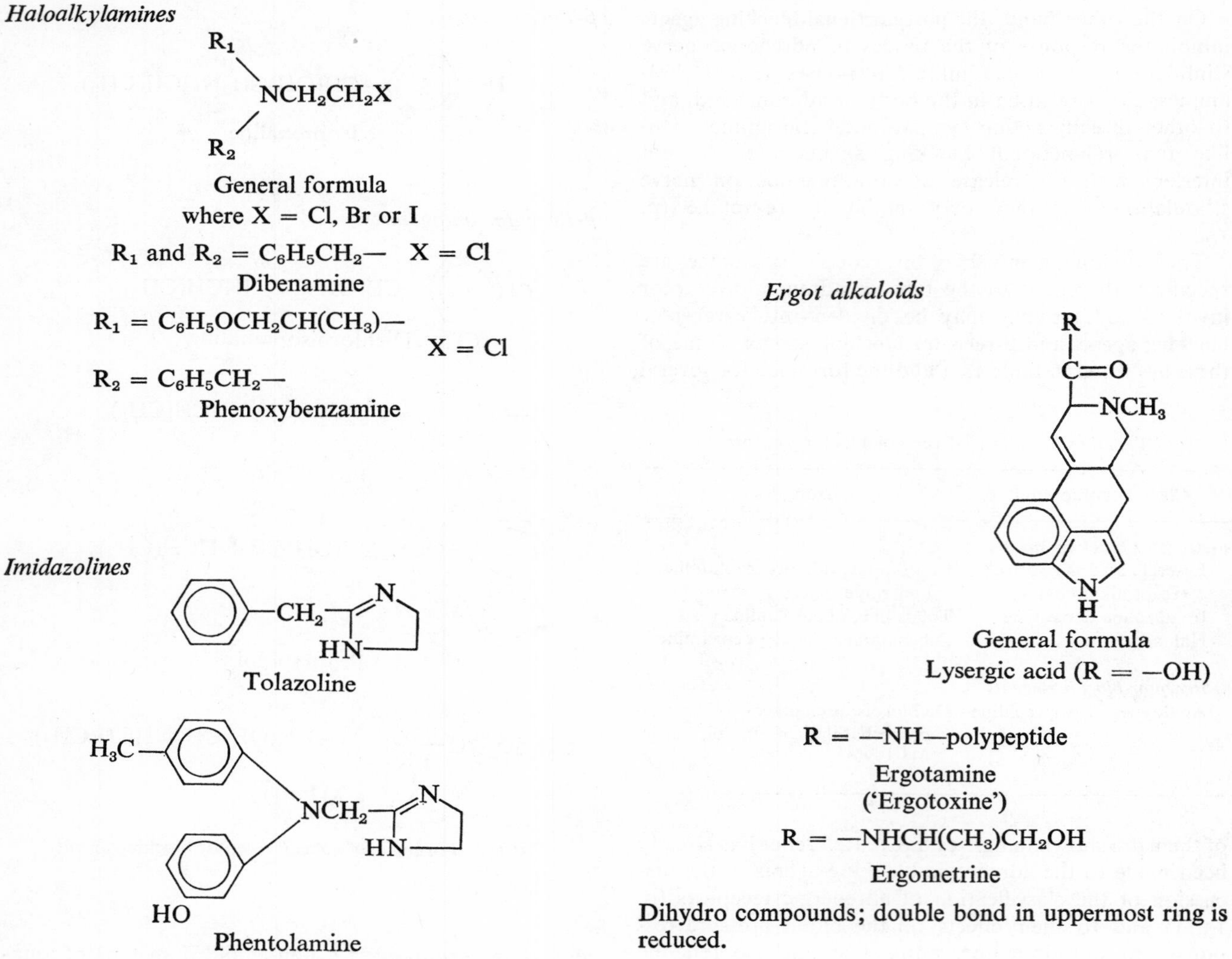

Haloalkylamines

$$R_1$$
$$\diagdown$$
$$NCH_2CH_2X$$
$$\diagup$$
$$R_2$$

General formula
where X = Cl, Br or I

R_1 and $R_2 = C_6H_5CH_2-$ X = Cl
Dibenamine

$R_1 = C_6H_5OCH_2CH(CH_3)-$
                                            X = Cl
$R_2 = C_6H_5CH_2-$
Phenoxybenzamine

Imidazolines

Tolazoline

Phentolamine

Ergot alkaloids

General formula
Lysergic acid (R = —OH)

R = —NH—polypeptide
Ergotamine
('Ergotoxine')

R = —NHCH(CH₃)CH₂OH
Ergometrine

Dihydro compounds; double bond in uppermost ring is reduced.

FIG. 15.9. Formulae of some α-receptor blocking agents

nictitating membrane, dilation of the pupil induced by nerve stimulation or by adrenaline and of the contraction of arterial strips to adrenaline or noradrenaline; in addition the response of the isolated rabbit uterus, which adrenaline contracts, becomes one of relaxation in the presence of an α-blocking agent.

A β-blocking action can be detected by the antagonism to the positive chronotropic action of isoprenaline on rabbit or guinea-pig isolated atria, the antagonism to the relaxant effects of isoprenaline or adrenaline on the isolated rat uterus and the antagonism to the tachycardia and vasodepressor action in anaesthetized animals.

CLINICAL PHARMACOLOGY OF POSTJUNCTIONAL BLOCKING AGENTS

As might be expected, these drugs have pharmacological properties in addition to their blocking actions which limit their clinical usefulness to varying degrees.

As α-blocking agents inhibit the vasoconstrictor response to sympathetic nerve stimulation, they might be expected to be of value in the treatment of hypertension. They have not proved satisfactory in this respect, however, because in the absence of β-blocking activity, reflex tachycardia and palpitations occur along with the hypotensive effect. The α-blocking agents are used to alleviate various peripheral vasospastic states and paradoxically in the treatment of some forms of shock where they inhibit the vasoconstriction induced by the hyperactivity of the sympathetic nervous system and which interferes with tissue perfusion.

Although they do not block the positive chronotropic and inotropic actions, the α-blocking agents inhibit cardiac arrhythmias which may be induced by adrenaline and other sympathomimetic amines, including those which occur due to sensitization to sympathomimetic amines under cyclopropane and the halogenated general anaesthetics such as chloroform. A major factor appears to be the suppression of the rise in blood pressure which sensitizes the heart to such arrhythmias and not to a direct inhibitory effect on the myocardium. β-Blocking agents are also of value in this situation.

The α-blocking agents are used in the diagnosis of phaeochromocytoma and in the control of the pressor effects produced by the hormones secreted by these tumours, before and during operation for their removal. The secretion may be paroxysmal or sustained, leading to paroxysmal or sustained rises in blood pressure. For diagnostic purposes, an intravenous injection of phentolamine (5 mg) may be given and this produces a sharp fall in the blood pressure. However, the test is not infallible. For various reasons false positive and false negative results may be obtained and the procedure should be supplemented by measurements of the urinary excretion of the catecholamines and their metabolites which are usually markedly increased.

With the introduction of effective β-blocking agents, it has been suggested that both types of blocking agent should be used to control the sympathomimetic responses in cases of phaeochromocytoma. The β-blocking drugs protect the heart from excessive stimulation by the catecholamines, an effect which is not prevented by the α-blocking agents. β-Blocking agents by themselves are obviously of no value in the control of the pressor effects resulting mainly from the vasoconstrictor action of the catecholamines secreted from the phaeochromocytoma, since this effect is not blocked and may, on the contrary, be potentiated by the inhibition of the vasodilator action (β-effect) of any adrenaline secreted.

In addition to preventing the response of the heart to sympathomimetic agents, the β-blocking drugs decrease the response to sympathetic nerve stimulation and thus reduce the increase in cardiac work and oxygen demand imposed on the heart, for example, by exercise and anxiety. They are thus useful in the treatment of some patients with angina pectoris. They are often effective in stopping various cardiac arrhythmias, including those occurring during anaesthesia and resulting from over-dosage with digitalis and allied drugs. It is controversial whether such anti-arrhythmic actions are due to β-blockade or to a local anaesthetic action or quinidine-

like depressant action on the heart, both of which these drugs possess.

These drugs may precipitate severe congestive heart failure in patients in mild failure or with low cardiac reserve because the β-blocking action removes the sympathetic drive to the heart upon which adequate cardiac function depends. They are also contraindicated in patients with asthma since their β-blocking action tends to produce bronchoconstriction and also prevents the bronchodilation induced by the therapeutic administration of adrenaline and other sympathomimetic amines.

α-BLOCKING AGENTS

The haloalkylamines
Dibenamine and **phenoxybenzamine** produce a slowly developing, but persistent block of α-receptors which is not reversible by even high doses of adrenaline or noradrenaline. This suggests that they form a particularly stable complex with the receptor. In neutral or alkaline solution, these substances give rise to a highly reactive ethylenimonium ion (fig. 15.10) and the molecular species which reacts with the receptor is probably the carbonium ion formed on opening the ring of the ethylenimonium ion. This reactive intermediate is capable of combining with various groups such as sulphydryl, carboxyl, phosphate and amino to form alkylated derivatives, and presumably this happens with one or more such groups on the α-receptor to give a stable covalently linked drug-receptor complex.

In their chemical structure and formation of reactive ethylenimonium intermediates, these compounds resemble the cytotoxic agents, the nitrogen mustards (p. 29.3).

The alkylating ability of these compounds is not confined to α-receptors, and they exert a similar type of blocking action on 5-HT, histamine and acetylcholine receptors. It is thus perhaps surprising that the β-adrenergic receptors escape. These other blocking actions appear to contribute little to the pharmacological actions of the haloalkylamines *in vivo*.

The development of complete α-blockade by the haloalkylamines slowly reaches a peak after about an hour when given intravenously, or when isolated tissues are treated *in vitro*, and this is probably due to the relatively slow formation of reactive forms of the drug. Owing to the high stability of the drug–receptor compound, the blockade once developed is persistent, a single dose *in vivo* producing an effect which lasts 48 hours or more.

In the early stages of the action of the haloalkylamines, the adrenergic receptor blockade has the characteristics of a competitive antagonism and can be overcome by increased concentrations of noradrenaline or adrenaline; this may be due to an initial combination of the drug with

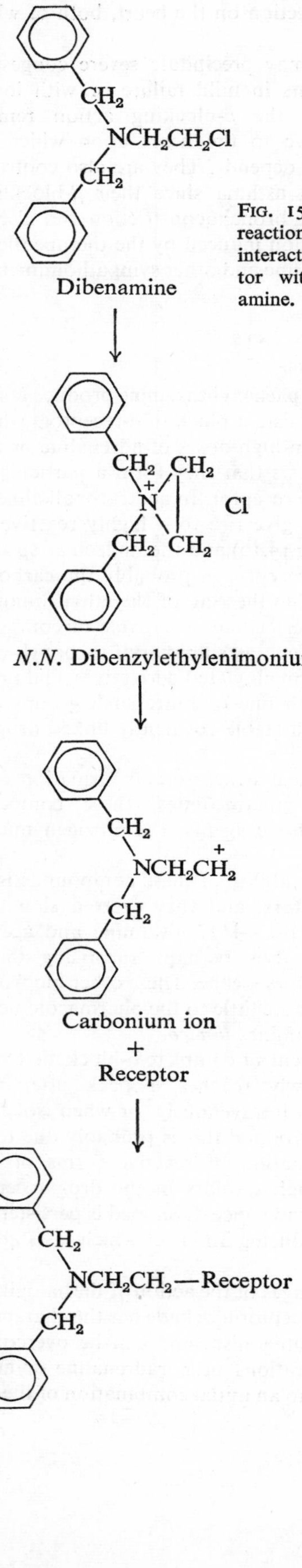

Dibenamine

FIG. 15.10. Sequence of reactions involved in the interaction of the α-receptor with a β-haloalkylamine.

N.N. Dibenzylethylenimonium ion

Carbonium ion
+
Receptor

the receptors by noncovalent bonding or to the slow reduction of the number of spare receptors available to the agonist by formation of the covalently linked complex (p. 3.10).

Phenoxybenzamine and particularly dibenamine are poorly and variably absorbed when given by mouth and they cause gastric irritation and nausea. They can be given intravenously, slowly and well diluted. By either route a blocking dose has little effect on the normal supine blood pressure but produces orthostatic hypotension. The blood pressure may fall in hypertensive patients in both positions.

Undesirable effects from α-receptor blockade include nasal stuffiness and miosis. Sedation, weakness and fatigue also occur. Because of many disadvantages, dibenamine is not now employed clinically. The daily dose of phenoxybenzamine varies from 20–100 mg.

The imidazolines

Tolazoline and **phentolamine** exert a relatively brief α-blocking action *in vivo*. They have many other pharmacological actions. They produce cardiac stimulation with tachycardia, usually ascribed to a direct action on the heart, and peripheral vasodilation by a direct action on the smooth muscle. Because of these effects, blood pressure responses to the drugs are variable but tolazoline usually produces a rise and phentolamine a fall in blood pressure on intravenous injection in man. Diarrhoea due to stimulation of the smooth muscle of the intestine is common. Gastric secretion is stimulated, an effect which is perhaps not surprising in view of the chemical relationship of these drugs to histamine.

Phentolamine is a more potent α-blocking agent than tolazoline and the other actions are somewhat less marked. Phentolamine (5–10 mg) by intravenous or intramuscular injection, is occasionally used for the diagnosis and the control of the hypertension associated with phaeochromocytoma. Tolazoline by mouth or by injection (25–75 mg/day) is mainly used for the treatment of vasospastic conditions because of its direct vasodilator action in addition to its α-receptor blocking action.

The ergot alkaloids

Ergotamine and ergotoxine (p. 13.8) possess α-receptor blocking properties. In these substances lysergic acid is combined with cyclic polypeptides through an amide linkage, and they are classified as amino acid alkaloids. The intense vasoconstrictor actions of ergotamine and ergotoxine, an example of their stimulant action on smooth muscle, lead to a rise in blood pressure. Ergometrine is not an α-blocking agent; it also has little vasoconstrictor activity. Reduction of the double bond in the lysergic acid moiety of ergotamine and ergotoxine yields dihydroergotamine and hydergine containing the three reduced alkaloids of ergotoxine. These dihydro derivatives show much less vasoconstrictor activity and greater α-adrenergic blocking activity than the parent substances.

Hydergine is sometimes used in the treatment of vascular spasm. It produces a fall in blood pressure due to peripheral vasodilation which is greater if the blood pressure is already raised. Other indications of peripheral vasodilation are a flushing of the skin and congestion of mucous membranes. These vascular effects probably arise from a depressant action on the vasomotor centre rather than from a peripheral α-blocking action.

The main therapeutic uses of the ergot alkaloids are as oxytocics (p. 12.15) and in the treatment of migraine. Again the effects are not related to α-blockade. The pharmacology of the ergot alkaloids is dealt with in more detail in chap. 13.

β-BLOCKING AGENTS

Dichlorisoprenaline, usually referred to as DCI, is closely related structurally to isoprenaline, differing from it in the presence of two chlorine atoms attached to the benzene ring in place of the two phenolic hydroxyl groups. This dichloro analogue of isoprenaline retains some power to activate β-receptors and in low doses it stimulates the heart, and produces vasodilation in voluntary muscle. However, in larger doses the initial activation of the β-receptors gives way to a blocking effect and the drug prevents responses of tissues to the catecholamines and sympathetic nerve stimulation which are mediated through activation of β-adrenergic receptors. The drug thus acts as a partial agonist (p. 3.10). DCI was the first compound discovered to exert a specific blocking action at β-receptors and has been much used in pharmacological investigations to identify the type of receptor present in tissues. The ability of the drug to activate these receptors before block develops has precluded its use in man. Modification of the isoprenaline molecule led to the discovery of **pronethalol**. This compound has a benzene ring in place of the two phenolic groups of isoprenaline. It is a more potent blocking agent than DCI, having much less ability to activate β-receptors. It has been used clinically in the treatment of conditions in which β-adrenergic block is advantageous. As the drug is carcinogenic, it has been withdrawn from clinical use. Its place has been taken by **propranolol** which is apparently not carcinogenic, and which, in addition, has a more favourable ratio of blocking action to unwanted effects, such as disorientation, incoordination, nausea and vomiting seen in man with pronethalol.

When given by slow intravenous injection, propranolol has little effect on blood pressure. Marked bradycardia and a sharp fall in blood pressure may occur if the drug is given quickly. With long-term administration by mouth, it causes a slowly developing hypotension, and its value in the treatment of hypertension is being investigated. In doses of 100–200 mg/day it also reduces the number and severity of attacks of pain in coronary insufficiency. Its use in the treatment of cardiac arrythmias is discussed on p. 15.25. Adverse effects are mostly referable to an action on the CNS, and they include giddiness, tiredness, mental depression, visual hallucinations, nausea and diarrhoea. They are infrequent and usually disappear on reducing the dose.

The danger of the β-blocking drugs in patients with incipient heart failure or with an asthmatic condition has already been mentioned.

The lower intensity and incidence of adverse effects on the CNS seen with propranolol than with pronethalol probably reflects the latter's more ready penetration through the blood–brain barrier.

MJ 1999 is a specific β-blocking agent which is less potent than propranolol. Local anaesthetic, quinidine-like, β-receptor stimulant action and effects on the CNS are relatively weak or nonexistent.

Methoxamine and its derivatives (fig. 15.11) form an interesting series of drugs because they block the hyperglycaemic and lipolytic actions of the catecholamines, and have β-blocking properties, the intensity of which varies with the different tissues.

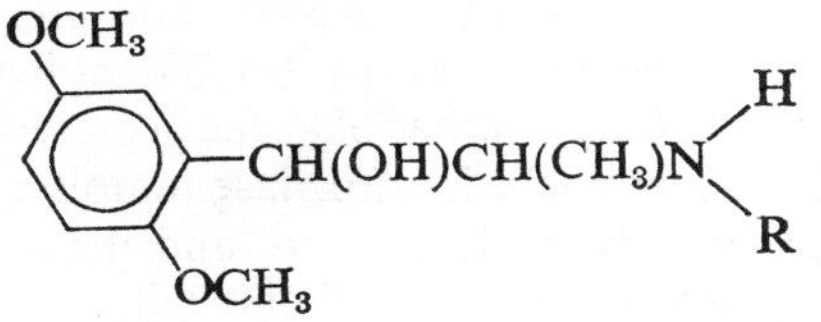

Methoxamine	R = H
Isopropylmethoxamine	R = —CH(CH₃)₂
N-Tertiarybutylmethoxamine	R = —C(CH₃)₃

FIG. 15.11. Methoxamine and its derivatives.

In particular they show little or no antagonism of the actions of the catecholamines in the heart. Methoxamine has strong α-receptor activating activity producing a rise in blood pressure by vasoconstriction and a reflex bradycardia *in vivo*. **Isopropylmethoxamine** has no intrinsic action at the α-receptors but acts *in vivo* like methoxamine because it is converted to this substance in the body. If a tertiary butyl group is substituted instead of the isopropyl, methoxamine is not produced *in vivo* and the compound does not give rise to sympathomimetic effects although it continues to exert metabolic blocking actions.

Drug inhibiting enzymes which synthesize catecholamines

INHIBITION OF DOPA DECARBOXYLASE
Inhibitors given to intact animals do not reduce the noradrenaline in the tissues or produce pharmacological effects; this indicates that the enzyme is present in the

tissues in excess of normal needs for noradrenaline synthesis.

INHIBITION OF DOPAMINE-β-HYDROXYLASE

Although benzylamine and benzylhydrazine derivatives are potent inhibitors of the enzyme *in vitro*, when given in tolerable doses they do not decrease significantly noradrenaline levels in the tissue.

Disulfiram is also a potent inhibitor of the enzyme *in vitro*. *In vivo* it reduces slightly the levels of noradrenaline in the tissues including the brain, and it raises the concentration of dopamine. In cats it decreases the responses of the nictitating membrane and spleen to stimulation of the sympathetic nerves. Under these circumstances dopamine is liberated from the tissues and may, therefore, act as a false transmitter.

The greater effectiveness of disulfiram *in vivo* compared with the other inhibitors may be due to their mechanisms of action. The benzyloxyamines and the benzylhydrazines act by competing with the substrate for the enzyme. Disulfiram apparently acts after reduction to diethyldithiocarbamate which inhibits the enzyme by chelating the copper which is the prosthetic group (p. 15.5). Other chelating agents also inhibit the enzyme *in vivo*.

Disulfiram is well known as an inhibitor of aldehyde dehydrogenase, another copper-containing enzyme, and is employed in 'aversion' therapy for alcoholism since it stops the metabolism of ethanol at the acetaldehyde stage (p. 5.72). Its dopamine-β-hydroxylase inhibiting property has only recently been discovered, and it remains to be seen whether it will prove useful clinically.

INHIBITION OF TYROSINE HYDROXYLASE

This enzyme catalyses the production of DOPA from tyrosine. Inhibition of noradrenaline synthesis might be most easily affected at this stage, which appears to be the rate limiting step. Analogues of tyrosine such as α-methyltyrosine, 3-iodotyrosine, 3:5-diodotyrosine and 3-iodo-α-methyltyrosine are competitive inhibitors of the enzyme *in vitro*. *In vivo* they decrease the catecholamines in the tissues. Because these inhibitors disappear from the tissues rapidly, repeated doses are needed to maintain adequate inhibition of synthesis while the catecholamines are depleted by utilization. α-Methyltyrosine, which has been studied most, does not inhibit noradrenaline storage or affect the uptake into stores.

Unlike α-methyl-*meta*-tyrosine, α-methyltyrosine, i.e. α-methyl-*para*-tyrosine does not give rise in the tissues to detectable amounts of the corresponding amine or β-hydroxylated amine, α-methyltyramine and α-methyl octopamine.

Very small amounts of α-methylnoradrenaline have been detected in animal tissues after α-methyltyrosine administration. Inhibition of aromatic amino acid decarboxylase does not prevent the depleting action of α-methyltyrosine, which is thus not dependent on metabolism of the amino acid to the amine. Further α-methyltyrosine lowers the rate of incorporation of ^{14}C-tyrosine into tissue dopamine and noradrenaline, but has no effect on the incorporation of ^{14}C-DOPA.

In animals, repeated administration of α-methyltyrosine produces some sedation and a reduction of motor activity possibly because of the reduced catecholamines in the brain. No hypotensive effect occurs, however, probably because depletion of noradrenaline in the peripheral adrenergic nerves is insufficient to produce a block of sympathetic nerve transmission.

In a few tests on patients with phaeochromocytoma with a rapid turnover of catecholamines in the tumour, α-methyltyrosine has produced sedation, lowered the blood pressure and decreased the urinary excretion of noradrenaline metabolites. No lowering of the blood pressure occurred in the cases of hypertension from other causes. Thus the inhibitors of catechol amine synthesis available at the present time are of little clinical use as antihypertensives. It remains to be seen whether new inhibitors more active *in vivo*, will be forthcoming.

Drugs inhibiting enzymes which metabolize catecholamines

Monoamine oxidase and catechol-*O*-methyl-transferase appear to be chiefly concerned with the inactivation by metabolism of the catecholamines and their inhibition might be expected to affect the intensity and duration of action of the catecholamines.

MONOAMINE OXIDASE

MAO, which is widely distributed in the body, can degrade many of the alkyl- and aryl-amines formed in or ingested into the body, e.g. tyramine, dopamine, adrenaline, noradrenaline, tryptamine and 5-HT. Many substances inhibit this enzyme and affect the disposition of these amines *in vivo*.

A discussion of the pharmacology of MAO inhibitors is given on p. 5.20. Consequently only a brief general consideration of their actions in so far as they are related to the catecholamines and other sympathomimetic drugs is given here.

It is currently believed that MAO in the mitochondria of neurones containing catecholamine is concerned with the intraneuronal inactivation of the amines synthesized in excess of storage capacity or released within the nerve either spontaneously or by drugs, e.g. reserpine. Consequently, administration of MAO inhibitors generally increases tissue catecholamine levels, e.g. in the heart and brain. However, this is not an invariable finding in all species. For example, in the mouse the noradrenaline content of the heart is not raised, but that of the brain is increased. In the cat and dog, neither in the heart nor in the brain are noradrenaline concentrations increased. In these cases where noradrenaline concentration fails to rise, the normal level of the amine is either not controlled to any significant extent by MAO or the balance between synthesis and inactivation is maintained by other systems when MAO is inhibited.

MAO inhibition has little or no potentiating effect on the responses to circulating adrenaline or noradrenaline or to sympathetic nerve stimulation. It is thus evident that the activity of the enzyme is not essential in limiting the response in these circumstances. Treatment with MAO inhibitors markedly potentiates the effects of non-catechol sympathomimetic amines, which do not carry a methyl group in the α-position in the side chain, e.g. phenylephrine and tyramine. When the enzyme in the liver and other tissues is inhibited, the rapid inactivation of the amines *in vivo* is diminished. More prolonged and more intense sympathomimetic effects result, whether these are produced mainly by direct action on α-receptors as with phenylephrine, or mainly by an indirect action depending on the release of noradrenaline from the neurones, as with tyramine. Potentiation by MAO inhibitors also occurs with sympathomimetic amines which contain an α-methyl group in the side chain, e.g. amphetamine, ephedrine, metaraminol, and are thereby not substrates of MAO. As described previously, these amines possess an indirect component of sympathetic action which depends on their releasing noradrenaline from adrenergic nerve endings. The potentiation of their actions by MAO inhibitors is probably due to increased release of noradrenaline, either because there is a supranormal amount of the transmitter available for release or because less of the noradrenaline released is inactivated intraneuronally and so more escapes to activate the receptors. Potentiation of the effects of these drugs may also arise because enzymes in the microsomal fraction, concerned in their metabolism in the liver, are inhibited by MAO inhibitors, particularly of the hydrazine type. Many other classes of drugs are potentiated by MAO inhibitors as a result of their action on the microsomal enzymes. The potentiation of the actions of noncatechol sympathomimetic agents is responsible for the severe hypertension with headache and vomiting and occasionally death from rupture of cerebral blood vessels which can occur in patients being treated with MAO inhibitors (p. 5.22).

Pretreatment with MAO inhibitors raises the amount of catecholamine, particularly of dopamine in tissues following administration of DOPA. In animals this results in signs of excitement and motor stimulation, presumably related to increased catecholamine levels in the CNS. As DOPA is found in broad beans, ingestion of this vegetable by patients on MAO inhibitors has led to pressor crises.

A dangerous drug combination in patients is that of MAO inhibitors with the tricyclic antidepressant compounds. Such combination can result in a severe hypertension, restlessness, hallucinations and hyperpyrexia. The effects have been attributed to raised levels of the catecholamines in the tissues as a result of the action of the MAO inhibitors coupled with the potentiating action of the tricyclic antidepressants on the effect of released amines (p. 5.22).

CATECHOL-*O*-METHYL TRANSFERASE INHIBITORS
O-Methylation of the catecholamines can be inhibited competitively *in vitro* and *in vivo* by several polyphenols such as pyrogallol and tropolone derivatives. In animals they reduce the rate of disappearance of injected catecholamines and prolong the duration of the biological responses. Responses to sympathetic nerve stimulation are also potentiated, indicating some involvement of the enzyme in the removal of the released noradrenaline. The catecholamine content of the tissues is not markedly affected by these inhibitors but they decrease the levels of *O*-methylated metabolites in tissues and in urine.

No clinical situation in which inhibition of catechol-*O*-methyltransferase might be of advantage can be envisaged and, as yet, no drug with this effect and suitable for administration to man has been found.

Drugs which block the release of catecholamines from neurones

The release of noradrenaline from site 4 on the nerve endings can be interfered with by a number of drugs. The result is a loss of sympathetic tone and such drugs are potentially useful for lowering the blood pressure in the treatment of hypertension (p. 8.8). Some of the adverse effects of these drugs when used clinically are due to interference with the sympathetic tone to organs other than the heart and blood vessels.

Important drugs which interfere with noradrenaline release are **bretylium, guanethidine, bethanidine** and **debrisoquine**, already mentioned as the prejunctional blocking agents (p. 15.22).

MECHANISM OF ACTION OF BRETYLIUM AND ALLIED DRUGS
These drugs decrease the response of tissues to postganglionic sympathetic nerve stimulation. This effect can be demonstrated on various tissues *in vitro* and *in vivo*, whether the response to nerve stimulation is excitor or inhibitor. Since they do not inhibit the actions of adrenaline or noradrenaline, their effect is not due to blockade of the receptor at site 6. In the intact animal, inhibitory effects on cholinergic transmission in autonomic ganglia, in the postganglionic parasympathetic system, at the neuromuscular junction and in the adrenal medulla are transient or nonexistent. These drugs evidently reduce the amount of noradrenaline released on sympathetic

nerve stimulation, but the precise mechanism of action is not known.

The blocking actions of these drugs are not dependent on a measurable depletion of the noradrenaline from the nerve endings although this can be produced with repeated high doses of bretylium, debrisoquine and bethanidine. A slow depletion occurs with a blocking dose of guanethidine, but the block in transmission occurs before depletion is detectable. Noradrenaline in the peripheral tissues may be reduced to low levels with repeated small doses of guanethidine and this may contribute in part to the blocking action under these circumstances. The depleting actions of guanethidine possibly result from a persistent release of noradrenaline from the nerve endings, and also to a decrease in reuptake. It has been suggested that the drugs block nerve conduction because they possess local anaesthetic properties and that the restriction of their action to postganglionic sympathetic nerves arises from the fact that they are selectively accumulated and retained there. Doses which are sufficient to produce neurone block, however, do not in fact prevent conduction in sympathetic postganglionic nerves; nevertheless it is suggested that conduction is blocked only in the fine terminals to the nerves. It has also been suggested that the mechanism of action is due to depletion of a small functionally essential pool of noradrenaline, the loss of which is not detectable. The matter is thus still undecided.

A further suggestion is that the site of action of these substances is in the cholinergic link in adrenergic transmission (p. 15.10). Like acetylcholine, they are strong bases and highly ionized at physiological pH, and so may interfere with noradrenaline release on nerve stimulation by replacing or blocking the action of acetylcholine which, according to the theory, is the mediator of the nerve impulse in noradrenaline release.

CLINICAL PHARMACOLOGY OF BRETYLIUM AND ALLIED DRUGS

In man these drugs produce a fall in blood pressure more evident in the patient suffering from hypertension than in the normotensive person. The effect is smaller in the supine position and the fall in systolic and diastolic blood pressure is mainly postural because, as a result of adrenergic neurone block, there is a reduction in the vasoconstriction which normally takes place when there is a change from the supine to the vertical position. For the same reason, postural hypotension leading to fainting may occur with exercise.

Bradycardia, nasal obstruction due to vasodilation in the mucous membrane, inhibition of ejaculation, increased frequency of micturition, are unwanted clinical effects also due to reduced sympathetic tone. Increased motility of the intestine which results in diarrhoea may also arise for the same reason. Diarrhoea is particularly troublesome with guanethidine, possibly because of additional stimulation of the intestine due to the release of 5-HT from the intestinal tract. Other unwanted effects include pain and tenderness in the parotid glands, most frequently seen with bretylium, and muscular weakness.

Because bretylium is a quaternary ammonium compound, its absorption from the gastrointestinal tract is poor and variable so that control of the blood pressure response was difficult. Furthermore, tolerance is produced rapidly so that the hypertension can no longer be controlled even by large doses. For these reasons it is no longer used as an antihypertensive drug.

Although a strong base, guanethidine is more reliably, if only partly, absorbed from the intestine. Once absorbed its clearance is slow, and there is danger of cumulation if the drug is given in too large doses. Consequently only small doses should be used at the beginning of treatment and adequate control of the blood pressure of a hypertensive patient may take some weeks to achieve. It is, therefore, useless if a rapid hypotensive effect is required. The duration of action of debrisoquine and bethanidine is shorter than that of guanethidine and therefore control of the blood pressure can be achieved more rapidly (p. 8.8).

Drugs depleting neuronal stores of catecholamines

The rauwolfia alkaloids are a group of drugs which by acting on site 2 on the membranes of the storage granules deplete the nerve terminals of transmitter. Reserpine is one of the alkaloids of *Rauwolfia serpentina* which have hypertensive and tranquillizing effects. They deplete the stores of catecholamines and 5-HT in the various tissues such as the heart, blood vessels, intestine and adrenal medulla. The catecholamines and 5-HT in the brain are also markedly reduced and the possible significance of this in relation to the centrally mediated effects of reserpine in inducing tranquillization, mental depression, and a syndrome like Parkinsonism in man is discussed on p. 5.31. The following discussion is restricted mainly to the effects on the peripheral sympathetic system.

MECHANISM OF ACTION OF RAUWOLFIA ALKALOIDS

After a suitable dose of reserpine in animals the noradrenaline content of the various tissues declines until, after several hours, only a relatively small amount is left. Thereafter the noradrenaline concentration remains low for one or two days after which there is a slow return to normal levels over the course of seven to fourteen days. In contrast to this prolonged effect, the reserpine disappears rapidly from the body, falling to undetectable levels in the tissues in a few hours. This finding has been taken to indicate that the drug produces some action, resulting in the noradrenaline depletion, which persists in the absence of the drug. However, experiments with ³H-reserpine show that minute amounts of the drug persist in the tissues for much longer time, and it is possible that this is responsible for the long lasting effect. Because of the long duration of action, repeated doses may have a cumulative effect.

With the loss of noradrenaline from postganglionic sympathetic nerves there is a decrease in sympathetic tone. This is not, however, evident until the noradrenaline concentration has been reduced to about 25 per cent of normal. After more intense depletion, restoration of function occurs before normal concentrations are again reached and parallels the recovery of the ability of the nerves to take up and store exogenous noradrenaline.

The mode of action of reserpine in causing depletion of noradrenaline from the postganglionic sympathetic nerves is controversial; the following explanation is put forward as reasonable, but it is not universally accepted. It seems possible that the depleting action is due to an inhibition of a transport mechanism which maintains the amine in high concentration within the storage granules against an adverse concentration gradient. In the absence of this pump, the spontaneous leakage of the amine is unopposed and the concentration in storage granules falls. The released noradrenaline is destroyed rapidly within the nerve by the mitochondrial MAO so that there is little or no release of the transmitter from the nerve endings. There is no evidence that reserpine interferes with the biosynthesis of noradrenaline, and it does not inhibit the re-uptake of released noradrenaline into the nerve, but, in the presence of reserpine, the amine is not stored. Reserpine has no ganglion-blocking action and it does not block the responses to adrenaline or noradrenaline.

CLINICAL PHARMACOLOGY OF RESERPINE
In experimental animals and man reserpine produces a slowly developing fall in blood pressure which is greatest when the pressure is initially high. The fall is due to a decreased peripheral resistance. In spite of a slowing of the heart, cardiac output is not significantly altered, although it may fall during long term treatment with the drug. The bradycardia is probably the result both of a decreased sympathetic tone and an increase in vagal effects. The latter appear to arise from central parasympathetic stimulation, which is also responsible for the miosis and increased salivary secretions noted in animals after administration of the drug.

Although reserpine produces sedation, the hypotensive effect does not appear to be due to a central depression of sympathetic outflow, which in animals is not reduced and may in fact be increased.

After adequate doses in animals reserpine depresses the reflex pressor response to such manoeuvres as carotid occlusion or stimulation of the sciatic nerve. When used as an antihypertensive agent in man, homeostatic cardiovascular reflexes are little affected, possibly because the extent of noradrenaline depletion produced by the very small doses employed is sufficient only to block the responses to low but not to high rates of firing in the sympathetic nerves (p. 8.9).

Drugs leading to the formation of false transmitters
Interference with the biosynthesis of noradrenaline in peripheral neurones is a possible way in which a drug could reduce transmitter stores, and so impair sympathetic function, and perhaps be of use in the treatment of hypertension.

α-Methyldopa, a competitive inhibitor *in vitro* of DOPA decarboxylase, is an effective antihypertensive drug in man. However, as more potent decarboxylase inhibitors are ineffective in this respect, inhibition of this enzyme is not the prime cause of the hypotensive action. Animal experiments show that α-methyldopa reduces the concentration of dopamine, noradrenaline and 5-HT formed by the action of the decarboxylase on 5-hydroxytryptophan in the brain and other tissues.

While the reduction in dopamine and 5-HT could be related to the duration of the decarboxylase inhibition, the reduction of noradrenaline persisted long after decarboxylase inhibition had ceased with the disappearance of the α-methyldopa from the tissues. Subsequently it was discovered that in fact L- (but not D-) α-methyldopa, could, like L- (but not D-) DOPA, serve as a substrate, albeit a poor one, of the decarboxylase leading to the formation of α-methyldopamine. *In vivo* this amine can be converted to α-methylnoradrenaline by the action of dopamine-β-hydroxylase and both these amines have been shown to be present in the tissues of various animals and in the urine of patients treated with α-methyldopa (fig. 15.12). Analysis of some tissues, e.g. heart and brain show that the missing noradrenaline is replaced by equimolar amounts of α-methylnoradrenaline. On sympathetic nerve stimulation α-methylnoradrenaline and noradrenaline, are released in the same proportions as occurs in the tissues, which indicates that both occupy the same stores in the adrenergic nerves. Both are also susceptible to release by drugs such as reserpine and tyramine. Administration of α-methyldopamine (by *in vivo* conversion to α-methylnoradrenaline) and α-methylnoradrenaline can also deplete noradrenaline in tissues by being taken up into the noradrenaline storage particles. It appears that α-methylnoradrenaline can compete, on a mass action basis, with noradrenaline for the binding sites in the storage particles. The relatively long persistence of α-methylnoradrenaline in these stores is probably related to the fact that, unlike noradrenaline, it is not

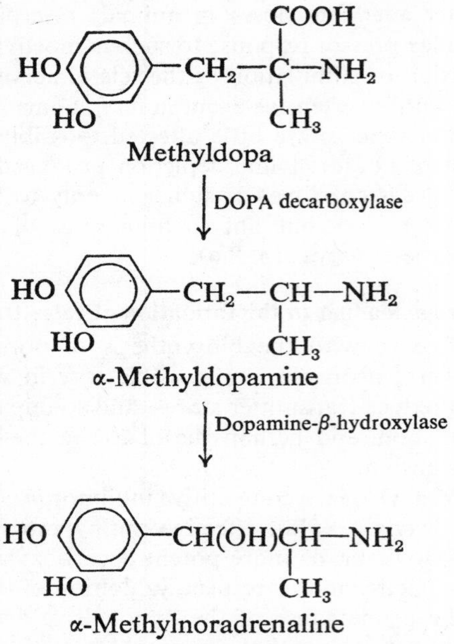

FIG. 15.12. Formation of false transmitter from methyl-dopa.

destroyed by MAO in the mitochondria because it contains the α-methyl group. Its eventual disappearance depends on slow spontaneous leakage and cumulative losses from the fraction not retaken up into the nerve following nerve stimulation.

In some tests, e.g. blood pressure responses, α-methylnoradrenaline is less potent than noradrenaline, generally by a factor of two to four. In other tests, e.g. bronchodilator action, α-methylnoradrenaline is the more potent.

On the basis of all these findings, it has been suggested the α-methylnoradrenaline, found in adrenergically innervated tissues after administration of α-methyldopa, acts as a substitute or **false transmitter**, replacing or partly replacing the noradrenaline normally released on nerve stimulation. In those tissues, e.g. the blood vessels, where it has a lower potency than the natural transmitter, the response to nerve stimulation is reduced. The false transmitter theory affords an explanation for the hypotensive action of α-methyldopa. It explains why no obvious signs of impairment of other sympathetic functions occur, such as miosis or relaxation of the nictitating membrane in cats or dogs. Similarly the responses to stimulation of sympathetic nerves are not blocked so markedly as they are with other inhibitors of synaptic transmission as in the ganglion or at the adrenergic neuroeffector junction.

Relatively large or repeated doses of α-methyldopa are required to produce an hypotensive effect, presumably because the α-methylamino acid is a relatively poor substrate for the decarboxylating enzyme and because it is cleared fairly rapidly (p. 8.9). **α-Methyl-*m*-tyrosine**, a closely related analogue of α-methyldopa, also behaves analogously. It is decarboxylated to yield α-methyl-*m*-tyramine, which in turn is converted to metaraminol, the corresponding β-hydroxylated derivative. The metaraminol is incorporated into the noradrenaline storage granules in adrenergic nerves with a concurrent displacement and depletion of noradrenaline. The metaraminol then functions as a false transmitter.

Metaraminol is a less potent pressor agent than noradrenaline or α-methylnoradrenaline in animals and in man. With parenteral administration, α-methylmeta-tyrosine has been shown to exert some antihypertensive effects in man and in animals made hypertensive by interfering with the renal circulation. In man it is not effective when given by mouth even in large doses, probably because the absorption from the gut is insufficient.

In conclusion it should be stressed that it has not been proven that the hypotensive actions of α-methyldopa and α-methyl-*m*-tyrosine are dependent on noradrenaline depletion and false transmitter formation, but the concept provides a useful working hypothesis for further investigation.

THE FALSE TRANSMITTER THEORY FOR THE
HYPOTENSIVE ACTION OF MONOAMINE OXIDASE
INHIBITORS

The formation of a false transmitter in adrenergic nerves has also been suggested to account for the sympathetic blockade and hypotension in man after long term administration of MAO inhibitors such as pargyline, which may be used as an antihypertensive agent. In animal experiments it has been found that after prolonged administration of MAO inhibitors there is an accumulation, in peripheral tissues, of octopamine, the β-hydroxylated derivative of *p*-tyramine, and this can be released on sympathetic nerve stimulation. Octopamine is a much weaker adrenergic receptor activator than noradrenaline and replacement by it of a portion of the noradrenaline released by nerve stimulation could result in a diminished response of the effector tissue. Tyramine is produced by decarboxylation of tyrosine but is normally rapidly destroyed by MAO. Under conditions of MAO inhibition it accumulates and some is converted to octopamine by the action of dopamine-β-hydroxylase in the noradrenaline storage granules in which it is retained.

Other mechanisms such as block in transmission in autonomic ganglia, and a bretylium-like action at postganglionic sympathetic nerve endings have been suggested to explain the hypotension action of MAO inhibitors, but it is doubtful if the true explanation is to be found in any one. A combination of several points of attack by the drugs is the probable answer. The pharmacology of the MAO inhibitors is dealt with on p. 5.20.

SUMMARY OF DRUG ACTION AT ADRENERGIC NERVE TERMINALS

The mechanisms of actions of the various drugs which affect the adrenergic neurone-effector cell complex are now summarized in relation to fig. 15.13, which is reproduced again.

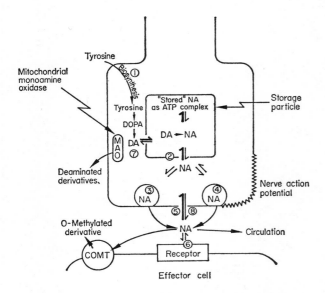

FIG. 15.13. Site of drug action at an adrenergic nerve terminal. NA, noradrenaline; DA, dopamine; MAO, monoamine oxidase; COMT, catechol-*O*-methyl transferase. For explanation see text.

(1) Synthesis may be blocked by enzyme inhibitors. This is most effective when the rate-limiting enzyme is inhibited, e.g. by α-methyl-*p*-tyrosine.

False transmitters formed from α-methyldopa or α-methyl-*m*-tyrosine substitute for noradrenaline at all points and compete with noradrenaline at sites of active transport.

(2) Active transport of catecholamines into storage particles may be blocked by reserpine. Released noradrenaline is then lost mainly by intraneuronal destruction by MAO and this leads to depletion of the store.

(3) Small amounts of noradrenaline are available for easy release by tyramine and other indirectly acting sympathomimetic amines. Tachyphylaxis to these amines is possibly due to preferential depletion of this store. Storage particles may be located in or close to the axonal membrane.

(4) Store from which noradrenaline is released by nerve stimulation; nerve function is not blocked when there is tachyphylaxis to sympathomimetic amines. Bretylium, bethanidine, debrisoquine and guanethidine block release of noradrenaline by the nerve action potential. Stores (3) and (4) run down after depletion of the main store by reserpine but are refillable by circulating noradrenaline.

(5) Re-uptake of released noradrenaline is by active transport through the axonal membrane and is blocked by cocaine. It is also inhibited by indirectly acting sympathomimetic amines which are transported.

(6) α- and β-receptors on an effector cell are activated by directly acting sympathomimetic drugs, e.g. adrenaline and blocked by α- or β-blocking agents.

(7) Inhibition of mitochondrial MAO, e.g. by phenelzine, causes a rise in noradrenaline concentration in the neurone.

(8) Finally there is probably a small spontaneous release of noradrenaline.

The picture of the adrenergic nerve terminal which has been presented, follows upon closely reasoned arguments about the findings of experimental pharmacologists. The picture should help physiologists to understand the mechanisms as an important site of homeostatic control; it should also help physicians to use accurately some of the powerful therapeutic weapons which they now possess.

FURTHER READING

AXELROD J. (1965) Metabolism, release and storage of catecholamines. *Recent Progr. Hormone Res.* **21**, 597.

IVERSEN L.L. (1967) *The Uptake and Storage of Noradrenaline in Sympathetic Nerves.* London: Cambridge University Press.

UDENFRIEND S. (1964) Biosynthesis of the sympathetic neurotransmitter, norepinephrine. *Harvey Lect.* **60**, 57.

VANE J.R., WOLSTENHOLME G.E. & O'CONNOR M., eds. (1960) *Adrenergic Mechanisms.* London: Churchill.

Chapter 16
5-Hydroxytryptamine

5-Hydroxytryptamine (5-HT) was first extracted from gut by Vialli and Erspamer in 1937 and given the name enteramine. Its structure was established in 1948, and at that time it was called serotonin on account of its vaso-constrictor properties. The amine has a ubiquitous distribution in nature. In the plant kingdom, bananas, pineapples and tomatoes have an especially high con- centration. In animals it has been reported in many species, ranging from the oysters and other edible mussels where it probably acts as a neurotransmitter, to man where its function is unknown.

Formation of 5-HT may differ in plants and in animals. Fig. 16.1 shows the accepted scheme in the higher animals and man. The starting material is the

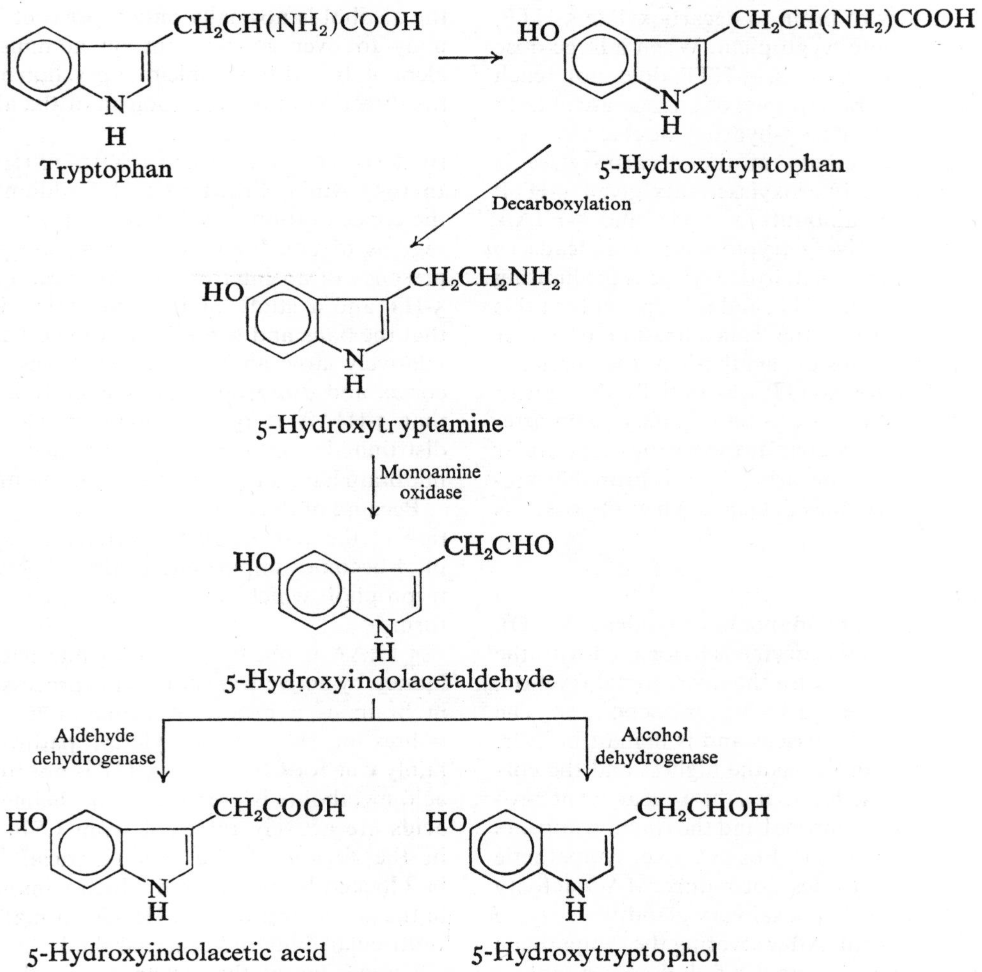

FIG. 16.1. Formation and inactivation of 5-HT.

16.1

essential aromatic amino acid tryptophan. In man about 1 per cent of the dietary tryptophan is converted to 5-HT. The first step is hydroxylation in position 5 to give the amino acid 5-hydroxytryptophan (5-HTP). The hydroxylase occurs in liver, gut and brain. In liver homogenates this enzyme is found in the cell supernatant fraction and it also hydroxylates phenylalanine to form tyrosine. In brain, however, it is in the mitochondrial fraction and is inhibited by phenylalanine.

Because hydroxylase activity in brain is relatively low it has been suggested that 5-HTP is formed at sites other than brain, such as the gut and, after being transported by the circulation, is converted in the brain to 5-HT. However, 5-HTP is not normally detectable in plasma. Weber carried out an ingenious experiment to test whether brain was capable *in vivo* of forming 5-HT from tryptophan. He eviscerated rats to eliminate extracerebral sources of 5-HTP and then perfused the brain with tryptophan via the carotid artery; the 5-HT in the brain rose above the level in animals perfused with saline alone. This experiment tested the ability of brain to decarboxylate 5-HTP, as well as to hydroxylate tryptophan. When a large dose of tryptophan is given to rats, 5-HTP does not reach detectable amounts in brain in spite of an increase in both 5-HT and its metabolite, 5-hydroxyindolacetic acid (5-HIAA). Since the activity of the decarboxylase is greatly in excess of the hydroxylase, rats given 5-HTP produce vastly greater amounts of 5-HT and 5-HIAA than they do after receiving tryptophan. This leads to the conclusion that tryptophan hydroxylase is the limiting enzyme in the synthesis of 5-HT, and it is probably at this point that feedback from the concentration of either 5-HT or 5-HIAA regulates the synthesis of the amine.

The decarboxylase for 5-HTP was initially thought to be in the cell cytoplasm, but this finding may be an artefact of the method used to separate the various subcellular components. In cells, the decarboxylase is probably present in particles but becomes detached when the tissue is homogenized.

DESTRUCTION

The amine is inactivated by monoamine oxidase (MAO). In liver, 70 per cent of this enzyme is associated with the mitochondria, and the rest with the microsomal fraction, but in brain it is located exclusively in mitochondria. The activity varies between the tissues and is highest in liver. In brain, the hypothalamus has the highest and the corpus callosum the lowest level. It is not clear what proportion of MAO is intraneuronal and the fraction appears to change from tissue to tissue. For example, sympathetic denervation of the heart does not reduce MAO activity whilst after denervation of the salivary gland the enzyme activity falls by 52 per cent. After severing the sympathetic nerve supply to the pineal there is a fall of 50 per cent.

The suggested role of MAO is to inactivate amine released within the neurones (p. 15.7). Brodie postulates that amines are maintained in a storage pool by active transport and that amine leaks out down a concentration gradient to the MAO. It is possible that the enzyme functions in a similar way for 5-HT. In the catecholamine pathway catechol-*O*-methyl transferase (COMT) is also responsible for the inactivation of noradrenaline released on nerve stimulation. There does not appear to be a generally distributed methylating enzyme fulfilling the same function for 5-HT. Whether MAO acts outside the neurones in the same fashion as COMT is unknown.

Monoamine oxidase converts 5-HT to 5-hydroxyindolacetaldehyde. At this point the pathway in the metabolism of the amine divides. The aldehyde may be converted either to 5-HIAA by aldehyde dehydrogenase or to 5-hydroxytryptophol by alcohol dehydrogenase. This latter pathway has been demonstrated *in vitro* and *in vivo* in liver and brain. The hydrogen donors in these two organs differ, $NADH_2$ being responsible in liver and $NADPH_2$ in brain. In man the extent of the pathway to the alcohol is normally only 2 per cent but rises surprisingly to over 40 per cent on administration of ethyl alcohol. It is also possible that psychotropic drugs change the direction of the metabolism of the aldehyde.

DISTRIBUTION IN BRAIN AND ELIMINATION

In 1953 Amin, Crawford and Gaddum were estimating the concentration of substance P (p. 17.3) in the various regions of dog brain. Using a bioassay they noted the presence of an interfering substance. This proved to be 5-HT and a study of its distribution in brain showed that the pons and medulla, and hypothalamus contained relatively large amounts whilst it was not detectable in cortex and cerebellum. Subsequently it was also shown that 5-HIAA is present in brain where it is unevenly distributed; the findings suggest that certain areas like midbrain have a higher turnover of the amine than others.

Because of the high turnover rate of 5-HT, the elimination of the end products 5-HIAA and 5-hydroxytryptophol becomes important. Little is known of 5-hydroxytryptophol which may be excreted in a conjugated form.

5-HIAA is one of several organic acids secreted by the kidney by active transport. This process probably occurs in brain as a means of eliminating one of the metabolites of the 5-hydroxyindol pathway. This is certainly true for CSF where 5-HT is not found although the acid metabolite is present. Pappenheimer has shown that acids are actively removed from CSF by a mechanism in the region of the 4th ventricle. This pump can be blocked by probenecid which eliminates the gradient in the concentration of 5-HIAA normally found between ventricular fluid and cisternal fluid.

Knowledge of the distribution of biogenic amines in brain was considerably advanced by a technique developed by Falk of Sweden. Slices of brain are frozen and dried. Subsequent exposure of the slices to an atmosphere of hot formaldehyde gas gives fluorescent condensation products of adrenaline, noradrenaline, dopamine and 5-HT (p. 5.17); the fluorescence of the catecholamines is green to yellow green, that of the 5-HT is yellow. On this basis the Swedish workers described both '5-hydroxytryptaminergic' and 'catecholaminergic' neurones in the CNS.

The catecholamines are much more easily visualized than 5-HT in spite of the high concentration of the amine in the regions examined, possibly because the terminals of the 5-HT neurones are too small to be seen by the light microscope or because the fluorescence of the 5-HT condensation product diminishes rapidly on irradiation with UV light. Pretreatment of the animals with nialamide, a MAO inhibitor, increases the fluorescence of the 5-HT neurones. These neurones have been demonstrated in the spinal cord and may arise from cells in the medulla. They descend in the cord and terminate in the ventral horn or the sympathetic lateral columns. Both 5-HT and noradrenaline terminals thus make intimate contact with motor neurones and autonomic nerve cells. A monosynaptic pathway from the reticular formation and midline region of the medulla to these cells has been suggested.

After transection of the spinal cord 5-HT accumulates above the transection and the fluorescence in the distal part of the nerves gradually fades with time. This has led to the theory that granular stores of 5-HT are made in the cell bodies and travel down the axon to the nerve endings. This theory fails to explain why the distal part of the cell retains its synthetic properties for some time after transection, e.g. fluorescence in this region can be increased by the administration of nialamide.

5-HT neurones in the brain have not been clearly demonstrated because of the difficulties mentioned. The medial forebrain bundle has fibres containing 5-HT derived from the midline region of the brain stem and midbrain central grey matter at the level of the superior corpora quadrigemina. They are distributed to the superior and cingulate cortex via the cingulum and to the hippocampus by way of the fornix. Section of the medial forebrain bundle diminishes the concentration of 5-HT in most areas of brain examined.

The subcellular distribution of 5-HT in brain has been studied by centrifugation of brain homogenates in isotonic sucrose (p. 5.15). Synaptosomes contain, besides 5-HT, histamine, noradrenaline and acetylcholine. Amines as well as acid metabolites are present in the supernatant but the extent to which it represents free amine in the intact cell or amine that is released after disruption is uncertain. The proportion found is 30 per cent in supernatant and 70 per cent in the particulate fraction of brain which includes the synaptosomes.

5-HT AS A NEUROTRANSMITTER

The evidence that 5-HT is a neurotransmitter in vertebrates is largely circumstantial. 5-HT appears to be released from isolated spinal cord of mouse, and the release is enhanced during nerve stimulation in the presence of nialamide. Prolonged stimulation of the medulla oblongata produces a fall in the noradrenaline and 5-HT content of the varicose nerve terminals of the cord as seen by fluorescence microscopy and biochemical analysis. Aghajanian stimulated the dorsal medial septal region of anaesthetized rats for long periods and then estimated the concentration of 5-HIAA and 5-HT in both whole brain and forebrain, the region to which the '5-hydroxytryptaminergic' neurones project. Compared with unstimulated controls, he found that as the concentration of 5-HT fell, that of 5-HIAA rose, thus confirming the view that 5-HT is released onto monoamine oxidase. The push–pull cannula has been used to apply very small doses of 5-HT to cells in the reticular formation or the amygdala and simultaneously to record action potentials. The results remain equivocal. In some cases 5-HT depresses and in some cases enhances response of cells in these areas. Many of the difficulties of this technique involve the electrical activity of the brain as a whole and hence both the preparation, e.g. the encéphale isolé, and the anaesthetic are important factors in determining the response of individual cells to the drug. It still remains to be shown by methods based on direct collection, that the amine or its metabolite is released on stimulation of tracts leading to the '5-hydroxytryptaminergic' terminals.

5-HT IN THE GUT AND BLOOD

5-HT has been found in the gut of all vertebrates examined where it is stored in the argentaffin cells of the intestinal mucosa (vol. 1, p. 30.21). Although the amounts of the amine are higher in gut than brain, the turnover is slower, being 11 hours in small intestine and about 1 hour in brain. 5-HT is released *in vitro* on distention of intestine and from the stomach on stimulation of the vagus nerve. The function of 5-HT in the intestine is probably concerned with motility; infusion of 5-HT in man produces spasm of the intestine and diarrhoea.

The effects of 5-HT on the cardiovascular system are complex and difficult to interpret. Further, it is doubtful whether the infusion of large quantities of 5-HT into the circulation where normally free 5-HT is scarcely detectable yields physiologically relevant information. Vasoconstriction due to direct action on the smooth muscle in the cutaneous and splanchnic vessels predominates and, in the kidney, afferent arteriolar constriction reduces renal blood flow and GFR. Arterioles in the skeletal muscle and the coronary vessels are dilated. A direct action on the heart increases the rate and force of contraction.

In whole blood the amine is present mostly in platelets. These actively concentrate 5-HT some thousandfold above the level in the surrounding medium. This process is inhibited by a variety of compounds including tryptamine, cocaine and imipramine and its analogues. 5-HT appears to be stored in electron-dense granules in the platelet from which it may be released rapidly by reserpine. The uptake process and its inhibition by drugs, is used as a screening procedure for drugs of the imipramine type, used in the treatment of mental depression; antidepressant activity correlates fairly well with inhibition of platelet uptake of 5-HT.

5-HT AND THE PINEAL

An interesting derivative of 5-HT is melatonin (vol. 1, p. 11.27). Lerner, investigating a pineal extract capable of lightening the skin of frogs used some 200,000 cattle pineals to isolate and identify the active substance which turned out to be *N*-acetyl-5-methoxytryptamine or melatonin. The relationships between the pineal and gonadal function had been investigated for many years but with few positive results. From studies of patients with tumours of the pineal and adjacent tissue it appears that a substance is secreted by the gland which depresses gonadal function (vol. 1, p. 24.36). In certain amphibia like the frog the gland is a photoreceptor or a primitive third eye. However, in higher animals and presumably man, although the organ is not a photoreceptor, it retains an interesting response to light. In the pineal gland, rhythmic changes occur in the concentration of 5-HT, and noradrenaline and the activity of an enzyme found exclusively in the pineal which limits the synthesis of melatonin, viz., hydroxyindole-*O*-methyltransferase (HIOMT). These changes are circadian and are of two kinds. The rhythm for 5-HT appears to be an endogenous one, triggered by some central biological clock which is synchronized by external light, and that for HIOMT seems to be completely dependent on the phasing of external light. The pineal is not affected directly by light, but the stimulus arises in the retina and passes into the sympathetic tracts via the superior cervical ganglion. In animals that respond to light by increased gonadal function (causing increased ovarian weight and accelerated oestrus cycles), the stimulus presumably acts by reducing the formation of melatonin and related compounds; these substances are themselves inhibitory, and it is possible that the timing of events such as oestrus or menstruation are brought about through this mechanism.

DRUGS AND 5-HT

Several drugs affect the synthesis and storage of 5-HT. Since these have a similar action on other biogenic amines, such as noradrenaline, it is difficult to draw conclusions concerning the role of 5-HT in behavioural responses. An exception is *p*-chlorophenylal-anine which seems to inhibit fairly specifically tryptophan hydroxylase causing a fall of 5-HT concentration in brain within 2–3 days. This comparatively slow fall when compared with the rapid turnover of the amine has been attributed to the formation of a metabolite of *p*-chlorophenylalanine as the active principal which takes about 24 hours to be maximally effective. Behavioral effects after *p*-chlorophenylalamine are not prominent although psychosis with hallucinations have been reported in man.

α-Methyldopa blocks the decarboxylation of 5-hydroxytryptophan. When rats are given a loading dose of tryptophan together with methyldopa, 5-hydroxytryptophan can be detected in brain. MAO inhibitors lead to large increases in body and brain 5-HT. In man paradoxically the 5-HIAA does not always fall in brain after their administration in spite of a rise in 5-HT, and it may be that inhibitors which contain hydrazine interfere with the active transport of the acid metabolite 5-HIAA from the brain.

Reserpine inhibits the capacity of cells to store 5-HT in granules and hence this drug leads to almost total depletion of 5-HT with a consequent rise in 5-HIAA as the amine spills out on to MAO.

Perfusion of the cerebral ventricles in rats with radioactive 5-HT leads to the accumulation of the amine in brain, probably by active transport. Study of its subcellular distribution has shown it to be associated with the synaptosomal fraction. The 5-HIAA was found only in the supernatant fraction. Fluorescence microscopy shows that after intraventricular injection of 5-HT the amine is taken up in very fine varicose nerve terminals and nerve cell bodies lying close to the ventricles. These are probably identical with the 5-HT nerve terminals. The catecholamine neurones do not accumulate 5-HT. Reserpine blocks accumulation of 5-HT by the nerve terminals, but when reserpine is given in combination with an MAO inhibitor 5-HT still enters the cells. Neither desmethyl imipramine nor amphetamine inhibit the process which therefore differs from that for noradrenaline. The evidence suggests that there is a central re-uptake mechanism for released 5-HT analogous to that for catecholamines which is not blocked by antidepressant drugs of the imipramine type. However in certain neuronal membranes, such as the sympathetic nerve to the ductus deferans of the guinea-pig, 5-HT behaves like noradrenaline and is taken up by active transport into the neurone. Imipramine and its analogues with antidepressant activity effectively block the uptake of 5-HT at this membrane while those without antidepressant activity do not.

Certain drugs such as LSD and methysergide antagonize the effects of 5-HT on many smooth muscle receptors although it is not clear whether they act centrally as antagonists.

THE ROLE OF 5-HT IN HEALTH AND DISEASE

5-HT has been implicated in many diseases such as hypertension, migraine, schizophrenia and depressive psychosis. However, conclusive evidence is lacking. Although the 5-HT antagonist methysergide appears to be an effective prophylactic drug in treating migraine, this does not mean that the amine has an aetiological role. The amine has been considered to be involved in schizophrenia because certain hallucinogens such as LSD and bufotenine, which occurs naturally and is found in the skin of the South American toad (*Bufo arenarum*), also possess the indole nucleus as part of their structure.

Reports of the identification of bufotenine in the urine of patients suffering from schizophrenia and depressive psychosis have been made but the evidence is conflicting. When patients with high blood pressure are treated with reserpine or methyldopa, both of which lower brain 5-HT, mental depression or even suicide may occur as a complication. Drugs that increase the concentration of the amine in brain, namely the MAO inhibitors, are used in the treatment of depression. These findings would, however, also support a similar role for noradrenaline in the illness. The finding that the imipramine and similar antidepressants affect the uptake of noradrenaline rather than 5-HT favours the view that noradrenaline is the more important amine. However, since there is evidence that 5-HIAA in the lumbar CSF reflects the concentration of 5-HIAA in brain, then a reduction in 5-HIAA found in depression provides indirect evidence for the hypothesis that 5-HT is functionally lower in depressive psychosis.

The carcinoid syndrome arises from tumours of argentaffin cells in the gastrointestinal tract and is characterized by flushing, diarrhoea and bronchoconstriction. Large quantities of 5-hydroxyindoles are secreted intermittently into the circulation. At first the symptoms were attributed to free 5-HT. However, apart from abdominal discomfort, it was not possible to reproduce these symptoms by infusion of the amine, and more recently bradykinin has been implicated as the cause of the flush and possibly other features (p. 17.3).

The release of 5-HT has also been thought to play a role in inflammatory and hypersensitivity reactions, but the evidence is much less satisfactory than for histamine. Pretreatment with 5-HT antagonists do not ameliorate the inflammatory reactions to thermal, chemical or irradiation injuries in experimental animals.

A physiological role for 5-HT is difficult to find. It would appear to play a part in sleep. Doses of tryptophan can induce the onset of rapid eye movement, hindbrain, paradoxical or dreaming sleep in susceptible individuals. This effect can be blocked by methyldopa and methysergide. Changes in the concentration of the amine in the pons in sleep have been found by Jouvet and there seems little doubt that amine has a role to play in this activity. Because the centrally acting sympathomimetic drugs such as amphetamine are able to block hindbrain sleep, it may be that catecholamines and 5-HT exert opposite effects within a balanced system which alternates between sleeping and waking.

Body temperature is controlled by mechanisms situated in the region of the hypothalamus. The hypothalamus is rich both in '5-hydroxytryptaminergic' and 'noradrenergic' neurones. This and the fact that 5-HT injected into the lateral ventricle causes a rise in body temperature in the cat, whilst noradrenaline causes a fall, led Feldberg and Myers to postulate that these amines had a thermoregulatory role. They suggested that the normal body temperature was determined by the relative proportions of these amines released in this structure. There are, however, species differences. In the rabbit 5-HT causes a fall and noradrenaline a rise in body temperature. Since these effects were obtained only by very large doses of the drugs, it is possible that they represent a direct action on blood vessels, so influencing blood flow and hence the activity of the thermoregulators in the hypothalamus.

At present, views of the role of 5-HT range from its being an important central neurotransmitter to a chemical remnant or legacy from our marine past. In spite of the enormous literature on the subject either view could be correct.

FURTHER READING

PAGE I.H. (1968) *Serotonin*. Chicago: Year Book Medical Publishers.
GARRATTINI S. & SHORE P.A. eds. (1968) Biological role of indolealkylamine derivatives, in *Advances in Pharmacology*, volume 6, part A. New York: Academic Press.

Chapter 17
Some pharmacologically active polypeptides

Many hormones are proteins or large polypeptides; there are in addition a number of polypeptides of low molecular weight which may act as local hormones and which have powerful pharmacological activity. These substances include the kinins and substance P, a peptide which has not yet been isolated, and angiotensin. The kinins and substance P appear to act mainly as local hormones, but angiotensin probably has both a local and general action (vol. 1, pp. 25.36 and 33.20). The role of kinins in the physiology of secretion has been discussed in vol. 1, pp. 17.6 and 30.5.

The kinins

The kinins are polypeptides of low molecular weight which occur in many tissues.

Investigations into the kinin-forming system began in 1926 when Frey showed that extracts of pancreas, pancreatic secretion itself and urine produced a fall in blood pressure when given intravenously to dogs. The active principle **kallikrein** (Greek, pancreas) owed its activity to the enzymic release of a substance, **kallidin**, from a plasma precursor. In 1949, a group of Brazilian workers described the release from plasma globulin by the action of snake venoms and trypsin of a hypotensive peptide which was named **bradykinin** because it caused a slow contraction of isolated guinea-pig ileum. They were then unaware that kallikrein had already been shown to

Bradykinin	Arg-Pro-Pro-Gly-Phe-Ser-Pro-Phe-Arg
Kallidin	Lys-Arg-Pro-Pro-Gly-Phe-Ser-Pro-Phe-Arg
Met-Lys-bradykinin	Met-Lys-Arg-Pro-Pro-Gly-Phe-Ser-Pro-Phe-Arg

FIG. 17.1. Structures of some kinins.

release kallidin from a plasma precursor. Bradykinin (fig. 17.1) was isolated in 1960, and its synthesis was soon achieved. A year later the original kallidin was shown to be a mixture of two peptides, the nonapeptide bradykinin and lysyl-bradykinin. The name kallidin now refers specifically to lysyl-bradykinin. Two other kinins have

been detected in mammalian tissue. Methionyl-lysyl-bradykinin is formed when pseudoglobulin is subjected to acid hydrolysis. Colostrokinin, a peptide having bradykinin-like activity, is formed by the action of saliva on colostrum.

In addition to the above kinins, bradykinin homologues and bradykinin-like activity are found in many parts of the animal kingdom, e.g. in wasp and scorpion venoms, in the skin of frogs and other amphibians and in the plasma of reptiles and birds.

KININ FORMATION

Specific kinin-releasing enzymes or kallikreins occur in plasma, urine, saliva, tears, sweat, lymph and CSF. They act on protein substrates, **kininogens** to release kinin peptides. Kininogens and kallikreins are present normally in plasma, as also is the kinin-inactivating enzyme, kininase. The plasma kallikreins are normally inactive (kallikreinogens) but are readily activated by dilution with saline, contact with glass or acidification; the exact mechanism of activation is not known. Blood contains several proteinase inhibitors, and in mammalian plasma there are at least two specific kallikrein inhibitors. These are large polypeptides and similar substances have been found at most of the sites where proteolytic enzymes occur. Inhibitor–kallikrein complexes readily dissociate at acid pH and this is possibly a factor in the acid activation of kinin release (fig. 17.2).

A complex relationship between release of plasma kinin and blood coagulation was brought to light by the observation that when plasma comes in contact with glass, a kinin-like pain producing substance is released. It was then shown that plasma from patients with the Hageman trait and deficient in Factor XII neither clots normally nor releases kinin on contact with glass. Factor XII is adsorbed on to the glass as the initial step of the clotting response. Glass carrying adsorbed Factor XII from normal blood is, however, capable of activating kinin-release in deficient plasma. Factor XII appears to be an activator for the formation of plasma kinin, not only as the result of contact with glass, but also for other activation procedures.

The picture is even more complicated since Factor XII

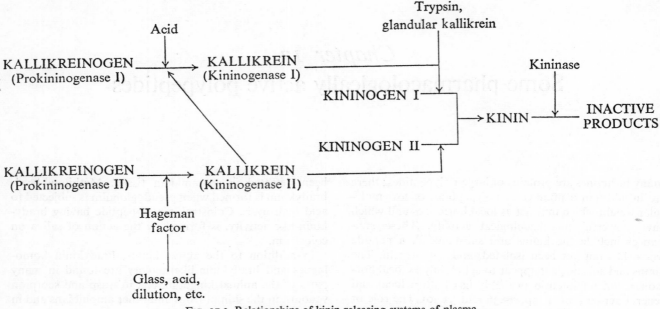

FIG. 17.2. Relationships of kinin-releasing systems of plasma.

also promotes fibrinolysis and may be involved in the activation of plasminogen. Plasmin itself can both activate plasma kallikrein and also release kinin by a direct action on kininogen. Glass activation causes depletion of only about 40 per cent of the total plasma kininogen, the remaining kininogen is susceptible to the action of trypsin and glandular kallikrein. As a result of this observation, it has been shown that plasma contains two distinct kinin-forming systems and two kininogens have been isolated from plasma. Fig. 17.2 shows the relationship between the two systems.

Although plasma and tissues contain readily activated kinin-forming enzymes and kininogens, free active kinin is rarely detected in biological fluids. Plasma and most tissues contain rapidly acting kininases, and can split the C-terminal arginyl bond common to both bradykinin and kallidin to form inactive products. As a result, free kinin in the circulation has an estimated half-life of less than 30 sec.

PHARMACOLOGY OF THE KININS

The pharmacological actions of bradykinin are typical of the kinins although there are some quantitative differences. Bradykinin contracts many smooth muscle preparations such as the guinea-pig ileum, the oestrus rat uterus and human uterine muscle strips but inhibits smooth muscles which show rhythmic activity and have a high resting tone, e.g. isolated rat duodenum. The actions on smooth muscles are often used to assay the kinins.

In the guinea-pig intravenous injection of bradykinin causes bronchoconstriction which is inhibited fairly specifically by analgesic antipyretic drugs such as salicylates (p. 5.54). Raised blood levels of bradykinin activity occur in animals during anaphylaxis and in man during severe asthma, and kinin may be in part responsible for bronchoconstriction in these conditions.

Bradykinin is one of the most potent vasodilators

TABLE 17.1 Pharmacological actions of bradykinin

SMOOTH MUSCLE
 Contracts many isolated smooth muscle preparations including guinea-pig ileum (concentration 1 ng/ml), oestrus rat uterus (concentration 0·1 ng/ml) and human uterine strip (1–10 μg/ml), and relaxes others such as rat duodenum (8 ng/ml).
 Generally relaxes human intestinal circular muscle, and inhibits peristalsis.
 Produces bronchoconstriction on intravenous injection in the guinea-pig.

CARDIOVASCULAR SYSTEM
 Intravenous injection (0·05–0·5 μg/kg) produces a fall in arterial pressure.
 Causes vasodilation in most vascular beds and a fall in total peripheral resistance.
 Intravenous injection of minute amounts causes cutaneous flushing in man.

NERVOUS SYSTEM
 Stimulates sympathetic ganglia and causes release of catecholamines from the adrenal medulla.
 Stimulates the pain fibres of an exposed blister base in man (0·1–1·0 μg/ml).

LOCAL ACTION
 Increases capillary permeability when injected intracutaneously (1–10 ng/ml).

known and a fall in arterial blood pressure is used in the assay of both kinins and kallikrein. In man, infusion of bradykinin causes a characteristic flush and increases skin blood flow in doses too small to produce detectable changes elsewhere. In the pulmonary circulation, however, bradykinin also acts as a vasoconstrictor. It also causes a marked local increase in capillary permeability, visualized by prior treatment with intravascular dye; on a molar basis it is some fifteen times more active in this respect than histamine. In man, intradermal injection of bradykinin produces a weal and flare, and topical application in dilute solution to an exposed blister on the human forearm causes transient pain.

Bradykinin releases catecholamines from the adrenal medulla and stimulates sympathetic ganglia. When given by arterial injection close to the cat superior cervical ganglion, the ipsilateral nictitating membrane contracts. This sympathetic stimulation could explain the inhibition of intestinal motility produced by the infusion *in vivo*. A summary of the pharmacological actions of bradykinin is given in table 17.1.

The role of kinins in disease

Although kinins might play a role in a number of pathological conditions, raised concentrations of free kinins have seldom been demonstrated. Since kinins cause pain, vasodilation and increase capillary permeability, they are possible mediators of inflammatory responses (p. 21.7). An increase in the free kinins and kinin-forming activity of lymph draining the limbs of animals subjected to various types of injury, including scalding, crushing and ischaemia, has been observed, and similar findings have been reported in man. Kallikrein may be released from tissues damaged by hypersensitivity reactions, and raised levels of plasma kinins have been detected in animals during anaphylactic shock and in patients during asthmatic attacks. Free kinins have been found in synovial fluid from patients with gout and other types of arthritis.

Kinins have recently been implicated in several disease processes associated with the gastrointestinal tract. The shock associated with acute pancreatitis has been attributed to kinin activation by proteolytic enzymes released into the circulation from the pancreas (p. 10.8). Carcinoid tumour tissue consisting of argentaffin cells has been shown to contain not only 5-HT but also kallikrein (p. 16.5). It has also been shown that intravenous injection of adrenaline, which provokes the carcinoid flush, simultaneously stimulates the release of kallikrein into the blood with the appearance of raised levels of kinin. The argentaffin cells of the small intestine contain kallikrein, as well as 5-HT. In patients with carcinoid tumours, typical symptoms are (1) increased bowel movement and diarrhoea, which may be due to the release of 5-HT and (2) flushing and difficulty with breathing (bronchoconstriction) which probably arise from the release of kinins.

After surgical removal of part of the stomach, patients sometimes suffer from attacks of sweating and flushing, weakness and occasionally fainting together with intestinal discomfort and explosive diarrhoea. These symptoms come on soon after a meal and are known as the dumping syndrome. Kinin activation has been shown to occur during the development of the syndrome. Kallikrein is present in duodenal and jejunal mucosae and may be released by hypertonic solution. Kinins and 5-HT may have a complementary role as local hormones modifying the vasomotor tone and motility of the intestine.

Substance P

Substance P (SP) was discovered in 1931 by von Euler and Gaddum while assaying acetylcholine in tissue extracts. They observed that alcoholic extracts of tissues, especially intestine and brain, produced a contraction of the rabbit's jejunum which was not abolished by atropine. The activity was dialysable and destroyed by trypsin and so was presumably due to a polypeptide of low molecular weight. Like the kinins, SP stimulates most smooth muscle preparations and is also a potent vasodilator.

The purification of SP and its chemical and pharmacological characterization have proved difficult; its precise structure is unknown. The minute amount in tissues is readily adsorbed to most materials used in peptide purification and large losses occur during isolation. The purest preparations are unstable. No specific chemical reaction for SP is known and bioassays are used to compare responses with a standard SP preparation. The amino acid composition of SP is very similar to that of kinin-like endecapeptides, eledoisin and physalaemin, which occur in certain amphibians and molluscs (fig. 17.3); the

Eledoisin   Tyr-Pro-Ser-Lys-Asp(OH)-Ala-Phe-Ile-Gly-Leu-Met-NH$_2$

Physalaemin   Tyr-Ala-Asp(OH)-Pro-Asp(NH$_2$)-Lys-Phe-Tyr-Gly-Leu-Met-NH$_2$

Fig. 17.3. Naturally occurring endecapeptides. (Greek, *endeca*, eleven)

purest known preparations of SP contain 21–27 amino acids.

SP has been found in all vertebrates so far investigated, but almost exclusively in the brain and intestinal tract. The content is generally low in the oesophagus and stomach, high in the duodenum and jejunum, but the ileum, colon and rectum contain moderate amounts. The muscularis mucosae contain a greater concentration than any other layer of the gut wall. SP is present in all parts of the mammalian CNS, although there are differences in concentration, even in closely neighbouring regions, and functional systems show significant differences. Thus apart from the retina, the concentration in the visual system is much lower than in the auditory system. The relatively high concentrations of SP in the sensory pathways are associated with only small amounts of acetylcholine or choline acetylase; this has led to the suggestion that SP may be a transmitter in the CNS. SP is also found in peripheral nerves, especially in autonomic nerves. In both the brain and peripheral nerves it occurs in bound form in granules present in the subcellular fractions containing nerve endings.

PHARMACOLOGY AND POSSIBLE
PHYSIOLOGICAL ROLES

Most of the studies on the pharmacology of SP have been carried out with impure preparations and hence many of the findings may be invalid. The main sites of action which have been so far investigated are the intestine, the circulation and the CNS. Substance P causes most extravascular smooth muscle to contract and has a powerful stimulating action on the intestine, increasing peristalsis, both in isolated preparations and *in vivo* when given intravenously to animals and man. Various intestinal preparations allow fairly specific bioassays. A clear distinction between the kinins and SP is provided by the isolated rat duodenum, which relaxes characteristically in the presence of the kinins and is contracted by SP.

The powerful stimulant action of SP on intestinal motility and its high concentration in the highly motile duodenum and jejunum suggest that it may be a physiological mediator of peristalsis. Hexamethonium blocks its action on peristalsis.

The purest preparations of SP are more active vasodilators than bradykinin, but, unlike bradykinin, it is not destroyed by the blood and this may account for the difference in potency. SP increases skin and muscle blood flow with a resultant fall in blood pressure, and causes bright red cutaneous flushing in man. The peptide is also as active as bradykinin in increasing vascular permeability and in producing pain.

Possible clues to a function of SP in the CNS have been sought through the examination of changes in concentration under different conditions. Increases in concentration have been found in the retina of cattle after closure of the eyes for 2 hours. In the brain of rabbit or rat the concentration falls when the animals are kept in the dark, and rises again on exposure to light. Elimination of the senses of smell or hearing reduces SP content of rat brain, while in the bat, elimination of tactile sense or the 'radar' mechanism produces an increase.

So far no clear evidence for a physiological role of SP has emerged, either in the CNS or in the gut. The characteristic distribution of the substance in these tissues, its great potency as a pharmacological agent and the changes in tissue concentration in different functional states all suggest a physiological role. What this role is, however, remains obscure.

Angiotensin

The angiotensins are small polypeptides and differ from the kinins in that they are among the most potent pressor agents known. Like the kinins they are released from an inactive protein precursor, angiotensinogen, occurring in the α_2-globulin fraction of plasma (vol. 1, p. 25.36). The enzyme which releases angiotensin from angiotensinogen was discovered in 1898 by Tigerstedt and Bergmann. They found a nondialysable, heat labile vasoactive substance which they called renin in extracts of kidney cortex (vol. 1, p. 33.21). Forty years later Braun-Menendez showed that the hypertensive action of renin was due to the secondary release of a heat stable principle, now known as angiotensin.

Angiotensins have now been isolated from several sources and synthesized (table 17.2). If angiotensinogen

TABLE 17.2. Naturally occurring Angiotensins.

Substance	Structure	Source
Tetradecapeptide (minimal substrate)	Asp-Arg-Val-Tyr-Ile-His-Pro-Phe-His-Leu-Leu-Val-Tyr-Ser-	Horse, pig
Angiotensin I	Asp-Arg-Val-Tyr-Ile-His-Pro-Phe-His-Leu-	Horse, pig
Angiotensin II	Asp-Arg-Val-Tyr-Ile-His-Pro-Phe-	Horse, pig
Val$_5$-angiotensin II	Asp-Arg-Val-Tyr-Val-His-Pro-Phe-	Cow

is degraded using trypsin, a tetradecapeptide is obtained, which is an effective substrate for renin. The tetradecapeptide has been synthesized, and its structure shows that renin by splitting the Leu–Leu bond yields the inactive decapeptide **angiotensin I** which is further degraded by another enzyme in plasma, the 'converting' enzyme to yield the pressor octapeptide, **angiotensin II**. Plasma and many tissues contain one or more enzymes capable of destroying angiotensin II. The stages in the release and inactivation of angiotensin are summarized in fig. 17.4.

PHARMACOLOGICAL ACTIONS OF ANGIOTENSIN

Intravenous injection in man of angiotensin I, in a dose of 0·1 μg/kg, leads to a rise in blood pressure lasting for several minutes. The action on blood pressure is not affected by ganglion-blocking drugs or adrenergic blocking agents (p. 4.7).

Like the kinins, angiotensins contract smooth muscle. The contraction of the isolated oestrus rat uterus by

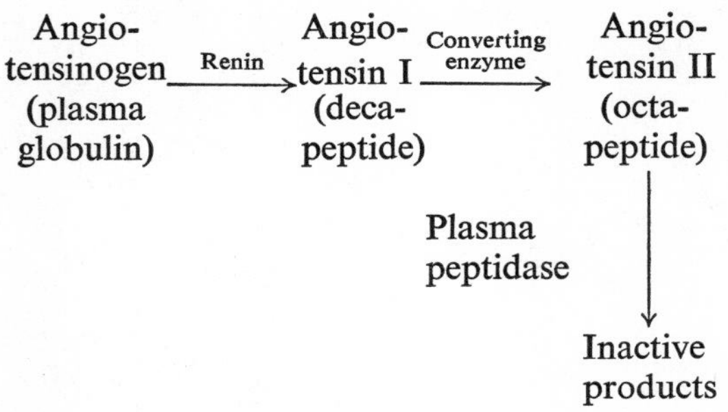

Angio- →Renin→ Angio- →Converting enzyme→ Angiotensinogen   tensin I   tensin II
(plasma   (deca-   (octa-
globulin)   peptide)   peptide)

Plasma
peptidase
↓
Inactive
products

Fig. 17.4. The renin–angiotensin system.

angiotensin appears to be due to a direct action on the muscle, but that of intestinal muscle is mediated partly by a cholinergic mechanism and may be partially blocked by atropine. In addition to this action on the parasympathetic nervous system, angiotensin has actions on the sympathetic nervous system. It acts on the adrenal glands to release catecholamines and part of its pressor response is due to this effect. Furthermore, angiotensin has been shown to be a potent stimulant of the cat superior cervical ganglion, acting directly on the ganglion.

As described in vol. 1, p. 33.20, angiotensin stimulates the release of aldosterone from the adrenal cortex and this effect may represent part of a volume control system. The increase in the excretion of aldosterone may be maintained for several days by the intravenous in-fusion of angiotensin. There appears to be a feedback relationship between aldosterone and angiotensin similar to that between cortisol and ACTH, since just as cortisol administration reduces ACTH secretion, so administration of aldosterone reduces the concentration of renin in the kidney and blood. It has also been suggested that angiotensin and renin act locally within the kidney. Renin may be released in response to reduced osmolality in the distal tubule; it may then activate the renin angiotensin system and so increase sodium conservation.

The powerful pressor effect of angiotensin has suggested its use in the treatment of hypotension due, for example, to blood loss. Angiotensin -II amide has been given by intravenous infusion in concentrations of 1 mg/l in isotonic saline at a rate of 1–10 μg/min in these circumstances. It suffers the same disadvantages as noradrenaline (p. 15.14), however, as it reduces the blood supply to the tissues and aggravates the defect in tissue perfusion, its use is not recommended.

FURTHER READING

Lewis G.P. (1968) Pharmacologically active polypeptides, in *Recent Advances in Pharmacology*, ed. J.M. Robson & R.S. Stacey. London: Churchill.

Schachter M. (1969) Kallikreins and kinins. *Physiol. Rev.*, **49**, 509.

Chapter 18
Bacteria, fungi and viruses

Before bacteria were first seen by van Leeuwenhoek, other workers had advanced hypotheses that diseases might be caused by living agents. Fracastorius in 1546, as a result of his studies on syphilis, then a new disease in Europe, suggested that a *contagium vivum* was the cause of some infectious diseases; his ideas were based on his records of the spread of epidemics in a community and not on the direct observation of any causal agent. His arguments included ideas about disease transmission that are now proven and accepted, e.g. he postulated that a causal agent could be deposited on inanimate objects such as clothing or cutlery from which infection could be acquired by another individual. Kircher claimed in 1659 that he observed minute 'worms' in the blood of plague victims, but it is doubtful whether he could have seen plague bacilli with the crude apparatus then available.

It is likely that the first person to observe microorganisms directly in various materials was Antonie van Leeuwenhoek (1676) of Delft. Not only was he scrupulously honest in reporting his observations, but he designed experiments to prove their validity. For example, he showed that rain water was devoid of his little animals until it reached some earth bound material, and he also noted that the little animals normally detected in scrapings from his teeth were immobilized after he had drunk hot coffee. Much of the scepticism regarding van Leeuwenhoek's work subsided when he was made a Fellow of the Royal Society; he died in 1723, and another century passed before Louis Pasteur was born, but during that century little if any advance was made in the study of van Leeuwenhoek's animalcules.

Van Leeuwenhoek's observations also sparked off further controversy regarding the validity of the doctrine of spontaneous generation which had held sway for many centuries; many notable individuals firmly believed that forms of life could come into being by the interactions of inanimate matter. Aristotle thought that eels developed in this way and Virgil in the Georgics described a method for the artificial production of insects.

The first to doubt this doctrine was Francesco Redi (1686) who showed that the maggots in putrid meat do not arise spontaneously; he found that if meat was held in paper or within a wire gauze of fine mesh to prevent the deposition of flies' eggs, it putrefied but remained free from maggots which hatched out on the protective coverings.

LOUIS PASTEUR

Spallanzani (1777) and Schulze (1836), among others, showed that fermentation of organic fluids was dependent on the introduction of live agents from the air, but the idea of spontaneous generation persisted until Pasteur finally despatched it. In a paper entitled *On the organized bodies which occur in the atmosphere; examination of the doctrine of spontaneous generation*, published in 1861, Pasteur reported experiments which in their simplicity and reproducibility were invulnerable. He introduced samples of urine and various liquids such as sugar solutions containing yeasts into open glass flasks, the necks of which were then drawn out in various ways that allowed entry of air but prevented the access of any organic material from the atmosphere. The contents of the flasks were then heated and boiled for several minutes; the contents remained sterile so long as the curved necks of the flasks were intact but became contaminated and showed evidence of fermentation within a day or two after the necks were snapped off (fig. 18.1).

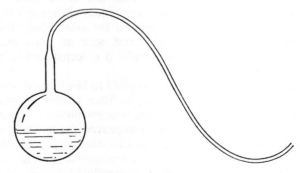

FIG. 18.1. Pasteur's swan-neck flask.

It is fascinating that Pasteur prefaced the presentation of these experiments by saying: 'The researches which I will report here are only a digression made necessary by my studies on fermentations'. This digression saw the birth of the science of microbiology, since he showed not only how to sterilize liquids but also how to maintain sterility. The development of sterilizing procedures was the first step towards the study of organisms in pure culture. Pasteur's work is commemorated daily in the provision of pasteurized milk.

ROBERT KOCH

In the same era Robert Koch had begun his study of infections in animals and man, and in his earliest observations on anthrax demonstrated the specificity of a particular organism for a given infection. Apart from his work on anthrax, tuberculosis and other infections, Koch is remembered chiefly because of his postulates. These were published in 1884 after he had completed his main research and stated the criteria to be met in relating a micro-organism causally to a given infection.

Koch's postulates are as follows:

(1) the organism must be observed in every case of the disease;

(2) the organism can be isolated in pure culture;

(3) the disease can be reproduced in a suitable experimental animal by introducing the pure culture, and

(4) the organism can be recovered in pure culture from the diseased experimental animal.

More will be said of these postulates, but it is clear that even today certain infections, e.g. leprosy, are regarded as being caused by specific micro-organisms although all the postulates have not yet been fulfilled. Nowadays, a fifth condition is often invoked to establish a causal relationship between organism and disease, namely that antibodies specific for the particular micro-organism should be demonstrated in the serum of the sick person.

There is no doubt that one of his teachers, Jacob Henle in the University of Göttingen, had a profound influence on the young Koch; Henle attempted to perform laboratory investigations on materials from infected patients and while the crude techniques then available did not meet all the strict criteria for establishing the association between causal agent and an infection, Henle's teaching of such principles is reflected faithfully in his student's postulates.

Staining methods had been applied to histological preparations for some time when in 1869 Hoffmann, the professor of botany in Giessen, first attempted to stain bacteria, but it was Koch who improved the techniques and laid the foundations for modern staining procedures in microbiology. In 1881 Koch introduced the idea of fixation of material by heat prior to staining, and in 1882 Ehrlich published his method of staining tubercle bacilli. With slight modifications by Ziehl, who employed carbolic acid as a mordant rather than aniline, and by Neelsen, who used sulphuric acid in place of nitric acid as a decolourizing agent, this method is still in use. The cloak of fame slipped from Ehrlich's shoulders in this instance since the technique is now known as the Ziehl–Neelsen method of staining.

Koch made advances also in the cultivation of bacteria; until he advocated the use of gelatin to produce solid transparent culture media, methods for *in vitro* isolation of bacteria in pure culture were time consuming and frequently ineffective. Koch demonstrated his method and medium in London at the International Medical Congress in 1881 before an audience that included Lister and Pasteur; the latter, meeting Koch for the first time and seeing his demonstration, exclaimed: 'C'est un grand progrès, Monsieur.' This prophetic statement was, within a few months, confirmed throughout the world.

The principles of Koch's methods of cultivation of bacteria on solid media have remained unchanged and unchallenged, but two improvements occurred within a short time. The first of these, the replacement of gelatin by agar as the solidifying agent, allowed incubation at 37°C, a temperature at which gelatin melts but which is the optimum temperature for growth of almost all bacteria pathogenic to man; this modification was made by Hesse in 1882 and stemmed from a suggestion made by his wife who incorporated agar in her jam.

Petri, an assistant with Koch, introduced **Petri dishes,** the second modification in 1887; the use of these covered glass dishes immediately superseded Koch's original method of pouring the medium onto glass slides which were then kept under a bell jar to reduce contamination.

Koch is regarded as the father of medical microbiology since he was the first medically trained person to concentrate on the science; Pasteur's training, although scientific, was not medically orientated. It is even more remarkable that van Leeuwenhoek, the Dutch founder of microbiology, had no training whatsoever, and throughout his long life managed a draper's shop and was also caretaker of the Delft Town Hall.

The relationship of microbiology to medicine

The vast majority of micro-organisms are **saprophytic**, i.e. they exist independently of living hosts and, in their natural habitat, they are involved in processes of decomposition of dead animal and plant material; these processes are essential to the natural economy of man and other living things. A minority of micro-organisms are **parasitic** and their survival depends on their presence in or on other living tissues or cells. Parasitic micro-organisms are further divided into **commensals**, which co-exist harmlessly with host cells, and **pathogens**, which damage host cells or the host organism in some way. However, the differentiation between commensal and pathogenic micro-organisms is by no means absolute; for example, certain types of bacteria are normally commensal in the human intestine, but they can cause infection if they are given access to the urinary tract. Moreover, some pathogenic species may be isolated from a healthy individual who at that point in time is suffering no ill effect from the organism; such **carriers** of potentially pathogenic micro-organisms may be sources of infection for other people.

While microbiology has applications in many fields, medical microbiology is directly concerned with the health of the individual and of the community. In veterinary microbiology the problems are different, as diseased animals, unlike patients, can be slaughtered to protect the remainder of the population.

There have been very many dramatic advances in medical microbiology in the last 60 or 70 years, but in spite of these the layman still tends to be careless or ignorant in matters of hygiene, and many silly notions persist; such attitudes displayed in previous centuries are inexcusable today. Not long ago it was commonplace for dirty drains to be held responsible for the occurrence and spread of diphtheria in a community, a view similar to that of Skene at Aberdeen, who stated in 1586 that the causes of plague were stink, corruption and filth and also clouds of smoke caused by burning coal on windless days.

It is apparent, however, that some of our forebears were more realistic, although perhaps without complete understanding. In 1647, Aberdeen Town Council passed regulations that 'poisone be laid for the destruction of myce and rattens' to reduce the spread of plague; in retrospect this measure may have been effective since the last indigenous case of plague in Scotland was reported in 1648. This act by a secular authority was perhaps more relevant than that by the Presbytery of Edinburgh more than 200 years later when in 1853 it requested that Royal Assent be given to a National Day of Prayer so that the Asiatic Cholera which was then sweeping the city might be abated. Palmerston, the Home Secretary, refused to grant the request and recommended that a more profitable course would be to improve the environment, particularly of the poor and overcrowded areas in the city; 'which if allowed to remain will infallibly breed pestilence and be fruitful in death, in spite of the prayers and fasting of a united but inactive nation'.

The natural result of the proof that bacteria were involved in causing certain diseases was a search for therapeutic agents to assist the patient's recovery, and for prophylactic agents to prevent disease. In 1881, Pasteur immunized sheep and cattle by inoculating them with attenuated cultures of *Bacillus anthracis* (p. 18.64).

ANTITOXINS

The first therapeutic advance was the discovery by Behring and Kitasato (1890) of diphtheria antitoxin. The antitoxin was produced within two years of Roux and Yersin's demonstration that the diphtheria bacillus produces toxin which has the same lethal effect as the diphtheria bacilli themselves. In 1891 the first patient to be treated with diphtheria antitoxin recovered, and antitoxin therapy became the accepted treatment for diphtheria. An antitoxin is a substance produced in the body of an infected individual or animal, that is antagonistic to the toxin of the causative organisms (p. 22.17).

ANAEROBIC ORGANISMS

Another infection for which antitoxin was early in use, both prophylactically and therapeutically, was tetanus. The causative organism, *Clostridium tetani*, is a strict **anaerobe**, i.e. it multiplies only in an environment from which oxygen is excluded, and it could not be grown *in vitro* until the introduction of adequate methods of ensuring anaerobic environments. Pasteur's report in 1861 that certain organisms could live and reproduce in the total absence of free oxygen caused quite a stir even in scientific circles, because it had been assumed that all living creatures depended on oxygen for their survival. In this context one may note that van Leeuwenhoek, in one of his numerous letters to the Royal Society, reported in 1680 that some of his animalcules could survive in a highly rarefied atmosphere.

By the beginning of the present century more than twenty methods of attempting anaerobic cultivation existed and their number indicates that most were inefficient and many were cumbersome; the introduction in 1916 of the anaerobic jar by McIntosh and Fildes provided a method for the growth of strictly anaerobic species.

WOUND SEPSIS

The problems of wound sepsis greatly concerned Lister who introduced the concept of antiseptic surgery in 1867 on the basis of Pasteur's observations. The credit for demonstrating that wound infection was due to micro-organisms must go to Ogston. In the early 1880's he employed Koch's culture methods to examine septic wounds and showed that **staphylococci**, as he named them, and **streptococci** played a major role in causation. Ogston's intense interest in bacterial infection of wounds could well serve as a model for many present-day bacteriologists and surgeons.

EPIDEMIOLOGY

Medical microbiologists are also deeply involved in investigations of the sources and modes of spread of infection and the term **epidemiology** was introduced to describe the study of the interacting factors which may result in infection; much epidemiological investigation took place before the discovery of micro-organisms, and the work of Fracastorius has already been mentioned. Similarly Budd's epidemiological analyses indicated that typhoid fever was caused by a microscopic living agent, long before the discovery of the typhoid bacillus. The basic function of the epidemiologist is to acquire sufficient knowledge of the causes of the spread of a disease to allow him to interrupt a chain of events and thus prevent the spread of the disorder. Snow investigated an outbreak of Asiatic cholera in London in 1848 and became convinced that the water pump in Broad Street (now called Broadwick Street), Soho, was the reservoir of infection (p. 35.2).

CHEMOTHERAPY

At the beginning of the present century, Paul Ehrlich dreamed of 'magic bullets' that would kill infecting organisms without damaging the patient. His exciting pioneer work saw the introduction of effective antimicrobial therapy. Domagk introduced the sulphonamide era in 1933–5, and Fleming's observations on penicillin were developed by Florey and Chain shortly thereafter. These stimulated a long series of deliberate attempts to find organisms producing antibiotics and Waksman in 1944 announced the discovery of streptomycin. In the subsequent decade chloramphenicol and the tetracyclines were added to man's antimicrobial armoury. These discoveries are described in chap. 20.

The introduction of chemotherapeutic agents and antibiotics has involved the medical microbiologist in their development and also in their clinical application and has created a new relationship with clinical colleagues. The use of such agents demands not only the isolation and identification of the causative organism but also *in vitro* tests of the organism's sensitivity or resistance to various antimicrobial drugs to provide a guide to their efficacy. The need for such guidance is increasing since many pathogenic bacteria originally sensitive to certain antimicrobial agents have acquired resistance to them (p. 20.6).

VIRUSES

Just as the study of bacteria had to await the introduction of the light microscope and suitable methods of cultivation, so did virology require the electron microscope and the introduction of tissue-culture techniques. However, as with bacterial infections, the presence of viruses was suspected long before proof could be offered. In 1884 Pasteur was able to transmit rabies from one animal to another by injecting pathological material in which he could not see an organism; he therefore postulated that the cause was an infinitely small micro-organism.

In 1886 Buist first saw under the light microscope the elementary bodies of vaccinia in calf lymph. Studies by Ivanowsky in 1892 and by Beijerinck in 1899 on tobacco mosaic disease of plants left no doubt that members of the plant kingdom are also afflicted by agents smaller than bacteria; the causative organisms could not be seen by the light microscope and could pass through filters that impeded the passage of any known bacterial species.

Animals and insects were found to suffer from infection by similar ultramicroscopic agents and during World War I, Twort and d'Herelle independently showed that bacteria themselves were subject to attack by viruses; the bacterial viruses, called **bacteriophages** by the latter worker, have since been extensively studied, and have been of great use in studies of microbial genetics (p. 18.57).

In the present-day practice of medicine, the microbiologist is one of a team that includes clinicians in hospital or general practice, public health officers and many others, and his commitment is to assist in the diagnosis, treatment and prevention of infections. So far as the individual is concerned, the microbiologist's role in **preventive microbiology** may go unseen, but his contributions to the diagnosis of infective conditions, and his value in planning correct therapy are apparent.

BACTERIOLOGY AND MYCOLOGY

CLASSIFICATION OF BACTERIA AND RELATED ORGANISMS

Bacteria do not produce disease by their mere presence in the tissues and their pathological effects in man are due to reactions of the host to specific bacteria and their products. For this reason the physiology and biochemistry of pathogenic organisms are considered in some detail so that quantitative knowledge of bacterial populations may be related to qualitative knowledge of the constitution and requirements of organisms involved in specific diseases. This kind of information is exploited in the development of antimicrobial therapy; it is also of use in classifying organisms and contributes to bacterial identification. In turn, the correct classification and identification of an infective agent provides the clinician with guides to the effective control of infection. It should also be noted that similar disease syndromes, such as those associated with diarrhoea or meningitis, may be caused by widely different organisms. The clinician is best equipped to deal with an infection when he knows the specific organism involved.

Cell organization as a basis for classification

In addition to the plant and animal kingdoms a third kingdom, **protista**, conveniently includes organisms of relatively simple organization, i.e. algae, protozoa, fungi and bacteria. Some basic facts apply to all cells, but since structure and function are related, it is helpful to have a system of classification that allows valid generalizations for particular cell types to be made. Cell types can be defined as being either procaryotic or eucaryotic.

Procaryotic cells are the more primitive and lack specific intracellular organelles concerned with the metabolic activities that are carried out by the mitochondria of mammalian cells and the chloroplasts of cells which perform photosynthesis. Instead, these functions are performed by processes that take place at cell membranes. Moreover, the nuclear apparatus of the procaryotic cell is thought to be a simple ring of double-stranded DNA devoid of any structural membrane.

Eucaryotic cells have an association of nuclear DNA with protein units which gives rise to the typical chromosome structure, and the genetic material is separated from the cytoplasm by a nuclear membrane. When division is about to occur, the mechanisms that produce sharing of the DNA in the eucaryotic cell are necessarily complex, and the cell contents may be seen to flow in a definite pattern; this does not happen in procaryotic cells. In addition, in those eucaryotic cells that have organs of motility, flagellar structure is more complex than the flagellar structure of procaryotic cells.

The more highly evolved eucaryotic cell is the essential unit of animal and plant tissues, and it occurs also among the higher protista in the fungi, protozoa and most algae. The primitive procaryotic cell type is found in the blue-green algae and in all bacteria and spirochaetes. Thus, the protista may be divided into a higher and a lower group on the basis of cell organization, and the links within the groups are closer than the historical development of the separately applied studies would suggest. The more primitive organization of the procaryotic cell allows a reduction in size and this tends to be accompanied by a formidable capacity for rapid multiplication. These are the characteristics of the lower group of the protista which contains the following subgroups,

(1) blue–green algae,
(2) myxobacteria,
(3) eubacteria,
(4) spirochaetes, and
(5) rickettsiae.

The only organisms of lesser size are the viruses (p. 18.93). The present section is concerned particularly with pathogenic members of the eubacteria, the spirochaetes and the rickettsiae; these organisms are unlike the algae in being devoid of chlorophyll-like substances, and they differ from the myxobacteria in their cell wall structure and their mode of motility. The eubacteria and rickettsiae possess rigid cell walls and some members possess simple flagella; the spirochaetes do not have rigid cell walls, and their motility is derived from an elastic axial filamentous structure or a modified fibrillar membrane. All of these organisms conform to the general pattern of the typical cell in having virtually all of their DNA in the nuclear apparatus and their RNA in the cytoplasm. The viruses differ fundamentally in that any one structural unit possesses only one form of nucleic acid, either RNA or DNA but not both.

Simple classification systems

Micro-organisms, like other living creatures, can be classified into orders, families, genera and species. However, there is at present no standard international classification of bacteria; although a biological classification, based on physiological, immunological and other characteristics is available, a simpler scheme, based primarily on cell morphology and staining reactions suffices for purposes of communication between medical microbiologists and clinicians.

The true bacteria or eubacteria are conveniently divided into a higher group that resemble the fungi in their morphology and a lower group of simpler organisms. The spirochaetes and rickettsiae form other separate groups.

THE HIGHER BACTERIA

These are filamentous organisms, often sheathed and frequently showing true branching and forming a mycelium; cells may show interdependence in that some are developed as specialized reproductive units. One family of the higher bacteria, **Actinomycetaceae**, comprises two genera, *Actinomyces* and *Nocardia*, both of which are pathogenic; the genus *Streptomyces* belongs to another family and contains no pathogenic members, but many species in this genus produce antibiotics that are of great clinical use.

THE LOWER BACTERIA

These simple unicellular structures are called **cocci** when the cells are spherical, **bacilli** when they are straight and cylindrical in shape, **vibrios** when they are curved and comma-shaped and **spirilla** when they are spiral, non-flexuous rods (fig. 18.2).

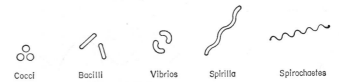

Cocci Bacilli Vibrios Spirilla Spirochaetes

FIG. 18.2. Typical morphology of some pathogenic bacteria. From Gillies R.R. (1968). *Lecture Notes on Bacteriology*. Oxford:Blackwell Scientific Publications.

Cocci are subdivided according to their reaction to the Gram stain (p. 18.16) and the spatial relationship of the cells to each other (fig. 18.3).

Staphylococci are arranged in irregular clusters, since successive cell divisions occur irregularly in a haphazard fashion; they are Gram-positive.

Streptococci are also Gram-positive, but the individual cocci adhere in chains since successive cell divisions occur in the same plane.

Diplococci are arranged in pairs or very short chains; they may be Gram-positive or Gram-negative.

Gaffkyae appear as flat plates of four cells, since consecutive planes of division are at right angles to each other; they are Gram-positive.

Sarcinae are seen as packets of eight cells because division occurs successively in three planes at right angles; they are also Gram-positive.

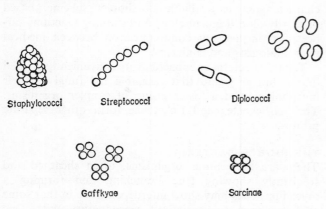

FIG. 18.3. Subdivisions of cocci according to the relationships of the cells. From Gillies R.R. (1968).

The further division of these morphological groups is dependent on cultural, biochemical and serological methods.

Bacilli (rod-shaped bacteria) are not so easily classified and are subdivided primarily according to their reactions when stained by Gram and Ziehl-Neelsen techniques (table 18.1, p. 18.8); Gram-positive bacilli may or may not form spores and may or may not grow under aerobic conditions. Recognition of genera within the non-sporing Gram-positive and Gram-negative groups requires further study of their physiological activities in artificial culture.

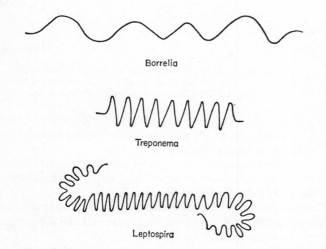

FIG. 18.4. Typical morphology of the three medically important genera of the spirochaetes.

SPIROCHAETES

These organisms are differentiated from spirilla since they show active flexion of the cell; in addition they are motile without possessing flagella. Their Gram staining reaction is rarely demonstrable because of their very slender filament diameter, but the larger species are Gram-negative. There are three genera of pathogenic spirochaetes (fig. 18.4). *Borreliae* are larger and more refractile than the others; they can be stained by ordinary methods and their coils are large with a wavelength of 2–3 μm. *Treponemata* are much slimmer with a coil wavelength of only half that of *Borreliae*; they are demonstrable by the light microscope only after staining by a silver impregnation technique unless dark-ground microscopy is used. *Leptospirae* are even finer, with a coil wavelength of 0·5 μm or less; one or both poles of the organism are hooked or recurved on the body so that under dark-ground illumination the actively motile, spinning organism may appear to have a button-hole at one or both extremities.

RICKETTSIAE

These are micro-organisms which range from spheres, 300–500 nm in diameter, to thin rods up to 2 μm in length and are regarded as intermediate between bacteria and viruses. They can be seen by the light microscope, do not pass filters that retain bacteria and have the principal structural features of bacteria. Rickettsiae have at least some of the enzyme systems of bacteria and contain both RNA and DNA. Moreover, they are susceptible to some antibacterial agents. On the other hand, almost all of the members of the group are obligatory intracellular parasites and can be grown in culture only when living cells are present.

MYCOPLASMAS

It is convenient to note at this point that a group of organisms initially designated 'pleuropneumonia-like organisms' (PPLO), and now included in the genus *Mycoplasma*, do not have a place in the taxonomic systems considered so far. These organisms are very small (50–300 nm in diameter) and they behave like bacteria but have no rigid cell wall. They therefore assume various shapes; they are very delicate and are nutritionally and physically exacting. They have much in common with bacterial L-forms (p. 18.11) and it has been suggested that they have evolved naturally from the bacteria as forms which have become deficient in synthetic cell wall mechanisms. The present weight of evidence is against this view; mycoplasmas incorporate cholesterol in their cell membrane and, although this occurs in fungi and yeasts, cholesterol is not known to occur in bacterial cell membranes. Further studies suggest that mycoplasmas are quite distinct from L-forms.

Classification of medically important bacteria

The micro-organisms of medical importance can be simply classified on an essentially morphological basis and subclassified on the basis of their nutritional requirements. A major differentiating feature is their behaviour in the Gram staining reaction which separates bacteria into two distinct classes. Many other characters show considerable correlation with the Gram reaction. For example, Gram-positive organisms, in general, have susceptibilities to various deleterious agents which differ from those of the Gram-negative bacteria; this is well illustrated in the different sensitivities of the two groups to antimicrobial drugs. An interesting exception to this general rule is seen in the behaviour of the Gram-negative pathogenic *Neisseria*; the gonococcus and the meningococcus seem to be Gram-negative by mistake.

Table 18.1 lists most of the genera and many of the species of bacteria that are pathogenic to man. According to international convention the names are given in Latin and printed in italics; for example, the species of streptococcus commonly associated with pus-producing (pyogenic) lesions is called *Streptococcus pyogenes*. Confusion may arise in the use of the word bacilli. This was introduced in the early days of bacteriology to designate micro-organisms shaped like rods and to distinguish them from round cocci. Official use now limits the word to describe a single genus *Bacillus*, of which only one species, *B. anthracis*, is pathogenic to man. Yet we continue to talk about tubercle bacilli, dysentery bacilli and diphtheria bacilli, and this older and broader use of the word is unlikely to drop out.

The list of pathogenic species given in the table is not complete. There are many bacteria with which man comes in contact, saprophytes in the environment and relatively benign parasites living on the skin and in the gut and respiratory passages, which are normally non-pathogenic. Of these a few become pathogenic under certain circumstances, and are listed, but to include all the many bacteria that have on rare occasions been reported to be pathogenic would be impractical. In addition, many bacteria are primarily pathogenic parasites of animals other than man, and men who come into close contact with the susceptible animals may become infected; several important human diseases are acquired in this way and are listed, but again it is impractical to include all bacterial infections that man on rare occasions has acquired from animals. Finally, like all other biologists, bacteriologists frequently disagree on the criteria that determine a species. For most of the species listed in the table there may be subdivisions of 'types' or 'variants'. Variations within a species may influence the nature of a clinical illness or the manner of spread of an epidemic, but it is impractical to list many of the possible variants.

The genera are grouped into **families** and **orders** by systematic bacteriologists; the details of these groupings do not concern the medical practitioner, but some groupings of genera are of practical value in medicine and these are indicated. Some of the terms are hallowed only by tradition and they rest on no sure scientific foundation.

THE STRUCTURE OF BACTERIA

The bacterial cytoplasm is contained in a cytoplasmic membrane which is encased by a relatively rigid cell wall (fig. 18.5). Outside this there may be an extracellular layer of slime, which in some species forms a definite capsule. Certain appendages, flagella and fimbriae, may also be present. There is no defined nucleus, but the cytoplasm contains nuclear bodies of DNA devoid of a nuclear membrane. Many different types of inclusion granules occur in the cytoplasm, and mesosomes (p. 18.14) and ribosomes can be defined. Some bacteria form well-defined spores (endospores) within the cytoplasm.

THE CYTOPLASMIC MEMBRANE

This membrane, known also as the plasma membrane, lies immediately inside and adjacent to the cell wall and is composed principally of lipoprotein. It is extremely thin, only 5–10 nm in thickness, has little mechanical strength and depends on the cell wall for support. It allows the selective absorption of nutrients into the cell and also the excretion of waste products, and it possesses several enzymes involved in cell respiration and in the manufacture of cell wall materials.

Whilst all the factors determining the cell's response to Gram's staining method are not understood, the porosity of the cytoplasmic membrane is involved and may differ in Gram-negative and Gram-positive species.

THE CELL WALL

This is relatively thick (10–25 nm) and has sufficient rigidity to give the various bacterial species their characteristic shapes, but it is permeable to molecules with a mol. wt. of less than 10,000. The strength of the cell wall may be judged by the fact that bacterial cells are not disrupted by intracellular osmotic pressures of several atmospheres; for example, it is estimated that the pressures inside staphylococci may be about 750 to 1000 mOsmols.

Bacterial cell walls contain a mucopeptide complex in which the amino sugars *N*-acetylglucosamine and *N*-acetylmuramic acid are linked alternately and the chains are cross-linked by peptides. *N*-acetylmuramic acid does not occur in mammalian cells. The existence of the unnatural isomers D-alanine and D-glutamic acid in the peptide links is another special feature of bacterial cell walls and, in addition, many bacterial cell walls contain diaminopimelic acid which does not occur naturally elsewhere (p. 20.10).

TABLE 18.1. Procaryotic micro-organisms that produce disease in man, and some of the diseases for which they are responsible.

Common group name	Genus	Species	Morphology and notable characters	Habitat or reservoir of infection	Common mode or vehicle of infection	Diseases produced in man
GRAM-POSITIVE BACTERIA						
	ACTINOMYCES	*A. israelii*	Branching filaments, micro-aerophilic	?Commensal in mouth	Apparently endogenous	Actinomycosis; abscess in cervico-facial region, occasionally in abdomen or chest
	NOCARDIA	*Noc. madurae*	Branching filaments	?Saprophytic and on skin	?Endogenous	Mycetoma; chronic ulcer seen in tropical countries
	LISTERIA	*L. monocytogenes*	Bacillus, often in pairs	Widely distributed in animals and man	Intrauterine in foetal infections	Foetal and neonatal mortality; meningo-encephalitis
THE ACID-FAST BACILLI	*MYCOBACTERIUM*	*Myco. tuberculosis* human type (1) *Myco. bovis* bovine type (2) *Myco. avium* avian type (3) etc.	Bacillus, acid-fast and alcohol-fast	(1) Lungs of man, (2) cows, (3) birds, sometimes pigs and cattle	(1) Airborne from human cases and via dust, (2) milk-borne, (3) human infection uncommon	Pulmonary tuberculosis; tuberculosis of lymph nodes, intestine, bones and joints; meningitis and genitourinary infections
		Myco. leprae	Bacillus, less acid-fast than *Myco. tuberculosis*, often occurring intracellularly	Lesion in skin and mucous membrane, e.g. nasal mucosa and internal organs	Prolonged human contact	Leprosy
	CORYNEBACTERIUM	*C. diphtheriae*	Bacillus, typically pleomorphic	Nasopharynx of case or carrier	Airborne, assisted by close contact	Diphtheria
	BACILLUS	*B. anthracis*	Bacillus, spore-forming	Anthrax in animals, especially cattle and sheep	Skin contact with spores in contaminated hides, bristles, bone-meal and sacking; occasionally, by inhalation of spores	Cutaneous anthrax (hide-porter's disease); pulmonary anthrax (wool sorter's disease)
THE SPORING ANAEROBES	*CLOSTRIDIUM*	*Cl. welchii* (*perfringens*) *Cl. oedematiens* (*novyi*) *Cl. septicum*	Bacillus, spore-forming, anaerobic	Intestinal flora of man and animals; spores widely distributed in soil and dust	Wounds contaminated with soil etc.; endogenous infection of wound is possible	Gas gangrene; also *Cl. welchii* food poisoning
		Cl. tetani	Bacillus, terminal spore-forming with drumstick appearance, anaerobic	Occurs in faeces of man and animals; widely distributed in soil and dust	Wounds contaminated with soil, dust, etc.	Tetanus
		Cl. botulinum	Bacillus, spore-forming, anaerobic	Occurs widely in soil and marine mud	Does not typically infect man; toxin is pre-formed in contaminated food	Botulism (form of food poisoning)
	LACTOBACILLUS	*L. acidophilus*	Bacillus, often micro-aerophilic	Human mouth and intestine. Related organisms are commensal in vagina	An association between dental caries and oral lactobacilli is postulated	?Dental caries

TABLE 18.1. *contd.*

Common group name	Genus	Species	Morphology and notable characters	Habitat or reservoir of infection	Common mode or vehicle of infection	Diseases produced in man
THE PYOGENIC COCCI	STREPTOCOCCUS	*Strept. viridans*	Coccus in chains	Commensal in mouth	Endogenous; bacteriaemic	Dental abscess; subacute bacterial endocarditis
		Strept. pyogenes	Coccus in chains; the β-haemolytic streptococcus	Nose and throat of case or carrier	Airborne dust and fomites or contact with a case or carrier	Acute tonsillitis; impetigo; wound infections; puerperal sepsis; otitis media; scarlet fever; rheumatic fever and glomerulonephritis
		Strept. faecalis	Coccus in short chains or pairs	Commensal of large intestine	Endogenous, sometimes exogenous	Urinary tract infections; wound infections; cholecystitis
		Strept. pneumoniae (Pneumococcus)	Coccus, in pairs (diplococcus)	Commensal of upper respiratory tract	Endogenous, or exogenous by airborne spread	Lobar pneumonia; infections of eye and ear; purulent meningitis
	STAPHYLO-COCCUS	*Staph. albus*	Coccus, in clumps; coagulase-negative	Commensal of skin and nasal vestibule; grows in sweat glands and follicles	Not typically associated with infection, but endogenous infection occurs	(See p. 18.70)
		Staph. aureus	Coccus, in clumps; coagulase-positive	Colonizes nasal vestibule and sometimes perineum of carriers; may also occur in groin, axilla, etc.	Endogenous or exogenous from case or carrier by direct or indirect routes	Superficial infections include boils and styes; wound infections; osteomyelitis etc; septicaemia, food poisoning
	GRAM-NEGATIVE BACTERIA					
	NEISSERIA	*N. meningitidis* (Meningococcus)	Coccus, in pairs	Commensal in nasopharynx	Endogenous; usually acquired by airborne spread from case or carrier	Acute meningococcal meningitis
		N. gonorrhoeae (Gonococcus)	Coccus, in pairs	Urogenital canal of human case	Acquired during sexual intercourse, or birth	Gonorrhoea; ophthalmia neonatorum
THE PARVOBACTERIA	HAEMOPHILUS	*H. influenzae*	Bacillus (typically slender)	Commensal in nasopharynx	Endogenous or acquired from carriers	Chronic bronchitis (not influenza); bronchopneumonia; acute purulent meningitis in children
		H. aegyptius (Koch–Weeks bacillus)	Bacillus	Conjunctiva of a case	Contact with a case	A form of conjunctivitis
		H. ducreyi	Bacillus	Genitalia	Acquired during sexual intercourse	Chancroid or soft sore
	BORDETELLA	*Bord. pertussis*	Bacillus (small coccobacillus)	Nasopharynx of a case	Airborne, assisted by close contact	Pertussis (whooping cough)
	BRUCELLA	*Br. abortus* *Br. melitensis* *Br. suis*	Bacillus (small coccobacillus)	Disease in cattle Disease in goats and sheep Disease in pigs	Contact with the infected animal or product (e.g. milk)	Brucellosis (undulant fever)
	PASTEURELLA	*P. pestis*	Bacillus, short, oval but pleomorphic	Disease in rats	Bite of infected rat flea, or airborne spread from a human case	Bubonic plague; pneumonic plague
		P. multocida (*septica*)	Bacillus, like *P. pestis*	Disease in animals	Bite of cat or dog	Wound sepsis following a bite

TABLE 18.1. *contd.*

Common group name	Genus	Species	Morphology and notable characters	Habitat or reservoir of infection	Common mode or vehicle of infection	Diseases produced in man
	VIBRIO	V. cholerae V. eltor	Vibrio, with darting motility	Endemic disease in India and East Pakistan	Water-borne and food-borne, assisted by close contact with cases and carriers	Cholera
	SPIRILLUM	Sp. minus	Spirillum, rigid, with darting motility	Rats	Bite of rat	Rat-bite fever
	PSEUDOMONAS	Ps. pyocyanea (aeruginosa)	Bacillus, resistant to many anti-microbial agents	Present in small numbers in intestinal flora; contaminates basins, slunge-areas, toilets etc.	Endogenous, or by contact with con-taminated areas or instruments	Infected wounds and burns; chronic otitis media, urinary tract infections, septicae-mia
THE ENTEROBACTERIA	ESCHERICHIA	Esch. coli	Bacillus	Commensal in large bowel	Endogenous, some-times exogenous	Wound infections; urinary tract infections; peritonitis, cholecystitis; septi-caemia; some strains cause infantile gastro-enteritis
THE ENTEROBACTERIA	KLEBSIELLA (Aerobacter)	K. aerogenes	Bacillus, typically capsulate	Saprophytic in water, also commensal in respiratory tract and intestine of man and animals	Endogenous, some-times exogenous	Urinary tract infections and other suppurative infections
THE ENTEROBACTERIA		K. pneumoniae (Friedländer's bacillus)	Bacillus, typically capsulate	Respiratory tract of man	?	Friedländer's pneumonia
THE ENTEROBACTERIA	PROTEUS	P. mirabilis and other species	Bacillus, pleo-morphic; swarming growth on agar media	Commensal in large bowel; widely distributed in soil	Endogenous, some-times exogenous	Urinary-tract infections; wound infections
THE ENTEROBACTERIA	SALMONELLA	S. typhi S. paratyphi A, B and C	Bacillus	Small bowel of cases and carriers; infected gall-bladder of carrier	Water-borne or food-borne by ingestion	Typhoid fever; paratyphoid fever (the enteric fevers)
THE ENTEROBACTERIA		S. typhimurium and other species, e.g. S. enteritidis, S. dublin	Bacillus	Disease in animals and man; important reservoirs of infection in cattle, rodents, pigs and poultry	Food-borne; ingestion after multiplication in food, especially meat products, egg products and milk	Salmonella food poisoning and other infective conditions
THE ENTEROBACTERIA	SHIGELLA	Sh. dysenteriae Sh. flexneri Sh. boydii Sh. sonnei	Bacillus	Human cases of bacillary dysentery and carriers; contaminated fomites in toilets	Ingestion by direct or indirect hand-to-mouth routes involving faecal contamination	Bacillary dysentery
THE BACTEROIDES-FUSIFORMIS GROUP	BACTEROIDES	Bact. fragilis and other species	Bacillus, pleo-morphic; anaerobic	Commensal in mouth and intestine of man and animals; present in vaginal flora	Endogenous	Appendicitis and peritonitis; wound infection; brain abscess; septicaemia
THE BACTEROIDES-FUSIFORMIS GROUP	FUSOBACTERIUM	F. fusiformis	Bacillus, spindle-shaped, anaerobic	Commensal in mouth and intestine	?Endogenous	Vincent's gingivitis and stomatitis is associated with this organism and Borr. vincentii

TABLE 18.1. *contd.*

Common group name	Genus	Species	Morphology and notable characters	Habitat or reservoir of infection	Common mode or vehicle of infection	Diseases produced in man
THE SPIROCHAETES →	BORRELIA	Borr. vincentii	Flexuous spirochaete, with 3–8 irregular coils, anaerobic	Commensal in mouth	Endogenous assisted by lowered local resistance; exogenous by kissing	Vincent's infection of gums or throat
		Borr. recurrentis (obermeieri)	As above	Blood and spleen of infected cases	Bite of infected body-louse	European (louse-borne) relapsing fever
		Borr. duttonii	As above	Infected cases and infected rodents	Contamination of scratch or tick-bite with infected excreta of tick	West African relapsing fever (African tick fever)
	TREPONEMA	T. pallidum	Spirochaete, with 6–12 very delicate coils having pointed ends	Infected human cases	Sexual intercourse	Syphilis
		T. pertenue	As above	Infected human cases	Direct contact with sores; probably also fly-borne	Yaws
		T. carateum	As above	Infected human cases	As above	Pinta
	LEPTOSPIRA	L. icterohaemorrhagiae	Spirochaete, numerous close coils, hooked ends	Disease in rats	Contact with rat urine or contaminated water etc.	Weil's disease (haemorrhagic jaundice)
		L. canicola	As above	Disease in dogs and pigs	Contact with dog's urine or infected pigs	Canicola fever
THE RICKETTSIAE	RICKETTSIA	R. prowazekii	Very small and variable in form; obligate intracellular parasites	Alimentary tract of blood-sucking arthropods; also disease in animals	Louse-borne	Epidemic typhus fever
		R. mooseri			Flea-borne	Endemic typhus
		R. rickettsii			Tick-borne	Tick-borne typhus
		R. tsutsugamushi			Mite-borne	Scrub-typhus (mite-borne typhus)
	COXIELLA	Cox. burnetii	Very small and variable in form; obligate intracellular parasite	Disease in cattle, sheep and goats	Ingestion or inhalation	Q fever

This table lists the important bacteria, spirochaetes and rickettsiae that are known to produce disease in man. There are inevitable omissions and generalizations. For example, many known pathogenic leptospirae are not listed. Moreover, the inclusion of the genus *Coxiella* in the Rickettsiae is not strictly correct. The table nevertheless provides a useful practical guide for further studies.

An interesting substance associated mainly with cell walls of Gram-positive bacteria is a polymer of teichoic acid which appears to be composed of ribitol or glycerol units linked by phosphodiester linkages. The mucopeptides provide the characteristic rigidity of the bacterial cell wall; the function of the teichoic acid residues has not yet been determined.

The lack of the mucocomplex in mammalian cell structure has been turned to great clinical advantage. Penicillin and some other antibiotics act by inhibiting mucopeptide synthesis and thus interfere with bacterial cell wall formation. Penicillin specifically interrupts the peptide cross-linkage mechanism and the rigidity of the structure is lost (p. 20.10).

PROTOPLAST FORMATION

Under highly selective conditions it is possible to remove the cell wall without rupturing the cytoplasmic membrane; the resultant body, the **protoplast**, then assumes a spherical shape, even if the original cell was rod-shaped. This type of alteration demonstrates the structural importance of the cell wall. The enzyme lysozyme (a muramidase) hydrolyses the N-acetylglucosamine linkage with N-acetylmuramic acid in some bacteria and produces protoplasts; these are extremely vulnerable to changes in osmotic concentration and must be held under strict environmental control if they are to survive.

L-FORMS

Among the eubacteria, errors in mucopeptide synthesis also occur naturally from time to time. The resultant cells are unusually variable in shape, and have other atypical properties that make them highly vulnerable to deleterious influences. They are particularly sensitive to changes in osmotic pressure. If they survive, they tend to revert to typical forms, but the atypical form is sometimes stable

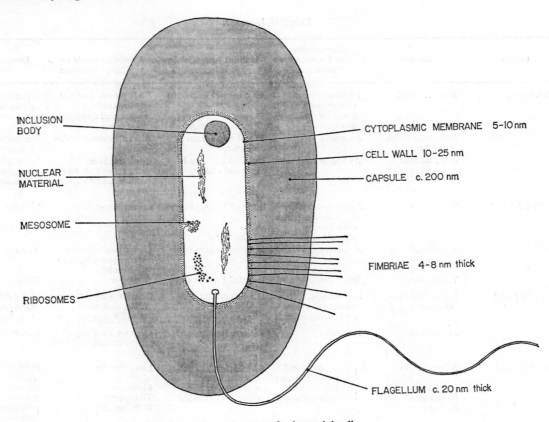

INCLUSION BODY

NUCLEAR MATERIAL

MESOSOME

RIBOSOMES

CYTOPLASMIC MEMBRANE 5-10 nm

CELL WALL 10-25 nm

CAPSULE c. 200 nm

FIMBRIAE 4-8 nm thick

FLAGELLUM c. 20 nm thick

FIG. 18.5. Diagram of a bacterial cell.

and can then be passed through repeated subcultures. These unusual eubacterial forms are called L-forms, and may be of importance as a mechanism of bacterial persistence in the presence of concentrations of penicillin that are lethal to normal bacterial cells. L-forms are also able to pass through filters that normally exclude rigid bacteria.

THE EXTRACELLULAR LAYER

Some species of bacteria are surrounded by a colloid material containing polysaccharides. This may form a water-soluble slime which disperses from the bacteria when they are grown in fluid culture media. When colonies of slime-producing bacteria are grown on solid media, however, they have a mucoid appearance and consistency. In some species the colloid material forms a definite **capsule**. Bacterial capsules are most clearly delineated by using the wet film India ink method with the phase-contrast microscope; it should be appreciated that the diffraction halo immediately outside the bacterial body is not the capsule but the highly refractile outline of the bacterium, and the capsule lies outside this. When capsules are less than 0·2 μm in width they are not visible under the light microscope and can be de-

tected only by indirect serological methods or by electron microscopy, when their presence is implied by the blurring of the usually crisp edge of the cell wall and a peripheral haze that makes the background less definite.

The capsule consists of a dilute solution of polysaccharide or sometimes polypeptide or protein; these, by acting as antigens or haptens (p. 22.4), give the bacteria highly specific immunological properties. This sometimes provides a basis for differentiation of types within a species, e.g. pneumococci; the capsule is made more visible when capsular antigen combines with specific antibody and this is sometimes referred to as the **capsule-swelling reaction**. Many saprophytic and parasitic bacteria produce capsules under suitable environmental conditions. Capsulation is not invariably related to virulence, but capsules tend to endow pathogenic organisms with enhanced resistance to phagocytosis and other antibacterial agencies, and so may be important in determining pathogenicity (e.g. p. 18.69).

THE APPENDAGES

Flagella act as organs of locomotion and can be visualized directly in the electron microscope, or by the light microscope after silver stains have been deposited on them; silver deposition increases the apparent width of the flagellum. Some of the possible distributions of flagella around the cell are seen in fig. 18.6, but in any

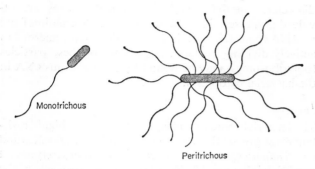

FIG. 18.6. Two examples of distribution of flagella around the bacterial cell.

one species there is usually only one pattern of distribution. Each flagellum is a thin, spirally-twisted filament, approximately 20 nm in width, usually longer than the cell from which it emerges. It consists of a protein, **flagellin**, which is related to muscle myosin.

Because of the technical difficulties of obtaining satisfactory silver-stained preparations and the time required to prepare material for viewing in the electron microscope, the presence of flagella is usually inferred by observing either motility in **hanging drop preparations** of fluid cultures under the microscope, or the spread of growth when the organism is inoculated into a tube of semi-solid agar. The latter method is preferable, since the inexperienced microscopist may confuse motility with Brownian movement. Furthermore, motility is intermittent and may be missed if frequent observations of hanging drop preparations are not made. The significance of motility to bacteria is not known, but it may allow escape from an unfavourable environment to areas where nutrients are more abundant.

Fimbriae are also filamentous appendages, but unlike flagella they are not associated with motility. They lack the spiral form of flagella and are usually more numerous, shorter and thinner (fig. 18.7); they therefore remain invisible under the light microscope even when attempts are made to increase their width artificially. Little is known of the function of fimbriae, but they may act by adhering to cell surfaces and so be of value in bringing bacteria into close contact with concentrated sources of nutrients. The affinities of different fimbriae for cells varies and while the adhesiveness of most fimbriae is readily inhibited by D-mannose, some are mannose-resistant. A few fimbriate species are devoid of all adhesive activity. Fimbriae occur in saprophytic and commensal bacteria as well as in pathogenic Gram-

negative micro-organisms, and they are apparently unrelated to any known mechanism of pathogenicity.

Fimbriae of several types are known to occur in different species of Gram-negative bacilli, but have not yet been found in other groups. They differ in their morphology and adhesive properties. Type-1 fimbriae are relatively thick; they confer haemagglutinating activity on the bacilli that bear them and, as this can be inhibited by mannose, are referred to as mannose-sensitive (MS). Type-2 fimbriae resemble type-1 fimbriae but they are non-haemagglutinating. Type-3 fimbriae are thin and confer mannose-resistant (MR)

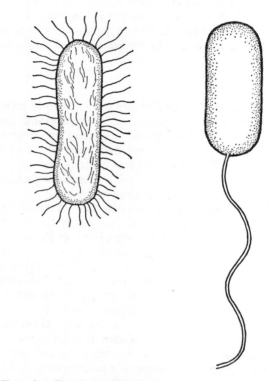

FIG. 18.7. Two bacterial cells at comparable magnifications to illustrate fimbriae and a flagellum.

haemagglutinating activity on the parent bacilli, but the red cells must first be treated with tannic acid before they are agglutinable. Type-4 fimbriae are very thin and have MR haemagglutinating activity for fresh red cells. Type-5 fimbriae are monopolar and have been observed in one *Pseudomonas* species, and type-6 fimbriae are very long and scanty structures observed in one *Klebsiella* species.

The F fimbria, **F pilus** or **sex fimbria**, resembles a type-1 fimbria, but a bacillus bears only 1–4 of these. The sex fimbria (p. 18.57) is long and flexible and possesses specific adsorption sites for certain bacteriophages that have affinity for this structure. It is involved in the transmission of genetic material from the donor cell to the recipient in the process of conjugation (p. 18.56).

NUCLEAR BODIES

These are only detectable in unstained bacteria by a special phase-contrast procedure; however, if the RNA content of the cytoplasm is first reduced by treatment with hydrochloric acid, it is possible to differentiate the DNA-containing nuclear bodies which then stain more deeply than the RNA-depleted cytoplasm. The nuclear apparatus does not possess a limiting nuclear membrane or nucleoli, and it is not seen as a nucleus; it consists of ovoid or elongated condensations of DNA which divide by simple fission, not by meiosis. Depending on the stage of the cell growth there may be one, two, four or even more nuclear bodies within a single bacterium.

INCLUSIONS

These, unlike nuclear bodies, are not constantly present in all bacteria, but several types of inclusion granule may be observed in many species, and they are generally thought to be reserves of nutrient materials. Polysaccharide granules are seen in some bacteria after staining with iodine; in other species, similar material is present in more diffuse form throughout the cytoplasm.

Lipid granules are recognized by their affinity for fat-soluble dyes, e.g. Burdon's method stains the granules black and counterstains the remaining cytoplasm red with basic fuchsin; since in Gram-stained films such granules remain unstained they may be mistaken for spores, but they are usually much smaller than spores and frequently more than one granule is present in a single bacterium. Lipid granules usually have polymerized β-hydroxybutyric acid as the main constituent, and this seems to be a store of carbon and energy.

Volutin granules are seen in several bacterial species but have a particular significance in the genus *Corynebacterium* since they are produced typically by the diphtheria bacillus. They contain polymerized metaphosphate and considerable amounts of nucleoprotein. Volutin granules are readily demonstrated by special staining procedures such as Albert's method (p. 18.16); their characteristic staining properties account for their alternative title of **metachromatic granules.**

MESOSOMES

These are intriguing structures formed by complex invaginations of the cytoplasmic membrane and seen in EM preparations of thin sections of most Gram-positive and some Gram-negative bacteria. They are thought to be involved in the formation of cross-walls in cell divisions or in the control of cell division, but other suggested roles for mesosomes include a mitochondrion-like function and

a site of attachment for replicating DNA. Bacterial spores are developed from mesosomal structures (see below).

RIBOSOMES

These are cytoplasmic granules, about 10–20 nm in diameter, containing protein and RNA. They are involved in transcribing protein sequence information from m-RNA to protein and they are particularly numerous in actively dividing bacteria. Aggregates of these particles (polyribosomes) may be bound by strands of m-RNA in the bacterial cytoplasm.

SPORES

The bacterial spore or **endospore** represents a highly resistant resting phase that develops particularly in *Bacillus* and *Clostridium*; spores can survive adverse environmental conditions that would kill ordinary vegetative cells of the species concerned. For example, most vegetative cells of the medically important bacteria are killed by exposure to moist heat at temperatures of 60–70°C for 10–15 min, whereas many sporing species must be exposed to temperatures of 100–121°C for a similar period before they are killed. The resistance of spores to deleterious agents is variously ascribed to the impermeability of the outer spore coat, the spore's low metabolic activity and its low content of unbound water, but there are valid objections to these simple theories. Another hypothesis is that condensation forces involved during contraction of the spore's internal structure help to stabilize bonds that would otherwise be broken by physical stresses that kill vegetative forms.

Each vegetative cell normally forms only one spore and each spore can germinate into only one vegetative cell; thus no multiplication is involved. In any one sporing species the size, shape and position of the spore in the parent vegetative cell are relatively constant and this assists in the identification of the species (fig. 18.8).

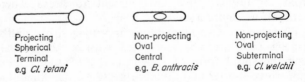

| Projecting Spherical Terminal e.g *Cl. tetani* | Non-projecting Oval Central e.g *B. anthracis* | Non-projecting Oval Subterminal e.g *Cl. welchii* |

FIG. 18.8. Shape and position of spores used in the identification of species. From Gillies R.R. (1968).

The cell committed to sporulation accumulates the necessary materials in the spore field and here the **forespore** becomes compartmented by a complex invagination of the cytoplasmic membrane. The spore is then developed as a mesosomal structure between a double membrane; the innermost **core** is invested in a thin **spore membrane** or **wall**; external to this is the **cortex** which can be shown to have a laminar structure, and this is protected by one or more **spore coats** of dense material. In some species, a thin **exosporium** forms the outermost layer and this may be patterned with complex folds and ridges (fig. 18.9).

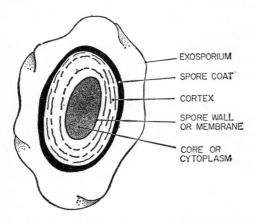

EXOSPORIUM
SPORE COAT
CORTEX
SPORE WALL OR MEMBRANE
CORE OR CYTOPLASM

FIG. 18.9. The structure of a mature bacterial spore in the free state, i.e. liberated from the remnants of the vegetative cell.

In unstained preparations, spores may be recognized within the vegetative cell by their high refractility, whereas in preparations treated with simple stains or by Gram's method the spore remains as an unstained clear area; the relative acid-fastness of spores allows their recognition by employing a modified Ziehl–Neelsen technique in which the concentration of the mineral acid used for decolourizing is lower than that used for strongly acid-fast structures.

Bacterial spores contain large amounts of calcium and equivalent amounts of dipicolinic acid (DPA) which does not occur elsewhere in nature. DPA appears to form a chelate with calcium which is involved in the characteristic heat-resistance of spores. The resistance of spores to chemicals and desiccation, on the other hand, seems to depend on the protection afforded by the tough spore coats. The sulphur content of the spore coat may contribute to the known radiation-resistance of spores.

Because of their power of survival in the outside environment separate from the human or animal host, spores play an important part in the epidemiology of diseases such as anthrax, tetanus and gas gangrene.

Microscopy

A modern light microscope can resolve structural detail down to about 0·25 μm with an oil-immersion lens system having a focal length of about 2 mm. The efficiency of a small lens working at such critical limits is largely dependent on the amount of light that it can gather and use without distortion. Much light is lost in such a system by refraction of oblique rays as they pass from the glass slide into the less dense air. The emerging light ray is bent towards the glass and passes wide of the front lens of the microscope objective. This loss is avoided by placing oil of a refractive index similar to that of glass, between the slide and the objective. The oil-immersion lens should be used in conjunction with a source of artificial light of adequate intensity.

The bacterial cell is a very feebly refractile structure and it is virtually transparent. Unless special optical effects are exploited, it is difficult to see the unstained cell with the light microscope; the experienced microscopist can visualize bacteria in wet films by suitable manipulation of the amount of light entering the microscope, but little detail can be seen. Examination of wet films has a useful but limited place in diagnostic work and stained smears or films are used as a routine.

The principle of **dark-ground microscopy** is of special advantage in studying some of the spirochaetes which are not readily stained (fig. 18.10). This reveals details of external morphology and motility but internal cell structure is not seen.

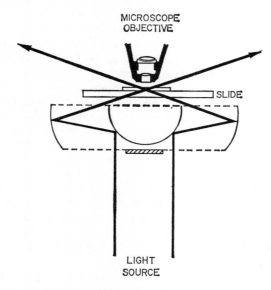

MICROSCOPE OBJECTIVE
SLIDE
LIGHT SOURCE

FIG. 18.10. The principle of dark-ground illumination. A cone of light is directed at the object in such a way that the individual rays pass obliquely through the slide. An object is thus seen as a brightly illuminated structure against a dark background.

Living, unstained cells can be clearly visualized by **phase-contrast microscopy**, which reveals some details of intracellular structure. A special system is incorporated in the microscope so that the retardation of the light rays as they pass through a cell in the field is augmented, and the ray is set maximally out of phase with that of the uninterrupted light path. When these two sets of light waves, the direct and the diffracted rays, pass through the microscope and converge, there is interference in proportion to the degree of phase variation. As the phase difference is augmented, the contrasts in the image are increased and an image of good quality is seen. The phase-contrast microscope is excellent for studies of gross cell structure and motility and it can be used to visualize living cells.

Measurement of the size of bacteria

Medical microbiologists seldom indulge in accurate measurement of bacteria, and ideas of size are usually communicated in a relative fashion. Cocci are known to measure about 1 μm in diameter whereas bacilli vary greatly in size from species to species; the anthrax bacillus is large in comparison with the bacillus of whooping cough.

The average cell size of any species, and particularly of rod-shaped bacilli, is affected by cultural conditions and many other factors. Distorted **involution forms** occur in old cultures or in the presence of various antibacterial agents. The dimensions of a bacterium observed in a heat-fixed stained smear may be considerably different from those of the cell in its natural environment.

Despite these reservations, methods for measuring bacteria can be of practical value and the earlier procedures have been largely replaced by EM techniques. Suspensions of the organism and of latex particles of known size, e.g. 0·1 μm, are mixed and after fixation the mixture is viewed in the EM and photographed; measurement of the organisms in relation to the latex particles gives an accurate estimation of bacterial size.

Of the older methods, the most exact again involves photography. A photograph at high magnification is taken of a smear of the bacterial culture on a slide. The slide is then replaced by a stage micrometer slide on which a millimetre scale graduated into 100 or 200 parts has been etched. The scale is photographed at the same magnification as the culture. From the prints thus obtained, the length of the bacterial cell is measured in relation to the micrometer scale.

As for blood cells, an electronic counter may be used for both counting and sizing bacteria.

Staining procedures

Bacteria in smears or tissue sections on slides are usually stained prior to microscopic examination. Very many staining procedures have been developed to facilitate studies of various morphological features and properties of the bacterial cell. The present description is restricted to three procedures that are in daily use for staining smears in diagnostic laboratories.

Gram's stain, of which there are now many modifications, was first described by Gram in 1884. A pararosaniline dye, e.g. methyl violet, is poured on to a prepared heat-fixed film and left for 5 min; this is followed by an iodine solution for 2 min. The film is then treated with acetone or another decolourizing agent for 5 sec and washed with water. Those organisms that retain the primary dye complex appear dark purple and are termed **Gram-positive**; those bacteria that are decolourized by the acetone take up a counterstain such as basic fuchsin applied for 30 sec and so appear pink and are termed **Gram-negative**.

Although the Gram stain has been in use for over 80 years and separates bacteria into two large groups, the difference in the chemical composition of these groups is not fully determined.

Gram-positive species contain a limited range of amino acids in their cell walls; in particular, aromatic and sulphur-containing amino acids are absent. These are present in the cell walls of Gram-negative species, which incorporate a range of amino acids similar to that in most common proteins. Moreover, the lipid content of the cell walls of Gram-negative organisms is very much greater than that of the walls of Gram-positive cells, yet paradoxically it appears to be the cell wall of Gram-positive bacteria that prevents the extraction of the primary methyl violet-iodine complex by the decolourizing agent.

Ziehl–Neelsen's stain was introduced by Paul Ehrlich and the modifications by Ziehl and Neelsen were minor (p. 18.2). Certain bacteria, notably tubercle bacilli, and also bacterial spores and the clubs of *Actinomyces*, can resist decolourization by strong mineral acids after they have been stained by a strong reagent such as carbol fuchsin, and are thus termed **acid-fast**. To demonstrate acid-fastness, a heat-fixed film is first stained for 5 min with carbol fuchsin which is heated intermittently during the process to assist the penetration of the dye; thereafter the excess dye is washed off with water and the preparation flooded with sulphuric acid. The concentration of acid used depends on the material that is being investigated; for tubercle bacilli it is 20 per cent, for leprosy bacilli 5 per cent, for actinomyces clubs 1 per cent and for bacterial spores 0·25–0·5 per cent. After the acid has acted for 1 min, it is washed off with water and fresh acid is successively applied at the appropriate concentration until adequate decolourization is achieved. After a final rinse in water, Loeffler's methylene blue is applied to the preparation for 15 sec. Any acid-fast material retains the bright red carbol fuchsin whereas non-acid-fast structures are counterstained light blue.

Albert's stain is one of several that may be used to demonstrate the presence of volutin granules in bacteria; in diagnostic practice the demonstration of such granules is restricted to the identification of different members of the Gram-positive genus *Corynebacterium*. It must be noted that Gram-negative bacilli frequently contain volutin granules so that a Gram-stained film must also be examined in parallel with an Albert-stained preparation. The technique consists of applying a mixture of toluidine blue and malachite green to a fixed film for 3–5 min; the slide is washed in water and blotted dry before an iodine solution is applied and allowed to act for 1 min. Finally the slide is washed in water and dried before being examined microscopically; any volutin granules show as black areas within the cell, which is itself coloured green.

MEDICAL MYCOLOGY

The great majority of the thousands of known species of fungi are saprophytic. They are involved in natural processes of decomposition in the soil and in vegetable and animal debris, and they include species of agricultural and industrial importance. Some, notably *Penicillium notatum* which produces penicillin (fig. 18.11), are of great benefit

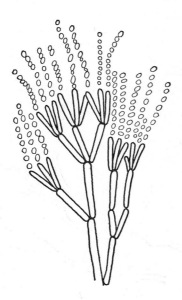

FIG. 18.11. *Penicillium* species.

to man. Other relatively harmless species are well known for the trouble they cause as contaminants of foodstuffs and of culture media in the laboratory. Many fungi cause disease in plants, but few are recognized pathogens of man and animals. However it is probable that the airborne spores of otherwise harmless species provoke more pulmonary reactions in man than is generally recognized at present (p. 23.6).

In man, fungal infections called **mycoses** are often superficial, involving skin, hair or nail tissue. The **superficial mycoses**, e.g. athlete's foot ('foot-rot'), are readily transmissible and are world-wide in distribution. In contrast, **deep** or **systemic mycoses** are relatively rare in some countries, e.g. Britain, but they are common in others, e.g. certain parts of the USA.

Classification of fungi pathogenic to man

The true fungi or *Eumycetes* can be classified into four groups on a morphological basis.

Moulds or **filamentous fungi** grow as branching filaments or **hyphae** that interlace to form a felted mass or **mycelium**; the hyphae are much larger than bacterial filaments and the main part of the vegetative mycelium grows into the material on which the mould is growing and absorbs nutrients. In contrast, the **aerial mycelium** rises into the air from the surface of the mould, and the hyphae give rise to various kinds of sexual spores which are readily disseminated into the atmosphere (fig. 18.12).

Yeasts or **unicellular fungi** are single round or ovoid cells that reproduce by bud formation and not by forming sexual spores; on solid culture media, yeasts form colonies similar to those of bacteria and unlike the fluffy or powdery colonies of moulds.

Yeast-like fungi also reproduce by budding, but grow either as round or ovoid cells, or as non-branching filaments or **pseudohyphae**; pseudohyphae can be further differentiated from true hyphae in that they do not give rise to spores but reproduce by forming buds at points where the filament constricts and divides. Thus, branching may seem to have occurred where two buds arise from the same end of a filament. On suitable solid media, colonies of yeast-like fungi are usually large, moist and creamy, similar to those of staphylococci.

Dimorphic fungi are those that grow in a yeast form (parasitic form) in animal tissues or *in vitro* when cultures are incubated at 37°C, but are present as a mycelial growth (saprophytic form) when incubated at 22°C or grown naturally in the soil.

The much more formal systematic classification of fungi depends essentially on the nature of their sexual processes and four classes are defined; it should be noted that the sexual stages are difficult to induce and are thus rarely observed.

CLASS I: PHYCOMYCETAE

Members of this class usually form non-septate hyphae; at the ends of the aerial hyphae indefinite numbers of asexual spores, **sporangiospores**, are contained within the sporangium or spore case; in addition sexual spores called **zygospores** are formed. These are large, thick-walled bodies produced when the tips of two hyphae come into apposition and their contents fuse.

CLASS II: ASCOMYCETAE

Genera in this class are characterized by the septate nature of the hyphae, and by the formation of various types of asexual spores and sexual ascospores; these latter occur usually as two, four or eight spores within a spore sac or ascus. Asexual spores produced in this class include **conidia** which are formed on special hyphae (conidiophores); they are produced by constriction of the conidiophore and become pinched off.

CLASS III: BASIDIOMYCETAE

Here again the hyphae are septate and sexual fusion produces a club-shaped basidium on the surface of which there are usually four sexual basidiospores.

CLASS IV: FUNGI IMPERFECTI

Most of the moulds, yeasts, yeast-like fungi and dimorphic fungi that are pathogenic to man belong to this class which includes all fungi in which a sexual stage does not occur or has not yet been observed. The class, therefore, encompasses those fungi that cannot be placed in one or other of the first three classes. Many *Fungi imperfecti* resemble *Ascomycetae* in morphology.

Since only a very few *Eumycetes* are pathogenic to man, a detailed classification of genera within the above four classes is not necessary. The following outline gives an account of some of the commonly occurring fungi with notes on the diseases which they cause. The main groups are dealt with according to the following subdivisions:

(1) fungi associated with superficial infections involving skin, hair and nails; these include the dermatophytes;

(2) pathogenic yeast-like fungi and pathogenic yeasts; these include *Candida albicans*, the cause of thrush and *Cryptococcus neoformans*, the cause of cryptococcosis:

(3) pathogenic dimorphic fungi include the causative organisms of North American blastomycosis, coccidioidomycosis, histoplasmosis, sporotrichosis and chromoblastomycosis;

(4) a miscellaneous group associated with maduromycosis, a chronic infection affecting the tissues of the foot;

(5) *Aspergillus* species associated with some conditions of medical interest;

(6) *Rhizopus* and *Mucor* species which cause phycomycotic infections.

Fungi associated with superficial infections affecting keratin include *Malassezia furfur* which causes a condition called pityriasis versicolor. This is a chronic infection of the skin characterized by the development of brownish desquamating macules over the trunk. Fungi and higher bacteria are also associated with relatively benign infections involving the hair of the axillary and pubic regions. *Pityrosporum ovale* (the bottle bacillus) is a commensal fungus often found on normal skin; it is seen in dandruff scales and may be causally related to seborrhoeic conditions of the scalp. In practice, the important fungi with affinity for keratin are those associated with ringworm infections and termed the dermatophytes. Drugs effective against fungi are described on p. 20.33.

The dermatophytes

The **ringworm fungi** produce superficial infections that spread peripherally from a focal point or a series of foci in the skin to give rise to ring-like lesions with an advancing active edge; infections of skin, hair and nails never extend deeper than the keratinous layer. The common dermatophytoses, called **ringworm** or **tinea**, are caused by various species belonging to one or other of three genera of *Fungi imperfecti*: *Trichophyton*, *Microsporum* and *Epidermophyton*; some species of these fungi infect primarily man and are termed **anthropophilic**, whereas others infect primarily animals and are termed **zoophilic**. Infections with anthropophilic species are usually acquired from human sources and the reaction to such an infection is generally less acute and more difficult to eradicate. Most of the dermatophytic fungi are found throughout the world, and many of them can be isolated from domestic pets and farm animals; transmission to children from dogs, cats and calves is common. **Geophilic** species in soil may also infect man. Some species fluoresce in ultraviolet light, and this can be of use in the detection of infected hairs.

When preparations of infected tissue are examined

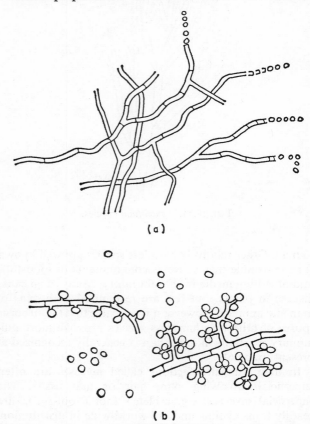

Fig. 18.12. (a) Septate branched hyphae forming a mycelium and showing the production of arthrospores by terminal segmentation. (b) Microconidia.

microscopically only two forms of the fungus can be seen, the vegetative mycelium and arthrospores, i.e. asexual spores derived from hyphae fragmenting into individual short, wide, thick-walled cells. Infection is transmitted to a new host by the resistant arthrospores which germinate and give rise to new hyphae when they are deposited on skin, especially if this is damaged by scratching or is moist, as in the webs of the toes.

The identification of genera and species of dermatophytic fungi depends on microscopic examination of the infected tissue, followed by cultivation of the material, allowing macroscopic examination of the resultant colonies; final identification is made or confirmed by microscopic examination of the sporing mycelium. This latter step allows the recognition of the size, shape and distribution of the various kinds of conidia. **Microconidia** are small, single-celled oval or round structures that occur on spore-bearing hyphae (fig. 18.12); they are often very numerous and are typically associated with *Trichophyton* species; they are generally scarce in *Microsporum* preparations and are typically not seen in cultures of *Epidermophyton*. **Macroconidia** are large, elongated, thick or thin-walled structures compartmented by transverse septa (fig. 18.13). The dermatophytes can be divided into the three genera noted above on the basis of macroconidial morphology; *Microsporum* produces large, fusiform macroconidia with generally thick walls and many septa; *Trichophyton* produces scanty, small, relatively thin-walled and irregularly

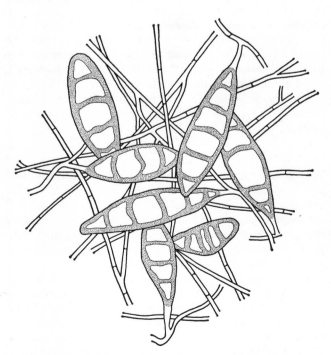

FIG. 18.13. Macroconidia of *Microsporum gypseum.*

cylindrical macroconidia, and *Epidermophyton* produces medium-sized, fairly thick-walled, pear-shaped structures (fig. 18.14).

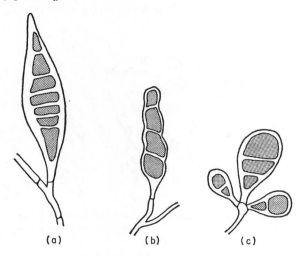

FIG. 18.14. Macroconidia typically produced by the dermatophytes; (a) *Microsporum*; (b) *Trichophyton*; (c) *Epidermophyton*.

Pathogenic yeast-like fungi and pathogenic yeasts

CANDIDA SPECIES

Candida albicans and other species of *Candida* are yeast-like fungi that occur commensally in man and animals. *C. albicans* (monilia) is encountered commonly as a human pathogen and it is usually involved in relatively benign superficial infections such as oral, oesophageal or vaginal **candidiasis** or thrush; the term derives from the speckled appearance on the mucous membrane. These consist of masses of mycelium and there is practically no inflammatory response in the tissue. The organism is a large Gram-positive cell, normally present in relatively small numbers in the gastrointestinal, respiratory and female genital tracts. In material from lesions in which it is associated with actual disease, it produces yeast-like cells and elongated processes that resemble hyphae (pseudohyphae, see fig. 18.15). It can be cultured readily on laboratory media and produces creamy soft colonies which initially resemble those of staphylococci. *Candida* organisms are resistant to most antibiotics and their growth is therefore favoured in a debilitated host if broad-spectrum antibiotic therapy is instituted (p. 20.9). The opportunist nature of candida infections is evident as the host is rarely attacked unless there is some predisposing factor; debility in early infancy is associated with oral thrush; patients with anaemia, diabetes and other conditions may develop oral or vaginal thrush; vaginal thrush is fairly commonly associated with pregnancy. Infection of the skin with *C. albicans* is usually limited to skin folds and other moist areas of the body surface; the infection can also involve the hands of people whose occupation involves prolonged immersion of the hands in water. If the nail bed becomes involved, the infection is difficult to eradicate.

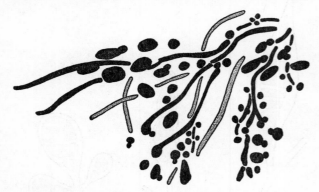

FIG. 18.15. *Candida albicans.* The typical large budding yeast-cell forms are seen, with elongated cells that form pseudohyphae.

In contrast to the usual surface infections, *C. albicans* also causes deep infections, when it may invade the respiratory tract, as in patients with chronic bacterial respiratory infections. Generalized candidiasis of the intestinal tract is sometimes associated with the administration of antimicrobial agents or immunosuppressive drugs and corticosteroids.

CRYPTOCOCCUS NEOFORMANS

This is a true yeast and reproduces by budding; it does not produce hyphae or pseudohyphae. *C. neoformans* can be isolated from bird droppings, from various animals and occasionally from faeces of healthy humans. **Cryptococcosis** occurs occasionally in Britain.

In human cases of infection, which are commonly fatal, cryptococcosis may be acquired endogenously or the source may be animal or avian; the disease usually runs a subacute or chronic course and, although the organism can be isolated from the skin and lungs of patients, it has a marked predilection for the brain and meninges and also the joints. The lesions consist of granulomata and may resemble tuberculosis. In the meninges, little inflammatory reaction may be seen, while in skin the lesions may be nonspecific abscesses.

The yeast has a characteristic microscopic appearance; it is ovoid, thick-walled, about 5–15 μm in diameter and surrounded by a thick capsule which can be clearly defined in an India ink preparation (fig. 18.16). A proportion of the cells may be seen to be budding. Like all other fungi, *Cryptococcus neoformans* is an aerobe; it produces mucoid colonies on suitable culture media. The organism was formerly known as *Torula histolytica* and the disease was referred to as torulosis or European blastomycosis.

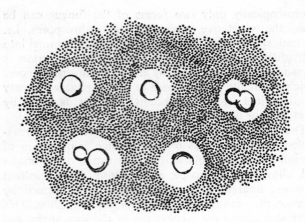

FIG. 18.16. *Cryptococcus neoformans*; budding cells with capsules defined by India ink.

Pathogenic dimorphic fungi

BLASTOMYCES DERMATITIDIS

This dimorphic fungus occurs as thick-walled, small budding spheres in infected tissues, and produces filaments when grown in cultures at room temperature. When grown on blood agar, the colonies are soft and wrinkled. On special glucose agar, brown colonies develop showing branching septate hyphae with round or pear-shaped spores. The organism causes **North American blastomycosis** which is a chronic granulomatous condition that may be localized in the skin or generalized throughout the body. The skin lesion is a pustule or irregular suppurating ulcer, and blood spread may affect many other organs. The organism usually enters the body through the respiratory tract and the disease may remain limited to the lungs, where the lesions consist of numerous small abscesses with intervening granulomatous areas.

The organisms may be seen in sputum, pus and biopsy material, or typical cultures can be grown on blood agar or glucose agar.

COCCIDIOIDES IMMITIS

This is the causative organism of **coccidioidomycosis** which is endemic in the south-west of the USA. In tissues, the dimorphic fungus occurs as large, thick-walled spherical organisms containing endospores. On culture, colonies are white and fluffy and contain hyphae that possess infective arthrospores; these are light and float in air with ease.

The disease follows inhalation of arthrospores which develop into the spherical organisms. The clinical features are usually respiratory and may be minimal or there may be an influenza-like illness. Usually the disease subsides, but in some cases hypersensitivity reactions such as areas of erythema develop a few weeks later in the skin. Thin-walled cavities may develop in the lungs, but they commonly disappear spontaneously. In a few patients a fatal generalized form occurs, called coccidioidal granuloma; this condition resembles disseminated tuberculosis clinically and histologically (p. 21.18).

Specimens of sputum, pus and biopsy material from suspected cases may be examined microscopically and cultured or inoculated into mice. Precipitating antibodies may be detected in the serum.

HISTOPLASMA CAPSULATUM

This is an ovoid budding organism which forms smooth white colonies on blood agar. In culture it produces filamentous forms, but in the tissues it assumes the yeast form (dimorphic fungus). On glucose agar the organism forms large spores, thick-walled and rounded, with small surface projections, and these are diagnostic of the organism.

H. capsulatum occurs in soil and dust; on inhalation it causes **histoplasmosis**, which is more common in the USA than in Britain. The infection is usually confined to the respiratory tract where it produces small granulomatous foci which may become calcified and simulate tuberculosis. A more serious form of the disease is associated with pneumonia. The organisms may be engulfed by macrophages; in a few cases, dissemination to other organs, especially liver, spleen, lymph nodes and intestine, may develop. Dogs and rodents may also be affected. In infected patients the organism is found inside macrophages.

The organism may be found in sputum or blood smears, or biopsies from infected organs. The serum gives positive complement fixation and precipitin tests. A positive skin test with histoplasmin, a filtrate of a broth culture of the organism, may also be demonstrable.

SPOROTRICHUM SCHENCKII

This normally saprophytic dimorphic fungus may be implanted in the skin following a minor injury and it produces a local pustule or ulcer from which lymphatic spread occurs to regional nodes with the formation of abscesses and subcutaneous lesions. The lesions of **sporotrichosis** are granulomata with central necrosis and surrounding chronic inflammation.

Organisms are not often seen in human material such as pus. Culture on glucose agar at 22°C produces characteristic firm colonies in which thin, septate, branching hyphae bear groups of pear-shaped conidia.

DIMORPHIC FUNGI ASSOCIATED WITH CHROMOBLASTOMYCOSIS

This condition is caused by *Cladosporium* and *Phialophora* species, and other organisms. It is a chronic granulomatous infection of the skin, often with lymphatic involvement. Over a period of months, small papillary growths appear on the skin, and may enlarge to form large nodules, usually on the leg. These are histologically granulomata and the causative organisms may be seen within macrophages. Lymphatic obstruction may cause enlargement of the limbs.

The organisms occur as dark brown septate forms which reproduce by splitting, and may be seen in tissue from the skin lesions. On glucose agar, colonies differ depending upon the organisms present, but are usually pigmented.

Miscellaneous fungi associated with disease in man

ORGANISMS CAUSING MADUROMYCOSIS

The condition occurs in tropical countries, particularly India and is known as **mycetoma** or Madura foot. It may be caused by several different filamentous fungi including *Monosporium apiospermum* (*Allescheria boydii*), *Madurella mycetomi*, *Madurella grisea*, and others; a similar condition is produced by *Nocardia* species (p. 18.60). The colour of the granules (microcolonies) which occur in the pus varies with the causative organism involved.

MONOSPORIUM APIOSPERMUM

This fungus produces septate hyphae with peripheral spores and forms yellow granules in tissue exudates. The organism is introduced by trauma into the subcutaneous tissue of the foot, and infective nodules or abscesses develop which often erupt on to the skin surface forming sinuses; muscles and bones are often involved. The lesions contain masses of necrotic and granulating tissue and there is much suppuration and reactive fibrosis. Fungal elements may be seen in smears prepared from crushed granules recovered from the pus. Culture of the pathological material may yield the organism; whitish fluffy colonies are produced on glucose agar and single conidia are typically borne on conidiophores.

ASPERGILLUS SPECIES

Aspergillus fumigatus is essentially a saprophytic fungus. It sometimes causes disease in birds and it may act as a secondary invader in human patients with serious diseases; this is especially so in chronic lung diseases such as tuberculosis or bronchiectasis. Under these circumstances, the fungus appears to colonize an already devitalized area of tissue and then spreads to form a large mycelial mass (mycetoma or aspergilloma); occasionally a type-1 hypersensitivity reaction leading to asthma occurs, as well as a bronchopulmonary Arthus-like reaction (p. 23.6).

Aspergillus species are involved also in opportunist infections, for example in the external auditory meatus (fungal otomycosis) when there has been an initial chronic bacterial infection. Microscopic examination of

Gram-stained or unstained films of sputum may reveal the organism (fig. 18.17). On culture of sputum the organism forms greenish colonies but interpretation is difficult because this is a common saprophyte and it frequently contaminates laboratory cultures. The patient's serum may contain specific precipitins.

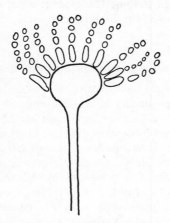

Fig. 18.17. *Aspergillus* species.

Aspergillus flavus produces a series of toxic products called **aflatoxins** which interfere with DNA synthesis and have mutagenic and carcinogenic properties. Groundnuts (peanuts) contaminated with aflatoxins have caused heavy losses in the turkey industry, but there is no record of any case of human poisoning.

RHIZOPUS AND MUCOR SPECIES

Certain species of *Rhizopus* and *Mucor* may produce infections called **phycomycosis** or **mucormycosis** in man. These organisms belong to the class *Phycomycetes*, and they more frequently affect animals. Spores are generally inhaled and may cause disease in debilitated patients with uncontrolled diabetes or receiving broad spectrum antibiotics or corticosteroids; fungal proliferation may involve blood vessels and produce thrombi and metastatic foci. Large non-septate hyphae are present in infected tissue.

Rhizopus and *Mucor* species, like *Penicillium* and *Aspergillus* species, may also be involved as secondary invaders in chronic infections of the external auditory meatus.

Saprophytic fungi and respiratory disease

Pulmonary hypersensitivity to inhaled actinomycete and fungal antigens has been reported in the last few years. The existence of a state of immunity has been confirmed by the finding of precipitating antibodies in the serum. The first of these disorders to be recognized was **Farmer's lung** in which precipitating antibodies could be demonstrated against fungal antigens derived from mouldy hay (*Microsporum faeni*). Subsequently, precipitins have been demonstrated against *Aspergillus clavatus* in maltworkers exposed to high concentrations of *A. clavatus* spores from contaminated barley, and against *Coniosporium corticale* in the serum of maple bark strippers. It is likely that following exposure to high concentrations of any of a variety of fungal spores, individuals would produce precipitating antibodies; thus this form of pulmonary hypersensitivity may be more widespread than has so far been identified. The hypersensitivity reaction induced by the presence of precipitating antibodies is the toxic complex or type 3 form (p. 23.6) and induces a diffuse pulmonary interstitial inflammation. Some of the antigens responsible for this form of hypersensitivity can also provoke the anaphylactic response in susceptible individuals and induce asthma.

Diagnostic mycology

Some pathogenic fungi may present typical microscopic appearances which can be recognized by direct microscopy of unstained or stained pathological material. In most cases, a definitive diagnosis rests on culture and identification of the causative organism. In general, the pathogenic fungi grow more slowly than bacteria and the optimum temperature for their growth is lower. Mycological cultures are incubated routinely at 20–28°C for periods ranging from several days to one or more weeks. Mycological media are often relatively rich in sugar and they may be acid; in addition, the incorporation of antibiotics or antibacterial chemicals inhibits the growth of bacterial contaminants. Sabouraud's glucose agar medium, commonly used in mycology, contains 4 per cent glucose in a peptone agar base at pH 5·4. Cultures are grown in Petri dishes or bottles, but fungi are always aerobic and air must be available. In some cases it is convenient to culture fungi on small blocks of agar medium mounted on a microscopic slide and covered with a coverslip; the exposed sides of the agar block can then be seeded with the culture and mycelial growth extends on to the glass of the slide and the coverslip. These can be examined microscopically and, at a suitable stage, the agar can be removed and the preparation stained for more detailed examination.

SPECIMENS FOR MYCOLOGICAL INVESTIGATION

Direct microscopy of hairs infected with dermatophytic fungi may provide a clue to the genus of fungus involved. *Microsporum* species and some *Trichophyton* species produce sheaths of arthrospores that lie outside the hair shaft (ectothrix infection) whereas in infections by other dermatophytes the fungus occurs within the hair shaft (endothrix infection). The affected hair should be removed with small tweezers with care to preserve the fragile infected area. In the case of infection with *Microsporum canis*, *M. audouini* and *Trichophyton schoenleini*, hair infection may be detected by examination under Wood's (filtered ultraviolet) light; the affected hairs usually fluoresce. When dermatophyte infections affect skin or nail tissue, it is necessary to proceed to culture of the fungus before identification is possible, and this is largely true in the case of hair infections also. Skin or nail scrapings from the active edge of the lesion may be examined microscopically after immersion in a warm aqueous solution of 10–20 per cent potassium hydroxide which renders the keratin more transparent; for this purpose, a fragment of the specimen is held for several minutes in a drop of the solution on a slide, but the process may require a much longer time if nail tissue is involved. Selected fragments of the specimen are also inoculated into suitable media and the fungus may be identified when growth occurs.

Clinical diagnosis of systemic fungal disease may be confirmed by recognition of the causative organism in specimens of pus, CSF or sputum or in tissue sections. The fungi associated with systemic mycoses can also be cultured on suitable media; this is still a specialist field and the procedure is not without danger in inexperienced hands. The dimorphic fungi are yeast-like in their parasitic phase in the tissues but they produce mycelial forms in artificial culture; *Coccidioides immitis* produces infective arthrospores under these conditions. Serological tests are available for the demonstration of precipitating or complement-fixing antibodies in sera of patients with systemic mycotic disease.

SOURCES AND MODES OF SPREAD OF MICROBIAL INFECTION

An **epidemic** of infection is said to exist when many cases arise within a short period of time in the same community. Epidemics may develop in a community where the infection is **endemic**, i.e. is occurring regularly, or alternatively an epidemic may arise by importation into a community in which the disease is not usually encountered; **pandemic spread** of infection implies transmission in epidemic proportions from country to country or continent to continent. Bacillary dysentery is a common endemic bacterial infection in Britain and annual epidemics occur with monotonous regularity; on the other hand, typhoid fever is no longer endemic in this country, having been eliminated by the provision of safe filtered and chlorinated water supplies. Occasionally epidemics occur following spread from individuals who have acquired their infection abroad or from imported foodstuffs. Pandemic spread of infection was in the past associated classically with the intercontinental spread of cholera, but nowadays the common pandemic disease is influenza.

The majority of infections that afflict mankind are acquired from other human beings, but a few, the **zoonoses**, are transmitted from animal sources and still fewer have their origins in the soil; all these are spoken of as **exogenous** in origin, i.e. the pathogen causing the infection has been derived from outside the patient's own tissues. Exogenous infections are frequently epidemic and call for swift preventive action in the community, as well as adequate treatment of individual cases in order to restrict or eliminate further spread.

Some infections are **endogenous**, i.e. the causal organism has been living in association with the host for a period of time as a commensal until some interference with the ecology allows it to assume a pathogenic role; frequently the infection develops at a site or in a tissue other than that in which the organism was commensal. Most endogenously acquired infections do not spread within the human community so that it is possible to concentrate on therapeutic aids for the individual patient; attempts to trace the source to another individual, or prophylactic procedures to protect the community are not then called for.

Endogenous infection

A classical example is subacute bacterial endocarditis for which the organism responsible is usually *Streptococcus viridans*. This is normally resident in the human mouth and throat where it leads a commensal existence; even in healthy people the organisms enter the blood stream on occasions but are destroyed rapidly. If a poor state of dental hygiene exists, bacteriaemia occurs more often and large numbers of organisms are involved; in the presence of certain predisposing congenital or acquired heart lesions, there is a risk of the heart valves becoming infected (p. 18.67). Hence in patients who are known to have such cardiac lesions, dental treatment should be undertaken only when the patient has been given prophylactic penicillin from just before until 48 hr after the dental attention.

Another and much more common example of endogenous infection is infection of the urinary tract with *Escherichia coli* or with enterococci (*Streptococcus faecalis*). In endogenous infection, the organisms almost always come from the patient's intestine and in many instances they become pathogenic in the urinary tract only when the latter is traumatized or when a mechanical abnormality interferes with the free excretion of the urine (p. 18.80).

Other infections which may be endogenous in origin are actinomycosis, Vincent's infection, periodontal disease, oral candidiasis (thrush) and some cases of puerperal and wound sepsis; when the balance between the host and his commensal flora is upset by antibiotic therapy, generalized candidiasis or staphylococcal enterocolitis may occur.

Exogenous infection

The man or animal from which an infecting micro-organism is derived may be suffering from an obvious clinical infection or may be a carrier of the pathogenic micro-organisms. Cases of infection acting as sources for fresh hosts may vary from fulminating, lethal illness through lesser degrees of severity to one so mild that medical advice is not sought; yet there is no evidence to suggest that the more severe the illness the greater is the risk to healthy people in the patient's environment. Indeed the mild, subclinical case is often a more dangerous source of infection than patients more obviously afflicted since an apparently fleeting indisposition may allow an individual to continue his daily labour and leisure pursuits, and thus be in contact with many more people than if he were sick enough to remain at home.

CARRIERS OF INFECTION

Human carriers constitute another source of infection and may be defined as individuals who are not ill but are excreting pathogenic micro-organisms. Two main types are recognized; **convalescent carriers** have suffered from an infection and recovered, but are still excreting the causative organism; **healthy carriers** are people or animals who are excreting a pathogenic organism but in so far as is known have not themselves suffered infection from it. Convalescent patients may be temporary or transient carriers when they excrete the pathogen for only a short time after clinical recovery, or alternatively may be regarded as permanent or chronic carriers if excretion continues for a long period.

The convalescent carrier should not be as great a risk to the community as the healthy carrier since he should be recognized before being discharged from hospital or allowed to mix with the community. On the other hand, healthy carriers can be detected only in surveys undertaken specifically to trace the possible source of an epidemic.

The significance of the carrier of pathogenic micro-organisms in transmitting disease depends on several factors. For example, the age of the carrier is often important; school children carrying group A haemolytic streptococci are more likely than adults to act as a source for other children with whom they mix during school hours, and in this way they may disseminate the infection to many families. The duration of carriage has an influence; at first sight it may appear that the longer the carriage continues the greater is the risk to others, but chronic carriers of *Streptococcus pyogenes* are less commonly the source of fresh infections than are temporary carriers, probably because with increasing duration of carriage the organisms produce less M protein, which is known to be closely associated with the virulence of such strains. The anatomical site at which the organism is carried is important in certain infections; thus it is known that nasal carriers of *Streptococcus pyogenes*, although much less common than throat carriers, are responsible for at least as many new cases of infection, probably because of the much greater number of organisms seeded into the environment (p. 18.67).

In some instances no discoverable association of carriers with other excretors can be made and here the best example is the meningococcus. Especially during epidemics of meningococcal meningitis, the meningococcus is frequently found in people without any known contact with cases or carriers and the organism apparently spreads widely in the community from person to person; thus it may be passed through several people without causing meningitis, but each person is capable of disseminating the organism to others among whom cases may occur. This explains the failure to establish continuity between successive cases which is a feature of many epidemics of meningitis (p. 18.71).

PREVENTIVE MEASURES

Only when the sources and modes of spread of exogenous infections are understood can intelligent action be taken to interrupt the chain of events. Early in this century when diseases such as typhoid fever and diphtheria were rife in Britain, rigorous measures were taken to stem epidemics when they arose and various techniques were introduced to reduce their endemic incidence. Where prophylactic measures can be applied at the community level, e.g. by the provision of a filtered and chlorinated water supply to reduce the hazard of water-borne disease, dramatic improvements follow swiftly. However, at present there are many infections, endemic and epidemic, that cannot be influenced by any method applicable to the entire community. Bacillary dysentery is an example of a disease that continues to increase throughout Britain; this is a reflection of low standards of individual personal hygiene and also indicates the inadequacy of toilets and facilities for hand-washing in many homes, schools, restaurants, hospitals and other public places.

ZOONOSES

What has been said regarding human cases and carriers acting as sources of infection for other individuals applies also to animal sources of infection. The human diseases which are acquired from animals, the zoonoses, are rarely transmitted from one human sufferer to another. Brucellosis, leptospirosis, rabies and pasteurella infections are zoonoses which do not usually spread from the patient to another human being; however salmonella infections from animal sources spread readily within the human community once a case has occurred.

ROUTES OF TRANSMISSION

In some infections, e.g. insect-borne blood infections and venereal diseases, transmission to a healthy individual is normally by a single mechanism, but usually infections are spread in a variety of ways. Sometimes the clinical picture depends on the avenue whereby the new host is infected; in anthrax the mode of infection most common in man is the implantation of the anthrax spore into the skin, frequently via a small abrasion. The almost invariable result is the development of a localized 'malignant pustule'; the term **cutaneous anthrax** is preferred nowadays since the lesion is rarely fatal and pus formation occurs only if the lesion is secondarily infected with a pyogenic organism. In the past, such lesions were commonly seen on the necks and shoulders of porters who unloaded animal hides containing anthrax spores; nowadays **hide-porter's disease** is rare since importation is legally restricted to one port, and unloading and movement of the hides is entirely mechanical until they have been treated chemically to remove or destroy spores. If, however, anthrax spores are inhaled, pulmonary anthrax develops; septicaemia frequently occurs, leading to death. This risk was not uncommon some decades ago when it particularly affected people engaged in wool-sorting and gave rise to **wool-sorters' disease**. This type of infection has been controlled by intelligent legislation and the introduction of mechanical handling combined with local exhaust ventilation to ensure that any spores in the raw wool are removed from the worker's environment. A third type of anthrax infection occurs when the spores are ingested by man; in this very rare form, primary symptoms are gastrointestinal, and the clinical picture is identical with that seen in the animal host (p. 18.64).

Venereal infections

The venereal diseases are transmitted almost exclusively by sexual contact, but primary syphilitic lesions may occasionally appear on sites other than the genitalia as a result of kissing or unusual sexual practices, or are acquired manually by the unsuspecting physician. There are two other classes of people who suffer gonococcal lesions transmitted by non-venereal contact. Babies may contract ophthalmia neonatorum, the eyes being infected directly from the mother during birth. This disease was once common, but rigorous screening of women during the antenatal period and the treatment of any found to be suffering from gonorrhoea has markedly reduced neonatal eye infections. Secondly, in children's nurseries or residential homes, cases of gonococcal ophthalmia or vulvovaginitis may arise by the spread of organisms on moist materials such as sponges or face towels, the source

being an attendant suffering from sexually acquired infection. The intimacy of contact required for transmission of the causative organisms of syphilis and gonorrhoea is due to the susceptibility of these organisms to drying. The smaller number of females than males suffering from venereal infection reflects the moral attitudes of the population, and the increasing use of the contraceptive pill may lead to a greater increase in the number of male cases since some mechanical methods of contraception afford a degree of protection against venereal infection (p. 18.72).

Transmission by blood

Here one immediately thinks of the spread of infection from an infected host to a healthy individual by blood-sucking arthropods, e.g. mosquitoes in the transmission of yellow fever and malaria, or the rat flea in the transmission of plague. Two other methods of blood spread of infection occur, first, congenital infection from mother to foetus, e.g. of the rubella virus and of the smallpox virus, and secondly transmission by syringe; although documentary evidence for the latter method is fragmentary, sepsis at the site of injection is probably the most common risk and occurs regardless of the material being injected. Similarly, although the incidence of serum jaundice or syringe-transmitted jaundice (p. 18.117) is not known, epidemics have occurred in some groups of patients receiving courses of injections or repeated blood investigations at clinics; these epidemics may be disastrous since therapeutic control is impossible after a patient has contracted the disease. Such iatrogenic calamities are readily avoided by ensuring that a separate sterile syringe and needle are used for each individual; the same holds good for needles or stylets used to obtain blood by finger puncture and the continuing occurrence of such infections is inexcusable (p. 18.117).

Respiratory tract infections

A large measure of control has been achieved with many communicable diseases. For example, the provision of safe water supplies and adequate methods of sewage disposal have reduced dramatically the incidence of many intestinal infections. However, most respiratory tract infections have defied control and, in the few instances in which this has been possible, success has generally been associated with the use of immunizing agents such as vaccines against tuberculosis, diphtheria and whooping cough. The causal organisms of respiratory tract infections are transmitted from a case or carrier in several ways; infected secretions may be transferred to the clothing, handkerchiefs and fingers of the patient, or expelled by spitting or noseblowing on to furniture, floors, bedclothing, and other surfaces in the environment where the organisms may survive in the dust for days or even weeks, provided that they are protected from direct sunlight. In addition, when the host talks, coughs, laughs or sneezes, small droplets are discharged which remain airborne for some time, although the larger droplets expelled at the same time fall rapidly on to surfaces and make their contribution to the dust population of organisms.

Thus anyone sharing the environment may be infected in two ways; **direct contact**, i.e. kissing is a common mechanism of transfer of organisms, and **indirect contact**, i.e. the transfer of organisms from inanimate objects to the recipient's nose or mouth via his fingers, is also efficient in spreading respiratory tract pathogens. When diphtheria was endemic in this country and its mortality sadly in evidence, it was commonplace for the parents, siblings and other relatives to kiss the child before it was removed to isolation and therefore the patient was not infrequently followed into hospital by several of the relatives after an interval of two or three days. Similarly, spread of diphtheria by indirect contact could be traced to the shared use of school pencils among pupils who put them in their mouths (p. 18.63).

SPREAD OF INFECTION BY DUST AND DROPLET NUCLEI

Dustborne spread of respiratory tract infections may occur by inhalation of infected particles in the air; these may have been redistributed by dusting of furniture, bedmaking or the like, or alternatively shed from the original host's clothing or handkerchief. Airborne spread is usually significant only within the rooms occupied by the host, but where inadequate or improperly maintained artificial ventilating systems have been installed in hospitals or other buildings, infected dust particles not only spread via the ventilating system to other rooms in the building but may in fact multiply in the humidifier tank and other moist warm parts of the apparatus or ducting; then the so-called clean air in circulation may be more heavily populated with micro-organisms than the used air entering the system.

Another method of spread of respiratory tract infection is by means of **droplet nuclei,** i.e. the minute particles, 1–10 μm in diameter, formed by immediate evaporation of small droplets; these remain airborne for long periods of time and are inhaled into the nose and throat and lungs. This is probably the least important method of spread since, because of their small size, few droplet nuclei are infected with bacteria. However, it is likely that some virus infections, e.g. measles and the common cold, are transmitted in this way, and perhaps also bacterial pathogens such as meningococcus which is rapidly killed outside the host tissues.

RESPIRATORY TRACT INFECTION IN HOSPITAL

This causes a great deal of anxiety; cross-infection all too often prolongs the patient's stay in hospital, and apart from adding many additional discomforts and hazards, affects the national economy by increasing the need for hospital beds and staff. Many attempts to reduce the number of micro-organisms in the hospital environment have been made, but only a few of the experimentally successful techniques can be put into practice; one of these, the oiling of floors and all fabrics such as bedclothes, pyjamas, etc., has been shown to reduce dramatically the number of dust-carrying particles released from these materials, with the result that cross-infection rates are reduced significantly. Of course, isolation of the infected patient, as practised in Infectious Disease Units, would effectively protect other individuals in the ward area, but this is rarely undertaken in general medical or surgical units for several reasons, including architectural difficulties and shortage of money for structural alterations in existing hospitals. On the other hand, there are certain categories of patients who must be isolated, not only to protect others but to prevent themselves from becoming infected; the latter include those with burns and patients under treatment with cytotoxic agents as a preliminary to or following organ transplantation. The sterilization or cleaning of the air in a general ward has not been achieved by procedures that are compatible with the patient's comfort and safety. Ultraviolet radiation has been used in operating theatres and also in experimental wards, but the lamps must be shielded or alternatively all occupants must wear protective clothing, caps and goggles; the technique is therefore not widely used.

Infections of skin and tissue surfaces

The origin of skin sepsis or infection of a wound or burn may on occasion be endogenous, but the hazards of exogenous infection are always present. Direct contact infection from a medical or nursing attendant is a risk that must be constantly kept in mind; the best safeguard is for all those who care for or visit the sick to be reminded frequently of the danger they constitute to their patients and of the precautions that they must take. For example, it is common sense to abstain from patient care when suffering from an infection, even if it seems to be apparently trivial, and it is inexcusable for anyone with a septic finger to participate in a surgical team. Indirect contact infection can arise easily if instruments and other materials used in theatres or wound dressing stations are not completely sterile.

Urinary tract infections

Although a proportion of such infections are truly endogenous (p. 18.23) it is with the exogenous group that epidemiologists and clinicians are most concerned. The anterior part of the healthy urethra is frequently colonized with various potentially pathogenic species; this probably explains the small but significant incidence of infections that follow catheterization with a sterile instrument under strictly aseptic conditions, since such organisms may be carried into the bladder. Obviously the introduction of a catheter or other instrument which is itself not sterile adds to the risk. Patients may require continuous drainage of the bladder by an indwelling catheter and the urine is collected in a bottle or other suitable container. Bacteria can travel up the tubing connecting the catheter to the receiving vessel and, if an open system is used, cross-infection is common; this risk is much reduced if a closed drainage method is employed. In the operating theatre, some of the methods by which infection may reach the bladder are similar to the contamination hazards associated with other operative procedures; instruments such as the cystoscope may transfer organisms from the urethra to the bladder.

Alimentary tract infections

Patients with gastrointestinal infections and carriers excrete pathogenic micro-organisms in the faeces and, in some cases of typhoid, in the urine. The methods of transmission to healthy subjects are various but in comparison with the majority of respiratory pathogens, intestinal pathogens are poorly resistant to drying and require moist surroundings for survival outside the human host. Infection of the gastrointestinal tract may be **waterborne**, through contamination of a water supply with excreta. This is the common method of spread of cholera and typhoid fever in countries where the water supply is neither filtered nor chlorinated. Many countries are as much in need of sanitary and water engineers as they are of modern methods of curative medicine; recently in Britain two separate epidemics of typhoid fever occurred which were judged to be foodborne, but the canned foods involved were contaminated by infected water at the processing plant in another country.

Even the most sophisticated water supply can be contaminated if a nearby sewage pipe fractures and human waste finds its way into the adjoining water mains; the organic matter may rapidly quench the residual chlorine and allow contaminating pathogens to survive and be distributed to households. Occasional epidemics of gastrointestinal infection occur in communities with 'safe' water supplies because of the wrong connection of waste pipes to water pipes when alterations are made.

Handborne spread of gastrointestinal tract infection occurs in even the most highly developed societies; where community methods of control have reduced the incidence of waterborne diseases, the proportion of those infections spread by poor personal hygiene rises. Patients and carriers with intestinal pathogens can contaminate their hands with traces of faeces when cleansing themselves after defaecation; organisms can readily pass through good quality toilet paper. Many flushing mechanisms produce infective aerosols. There are therefore many opportunities for the spread of infection when patients or carriers flush the toilet and turn on taps before washing their hands; if facilities for handwashing are not in the same room as the toilet, they also contaminate the door handle when leaving. The next person to touch either tap or handle can easily pick up the organisms and transfer them to his mouth. Similarly, nurses and hospital cleaners can contaminate their hands when touching bedpans; apart from infecting herself, the nurse may then handle food and spread the pathogens.

When one considers the frequency with which we touch our mouths with our hands, it is easy to appreciate the danger of transferring pathogens acquired from other people via every object in our environment.

Foodborne infection occurs under various circumstances and from several sources; when a **foodhandler** is a carrier of an intestinal pathogen or is suffering from an infection he has innumerable opportunities to contaminate foodstuffs at various stages in their preparation or distribution. The use of infected water for washing food may be a source of epidemic spread in a community and this is still a common method of spread in those areas of the world that lack a safe water supply. In areas where sewage disposal is primitive or nonexistent, filthy, faecal-feeding flies can contaminate unprotected foods after feeding on human refuse.

Bacterial food poisoning occurs throughout the world, and it may arise as a result of contamination of meat or other animal products which till that point were entirely wholesome; alternatively, the food or an ingredient may be derived from an infected animal or poultry source. It is obvious that in abattoirs or wholesale or retail premises, only one infected carcase need be processed to contaminate handlers, implements and the carcases that follow. The increase in communal feeding in canteens, hotels and other establishments has added to the food poisoning problem; in the home, only one person is initially infected from an egg containing salmonellae, whereas a contaminated egg compounded with others or with other materials in the preparation of some communal dish can infect many people.

One of the problems in controlling food poisoning is the need to ensure adequate cooking and storage of food; all too often, investigation of an outbreak reveals that the incriminated material has been cooked some hours or even a day or two before consumption and has then lain at room temperature, thus allowing multiplication of the causal organism so that the challenge dose (fig. 18.18c) is increased enormously.

MICROBIAL PATHOGENICITY

The relation between man and his microbial parasites, the **host–parasite association**, may range from that of harmless commensalism with varying degrees of symbiosis to flagrant aggression with interacting offensive and defensive systems.

The production of clinical infection in a patient is thus a stage in a series of interactions between the host and the aggressive pathogen. The steps in the initiation of an infection have many parallels with traditional patterns of warfare; the aggressor first mounts an adequate attacking force from a **source** or **reservoir of infection** and the adequacy of this force may be judged qualitatively and quantitatively. There is next a stage of transmission of the infecting agent which establishes and exploits an initial break in the host's defences. The latter stage reflects the infectivity of the pathogen. The organism may then overwhelm the host by massive invasion producing a generalized infection, or it may remain in a localized focus of infection and upset the host's economy by elaborating diffusible exotoxins that have selective affinity for vital host systems (p. 18.30).

In general, mechanisms of microbial pathogenicity appear to depend upon:

(1) **transmissibility**, the transfer of an effective challenge dose from a source of infection to a susceptible host;

(2) **infectivity**, the ability to overcome host defence mechanisms and to establish an effective challenge; and

(3) **virulence**, the capacity to inflict damage on the host. Virulence may involve **invasiveness** or **toxigenicity**; some pathogenic organisms are typically invasive, e.g. the causative organisms of typhoid fever, and some are typically toxigenic, e.g. the causative organism of tetanus; some organisms such as *Streptococcus pyogenes* exhibit both components of virulence.

This concept of pathogenicity provides a useful framework, though it is clear that the traditional terms are not well defined. While insufficient knowledge does not permit a more precise definition of the terms some of the interacting factors that influence the outcome of a microbial challenge in man are being elucidated. Thus the development of a specific infection depends on the following:

(1) the nature and number of the infecting organisms,

(2) the route or avenue of infection, and

(3) the state of the host's defence mechanisms and reactions.

Host defence mechanisms are discussed in chap. 22; the present account is concerned with mechanisms of microbial attack and defence which influence microbial pathogenicity.

Avenues of infection

The route by which a microbial challenge is presented may determine whether infection results, e.g. the spread of anthrax bacilli (p. 18.25). Staphylococci may cause pyogenic infections in the skin and in other tissues, but these organisms do not generally cause trouble if they are ingested. If they have grown in food, they may produce a toxin which is harmful on ingestion but this does not represent a direct infective process. The vibrios of cholera, which give rise to severe acute gastrointestinal symptoms after ingestion, are harmless if they are applied to the skin or injected subcutaneously in man. Similarly, gonococci produce primary lesions only when they are implanted in the genitourinary tract or conjunctiva.

Challenge doses

The size of the dose of organisms delivered to the susceptible host usually diminishes on its way from the

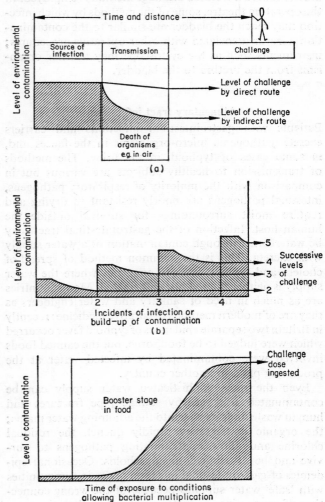

FIG. 18.18. Mechanisms which influence the level of challenge (a) by reduction of the dose during transmission; (b) by cumulative increase in the level of contamination and (c) by great increase of the dose as a result of bacterial multiplication in food.

source of infection (fig. 18.18a). Thus, the viability of an organism is of considerable importance and this is subject to marked variation. The gonococcus is highly vulnerable and dies rapidly if it is separated from its host. The tubercle bacillus is protected *en route* by its waxy coat. The pneumococcus is protected by a capsule and can resist the hazards of desiccation and phagocytosis. The organisms of anthrax and tetanus rely on their capacity for sporulation to retain their viability in soil and dust. The arboviruses (p. 18.114) are injected by insect vectors and are thereby protected against loss in transit. The virus of measles does not have this insurance and is transmissible by an airborne route; it is therefore, effective only when a suitably large dose is delivered from a person incubating the infection to a nearby susceptible individual.

In some cases, the size of the dose of organisms is gradually built up in the environment (fig. 18.18b). The populations of staphylococci and pseudomonas organisms which tend respectively to colonize hospital staff and to develop in wet washing-up areas, present a sustained challenge to susceptible hosts.

There are circumstances in which the challenge dose may be boosted enormously (fig. 18.18c). For example when contaminated food is kept under conditions favourable for the bacteria, they multiply. The victim then ingests a greatly augmented dose of the bacteria and an **infective dose** is ensured.

Infective and lethal doses

The number of organisms that reach the host seems to be of crucial importance for the success of many microbial challenges. Healthy tissues normally resist attack by a small number of organisms of moderate virulence. Experimental animals given graded doses of a pathogen often show graded responses; there may be local lesions, general disease or a fulminating lethal infection. However, individual responses are extremely variable and, although it may be possible to make a rough estimate of the **minimum lethal dose** (MLD) of a particular pathogen for the test animal species, it is more accurate to work in terms of the dose that is lethal for 50 per cent of the test group (LD50) (p. 20.3). This applies also to determinations of the infective dose (ID) and the ID50. It then becomes evident that the LD50 and ID50 of a microbial species for a susceptible host are influenced by many factors such as the strain of the organism, the age of the culture, the culture medium and the suspending agent in which the challenge is delivered. Moreover, many host factors are also critical; these include the species and age of the host and the avenue of infection.

With the above reservations, it is nevertheless true that the level of the infective dose required to produce certain infections in man is relatively low, whereas other infections are typically associated with a high infective dose.

For example, relatively small numbers of dysentery bacilli or typhoid bacilli appear to produce their respective diseases when they are ingested by man, but very large numbers of organisms are thought to be involved in the challenge dose that precipitates salmonella food poisoning in man. Thus, a differentiation can sometimes be made between species of high and low infectivity.

Virulence

Bacterial virulence, i.e. the capacity to damage or kill the host, is dependent on many factors which include the organism's invasiveness and toxigenicity.

Invasiveness, the capacity to produce a generalized infection in the host, is a typical feature of some virulent pathogens of man. Pneumococci cause acute lobar pneumonia by overwhelming local defence mechanisms in the lung; they sweep through the tissue on a wave of rapid multiplication that is limited only by the anatomical boundaries of the affected lobe. Even then, the organisms are liable to spill into the blood stream and a **bacteriaemia** may result. The virulent pneumococci are protected from host phagocytes by a polysaccharide capsule and it can be shown readily that noncapsulate pneumococci are nonvirulent.

Virulent streptococci similarly have a protective surface component called M-protein which is associated with pathogenicity, and virulent anthrax bacilli are protected by a polypeptide capsule. When anthrax bacilli have established a local infective focus, they may then enter the blood stream. The initial bacteriaemia, a passive state of **haematogenous spread**, gives way to a state of **septicaemia** in which the normally effective bactericidal mechanisms of the blood stream are inadequate to cope with the number of organisms from the infective focus. Whereas bacteriaemia is a natural and clinically accepted phase of some infections in man, septicaemia indicates that the host is being overwhelmed.

Although capsulate organisms provide good examples of invasiveness, capsulation is not an invariable criterion of pathogenicity and is not essential for invasiveness; many capsulate saprophytes are harmless for man, and many invasive pathogens are devoid of recognizable capsules. The waxy coat of the noncapsulate tubercle bacillus may not protect it against phagocytosis, but it seems to protect it from digestion when it has been phagocytosed and the organism can subsequently escape by multiplying and killing its captor. Similarly, the small Gram-negative organisms of undulant fever (brucellosis) are able to escape normal phagocytic clearing systems and they survive intracellularly to produce recurring disease in man.

Salmonella typhi, the causative organism of typhoid fever, is highly invasive and noncapsulate. After an infective dose has been ingested, an initial focus of infection in the lymphoid tissue of the small intestine is followed by a bacteriaemic phase. The resulting haematogenous spread results in a generalized infection and bacteria may be isolated from many organs and tissues. It is thought that the lipopolysaccharide and other superficial components of the cell wall of the typhoid bacillus are involved in protecting it from phagocytic mechanisms; it is possible that under these circumstances, phagocytes may perform a disservice to the host by carrying organisms into areas that would otherwise be inaccessible to the invaders.

VI ANTIGEN

The difficulties in interpreting the value to bacteria of 'aggressive mechanisms' and in translating experimental results obtained with laboratory animals to the natural infective process in the human host are illustrated by the **Vi (virulence) antigen** of *Salmonella typhi*. Strains of *S. typhi* that possess this surface antigen are much more lethal to mice than otherwise identical strains lacking it; similarly mice passively or actively immunized against Vi antigen have greater power of survival when challenged by Vi-containing strains of the typhoid bacillus than mice not so protected. However, these results in mice do not reflect the natural history of typhoid fever in man, since controlled trials conducted on a large scale have shown that individuals actively immunized with typhoid vaccine containing the Vi fraction receive less protection than others immunized with a similar vaccine which lacks the Vi component.

Toxigenicity

Many bacteria produce substances that damage host tissues or upset systems that are vital to the host; the substances are referred to as **toxins** and some have been chemically defined. Unfortunately, the word toxin has been used loosely to denote mixtures of substances that occur in culture products, and it is sometimes applied wrongly to a product that may enhance the pathogenic effect of an organism although not itself demonstrably toxic; the latter type of product is better termed aggressin.

Bacterial toxins are conveniently classified as **exotoxins** and **endotoxins** but the differentiation is not always simple.

EXOTOXINS

These are highly toxic soluble proteins liberated from bacterial cells which may remain viable. They have specific affinities for particular host systems; for example, diphtheria toxin poisons cardiac muscle and nervous tissue, and tetanus toxin specifically affects motor nervous pathways. The lethal dose of some of the exotoxins is exceedingly small and the toxin of *Clostridium botulinum* is one of the most toxic substances known (p. 25.20). Exotoxins are generally thermolabile at 60–70°C and, if they are heated gently in the presence of formaldehyde,

they lose their toxic properties but retain their specific antigenic properties; in this state they are termed **toxoids** and are used in vaccines to stimulate the production of antitoxins (p. 22.6). An antitoxin specifically neutralizes the effect of the homologous toxin, and antitoxins have important applications in medicine.

Exotoxins are typically associated with Gram-positive bacteria and the most potent are produced by the diphtheria bacillus and the clostridial group which includes the causative organisms of botulism, tetanus and gas gangrene. The exotoxins are mainly responsible for the clinical features of these diseases. The pathogenic staphylococci and the streptococci that cause tonsillitis and scarlet fever also produce exotoxins, but these organisms produce such a multiplicity of toxins and aggressins that it is difficult to attribute their pathogenicity to any single agent.

Some exotoxins produce demonstrable effects and they may be named accordingly, but it should be noted that a single substance may produce more than one effect. Thus the principal toxin produced by *Clostridium welchii* is lethal on injection into mice, haemolytic to red cells *in vitro*, and causes necrosis of the skin on intradermal inoculation into guinea-pigs. The mode of action of exotoxins in cell injury is discussed on p. 25.20.

Some toxigenic bacteria may produce nontoxigenic mutants that are harmless. The toxigenicity of the diphtheria bacillus is dependent on the presence of a particular bacteriophage (p. 18.63) in the organism; in the absence of the phage, it seems that the diphtheria bacillus is nontoxigenic.

ENDOTOXINS

These are substances which are structurally associated with the bacterial cell and are liberated only when the cell disintegrates. They are poorly characterized but endotoxin activity is associated particularly with the molecular complexes containing protein, lipid and carbohydrate that can be isolated from cell walls of Gram-negative bacteria. Substances with similar pharmacological activity have more recently been obtained from Gram-positive bacteria. Bacterial endotoxins are less specific and much less potent than the classical exotoxins, but they nevertheless produce marked clinical effects when they are injected into experimental animals. Typical features of endotoxic reactions in the host are pyrexia and malaise; there may be vasomotor disturbances leading to shock which is sometimes fatal. A similar clinical picture is seen in some patients with bacteriaemia or septicaemia; this is described as **bacteriogenic**, endotoxic or septic shock. The synonym endotoxic shock indicates the mechanism that is assumed to be involved in these cases and the endotoxin is thought to stimulate the release of histamine in the host.

Bacterial endotoxins are thermostable at 100°C. They are poorly antigenic and cannot be made readily in toxoid form; thus vaccines against endotoxic mechanisms are not generally available.

When an invasive organism multiplies in the tissues of the host, it is reasonable to ascribe some of the observed signs and symptoms to the release of endotoxin and other bacterial products. The host may also react to toxic breakdown products released by bacterial action on host tissue.

SHWARTZMAN REACTION
Polymorphonuclear leucocytes possess cytoplasmic lysosomes which are probably responsible for the ability of these cells to digest bacteria and other foreign matter. Studies with animals have shown that virtually no damage is caused to the ingesting cells when macrophages phagocytose the granules of polymorphs. However, if bacterial endotoxin is then administered intravenously, the lysosomal membranes break down and the macrophages are killed. It has been suggested that this phenomenon is the general basis for the Shwartzman reaction.

This reaction is at present known to occur only in the experimental model. There are two types, the localized Shwartzman reaction results when an intradermal injection of endotoxin is followed 12–36 hours later by an intravenous injection of endotoxin, which may be derived from the same or a different source. There is rapid necrosis of tissue at the site of the first injection. The generalized Shwartzman reaction is elicited by giving an intravenous injection of endotoxin or organisms containing endotoxin, followed 24 hours later by another intravenous dose of endotoxin or endotoxic organisms. There is collapse with shock and the test animal usually dies. At autopsy, small vessels throughout the body are found to be blocked by fibrinoid material (p. 30.3) and there are related lesions such as infarcts and partial bilateral cortical necrosis of the kidneys.

Although the Shwartzman reactions were previously thought to be mediated by hypersensitivity, the mechanism is now attributed to the activities of the enzymes of cellular lysosomes in the inflammatory state. No circulating antibodies seem to be involved and there are similarities between the features of this reaction and those of bacteriogenic shock.

Noninvasive, nontoxic infections
The concept of invasiveness and toxigenicity as components of virulence is not readily applicable to infections such as cholera and the common forms of bacillary dysentery. The causative organisms of these diseases do not produce recognized toxins and, although they may cause overwhelming infections, they attack the intestinal mucosa superficially and are not truly invasive. The common dysentery bacilli are locally invasive in the gut, but the cholera vibrio produces no visible lesion in the intestine. The reader may hold that such a distinction is contrived and that aggression across a tissue plane constitutes invasion; nevertheless, the pathogenic effects remain unexplained. It is thought that unrecognized toxic mechanisms may be active in these diseases and the cholera vibrio is the subject of much research along these lines (p. 18.78). It is also of interest that certain strains of the commensal *Escherichia coli* produce severe cholera-like gastroenteritis in children. There is no invasive process and, although enterotoxic substances have been described, no recognized toxin has been characterized; nevertheless these diseases undoubtedly demonstrate their lethal potential on frequent occasions. It is possible that in gastroenteritis caused by *Esch. coli*, the severe clinical features may be a hypersensitivity reaction (p. 23.1).

Variations in virulence
There is much variation in the degree of damage that a pathogenic organism may produce in different host species. Many pathogenic organisms display marked **species specificity**; although they may cause severe disease in one species, they may be virtually nonpathogenic for another. For example, the three main types of tubercle bacillus, human, bovine and avian (p. 18.61), have been named in accordance with their natural hosts; the human type can cause obvious disease in man and some animals including the guinea-pig, but in comparable doses it does not produce disease in the rabbit.

When a pathogen is transmitted serially (**passaged**) through susceptible members of the same species, its virulence may become enhanced or exalted. On the other hand, serial artificial subculture of an organism in the laboratory frequently results in diminished or **attenuated virulence**. These changes may be paralleled by gain or loss of demonstrable virulence factors such as capsulation and toxin production, but many unknown factors are involved. Man's increasing tendency to live in crowded communities obliges him to depend increasingly upon the preventive aspects of microbiology and he is already committed to the widespread use of vaccines. A vaccine is unlikely to stimulate the production of protective antibodies unless it contains the proper virulence factors which are thus sometimes paradoxically regarded as **protective antigens**; it is clearly in our interest to investigate the components that make pathogens dangerous. An alternative approach is to produce organisms of attenuated virulence for 'live vaccines'.

Since the time of Pasteur, it has been possible to reduce the virulence of micro-organisms. Several methods can be used, e.g. growing a virulent strain *in vitro* at abnormal temperatures or in the presence of mildly antagonistic substances, or passing a pure culture of the virulent strain through a series of animal hosts other than the host for which the species is naturally virulent. Such attenuated living cultures can be used for immunization against several infections (p. 22.22).

Attenuation can also be observed indirectly *in vivo*; it has been shown, for example, that carriers of *Strept. pyogenes* become less dangerous as a source of infection for other people the longer the carrier state lasts; this epidemiological observation can be explained by the fact that with increasing carriage the strain produces more M proteinase and in consequence contains less M protein, the factor responsible for its virulence (p. 18.67).

Comparative studies made *in vitro*, although allowing chemical analysis of bacterial products, must be interpreted with extreme caution, since it is impossible to reproduce the complex and dynamic environment provided by the living host; reference has already been made to the pathogenicity of human tubercle bacilli for guineapigs and their relative nonpathogenicity for rabbits. Rabbits, however, are very susceptible to bovine tubercle bacilli. Quantitative studies have shown that when rabbits are inoculated with either human or bovine tubercle bacilli, the organisms multiply in the tissues with the same ease and rapidity; one must assume that rabbit tissues provide all that is required for the growth and reproduction of human tubercle bacilli. During the first two or three weeks after inoculation, the number of tubercle bacilli harvested from various organs increases; thereafter the recovery of human bacilli from rabbit tissues declines rapidly until by the 12–16th week all have been destroyed. Obviously, infection with human bacilli promotes in the rabbit tissues some alteration that eliminates the organism, whereas bovine infection is progressive and fatal. Such findings serve to emphasize the dangers and difficulties of considering bacterial factors involved in infection in isolation from response mechanisms of the host, but they also direct our attention to useful areas for further research (p. 22.1).

Enhancement of virulence

An **aggressin** is a bacterial product which, although not toxic *per se*, may contribute towards the virulence of the pathogen that elaborates it. Among the earliest of such substances to be described was the spreading factor hyaluronidase, which catalyses the breakdown of intercellular substance and therefore facilitates penetration of tissues.

HYALURONIDASE
The role of hyaluronidases in promoting the spread of bacterial invaders within the tissues of the host is not yet clear; there are many highly invasive species, e.g. *Brucella melitensis*, which do not produce the enzyme in large quantities. Even when hyaluronidase production assists a particular species to produce a spreading lesion, other factors may determine the final effect. The

spread of a lesion may dilute a small bacterial population sufficiently to allow host defence mechanisms to prevail and the lesion may then quickly regress, whereas localized multiplication of the same bacterial population in the absence of hyaluronidase could ensure persistence of the infection.

The picture is even more clouded since some strains of *Streptococcus pyogenes* produce hyaluronidase but also possess capsular material containing hyaluronic acid; the virulence of such strains may decrease as they multiply and produce more enzyme. Indeed, hyaluronidase has been shown experimentally to have a protective effect in infections caused by streptococci that possess hyaluronate capsules.

FIBRINOLYSIN
Some of the pathogenic streptococci also produce a factor which digests human fibrin; this enzyme, streptokinase (streptococcal fibrinolysin) is similar to fibrinolysins produced by several other species, particularly staphylococci. Streptokinase is produced in larger quantities by strains freshly isolated from acute suppurative lesions than by strains obtained from carriers, but its role in the spread of the infection in the human host is not clear. The clinical use of streptokinase is described on p. 7.13.

COAGULASE
There is much more evidence to incriminate the enzyme coagulase as a virulence factor produced by pathogenic staphylococci. The enzyme coagulates citrated plasma, and its production greatly enhances the resistance of staphylococci to phagocytosis in an artificial system containing coagulable plasma; strains which do not produce coagulase can be made resistant to phagocytosis by the adsorption of coagulase to their surface. Moreover, anticoagulase antibodies afford protection to rabbits challenged with coagulase-positive staphylococci (p. 18.70).

MUCINASES
Many bacteria produce enzymes which catalyse the decomposition of various mucins that occur in or near mammalian cell surfaces. It is thought that bacterial mucinases may be involved in mechanisms of cell surface attack, or they may simply ensure that a bacterial cell is not separated from a nutrient source at the host cell surface. Neuraminidase is an important mucinase produced by many bacteria and some viruses; the enzyme attacks mucoproteins that occur at various cell surfaces.

OTHER BACTERIAL EXOENZYMES
Bacterial exoenzymes are of great interest in medical microbiology as they are often involved in the breakdown of substrates that are to be found in mammalian tissues.

Potent bacterial **proteinases** and **collagenases** decompose muscle tissue and collagen. Bacterial **lipases** are active against mammalian lipids. **Deoxyribonucleases** can be detected by their effect on cell nuclei; they merit more study than they have received. The **lecithinase** of *Clostridium welchii*, which causes gas gangrene, breaks down cell membranes and interferes with mitochondrial function (p. 25.20). With the possible exception of the *Cl. welchii* lecithinase, the contribution made by these biochemically active bacterial products to known mechanisms of pathogenicity has not been defined.

Mixed infections

A simultaneous or sequential attack by two separate species may produce an unusually severe disease. Virus influenza is not usually fatal, but a superadded respiratory infection with staphylococci or other bacteria may result in a fatal pneumonia. It is possible that pathogens operate in concert against man more frequently than is recognized at present. On the other hand, man's commensal flora is protective. For example, commensal salivary streptococci produce substances which are inimical to diphtheria bacilli; the suppression of the normal bacterial flora of the gastrointestinal tract by prolonged broad spectrum antibiotic therapy renders the patient vulnerable to invasion by yeast-like fungi and staphylococci, and the normal commensal flora of the vagina maintains an acid environment which resists colonization by potential pathogens.

Sites of predilection

Although some generalized infections may involve most of the tissues of the host at some phase of the disease, a pathogenic species often shows a tendency to localize in specific tissues. Thus, the meningococcus may produce a bacteriaemia in man, but typically infects the meninges; the pneumococcus can also produce a meningitis and a bacteriaemia, but it characteristically attacks lung tissue. The typhoid bacillus has a predilection for lymphoid tissue and, although it is notoriously ubiquitous in the infected host, it has a tendency to linger in the gall bladder of a convalescent. In some cases, the avenue and mode of infection clearly selects the site of localization; the airborne human tubercle bacillus naturally produces a focus of infection in the lungs of the new host, whereas the bovine tubercle bacillus in ingested milk may understandably give rise to abdominal tuberculosis. However, the bovine organism may give rise to tuberculosis of bones and joints and these particular sites of localization are less readily explained. *Brucella abortus* localizes in the placental tissue of cattle and causes abortion. The bovine placenta is rich in erythritol which is a growth factor for the brucella organism. Here we have an acceptable explanation for a particular organism's preference for a particular site, but there are many other examples of **tissue specificity** which cannot be explained at present.

STERILIZATION AND DISINFECTION PROCEDURES

Sterilization means the removal or destruction of all living organisms, including viruses, spores and vegetative forms. There are no degrees of sterility; the term is absolute and implies the loss or death of every cell. A few cells surviving an attempted sterilization procedure provide the basis for a new microbial population. For example, since pasteurization does not inactivate spores present in milk, the process is not one of sterilization.

With dependable methods of sterilization it is usually possible to predict a degree of exposure that carries a virtually absolute insurance of sterility, but this demands attention to detail and the methods in common use incorporate exposure periods to provide safety factors. It is usually not practicable to extend the period unduly without damaging the item to be sterilized. In some cases, a minimal exposure consistent with sterilization is required, e.g. in the inactivation of vaccines. The distinction must also be made between,

(1) a minimal exposure that achieves sterilization and is subjected thereafter to a careful check, and

(2) a routine exposure that experience shows to be adequate with intermittent checks that test the system up to limits exceeding those likely to apply in practice.

It is not always possible or practicable to rid every article of all living organisms; for example, living skin cannot be exposed to damaging sterilizing agents and procedures to sterilize a toilet are costly. Then the aim is usually to destroy as many potential pathogens as possible and for this purpose disinfectants or antiseptics are used. **Disinfection** is the freeing of an inanimate object from vegetative micro-organisms but not necessarily from spores. Disinfectants are mainly bactericidal in action; they are generally used at concentrations that would damage living tissues. **Antisepsis** implies the use of primarily bacteristatic agents for the local removal of pathogenic bacteria from tissues. The application of antiseptic agents to the skin is sometimes called skin disinfection. The degree of success of any agent in killing a population of bacterial cells is measured by estimating the number of bacteria that survive. Commonly used tests to determine the efficacy of the antimicrobial process measure the ability of any remaining organisms to grow on various culture media.

Bacterial spores are highly resistant to all sterilizing agents. Vegetative bacteria are more readily killed, but they vary in their susceptibility to different agents. Viruses are more resistant than bacteria to some chemicals. Tubercle bacilli are relatively resistant and they are further protected when they are suspended in sputum.

The time required to effect sterilization varies with the size of the initial microbial population. There is progressive inactivation of this population during the time of exposure to the inactivating agent and, in general, time and temperature are inversely related. Thus, the graph of survivors plotted in relation to time is essentially linear, until the area of 100 per cent kill is approached. At this point, the graph shows a 'tail' of survivors that seem to disobey the exponential rule (fig. 18.19). This may

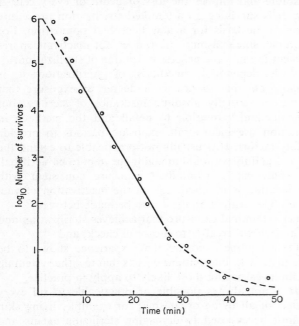

FIG. 18.19. The progressive inactivation of a sporing culture of bacteria at 100°C in water (pH 7·2). There is a 'tail' of survivors as 100 per cent inactivation is approached.

be attributable to nonhomogeneity of the cell population or to the presence of a few mutant cells; in addition, as bacteria are killed, they release materials which may afford some protection to the surviving cells. The 'tailing' effect is a source of anxiety when absolute sterility is essential and in most sterilizing procedures extra times of exposure are added to provide the necessary safety factor.

The constituents of the suspending medium greatly influence the efficacy of many sterilizing agents. For example, moist heat at sterilizing temperatures is much more rapidly effective if the environment is acid or alkaline than at neutral pH. The presence of protein and some carbohydrates protects organisms against inactivation by heat or by some chemicals.

The cardinal rule of sterilization derived from the above observation is that, whenever practicable, an article to be sterilized for surgical use should first be thoroughly clean.

The following methods are available for the destruction or removal of micro-organisms:
(1) exposure to heat,
(2) filtration,
(3) exposure to irradiation, and
(4) exposure to chemical agents.

Sterilization by heat

Both dry and moist heat are employed to kill micro-organisms. Moist heat is much more effective as it sterilizes at lower temperatures for any given exposure time.

DRY HEAT

Dry heat kills organisms by oxidation and charring of the cell constituents. There are four methods in which dry heat is employed.

(1) The common bacteriological practice of heating nichrome or platinum wire inoculating loops in a bunsen flame to **red heat** is a certain method of ensuring sterility. An unreliable modification of this procedure is to dip instruments such as scalpels and scissors into spirit which is then burned off. This has the disadvantages of uncertain sterilization and of rapidly blunting the cutting edges.

(2) The **hot air oven** consists of a closed metal chamber, the air in which is heated by gas or electric elements. Articles are subjected to a temperature of 160°C for 1 hour, which ensures sterilization. To promote even distribution of hot air within the chamber, a fan is normally fitted. Articles which can be sterilized in a hot air oven include glassware (all-glass syringes, culture plates, pipettes, etc.), metal instruments (scalpels, bowls, etc.), various powders and oils which cannot be sterilized by moist heat due to their impermeability to moisture, cotton-wool swabs and paraffin gauze dressings. To avoid breakage of glass it is essential that the oven is loaded when cold and is not opened after sterilization until it has cooled.

(3) Articles such as all-glass syringes are loaded on a conveyor belt and carried beneath a source of **infra-red radiation**. Sterilization is more rapid than with the hot-air oven, the usual sterilizing cycle taking 22 min at a temperature of 180°C.

(4) Another method employs an electrically heated aluminium block in which syringes for sterilization are inserted and heated to 180°C for 18 min.

MOIST HEAT

Moist heat kills organisms by coagulation and denaturation of the cellular proteins. A temperature of 120°C kills all pathogenic spore-bearing bacteria within 12 min. However, moist heat is often employed at lower temperatures than this; if so, the articles cannot be properly described as sterilized. The following methods employ moist heat.

(1) Vaccines that contain vegetative organisms and no sporing forms may be inactivated in a **vaccine bath** by

exposure to 60–70°C for one hour only; they are treated under rigidly controlled conditions and there are subsequent checks of sterility. This is, therefore, a special case and provides no guide to the amount of heat that is required to effect sterilization in normal practice.

(2) **Boiling in water** has a restricted use as a method of sterilization. Although vegetative cells are killed at 100°C in 10 min, some spores can withstand hours of exposure to this temperature. Another disadvantage is that wet articles are very liable to recontamination when removed from the boiler. Articles for sterilization such as syringes, needles and other metal instruments should be boiled for a minimum of 5 min, and they should then be held in a perforated tray clear of the water to drain before they are handled. The addition of 2 per cent sodium carbonate to the water aids in the prevention of rust and markedly enhances the sterilizing effect. Although boiling water retains a practical place in sterilization, especially in general practice, there are powerful arguments for the preferential use of sterile disposable instruments and syringes whenever possible.

(3) **Pasteurization** is employed widely for the heat treatment of milk supplies, e.g. 63°C for 30 min or 72°C for 20 sec, to ensure the destruction of vegetative bacterial cells of species such as *Mycobacterium bovis*, *Brucella abortus*, and *Staphylococcus aureus*. Some milk supplies intended for storage are subjected to greater heat (100°C for 1 hour), but this alters the taste of the milk. **Hot-water pasteurization**, which involves exposure to

water at 75°C for at least 10 min, is sometimes used for disinfection of instruments that cannot withstand higher temperatures; some nonboilable cystoscopes and bronchoscopes, specula and items of anaesthetic equipment are treated in this way. While some articles may be justifiably dealt with in such a manner and admitting that it is important to preserve a sense of proportion, it is essential that the limitations of the procedure should be appreciated.

(4) Exposure to **steam at 100°C** for 90 min in a closed cabinet is used for the sterilization of some bacteriological culture media such as sugar media and gelatin-containing media which are altered at high temperatures. The steam is not pressurized and is referred to as free steam.

(5) **Tyndallization** involves exposure to steam at 100°C for 30 min on each of three successive days. The first steaming kills all vegetative cells that may be present in the media but has little or no effect on spores. These are allowed to germinate overnight and the vegetative cells thus formed are killed during the second steaming. The third steaming is purely a precautionary measure. As the germination of spores is not dependable, the method is unreliable, but it may be used in the controlled preparation of bacteriological media.

(6) **Pressurized steam** in the autoclave (fig. 18.20) affords a most effective method of sterilization provided that those who use the autoclave understand the principles involved. Responsibility for the proper use and main-

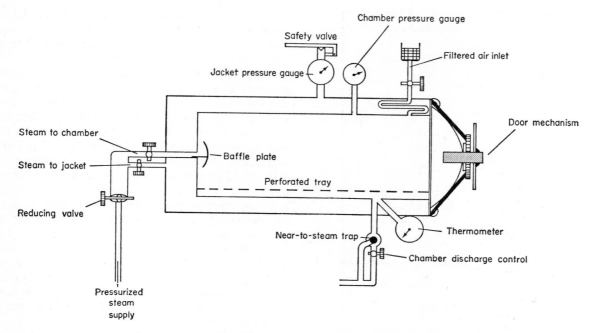

FIG. 18.20. A simplified diagram of an autoclave. The detailed steam supply mechanism, steam trap devices, vacuum discharge and other important systems in a modern autoclave are not shown here.

tenance of sterilizing equipment is frequently improperly delegated and this may have serious consequences for the patient.

There have been recent improvements in the design of autoclaves and it is probable that more will follow.

Principles of sterilization with steam

Water boils when its vapour pressure equals atmospheric pressure. Normally this occurs when the temperature of the water reaches 100°C. When the pressure exerted on the surface of the water is artificially increased, the temperature at which the water boils rises to above 100°C. Correspondingly, the temperature of the pressurized steam formed from the pressurized boiling water also rises in parallel with the water temperature. This is the principle of the domestic pressure cooker and the autoclave.

STEAM

When water is heated sufficiently to boil, some of the energy is stored as latent heat in the steam which is produced; the actual temperature of the steam does not rise immediately above that of the water from which it was produced, and the steam is just on the borderline or **phase boundary** that separates water and steam (fig. 18.21). In this state it is referred to as saturated and if no drops of condensate are present, it is said to be dry. Dry saturated steam is essential for the proper functioning of the autoclave.

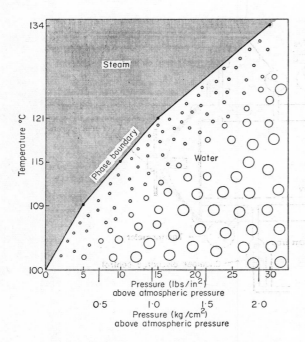

FIG. 18.21. The phase boundary that separates water and steam.

One ml of condensate can be formed from every 865 ml of steam at 1·05 kg/cm² (15 lb/in²) and in the process much energy is released as latent heat. It is this extra output of energy associated with wet heat at 121°C that makes pressurized steam in the autoclave such an efficient sterilizing agent. When dry saturated steam strikes a cool surface, such as that presented by a bundle of dressings, it condenses to wet the object with a film of water and conveys its latent heat to the material. The condensation creates a vacuum effect that pulls in more steam to penetrate the load.

If the steam supplied to the autoclave is already mixed with wet condensate, this soaks the load, gives up no latent heat, and produces no vacuum effect. If the steam is mixed with air when the autoclave is operating, the partial pressure of the air results in a decreased chamber temperature at the selected pressure. If the steam is heated excessively (superheated), it is in effect a form of dry heat and lacks the sterilizing efficiency of saturated steam.

GRAVITY DISPLACEMENT AUTOCLAVE

An autoclave (fig. 18.20) consists of a horizontal cylindrical chamber into which steam is introduced at above-atmospheric pressure. There are usually two concentric cylinders and the intervening space is filled with steam to provide a steamjacket. A swing door is fitted with a steam-tight seal. Steam at high pressure (4·2–5·6 kg/cm²; 60–80 lb/in²) is supplied from a central boiler and passes through a steam regulator that reduces the pressure to about 1·2 kg/cm² (17 lb/in²). This steam first supplies the jacket which acts as a lag to prevent loss of heat from the chamber. The jacket steam pressure is set to 1·05 kg/cm² (15 lb/in²), and maintained at this level throughout the day.

The articles to be sterilized are placed within the chamber in a manner that ensures free circulation of the steam to all parts of the load. After the door is secured, steam is allowed to enter the chamber. Steam, being less dense than air, at first floats at the top of the chamber; as more steam is run in, the residual air and any condensate in the chamber and within the load is displaced through a chamber drain at the bottom of the autoclave. While the emerging pressurized steam contains air, the temperature of the mixture is less than 121°C but the passage of pure steam at 1·05 kg/cm² (15 lb/in²) pressure through the drain will raise the temperature to 121°C. A thermostatically controlled valve (the near-to-steam trap) on the chamber drain remains open until this temperature is reached. Thereafter, if the temperature drops as a result of the release of air trapped in the load or following the accumulation of condensate, the valve opens and blows off until pure steam is expelled.

The displacement of air from the centre of fabric loads involves many variables that are more reliably dealt with by high prevacuum autoclaves (see below). With gravity-displacement machines, a period of 10–15 min is allowed for the steam to penetrate. Sterilization begins when the thermometer registers 121°C and is then achieved within 12 min (the holding period), but a 50 per cent safety factor is applied and the normal sterilization period is therefore 18 min at 1·05 kg/cm² (15 lb/in²), at a temperature of 121°C.

When the sterilization period has been completed the supply of steam to the chamber is stopped. The load cools by loss of heat via the unjacketed door, and the steam pressure falls accordingly. Moisture within the load evaporates, and evaporation is hastened by the heat of the steam retained in the jacket. In many cases it is possible to apply a vacuum to remove steam from the chamber at this stage. Filtered warm sterile air may then be introduced to hasten still further the drying and cooling of the load.

Autoclaving is highly effective since it sterilizes completely with minimal damage to the material being treated. In hospital practice, autoclaves have largely eliminated the need to retain boiling-water sterilizers. In general practice, the ordinary pressure cooker should replace simple boilers wherever possible.

Many items can be sterilized in the autoclave, but important exceptions include water-impermeable fats, greases, oils and powders which can be sterilized by hot air if they are thermostable. Sealed ampoules containing aqueous fluids may be sterilized satisfactorily in an ordinary autoclave, but not in an autoclave in which pre-evacuating systems are employed.

CAUSES OF FAILURE TO ACHIEVE STERILIZATION

Errors in loading the autoclave are many, and include overloading, incorrect positioning of the load, and the use of impervious wrapping materials and containers. Surgical dressing drums must be positioned on their sides so that the louvres allow entry of steam and displacement of air; they must not be packed tightly. Articles for all sterilization procedures should be rendered as clean as possible, and must not contain any trace of pus or blood, or other proteinaceous fluid which harbours bacteria and protects them from the wet heat. Wrapping material should be tear-resistant, permeable to steam and impermeable to bacteria. Kraft paper is satisfactory but is easily damaged in handling.

Faults in the autoclave are most often the result of failure to use pure saturated steam. Occasionally there may be a fault in a recording gauge, and it is important to check both temperature and pressure readings.

After proper sterilization, the load may still be subject to contamination. Improper handling of the load on removal from the autoclave, the placing of still moist sterilized paper-wrapped articles on wet unclean surfaces,

and the presence of an inadequate air filter, are factors which may account for this.

HIGH PREVACUUM AUTOCLAVE

This is an important development in which 98 per cent of the chamber air is evacuated by pumps before steam is admitted. The procedure greatly accelerates removal of air from fabric loads and allows virtually instantaneous penetration of steam to all parts of the load. An initial evacuation procedure overcomes problems associated with the development of pockets of air that may avoid gravity displacement. The process is designed for sterilization of hospital items that include fabrics, e.g. preset instrument trays and dressings for surgical use; it is not suitable for bottled fluids. After the prevacuum period, pressurized steam is admitted to the chamber for the sterilizing period; steam at 121°C (1·05 kg/cm²; 15 lb/in² for 15 min) or at 134°C (2·1 kg/cm²; 30 lb/in² for 3 min) may be used. The load can then be dried rapidly by drawing a second vacuum when sterilization is completed, and air is finally admitted through a sterilizing air filter.

As this autoclaving procedure allows more complete steam penetration, more rapid sterilization and more rapid drying of fabric loads, it can contribute greatly to the efficiency of a sterilizing team. The temperature and pressure of the steam in the chamber are recorded on gauges. Especially with associated automation, there is a marked reduction in the sterilization cycle time with a greater ensurance of steam penetration of fabrics. However, any failure in the prevacuum process is critical and the high prevacuum autoclave, therefore, demands even greater maintenance and more constant checking than the simpler machine. Important checks include the use of thermocouples and the Bowie–Dick test.

CONTROLS OF ADEQUACY OF STERILIZATION

When the autoclave chamber has been held at the recommended temperature and pressure for the required time, it does not follow that all parts of the load have been subjected to these conditions. Moreover, human errors in timing the various periods of the sterilizing cycle are common. A reliable check on the efficiency of sterilization should ideally be incorporated with each load. In practice, a screening check usually accompanies each load and regular test loads are used to monitor the autoclave.

Tests in the past have included the use of spore-impregnated papers that were subsequently cultured, but these have been replaced by strips of autoclave tape on which diagonal grey shaded lines are superimposed. These lines change to a dark colour when exposed to a given amount of heat. In the **Bowie–Dick test,** which was designd for the regular checking of an autoclave, such tapes are distributed in a standard test load of fabric dressings. If steam penetration, and therefore heat transfer, is impaired by air retained in the bundle or by any other fault, the marked lines fail to change colour.

Monitoring and timing equipment is sometimes available. For example, a thermocouple inserted in a test article within the load may be electrically connected to a potentiometer outside the autoclave. A mechanism for the timing and control of the whole sterilization cycle is incorporated in the design of many modern autoclaves which may also be fitted with a recording thermometer to give a continuous graphic record of the chamber temperature.

Removal of bacteria by filtration

Filtration as a means of removing bacteria from fluids such as culture media and serum has long been used in laboratories. For the community, filtration of water through sand filters or metal micromesh filters prior to chlorination is an essential procedure in the provision of water supplies that are safe and free from pathogenic bacteria. It is important to note that viruses were initially described as filter-passing agents; they are not retained by many filters in general use and, unless a special filter system is employed, filter-sterilized fluids cannot be regarded as virus-free.

Fluid filtration using older 'candle' filters made of porcelain (Chamberland) or diatomaceous earth (Berkefeld) have now been largely replaced for laboratory use by other types. Filtration through an asbestos pad (Seitz) or through sintered (fused) glass is often employed. Even these methods have disadvantages such as absorption of the filtrate and uneven pore size.

For more accurate work, membrane filtration is the method of choice. Membrane filters are made of cellulose acetate and can be obtained with a variety of pore sizes ranging from 0.45 μm to 10 nm. Such filters can be autoclaved prior to use, and have been employed extensively for the bacteriological analysis of water, and for the grading of virus particles by size. As with other filtration methods, the flow may be assisted by positive or negative pressure. It is necessary to use filters with mean pore diameters of less than 0.25 μm to exclude bacteria.

Air filtration is the most practicable method of removing bacteria from the air of operating theatres and other rooms where aseptic techniques are employed, as in pharmaceutical laboratories. Filters may be made of various materials; 'paper absolute filters' remove over 99 per cent of particles between 0.1 μm and 0.5 μm diameter; if used along with prefilters to remove gross dust, they have a life of about 3 years.

Another method of air filtration involves the use of electrostatic precipitation.

Sterilization by irradiation

There are two forms of radiation that are used in sterilization, non-ionizing and ionizing.

NON-IONIZING RADIATION

Ultraviolet rays used in sterilization have a wavelength in the range of 330 nm to 240 nm. These ultraviolet rays induce a chemical alteration in the cellular DNA.

The sun is a natural source of ultraviolet rays; in the laboratory and in hospitals, mercury vapour lamps emitting rays of 253.7 nm are used. Such waves possess low electromagnetic energy and have relatively poor penetrating powers compared with ionizing radiation.

Ultraviolet radiation is used mainly for rendering clean the air of operating theatres, wards, bacteriological inoculating cabinets, and culture preparation rooms. In industry, it is used to disinfect the air of special processing plants such as those involved in the packaging of drugs, etc. Ultraviolet radiation may also be employed to provide sterile water for microbiological and pharmaceutical laboratories.

IONIZING RADIATION

Two forms of ionizing radiation are employed, high energy electrons, and electromagnetic radiation of short wavelength, sometimes termed γ-rays or X-rays.

High energy electrons

These electrons are emitted from the cathode when a high voltage potential is set up in an evacuated tube and they are known as cathode rays. The rays may be accelerated by electrostatic forces and can be directed through an aluminium window on to the articles to be sterilized. Two types of electron accelerators are in use, the microwave linear accelerator and the Van de Graaff electrostatic accelerator. The doses used in sterilization are measured in rads. A rad is a dose corresponding to the dissipation of 100 ergs/g. Electrons possess poor penetrating powers but have a high energy content.

Electromagnetic γ-rays

These are similar to short-wave X-rays, and are emitted from radioactive material such as ^{60}Co. The ^{60}Co source is usually stored within a thick steel–concrete container and the articles to be sterilized are exposed to radiation on a conveyor belt. Doses for sterilization are measured in M rads, or in kilocuries (1 curie is the amount of isotope that has an activity of 3.7×10^{10} disintegrations per sec). γ-Rays have good powers of penetration but are of low energy yield.

Advantages and disadvantages of ionizing irradiation

Both methods are very efficient sterilizing agents, and produce a negligible rise in temperature of the article that is treated. Articles may also be packed and sealed prior to sterilization. High energy electrons achieve complete sterilization in seconds.

The main disadvantages include the long sterilization period required with γ-rays (up to 60 hours), the loss of tensile strength of glassware and textiles, and the tendency to spoil the flavour of foods. The activity of some drugs (sulphonamides, barbiturates, steroids) may be affected.

The uses of ionizing irradiation include the sterilization of surgical sutures, gloves, catheters, dressings, culture plates, syringes, bone grafts, plastic prostheses, foods and some drugs.

Antimicrobial chemical agents

These have a long history and are inseparably associated with the name of Lister and the development of antiseptic surgery. Chemicals which are too toxic for application to human tissues are referred to as **disinfectants**, whereas those which are less irritant and injurious to living tissue cells are called **antiseptics**. Unfortunately, there is no single chemical agent that will serve the purposes of disinfection, antisepsis and sterilization.

The assessment of a chemical agent for disinfection or antisepsis must take into account the following factors.

Bactericidal activity

The only sterilizing agents which are sporicidal are chlorine, iodine, formaldehyde and ethylene oxide. *Mycobacterium tuberculosis* is resistant to most agents though immersion for several hours in a solution of phenol kills these organisms. Gram-negative bacilli, especially *Pseudomonas pyocyanea*, tend to be more resistant to the action of some chemical agents than Gram-positive organisms. Viruses are more resistant than bacteria; chlorine, chlorine-liberating compounds and formalin are the most useful agents for the chemical destruction of viruses.

Bacteristatic activity

Mercurials and quaternary ammonium compounds act by inhibiting multiplication of bacteria and have no lethal effect. Blood neutralizes the action of mercurials, so bacteria can withstand the toxic effects of locally applied mercury salts for many hours if there is blood present.

Speed of action

Most chemical agents take hours to achieve their effect. This slow activity can be accelerated by raising the temperature, by increasing the concentration of the agent, and by employing agents which possess good powers of penetration through blood, pus, faeces, grease, etc.

Quenching effect

Proteinaceous material, such as blood, faeces and pus, has a quenching effect on the action of chlorine compounds, iodine and quaternary ammonium compounds.

Toxicity and other factors

The suitability of a given chemical agent may be limited by its toxicity to living tissue cells, its irritable vapour, corrosive action on instruments or textiles, staining effects, poor keeping properties and cost.

STANDARDIZATION OF DISINFECTANTS

The classical test is the **Rideal–Walker test**, which compares the power of the test substance with that of phenol to kill a standard culture of *Salmonella typhi*. The **phenol coefficient** expresses the ability of the test disinfectant to kill the organisms when compared with phenol. Nowadays this test is seldom employed in hospitals. Its drawbacks are that distilled water is used as the suspending medium, no account of the quenching power of proteins is taken, the contact with the disinfectant is only a few minutes, and the action of the test substance against other organisms is not evaluated. The **Chick–Martin test** was introduced to overcome some of the disadvantages. Organic matter in the form of a suspension of yeast or sterile faeces is added to the test medium; longer exposure times are employed, and the disinfectant is tested against other organisms.

More realistic tests have since been developed to assess disinfectants and antiseptics for specific applications. **Use-dilution tests** involve a parallel study of the bactericidal efficiencies of compounds applied to artificially contaminated test objects. Another type of test measures the capacity of various compounds to disinfect after repeated additions of a suspension of the test organisms. The **in-use test** is most suitable for day-to-day use in hospital. Samples of contents of mop-buckets, liquid expressed from mops, disinfectant from storage containers, etc. are diluted in Ringer solution and inoculated on suitable agar media. The disinfectant fails this test when more than half the samples yield viable bacteria.

When surviving bacteria are enumerated by viable counts in these studies, it is most important that an appropriate neutralizer of the test compound should be incorporated at the enumeration stage lest carry-over of the test disinfectant into the culture medium should produce falsely favourable results.

MODES OF ACTION OF CHEMICAL AGENTS

Disruption of cytoplasmic membrane

Some agents, such as detergents, concentrate in the membrane and so alter its physicochemical properties. This leads to cell death or to inhibition of cell function. However, most chemical agents must first penetrate the cytoplasmic membrane to achieve their effect.

Alteration of SH groups

Many cell enzymes cannot function unless their SH groups remain free and in a reduced state. Oxidizing agents, such as chlorine, iodine, peroxides, act on these free SH groups, resulting in widespread cell damage leading to cell death.

Coagulation of protein

Most enzymes in the cell exist in a colloid state. If these proteins are coagulated and precipitated they become inactive and the cell dies.

CLASSIFICATION OF CHEMICAL AGENTS

A short review of the more commonly used chemical agents is now presented.

Phenols

These substances act by coagulating protein. Phenol itself (carbolic acid) was used by Lister to control surgical wound infection, so laying the foundation of antiseptic surgery. It is effective against bacteria and viruses, but is no longer used as a disinfectant because it is expensive (it is now used extensively in the manufacturing of plastics) and it is toxic. Cresols are alkyl phenols and are obtained from the distillation of coal tar. Lysol and Sudol are solutions of cresols in soap. Lysol is used in labora-

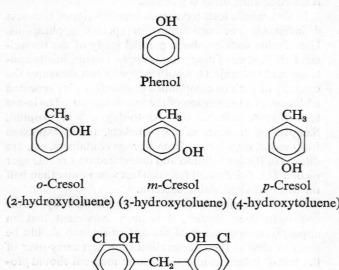

Phenol

o-Cresol   *m*-Cresol   *p*-Cresol
(2-hydroxytoluene) (3-hydroxytoluene) (4-hydroxytoluene)

Hexachlorophane

Fig. 18.22. Cresols are hydroxyl derivatives of alkyl benzenes with disinfectant properties.

tories for the disinfection of contaminated glassware and specimens of faeces, sputum, etc. It is irritant to the skin. Sudol is less toxic, and in 0·75–1 per cent solution is used extensively for the coarse disinfection of floors, benches, bedpans, lavatories, etc. Cresols have the advantage of not being quenched by organic material. Xylenols are methyl cresols, and Dettol, a chlorinated xylenol, is probably the most widely used disinfectant and antiseptic for domestic purposes. It should not be used for coarse disinfectant purposes. It is not irritant, but has

the drawbacks of being easily quenched and of being inactive against *Pseudomonas pyocyanea*. In fact, Dettol is sometimes used in culture media as a selective agent for *Ps. pyocyanea*. Hycolin is a chlorinated xylenol similar to Dettol, and may be used for skin antisepsis as a 5 per cent solution. Hexachlorophane is a complex chlorinated diphenyl phenol. It has a bacteristatic action and is more active against Gram-positive cocci; it is only weakly active against Gram-negative bacilli. It should be used repeatedly for it possesses a cumulative action; a single application is virtually useless. Its main use is for skin antisepsis, either as a surgical scrub or for bathing of infants or for use in baths, and it is employed primarily to remove *Staph. aureus* from the skin. Proprietary preparations include Phisohex (3 per cent hexachlorophane in a detergent cream base), Ster-Zac dusting powder (containing 0·33 per cent hexachlorophane), Ster-Zac liquid soap (containing 3 per cent hexachlorophane) and a bath concentrate containing 10 per cent hexachlorophane.

Alcohols

Ethyl alcohol, or better **isopropyl alcohol**, are used for rapid skin disinfection and are probably the best substances for this purpose. A 70 per cent concentration in water is the most effective. These alcohols coagulate cell proteins and kill bacteria and some viruses. They are rapid in action, but they do not readily penetrate organic matter.

Oxidizing Agents

Hydrogen peroxide and **potassium permanganate** act by oxidation of free SH groups. These agents have limited clinical use and are easily quenched.

Halogens

Chlorine, iodine, and compounds which release chlorine, such as **sodium hypochlorite**, are lethal to bacteria, viruses, fungi and spores. Thus they may be truly regarded as sterilizing agents but in practice they are used primarily as disinfectants or antiseptics and they have limited applications. Their mode of action is to oxidize SH groups. The main disadvantage to their use is their susceptibility to quenching by organic matter.

Chlorine and hypochlorite are used widely for the disinfection of drinking water and swimming baths. Sufficient must be added to give not less than 0·1 parts per million residual chlorine, and in the case of swimming baths continuous chlorination is necessary. Hypochlorite is used for the disinfection of relatively clean items (feeding bottles, baths, glassware, etc.). **Eusol**, a 0·3 per cent solution of hypochlorous acid, is useful for local application to ulcers and bedsores.

Iodine, as a 2 per cent solution in isopropyl alcohol, is an excellent skin disinfectant, but must not be used where the skin surface is breached. Some people are susceptible to iodine and may suffer severe skin sensitization.

Iodophors are solutions of iodine in a non-ionic surface active detergent. Betadine is a well-known proprietary preparation and contains 0·75 per cent available iodine. Iodophors are quite widely used for skin disinfection as they are less irritant than iodine. They are, however, poorly resistant to quenching effects.

Metallic salts

Salts of mercury, silver and copper have had their vogue in chemical disinfection and are little used today. They act by coagulating protein, and also by combining with free SH groups. These salts are predominantly bacteristatic, slow in action and readily quenched. Mercuric perchloride is the most active inorganic mercury salt but it

$$C_2H_5HgS \langle \bigcirc \rangle$$
$$COONa$$
Merthiolate

has no place in modern surgical practice. **Merthiolate**, a proprietary organic mercurial, is used as a preservative of serum and serological reagents. Silver nitrate was extensively employed in the past in prophylaxis against gonococcal infection in neonates and now has a place in the control of infection in burns; colloidal silver (argyrol) is still of use in ophthalmic care.

Dyes

Aniline dyes, e.g. gentian violet, brilliant green, are active against some Gram-positive organisms and are relatively nontoxic to the skin tissues. A 1 per cent gentian violet solution is sometimes used topically for the treatment of oral yeast infection (thrush). *Myco. tuberculosis* and *Strept. pyogenes* are resistant to these dyes. The main disadvantages to their use are their skin staining properties and their susceptibility to protein quenching.

Acridine dyes, e.g. proflavine, acriflavine, are more active than aniline dyes against Gram-positive bacteria, and are also active against Gram-negative bacilli. They are nontoxic, resist quenching and are bactericidal. These dyes are of use as a 0·1 per cent solution for application to cuts, burns and grazes.

Soaps

Soaps possess a weak disinfectant activity and are active against *Strept. pyogenes*, *Strept. pneumoniae*, *H. influenzae* and the influenza virus, but they have no action on *Staph. pyogenes*, *Myco. tuberculosis*, or Gram-negative bacilli. The main effect of washing with soap is a mechanical one and soaps are useful for the removal of transient skin flora. Soaps act by disrupting the cytoplasmic membrane.

Detergents (surface-active agents)

Anionic detergents and **non-ionic detergents** are cleansing agents with poor disinfecting activity. Anionic detergents include soaps.

$$\begin{array}{c} CH_3 \\ | \\ C_nH_{2n}-N^{\pm}-CH_2 \langle \bigcirc \rangle \quad Cl^- \\ | \\ CH_3 \end{array}$$
Benzalkonium chloride

Cationic detergents include the quaternary ammonium compounds benzalkonium chloride (Zephiran, Roccal) and cetyltrimethylammonium bromide (Cetavlon, Cetrimide). These are good cleansing agents for inanimate surfaces as well as the skin, and possess disinfectant powers. They are active against Gram-positive cocci but they are of no value against *Myco. tuberculosis*, spores or viruses. Bacteristatic in action, they are easily quenched and are incompatible with soap. Their usefulness is restricted by the resistance of Gram-negative organisms. Thus *Ps. pyocyanea* has been shown to multiply in the corks of bottles containing the disinfectant. Quaternary compounds are readily absorbed to textiles, which is a drawback. In one instance cotton wool swabs stored in Zephiran absorbed the disinfectant, and allowed *Ps. pyocyanea* to grow freely in the storage fluid. When these swabs were subsequently used for treating the skin prior to intravenous manipulations, a severe epidemic of *Ps. pyocyanea* septicaemia followed. This illustrates a disadvantage of quaternary ammonium compounds, but swabs should not be used in this way with any disinfectant.

The mode of action of detergents is similar to that of soap.

Chlorhexidine

Chlorhexidine (Hibitane) is a chlorinated phenyl diguanide with bactericidal and bacteristatic properties. It is more active against Gram-positive bacteria, including *Myco. tuberculosis*, but it has a useful degree of activity against some Gram-negative bacteria. Spores and viruses are resistant. It is well tolerated by tissues and is widely used as an antiseptic; chlorhexidine possesses low toxicity, is not readily quenched, but is incompatible with soap. Cork bark contains tannins which interfere with its antibacterial action, and it should not be stored in containers with corks or cork-lined caps.

A 0·5 per cent solution of chlorhexidine in 70 per cent isopropyl alcohol in water is useful as a preoperative skin disinfectant; it is equivalent in activity to a 1 per cent solution of iodine in alcohol, and sensitivity reactions do not occur. The solution may be used also for disinfecting ward thermometers, but it is not antiviral. Aqueous preparations of chlorhexidine have many applications in hospital and general practice. Chlorhexidine possesses greater activity in combination with Cetrimide (p. 18.41) than when used alone. The mixture is commercially available as Savlon hospital concentrate (ICI); at the recommended dilutions, this mixture can be used in aqueous solution for

Chlorhexidine: 1,6 *di-(N-p-chlorophenyldiguanido) hexane*

antiseptic and disinfectant purposes ranging from the treatment of wounds to surface disinfection of tables; alcoholic solutions provide rapid and efficient skin cleansing and skin disinfection.

Chlorhexidine ointment or cream, e.g. Hibitane 1 per cent, is used in surgical and obstetric work, and this is a useful first-aid application which should replace many traditional ointments that still linger in first-aid boxes and medical cabinets. Combined with neomycin, chlorhexidine is used in ointment form to suppress nasal carriage of *Staph. aureus*.

Formalin

Formalin is a 40 per cent solution of formaldehyde in water. When diluted to 10 per cent, it remains a true sterilizing agent and is lethal to bacteria, viruses, fungi and spores. However, it is slow in action and may require up to 24 hours to achieve its maximum effect. It possesses an irritant vapour and has poor penetrating power in the presence of organic matter. Formalin is used in the treatment of wools and hides to kill anthrax spores. Its use as a vapour is described below.

Glutaraldehyde

As a 2 per cent aqueous solution buffered at an alkaline pH, this aldehyde is more rapid in action than formalin and is less irritant. It is marketed as Cidex, and is widely used for the sterilization of objects not suitable for autoclaving, e.g. plastic prostheses, thermometers, pacemakers, anaesthetic equipment and endoscopes. Items treated with glutaraldehyde must be washed with sterile water to remove traces of the chemical before use. In the acid state, glutaraldehyde solution is stable for long periods if kept cool and in a closed container; aqueous solutions are mildly acid and stable, but they are much more potently antimicrobial and sporicidal when they are made alkaline. The alkaline solution then gradually polymerizes and begins to lose activity after 2 weeks. Cidex is therefore supplied as a stable acid solution; the activated solution is prepared by adding a powder supplied with the solution and this adjusts the pH to alkalinity and incorporates a rust inhibitor.

GASES AS STERILIZING AND DISINFECTING AGENTS

Sterilization with gaseous agents has the advantage of leaving the articles undamaged, and, with the exception of formaldehyde, penetration is good. Expense, lengthy sterilization times, and the necessity of a humid environment are the main drawbacks. γ-Irradiation is superseding gaseous methods.

Formaldehyde vapour

This gas is used for the disinfection of rooms and bulky items such as blankets and mattresses. It is the most effective agent for room disinfection and may be employed after a room has been occupied by a patient suffering from smallpox or tuberculosis. For this purpose, formalin is boiled in an open container.

The room must be sealed and water should be sprayed on the floors and walls to raise the humidity to 50 per cent. After exposure to the formalin vapour for 24 hours, the room is aired or exposed to ammonia vapour to rid it of toxic paraformaldehyde which forms when formalin boils.

Disinfection of mattresses, blankets, pillows, toys, etc. may be achieved in a closed chamber such as an autoclave. Penetration of formaldehyde is improved when the humidity is over 50 per cent, the temperature over 50°C and in the presence of a partial vacuum. Nevertheless, this method is not wholly reliable, as penetration of formaldehyde into fabrics is uncertain. For the sterilization of such bulky items formaldehyde in association with steam at subatmospheric pressure is preferred (p. 18.44).

Ethylene oxide

This agent is in gaseous form at room temperature, and forms an inflammable mixture with air. Consequently it is normally mixed with CO_2 or nitrogen. The risk of explosion is avoided if the ethylene oxide contributes no more than 12 per cent of this mixture. A specially designed chamber is used into which water is first introduced to raise the humidity to 50 per cent. The gas is then admitted and the temperature raised to 50°C to accelerate sterilization. Alternatively the article to be sterilized is enclosed in a plastic bag which is then exhausted of air and inflated with ethylene oxide. The former method takes 3 hours and the plastic bag method 12 hours to achieve sterilization.

Ethylene oxide gas has diverse uses. Heart–lung apparatus, plastic disposable items (transfusion sets, syringes), catheters, artery and bone grafts, cystoscopes, bedclothing, clothes, books, toys and pharmaceutical products may all be sterilized by it. It has been used for the sterilization of rooms (provided the room is thoroughly aerated afterwards), and it has even been used to treat rockets for space travel.

Ethylene oxide in liquid form, i.e. at less than 10·7°C, may be employed for sterilizing fluid culture media and vaccines.

Advantages of ethylene oxide are its rapid penetration through paper, fabrics and plastics, and its solubility in oils, rubber and plastics. Its main disadvantages are its explosiveness in air, and its toxicity for the skin and on inhalation. Skin irritation is shown by the development of vesicles. Mutagenic properties have been ascribed to this agent. Rubber tends to retain the gas for several hours and should not be handled for 24 hours after exposure. A humid environment is necessary, for bacteria in a dry state are very resistant to the gas.

β-Propiolactone

This gas produces rapid sterilization of such materials as serum and grafts. Due to its alleged carcinogenic properties its use is limited.

Notes on sterilization or disinfection of special articles or sites

STERILIZATION OF BOTTLED FLUIDS

Fluids for intravenous use and sterile water for the operating theatre are autoclaved. The holding period need be only 12 min at 121°C. Bottles should be filled to four-fifths and loosely stoppered to avoid breakage. The cooling period must be over 30 min.

STERILIZATION OF SURGICAL AND WRAPPED DRY MATERIALS

Two essential requirements are the complete removal of air from the autoclave chamber during the sterilization period, and proper drying of the load before removal from the autoclave.

The load should not be tightly packed and must not be placed in containers impervious to steam. It is preferable to pack all materials for autoclaving in a double wrapping of Kraft paper. Surgical dressing packs must not exceed 30 × 30 × 50 cms (12 × 12 × 20 ins). Rubber gloves should be powdered and packed in muslin. Tubing should be wetted internally, and instruments freed from grease. Completely dry cloth or rubber should never be autoclaved as charring may occur.

Holding periods vary according to the size of the load and the type of autoclave.

Drying of the load is achieved by allowing the rapid escape of steam, together with the heating effect of steam in the jacket and the entry of warm sterile air into the chamber. This process may take 25 min, but the use of high prevacuum autoclaves greatly speeds sterilization, only 17 min being required to complete the whole process. On removal from the autoclave, wrapped packs must not be placed on a cold surface as condensation of moisture allows bacteria to gain entry through the wrap-

ping. Such packs should be sterilized in cardboard containers. The storage life is several weeks.

STERILIZATION OF SURGICAL INSTRUMENTS

Boiling is not recommended. Autoclaving as described above is the best method, or the hot-air oven, when instruments are packed in impermeable containers.

With instruments which may be damaged at high temperatures (some cystoscopes and bronchoscopes), other methods must be used, but some are not sterilizing. Nonsterilizing procedures include steam at sub-atmospheric pressure, hot water pasteurization, boiling in sterile water for 3 min, and immersion in alcoholic chlorhexidine. Prolonged immersion in 2 per cent buffered glutaraldehyde (Cidex) or exposure to ethylene oxide gas may achieve sterilization if the article is clean initially.

STERILIZATION OF SYRINGES

The use of sterile disposable syringes solves many problems.

All-glass syringes

Boiling in water for at least 5 min with the syringe dismantled may be used in emergencies; the syringe should be used at once and not stored in a 'germicidal solution'.

For sterilization in the hot-air oven, the piston and inside of the barrel must be smeared with liquid paraffin. The assembled syringe and needle are packed in a glass or aluminium tube, and remain sterile indefinitely after exposure to 160°C for 1 hour. If the autoclave is preferred, paraffin lubrication is avoided and the syringe is dismantled (but may be assembled if the high prevacuum type of autoclave is used).

After each use the syringe and needle should be washed through with cold 2 per cent Lysol, then brushed with soap and water and very thoroughly rinsed. A stilette should be used to clear the needle bore.

Glass–metal syringes

These cannot be sterilized unless dismantled. Sterilization is as for all-glass syringes except that the hot-air oven is to be avoided, as the high temperature may cause the solder to melt.

DISINFECTION OF ANAESTHETIC APPARATUS

Endotracheal tubes, face pieces and airways should be autoclaved, or treated by special procedures as advised by the hospital bacteriologist. The disinfection of corrugated tubing, rebreathing bags and absorber canisters presents similar problems. Heat-sensitive valves should be dismantled, cleaned and then sterilized by steam if practicable, or treated with 70 per cent alcohol. Ventilators should be sterilized with ethylene oxide after each use by an infected patient.

STEAM AT SUBATMOSPHERIC PRESSURE
(high vacuum low temperature steam)

Steam at a temperature of 70–80°C has been employed in recent years for the disinfection of materials liable to damage if subjected to repeated exposures to higher temperatures. Thus, contaminated cystoscopes, bronchoscopes, electrical equipment, fabrics, rubber goods, plastics and bulky items such as blankets and mattresses can be treated by this method.

The method is first to evacuate the loaded autoclave to less than −500 mm Hg pressure. Steam is then allowed to enter the chamber where it expands rapidly and so loses heat. The steam supply is stopped when the chamber pressure equals −250 mm Hg pressure; the steam at this pressure is at a temperature of 70–80°C. Penetration of the load by the steam is rapid and articles are disinfected but not necessarily sterilized in 15–30 min. Sterilization may be achieved by introducing formaldehyde into the chamber and this added procedure kills spores in 1–3 hours.

DISINFECTION OF THE SKIN

A good skin disinfectant (antiseptic) must be non-irritant, have a wide spectrum of antimicrobial activity, be rapidly bactericidal and possess a prolonged action.

Preoperative preparation
Where clostridial infection is likely, e.g. operation sites on the leg or in the perineal region, the area should be thoroughly cleaned several times with a detergent such as Cetavlon and a Betadine compress then applied for 30 min. This procedure helps to rid the site of sporing bacteria.

Preoperative skin antisepsis
Either 2 per cent iodine in 70 per cent isopropyl alcohol or 0·5 per cent chlorhexidine in 70 per cent alcohol are the agents of choice. For cleansing of skin over the site of venepuncture, 0·5 per cent alcoholic chlorhexidine is recommended.

Disinfection of hands
For general ablution purposes either Phisohex or Betadine is recommended. Betadine is preferable for a single wash as Phisohex must be used repeatedly to achieve its maximum activity. As a surgical scrub, a wash with either of these agents is advised, followed by immersion of the hands in 0·5 per cent alcoholic chlorhexidine.

ANTISEPTICS IN THE CONTROL OF CROSS-INFECTION

In maternity nurseries infants may be bathed after birth and then daily with Phisohex. The staff may wash with Phisohex after handling each infant. Savlon may be employed for washing floors, walls, furniture, etc. Acetic acid (0·5 per cent) may be added to incubator water tanks and the incubator washed with Savlon.

Phisohex or Betadine for handwashing, and the instillation of a powder containing chlorhexidine into wounds are of use for the control of cross-infection in wards.

Cases of urinary infection following surgery may be controlled by the employment of closed bladder drainage and the preoperative disinfection of the urethra with chlorhexidine jelly. After catheterization, 1 in 5000 aqueous chlorhexidine may be instilled into the bladder.

For skin treatment in cases of recurrent boils and 'spreaders' or dispersers of staphylococci, hexachlorophane preparations are of use; Phisohex should be used in the hospital and at home for handwashing. This should be supplemented by daily baths for 4 weeks using Ster-Zac bath concentrate, and Ster-Zac powder should be dusted twice daily on the axillae, groins and perineum.

THEATRE SERVICE CENTRES
Centralized bulk sterilization of ward and theatre instruments, dressings and apparatus reduces the risk of infection from failure in sterilization.

In the past, much waste of labour, time and apparatus was expended when each ward or theatre unit was responsible for the provision of its own sterile materials. The past few years have seen the introduction of units in which the sterilization of instruments and other hospital equipment is centralized. Such units or departments now serve the needs of several wards and theatres, or may even supply sterilized materials to a group of hospitals.

The basic equipment for central sterile supply departments consists of an autoclave (usually of the high pre-vacuum type) and at least one hot-air oven of the conveyor belt type. Each department should have a manager responsible for production (often the hospital pharmacist), and the methods employed in the unit should be under the control of the hospital bacteriologist. The supervision of the whole unit and the checking of priorities of sterilization should be undertaken by an infection control committee comprising various members of the hospital medical and nursing staff and convened by the hospital bacteriologist.

BACTERIAL METABOLISM AND NUTRITION

The bacteria may be divided into
(1) simple nonparasitic **autotrophs** which utilize CO_2 and inorganic compounds, and
(2) **heterotrophs**, which include all parasites and require organic nutrients. The more exacting of the heterotrophs require ready-made amino acids and essential growth factors.

Another classification is recognized:

(1) **Phototrophs** utilize mainly solar radiation as an energy source and are subdivided into **photolithotrophs** which oxidize inorganic compounds for growth, and **photo-organotrophs** which oxidize organic compounds for growth.

(2) **Chemotrophs** obtain their energy from chemical compounds; **chemolithotrophs** obtain energy from oxidation-reduction reactions involving inorganic compounds, and **chemo-organotrophs** oxidize or ferment organic compounds to provide energy.

Bacterial metabolism

Mammals and their bacterial parasites are chemo-organotrophs. They obtain their energy mainly by the oxidative breakdown of carbohydrates, fats and proteins; some bacteria, like many mammalian tissues, may also obtain energy from the anaerobic breakdown of carbohydrates and a few species are obligatory anaerobes. In general, parasitic bacteria and mammalian tissues use the same intermediary pathways for the breakdown of carbohydrates, fat and proteins. Bacteria also have to synthesize structural protein and lipid and to maintain small stores of energy in the form of triglyceride and polysaccharide. Again, for these purposes, parasitic bacteria and mammalian tissues use the same chemical pathways. Thus the greater part of the account of general biochemistry which is presented in Volume 1 is applicable to both mammalian and bacterial cells. Some parasitic bacterial species, like some types of specialized mammalian cells, have acquired new chemical pathways for the synthesis or breakdown of specific chemical substances; others, e.g. the obligatory anaerobes, have lost certain specific chemical mechanisms. The metabolism of individual bacterial species is considered later in this chapter, but only when a knowledge of these metabolic properties helps to explain the spread of the organism within the human body or its survival and spread in the environment; a knowledge of metabolic differences between bacteria is also useful in the identification of bacterial species and subtypes.

BACTERIAL ENZYMES AND THEIR CONTROL

The enzymes formed by a bacterial cell may be divided into two types. First there are **constitutive enzymes** and these are present whatever the environment or conditions of growth. Secondly there are **inducible enzymes** which are not normally present in significant or detectable amounts but are developed by the cell when a specific inducing agent is present. The inducer is usually the specific substrate for the induced enzyme. The process of induction may occur sequentially; substance A induces enzyme EA which leads to the production of intermediate B which induces enzyme EB, and so on. Alternatively, the initial inducer may bring about the production of a whole set of

enzymes required for a particular series of steps on a metabolic pathway (fig. 18.23). In the absence of the inducer, an inducible enzyme is held in check by intracellular **repressor mechanisms** acting via the nuclear apparatus and inhibiting synthesis of the specific enzyme. A similar system involving negative feedback control

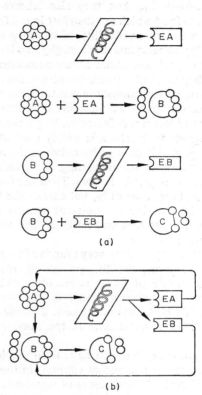

FIG. 18.23. Simplified concepts of enzyme induction. (a) The inducer A induces production of enzyme EA, and the intermediate B induces enzyme EB to produce end-product C. (b) The inducer A induces EA and EB directly to produce C.

operates within the cell to regulate the production of the appropriate biosynthetic enzymes in the presence of excess amounts of the normal end-product of their activity. These complex control mechanisms are discussed further on p. 18.53.

Nutrients

Parasitic bacteria are limited in their synthetic ability and require organic material to enable them to grow and survive. Many of them are less exacting than mammals in their needs for essential amino acids, but certain species require individual amino acids, e.g. tryptophan and leucine, and in some cases preformed purines are also necessary. Bacteria vary in their ability to synthesize vitamins and in many species an external supply of one or more of the B group of vitamins is essential. In some instances, mammalian and bacterial cells may compete for a limited supply of a vitamin present in the environment and some antibacterial drugs act by blocking the action of a vitamin essential for bacterial growth (p. 20.2).

Bacteria in the gut of man synthesize significant amounts of vitamin K, riboflavine, nicotinic acid, folic acid and vitamin B_{12}, but they also absorb vitamins ingested in the food which are then lost in the faeces. The overall effect on the availability of vitamins in healthy persons taking an adequate diet is negligible. However, in some forms of gastrointestinal disease associated particularly with stagnation of intestinal contents, the number of bacteria increases enormously in certain areas of the gut and their consumption of vitamins contributes to the development of vitamin deficiencies. The feeding of antimicrobial agents to livestock is widely used to improve growth and probably does so by reducing the number of bacteria in the gut and increasing the availability of vitamins and other growth factors. Their use for this purpose is valuable economically, but carries the hazard of increasing the number of resistant strains (p. 20.6). There is no evidence that oral antimicrobial therapy improves nutrition in man.

Some bacterial species are very exacting in their growth needs. For example, for the growth of *Haemophilus influenzae* a supply of haem is essential and *Brucella abortus* requires erythritol which is abundant in the placenta and foetal tissues of the cow. Bacteria also have requirements for mineral salts in the same manner as mammals.

Exacting strains of bacteria have been much used for the bio-assay of the B group of vitamins in foods, blood and urine. Microbiological assays of vitamins are largely replaced by chemical methods, but are still the best means available for assaying folic acid and vitamin B_{12} in foods and other biological material.

TRANSPORT OF NUTRIENTS

Bacteria take up nutrients from the environment in aqueous solution. The concentration of solutes inside the cell often far exceeds that outside; hence molecules of water tend to enter and dilute the cell contents. If this were not checked, the cell membrane would expand and rupture, killing the organism. To withstand the large osmotic pressure, the membrane is supported by the cell wall, which is relatively rigid (p. 18.7).

Passage of nutrients through the cytoplasmic membrane may be either active or passive. Active transport is assisted by **permeases**, enzymes present in many bacteria which transfer specific substrates across the cell membrane against concentration gradients.

Most of the enzymes of the bacterial cell are intracellular **endoenzymes**, but bacteria also produce **exoenzymes** which are excreted into the environment. They are mostly hydrolases, concerned with the breakdown of macromolecules into small fragments which can be taken into the cell as nutrients. For example, many bacterial proteases, lipases and carbohydrases are known.

THE CULTIVATION OF BACTERIA

Environmental factors

Important environmental factors which must be provided to ensure the successful cultivation of bacteria are now considered.

ATMOSPHERIC REQUIREMENT FOR GROWTH

Many pathogenic bacteria can grow either aerobically or anaerobically, i.e., in the presence or absence of free oxygen, and are described as **facultative anaerobes**. Some species, e.g. tubercle bacilli, will grow only in the presence of free oxygen and are termed **strict (obligate) aerobes**; other species, particularly members of the genus *Clostridium* and the genus *Bacteroides*, are strictly **anaerobic** and must be provided with an environment from which all traces of free oxygen have been removed. An important characteristic of a strict anaerobe is that it cannot initiate growth from a small inoculum unless the oxidation-reduction potential (Eh) of its environment is low. These requirements are met in the necrotic tissue of some infected lacerated wounds, especially if fragments of debris or soil particles are present, and such wounds are thus associated with a risk of anaerobic infections which include tetanus and gas gangrene. In the laboratory, several methods are available for the production of anaerobic environments, but the most convenient, effective and widely used is the McIntosh and Fildes anaerobic jar or some modification of it. Most of the air is removed by evacuation; any residual oxygen is eliminated by introducing hydrogen into the jar; an electrically heated catalyst or a cold catalyst within the jar catalyses the union of hydrogen and residual oxygen so that an oxygen-free atmosphere is obtained.

A few species of bacteria do not grow in the presence of normal atmospheric concentrations but require trace amounts of oxygen. These **microaerophiles** often prefer a concentration of CO_2 that is higher than normal, e.g. 5–10 per cent. The growth of some aerobic and anaerobic species may also be greatly improved by added CO_2 and some organisms have a clear requirement for CO_2.

TEMPERATURE

It has long been customary to divide micro-organisms into three groups depending on the optimum temperature for their growth *in vitro*, which reflects approximately the temperature of their natural habitat. Bacteria parasitic for warm-blooded hosts usually grow best at about 37°C. Such parasitic species and many saprophytes are **mesophiles** with an optimum temperature for growth in the range 25–40°C. **Thermophilic** bacteria belong to a group which grow best at temperatures greater than 40°C, whereas those which grow best at temperatures lower than 20°C are termed **psychrophilic**. These are generally nonpathogenic to man, but they can cause spoilage of refrigerated food. Thermophilic species can spoil canned foods unless the processing of the latter is sufficient to destroy the bacteria and the highly heat-resistant spores that many thermophiles can produce.

Sterilization procedures aimed at ridding materials of all forms of microbial life are described on p. 18.33. Bacteria are always killed by exposure to sufficiently high temperatures but not necessarily by exposure to low temperatures (see fig. 18.24). Species differ in their resistance

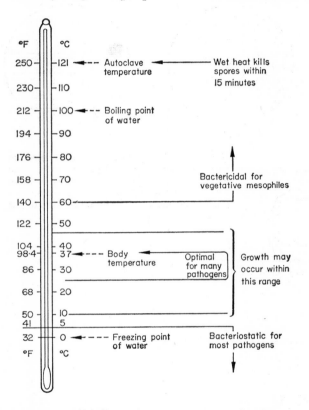

FIG. 18.24. The effect of temperature on the (mesophilic) pathogenic bacteria of man.

to heat and cold. Spores are generally much more heat-resistant than the vegetative cells. A practical index of heat-sensitivity or heat-resistance is provided by the **D value** or **decimal reduction time**; this is the time of exposure (minutes) at a given temperature that results in a ten-fold reduction in numbers of a test bacterial suspension under standard conditions. Some species of bacteria die rapidly when exposed to temperatures of 0° to −2°C or lower, but many bacteria survive for long periods in the cold provided that they are held in a suitable medium.

Rapidly freeze-dried cultures can be maintained for very long periods without the need for subcultivation.

HYDROGEN-ION CONCENTRATION
The bacteria that parasitize man grow best within a fairly restricted range of pH between 7·2 and 7·6 although the absolute limits of hydrogen ion concentration for growth generally are wider, viz. 4·0–9·0. Some bacteria, however, grow best at a low pH value and are termed **acidophilic**, e.g. *Lactobacillus acidophilus*, whereas others such as *Vibrio cholerae* are intolerant of an acid environment and flourish at pH 8·5. The resistance of tubercle bacilli to strong solutions of acids and alkalis allows us to employ 4 per cent caustic soda for the treatment of material like sputum; this destroys other bacteria whilst the tubercle bacilli survive. The treated material can then be cultured or inoculated into animals for diagnostic purposes and the test is uncomplicated by contaminants. However, the material is neutralized before these steps are undertaken and there is a difference between acid-tolerance in culture (*Lactobacillus*) and acid-resistance prior to culture (tubercle bacillus).

LIGHT AND OTHER RADIATIONS
A dark environment is the most favourable for the growth and reproduction of bacteria parasitic on animal hosts; phototrophic species require sunlight for their metabolic processes. Bacteria parasitic on man are susceptible to ultraviolet radiation from natural or artificial sources.

Ionizing radiations, X-rays and γ-rays, are also lethal to bacteria and of practical use in sterilization (p. 18.38).

INFLUENCE OF MOISTURE
About 80–90 per cent of the weight of bacterial cells is accounted for by water; drying in air prevents growth and reproduction and results ultimately in the death of vegetative bacteria. The effect of desiccation varies from species to species. For example, highly parasitic species such as gonococci die extremely rapidly under natural conditions when they are separated from a susceptible host. Hardier nonsporing bacterial species such as tubercle bacilli and staphylococci can survive drying in dust for weeks or even months provided that they are not subjected simultaneously to other naturally lethal agents such as sunlight. The remarkable resistance of bacterial spores to desiccation is well recognized. For example, anthrax spores have been shown to survive for at least 50 years when dried on cloth.

Laboratory media
Bacteria are commonly grown in the laboratory in various culture media which range from simple aqueous suspensions of salt, peptone and meat extract (nutrient broth) to

complex media enriched with special growth factors. Peptone is a commercially available powder prepared by proteolytic digestion of meat and it is a convenient crude source of polypeptides, amino acids, mineral salts and growth factors required by relatively undemanding pathogens. Casein hydrolysate is a useful alternative to peptone. Meat extract contains the water-soluble substances of meat extracted by hot water and subsequently concentrated to produce a dark paste; it is rich in many peptide and nitrogenous nutrients and contains minerals and growth factors. Yeast extract is sometimes used in place of meat extract. Nutrient broth may be enriched with carbohydrates, to make 'glucose broth', or it may have meat particles added to make 'cooked-meat broth'. The meat in cooked-meat broth contains reducing substances, e.g. glutathione, which maintain anaerobic conditions at the bottom of the tube and this medium supports the growth of both aerobes and anaerobes.

CULTURE ON SOLID MEDIA

The growth of organisms in fluid culture has the disadvantage that mixtures of species are not readily separated into pure cultures. This difficulty is overcome by culture on the surface of solidified media when individual bacteria or viable particles give rise to **colonies** after incubation. A colony is often derived entirely from one cell and usually allows a pure culture to be picked off and subcultured. Different bacterial genera produce colonies with different characteristics and **colonial morphology** gives the bacteriologist an indication of the probable genus or sometimes the species involved. Thus, a mixed culture present in a specimen of pus from a wound or obtained from a subculture in the laboratory can be resolved into its component pure cultures by 'plating out' procedures which ensure colonial development from individual cells on solid media (fig. 18.25). The solidifying agent is usually 1–2 per cent agar-agar which is an inert polysaccharide obtained from varieties of seaweed. Nutrient agar is nutrient broth solidified

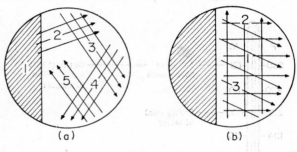

FIG. 18.25. Plating out (a) on normal medium with successive series of strokes (2–5) from the well or reservoir (1); (b) on selective medium with a cross-hatching procedure that ensures a graded but more concentrated seeding of the plate.

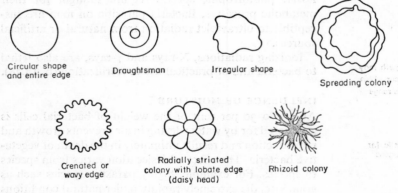

Circular shape and entire edge

Draughtsman

Irregular shape

Spreading colony

Crenated or wavy edge

Radially striated colony with lobate edge (daisy head)

Rhizoid colony

ELEVATION

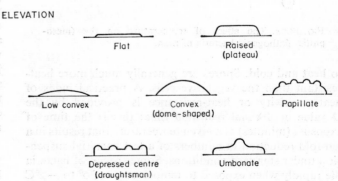

Flat

Raised (plateau)

Low convex

Convex (dome-shaped)

Papillate

Depressed centre (draughtsman)

Umbonate

FIG. 18.26. Bacterial colonial morphology.

with agar; it is frequently enriched with blood to make 'blood agar'.

Some of the various colonial appearances of bacteria are illustrated in fig. 18.26. These are of considerable importance to the clinical bacteriologist, but they are not discussed in detail here. An important variation that may occur in colonial morphology is referred to as **smooth-rough (S-R) variation** (fig. 18.27). This reflects a change in the somatic antigen of the organism and the 'rough variant' may produce atypical reactions in laboratory tests. The change is associated also with loss of virulence in some species.

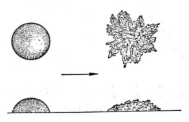

FIG. 18.27. Smooth-rough variation.

A culture medium may be rendered **selective** for a particular group of organisms by incorporating a substance which is inhibitory for other species that are likely to be encountered. Thus, the addition of 4–10 per cent of NaCl to a medium inhibits the growth of most pathogens and commensals excepting staphylococci which are salt-tolerant. Similarly, the growth of staphylococci in a medium can be inhibited by concentrations of crystal violet which allow the growth of streptococci. Many selective agents are incorporated in culture media used for diagnostic purposes in clinical microbiology.

Indicator media contain substances or systems that give visible indications of significant reactions. For example, a medium containing lactose and a trace of neutral red gives rise to pink colonies if the bacteria involved produce acid by fermenting the lactose. This contrived mechanism should not be confused with natural colony pigmentation attributable to pigment production by some species of bacteria. Blood agar has an indicator effect useful in distinguishing some species from others. Diffusible substances produced by colonies of certain bacteria grown on blood agar give rise to various clearing or haemolytic effects in the surrounding medium. **β-haemolysis** is the term used to describe complete haemolysis in which all the surrounding red cells are lysed and the zone is entirely clear. A greenish and less complete effect is termed **α-haemolysis**. The haemolytic effects are markedly influenced by the species of blood used in the medium. Horse blood is commonly employed. Other indicator effects are observed when colonies are grown on media containing specific substrates which may be decomposed or altered. For instance,

phospholipase-C enzymes are produced by some bacteria; colonies of these organisms grown on egg-yolk media are surrounded by zones of opacity caused by breakdown of stabilizing phospholipoproteins in the egg-yolk emulsion.

Pathogens, commensals and contaminants often co-exist in specimens submitted for investigation. The serial and combined use of selective and indicator media greatly facilitates the detection and isolation of the significant pathogens from mixed populations in pathological material.

BACTERIAL MULTIPLICATION AND SYNTHESIS

The term 'bacterial growth' is used loosely to denote the growth of bacterial populations. The actual growth of a bacterial cell is accomplished by a series of integrated enzymic reactions which provide the energy and accumulate and align the materials required for building the new bacterial cell components. In an actively growing bacterial population, the mechanisms of cell synthesis and reproduction proceed together; the individual cells normally achieve a relatively constant size and promptly divide into two progeny cells by simple **binary fission**.

In the microbial world, generation times are scaled down. Given optimal conditions of atmosphere, temperature, moisture, energy-source and nutrition, and protection from deleterious influences, a typical bacterial cell may divide within 15–20 min and the single cell may give rise to 8–16 bacteria within the first hour of active division. These cells in turn grow and divide also. If the cells take a certain time T to complete the growth cycle and divide, the growth in numbers of the whole population proceeds as follows: if there are N_0 cells at time 0, there will be $2N_0$ cells at time T, $4N_0$ cells at time $2T$, $8N_0$ cells at time $3T$. Generally the number of cells N at time t is given by the equation:

$$N = N_0 \times 2^{t/T}$$

The increase in numbers follows an exponential curve as long as the environment can continue to support growth without restriction. Within 24 hours, the hypothetical potential of 10^{20} cells would be reached from a single cell dividing every 20 min and the resultant bacterial mass would weigh several thousand tons. It is clear that, in practice, limiting factors come quickly into operation and these dictate the size of bacterial populations; under laboratory conditions bacterial cells can be shown to be capable of indefinitely prolonged exponential growth. Chemical and physical changes are linked with bacterial growth mechanisms and increasingly alter the bacterial environment. For example, the accumulation of metabolites influences the pH and Eh of the system; moreover, the supply of essential growth factors, available oxygen, or a suitable energy source, may become exhausted. Even in controlled experimental systems, all the bacterial cells do not divide for more than a few generations. In simple cultures, multiplication proceeds rapidly for perhaps fifteen to twenty generations before a significant check occurs. Under natural conditions, similar limitations may appear rapidly and restrict the increase in numbers, or slow the growth cycle to such an extent that other processes such as the death of individual cells balance the residual growth. The growth cycle time of a bacterial cell may be short or long, and there appears to be no limit to the length of the cycle. However, a slowly growing cell makes less efficient use of the available nutrients, since it has to provide energy and materials merely to maintain its structure in a viable state, leaving less nutrient for further growth. One of the slowest observed growth rates is that for *Mycobacterium leprae*, each cell taking about 12 days to grow and divide in a natural host.

Although the infective dose of a single bacterial species may vary widely, small challenge doses of some pathogens are generally dangerous, whereas others are unlikely to cause trouble unless delivered by a particular route in relatively large numbers (p. 18.28). For example, the bacterial challenge delivered in a freshly sustained wound can become a much greater threat if treatment is delayed for a few hours. It is therefore useful to understand some of the dynamics of growing bacterial populations if microbial infections are to be prevented and treated intelligently.

A parallel may be drawn between the growth of bacteria in a liquid medium and the rapid development of a systemic bacterial infection. Similarly the growth of a bacterial colony on a solid medium resembles the development of a localized bacterial infection. In the first case, growth proceeds until the environment changes to limit it; in the second case, growth is always restricted by the necessity for the nutrients to diffuse to the cells, and, as numbers increase, the only cells capable of rapid growth may be those at the periphery of the colony.

The bacterial growth curve

When a small inoculum of a single species of bacterium is cultured under suitable conditions in a fluid medium, four distinct phases of growth of the bacterial population may be demonstrated by estimating the number of cells present in samples taken at intervals. The numbers of bacteria, plotted against time, give a growth curve. The shape of the curve drawn for the total numbers of bacteria differs from the plot obtained if only viable cells are enumerated; typical graphs are shown in fig. 18.28.

LAG PHASE

When bacteria are inoculated into a fresh fluid medium there is little or no increase in their number for a period; the length of this lag phase varies not only with the bacterial species but with the nature of the new medium. It also is likely to be shorter if the fresh medium is identical with the original culture medium and longer if

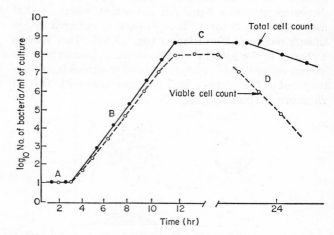

FIG. 18.28. A bacterial growth curve. A, lag phase; B, logarithmic or exponential phase; C, stationary phase; D, decline phase.

the new medium is different from that of the bacterial inoculum. Although there is virtually no increase in the bacterial population during the lag phase, individual cells usually show a marked increase in size and in metabolic activity.

For example, when spores are placed in a growth medium the phase during which the spores germinate appears to be a lag, although it is full of intense metabolic activity. Where vegetative cells are used as the inoculum, there are two likely explanations for the lag, one general and the other specific. The general case is one of an unbalanced internal environment. An actively growing cell continuously uses and regenerates ATP, NAD and NADP. If this cycle is interrupted, the cell may be unable to resume normal growth even if the external environment is favourable. The recovery of these substances to concentrations needed for normal growth may be a slow process, giving a lag. The loss of any pool of intermediates can cause a lag but those involved in cyclic transfers are the most vital.

The specific reason for a lag arises when a cell is placed in a medium containing nutrients to which it has not been adapted during its previous growth. Adaptation, the mechanism of which is considered on p. 18.45, is an alteration of the phenotype of a cell in response to its environment and in this case may be regarded as a device by which the cell spares itself the task of manufacturing enzymes for which it has no immediate need. Thus cells adapted to use glucose, when provided with fructose, may fail to contain the enzymes required for its metabolism.

Under these conditions, a cell with no source of energy immediately available from its environment must synthesize new enzymes to obtain them; the synthesis of enzymes, however, requires both energy and suitable intermediates. The cell escapes from this impasse by a process of autodigestion; a trickle of energy and of free amino acids is obtained by degradation of the existing cellular proteins. Once the cell has synthesized even a little of each of the new enzymes it needs, it begins to use the new nutrient, and the block to normal growth is overcome.

EXPONENTIAL (LOGARITHMIC) PHASE

Towards the end of the lag phase, the rate of cell division accelerates rapidly and soon the cells divide at a constant rate; the increase in numbers becomes exponential and there is a straight line relationship between the logarithm of the number of cells plotted in relation to time. This exponential or logarithmic phase of growth ends only when there is exhaustion of nutrient material and/or accumulation of toxic metabolites. The culture then enters the stationary phase.

STATIONARY PHASE

During this phase, the number of cells remains virtually constant.

DECLINE PHASE

This phase is characterized by the death and autolysis of cells. The speed with which the population of living cells is decimated is dictated *inter alia* by the concentration of toxic metabolites in the medium; in many instances during the decline phase the total bacterial count may remain unaltered, but with species particularly subject to autolysis it may fall rapidly. During the decline phase, cells show varying degrees of change in size and shape; Gram-positive cells frequently degenerate into Gram-negative involution forms.

Indices of bacterial cell synthesis

The use of estimates of 'total cell numbers' or 'viable cell counts' as indices of the growth of a bacterial population does not find favour with mathematicians or cytologists who justifiably point out the errors involved in making these estimates and in equating counts of viable particles with counts of single cells. Alternative indices of growth include:

(1) spectrophotometric or turbidimetric measurements which indicate increasing optical density of the growth medium,

(2) the wet weight or dry weight of the bacterial mass produced, and

(3) the nitrogen content of the washed bacterial yield.

As the nature of the culture medium markedly influences the composition and structure of the bacterial cell, many variable factors tend to reduce such studies to academic exercises unless complicated control systems are employed. More elegant methods may make it possible to relate observations made *in vivo* to results obtained *in vitro*. Moreover, detailed studies of microbial cell synthesis have yielded information of great interest in general biology.

BACTERIAL CELL DIVISION

The growth cycle of a single bacterial cell is accompanied by an approximate doubling of all the cellular components, followed by partition of these into the daughter cells (fig. 18.29). Studies using specific antibodies tagged

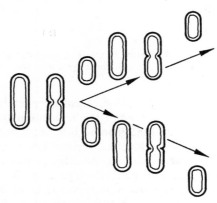

FIG. 18.29. Bacterial cell division. Binary fission with cross-wall formation.

with a fluorescent dye show that the surface layers of the bacteria, principally the cell wall, grow either by intercalation of new material into the existing structure at many points, or by the new material forming a separate region as a girdle around the organism. The appearance of the division furrow serves to determine the partition of the existing cell wall and membrane, but the cytoplasm remains connected and able to diffuse until the cross-wall is closed. The partition of the nuclear material must precede the closing of the cross-wall, and hence replication of the DNA has to be completed even earlier. The DNA or **genome** is a condensed mass within the cell, continually in motion and eventually splitting into two bodies. Nuclear replication and division in bacteria has no discernible stages as in mitosis; no nuclear membrane is present, and no structures resembling centrioles or spindles are seen. The replication of bacterial DNA has been the subject of much interest in recent years, and current observations may be summed up as follows.

(1) DNA synthesis can occur throughout the cellular growth cycle.

(2) Initiation of the replication process is triggered by factors that in some way are related to the size and state of the cell. The process leads to the formation of a complex of enzymes which unwind the parental DNA strands and synthesize new strands, using the old ones as templates. This occurs at a replication point which travels along the DNA in one direction, presumably from beginning to end of the genome if it is a linear structure (fig. 18.30a). If the

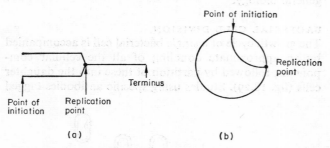

FIG. 18.30. Branched appearance of a bacterial genome undergoing replication; (a) linear genome; (b) circular genome.

genome is circular (e.g. as in *Esch. coli*), replication starts at one point and ends when the replication point has completed one tour of the genome, bringing it back to the point of origin (fig. 18.30b). Circular DNA structures are found in bacteria, viruses and other genetic elements such as F factors and plasmids (pp. 18.56 & 59). In a circular genome, the two strands of the DNA molecule can each be linked into a continuous loop; then it is necessary to break one of the strands before they can untwist and separate into the two progeny circles.

(3) The speed of replication is determined by the availability of the nucleotide precursors of the DNA, and also by the ability of the replicating enzymes to incorporate them. Under good growth conditions, the replicating enzymes work at their maximum rate, and this determines

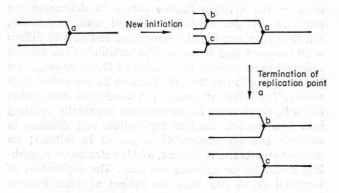

FIG. 18.31. Multiple initiation and replication of linear genome leading to multibranched genomes. Branched structure is exactly replicated in the time it takes a replication point to travel half the length of the genome.

the minimum time for one replication point to travel the length of the genome. This is not necessarily the shortest time for a cellular growth cycle; paradoxically, a cell may go through its growth cycle and divide into two identical progeny in less time than this minimum period. This is achieved by initiating a second replication before the previous replication point has completed its round. The DNA is therefore in process of replication at more than one independent replicating point (fig. 18.31) and has a multi-branched structure.

Relationship between the genotype and the phenotype of an organism

Although mentioned in vol. 1, chap. 12, information concerning the regulation and control of bacterial genes is discussed here in more detail.

A growing bacterial cell expresses much of its available genetic information; in contrast, a mammalian cell, although it may be no more complex than a bacterial cell, contains the genetic capability of producing any one of the differentiated forms found in the whole organism. The phenotype of a bacterial cell is variable within narrow limits as the cell responds to its environment; the phenotype of a mammalian cell is determined primarily by the factors that bring about its differentiation, and subsequently within only narrow limits by environmental factors. Bacterial regulation systems are understood in far greater detail than those in mammalian cells, and they illustrate the principles by which the genetic material functions in higher organisms.

Aside from its self-replication, the only known function of DNA is to allow the synthesis of RNA molecules of specific base sequences. Some of the molecules find a role as transfer RNAs, or as components of ribosomes; others, known as messenger RNAs, convey information that is translated into the polypeptide sequences of the proteins of the cell. The region of the DNA carrying the information for a complete polypeptide is called a **structural gene**; evidence from genetic analysis suggests that changes (mutations) in other genes may specifically affect the expression of a structural gene, measured as the amount of protein end-product formed.

The phenomenon of enzyme adaptation stems from the activity of **regulatory genes** (vol. 1, p. 38.2) which determine the expression of one or more structural genes. The mode of action of regulatory genes has been interpreted by Jacob and Monod in a model system which accounts for the properties of many bacterial regulatory systems and of the mutants derived from them. The model explains the behaviour of an inducible enzyme system in the following way (fig. 18.32). The product of the regulatory gene must determine whether or not the structural gene is expressed by physically interacting with the DNA of the structural gene (or some region close to it); in this way it prevents the RNA polymerase molecule from attaching to the DNA and forming the messenger RNA molecule coding for the polypeptide. The regulatory gene is always expressed; copies of its product are present in the cell, blocking the expression of the structural

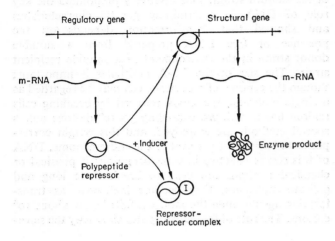

Fig. 18.32. Model of genetic regulation proposed by Jacob and Monod.

gene. This is called **repression**, and the regulatory gene products are **repressors** (vol. 1, p. 38.2). The model then supposes that the repressor combines with some other molecule (inducer) as a result of which it can no longer bind to the DNA and block expression of the structural gene. The **inducer** stimulates the formation of the protein. In the best studied case, the natural inducers of the enzyme β-galactosidase in *Esch. coli* are compounds such as lactose which this enzyme splits into glucose and galactose, both sugars that the cell can then utilize. The regulation extends at the same time to the other enzymes concerned with the metabolism of lactose, and the structural genes for these enzymes are adjacent to that for β-galactosidase itself. It seems that when the RNA polymerase transcribes the gene for β-galactosidase it can carry on along the DNA transcribing the other genes at the same time, so producing one large messenger RNA molecule carrying all this information.

This regulation is an economical process, conserving the cell's resources when there is no use for the gene product, at the expense of a steady expression of the regulatory gene itself. The active product of this gene is believed to be not the primary product (RNA) but the secondary product (the protein) derived from it. Proteins such as enzymes have astonishing ability to interact with specific molecules; a protein with the ability to recognize a sequence of bases in the DNA on the one hand and an inducer molecule on the other would act as a relay of information to the DNA, affecting the behaviour and phenotype of the cell directly in response to specific

information from the environment. Proteins with the required properties, e.g. a high affinity for DNA and for the inducer in the case of the β-galactosidase regulatory system, have been isolated for several systems.

The model proposed by Jacob and Monod is not restricted to inducible systems; by reversing the roles of the repressor and the repressor-inducer complex, so that the free regulator gene product does not bind to the DNA but the complex does, the cell produces the protein unless the external molecule is present. That is to say, the formation of the enzyme is repressed by this external molecule; an example of this type of regulation is the formation of alkaline phosphatase by *Esch. coli*, which is repressed by inorganic phosphate ions. Similarly, the formation of sets of enzymes required to synthesize an amino acid (e.g. histidine or tryptophan) is regulated and repressed by supplying the amino acid to the environment of the cell.

BACTERIAL VARIATION AND MUTATION

Variation in bacteria can be **phenotypic** or **genotypic**. The adaptation of bacterial metabolism to the environment depends on phenotypic variation. An example is the effect of lactose in the medium on the enzymes present in *Esch. coli*. A second type of variation appears in the phenomenon of 'phase variation' in *Salmonella* and a number of other related phenomena. In this case, the flagellar structure can be of two distinct types coded by at least two different and unlinked structural genes. The flagella on a cell may be of either type, but when the cell grows and divides there is a faint possibility of a switch occurring, repressing the formation of one flagellar type and allowing that of the other. Expression of both at the same time does not appear possible. While a model can be constructed along the lines of the Jacob–Monod model of regulation described earlier to give such a bistable state, evidence is lacking to give a more precise explanation. What causes the switching is unknown; no permanent genetic change has occurred.

Genotypic variations

These are stable heritable variations arising from alterations to the DNA of the cell. Alteration, addition or deletion of bases in the original DNA may change the structure of the gene product (vol. 1, chap. 12); if the gene is regulatory, then the expression of the genes under its control may be entirely altered. In the scheme advanced by Jacob and Monod (fig. 18.32) a mutation affecting the regulatory gene product, the repressor, by destroying its binding capacity to the DNA, would lead to continuous and unrestricted expression of the structural gene; this is a **constitutive mutant**. A mutation that destroys the ability of the repressor to interact with the inducer never allows expression of the structural gene, and is called a super-repressed mutant. Many variations of these properties are possible as a result of mutations.

In general, mutations usually bring about a loss of function or a loss of control. It is not possible to develop a new function simply as a result of a single mutation; the amount of genetic material that must be altered is much greater than that changed in the DNA by any simple mutation. However, a qualification should be added; it is possible to produce modifications to structures or regulatory mechanisms which become damaged, but yet have some new secondary property that can be recognized. For example, insensitivity to an antibiotic may arise in this way; resistance to streptomycin can be produced as a result of mutation affecting the structure of a ribosomal component, rendering the protein synthetic machinery free from inhibition by the drug.

Transmission of genetic information between cells

Bacteria divide by binary fission and, in the absence of mutation, each daughter contains an accurate copy of the genetic material. Transmission of any mutation is therefore directly to the lineal descendants of the first mutant cell.

It is possible to detect three other types of transmission in which genetic information is passed between genetically distinct organisms. These have profound implications, for the evolution of bacteria is not then restricted to the emergence of a 'super' strain as a result of multiple genetic changes occurring sequentially within a single successful line of organisms. Instead, genetic events occurring in different lines can be brought into a single organism in random fashion, allowing the emergence of the 'best' combination of genetic characters to proceed more rapidly. Genetic information in an 'unsuccessful' organism is not lost until none of its descendants is alive, for any one of these may transmit the genetic information to another line by means of these transfer methods. The three methods are transformation, conjugation and transduction.

TRANSFORMATION

Transformation, the first of these methods to be detected, was observed by Griffith in 1928. The agent responsible for it, however, was not identified until 16 years later by Avery, MacLeod and McCarty in 1944. Griffith's original observations were made during a study of the virulence of different strains of pneumococci in mice. He injected an avirulent variant giving a rough colonial form, together with a suspension of dead organisms of the virulent strain giving a smooth colony, and noted that some of the mice died. From these mice, cultures of the smooth colonial virulent pneumococcus were obtained. The difference between the smooth and the rough forms of the organism lies in the capsular polysaccharide produced by the smooth form. The experiment was repeated in the test-tube and it was possible to identify the agent responsible for the conversion of the rough strain into the smooth strain as the DNA of the smooth strain. This discovery pinpointed the key role of DNA in determining genetic characteristics and showed that transformation depends on the presence of free DNA prepared from a suitable donor strain in the environment of a suitable recipient strain. The size of the DNA molecules is important; though the genome of a bacterial cell may be regarded as a single molecule, the DNA released by breaking cells seldom has a mol. wt. exceeding 5×10^6 daltons unless special methods are employed, and this weight corresponds to less than 1 per cent of the entire genome. DNA of this size is effective in transformation; if physical or chemical methods are used to break these long and delicate molecules, they become ineffective as transforming agents when the mol. wt. falls below about 10^6 daltons. The role of free DNA is also shown by the sensi-

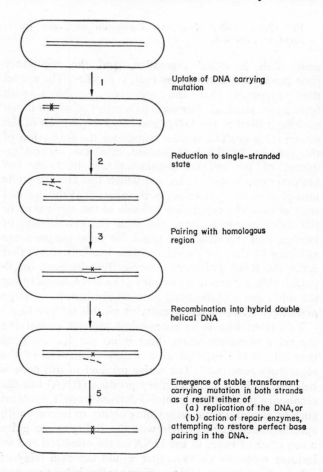

1 Uptake of DNA carrying mutation

2 Reduction to single-stranded state

3 Pairing with homologous region

4 Recombination into hybrid double helical DNA

5 Emergence of stable transformant carrying mutation in both strands as a result either of
(a) replication of the DNA, or
(b) action of repair enzymes, attempting to restore perfect base pairing in the DNA.

FIG. 18.33. Stages in the transformation of a competent bacterial cell.

tivity of the transforming agent to deoxyribonuclease, which degrades DNA to fragments of low mol. wt. Cells absorb labelled DNA which then becomes no longer sensitive to deoxyribonuclease. The double helical DNA is broken down inside the cell to one single-stranded molecule and small degradation products, and the transformation is completed when the single-stranded DNA pairs with a complementary region in the recipient genome and is incorporated into a double helical DNA molecule (fig. 18.33.) If the DNA coming into the recipient cell carries a genetic marker distinguished by a mutation, the transformed cell exhibits the new character instead of its original allele. The more differences there are, the greater becomes the chance of finding a hybrid cell emerging with mixed characteristics arising from both parental types. However, transformation for multiple markers occurs very infrequently, since it results from the transformation of one cell by a number of different DNA fragments from the donor on a random basis. Exceptionally, multiple transformants occur as a result of the incorporation of one transforming DNA molecule. These genetic markers show linkage. The degree of linkage reflects their proximity in the DNA molecule, and is limited by the occurrence of the break in the transforming DNA molecule, and by the termination of the incorporation process, which does not necessarily place the whole single-stranded DNA molecule into the newly trans-

formed genome. By this means, information can be obtained about the short range mapping of large numbers of genes in transformable bacteria.

Since transformation was discovered in pneumococci, it has been found to occur with *H. influenzae*, *B. subtilis*, *B. licheniformis* and other organisms. All these bacteria show similar features with respect to the state of the recipient cells. A transformable strain of bacterium may take up DNA and produce transformants only during a limited phase of growth; typically this is towards the end of the exponential or log phase, or during the early lag phase. This state is called **competence**, and its development in some organisms is associated with the action of enzymes attacking the cell wall of the bacterium. Penetration of the DNA into the cell may therefore be a major factor; strains that appear to differ only in their surface properties often differ in their ability to be transformed by a factor as large as 10^6. Even in a good recipient strain, the competent cells may be only a small percentage of the total.

The role of transformation under natural conditions is apparent when two strains of *B. licheniformis* are grown together for a short time since recombinants are formed. In this case, transformation must be the mechanism of genetic transfer, since it is blocked by the addition of deoxyribonuclease to the mixed culture; this has no effect on growth. It follows too that, under ordinary

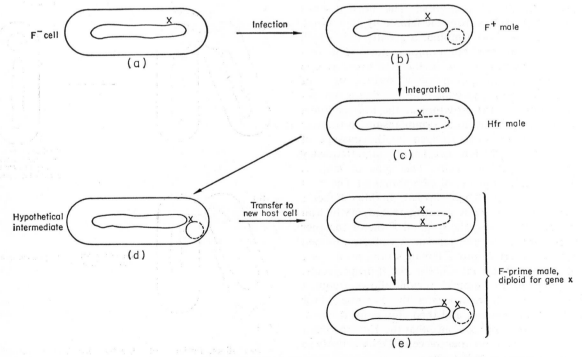

FIG. 18.34. Classes of bacterium involved in conjugation in *Esch. coli*. Chromosome is the continuous line and the F factor is shown as a dotted line.

growth conditions, the organisms must release DNA in quantities and of such a quality that transformants can be produced.

CONJUGATION

This method of genetic transfer was discovered in 1946 by Lederberg and Tatum in strains of *Esch. coli*; on mixing genetically distinct strains, hybrid bacteria were produced which could have arisen only as a result of a transfer of genetic material from one strain to the other. This process is not sensitive to deoxyribonuclease, and no extracts from either strain can bring about hybrid formation.

Direct cell-to-cell contact is required. When the strains are mixed they form pairs which become physically joined by a tube called the **conjugation bridge**. The formation of hybrid strains is polarized so that one strain acts as the donor, and the other only as a recipient. The strains are called male and female, and the process likened to classic zygote formation and termed **bacterial sexuality**. The pattern of behaviour that emerges from possession of the **sex factor** shows three related classes of male strains, illustrated in fig. 18.34. It was discovered that a male strain that had lost its ability to act as a donor would be restored to the fertile state on contact with a normal male strain; i.e. a genetic element conferring fertility (F^+) is transferred by conjugation at high efficiency into non-fertile cells (both defective male strains and natural female strains called F^-) without any transfer of genetic markers on the chromosome. The normal male strain (fig. 18.34b) differs from the female by containing, independent of the host genome, a genetic unit which replicates itself in this autonomous state. The formation of the hybrid strains in the first cross is due to the occasional formation of a second type of male strain (fig. 18.34c) in which the F^+ factor has become combined into the structure of the host genome. Conjugation with this strain as donor results in transfer of the donor chromosome (judged by the passage of genetic markers into the female cells) at a high frequency giving many recombinant cells. This type of male is called Hfr (for high frequency of recombinants). The third type of male strain (fig. 18.34e) carries a modified F factor derived from an intermediate state (fig. 18.34d) in which an Hfr strain has eliminated the original F factor together with a region of the bacterial genome. This factor, termed F-prime, when inserted into a female strain, produces a cell diploid for the bacterial genes in the F-prime factor. The homology in the diploid region allows frequent recombination, which incorporates the F-prime factor into the bacterial genome, and then eliminates it again. This behaviour provides evidence that the F-factor has a circular structure since no open piece of DNA is likely to produce this pattern of behaviour.

A male strain produces characteristic pili or fimbriae

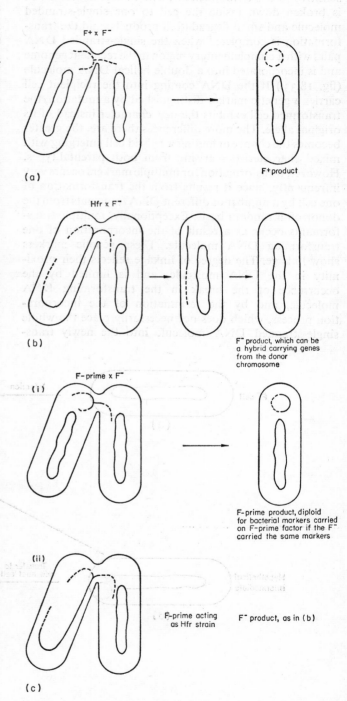

FIG. 18.35. Patterns of gene transfer during conjugation given by the male types of *Esch. coli*. Replication of the nucleic acid accompanies the transfer.

not produced by females, called **F-pili** or **sex fimbriae.** These play a role in the pairing process and, since they are hollow, it is possible that the transfer of genetic material takes place through them instead of the tube that can also be demonstrated joining pairs of cells. The establishment of the bridge triggers the transfer of genetic material from male to female cell. The DNA that is transferred is newly synthesized and the process of replication may provide a driving force to extrude one of the daughter copies into the female cell (fig. 18.35).

On this basis (fig. 18.35a), it can be seen that an F$^+$ male cell can infect F$^-$ cells as often as it can conjugate and replicate the F factor. Pairs of cells probably break apart from random buffeting in the solution, freeing the cells for further matings; the new male cell now replicates the F factor and grows F-pili until it in turn is able to conjugate and infect other F$^-$ cells. The conversion can sweep through the bulk of an F$^-$ population within an hour.

The behaviour of the Hfr strains (fig. 18.35b) stems from the same pattern of transfer of a newly replicated copy of the genetic material into the female cell. In this case the results are strikingly different, however. The transfer starts with a small piece of the F-factor, followed by the bacterial genes in a fixed order determined by their position on the genome. When all of these have been transferred, the remaining piece of F-factor terminates the process. This has transferred the entire genetic content of the Hfr strain into the F$^-$ strain, which now becomes Hfr also. This model transfer is, however, exceedingly rare; complete transfer takes about 90 min and breakages in the DNA can stop the transfer at any time. The common occurrence is partial transfer of the leading bacterial markers at high efficiency and soon after conjugation starts. The failure to transfer the terminal part, carrying the rest of the F factor, leaves the recombinant cells F$^-$ and still able to act as recipients in further crosses. The ordered transfer of genetic markers allows detailed mapping of the genome of *Esch. coli* in this region. The discovery that there are various Hfr strains that differ in the point at which they initiate transfer of the bacterial markers, and also in the direction of transfer, has extended detailed mapping to the entire circular genome of *Esch. coli*.

The third class of male, the F-prime, behaves both as an Hfr and as an F$^+$ in mating experiments (fig. 18.35c), because of the ease with which the F-prime factor is switched from the free autonomous state to the integrated state. It therefore transfers bacterial markers readily as well as infecting the female cells with the free F-prime factor.

The formation of a partial diploid, in a cell carrying an F-prime factor, has been of enormous value in understanding how genes work, since the interaction of two alleles of the same marker can be studied very simply. Much of the evidence used by Jacob and Monod to develop their theory of gene regulation was obtained

13

from a study of such diploids in the genetic region concerned with lactose utilization.

Though the F-factor appeared unique when it was first discovered, a number of other genetic elements have similar properties, and consist of a 'transfer' factor (analogous to F) and some other characters which do not have equivalent characters in the host genome. Some of these are then similar to F-prime factors in a host cell which carries no equivalent to the markers acquired by the original F factor. Some of these factors carry markers that produce colicines, agents that kill cells of *Esch. coli*, but the most important class are called **resistance transfer factors** (RTF), and transfer genes conferring resistance to antibiotics. These factors behave as highly infectious agents like the F factor, and may accumulate multiple markers—one isolated from *Salm. typhimurium* carried resistance to seven different antibiotics.

The resistance transfer factors and the F factor unfortunately share another property. The F factor can be transferred by conjugation from *Esch. coli* to other bacteria such as *Salmonella*, *Shigella*, *Proteus*, *Pseudomonas* and *Serratia* species. Since *Esch. coli* is a normal commensal in the gut, it can act as a reservoir for resistance transfer factors, and pass them to pathogens, raising great difficulties in treatment. The incidence of drug-resistant strains of *Salm. typhimurium* where the resistance is carried on a RTF was over 60 per cent of isolates referred to the Enteric Reference Laboratory by the end of 1964, and has probably increased since then. Resistance transfer factors represent a world-wide problem which is becoming increasingly serious (p. 20.7).

TRANSDUCTION

The final method of genetic transfer has certain features in common with both transformation and the role of the F factor in conjugation. The general process involves transfer of genetic material through the agency of a bacterial virus, or bacteriophage (p. 18.99). A phage particle attaches to a bacterial cell and injects its nucleic acid into the interior. Replication of the nucleic acid and synthesis of viral components follow, leading to assembly of new viral particles which incorporate the nucleic acid, and ultimately the progeny virus particles are released from the cell which is killed. The first type of transduction arises from progeny phage particles that do not carry a complete phage genome (and are therefore defective and non-reproductive) but which have in error picked up some of the bacterial DNA instead (fig. 18.36). After injection into a host cell, the bacterial DNA from the defective phage can undergo pairing with homologous regions of DNA in the host, and recombination then completes the genetic transfer with the formation of new hybrid genomes. In this transfer the hybrids that emerge can be derived from any piece of bacterial DNA picked up by the defective phage particle, and the process is called

GENERALIZED TRANSDUCTION

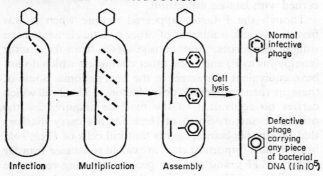

(a) Normal lytic cycle of bacteriophage

SPECIALIZED TRANSDUCTION

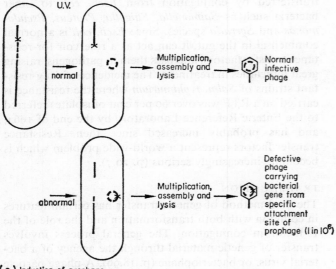

(c) Induction of prophage
This mixture of phage particles transduces gene x better than any other bacterial gene and is called a LOW FREQUENCY TRANSDUCING LYSATE

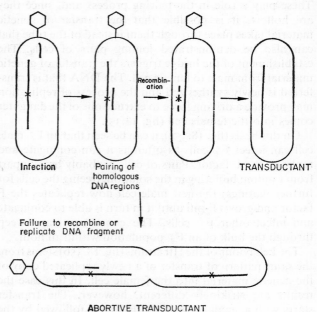

(b) Transduction by defective phage produced in (a)

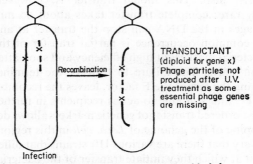

(d) Transduction by defective phage produced in (c)

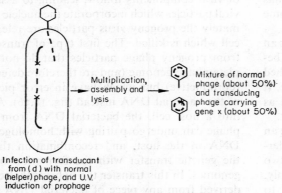

(e) Preparation of HIGH FREQUENCY TRANSDUCING LYSATE

FIG. 18.36. Patterns of behaviour leading to the formation of transductants at low and high frequency. Bacterial chromosome shown as solid line; phage chromosome shown dotted.

generalized transduction. After the insertion of the DNA into the host cell its fate matches that of transforming DNA. DNA transduced by a phage is longer than that entering a cell during transformation, and linkage between different markers is retained on transduction which is lost in transformation.

In generalized transduction the proportion of defective phage to normal phage is very low, perhaps 1 in 10^6 or less. A large number of cells must be exposed to the phage to be sure of obtaining a transductant, and the remainder are killed if they are susceptible to the phage.

Occasionally the incoming DNA does not complete the integration, but its genes may be expressed. The DNA does not replicate and, though division occurs, only one cell retains this DNA. This is **abortive transduction.**

A special case occurs when the phage genome has been recombined into the bacterial genome. This rare event resembles the fate of the F factor which after integration to the Hfr state becomes an F-prime. If the phage genome emerges carrying a bacterial gene or region of DNA, the phage particle carrying this is again defective, but on injection of the DNA into a bacterium the bacterial genes carried by the phage can pair with the homologous genes in the cell. A recombination is very likely, leading to a heterogenote diploid for these genes, with the viral genes forming part of the bacterial genome and being replicated as the bacterial DNA replicates. If another phage infects the cell, its DNA supplies information for all the phage components, some of which was lacking in the first defective phage. As the infection proceeds and viral DNA replicates, any of the first viral DNA that is freed from the bacterial genome can be replicated too, and incorporated into new phage particles; release of the viral DNA is stimulated by a dose of UV to the cells. A large proportion of the progeny phage are now transducing particles, carrying only one specific region of the bacterial genes. This is called a **high frequency transducing lysate.** The addition of the second (or helper) phage is unnecessary if the cell carries a normal phage genome in the prophage state, i.e. also integrated into the bacterial genome and so restricted from producing phage components as a consequence. This is induced by UV into a state where phage production and multiplication of phage DNA proceed as fast as in a normal lytic infection.

Phage can transduce DNA other than from the bacterial genome. Some plasmids (genetic elements that are self-replicating and need not integrate with the host genome) can be transduced, and in *Staph. aureus* the plasmids carry resistance markers to a number of antibiotics. Though the donor cell producing the phage is killed in this case, the transduced plasmid may enter a cell already carrying a variant plasmid, and undergo recombination leading to a reassortment of the genetic markers. When recombination does not occur immediately, the two plasmids may enter a new state if they recombine once and form a linked structure. This can multiply with the cells, giving an enhanced chance of a recombinant with survival value to the cell. Eventually a second recombination separates the plasmids which segregate out into the progeny cells. In the case of the plasmid carrying the genes for penicillin resistance in *Staph. aureus*, this is the only method of transfer known; these strains have such survival value that they form the majority of isolates of *Staph. aureus* from infections acquired in hospitals.

BACTERIA AND RELATED ORGANISMS OF MEDICAL IMPORTANCE

THE ACTINOMYCETES

A group of 'higher bacteria' possesses properties intermediate between fungi and bacteria. They grow as branching filaments that interlace to form a mycelium. Fragmentation of the filaments occurs and gives rise to forms resembling bacilli and this is seen most readily in culture. In their bacillary form, and in the staining properties of some species, they resemble corynebacteria and mycobacteria. The organisms are Gram-positive, nonmotile, nonsporing and can grow on ordinary media.

The two genera in the family are *Actinomyces* and *Nocardia*.

Actinomyces

ACTINOMYCES ISRAELII

This is the only species pathogenic to humans. It may be found as a commensal in the mouth in about 5 per cent of persons, particularly in the tonsils or around carious teeth.

Morphology and staining properties

In the tissues, *A. israelii* forms a dense felted mass of Gram-positive mycelium (plate 18.1e, facing p. 18.62). Mycelial masses appear in the pus from a lesion in the form of yellow granules about 0·2–2·0 mm diameter (sulphur granules). Club-shaped swellings, which stain Gram-negatively and are slightly acid fast, are sometimes arranged radially around the periphery of the mycelial mass; they contain lipid and are believed to be deposited by the host's tissue cells as a reaction to the presence of the organism. The histological appearance of the mycelium with its radiating clubs has led to the name of 'ray fungus' for this species.

After anaerobic incubation for 3–4 days on agar or glucose agar, light grey colonies develop up to 1·0 mm in diameter. The presence of 5 per cent CO_2 aids growth.

An alternative method of culture is to inoculate a tube of melted serum agar (shake culture). Growth occurs as a band of colonies appearing 10–20 mm below the surface of the medium, i.e. in a microaerophilic environment.

Actinomycosis is an initially suppurative inflammation which progresses to a chronic granulomatous abscess (p. 21.15). Lesions are seen most often in the cervicofacial region, but also occur in the oesophagus and mediastinum, and in the appendix and caecum. A subdiaphragmatic abscess may develop.

A. bovis is often present in the mouths of cattle and may cause local lesions but does not infect man.

Trauma is associated with the development of actinomycosis. Thus dental extraction and appendicectomy are precipitating factors. Tissue hypersensitivity to the organism is also believed to play a part in the initiation of the infective lesion.

Actinomycosis is endogenous in origin, i.e. the infecting organism is present as a commensal in the patient's mouth or intestine. Exogenous infection with *A. israelii* cannot occur as it is a strict parasite for man and does not exist saprophytically.

Males are more often infected than females, and the usual age incidence is 10–30 years.

Pus or sputum is examined for sulphur granules which can be washed in saline, crushed between two microscope slides and examined for the presence of Gram-positive branching filaments. If no sulphur granules are found, the presence of Gram-positive branching filaments and rods in the pus is suggestive of actinomycosis.

Culture of the washed sulphur granules should be made whenever possible in preference to culture of the pus, sputum or other material.

Tissue stained by the Gram method may show mycelia and clubs (ray fungus). A modified Ziehl–Neelsen stain demonstrates the acid-fast nature of the clubs.

Nocardia

There are over forty species of *Nocardia* most of which are saprophytic. Two species infect man rarely, *Noc. asteroides* and *Noc. madurae*. Nocardiae resemble actinomycetes in their mycelial morphology though the filaments are narrower (0·5 μm) and in some species are acid fast. Clubs also occur *in vivo*. Pigmentation of the mycelial granules is a characteristic feature and red, yellow or black granules may be seen in pus. Nocardiae are obligatory aerobes (cf. *A. israelii*) and give rise to red or yellow colonies on ordinary media especially in old cultures. The typical clinical lesion is of a chronic granuloma.

Nocardiosis due to *Noc. asteroides* is often associated with some underlying disease and is not generally communicable. The source of *Noc. asteroides* is from the patient's skin or respiratory tract where it may lead a commensal existence. The source of *Noc. madurae* is usually the soil.

NOCARDIA ASTEROIDES

This species causes a systemic infection in the lungs and sometimes spreads by the blood stream to the brain and other organs. Diffuse suppuration occurs in the lungs and *Noc. asteroides* may be isolated from the sputum; this infection resembles pulmonary tuberculosis. Microscopy of granules from infected material reveals the typical branching mycelium. The filaments are acid-fast to 1 per cent sulphuric acid. On agar medium, white, dry, star-shaped colonies are seen, hence the epithet 'asteroides'; they are usually composed of Gram-positive bacillary forms, some of which may show branching.

NOCARDIA MADURAE

This organism is one of the causative agents of **mycetoma**, a chronic suppurative granuloma of the foot seen in tropical countries (Madura foot). The infection may spread by direct extension to involve the bones of the foot and results in gross deformity with multiple loculated abscesses discharging pus containing yellow granules through external sinuses. The laboratory diagnosis consists in the demonstration of Gram-positive mycelial elements in the granules. These mycelia are not acid-fast. Growth on agar medium is slow, with the development of round, smooth, yellow colonies that later assume a worm-cast appearance and are very adherent to the medium. Other causes of mycetoma are given on p. 18.21.

THE ACID-FAST BACILLI

Mycobacterium

This genus includes the causative organisms of **tuberculosis** and **leprosy**. These bacteria produce chronic inflammatory lesions and the interactions between parasite and host often proceed slowly over many years. In human patients the battle with these diseases may continue for 50 years or more; episodes of parasitic aggression alternate with long periods of quiescence and death may be precipitated finally by some other disease.

The mycobacteria are straight or slightly curved rods which are nonmotile, noncapsulated and nonsporing. They are Gram-positive, but many are not readily stained because they have a waxy substance in their cell walls. Ziehl–Neelsen's stain is used as a routine for the microscopical detection, and exploits their characteristic resistance to decolourizing agents such as acid or alcohol, once a stain has been successfully incorporated in the cells. The mycobacteria are therefore called **acid-and-alcohol-fast bacilli**, but the different species vary in this respect. The pathogenic members of the genus include *Myco. leprae*, the cause of leprosy, and five species of 'tubercle bacilli', human, bovine, avian, murine and piscine. Only the human, bovine and avian species are recognized causes of tuberculosis in man. The human species is called *Myco. tuberculosis*, the bovine species is now termed *Myco. bovis*, and the avian *Myco. avium*. The so-called anonymous mycobacteria include a few pathogens of man.

MYCOBACTERIUM TUBERCULOSIS

This is a thin, often slightly curved rod (1–4 μm × 0·2–0·5 μm). Highly virulent strains produce cords or parallel lines of bacilli. Mycolic acid is a component of the waxy substances in the cell walls which make them acid-fast and alcohol-fast (plate 18.1c, facing p. 18.62). Fluorescent staining with auramine sometimes helps to detect tubercle bacilli in smears prepared from sputum, and especially in screening tests in which many specimens are examined.

Myco. tuberculosis is a strict aerobe and grows best at 37°C, and more slowly than many other pathogens. On coagulated egg media containing glycerol, e.g. Lowenstein–Jensen medium, the colonies are dry, raised, buff-coloured and wart-like (plate 18.1d, facing p. 18.62), and take at least 2 weeks to develop. Cultures should be observed for up to 8 weeks before being discarded as negative. Subcutaneous inoculation of *Myco. tuberculosis* produces a progressive and lethal disease in guinea-pigs, but not in rabbits. The organism survives desiccation in dust for several months and is very resistant to disinfectants; this latter property is attributable to the high lipid content of the cell wall which renders it relatively impermeable to water. Sputum also protects the organisms against disinfectants.

Tuberculoproteins or tuberculins of the cell wall are of importance in the Mantoux, Heaf and other skin tests which demonstrate a patient's hypersensitivity and indirectly indicate his relative immunity to tubercle bacilli (p. 21.17).

There are no serological tests for the diagnosis of tuberculosis. Since detection by microscopy and cultural methods is all-important, concentration procedures are used to increase the chances of finding the organism in pathological specimens. Dramatic reductions in the tuberculosis mortality rates during the last 30 years in Britain (p. 34.11) are attributable to raised standards of living, specific antibiotic therapy, community tracing of disease (mass radiography) and effective prophylactic vaccination with BCG vaccine (see opposite).

MYCOBACTERIUM BOVIS

This tends to be shorter and thicker than *Myco. tuberculosis*. Growth is much less luxuriant on Lowenstein–Jensen media with flat, whitish, smooth, moist colonies (plate 18.1d, facing p. 18.62). The organism is lethal for both guinea-pigs and rabbits when inoculated subcutaneously. It is a natural pathogen of the cow; **bovine tuberculosis**, which affects cervical lymph nodes, the alimentary tract and the mesenteric lymph nodes and spreads to involve meninges, kidneys, bones and joints, is transmitted especially to children by drinking raw milk from infected cows. It has virtually disappeared from Britain, as a result of the pasteurization of milk and, later, the formation of tuberculosis-free dairy herds. A living attenuated strain of *Myco. bovis* was used by Calmette and Guérin to produce **Bacille Calmette Guérin, BCG vaccine**. Killed tubercle bacilli and tuberculoprotein are unable to stimulate immunity to primary tuberculosis, but the living attenuated BCG affords protection to about 80 per cent of those immunized. The vaccine and its use are described on p. 22.22.

ANONYMOUS MYCOBACTERIA

These are a group which cannot be identified as *Myco. tuberculosis* or *Myco. bovis* but some members are associated with human disease. They are classified on the basis of colonial pigmentation (red, orange and yellow) and speed of growth in culture varying from as little as 3 days up to several weeks. Almost all of them are resistant to antituberculous drugs (p. 20.31). The above definition also includes *Myco. avium*, which is involved occasionally in human pulmonary infections.

The reaction of the body to tubercle bacilli and their methods of spread throughout the body are discussed on p. 21.16.

MYCOBACTERIUM LEPRAE

There is no reasonable doubt that this is the causative organism of **leprosy**, but it cannot be grown in laboratory media and so Koch's postulates have not yet been fulfilled. It is morphologically not unlike *Myco. tuberculosis*, but it is not so markedly acid-fast, is not alcohol-fast and stains readily Gram-positive in tissue sections. The bacilli can sometimes be grown in tissue culture, and may multiply if inoculated into the footpad of the mouse.

The acid-fast bacilli can be seen densely packed and often intracellularly in stained sections of the granulomatous lesions that occur in nodular leprosy and in skin snips and nasal secretions from affected patients. The infectivity of leprosy is low and prolonged contact with lepers is usually regarded as essential before transmission occurs. Even so, most doctors and nurses working for years amongst lepers have remained free from the disease.

THE DIPHTHERIA BACILLUS AND DIPHTHEROID ORGANISMS

Corynebacterium

Corynebacteria are small Gram-positive rods, often having an expansion of one pole which may make them look like a club. The organisms stain irregularly and do

PLATE 18.1 Bacteriology.

(a) These two photographs are of the same pure culture of *Corynebacterium diphtheriae*; the upper preparation has been stained by Gram's method and the lower by Albert's staining method to demonstrate the presence of volutin granules (× 1000).

(b) Tellurite blood agar medium which had been inoculated with *C. diphtheriae* var. *intermedius* 36 hours previously and incubated at 37°C. This medium is very selective for diphtheria bacilli and allied species; on it the three biotypes of *C. diphtheriae* give rise to different colonies that an experienced bacteriologist can distinguish.

(c) Film of a concentrated specimen of sputum stained by the Ziehl–Neelsen method; acid- and alcohol-fast bacilli can be noted against the background debris which has been counter-stained with methylene blue (× 1000).

(d) Lowenstein–Jensen egg medium. On the left is the appearance of human type tubercle bacilli, *Mycobacterium tuberculosis*, after 8 weeks incubation at 37°C; such growth is often described as being 'rough, tough and buff' in comparison with the smooth, friable and whitish appearance of bovine type bacilli, *Myco. bovis*, as shown on the right. The latter culture had been incubated under identical conditions and illustrates the slow growth of these mycobacteria even on rich media. By courtesy of E. & S. Livingstone Ltd.

(e) This Gram-stained preparation is from a culture of *Actinomyces israelii*, the causal organism of human actinomycosis; the long branching filaments, showing some fragmentation, emerge from a dense mycelium (× 1000).

(f) Film from a pure culture of *Clostridium tetani* and stained by Ziehl–Neelsen's method modified by using a weaker strength of H_2SO_4 (0·5 per cent) for decolourization; the terminal, spherical and projecting spores produce the typical appearance of 'the drum-stick bacillus' (× 1000).

(g) Blood agar plate viewed by oblique illumination in an endeavour to show the very fine, diaphanous film of spreading growth characteristic of *Cl. tetani*.

(h) Preparation of *Clostridium welchii* showing capsules; this India Ink film was dried, fixed with methanol and then stained with methyl violet for 2 min. For normal purposes, India Ink films are viewed in the wet state.

(i) Film stained for 10 min with 1 in 10 carbol fuchsin; the film was from a case of gingivostomatitis and shows large numbers of *Fusiformis fusiformis* (cigar-shaped bacilli) and *Borrelia vincentii* (spirochaetes) (× 1000).

(j) Carbol fuchsin-stained film of blood from a white mouse that had been infected with *Borrelia duttonii*, the cause of West African relapsing fever (× 1000).

(k) Coagulase tests. Both tubes contained citrated rabbit plasma, diluted 1 in 10 in sterile saline; the upper tube received five drops of an overnight broth culture of a nonpathogenic staphylococcus and the lower tube received a similar volume of an broth culture of a staphylococcus isolated from an infected wound. The tubes were then incubated overnight at 37°C for 6 hours. The contents of the upper tube remained fluid, whereas the plasma in the lower tube has been gelled; thus the staphylococcus inoculated into the latter tube was coagulase-positive.

(l) Nagler's reaction on egg-yolk medium. Three drops of *Clostridium welchii* type-A antiserum were spread over one-half (upper part of plate) of the medium; a culture of *Cl. welchii* was then streaked on the medium and two spot inoculations were also made. After anaerobic incubation at 37°C for 20 hours, the organisms grew on both halves of the plate. On the antitoxin-free half, lecithinase activity produced zones of opacity but this activity has been inhibited by the antitoxin present on the upper half.

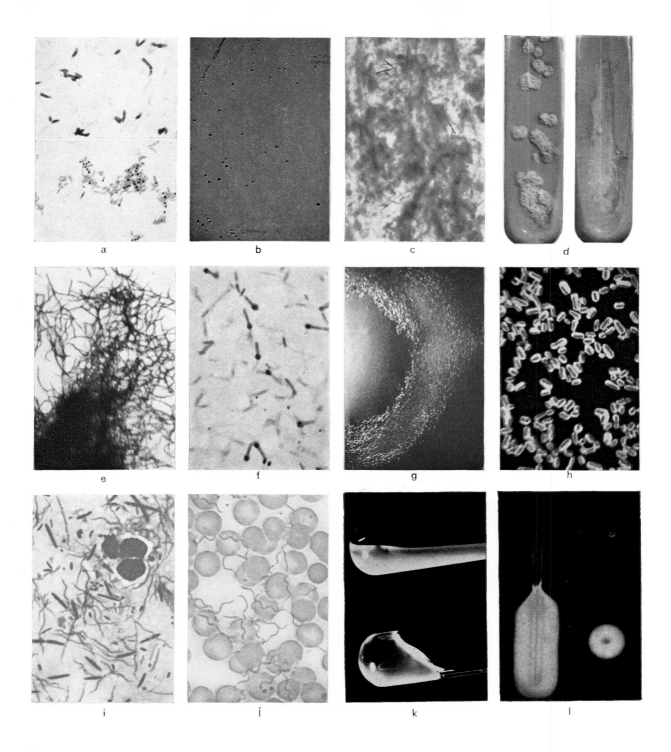

a

b

c

d

e

f

g

h

i

j

k

l

not separate completely after fission and this leads to a characteristic angular 'Chinese lettering' appearance (plate 18.1a, facing p. 18.62). They are nonmotile and nonsporing, but some members of the group produce polar granules (volutin granules) of material containing high-energy polyphosphates and these stain characteristically with Albert's stain (p. 18.16) (plate 18.1a, facing p. 18.62). Some corynebacteria produce disease in animals and several members of the group are commensals of man; the general term for unspecified corynebacteria is diphtheroids. Commensals of man include *Corynebacterium hofmannii* which is harboured in the throat, *C. xerosis* which is often present in the healthy conjunctival sac, and *C. acnes* which is found on the skin in association with acne though it is not the cause of the disease. The important pathogen of man is *C. diphtheriae*, the causative organism of **diphtheria.**

In diphtheria, the bacteria multiply locally in the nasopharynx and upper respiratory passages and produce a potent exotoxin. This causes necrosis of the mucous membrane with the formation of grey sloughs. There may be much swelling of the surrounding tissues, which together with a separated slough may block the larynx and asphyxiate a child. The bacteria remain at the site of the infection but the exotoxin diffuses out to produce widespread effects, particularly on the heart and peripheral nerves. Although diphtheria bacilli are sensitive to antibiotics, the prompt administration of antitoxin is of paramount importance in the treatment of the disease. In the rare form of **cutaneous diphtheria,** the organisms are found in ulcerative lesions of the skin where exotoxin is produced and may cause peripheral neuritis.

CORYNEBACTERIUM DIPHTHERIAE

Three types of *C. diphtheriae* exist, *gravis*, *mitis* and *intermedius*, which can be differentiated by their cultural appearances (plate 18.1b, facing p. 18.62) and biochemical properties. The organisms cannot be identified with certainty by their microscopic appearances because, although most of the commensal diphtheroids are shorter and stumpier than *C. diphtheriae*, the genus is typically pleomorphic. It is therefore necessary to confirm a provisional diagnosis by culture of the organism and to demonstrate the toxigenicity of the strain. The clinician must not meanwhile postpone giving life-saving antitoxin if diphtheria is suspected on clinical grounds, but there are important epidemiological reasons for confirming the diagnosis in the laboratory. Cultures are prepared from throat swabs and the toxigenicity of a suspected strain is confirmed by antitoxin-controlled tests in guinea-pigs or by an *in vitro* precipitin reaction in a gel-diffusion system.

Diphtheria toxin is a protein and a lethal dose for a guinea-pig may be as low as 0·4 μg/kg. The toxic reaction appears to depend on inactivation of an enzyme system involved in the transfer of amino acids from t-RNA to peptide chain synthesis at the ribosomal level. Only those diphtheria bacilli that harbour a particular phage (β-phage) or a closely related phage in the lysogenic state appear to be toxigenic and this finding is of great interest as it thus appears that the exotoxin is phage-specified. In addition, the concentration of iron in the culture medium markedly influences the amount of toxin produced.

When toxin is held at 37°C in an aerobic environment, especially if formaldehyde is present, it loses its toxic activity but it retains its specific antigenicity and it is then referred to as (formol) toxoid; this is a good antigen and stimulates the production of specific antitoxin when it is injected parenterally. Diphtheria toxoid is an important immunizing agent. Its general use since 1940 has virtually eradicated diphtheria from Britain, although sporadic cases of the disease occur and these may be fatal in unvaccinated patients.

The intradermal injection of a minute dose of diphtheria toxin causes an erythematous reaction with local swelling in a person devoid of circulating antitoxin. This is the basis of the **Schick test** which is used to detect those who may be vulnerable to the disease. Some people react to other constituents of the toxin preparation, and it is therefore necessary to inject a test dose of the toxin in parallel with another injection of the same preparation inactivated by heat. The control injection is given into the skin of one forearm, and the test dose into the other.

Diphtheria is spread by infected patients and carriers of virulent organisms who may or may not have suffered from a recent clinical infection. Direct contact involved for example in kissing and cuddling the infected child by parents and siblings before removal to hospital, may well have spread the disease when diphtheria was rife in this country and when parents were well aware that the chances of survival for a sick child were not high. The disease has been responsible for large numbers of deaths of children in early childhood and, although it is now much reduced in incidence and almost completely controlled in some countries, it remains an important cause of death in some developing countries. Eradication has followed the detection and treatment of carriers, the investigation of the general immunity by Schick-testing, and efficient immunization campaigns.

THE AEROBIC SPORE-FORMING BACTERIA

Bacillus

The genus *Bacillus* contains only one species pathogenic for man; this is *B. anthracis*, which causes **anthrax,** primarily a disease of herbivorous animals, but occasionally infecting man. The genus is otherwise associated with a saprophytic existence and the organisms are widely distributed in soil, dust, water and air. They all form spores that can persist for a long time in an unfavourable environment. As the spores are ubiquitous, members of this genus are common contaminants of culture media and species such as *B. subtilis* and *B. cereus* are well known to bacteriologists on this account. *B. cereus* is also of note as a penicillinase producer.

Bacillus organisms are Gram-positive rods of varying size. Spores may be central, subterminal or terminal. Some species are motile. The organisms grow readily under aerobic conditions on simple media.

BACILLUS ANTHRACIS
This is a large rectangular Gram-positive rod and it tends to form long chains. A well-defined polypeptide capsule is produced *in vivo*. When the organism is outside the host, spores form and they are usually oval and lie centrally within the cell. Under low power magnification, the wavy margins of colonies of bacilli may resemble locks of hair and have earned the name 'Medusa head'.

Anthrax has an important place in medical history. In 1881, Pasteur demonstrated in field trials in France that administration of an anthrax vaccine protected sheep and cattle subsequently challenged with anthrax. This was the first occasion on which a vaccine prepared from bacterial cultures was successfully used.

In herbivores anthrax is a serious disease in which the organisms, probably ingested as spores, produce an overwhelming septicaemia and spread to all the organs of the body. They are present in the urine and faeces of the moribund animal and pastures are readily contaminated. The organism does not produce spores *in vivo*.

It is illegal to conduct a full post-mortem examination of an animal thought to have died of anthrax in Britain, because spores are formed when the bacilli are exposed to air and dissemination is likely to occur.

How man may become infected with anthrax by contact with sick animals or infected animal products is described on p. 18.25.

The anthrax organism produces several toxic factors when it multiplies *in vivo* and these together with its capsule, determine its invasiveness and its formidable virulence for the host.

Anthrax has been considered as a disease that might be exploited for purposes of microbiological warfare. Aerosols of infective spores can be produced cheaply in great amounts, but the weapon would be of danger to the aggressor as well as the defender since the spores would persist in the contaminated ground for many years.

THE ANAEROBIC SPORE-FORMING BACTERIA
Clostridium
The clostridia are primarily saprophytic organisms that live in decaying matter but some occur in the large intestine of man and many animals. They play an important role in the decomposition of dead animals and plants. Important clostridial diseases of man are **gas gangrene**, **tetanus** and **botulism**. Gas gangrene and tetanus took a heavy toll of the wounded in the fighting in 1914 in the heavily manured fields of Flanders. The introduction of new methods of prophylaxis and treatment based on bacteriological studies greatly reduced these complications. In many countries, the decline in the use of farm manure and in the number of horses and farm workers employed on the land has led to a decline in the incidence of gas gangrene and tetanus; this has been accelerated by active immunization against tetanus and by better facilities and techniques for wound treatment. Nevertheless tetanus continues to be an important cause of mortality in many areas of the world.

Anaerobiosis
Three properties of the clostridia determine the circumstances and nature of the diseases that they produce. First, they are anaerobes. Oxygen inhibits their growth and they cannot multiply in healthy tissue with a good blood supply. The presence of necrotic tissue, foreign bodies in a wound and secondary pyogenic infection all encourage their growth. Hence, careful cleaning of a wound and surgical removal of devitalized tissue and chemotherapy are likely to prevent the growth of clostridia. If they multiply in a tissue, some release gas and give the tissue the characteristic appearance and feel of gas gangrene.

Sporulation
Second, the clostridia form spores which are widely distributed in dust, soil, water and air. They are also present in faeces and frequently contaminate skin.

Production of exotoxins
Third, the pathogenic clostridia produce powerful exotoxins and aggressins that are largely responsible for their lethal effects. Some of the exotoxins produced when the organisms are grown in culture have been concentrated and purified. Lethal doses of tetanus and botulinum toxins for mice are 4 ng/kg and 1·3 ng/kg respectively; these toxins kill by specific actions on the nervous system and the toxin of *Cl. botulinum* is perhaps the most toxic substance known. Most of the toxins associated with the gas gangrene group of organisms have more general effects. Some are phospholipases and lipases, and

these damage mitochondrial and other cell membranes; although intensely toxic, they are a little less potent than the neurotoxins described above (p. 25.20).

The bacilli are typically Gram-positive, though Gram-negative forms are often seen in cultures more than a few hours old. Depending on the species, the vegetative cells possess different shapes, and the spores may be either central or at one end. The terminal spores of *Cl. tetani* give a characteristic drumstick appearance to the rods (plate 18.1f, facing p. 18.62). Infection may arise in a wound when spores of a pathogenic *Clostridium* species are introduced under suitably anaerobic conditions that allow germination and outgrowth of the organisms.

Cultural characteristics

The pathogenic clostridia are not homogeneous in their biochemical activities. Some are predominantly saccharolytic in culture and produce much gas if a fermentable carbohydrate is available. Others are proteolytic and their cultures evolve unpleasant odours. Many clostridia possess both saccharolytic and proteolytic activities. The members of the genus are typically motile and produce spreading growth on solid media (plate 18.1g, facing p. 18.62), but *Cl. welchii* (*Cl. perfringens*) is nonmotile; this species is also atypical in being capsulate (plate 18.1h, facing p. 18.62) and, although it has the ability to spore, it does not do so readily in artificial culture.

Serological types

The serology of the clostridial exoproteins is interesting and there are good practical reasons for being informed in this field. For example, although ten different serotypes of *Cl. tetani* can be differentiated on the basis of flagellar antigens, they all produce an immunologically identical toxin and tetanus antitoxin is protective against the product of all of these types. On the other hand, different strains of *Cl. botulinum* produce six antigenically different toxins and it is necessary to have the correct antitoxin to confer specific protection. *Cl. welchii* is an example of an organism that produces a wide range of toxic products and aggressins; more than half the Greek alphabet has already been used to denote the individual exotoxins. The product that seems to be primarily associated with the organism's pathogenicity is a phospholipase-C which produces opacity in egg yolk or serum media (Nagler reaction, plate 18.1l, facing p. 18.62) and this reaction is exploited for the rapid detection of the species in the laboratory. The *Cl. welchii* group of organisms produces much disease in animals and there are five main types (A–E) differentiated on the basis of the production of various permutations of exoproteins. Type A is the common human pathogen, and it also occurs as a commensal in the intestine of man and animals.

CLOSTRIDIAL INFECTION OF WOUNDS

The clostridia that may be individually or collectively involved in **gas gangrene** include *Cl. welchii* (*Cl. perfringens*), *Cl. oedematiens* (*Cl. novyi*) and *Cl. septicum* (*Vibrion septique*). There are many other species that have been associated less commonly with the condition. The causative organisms are present as spores in soil and frequently in faeces and the condition arises as a result of contamination of a wound under conditions that allow the spores to germinate. Specific antitoxins are available and may be of clinical use, but until the causative organism is identified bacteriologically the clinician is obliged to give polyvalent antitoxin prepared against the three most common clostridia involved. The best preventive measure is prompt and adequate surgical attention to any wound so that anaerobic conditions in which the organisms flourish are avoided.

Tetanus may arise when a wound is contaminated with spores of *Cl. tetani* which occur in the soil and dust. Tetanus bacilli can be isolated from faeces of animals such as the horse, cow and dog. *Cl. tetani* is much less commonly found in human faeces, though the incidence varies markedly in different populations. It causes no trouble to the host when it occurs in the intestine. In contrast with the gas gangrene organisms, the tetanus bacilli multiply only at the site of introduction in the tissues and they do not extend from this focus. However, they elaborate tetanospasmin which is so potent a neurotoxin that severe and even fatal tetanus may follow a trivial injury contaminated with tetanus spores. The toxin diffuses slowly up the motor nerves to reach the spinal cord where it interferes with the normal inhibitory control of the lower motor neurones by the higher centres. Affected muscles in a patient with tetanus are hypertonic and violent spasms are triggered by trivial stimuli. In addition to the protection afforded by proper attention to all wounds, specific protection is provided by a course of active immunization with tetanus toxoid; the resulting immunity lasts for more than 5 years (p. 22.23). Injured patients considered to be at risk with respect to tetanus can be protected passively with antitoxin; this is usually given as a preparation of equine serum and, in addition to the disadvantage of its rapid elimination within a week or two, the heterologous serum produces hypersensitivity reactions in some patients. In occasional cases, severe and even fatal anaphylactic shock occurs (p. 23.1). Accordingly, there is much to commend the increasing use of 'homologous antitoxin' prepared from human serum.

CLOSTRIDIAL FOOD POISONING

Botulism is a severe form of food poisoning caused by a powerful toxin in food in which *Cl. botulinum* has had the opportunity to grow. *Cl. botulinum* occurs widely in nature as a saprophyte in soil; it can be recovered from vegetables and from fish and marine products and it is able to grow and to produce toxin at low temperatures, provided that anaerobic conditions are assured. The spores are markedly heat-resistant and, if they are protected by the presence of protein, may survive boiling for several hours. The potent toxin is not inactivated on ingestion and it is absorbed from the gastrointestinal tract; it has affinity for the central nervous system and interferes with mechanisms of acetylcholine release, producing symptoms such as difficulty in swallowing, ocular paresis, respiratory embarrassment and cardiac arrest (p. 4.5).

Six types of *Cl. botulinum* are differentiated on the basis of the serologically different but pharmacologically similar toxins that they produce; types A, B and E are associated with disease in man and the type-E strains are generally of marine origin. *Botulus* is the Latin word for a large sausage of the German variety within which no doubt anaerobic conditions can be found. Large hams may also be internally anaerobic, and home-canned vegetables can support anaerobic growth. Liver paste and specially fermented fish dishes are also associated with the risk of botulism. The most famous tragedy occurred in 1922 when a fishing party set out from a well-known hotel on Loch Maree in Scotland. Within 24 hours, eight of the party had died and the trouble was traced to wild duck paste in the sandwiches provided for lunch. The food industry is well aware of the danger of botulism and, with a notable exception in which the first cases presented in Montreal in 1967, botulism is not usually associated with industrially processed foods.

A much more common and much less dangerous form of clostridial food poisoning is associated with *Cl. welchii*. When this organism is consumed in large numbers in food in which it has grown, it causes abdominal cramps and diarrhoea that last for a day or two. The condition is typically associated with meat foods that have been precooked on the previous day and allowed to cool under conditions that allow multiplication of the organism in an anaerobic environment. Anaerobiosis is ensured by the heating of the food and it is sustained by the reducing agents in the meat. Spores of some strains of *Cl. welchii* are particularly heat resistant and these strains, because of their resistance to cooking procedures, are characteristically associated with this form of food poisoning. The spores of these strains occur widely and can be recovered from dust, faeces, flies and raw meat. They are protected if meat is cooked in bulk and the spores are actually activated by heat so that their subsequent germination is ensured. Their growth is allowed by the anaerobic state of the environment and is enhanced by the prolonged cooling period that is often involved with bulk-cooked food. The population at risk is usually a large number of diners in a works canteen or members of a semi-closed community such as a hospital, and consequently many people may be affected.

THE ACIDOPHILIC BACILLI

Lactobacillus

This genus contains a number of species with many varieties which inhabit the intestinal tract of animals including man. They are Gram-positive nonsporing bacilli and they can grow under acid conditions. The best known species are *Lactobacillus acidophilus*, commonly found in faeces, the mouth and in milk; *L. bulgaricus*, was isolated long ago from yoghurt, and *L. bifidus* is found in large numbers in the faeces of breast-fed infants. *L. odontolyticus* is closely allied to *L. acidophilus* and found frequently in the mouth. These bacilli have probably been more productive of controversy than disease. In 1905 Elie Metchnikoff, the Russian bacteriologist and philosopher, put forward the view that to achieve a long life with a healthy old age, it was necessary to establish the Bulgarian bacillus firmly in one's colon. The idea attracted much support and for the next 25 years was the basis of a school of thought which did not lack doctors of eminence; it then died. *L. bifidus* the predominant organism in the faeces of a breast-fed infant in the early days of life is readily displaced by other organisms when any form of artificial feeding is instituted. The microbiological change may or may not be responsible for the diminished absorption of nutrients that often accompanies a change of diet in the very young. As long ago as 1890, Miller who worked in Koch's laboratory in Berlin suggested that acid produced by the fermentation of sugars in the mouth by *L. acidophilus* might dissolve calcium salts in dental enamel and contribute to the aetiology of dental caries. This view went into oblivion for 50 years, but it has become fashionable again, and there is now much interest in the possible role of *L. odontolyticus* in dental caries. A lactobacillus known as **Doderlein's bacillus** is found in the vagina. If this organism is suppressed by antibiotic drugs, yeasts and other bacteria may multiply and cause a vaginitis.

There is no quantitative experimental evidence that lactobacilli maintain the normal chemical environment within the mouth, the colon or the vagina. Without this there can be nothing but sterile speculation and controversy, which readily leads to cynicism. Metchnikoff was an imaginative genius, and future studies may show that lactobacilli are more important to our health than the textbooks of today indicate.

THE PYOGENIC COCCI

Streptococcus

This large group of Gram-positive cocci derives its name from the tendency of the organisms to occur in chains; long chains are typical of most species, e.g. *Strept. pyogenes*, but in *Strept. pneumoniae* two cocci (diplococci) are typically attached together (plates 18.2c & 2e, facing p. 18.68). A practical if over-simplified classification of the species pathogenic to man is made by subdivision according to the haemolytic effect produced when growing on horse blood agar. A colony of the *Strept. viridans* group, which are typically commensals living in the mouth, is surrounded by a zone of greenish discoloration associated with partial haemolysis. A colony of *Strept. pyogenes* produces a zone of complete haemolysis. Other streptococci do not produce any haemolysis on blood agar. The viridans effect is **α-haemolysis** and the complete effect is **β-haemolysis** (p. 18.49) (plate 18.2d, facing p. 18.68); *Strept. pyogenes* is also called the β-haemolytic streptococcus. The most common member of the nonhaemolytic group is *Strept. faecalis*, a commensal of the large bowel. The above classification takes no account of *Strept. pneumoniae* and the anaerobic streptococci; these important organisms are discussed on p. 18.69.

The streptococci of medical importance are nonmotile and nonsporing. Some strains produce capsules. They often grow on simple media, but some varieties grow much better on enriched media such as blood agar. The streptococci are more resistant than the staphylococci to the antibacterial effect of crystal violet and this dye may be incorporated in a selective blood agar medium for streptococci.

STREPTOCOCCUS VIRIDANS

This organism is present in large numbers in the mouth and throat of man. It may be found in the blood stream in small numbers from time to time, perhaps as a result of vigorous chewing, but this has no serious consequences in the normal person. However, if there is a previously damaged heart valve, the organism may gain access to it and a condition known as **infective endocarditis** follows; this is the classic role of *Strept. viridans* as a pathogen. The organism may also be involved in apical **dental abscesses**.

STREPTOCOCCUS PYOGENES

This organism is the common cause of sore throat and **tonsillitis,** and quinsy or tonsillar abcess may be a complication. The infection may spread to adjacent tissues and cause **adenitis, mastoiditis** and **otitis media.** In some individuals, a characteristic punctate erythematous rash develops as a sequel to the throat infection and this is called **scarlet fever** (scarlatina). *Strept. pyogenes* may infect **burns** and other wounds sustained accidentally or surgically. The organism is also associated with superficial spreading cutaneous infections such as **impetigo** and **erysipelas** or subcutaneous infections such as **cellulitis.** *Strept. pyogenes* is also the important cause of **puerperal fever** which used to be a common cause of maternal mortality. **Acute rheumatic fever** and **acute glomerulo-nephritis** are closely associated with streptococcal infections; although streptococci are not normally found in the heart or in the kidneys in these diseases, hypersensitivity reactions to streptococcal antigens present in the tissues are thought to be responsible (p. 23.6).

Students at Edinburgh pass every day a bust of Archbishop Tait which marks the site of his family home, demolished to make space for the Anatomy Department. Few of them know his family tragedy. At the beginning of March 1856 he was living with his son and his six little daughters in the deanery at Carlisle. Scarlet fever in its virulent form broke out in the city and, one by one between March 6th and April 8th, the five older girls died; only the two-month-old daughter and his son survived. Such tragedies were frequent in Victorian homes where scarlet fever was a dreaded infection. However, there was always an extraordinary variability in the severity of the outbreaks; they gradually became milder and in England and Wales in 1928 there were just under 600 deaths, compared with 12,000 in 1883. This variation in virulence is a feature of the natural history of streptococcal infections. Although much is now known about the properties of the organism, a full understanding of this important feature is lacking.

Strept. pyogenes produces a wide range of extracellular products in culture and these include an oxygen-stable haemolysin (streptolysin S) and an oxygen-labile haemolysin (streptolysin O), a fibrinolysin (streptokinase, p. 18.32), a hyaluronidase that probably facilitates the spread of bacteria in tissues, a deoxyribonuclease (streptodornase) which lowers the viscosity of purulent exudates, an NADase, and an erythrogenic toxin that is produced by strains capable of causing scarlet fever. The role played by each of these products in the pathogenicity of the organism is not easily assessed and *Strept. pyogenes* provides a striking example of a species that is associated with an impressive number of widely different clinical syndromes. Strains of *Strept. pyogenes* that produce erythrogenic toxin are lysogenic for a particular bacteriophage. This is an interesting parallel to a similar phenomenon observed with *C. diphtheriae* (p. 18.63).

There are actually many antigenically different members of the β-haemolytic streptococci and, on the basis of specific carbohydrate haptens (C antigens) present in the cell wall, they can be differentiated by precipitin reactions into groups originally devised by Lancefield and now extending from A–S. The β-haemolytic streptococci that are pathogenic for man belong predominantly to Lancefield's Group A, and these can be further subdivided into almost 50 different types according to their specific M-protein which is a surface antigen associated with virulence. The situation is complicated by the occurrence of other streptococcal antigens (T and R), but these will not be discussed further. A patient exposed to one type develops type-specific antibodies. Only a relatively

PLATE 18.2. Bacteriology.

(a) Film of pus containing staphylococci showing the characteristic arrangement. Gram stain (× 1000).

(b) Blood agar plate seeded with pus and incubated at 37°C for 18 hours; a pure and profuse growth of *Staphyloccus aureus* is seen. These proved to be coagulase-positive (plate 18.1k); the colonies should be contrasted with the smaller, nonpigmented colonies of streptococci (d).

(c) Film of pus containing *Streptococcus pyogenes*. Chains of varying length are apparent, but the chain length is no guide to the cultural type of streptococcus. Gram stain (× 1000).

(d) Blood agar plate seeded with a throat swab and incubated for 18 hours at 37°C. Two colonial types of streptococci are present; these are identical in size but β-haemolysis around the colonies of the pathogenic *Strept. pyogenes* makes them more obvious than the colonies of commensal *Strept. viridans* which form a series of α-haemolytic spots in the background.

(e) Film of sputum from a case of lobar pneumonia. The pneumococci occur in pairs; the capsules are not demonstrated by the Gram stain (× 1000).

(f) Blood agar plate seeded with a pure culture of pneumococci and incubated for 36 hours at 37°C; the colonial size after 18 hours was identical with that of *Strept. viridans* (d) and the associated α-haemolysis was similar.

(g) Film of urethral discharge from a case of gonorrhoea; two polymorphs are packed with Gram-negative diplococci. This intracellular appearance is characteristic of the pathogenic neisseriae (× 1000).

(h) Chocolate blood agar medium seeded with urethral discharge and incubated for 48 hours at 37°C in air with 5 per cent CO_2. The white, pigmented colonies were shown to be coagulase-negative staphylococci; the lower photograph was taken 5 sec after oxidase reagent had been flooded over the plate. The colonies that then became purple belong to the genus *Neisseria* and biochemical tests showed that they were *N. gonorrhoeae*.

(i) Gram-stained film of a pure culture of *Escherichia coli;* these are indistinguishable from other enterobacteria by Gram staining.

(j) The culture medium employed here is that of MacConkey which contains lactose and phenol red indicator; in the upper half is a mixed culture of *Esch. coli* showing pink, lactose-fermenting colonies with pale, lactose nonfermenting colonies which proved to be *Shigella sonnei*. In the lower part are colonies of *Klebsiella aerogenes* which have also utilized the lactose; this species produces large amounts of extracellular slime which endows the colonies with a mucoid appearance and also allows adjacent colonies to coalesce.

(k) This blood agar plate was stab-inoculated with a pure culture of *Proteus vulgaris* and then incubated at 37°C for 18 hours; successive waves of spreading growth can be seen. The swarming nature of *Proteus* species frequently delays the isolation of other species in mixed culture but can be prevented by incorporating various substances, e.g. chloral hydrate (1 in 500), in the medium.

(l) This nutrient agar plate was seeded with a swab from an infected burn and then incubated at 37°C for 18 hours; the natural light straw colour of the medium has been altered by pyocyanin pigment produced by the organism.

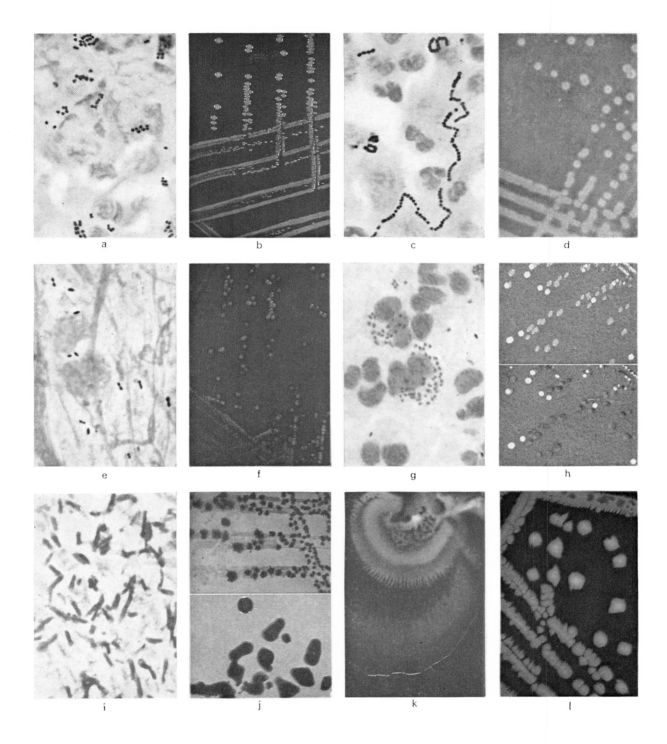

a

b

c

d

e

f

g

h

i

j

k

l

small number of types is associated with glomerulonephritis (p. 23.6). These nephritogenic strains include types 12 and 49 particularly. No specific antigenic types appear to be responsible for acute rheumatic fever (p. 30.10).

Sources of infection include patients suffering from disease caused by *Strept. pyogenes* and healthy carriers who may harbour the organism in the throat or nose. Throat carriers are the most common (10–20 per cent), but spread from nasal carriers is more likely to occur. *Strept. pyogenes* has not developed resistance to penicillin which remains the antibiotic of choice for the control of infections caused by this organism. Tetracycline-resistance is commonly encountered with strains of *Strept. pyogenes*.

STREPTOCOCCUS FAECALIS

This is the name given to a group of bile-tolerant streptococci commensal in the large intestine and sometimes referred to as enterococci; they cause no trouble in the healthy gut, but may participate in local inflammatory reactions such as **appendicitis**. If they gain access to tissues beyond the intestine, they may be involved in pelvic sepsis, **cholecystitis** or **peritonitis**. *Strept. faecalis* is a common pathogen in the urinary tract and it may give rise to **cystitis** and **pyelonephritis**, often in combination with *Esch. coli*. Although the faecal streptococci are typically associated with sepsis at the abdominal or pelvic level, they may participate in pyogenic infections elsewhere in the body; they are occasionally carried in the blood and may also be responsible for **infective endocarditis**.

STREPTOCOCCUS PNEUMONIAE

These are the pneumococci and, as they occur in pairs, used to be known as *Diplococcus pneumoniae*. The cocci are lanceolate and the pairs have their rounded ends apposed; short chains are common. They are nonmotile and nonsporing, but capsules are present in pathogenic strains recently isolated. *Strept. pneumoniae* is associated primarily with **lobar pneumonia**, but may be responsible for pyogenic infection elsewhere in the body; pneumococci may therefore cause **meningitis, otitis media, conjunctivitis, sinusitis, pericarditis** and even **peritonitis**. Pneumococci are common commensals of the upper respiratory tract and in addition to their classical association with lobar pneumonia they are often involved as secondary invaders in **bronchopneumonia** and other inflammatory conditions of the respiratory tract.

The virulence of the pneumococcus is associated primarily with the presence of a capsule. This is composed of polysaccharide and different types of pneumococci can be differentiated on the basis of the specific polysaccharide involved. In association with the bacterial cell protein, the capsular polysaccharide acts as a hapten so that type-specific antibodies can be produced. When a specific antiserum is mixed with a suspension of the homologous pneumococci, the capsule becomes more clearly defined on microscopical observation, due to changes in its optical properties and also probably to actual capsule-swelling. When specific serotherapy was used in the treatment of lobar pneumonia, typing of the organism by this method was important, but the advent of chemotherapy and antibiotics replaced serotherapy and removed the necessity for typing; the success that the physician now achieves in the treatment of primary lobar pneumonia makes it easy to forget how dreaded the disease was in the recent past.

The capsule of *Strept. pneumoniae* has important associations with the study of microbial genetics, particularly in relation to early observations on transformation (p. 18.54). Virulent pneumococci are capsulate; loss of the capsule results in loss of type-specificity and loss of virulence, and the colonies of non-capsulate strains are not smooth but appear to have a rough surface (S–R variation, p. 18.49).

Capsulate pneumococci are very invasive in the lung and sweep through the tissue of an affected lobe until they are limited by an anatomical boundary. The organisms produce hyaluronidase and neuraminidase, and although a haemolysin related to the oxygen-labile haemolysin of *Strept. pyogenes* is produced *in vitro* no soluble product is directly associated with their pathogenicity (p. 23.1).

In culture on blood agar, young colonies of *Strept. pneumoniae* resemble those of *Strept. viridans*; older colonies of *Strept. pneumoniae* tend to develop flat tops and concentric furrows and they are referred to as 'draughtsman colonies' (plate 18.2f, facing p. 18.68). Early differentiation is not straightforward and various tests are used to identify isolates; one such test is based upon the sensitivity of pneumococci to ethyl dihydrocuprein hydrochloride (optochin), and another depends on the solubility of pneumococci in solutions of bile salts.

The anaerobic cocci

A large group of Gram-positive and Gram-negative cocci includes various commensal and pathogenic organisms of man which have the common property of being obligate anaerobes. This poorly characterized and heterogeneous collection includes Gram-positive cocci that are typically arranged in chains, and also Gram-negative and Gram-positive cocci that occur in clumps. These organisms have been classified into nine groups on the basis of their morphology and biochemical properties. The most distinctive is Group 1 which corresponds with *Strept. putridus* of the older terminology.

In general, the anaerobic cocci occur as commensals in the vagina and in the upper respiratory tract, and may be involved in inflammatory conditions in these areas. For example, anaerobic streptococci may cause **puerperal sepsis** and they may be isolated from **lung abscesses.** They have also been isolated from infected wounds and brain abscesses and are often found in association with other pathogens.

Staphylococcus

The staphylococci form a large group of Gram-positive cocci; they occur widely in nature and can be isolated from man and animals and from soil, water, air and dust. The pathogenic staphylococci are typically associated with pus formation and circumscribed infections; they are the usual cause of sepsis of abrasions or wounds and are often involved in septic spots on the skin, including the 'stye' of an infected eyelid. The organisms vary in their invasiveness; a typical staphylococcal lesion is localized in the form of a **boil, carbuncle** or **abscess,** but staphylococci may cause spreading infections in the skin, e.g. **impetigo,** and the organisms may spread also by the blood stream to cause **septicaemia** and infections such as **osteomyelitis, multiple pyogenic abscesses** or **endocarditis.**

The cocci are small and spherical; they occur in irregular clusters of varying size, resembling bunches of grapes (plate 18.2a, facing p. 18.68). They are nonmotile and nonsporing. A few strains produce capsules. The staphylococci grow well on ordinary culture media and the colonies develop characteristic colours which range from white to gold (plate 18.2b, facing p. 18.68). The golden *Staph. aureus* is usually responsible for infections and the white *Staph. albus* and other pigmented strains such as the lemon-yellow *Staph. citreus* are commensals and much less frequently pathogenic. Some strains which do not produce the golden pigment masquerade as apparently harmless *Staph. albus* strains and possess the pathogenic characteristics of *Staph. aureus*; this complicates the work of the bacteriologist. However, virtually all pathogenic staphylococci produce coagulase, an enzyme which clots citrated plasma *in vitro*. The correlation between coagulase production and pathogenicity is of great use in differentiating potentially dangerous from commensal strains (the coagulase test) (plate 18.1k, facing p. 18.62). *Staph. albus* is such a common resident on the skin that it has been termed *Staph. epidermidis albus*; these coagulase-negative strains may occasionally cause trouble.

STAPHYLOCOCCUS AUREUS
The potentially pathogenic coagulase-positive *Staph. aureus* has been found in nasal swabs from 20–30 per cent of persons in apparently healthy populations and also in the perineal region of some people. Since healthy carriers of potentially dangerous staphylococci are relatively common, staphylococcal infection may arise from either an endogenous or an exogenous source. Exogenous infection is common in hospital because the inmates, both

patients and staff, are likely to include a large number of carriers of virulent staphylococci. There are a number of phages with specific affinities for different staphylococci and it is therefore possible to identify strains of staphylococci by their phage-sensitivity patterns. This is the basis of phage-typing which is of great use in the investigation of outbreaks of staphylococcal sepsis.

Most strains of staphylococci associated with epidemic and endemic disease in hospitals are notoriously resistant to penicillin, and penicillin-resistant staphylococci produce penicillinase which decomposes the antibiotic (p. 20.7). These staphylococci are frequently resistant to other antibiotics in addition to penicillin; for example, most strains that cause surgical sepsis are tetracycline-resistant, and they also carry a related resistance to mercury salts. This does not imply that mercury salts have a place in modern surgical antisepsis, but the relation is an interesting example of a linked character (vol. 1, p. 38.5).

In addition to coagulase, other toxins and aggressins are produced by *Staph. aureus*; these include four immunologically distinct haemolysins, a leucocidin, a fibrinolysin and a hyaluronidase, but how these contribute to the pathogenicity is unknown. Another product, the enterotoxin, is elaborated by some strains which may cause **staphylococcal food poisoning.**

Food contaminated by staphylococci may serve as a culture medium, in which enterotoxin may be produced. If such food is subsequently ingested, the toxin gives rise, usually within a few hours, to acute food poisoning with giddiness, vomiting and diarrhoea; the reactions are often severe, but patients generally recover within a day or two. This is an intoxication and not an infective condition.

The pathogenic staphylococci are serologically heterogeneous; no effective vaccine has been prepared and there is no routine method for their serological grouping. Toxoid preparations of the α-haemolysin are sometimes used to enhance resistance of patients who suffer from recurrent staphylococcal infections, but their value is not established.

Prevention of staphylococcal infection depends primarily upon measures to control transmission of the organism. Hands transfer the organisms from carrier sites and there are innumerable opportunities for endogenous and exogenous infection. Transfer of staphylococci from the skin to the environment is a normal process, but some people seem to shed organisms readily and are referred to as **dispersers.** The sustained and repeated local application of antibacterial agents such as neomycin and chlorhexidine to the anterior nares sometimes controls the carrier state, but re-colonization occurs (p. 18.42) Almost all healthy infants born in hospital are colonized with staphylococci within 1–2 weeks and they constitute an important reservoir of hospital staphylococci before they leave. The sustained use of hexachlorophane preparations for skin disinfection (p. 18.40) in neonatal units and in surgical units has been successful in controlling staphylococcal sepsis.

Staphylococci are remarkably resistant and survive for long periods in the environment. They can remain viable in the dry state in dust and on textiles for months. They are salt tolerant and grow in the presence of concentrations of salt which are bacteristatic for most other pathogenic bacteria; thus they can multiply on salted cooked and processed meats which may be associated with food poisoning. They also grow well in milk and milk products; pasteurization ensures the safety of milk in this respect, but it may be recontaminated in the kitchen.

Neisseria

Two species of neisseriae are pathogenic to man; *N. meningitidis* (meningococcus) and *N. gonorrhoeae* (gonococcus); some of the others, e.g. *N. catarrhalis*, are normal commensals.

The neisseriae occur as pairs of Gram-negative kidney-shaped cocci with their apposed surfaces flattened. They are nonmotile and nonsporing, and some species are capsulate. Capsules are not seen on direct microscopy but they may be demonstrated by capsule-swelling reactions with specific antisera. Neisseriae are obligatory aerobes. All species possess cytochrome oxidase, which is demonstrated by the oxidase test using tetra-methyl-*p*-phenylene diamine solution (oxidase reagent). Cytochrome oxidase catalyses the oxidation of reduced cytochrome and the transport of electrons from bacterial electron donors to the oxidase dye which is reduced to a violet colour. Both species possess toxic nucleoproteins which may account for their toxic effects.

N. MENINGITIDIS

N. meningitidis is a not uncommon temporary commensal in the nasopharynx and has been found in 10 per cent of healthy populations. Between epidemics of meningitis these commensal strains are usually of groups B or C; group A strains are rarely found as commensals.

After reaching the nasopharynx, meningococci may be established as temporary commensals or may cause a **nasopharyngitis**. The infection is usually arrested at this stage, but meningococci may invade the blood to produce an acute bacteriaemia with fever, muscle pain and a petechial rash, though the rash is by no means always observed. There is usually a polymorph leucocytosis, and the organism can be recovered from the blood. The acute bacteriaemic stage may be arrested or systemic lesions may follow, of which **meningitis** is by far the most common. Meningococcal meningitis is usually seen in children and young adults and is relatively rare after the age of 25.

Sporadic meningitis in infants and young children is usually caused by meningococci of groups B or C.

Epidemic meningitis is caused by group A organisms, and is most likely to occur in those sleeping in dormitories or barracks. Not only do cases of meningitis harbour the organism in their nasopharynx, but healthy contacts may acquire meningococci and be a source of danger to others. A nasopharyngeal carrier rate of Group A strains in over 20 per cent of the population points to an impending epidemic. Less than 1 per cent of persons who harbour the organism in their nasopharynx develop meningitis. During epidemics, up to 90 per cent of contacts may be carriers.

Transmission is by droplet spray through coughing and sneezing. Fomites and dust cannot be implicated, as meningococci are very sensitive to drying. The sources of infection may be healthy or convalescent carriers. Meningococcal meningitis diagnosed early usually responds to antimicrobial therapy, and recovery is rapid and complete. If untreated, the disease is often fatal, or chronic inflammation may lead to hydrocephalus and other severe cerebral damage. Nowadays only sporadic cases are seen in most countries, but very large epidemics continue to occur in parts of Africa. These arise in the dry season and stop abruptly when the rains come.

The meningococcus is a delicate organism and is killed within an hour or two by drying. Where practicable, specimens of CSF should be kept at 37°C during transit; they must not be refrigerated and should be dealt with promptly in the laboratory.

Laboratory diagnosis

Lumbar puncture is essential for the diagnosis of meningitis. In an established case the fluid is turbid due to the presence of large numbers of polymorphs. Meningococci are seen in the Gram-stained deposit, lying within the polymorphs and also free in the fluid. The organisms rapidly undergo autolysis and a turbid CSF containing many pus cells but no observable bacteria is nearly always meningococcal in origin. Neutral red is the best Gram counter-stain as it delineates meningococci well.

To culture the organism a centrifuged deposit is inoculated on blood agar, incubated aerobically and anaerobically, and on 'chocolate' (heated blood) agar incubated aerobically in 5–10 per cent CO_2. Blood agar media are used for the detection of other organisms which may be the cause of the meningitis. Blood culture should not be omitted in a case of meningitis. Recovery of meningococci from the blood is the sole means of establishing a diagnosis of chronic meningococcal bacteriaemia.

Four antigenic groups (A–D) are based on agglutination reactions. The group-specific antigens are polysaccharides and are probably located in the capsule. For final confirmation, tube agglutination tests with monospecific antisera may be performed. A rapid precipitin test for diagnosis is done by layering some CSF supernatant onto polyvalent antimeningococcal serum in a tube. A ring of precipitation indicates the presence of *N. meningitidis* antigen in the CSF.

N. GONORRHOEAE

N. gonorrhoeae is indistinguishable from the meningococcus in its morphology and staining reactions; both are Gram-negative diplococci (plate 18.2g, facing p. 18.68).

The gonococcus is a strict human parasite, and animals cannot be infected. It is always pathogenic and never assumes a commensal existence.

Gonococci are delicate organisms. Unless maintained at 37°C in a moist atmosphere, they die within 2–3 hours, being very susceptible to drying, and they cannot live for any length of time outside the body, e.g. on lavatory seats, etc. An exception occurs where gonococcal pus has soaked fabrics; then the organism is protected by protein and may remain viable occasionally for up to 3 days.

In the vast majority of cases, therefore, **gonorrhoea** is venereally acquired; sexual intercourse allows transmission of an infective dose of the delicate organism to susceptible epithelial cells in the new host. After exposure to infection, the gonococci multiply on the surface of the urethral epithelium and on the cervix. The surface epithelium is attacked and there is hyperaemia and emigration of leucocytes in the underlying submucosa. Polymorphs escape on to the inflamed surface and phagocytose the gonococci. The organisms also penetrate between the epithelial cells to the submucosa. In favourable cases the inflammatory process resolves, but where the infection is severe with much tissue damage, healing occurs with extensive fibrosis and cicatrization, and a fibrous stricture surrounding the urethra is produced. Gonococcal infection can lead to severe and permanent damage to the urinary tract and also cause sterility. It is a serious disease.

Neonatal ophthalmia is acquired when the eyes of the child are exposed to infected tissues during birth, and **gonococcal vulvovaginitis** may occur in young children from contact with infective discharge on wet towels. In contrast to the adult vaginal squamous epithelium, the prepubertal vagina is lined by columnar epithelium which is susceptible to gonococcal infection. In addition, the absence of glycogen in these columnar cells and the scarcity of lactobacilli results in a higher vaginal pH (about 7·0) than is observed in adults. This neutral pH permits the free multiplication of gonococci.

Public health aspects

Gonorrhoea is now one of the most common infectious diseases in the United Kingdom. A rapid decline in the annual incidence of infection occurred after World War II, but since 1954 there has been a steady increase in the number of new infections seen each year at venereal disease clinics (table 18.2).

TABLE 18.2. New cases of gonorrhoea attending venereal disease clinics in England and Wales

Year	Number of cases
1941	22,900*
1946	47,300*
1954	17,536
1961	37,107
1965	36,691
1966	37,483
1967	41,829

* To nearest 100 cases.

In general, males outnumber females by approximately three to one. Many venereologists consider that these figures represent only four-fifths of the true incidence of gonorrhoea.

The extent to which the increase in gonorrhoea is related to promiscuity is shown by the remarkable correlation between the number of illegitimate births and the number of new infections occurring in any one year. The sharp fall in the incidence of gonorrhoea that occurred between 1946 and 1954 was due largely to the return to peacetime conditions and also to effective antibiotic control of infection in persons exposed to risk. However, recent figures for infection rates show that the ground gained in the control of gonorrhoea by therapeutic means is now virtually lost. Gonorrhoea is one of the world's most urgent health problems, and we are now faced with the third 'epidemic' of venereal disease this century, but without the stresses of war to account for it.

Failure to control gonorrhoea has been attributed to difficulty of diagnosis in females, insufficient awareness of its seriousness, difficulties in tracing contacts, widespread travel with its increased chances of the spread of infection, and above all, to the freedoms that a permissive society confers. Immunity following infection does not occur.

Laboratory diagnosis

Smears are made of pus from urethral or cervical discharges and stained by the Gram method with neutral red as the counter-stain. The pus should be obtained preferably with a wire loop and direct smears made, along with inoculation of the pus on to culture media. Pus cells in large numbers together with intracellular or extracellular Gram-negative diplococci provide a tentative diagnosis.

To culture gonococci, the exudate is inoculated on blood agar and chocolate agar which are incubated at

37°C in 5–10 per cent CO_2. The oxidase test (plate 18.2h, facing p. 18.68) and sugar fermentation tests confirm the nature of the organism. Cultural methods often succeed where microscopy is negative, especially in specimens from females. A special transport medium should be used where there is a delay in the transport of swabs.

Colonial growth on blood agar or chocolate agar (pH 7·4) is enhanced by the addition of 5–10 per cent CO_2. A useful selective medium (Thayer–Martin) is a chocolate agar enriched with yeast extract and haemoglobin, to which the antibiotics vancomycin, colistin and nystatin have been added to suppress growth of contaminant organisms. The use of heavily contaminated material (urethral discharge, cervical and rectal swabs) with such a medium often yields *N. gonorrhoeae* when other cultural methods have failed.

Serological studies have divided the organism into two groups, I and II, based on their polysaccharide capsular antigens but the separation of gonococci into these two groups has no diagnostic value. Cross-antigenicity exists between the gonococcus and the meningococcus. However, a gonococcal complement fixation test (GCFT) is of value in diagnosis. The test is negative in acute gonorrhoea when infection is limited to the anterior urethra, but may become positive when the posterior urethra is involved. Its main value is in chronic gonococcal infection where complications have occurred, e.g. arthritis, prostatitis, and in gonococcal endocarditis.

In chronic gonorrhoea, gonococci are usually scarce. In the male, probably the best chance of recovering the organism is after prostatic massage. The patient is requested to urinate and to interrupt the flow of urine before the bladder is emptied. The prostate gland is massaged per rectum and the patient then completes micturition. This latter specimen is examined microscopically and by cultural methods. Alternatively, the centrifuged deposit of an early morning urine may be examined. In the female, swabs are taken from the cervix.

In both sexes the discharge in the later stages of infection may contain streptococci, staphylococci, diphtheroids, and other organisms besides the gonococci. In females this mixed flora may occur even in the early infection, and an independent leucorrhoea or superinfection with yeasts or trichomonas organisms may add to the difficulty in recovering gonococci.

OTHER NEISSERIAE

In addition to the two pathogenic neisseriae, other species are often recovered from human material. Neisseriae constitute part of the normal commensal flora of the upper respiratory tract, and *N. catarrhalis* or *N. pharyngis* are present in the nasopharynx of almost all healthy persons. Commensal neisseriae flourish also in other sites (vagina, urethra) and care must be taken to distinguish them from gonococci in doubtful cases.

Classification of the commensal neisseriae is unsatisfactory, but a tentative separation of the species may be made on the basis of their fermentation of sugars and their production of yellowish pigmented colonies.

All commensal neisseriae grow on nutrient agar at room temperature. This distinguishes them from the pathogenic neisseriae.

THE PARVOBACTERIA

Haemophilus

This genus contains three species pathogenic to man, *H. influenzae*, *H. aegyptius* and *H. ducreyi*. They are small, nonmotile, Gram-negative rods. Pleomorphism is a characteristic feature; many organisms are very short and ovoid (coccoid forms), but filamentous forms are often seen in old cultures and in specimens from patients receiving antibiotics. The frequent appearance of rods and coccoid forms occurring together has led to the morphological description of *Haemophilus* spp. as Gram-negative coccobacilli. These are aerobic bacteria and most varieties require both haematin and NAD as growth factors. Although *Haemophilus* grow on blood agar, their growth is promoted if the blood is first heated at 80°C to make chocolate agar in which the haematin is more readily available. The colonies are small with greyish blue translucency. Colonies growing in the vicinity of a *Staph. aureus* colony are larger than those elsewhere on the medium, due to the synthesis of NAD by *Staph. aureus*. This phenomenon is known as satellitism.

HAEMOPHILUS INFLUENZAE

This species was so named because it was once believed to be the cause of influenza. Indeed it may be recovered frequently from the sputum and nose of patients with influenza but now the myxoviruses are the proven cause of the infection (p. 18.104). *H. influenzae* may be found as a commensal in the nasopharynx and throat of 25–75 per cent of healthy persons. About 1–2 per cent carry capsulated strains. In infections it often acts as an opportunist pathogen. Thus virus infections, e.g. influenza and measles, may pave the way for infection with *H. influenzae*, and **sinusitis, bronchitis, bronchopneumonia** and other pulmonary complications of influenza are not uncommonly attributable to this organism. It can exacerbate chronic bronchitis and infection in bronchiectasis. Along with pneumococci it occurs in large numbers in the sputum during exacerbations, and effective treatment rids the sputum of both organisms and improves the clinical state. Fully virulent strains are capsulate, but those found in chronic bronchial disease are sometimes noncapsulate. *H. influenzae* is classified into six Pittman types (*a–f*) based on the capsular polysaccharide fractions. Type *b* is most common; it is almost always associated with meningitis. Type *a* predominates in sinusitis and types *e* and *f* in some respiratory infections. In culture, S-R colony variation occurs with the loss of capsules, and there is usually a parallel loss of virulence and serological specificity. Typing is performed by the addition of type-specific antisera to the organisms when identification is shown by capsular swelling (p. 18.12). The organisms are delicate and die rapidly in specimens sent for examination, which should be performed as soon as possible. Refrigeration is useless as the organisms die at 4°C.

H. influenzae Pittman type *b* causes **meningitis** in children under 3 years of age. The CSF shows organisms lying free or within the polymorphs. Filamentous forms may occur and this is a useful distinguishing feature from meningitis caused by enterobacteria, unless the patient has received antibiotics. Spread is from the nasopharynx to the blood and thence to the meninges.

Blood stream dissemination may lead to infections of joints and to **subacute endocarditis**. Local extension from the nasopharynx may result in **acute epiglottitis** and in **laryngotracheitis** in young children. Both conditions may be so severe as to require urgent tracheostomy.

OTHER HAEMOPHILUS SPECIES
H. aegyptius, also known as the Koch–Weeks' bacillus, is similar to *H. influenzae*. Both are associated with **acute infectious conjunctivitis**. In conjunctival exudate the organisms can often be seen lying within polymorphs.

H. ducreyi is the cause of a venereal disease known as **chancroid** or **soft sore**. Painful sores develop on the genitalia, the inguinal lymph nodes enlarge (buboes) and suppuration occurs with abscesses in these nodes. Discharge of pus may occur through an external sinus. Gram negative coccobacilli arranged in pairs or chains can be seen in this pus or in aspirated juice from a bubo.

Bordetella

Two species, *Bord. pertussis* and *Bord. parapertussis*, each cause whooping cough; *Bord. pertussis* is commoner and gives rise to more severe infections. These organisms resemble *H. influenzae* in morphology, but do not require the same growth factors. They can be distinguished by biochemical and serological methods.

Whooping cough occurs in children under the age of 5 years and mostly under 1 year. Second attacks are rare. The disease is endemic throughout the world and the highest mortality occurs under 1 year. Thirty years ago the disease annually accounted for over 350 deaths of English children under 1 year, but in the last decade the annual number has been as low as 20.

The disease is highly infectious and about 90 per cent of unvaccinated child contacts acquire the infection. Particularly susceptible are babies up to 3 months, as they possess little passive immunity from maternal antibodies. Spread of the infection is from other patients in the catarrhal stage of the disease. *Bord. pertussis* may occur as a commensal in the upper respiratory tract, but this is uncommon. Transmission is by direct droplet spray.

LABORATORY DIAGNOSIS
The organism does not survive long outside the body, and early inoculation of culture media is essential for its recovery from human material. It is a small Gram-negative rod. Films of specimens or young colonies show capsulated rods often arranged in small groups ('thumb-print' distribution). For culture, Bordet–Gengou blood-starch-glycerol agar is used, to which penicillin and diamido-diphenylamine hydrochloride are added to suppress the growth of contaminant organisms. Charcoal agar may also be used for the primary isolation. The charcoal absorbs oleic acid present in ordinary media, which suppresses the growth of *Bord. pertussis*.

Antigenic analysis and diagnosis
The antigens of this organism are very complex and four classes have to be considered.

(1) Capsular antigens may be demonstrated by agglutination reactions.

(2) A haemagglutinating antigen is also located in the capsule and appears in culture filtrates.

(3) Cell wall antigens include the somatic antigens, a protective antigen and a histamine-sensitizing factor. The somatic antigens are similar to those found in the enterobacteria in that they are heat-stable complexes which behave as endotoxins. The nature of the protective antigen is not known; it occurs mainly in virulent capsulate strains, stimulates production of protective antibodies and is involved in immunizing procedures against whooping cough. The histamine-sensitizing factor, when inoculated into mice, renders them hypersensitive to histamine; it may be identical with the protective antigen.

(4) Cytoplasmic antigen is a heat-labile endotoxin of protein nature. Inoculation into animals fails to stimulate the production of anti-endotoxin and its function is obscure.

Diagnosis of whooping cough depends primarily upon isolation of the causative organism. This may be attempted by two procedures.

(1) A plate of Bordet–Gengou medium with added antibiotics is held 10 cm in front of the patient's mouth during a paroxysm of coughing. After 3 days at 37°C the plate is examined for the typical 'pearly' colonies of small Gram-negative rods; agglutination by type 1 antiserum confirms the diagnosis.

(2) A prenasal or postnasal swab is inoculated on Bordet–Gengou medium. Incubation and examination is as for cough plates. Swabs are superior to cough plates

for the recovery of *Bord. pertussis*, provided inoculation on to culture media is done at once, i.e. at the bedside.

Both methods should be employed during the catarrhal stage and in the first few days of the paroxysmal stage, when the chance of isolating the organism is maximal. Examination of direct smears by the fluorescent antibody technique is useful in some cases.

Serological tests are of some value after the first week of the paroxysmal stage, but by this time the diagnosis has usually been made by other means. A slide agglutination test with the patient's serum and fresh living organisms is probably the best method.

Immunization

Immunization with formalin-killed *Bord. pertussis* has given excellent protection for many years. Three doses, each of 20,000 million organisms, are given at four week intervals within the first year of life. Immunization is normally combined with prophylaxis against diphtheria and tetanus in the DPT triple vaccine (p. 22.23).

Mild reactions to whooping cough vaccine are common, and redness and swelling at the site of inoculation occur in 75 per cent of cases. Severe reactions are very rare. Encephalopathy has been recorded in over 100 cases, of whom more than half have recovered completely; but there have been at least sixteen deaths. Immunization, should be avoided during any illness and within 3 weeks of a small-pox vaccination.

Brucella

Brucella organisms are the cause of **undulant fever** (brucellosis) in man. The disease usually results from drinking the unpasteurized milk of infected cows or goats. The three species, *Br. abortus*, *Br. melitensis* and *Br. suis*, cause infection in cows, sheep and goats, and pigs respectively.

Undulant fever caused by *Br. abortus* (abortus fever) is prevalent throughout the world and is indigenous in Britain. In cows the organism usually establishes itself in the udder and is excreted in the milk. Infection also involves the uterus, and the organism can be recovered from the uterine discharge and also from the urine and faeces. Epidemics of abortion may follow the initial infection of a herd, but thereafter sporadic abortions are uncommon. Transmission of infection from cattle to man is usually by drinking contaminated milk or cream, but persons at special risk (veterinarians and farmers) may acquire brucellosis from contact with infected uterine discharges or urine. The frequent occurrence of brucellae in the bovine placenta is due to the presence of erythritol which promotes their growth. Erythritol is absent from the human placenta.

Br. melitensis causes a similar infection in goats and is common in Mediterranean countries. In man it gives rise to a severe form of undulant fever called Malta fever, acquired from drinking raw goat's milk. Sheep may become infected from contact with goats, the infection being then transmitted from sheep to man via contaminated discharges. *Br. suis* causes infection in swine and is common in parts of the USA. Man acquires the disease by direct contact with infected raw pork.

UNDULANT FEVER

Following an incubation period of about 2 weeks the acute infection is ushered in with headache, general malaise and drenching sweats. In Malta fever the temperature is remittent and rises generally over several days to fall slowly to normal in 2–3 weeks. After a period of quiescence the fever appears again, and this cycle may recur over several months; hence the name undulant fever. The disease may become chronic with periodic exacerbations of sweating, joint pains and general ill-defined malaise. Abortus fever is similar to Malta fever in its clinical features, though usually less severe. Latent or subclinical infections are probably much more common than is realized.

Following their entry into the host, brucellae are conveyed by the lymphatics and blood stream to the reticuloendothelial system (lymph nodes, spleen, liver, marrow) where they multiply intracellularly to produce granulomatous lesions. Organisms are also found inside reticuloendothelial cells within other organs. Their characteristic intracellular habitat tends to protect brucellae from the effects of antimicrobial drugs and specific antibodies (p. 22.17).

Although several humoral antibodies are produced as a result of infection and these can be detected in relatively large amounts, spontaneous recovery is associated with the development of cellular immunity. This may be demonstrated by delayed-type hypersensitivity skin tests, e.g. brucellin test. Natural immunity to infection appears to be associated with the absence of a serum factor which suppresses R variants and allows S virulent strains to proliferate.

The laboratory diagnosis of brucellosis in man rests upon blood culture and serological tests. A special blood culture medium (Castaneda) may be used. In the acute stage of infection, agglutinating IgM- and IgG-globulins are detectable. In some cases a prozone phenomenon interferes with the reaction (p. 22.15).

In chronic brucellosis, agglutination tests may be negative, but IgG- and IgA-antibodies are present. To detect these nonagglutinating antibodies the antihuman globulin test (Coombs test) is used (vol. 1, p. 26.18). The presence of IgA-antibody is associated with the skin hypersensitivity that develops during chronic brucellosis.

Antibodies of IgG-type are readily demonstrated by a complement-fixation test (CFT). These antibodies may be of either the agglutinating or sensitizing type and the CFT identifies these globulins in both the acute and chronic stages of brucellosis. The CFT is, therefore, the most suitable test for the diagnosis of brucella infection.

There is some cross-antigenicity with *Salmonella* spp. which may cause difficulty in interpretation of laboratory agglutination tests.

CULTURAL CHARACTERISTICS

Brucellae are small, noncapsulate, nonmotile, Gram-negative coccobacilli. They are obligatory aerobes and are best grown on liver extract or serum agar. *Br. abortus* requires an atmosphere containing 10 per cent CO_2, but the other two species are not demanding in this respect. Growth is slow, often taking 48–72 hours to appear; colonies are 0·5–1·0 mm in diameter, translucent, colourless, smooth and soft. The organisms are readily killed by exposure to heat and pasteurization of milk destroys them effectively. However, viability is maintained for several months in dead bovine foetal material, and in dust unless exposed to direct sunlight.

Inoculation into guinea-pigs reproduces the natural disease from which the animal usually recovers.

The tests used in differentiating the species are (1) H_2S production, and (2) ability to grow in the presence of the dyes basic fuchsin and thionin. *Br. abortus* and *Br. suis* both produce H_2S for at least 3 days whereas *Br. melitensis* does not. *Br. abortus* grows on media containing basic fuchsin, *Br. suis* on media containing thionin, and *Br. melitensis* grows in the presence of either dye.

ANTIGENIC STRUCTURE

Brucellae possess two antigens, A and M, which are present in the different species in varying amounts. In *Br. abortus* and *Br. suis* the A antigen, and in *Br. melitensis* the M antigen, is dominant. Antisera to *Br. abortus* agglutinate this organism and *Br. suis* to a high titre and *Br. melitensis* to a much lower titre. Similarly, *Br. melitensis* antisera agglutinate the homologous organism to high titre, and the other two brucellae to low titre.

BRUCELLIN SKIN TEST

Intradermal inoculation of extracts of brucella organisms (brucellin, brucellergin) results in a Mantoux-type reaction in individuals with active, latent, chronic or subclinical infection. The value of this test is limited by its variability, and it has the disadvantage of stimulating antibody production in man and animals.

No satisfactory, safe method of immunizing man against brucellosis has been generally introduced. In the USSR a living vaccine has been employed during the past 15 years, but it may provoke serious hypersensitivity reactions.

A live attenuated vaccine of *Br. abortus* strain S19 is used for the immunization of calves in Britain. Two disadvantages of its use are, first, that the stimulation of agglutinins in the animal makes the diagnosis of suspected infection difficult, and second, that veterinarians may become infected.

The control of brucellosis is generally directed towards the elimination of the endemic reservoir in animals by the development of brucellosis-free herds, and to milk pasteurization.

Pasteurella

The *Pasteurella* group includes *P. pestis*, the cause of **bubonic plague**, and a few less well known pathogens of man.

P. pestis is a short Gram-negative coccobacillus with rounded ends; the poles stain more deeply with methylene blue than the central zone (bipolar staining). It is nonmotile and does not form spores, but capsules are present when the bacillus is seen in the tissues and on first isolation. The organism grows readily on ordinary media over a temperature range of 14–42°C. The optimum temperature is 27°C. Pleomorphic forms are often encountered in cultures.

Plague is primarily a disease of rodents, particularly of rats, and the organisms are conveyed from rat to man by fleas (p. 19.49). Thus an epidemic of human plague involves a complex ecological relation between a bacterium, an insect and two species of mammal. Plague bacilli are inoculated into man when an infected flea bites. Infection is first limited by the neighbouring lymph nodes, which form the primary bubo or focus of infection, hence bubonic plague. Buboes may suppurate and become necrotic; they then appear as blackened areas, from which the Black Death derived its name. Infection may spread rapidly into the blood stream, leading to septicaemia, toxaemia and death. The mechanism of pathogenicity is incompletely understood, but it is known that the plague bacillus contains antiphagocytic substances in its capsular material and also in a lipoprotein antigen; in addition, the organism contains endotoxin. Infection in bubonic plague does not usually spread directly from man to man. In an epidemic, fresh cases are infected by rat fleas. If septicaemia leads to pulmonary infection in a patient, others may acquire pneumonic plague by direct inhalation of infected droplets or particles contaminated with infected sputum.

Plague has been the most terrifying of all human diseases. The famous Black Death that broke out in the middle of the fourteenth century destroyed a quarter of the population of Europe, and it continued to be a dominating influence in the social and economic life of Europe until the end of the seventeenth century when it rapidly declined. In 1896, an outbreak of plague in India reached epidemic proportions and was responsible for over 8 million deaths within the following 15 years. In recent years there has been a steady decline in the incidence of plague, but there are large reservoirs of rodent infection in many parts of the world and outbreaks still occur.

The prevention of plague involves essentially control of the rat population which harbours the disease and this is often a difficult technical problem. Protective clothing and insecticide preparations are important items of equipment in antiplague campaigns. Prophylactic plague vaccines have been widely used, but their value has not been adequately established; prophylactic chemotherapy with sulphonamide drugs has been successful during an epidemic.

OTHER PASTEURELLA SPECIES

Other pasteurellae, usually associated with disease in animals, may cause disease in man. *P. pseudo-tuberculosis* is carried by wood pigeons and causes chronic infections in rats and guinea-pigs; the disease may be introduced into an animal house by feeding contaminated cabbage leaves to the animals. This organism occasionally gives rise to **mesenteric adenitis** in man and the clinical picture may be mistaken for appendicitis, or may present as a typhoid-like illness.

P. tularensis produces a plague-like disease in wild rodents and the infection is transmissible to man, when it is termed **tularaemia**. This is a continued fever that in some areas affects hunters and others who handle the skins or carcases of infected animals. *P. multocida* (*P. septica*) occurs as a commensal in the mouths of animals, and it causes many systemic diseases in animals; the organism may cause local sepsis associated with animal bites in man.

SPIRILLACEAE

This family contains two important species pathogenic to man: *Spirillum minus* and *Vibrio spp.*

Spirillum

SPIRILLUM MINUS

This causes **rat-bite fever**. It is spirally shaped, 2–5 μm in length, and bears a close resemblance to a spirochaete. It differs from the latter in possessing flagella at either pole and in having a rigid body. It can be seen by dark-ground microscopy and also stains with the Gram or Leishman method, being Gram-negative.

Rat-bite fever may follow the bite of a rat, cat, mouse or ferret. The wound heals at first, but characteristically breaks down 3–4 weeks later, with local lymphadenopathy, fever and a rash. The fever is remittent and lasts for 5–7 days. Relapses are frequent and may continue for years. Often the presenting clinical features resemble influenza and early antibiotic therapy may mask the true diagnosis. Diagnosis is by microscopical examination of tissue or serum from the wound, lymph node juice or the blood. After intraperitoneal inoculation of these materials into mice or guinea-pigs, spirilla can be seen in the blood 14 days later. Guinea-pigs often suffer a severe infection, with alopecia and eye lesions, but mice are unharmed. A similar syndrome may follow a rat bite when the causative organism is *Streptobacillus moniliformis* (Haverhill fever).

Vibrio

The two species important in human disease are *V. cholerae* and *V. eltor*. The latter is named after the Egyptian quarantine station at El Tor where it was discovered in 1905. Both vibrios produce **cholera**, but whilst *V. cholerae* is becoming less frequent, *V. eltor* has spread widely during recent years. *V. cholerae* may be taken as the type species and *V. eltor* is discussed only where it differs from *V. cholerae*.

Cholera is characterized by a profuse diarrhoea (rice-water stools) causing marked dehydration and loss of electrolytes. In the absence of appropriate treatment, there is a high mortality. Cholera has been endemic in Bengal and S.E. Asia for over a thousand years, but not until the nineteenth century did it spread to Africa, Europe and America, causing big epidemics with high mortality rates in all these continents. Today it remains an important disease in Bengal, but the introduction of safe water supplies has eliminated it from most other countries.

The main method of spread is by contamination of the water supply and the vibrios can grow well at temperatures of 25–30°C, as commonly found in the water tanks in Bengal. Man is the only host. The disease is usually spread by patients infecting the water supply. Chronic carriers of the classical *V. cholerae* have never been found; the carrier state appears to be much more common in the case of *V. eltor*.

In an epidemic the great majority of cases can be recognized easily and a bacteriological diagnosis is often not required for clinical purposes. However, accurate identification of vibrios is essential in epidemiological studies and for the control of the disease.

VIBRIO CHOLERAE

This organism, also called the comma bacillus because of its curved appearance, is Gram-negative, motile by means of a single polar flagellum, and noncapsulate, measuring 1–5 × 0·3 μm. Occasionally S-shaped and C-shaped forms occur due to pairing of the bacilli or to rapid growth prior to division. Older cultures show marked involution forms with club-like appearances.

V. cholerae is a facultative anaerobe and grows well on simple media. Characteristically it withstands a strongly alkaline environment (pH 8–9·2). For selective culture, Monsur's medium (bile–gelatin–tellurite agar), or alkaline agar (pH 8·2), and alkaline peptone water (pH 9·0) are used. Colonies on agar are translucent, smooth, glistening and soft, and appear bluish with transmitted light. Although S→R variation occurs, R colonies do not appear rough. The organism survives drying for only 3–4 hours, but may remain viable for up to 10 days in stagnant alkaline water.

V. cholerae does not ferment lactose, but forms both indole and nitrites in peptone water media; this may be shown by the addition to a 24-hour-culture of H_2SO_4 which colours the culture red (cholera-red reaction). The oxidase reaction is positive. *V. eltor* produces a haemolysin for sheep cells which is of value in differentiating it from *V. cholerae* (Greig test).

Classification of *V. cholerae* and the cholera-like vibrios is made on the basis of their antigenic structure (fig. 18.37).

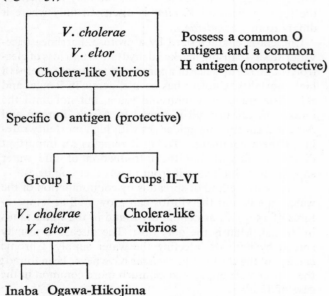

FIG. 18.37. Antigenic classification of cholera and cholera-like vibrios.

Group I, which includes *V. cholerae* and *V. eltor* has a specific O antigen in common. Vibrios not agglutinable with O group I antiserum are placed in Groups II–VI and are the cholera-like vibrios, also known as non-agglutinable (NAG) vibrios. These may produce diarrhoea with rice-water stools, but are not usually associated with severe illness. Group I vibrios can be further differentiated into Inaba and Ogawa–Hikojima subtypes. With all vibrios the transformation S→R results in the loss of specific O antigens.

Mukerjee has differentiated five *V. cholerae* bacteriophage types according to the patterns of lysis obtained with four specific phage lysates (I–IV). Types 1 and 3 were the commonest endemic strains.

It has not been possible to reproduce true cholera in animals but the baby rabbit has proved an experimental model. Intraperitoneal inoculation of *V. cholerae* into guinea-pigs is rapidly lethal, and a suspected strain that produces no disease in these animals is not *V. cholerae*.

Pathogenesis of cholera

V. cholerae (and *V. eltor*) multiply in the lumen of the small intestine and are excreted in enormous numbers in the faeces. Penetration of the intestinal mucosa occurs only as far as the basement membrane, and bacteriaemia probably never results.

Vibrios rapidly undergo autolysis within the gut lumen. How the endotoxin, or possibly some other toxic bacterial metabolite, produces the irritation of the intestine is not known, but it has been postulated that the sodium pump of the intestinal mucosal cells becomes impaired, leading to an excessive loss of water and electrolytes into the gut lumen. This in turn results in the severe depletion of water and electrolytes that occurs in an established case with consequent renal failure and death. The penetration of a toxic metabolite into the intestinal mucosa may be facilitated by a mucinase produced by cholera vibrios, which dissolves the surface mucus and so exposes the surface epithelium. An enterotoxic factor which may be involved is known as choleragen and is produced by *V. cholerae* in culture; this is possibly the same as a factor that has marked vasodilatory properties (skin toxin).

V. cholerae produces another mucinase (neuraminidase) which hydrolyses *N*-acetylneuraminic acid in mucoproteins present in human plasma and in mucus; the particular mucoproteins are major constituents of red blood cell and respiratory tract cell surface receptors for myxoviruses. Because of the ability of neuraminidase to disrupt cell receptors it has also been called receptor-destroying enzyme (RDE).

Prophylaxis

Cholera will be eradicated only when it is possible to separate faeces effectively from drinking water in the endemic areas.

A killed vaccine is available for the immunization of all persons travelling to an endemic area, and for use in large-scale immunization programmes to assist in terminating an epidemic. The protection afforded by the vaccine is of short duration and lasts for less than a year.

VIBRIO ELTOR

The main features that distinguish El Tor species from *V. cholerae* are summarized in table 18.3.

TABLE 18.3. Differential tests for *V. eltor*.

Test	*V. cholerae*	*V. eltor*
Voges–Proskauer*	−	+
Oxidase production	+	−
Haemolysin production	−	+
Agglutination of chicken red cells	−	+
Sensitivity to *V. cholerae* phage IV	+	−
Sensitivity to polymyxin	+	−

* acetylmethylcarbinol formation

PSEUDOMONADACEAE

Pseudomonas

These are common saprophytes in water and soil. They characteristically produce a variety of pigments. A few species are pathogenic for plants and some cause disease in animals. The only one that is pathogenic to man is *Pseudomonas pyocyanea* (*Ps. aeruginosa*). Formerly it received little attention, but was known to be associated with 'blue pus' and many strains were shown to produce blue, green, red and brown pigments, when grown on agar (plate 18.2l, facing p. 18.68). The organism's potential as a pathogen is related to its ability to to resist many antimicrobial agents, notably antibiotics, and to flourish at relatively low temperatures.

Ps. pyocyanea is a nonsporing, motile Gram-negative bacillus with polar flagella. It grows readily on simple media over a wide temperature range. The organism is found in the intestine and on the skin of healthy man. It may cause secondary infection in association with pyogenic cocci and it is sometimes a primary pathogen, especially if the host is debilitated or if the balance is tipped in the organism's favour by circumstances that lead to an overwhelming bacterial challenge or entry into susceptible tissues. *Ps. pyocyanea* is now an important cause of infection acquired in hospital. This has followed the introduction of antibiotics, to many of which the organism is resistant. Moreover, it is also resistant to some of the common hospital disinfectants. Pseudomonas organisms are readily isolated from drains, sinks, slunge areas and pails, and the organism not uncommonly contaminates apparatus such as respirator equipment, masks and flexible tubing. It is a frequent threat to patients with **genito-urinary disease** and **severe burns**. Infection may be localized to a wound or burn or to the urinary tract, but in patients already debilitated by a long illness as a result of multiple injuries or cytotoxic therapy, fatal **septicaemia** may develop. The challenge presented by *Ps. pyocyanea* is related to its resistance and persistence; these properties make it a formidable pathogen when it is established in a patient. Bacteriological monitoring is useful in detecting its presence, but it is so common that quantitative assessment is required, unless the source is normally sterile. Quantitation of a highly motile organism that spreads over culture media is technically difficult. Tracer techniques that exploit the bacteriocine-production (p. 18.90) of *Ps. pyocyanea*, a procedure known as **pyocine typing**, help in defining the links in a chain of infection in hospital.

THE ENTEROBACTERIA

This large family of nonsporing Gram-negative bacteria includes groups of organisms commonly found as commensals in the gut of man and animals and some that are free-living saprophytes. The disease-producing enterobacteria include well known intestinal pathogens such as the genus *Salmonella* which contains the causative organisms of the **enteric fevers** (typhoid and paratyphoid) and of a common form of **bacterial food poisoning**; the genus *Shigella* is responsible for **bacillary dysentery**. Two other large genera, *Escherichia* and *Proteus*, contain species that are saprophytic and inhabit the large intestine of man and animals where they are not normally pathogenic. However, they may be responsible for **urinary tract infections** and **wound infections** and occasionally **septicaemia**, especially in debilitated or very young patients. Some strains of *Esch. coli*, a very common commensal of the gut, produce severe **gastro-enteritis** in young children.

The classification of this extensive family is confused and confusing. The various members cannot be defined sharply, but accurate diagnosis of conditions caused by the pathogenic members is essential before proper treatment can be instituted and, for practical purposes, the recognized genera are based on characters of representative strains that are homogeneous biochemically and related serologically.

All the enterobacteria are Gram-negative rods (plate 18.2i, facing p. 18.68) which grow well on ordinary media. They ferment a variety of carbohydrates with the production of acid and usually gas, and these reactions help in identifying species. Among the intestinal pathogens, the non-fermentation of lactose is a typical feature and, as the commensal *Esch. coli* ferments lactose, this is a useful marker (plate 18.2j, facing p. 18.68). However, it is sometimes assumed wrongly that lactose-fermentation is synonymous with nonpathogenicity and this is not the case. For example, enteropathogenic strains of *Esch. coli* and those involved in urinary tract infections are lactose-fermenting; this property is a characteristic of the genus. However, the pathogenic *Salmonella* and the *Shigella* are non-lactose fermenters, and the isolation of these organisms from the gut calls for attention. The non-lactose-fermenting *Proteus* group and others, not usually associated with pathogenicity in the intestine, have to be differentiated from suspected pathogens. As the various enterobacteria look alike and are frequently pleomorphic, they cannot be distinguished by their microscopic appearances and their colonial morphology on ordinary media is usually of little help.

Escherichia

Many strains of *Esch. coli* exist and they are generally thought to be the predominant organisms in the healthy large intestine, though they are heavily outnumbered by *Bacteroides* species that do not grow aerobically. They are usually motile and many strains produce fimbriae. The ability to ferment lactose usually distinguishes them from the *Salmonella* and *Shigella* species. *Esch. coli* possesses both O (somatic) and H (flagellar) antigens and, in addition, most strains produce a group of K antigens associated with superficial capsules or envelopes and designated L, A or B; these may block the normal reactivity of the somatic O antigen in test systems and allow the organisms to be subdivided serologically into a large number of types. Several of these may be present at any one time in the flora of a healthy person and the types present may vary from time to time. The K antigens seem to be associated with potential pathogenicity *in vivo*.

Esch. coli is a common cause of **infection in the urinary tract**, especially when there is an associated structural defect leading to incomplete elimination of urine. Infection is usually acquired endogenously and the shortness of the female urethra renders it vulnerable to ascending infection, for example in the development of the common 'honeymoon cystitis' (vol. 1, p. 47.4). Infection may be introduced also by catheterization and this procedure carries a risk that merits consideration before it is employed. The common association of *Strept. faecalis* with *Esch. coli* in infections of the urinary tract indicates the source of the organisms. Some strains of *Esch. coli* are associated with severe **gastroenteritis** which affects predominantly children below the age of 2 years. Bottle-fed children are particularly at risk and when the infection arises in a hospital the outbreak may spread rapidly. It is possible that enteropathogenic strains of *Esch. coli* cause more trouble in older age groups than is generally realized; they can certainly cause diarrhoea in adults.

Esch. coli may be involved in infections such as **appendicitis, cholecystitis, wound infections** and bedsores. In the neonatal period an overwhelming challenge may lead to **septicaemia** or **meningitis** and *Esch. coli* septicaemia is seen also in debilitated patients, sometimes as a terminal event. The presence of *Esch. coli* and related organisms in the blood stream may precipitate bacteriogenic shock (p. 18.30).

As *Esch. coli* is a bowel commensal, its presence in water is regarded as an index of faecal contamination and quantitative and qualitative tests are performed as a routine check on water supplies. Since the organism can contaminate a urine sample without necessarily being the cause of infection, the quantitation of *Esch. coli* and other urinary tract pathogens is of diagnostic value in determining whether an apparent bacteriuria indicates infection or is simple contamination. **Significant bacteriuria** is present when a properly taken midstream sample (p. 18.92) is promptly examined and found to contain more than 10^5 organisms/ml.

Klebsiella and related organisms

There are many enterobacteria with which a medical bacteriologist must be familiar in order to distinguish them from known pathogens. A large group share with the *Escherichia* the common features of being frequently saprophytic, sometimes commensal and occasionally pathogenic to man. The group is known as the **coliform bacteria** and sometimes loosely referred to as 'the coliforms', though this term could be applied also to any aerobic Gram-negative rod-shaped bacterium; a more restrictive term is 'the coli–aerogenes group'. The latter term embraces the genus *Klebsiella*. *K. aerogenes* (formerly *Aerobacter aerogenes*) is typically nonmotile and capsulate. It is a saprophyte found in water and occurs commensally in the human intestine. Like *Esch. coli*, it may be responsible for **urinary tract infections** and occasionally infects **wounds**. In culture, its colonies are particularly mucoid (plate 18.2j, facing p. 18.68). *K. pneumoniae*, formerly known as the Friedlander bacillus, is a commensal in the upper respiratory tract and is responsible for a very small proportion of cases of **acute bacterial pneumonia**; the disease is dangerous when this organism is involved, because it does not respond to penicillin (p. 20.26). *K. pneumoniae* is also well recognized as a secondary invader in cases of chronic disease of the respiratory system and it may prove difficult to eradicate.

Other medically important members of the *Enterobacteriaceae* are described below, but less important groups that may be of medical significance such as the *Alkalescens-Dispar*, *Citrobacter*, *Enterobacter*, *Hafnia*, *Providencia* and *Arizona* groups are not included in this outline.

Proteus

This genus is commonly represented in the faecal flora of animals and man and in the soil. In Greek legend, Proteus changed his shape and form to elude those who pressed him to predict future events; the genus merits the name on account of the characteristic pleomorphism of the bacteria, though it is not unique in this respect. These organisms produce typical 'swarming growth' on agar media (plate 18.2k, facing p. 18.68) and are therefore a nuisance when attempts are made to separate discrete colonies of different bacteria from a mixed culture. Four types are differentiated on the basis of biochemical reactions and they form the species *Pr. vulgaris*, *Pr. mirabilis*, *Pr. morganii* and *Pr. rettgeri*. All of them produce urease.

Certain strains of *Pr. vulgaris* possess O antigens which by chance share a relationship with antigens present in rickettsial species that cause typhus fever. In consequence, the serum of a patient with typhus fever contains agglutinins for some of these *Proteus* strains, depending upon the form of typhus fever involved. This is the basis of the Weil–Felix reaction, employed in the diagnosis of typhus, but there is no evidence that *Proteus* has any causal relationship to the disease (p. 18.86).

Infections with *Proteus* species in man are usually caused by *Pr. mirabilis* which is not normally a virulent organism, unless the patient is debilitated. However, it can cause **acute infection in the urinary tract** and it is not uncommonly involved, often as a secondary invader, in **wound infections.** *Proteus* infections are often resistant to antimicrobial therapy.

Shigella

In 1897 the Japanese bacteriologist, Kiyoshi Shiga, discovered the dysentery bacilli. It then became possible to subdivide the 'bloody fluxes' into amoebic dysentery and **bacillary dysentery** and this is of great importance in the therapeutic approach to these conditions. The dysentery bacilli, now constituting the genus *Shigella*, are subclassified largely on the basis of their carbohydrate fermentation reactions and the main species are *Shigella dysenteriae* (formerly *Sh. shigae*), *Sh. flexneri*, *Sh. sonnei* and *Sh. boydii*. Epidemics with many severe cases have nearly always been due to *Sh. dysenteriae* which, in addition to its inherent endotoxin, produces a soluble neurotoxin called Shiga toxin. The prevalent species in Britain at present is *Sh. sonnei* and this tends to produce relatively mild forms of the disease, though patients can be seriously at risk with *Sh. sonnei* dysentery and the condition is not trivial. *Sh. flexneri* infections are often of intermediate severity.

The *Shigella* genus is typically nonmotile. *In vivo*, the organisms are not truly invasive and they remain localized in the gut. Humoral immune mechanisms do not appear to be involved significantly in the host response and the detection of antibodies in the patient's serum plays no part in the laboratory diagnosis of the disease, which rests upon the isolation and identification of the causative organism from the faeces.

The dysentery bacilli are parasites of man; with insignificant exceptions, natural infection does not occur in animals and it has so far proved impossible to infect laboratory animals. Infection arises from the faeces of human cases or carriers and the disease appears to spread from person to person by passage of dysentery bacilli from human faeces to human mouth. The organisms are abundant in the faeces of a patient suffering from dysentery; they are less abundant in the faeces of a carrier, who may be convalescent from a clinically recognized infection or who may have had no obvious disease. It is significant that bacillary dysentery has a high incidence among young children in day nurseries and among mentally handicapped patients in institutions. In both cases, difficulty in coping with a diarrhoeal disease increases the environmental contamination.

There are two important vehicles of infection in bacillary dysentery. The first is the human hand. Despite the generally high level of domestic sanitation in Britain, cases of dysentery have been reported in steadily increasing numbers in the last 30 years. Fortunately, most are due to *Sh. sonnei*, and the illnesses are relatively mild. They occur most commonly in school children, but all ages may be infected, including the very young and the very old, in whom the consequences are sometimes more serious. Sanitary arrangements in many schools and institutions still leave much to be desired. The soiled hands of a mild case or carrier may transmit infection directly to the hands of another person or more probably indirectly as a result of the contamination of toilet fixtures, communal towels and door handles. Improved personal hygiene and better facilities for washing hands would reduce the incidence of dysentery in Britain.

The second vehicle of spread is the house fly. In tropical and semitropical countries, where methods for disposal of faeces are primitive, flies move easily from infected faeces, carrying the *Shigella* on their legs, to vegetable and meat markets, pastry shops, cookhouses, and restaurants and dining rooms.

Absence of a modern sanitary system and the prevalence of house flies leads almost inevitably to outbreaks of dysentery. House flies were almost certainly responsible for outbreaks of dysentery common in Britain many years ago, but they are unlikely to be an important vector now. Although a dangerously high dose of dysentery bacilli would be transmitted as a result of their multiplication in food, this does not appear to be a common occurrence. However, the organisms can be passively transferred from the hands of a carrier to a new victim by contamination of plates or utensils or by food that has been contaminated.

Epidemiological study of the spread of *Sh. sonnei* has been handicapped by the fact that the organism is serologically homogeneous. By means of **colicine typing,** seventeen types of *Sh. sonnei* have been identified, and this will facilitate the study of future epidemics (p. 18.90).

Salmonella

The salmonellae are parasites of man and animals. These Gram-negative rods are nonsporing and noncapsulate; they are frequently motile and they may be fimbriate. The general cultural and morphological characteristics of *Salmonella* are typical of those already described for the enterobacteria, but the organisms of this group have distinctive biochemical and serological characteristics. They do not survive desiccation unless protected by incorporation in protein, e.g. dried egg, but they can survive for weeks in water. There are two main types of human infection. First, the **enteric fevers,** typhoid and paratyphoid, are caused by *Salmonella typhi* and *S. paratyphi A*, *B* and *C*. Human cases and carriers are recognized sources of infection for these diseases; *S. typhi* is associated with infection in man only and the disease is usually spread by contamination of water supplies or foodstuffs. Secondly, *S. typhimurium* and a vast number of allied species are responsible for **salmonella food poisoning**. These organisms are parasites of a large number of animal species including cattle, rats and mice. There is thus a large reservoir of infection and food may be contaminated in many places such as slaughter-houses, markets, food-processing factories, shops, catering premises, kitchens and warehouses.

There are distinctions between the clinical features of the disease resulting from the two types of infection. Typhoid and paratyphoid fever usually present as a continued fever with toxaemia which is consequent upon bacteriaemia. Although enteritis may be severe and sometimes causes death from haemorrhage or perforation, it is not a constant feature and a case of typhoid with severe septicaemia may show little evidence of enteritis. In the case of salmonella food poisoning, on the other hand, infection is usually limited to the gut; bacteriaemia is often absent and involvement of other organs and tissues is unusual. It is also characteristic of all forms of salmonella infection that there is a great variation in virulence. In the same outbreak, one man may suffer an overwhelming infection, another may have a disease of moderate severity and a third may be a carrier of the organism for some weeks with only trivial symptoms. In general, the organisms responsible for salmonella food poisoning are less invasive in man and cause less severe human illness than does *S. typhi*. The reverse is true for animals; *S. typhi* does not produce a natural infection in animals whereas *S. typhimurium* is regularly lethal for mice.

ENTERIC FEVER
In the acute stage of typhoid fever, within the first 10 days of infection, the organisms may be isolated from the blood and from the faeces. After ingestion, the typhoid bacilli tend to settle in the lymphoid tissue of the small intestine and following multiplication in the mesenteric nodes they enter the blood stream. This bacteriaemic phase disseminates the organisms widely to organs such as the kidneys, bone-marrow, spleen, liver and gall-bladder; from the latter, there is a renewed invasion of the small intestine and the organisms multiply in the Peyer's patches and other areas of lymphoid tissue. Typhoid bacilli then begin to disappear from the blood stream, but they are present in the faeces at this stage and they may also appear in the urine. In about 2–5 per cent of cases, the infection tends to linger in the gall-bladder and a chronic carrier state results.

Laboratory diagnosis
As enteric fever may present in various atypical ways, it follows that blood culture is essential in diagnosis and is often employed in the investigation of an obscure pyrexia of uncertain origin. A useful procedure when facilities for blood culture are limited is to culture clotted blood in a tube; the serum can be used for serological studies. Later in the infection it is important to culture the urine and to continue to culture the faeces in order to ensure that the patient does not leave hospital before he has ceased to excrete pathogenic organisms.

Specific agglutinins are developed during the course of enteric fever and the agglutination test employed to detect these is the **Widal test** (p. 22.15). A sample of the patient's serum is obtained by separation from a blood specimen and a laboratory suspension of typhoid bacilli is added to serial dilutions of the serum. Similar tests are done in parallel with suspensions of paratyphoid bacilli of types A and B; type-C infections are not usually encountered in Britain. The procedure is actually more complicated than is indicated above, because in each case a bacillary suspension is prepared so that it indicates the somatic (O) or flagellar (H) component of the response; a formalin-treated suspension retains H-specificity and a boiled suspension retains O-specificity. Thus, the patient's antibodies to *S. typhi* (O and H) and *S. paratyphi* A (O and H) and B (O and H) are determined. If a specimen of blood is examined early in the disease and another tested during the second week, a rising titre of antibodies for the specific organism may be detected. A knowledge of the O and H components of the antibody response is useful because the serum of a normal person often reacts weakly with the antigens and the situation is even more complex if the person has been previously immunized with TAB vaccine (see below). In general, O agglutinin responses are more likely to be associated with a recent experience of the organism. In addition to the O and H antigens, the typhoid bacillus produces a Vi antigen which is associated with the virulence of the organism for mice. The presence of antibodies to this component is thought to imply that the organism is still harboured by the patient and the Vi agglutination test is used in the detection of the carrier state.

Prevention
Enteric fever arises when a water supply or food becomes contaminated with infective excreta. In countries in which sewage and drinking water have been successfully kept apart, enteric fever has become a rare disease. There are still many parts of the world in which the separation is far from reliable and enteric fever remains common in these areas. Immunization with a killed suspension of the typhoid and paratyphoid A and B organisms (TAB vaccine) affords some protection and this is often given to travellers before they visit countries in which enteric fever is endemic.

SALMONELLA FOOD POISONING
The three common causes of bacterial food poisoning are *Salmonella*, *Clostridium welchii* and *Staphylococcus*

aureus; of these, salmonella species are by far the most important single cause and the salmonella problem is worrying. Direct case-to-case infection with salmonella organisms is known to occur, but there is much evidence that food or drink is the common vehicle of salmonella gastroenteritis and the majority of cases follow consumption of materials associated with infection of an animal or man. Salmonellae have been isolated from species as varied as man, cattle, pigs, ducks, hens and chickens, turkeys, cats, dogs, rats, mice, lizards, turtles, canaries, cockroaches and a Persian crow. This list is far from complete and, as each new serotype has been given species rank, the catalogue of the different species of salmonellae is enormous.

The modern tendency to bulk or pool supplies of egg, raw milk and processed meat in commerce is conducive to dissemination of salmonellae throughout the population. Subsequent manipulation of these products frequently allows multiplication of their bacterial content at some stage of the process. Although the dose of salmonellae required to produce food-poisoning seems to be high, conditions may permit a small initial contamination to be boosted until a significantly high bacterial challenge builds up in the food. The food involved is frequently not subjected to high temperatures before it is consumed. Raw meat is not uncommonly contaminated with salmonellae. This food is, of course, heated before consumption, but it may introduce salmonellae into the kitchen to contaminate processed foods and allow the salmonellae to multiply there.

The species most commonly involved in salmonella food poisoning is *S. typhimurium*, the cause of mouse typhoid. Rodent-proofing of food stores and catering premises is clearly advisable, but the organism can produce disease in other animals. Other species of *Salmonella* that commonly cause trouble in Britain are *S. enteritidis*, *S. thompson*, *S. newport*, *S. heidelberg* and *S. dublin*. Cattle and pigs constitute important reservoirs of infection and there are many opportunities for exacerbation of a latent infection or for cross-infection during transit to market and while awaiting slaughter in crowded abattoirs. Strains of salmonellae in animals receiving antibiotics in clinical use may develop multiple resistance to antibiotics, due to the action of transfer factors (pp. 18.57 & 20.7).

Until recently, imported raw egg products were a common source of salmonellae and the legal requirement for pasteurization of these products is well justified. The continuing problem of salmonellosis in cattle provides a further strong argument for the pasteurization of all milk destined for human consumption.

The bacteriological diagnosis of salmonella food-poisoning rests upon the isolation of the causative organism from the faeces of cases and from a sample of the suspected food or drink. The steps involved are technically complex, but the procedures are now highly developed and the bacteriological evidence is frequently obtained if the epidemiological clues are followed adequately and promptly. Much depends upon close co-operation between the general practitioner, the Public Health authorities and the bacteriologist. When a case or a carrier of salmonella infection is found, it is most important that he or she should be excluded from any aspect of food preparation, food distribution or catering until the organism is eliminated.

THE GRAM-NEGATIVE NONSPORING ANAEROBES

The Bacteroides-Fusiformis group

This group includes many Gram-negative nonsporing bacteria that are anaerobic and typically parasitic in animals or man. They have been variously classified as *Bacteroides*, *Fusobacterium*, *Fusiformis*, *Dialister* and *Sphaerophorus* and they are common commensals in the mouth, intestine and genital tract of healthy people. They are particularly numerous in the intestine where they outnumber the *Esch. coli*. They may be involved in pyogenic infections, often in association with other bacteria such as anaerobic cocci, and they are not infrequently associated with localized inflammatory conditions in the pelvic or abdominal areas. Sometimes they are carried in the blood to produce a brain abscess and they may be associated with bacteriaemia or septicaemia in debilitated patients and cause bacteriogenic shock. Many strains are extremely oxygen-sensitive and their isolation requires more than ordinary care and experience; in consequence, the role of this group of bacteria in disease is probably underestimated.

The association of fusiform bacteria with Vincent's infections in the oropharynx is discussed on p. 18.84.

THE SPIROCHAETES

Spirochaetes are slender flexuous organisms. Their structure differs from that of bacteria in that each cell is spiralled around one to twelve axial filaments which run longitudinally from end to end. These filaments hold the organisms in their characteristic shape and are probably responsible for their movements. There are many different spirochaetes and most of them are free-living, but three genera include pathogens of man.

Borrelia

These are flattened organisms, 10–20 × 0·3–0·5 μm in size, with three to eight loose coils (p. 18.6). They are strict anaerobes and are difficult to grow in culture, but stain readily with Romanowsky stains and can then be seen with the light microscope.

Borrelia recurrentis is the cause of **relapsing fever** which is transmitted from patient to patient by lice. This used to be responsible for many deaths in Europe and it was common in Ireland in the eighteenth and nineteenth centuries. Known as famine fever, it was associated with poverty and squalor which produce favourable conditions for lice (p. 19.43). Relapsing fevers caused by *Borrelia* continue to occur in many parts of the world. The disease is still important in parts of North Africa and India where the louse is the vector. In West Africa, transmission is by ticks and the organism responsible is *Borr. duttonii* (plate 18.1j, facing p. 18.62). Louse-borne and tick-borne forms of the disease are encountered also in the USA and in Central and South America.

The spirochaetes are readily seen in the blood during the febrile stage of the illness. Characteristically, there are two or three and sometimes four or five bouts of fever at intervals of a week or more.

During intermission of fever, the organism is suppressed by the host's antibody response and reticulo-endothelial activity, but, as Cunningham showed in India in 1934, antigenic variants of the organism then arise and are able to present a slightly different challenge to the infected host. There is therefore a human reservoir of infection and in addition there may be a reservoir in rodents and other small mammals acting as carriers, but lice and ticks are probably the definitive hosts.

Borr. vincentii is a spirochaete which occurs in small numbers in the healthy human mouth, often in association with a fusiform bacterium which is a member of the *Bacteroides–Fusiformis* group (p. 18.83). These organisms may be present in greatly increased numbers when oral hygiene is poor or when periodontal conditions lower local resistance. A gingivitis is then common and the two species can be seen in large numbers in stained smears of the exudate (plate 18.1i, facing p. 18.62). The organisms also cause inflammation of the fauces and severe painful throat infection (Vincent's angina).

Treponema

Treponema pallidum is the cause of **syphilis**. This spirochaete is a fine slender structure with six to twelve regular coils which are so delicate as to be invisible with the light microscope unless dark-ground illumination is employed. The organisms can be seen in the tissues after their size has been increased by silver impregnation. *T. pallidum* cannot be cultured on a laboratory medium, and it does not cause a true infection in any animal except man. Strains can be maintained artificially in the laboratory by inoculating them into the testes of rabbits.

T. pallidum dies rapidly outside the human body and syphilis is almost always contracted by sexual intercourse. The primary lesion (the chancre) typically appears on the external genitalia (p. 21.19); occasionally it may be found on the lips of a patient who has kissed an infected person.

The spirochaetes from the primary lesion can be seen in exudates examined by dark-ground microscopy; their typical motility and delicate morphology distinguish them from commensal spirochaetes.

Clinically the condition occurs in three stages. The primary lesion or chancre is usually accompanied by enlargement of lymph nodes draining the sites. It heals in 4–6 weeks and in the secondary stage the spirochaetes are disseminated all over the body. There is fever and there may be skin eruptions with lesions on mucous membranes and in lymph nodes. In the third stage, the lesions may occur in any part of the body, including blood vessels and nervous tissues. The spirochaetes can readily cross the placenta and cause congenital infection of the foetus.

The natural history of syphilis varies greatly and almost certainly depends on the strain and on the population involved. It is possible that the disease was brought from the New World to the Old World by Spanish sailors arriving from Haiti. It caused havoc in the French and Italian armies fighting around Naples in 1493, and it was then a severe febrile illness with marked pustular eruptions. In 1494 it was referred to in Paris as the greater pox (la grosse verole) in contrast to smallpox (la petite verole). There can be no more striking example of a disease that has changed its character with the passing of time. In many countries it is now a chronic disease in which the secondary stage may be mild and the patient in apparently good health for a decade or two before the third stage becomes manifest.

T. pallidum is very susceptible to antibiotics. In Western countries most persons seek advice after contracting a primary infection and so usually receive some treatment; hence the secondary stages of syphilis are seldom seen, although they may be common in other parts of the world. However, tertiary syphilis may develop in cases in whom treatment has been adequate to suppress the secondary manifestations but inadequate to effect a complete cure.

As the organism cannot be cultured, laboratory diagnosis depends upon:

(1) microscopic identification of the spirochaete, usually practicable only in the primary lesion, and

(2) serological tests which include flocculation (precipitin) tests such as the Kahn test and a well known complement-fixation test, the Wassermann reaction. Another procedure, the treponemal immobilization (TPI) test, is more specific and depends upon the immobilizing effect of specific antibody on laboratory preparations of motile treponemata which are maintained intratesticularly in rabbits. Other serological tests include an indirect fluorescent antibody (FTA) procedure which detects treponemal antibodies in serum (p. 22.16).

PINTA, BEJEL AND YAWS

In many remote rural areas of the world, it is still

possible to see syphilis in its florid forms and there are also diseases caused by spirochaetes indistinguishable from *T. pallidum* which are not true syphilis. Pinta is a disease which is not uncommon in the Caribbean and Central America; it resembles syphilis in having a primary, secondary and tertiary stage. The spirochaetes found in the primary lesion are morphologically identical with *T. pallidum*, but the primary lesion is extragenital and is not venereal. This condition is spread by direct contact and also by flies.

Bejel is a condition closely resembling secondary syphilis found in Bedouin Arabs, and it occurs in young children. Similar diseases, sometimes referred to as endemic syphilis, have been reported in South East Europe, in India, West Africa and Rhodesia.

Yaws was formerly a common disease in many parts of the tropics, in Africa, Asia and the Caribbean. Multiple granulomata appear on the skin and exude a serous fluid which contains spirochaetes. The causative organism is *T. pertenue*, and this is also morphologically indistinguishable from *T. pallidum*, but it is possible to infect monkeys by inoculation of the infective material. Yaws is clinically difficult to distinguish from severe secondary syphilis. *T. pertenue* is particularly sensitive to penicillin and a single injection cures a child of a revolting skin disease; subsequent relapse is unusual. The disease primarily affects primitive people living in remote villages and it has been eradicated completely in many areas by World Health Organization teams, who have sought out and systematically treated all cases. The success of the United Nations in eradicating yaws from many areas has received too little publicity.

Leptospira

This large group of spirochaetes includes many saprophytic organisms, but others are parasites of many species of animals, especially rodents and other small mammals; as their distribution differs geographically, the diseases they cause are given different local names. It is debatable whether the leptospirae should be regarded as separate species or as related serotypes. Two species represent the pathogenic range of the genus for man, but there are many immunologically distinct strains. *Leptospira icterohaemorrhagiae* is the cause of infective jaundice or **Weil's disease**, which is frequently severe, and *L. canicola* causes **canicola fever** which is often associated with a clinically mild or even unrecognized infection.

Weil's disease is liable to occur wherever man comes into contact with the urine of rats. Isolated cases and small outbreaks may arise in miners, fishgutters, sewage workers and others who work in damp, rat-infested places, such as Australian sugar cane fields. The disease may be contracted also by bathing in canals, rivers or ponds in areas populated by rats.

L. icterohaemorrhagiae has numerous coils (p. 18.6)

close-set and so small that they are obscured in stained preparations. They are well seen by dark ground illumination and the organism has characteristically recurved ends which give it a double-hooked appearance.

L. canicola is morphologically identical. This organism is a parasite of dogs and pigs and it spreads to man from contact with dog or pig urine. Thus, piggery workers and farmers, and abattoir workers have an occupational hazard. Canicola fever is usually mild, though it may be associated with meningitis.

The pathogenic leptospirae can be cultured in the laboratory and this is of help in the diagnosis if the correct specimens are taken at a suitable stage of the illness. For example, blood culture may be successful but only if special procedures are employed. Although the organisms may be present in the urine, they are quickly killed when it is acid and precautions must be taken to avoid this. Serological diagnosis is a useful clinical aid; there are cross-reacting antigens in *L. icterohaemorrhagiae* and *L. canicola*, but other components allow a distinction to be made.

RICKETTSIAE AND RELATED ORGANISMS

Rickettsia

The micro-organisms in this family range from spheres, 300–500 nm in diameter, to thin rods up to 2 μm in length, and are regarded as intermediary between bacteria and viruses. They can be seen by the light microscope, do not pass filters that retain bacteria and have the principal structural features of bacteria. Rickettsiae have at least some of the enzyme systems of bacteria and contain both RNA and DNA. Moreover, they are susceptible to some antibacterial agents. On the other hand, almost all of the members of the group are obligatory intracellular parasites and can be grown in culture only when living cells are present.

TYPHUS FEVER

The rickettsiae are the causative organisms of typhus fever which is one of the great pestilences of man. The micro-organisms spread rapidly throughout the body, causing a severe and often fatal infection, and they frequently settle in endothelial cells of small blood vessels in the skin, brain and heart. There are several different rickettsiae, distinguished by the insect vectors that effect their transfer from man to man and possibly from an animal host to man (p. 19.51). The organisms stimulate the production of complement-fixing antibodies which react with specific rickettsial antigens in the laboratory. In addition, antibodies are produced which happen to react with the O antigen of certain *Proteus* strains, and as the particular strains of *Proteus* involved differ with the various forms of typhus, detection and quantitation of these antibodies (the Weil–Felix reaction) allows the diagnosis of the different forms of the disease.

Rickettsia prowazekii is responsible for **epidemic typhus**, which is transmitted by lice. *R. mooserii* causes the milder **endemic murine typhus**, primarily a disease of rats, amongst which it is spread by the rat flea. *R. tsutsugamushi*, responsible for **scrub typhus**, an infection acquired in tropical scrub country or jungles, is transmitted by mites. *R. rickettsii* causes **Rocky Mountain Spotted Fever,** and *R. conori* causes South African tick fever and Mediterranean fever; these are carried by ticks. The manner in which these insects spread the different forms of typhus is described on p. 19.51.

With the exception of endemic typhus caused by *R. mooseri*, the diseases may spread from man to man, via the insect vector, without an intervening alternative mammalian host, and this is the normal way in which an epidemic spreads. These rickettsiae all cause infection in laboratory guinea-pigs and mice when they are injected in blood taken from an infected patient, but the role of small animals as a potential reservoir for these infections between epidemics is uncertain.

Other rickettsiae have been held responsible for outbreaks of febrile disease, usually localized, in many parts of the world. Of these, Trench fever was common in soldiers in World War I, but the taxonomy of the causative organism, *R. quintana*, is at present in doubt.

Typhus can be treated by tetracyclines, and it can be prevented by attention to hygiene and control of the insect vector. DDT is effective if correctly used, and it can stop an outbreak of louse typhus. Dimethyl phytate is a miticidal agent that can be effective against other forms, but the prevention of scrub typhus is difficult and less certain. Active immunization against typhus is commonly carried out with a vaccine prepared from cultures of rickettsiae grown in the yolk sac of chick embryos.

Coxiella

Q fever is an acute febrile illness associated with pneumonia. The Q is not for Queensland, where it was first recognized, but stands for 'query', because the cause of the disease was unknown. Q fever is now known to be caused by *Coxiella burnetii* which is enzootic among domestic and farm animals and can be isolated from ticks, lice, mammals and birds in many parts of the world. Infection is transmitted from animal to animal by ticks, but man contracts the disease usually by drinking contaminated milk or by inhaling infected dust. The organism sometimes causes an endocarditis in man.

Cox. burnetii resembles *Rickettsia* in many ways, but it differs in being remarkably resistant to desiccation, and it can survive for long periods. Q fever differs from typhus fever in that it is not transmitted to man by insects.

OTHER INFECTIVE AGENTS

Bedsonia (Chlamydia)

Psittacosis is a febrile illness, usually associated with a pneumonitis, which is often mild, but sometimes severe and occasionally fatal. The disease is primarily an infection of parrots, cockatoos and budgerigars, and it occurs not uncommonly in fanciers and others who keep these birds.

Lymphogranuloma venereum is a venereal infection. It involves the inguinal lymph nodes, which may suppurate.

Trachoma is a keratoconjunctivitis, often mild, but which may be very severe with blindness resulting from ulceration with associated scarring. Formerly widespread throughout the world, it is still seen in many poor countries. The infection spreads readily in undernourished children living in unhygienic conditions. Flies are probably important in carrying it from child to child.

Clinically and epidemiologically, the above diseases have little in common, but the causative bedsoniae are related although their classification continues to be a matter for debate. The organisms are about 250 nm in diameter and they are thus larger than viruses but smaller than bacteria. Unlike rickettsiae they have no insect vector and transmission occurs by close contact between humans or by close association with birds. The organisms possess cell walls composed of mucopeptides, and they are sensitive to antibacterial antibiotics that interfere with mucopeptide synthesis. In addition, as they possess both RNA and DNA, they are not viruses.

These organisms can be seen as inclusion bodies within the cells of the host, and they pass through a sequence of structural changes which can be followed in the electron microscope; they appear to reproduce by fission or by a process analogous to budding. They do not grow on bacteriological culture media, but can be cultured in the yolk sac of the chick embryo.

Mycoplasma

The genus *Mycoplasma* includes a group of organisms which are unusual in lacking a rigid cell wall and which therefore assume many different shapes and sizes; small forms can pass through filters that retain bacteria and are comparable with medium-sized viruses (about 150 nm). They can be grown on artificial media enriched with serum and have a characteristic requirement for cholesterol or related steroids. On solid media they form very small transparent colonies which become visible after incubation for periods ranging from 2–10 days.

The mycoplasmas include the causative agent of a disease of cattle called pleuropneumonia which has been recognized for centuries, and the group was formerly referred to as the pleuropneumonia-like organisms (PPLO). Related organisms have been isolated from animals in which they may be commensal or pathogenic, and some appear to be saprophytic in soil and water. Mycoplasmas have been isolated from the mouth and upper respiratory tract and from the genito-urinary tract of man. The species obtained from human sources include *M. hominis, M. salivarium, M. orale, M. fermentans* and *M. pneumoniae*. Although several pathogenic roles have been suggested for these organisms, such as nonspecific or nongonococcal urethritis in the case of those species isolated from the urethra, only *M. pneumoniae* has a definite association with human disease.

M. pneumoniae (Eaton's agent) causes a febrile respiratory illness often with severe cough and with patchy consolidation in the lung. It does not respond to treatment with sulphonamides or penicillin, and the illness is often referred to as **atypical pneumonia**. During the course of the infection, the patient develops specific antibodies which can be detected by serological tests, including an immunofluorescence test; in addition, the titre of cold agglutinins (vol. I, p. 26.18) is raised. Some patients develop antibodies to the aetiologically unrelated α-haemolytic *Streptococcus MG*, which may share a common antigen with the causative mycoplasma. *M. pneumoniae* may be isolated from the sputum of a patient with atypical pneumonia by selective culture methods. The organism is sensitive to tetracycline and some other antibiotics.

THE COMMENSAL BACTERIAL FLORA OF MAN

Very many bacteria colonize man and this state of peaceful co-existence persists until something happens to disturb the delicate balance of commensalism. Man's skin, nasopharynx and mouth have an abundant microbial flora. The acid barrier of the stomach inhibits bacterial growth, and inadequately understood antibacterial mechanisms are effective in maintaining the jejunum and upper ileum relatively free from resident bacteria. However, there is an established intestinal bacterial population in the lower part of the ileum and an abundant flora in the caecum and colon where numerous species are present in numbers that approach or exceed hundreds of millions/g of faeces.

On the other hand, bacterial access to deep tissues, the blood stream and the mucous surfaces of some special organs is transient and countered effectively in health. Thus, the CSF is normally sterile and bacteria are not usually found in muscle, bone or connective tissues. Joints are sterile; the lower bronchi are kept virtually bacteria-free, and the blood, kidneys, urinary tract, liver and spleen have efficient clearing mechanisms.

Staph. albus and some other staphylococci, diphtheroid organisms, lactobacilli and various micro-cocci, some of them obligate anaerobes, colonize the skin and are harboured in sebaceous glands, and hair follicles. These organisms constitute the resident flora which can be distinguished from bacteria transiently acquired on the skin. The commensal bacteria of the upper respiratory tract include commensal *Neisseria* species, streptococci and pneumococci, some staphylococci, *H. influenzae*, diphtheroid organisms and micrococci. *Staph. aureus* and *Staph. albus* are regularly harboured in the anterior nares. *Strept. viridans* is very numerous in the mouth, and the abundant flora here includes commensal micrococci, staphylococci, spirochaetes, *Bacteroides–fusiformis* species, lactobacilli, mycoplasmas, yeast-like organisms such as *Candida, Actinomyces* species and fungi. Organisms of the *Bacteroides–fusiformis* group are probably the predominant bacteria of the intestine; the gut commensals include also lactobacilli, *Esch. coli* and many related organisms, *Proteus* and *Pseudomonas* species, *Strept. faecalis, Cl. welchii* and staphylococci. The biochemical potential of the gut flora is enormous and is perhaps not adequately recognized at present. Lactobacilli are predominant in the commensal flora of the adult vagina, which is acidic in health and also harbours streptococci, diphtheroid organisms, yeasts and fungi, *Bacteroides* species and mycoplasmas.

Commensal bacteria play a part in denying pathogens an opportunity to colonize, and this is well illustrated when the normal pattern is upset by some antimicrobial drugs which allow relatively nonvirulent resistant opportunists to take advantage of the situation. Moreover, the clinical use of immunosuppressive drugs, corticosteroids and cytotoxic agents may render the patient vulnerable to invasion by organisms with which he otherwise lives on peaceful terms.

CLINICAL BACTERIOLOGY

In normal practice, detailed bacteriological analysis of every specimen is not feasible, but accuracy and speed in detecting significant pathogens and in reporting the findings are of paramount importance. An outline of the procedures commonly undertaken to identify an organism present in pathological material is shown in fig. 18.38; all of these investigations are not necessary in every case since some pathogens are more readily recognized than others, whereas some share common characters with harmless commensals and require more diligent detection.

MICROSCOPY

Direct microscopy is of great value as a means of characterizing bacteria according to their morphology and staining reactions. It is also useful in determining whether the material taken from a patient shows

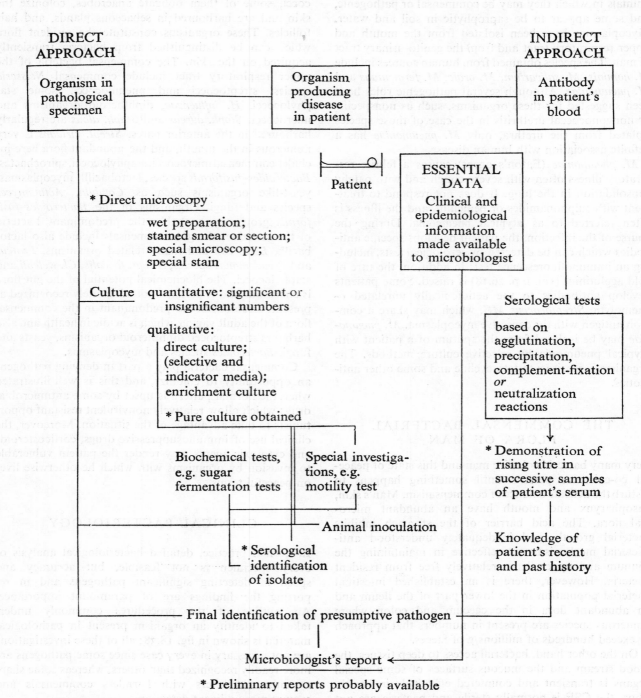

FIG. 18.38. An outline of the components of direct and indirect bacteriological diagnostic procedures.

evidence of a cytological response which itself may be of diagnostic assistance. Only occasionally, however, does direct microscopy of an exudate provide a firm diagnosis. Microscopy of a stained smear of sputum from a patient with advanced pulmonary tuberculosis often establishes the diagnosis beyond reasonable doubt; even then it is advisable to isolate the causative organism in pure culture so that *in vitro* tests of sensitivity to antimicrobial drugs can be undertaken.

There are a few infections for which microscopy is the only practical method of diagnosis; e.g. leprosy and Vincent's gingivitis. In other infections a rapid provisional diagnosis can sometimes be based on special morphological features, e.g. the CSF in acute purulent meningitis.

Special microscopic techniques may also quickly yield information of particular value, e.g. *T. pallidum* can be seen in an unstained wet preparation of exudate from a primary chancre viewed by **dark-ground microscopy**. A combination of serological and microscopic methods, **immunofluorescent microscopy**, involves staining an organism with a fluorescent preparation conjugated to a specific antiserum; the organism then fluoresces when viewed by ultra-violet light. This special procedure has only limited application in diagnostic work at present.

However the commensal flora are often microscopically identical with pathogenic species which may infect an area of the body. Moreover, different pathogens that produce different syndromes and respond differently to antibiotics are sometimes morphologically indistinguishable. Hence more elaborate methods are required for diagnosis.

CULTURAL CHARACTERISTICS
Colonial features such as size, shape, elevation, pigmentation and consistency are useful aids to identification, as are the cultural requirements, e.g. the success or failure of growth on simple or enriched media and in the presence or absence of oxygen; changes produced in the medium around the colony may be detected, e.g. streptococci are subclassified by their haemolytic activity on blood agar (p. 18.67).

When a suspected pathogen is isolated in pure culture, the organism's special features may be examined microscopically after suitable staining and its behaviour in special culture media may reveal differentiating characters such as motility or pigmentation. Knowledge of distinctive biochemical and serological reactions is then applied to identify the organism more definitely (see below).

In some circumstances, **quantitative cultural procedures** aid diagnosis and this approach is likely to be extended in the future. These are of particular use in the investigation of infections of the urinary tract. Although the urinary tract is sterile in health, a sample of urine is often contaminated with the bacterial flora that are present in the terminal part of the urethra. Such a specimen is likely to

14

contain relatively insignificant numbers of a variety of bacteria. On the other hand, urine from a patient with a urinary tract infection usually contains significantly large numbers of one or perhaps two pathogenic species. Bacteria multiply readily in urine and if a contaminated sample is not examined promptly, it may simulate an infected specimen. Provided that the specimens are examined promptly, however, the quantitative and qualitative differences between urine that has been contaminated and **significant bacteriuria** is readily apparent (p. 18.80).

BIOCHEMICAL TESTS
The biochemical activities of pure cultures are commonly employed to separate pathogenic species of a genus from each other and from commensal members of that genus, especially when differences in colonial appearances are small or indeterminate. Commonly, fermentation tests are used for this purpose; a pure culture of the organism is inoculated into tubes of peptone water, each containing a small quantity of a test carbohydrate. The utilization of the carbohydrate is detected by production of acid and perhaps gas. **Sugar reactions** are used regularly to identify the intestinal pathogens of the genus *Shigella* and the genus *Salmonella*.

Other biochemical tests are used in differentiating species. In some cases a specific enzymic reaction is employed; for example, pathogenic staphylococci produce coagulase, which brings about the coagulation of citrated plasma, and organisms of the *Neisseria* and *Pseudomonas* groups elaborate oxidases which produce a rapid change of colour in a freshly prepared test solution of tetramethyl-*p*-phenylenediamine (p. 18.71).

An outline of the use of these methods in a specific case may be helpful. When a sample of faeces from a case of gastroenteritis is submitted for bacteriological examination, the colour and consistency of the specimen are noted and the presence of mucus or blood is recorded. A wet unstained film of the specimen is then examined microscopically to determine whether ova or protozoa are present; however a Gram-stained preparation is of no value in determining whether or not the patient is suffering from bacillary dysentery or salmonella infection, since by this means these bacteria are indistinguishable from each other and from the commensal coliform flora.

The specimen is therefore emulsified in sterile isotonic saline and plated out directly on suitable selective and differential media such as MacConkey medium and desoxycholate citrate agar (DCA). Fluid enrichment media may allow small numbers of pathogens to overgrow commensals. After a period of incubation, the fluid cultures are plated on selective media, from which suspected colonies of pathogenic species can be harvested, free from the commensals.

Colonies on solid MacConkey or DCA media which

have not fermented lactose are possibly those of shigellae or salmonellae; these therefore are subcultured in fluid media to determine their ability to produce acid and perhaps gas. Simultaneously, motility in pure culture is examined either by a hanging-drop preparation or preferably by a cultural method using semi-solid agar (fig. 18.39). The organism's ability to produce indole

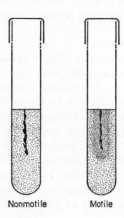

Nonmotile   Motile

FIG. 18.39. Stab-cultures of nonmotile and motile organisms in semi-solid agar medium. The motile organism produces a zone of turbidity as it grows away from the needle track.

and/or H$_2$S is also determined. On the results of the biochemical tests, the organism can be regarded provisionally as a recognized pathogen or discarded as being nonpathogenic. The biochemical results often indicate the genus involved. The final establishment of generic identity and type identity within the genus is based on serological procedures.

SEROLOGICAL IDENTIFICATION

Many stock or standard antisera, i.e. sera containing antibodies to specific organisms, are available for the antigenic characterization of bacteria; these antisera are prepared by injecting pure cultures of inactivated bacteria into rabbits or other animals and subsequently withdrawing serum. The sera then react demonstrably and specifically *in vitro* with the specific bacterial antigens. For example, when an organism with the cultural and biochemical attributes of *Shigella* is isolated from faeces, it can be tested with four standard antisera developed against each of the four species of the genus (p. 18.81); after allocation to its particular subgroup, its actual serotype can then be determined by testing the organism against type-specific antisera prepared against specific serotypes within the subgroup. Similarly, β-haemolytic streptococci can be grouped by antisera prepared against the various group-specific

carbohydrate antigens, and if the isolate belongs to group A, it can then be typed by employing antisera separately developed against the highly specific M-protein antigens possessed by this group of streptococci.

ANIMAL INOCULATION

In the diagnosis of certain infections, inoculation of pathological material into a susceptible animal offers a more sensitive and reliable method than cultural procedures. An instance is the detection of tubercle bacilli in the urine of a patient with suspected early tuberculosis of the renal tract, when the organisms may be scanty. Early diagnosis is here of great importance and the organisms may be missed if reliance is placed solely on microscopic examination or cultural procedures. The use of experimental animals for diagnostic purposes is limited and strictly controlled in Britain.

EPIDEMIOLOGICAL MARKERS

Although precise identification of the strain of a pathogen is often unnecessary for clinical purposes, it is of great value when there is the possibility of an epidemic of infection in the general population or in a semi-closed community such as a residential nursery or a hospital. Identification of the type helps to determine the relationship between the different cases and the source of infection, and so indicates appropriate preventive measures.

Although many of the available serological methods facilitate the identification of a group or species there are nonserological procedures that allow more detailed subclassification in certain cases. A typing method for tracing staphylococci exploits the specific affinities of staphylococcal bacteriophages (p. 18.70). **Bacteriophage typing** has been applied also to the subdivision of some salmonella serotypes so that, for example, it may be possible to show that a patient who develops typhoid in Edinburgh was infected with a strain of the organism known to be causing trouble in a continental holiday town from which he recently returned (p. 18.102).

Another technique of value for epidemiological tracing depends on the ability of certain bacteria to produce **bacteriocines**; these are naturally occurring substances with antibiotic activity effective mainly against other strains of the same genus. When a test strain has produced bacteriocines on a solid culture medium, a number of passive indicator strains are inoculated in a standard fashion on to the plate and different patterns of inhibition may occur. The producer strain is given a type number in accordance with the pattern that is produced. Bacteriocine typing has proved particularly useful in subdividing *Shigella sonnei*, which commonly causes bacillary dysentery, into subtypes; this is impossible by serological or biochemical methods (p. 18.81).

Indirect methods of diagnosis

The diagnosis of an infective condition is usually best achieved by identifying the causative organism directly. Moreover, the isolation of the organism is often an essential step in deciding the most effective therapy, especially when the particular strain is resistant to the commonly used antibiotics. In some cases, however, this is not possible. For example, a patient may seek medical help at a late stage of an infection when the causative organism is difficult to isolate; this is often the case in subacute or chronic stages of generalized infections which smoulder as multiple small foci in the deeper tissues. In addition, an acute infective focus in which a primary pathogen was originally predominant is often infected by secondary invaders derived from nearby commensal flora. These opportunist pathogens obscure the primary pathogen and render difficult its isolation and identification. Under these circumstances indirect methods of diagnosis must be employed. As it is frequently impossible to predict at the outset the success of either direct or indirect procedures, they are frequently initiated in parallel.

DIAGNOSTIC SEROLOGY

When a pathogenic organism multiplies in the tissues, the microbial antigens frequently stimulate the production of antibodies which become detectable in the serum. When the patient recovers from the infection, the antibodies persist for a period and then gradually decrease. The antibodies are specific for the infecting organism and the two can be shown to interact in various ways. The nature of antibodies and the laboratory procedures commonly used for their demonstration in patients' sera are described on p. 22.14.

The basis of these diagnostic tests is that serial dilutions of the patient's serum are tested in the reaction system to determine the maximum dilution that gives a positive result. This is loosely referred to as the titre. A simple example is the Widal agglutination test in which agglutinating antibodies produced by the patient against the typhoid organisms are detected by adding

suspensions of typhoid organisms to graded dilutions of the patient's serum (fig. 18.40). Of course, in many instances an individual may possess antibodies against a particular pathogen at the time of testing although his present illness is not attributable to that pathogen. For example, a patient with detectable antibodies against typhoid organisms may have been immunized artificially against typhoid or he may have acquired a degree of natural immunity during an unrecognized subclinical infection. **Anamnestic factors**, i.e. previous known infection or immunization, should always be sought when the patient's history is taken and the information should be given to the microbiologist. The serological diagnosis of infection is most convincing when a significant rise in titre of antibody can be demonstrated. Thus, as soon as symptoms or signs meriting such an investigation develop, an early sample is forwarded to establish a baseline and, after 7–10 days, a second sample is likely to contain a significantly increased amount of antibody (fig. 18.40).

Many diagnostic tests are done with doubling dilutions of the test serum. Thus, a difference of one tube in a parallel series will change a reading of 1 in 60 to one of 1 in 120 and this is often within the range of experimental error. It is therefore advisable to regard nothing less than a fourfold change in titre as a significant rise or fall. If the patient is already at an advanced stage of an infection when his serum is first tested, any titre may already be relatively high. In this case, a second sample taken some weeks later may show a significant fall in titre and this may be of value in retrospective diagnosis.

Many other factors need to be taken into account in the interpretation of serological results. Not uncommonly, an infection temporarily raises levels of antibodies that are unrelated to the causative organism. This effect is seen, for example, with some serological tests for syphilis in nonsyphilitic patients suffering from malaria, leprosy or tuberculosis. It is clear that the correct interpretation of serological tests requires experience and a full knowledge of the patient's history.

Similarly, results of direct microbiological diagnostic procedures cannot be accepted unreservedly. If an accepted pathogen is isolated from tissues or body fluids which are normally sterile in health, e.g. blood or CSF, the finding in conjunction with the clinical features may make the diagnosis obvious. It is also true that the isolation of pathogens such as tubercle bacilli, gonococci or anthrax bacilli is unequivocal evidence of specific disease activity. However the diagnosis may be less straightforward. A vaginal swab from a patient with a puerperal fever may yield *Cl. welchii* or *Esch. coli*; while these organisms may be involved in a serious inflammatory process, their presence is more commonly attributable to contamination of the swab or the

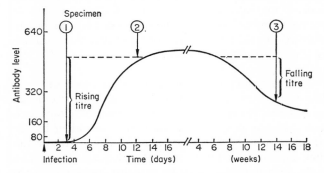

FIG. 18.40. Diagrammatic representation of a rising and falling titre of antibody.

swabbed area with faecal flora and is not of pathogenic significance.

Specimens for bacteriological investigation

Attention to detail in taking a bacteriological specimen and in submitting it to the laboratory are important. Moreover, the time of taking a particular specimen may be influenced by understanding the pathogenesis of the suspected disease; for example, blood culture is likely to yield the causative organism of a case of typhoid if it is undertaken within the first 10 days, but it is less likely to do so in the third week of the disease, when the organisms are often abundant in the faeces.

Samples of pus and purulent exudates

These samples are frequently submitted to the laboratory on sterile swabs. The swabs should be prepared specially for the purpose, as some batches of cotton wool contain antibacterial substances. It is important to ensure that the swab is well soaked with the exudate and it should not be allowed to dry in transit. An accompanying heat-fixed smear on a glass slide often yields more microscopic evidence than a smear subsequently prepared from the swab. This is important, for instance, in cases of gingivitis in which the causative organism is not readily cultivated, and also in suspected cases of gonorrhoea. In general, it is better to send a specimen of actual exudate in a sterile bottle, if there is an adequate amount, for this allows the bacteriologist to extend his range of investigations. In special cases, even small amounts of exudate are better sent in a small capillary tube than on a swab; for example, this procedure allows dark-ground examination of the exudate from a primary syphilitic chancre, whereas a swab is useless in such a case.

Samples of urine

Special precautions must be taken in collection. In male patients, a midstream specimen usually suffices; in females, a 'clean-catch' midstream specimen is taken so that contamination with commensal flora is avoided. These procedures are of special importance if quantitative and qualitative results are to be correctly interpreted. For routine investigation for pyogenic organisms a volume of 10–20 ml is adequate. Larger volumes are required in investigation for tubercle bacilli. The passing of a urethral catheter is associated with a risk of introducing infective organisms into the bladder and this procedure is not now recommended as a method of obtaining a clean specimen of urine for bacteriological investigation.

Samples of faeces

A wide-mouthed and properly sealed container should be used. It should not be over-filled and the patient should be asked to ensure that it is not soiled externally. It is also worth while ensuring that the specimen is obtained free from disinfectant which may have been present in a chamber-pot. The use of a rectal swab avoids many difficulties when examination of faeces is wanted, but the swab must be taken properly and in some cases it is not a reliable alternative, e.g., in the case of an infection which predominantly involves the small intestine. A swab of a suitable portion of a specimen of faeces, a faeces swab, is often a useful compromise.

Samples of sputum

The patient must be advised that a sample of saliva is of no use.

Samples for blood culture

Blood culture is a most useful aid to the diagnosis of infections that have a bacteriaemic phase or in which septicaemia has developed. The skin over the venepuncture site must be cleansed and disinfected carefully, otherwise the investigation is vitiated by the presence of contaminating commensal organisms. The sterility of the syringe must be beyond doubt. About 5–10 ml of blood is introduced into a blood culture bottle, which is a 100 ml flat bottle containing about 50 ml of nutrient broth. The metal cap is drilled so that the syringe needle can be introduced directly by puncturing the rubber seal. The outfit is usually distributed with a plastic seal and a release mechanism so that the sterile top of the bottle is protected in storage and requires no swabbing before use. Blood culture bottles may be supplied with various media for special purposes and the laboratory staff should be consulted; for example broth containing *p*-amino benzoic acid may be supplied if it is known that the patient has been receiving sulphonamides, or penicillinase-containing broth can be used for the culture of blood from a patient who is receiving penicillin.

Samples of cerebrospinal fluid

The bacteriological examination of CSF may be an emergency procedure, as useful information may be obtained from direct microscopic examination of a wet film and a stained smear of the exudate, if carried out at once. If the patient's condition is sufficiently serious to warrant lumbar puncture, the clinician and the microbiologist should co-operate to ensure that the specimen of CSF is properly examined.

The quality of the specimen and its transport

The success or failure of a diagnostic bacteriological procedure is often determined by the quality of the specimen and this frequently reflects the care taken by the clinician. A suitable specimen must be taken at the proper time and forwarded promptly with adequate information if the microbiologist is to be properly employed in the patient's interests.

In some instances, microscopical examination of the specimen reveals numerous organisms but attempts at cultivation are persistently unsuccessful. This may be due to feeble viability of the organisms outside the host, but it is often the result of delay in transmission of the specimen to the laboratory. Another cause is the presence of an antimicrobial drug in the sample sent for investigation. When the clinician suspects that the causal organism may be delicate, or when he knows that some delay in transmission is unavoidable, special care should be taken to prolong the survival of the organism; special transport media are available for delicate pathogens such as the gonococcus, or alternatively the diagnostic medium may be brought to the patient so that the specimen can be seeded directly on to it. The survival of other pathogens can be prolonged by simple means such as the use of special swabs. If a swab dries in transit, it may yield little material to a culture medium and it becomes impossible to prepare a smear for direct examination. On the other hand, urine is a good culture medium and delay in processing permits multiplication of any organisms present. This may result in an overgrowth of contaminants originally present in insignificantly small numbers, or misleadingly large numbers of potential pathogens may be isolated per unit volume and a wrong diagnosis may be made. Thus, urine should either be examined promptly or it should be refrigerated until it can be transported in a container which keeps it chilled. These observations do not apply to bulk collection of urine in cases of suspected renal tuberculosis. All specimens should be submitted for bacteriological investigation accompanied by a request form on which the relevant clinical details are given. For example, it is well known that knowledge of a patient's recent antibiotic therapy or past immunization history is essential for the interpretation of microbiological findings, but it is not always appreciated that awareness of these facts may also influence the design of the investigation.

VIRUSES

Infectious virus particles or **virions** consist of a strand or strands of either DNA or RNA, but not both, surrounded by a protein coat or **capsid**. As viruses do not possess ribosomes and are dependent on those of their host cell, they are strict intracellular parasites. They can be distinguished from bacteria, rickettsiae and related organisms by their lack of muramic acid, their single nucleic acid content, their mode of replication (p. 18.103) and their resistance to antibiotics (p. 21.34). Most viruses are too small to be seen with the light microscope.

More than 300 different viruses have been isolated from animals; some appear to be harmless, but others are responsible for many important diseases in man and animals. Of the five great pestilences, smallpox and yellow fever are caused by viruses, typhus is a rickettsial infection, and plague and cholera are caused by bacteria. Until the development of vaccines that protect against poliomyelitis, the poliovirus was greatly feared, especially in modern cities. The most troublesome viruses today are those responsible for the majority of infections of the upper respiratory passages.

There are also large numbers of plant viruses. None of these can infect man or other animals, though they may ruin his crops. Plant viruses, such as tobacco mosaic virus (TMV), are more easily studied than animal viruses and they have been the source of much fundamental knowledge of virology.

Bacteria may also be attacked by viruses, known as **bacteriophages** or **phages** (p. 18.101), which in some cases lyse the host cell. After their discovery in 1915, there were hopes that phages might be used to control and treat bacterial diseases like cholera and plague but these have not been fulfilled, and phages have no place in therapeutics. However, their dependence on specific hosts allows typing and identification of many strains of bacteria, and this can be useful in studies of the spread and control of some bacterial infections. Bacteriophages are of great value in the study of biology and in particular in the elucidation of fundamental processes involved in parasitism and genetic transfer mechanisms.

CLASSIFICATION AND NOMENCLATURE

Viruses were first classified as dermotropic and neurotropic, depending on the tissues which they tended to affect, but this led to false associations; for instance both smallpox virus and Coxsackie A16 virus localize in skin but they share no other common characteristic. In addition, such a classification could not include plant and bacterial viruses and therefore a more fundamental approach was sought. The use of a Latin binomial system has been discouraged, as sufficient information on the relationships of viruses is not yet available and therefore the terms genus and species cannot be applied. The present classification of animal viruses is based primarily on four characters:

(1) the type of nucleic acid present,
(2) the structure of the capsid,
(3) the presence or absence of an envelope, and
(4) the stability of the virus in the presence of ether.

Table 18.4 shows this classification in which there are twelve different groups. Such a system can be extended to include both plant and bacterial viruses.

Picornaviruses (Portuguese, *pico*, small; RNA viruses) include the entero- and rhinoviruses. Polioviruses 1, 2 and 3, Coxsackie A and B viruses and Echoviruses, are frequently recovered from faeces and so are grouped to-

TABLE 18.4. The classification of viruses.

Type of nucleic acid	Structure of capsid	Presence of envelope	Sensitivity to ether	Group	Examples of viruses	Examples of diseases produced
RNA	I	−	−	PICORNAVIRUSES	Subgroup A of human origin Enteroviruses Poliovirus (3) Coxsackie A (20) Coxsackie B (6) Echovirus (30) Rhinovirus (60) Subgroup B of animal origin Foot and mouth disease	 Poliomyelitis Aseptic meningitis Pleurodynia; myocarditis Aseptic meningitis; diarrhoea Common cold Foot and mouth disease
RNA	I	−	−	REOVIRUSES	(3)	No proven connection with disease
RNA	I	+	+	ARBOVIRUSES	Group A (17–19) Group B (33) Group C (9) Ungrouped (?)	Encephalitis Yellow fever; dengue fever; louping-ill; encephalitis Encephalitis
RNA	H	+	+	MYXOVIRUSES	Influenza A (3) Influenza B (2) Influenza C (1)	Influenza Influenza Influenza
RNA	H	+	+	PARAMYXOVIRUSES	Parainfluenza (4) Mumps	Respiratory tract infection Mumps
RNA	H	+	+	RHABDOVIRUSES	Rabies	Rabies
RNA	Uncertain	+	+	FOWL LEUKOSIS VIRUSES	Rous sarcoma virus	Rous sarcoma in hens
RNA	Uncertain	+	+	MOUSE TUMOUR VIRUSES	Bittner agent	Mouse mammary cancer
DNA	I	−	−	ADENOVIRUSES	Human types (28)	Upper respiratory infections; keratoconjunctivitis; pharyngo-conjunctival fever
DNA	I	−	−	PAPOVAVIRUSES	Papilloma viruses Polyoma virus Vacuolating agent	Human wart; rabbit papilloma Tumours of mice Latent infection of monkeys
DNA	I	+	+	HERPESVIRUSES	Herpes simplex (2) Varicella virus Herpes B Cytomegaloviruses	Stomatitis; cold sores; keratoconjunctivitis; genital herpes Chickenpox; herpes zoster Latent disease of monkeys; fatal disease in man Cytomegalic inclusion disease
DNA	Uncertain	+	?±	POXVIRUSES	Variola (2) Vaccinia Molluscum virus Orf virus	Smallpox Vaccinia Molluscum contagiosum Pustular dermatitis of lambs

RNA, ribonucleic acid; DNA, deoxyribonucleic acid; I, isometric; H, helical; figures in brackets are the number of subtypes.

gether as the enteroviruses. Coxsackie viruses are named after the place in New York State where they were first isolated. Echoviruses derive their name from enteric, cytopathic, human, orphan. These viruses, which can be isolated from human faeces, produce a cytopathic effect in tissue culture (p. 18.101) and were called orphan because initially they were not associated with any clinical syndrome. Rhinoviruses cause the common cold and multiply in the nasal mucous membranes. Viruses from these different groups may be distinguished by a number of properties, including their serological reactions, pathogenicity for mice and growth in tissue culture.

Reoviruses, whose name is derived from respiratory, enteric, orphan, can be isolated from respiratory and enteric secretions, but their presence is not related to any clinical syndrome and so their role in human disease is uncertain. Three types may be distinguished by serological techniques.

Arboviruses, whose name derives from their being **ar**thropod **bo**rne **viruses**, are transmitted by blood-sucking arthropods to further hosts of the same or different species. Three main groups, A, B and C, may be distinguished by serological reactions, but other smaller groups exist.

Myxoviruses are so called because of their affinity for mucoproteins (Greek *myxo*, mucus). Human myxoviruses may be divided into three subgroups, each responsible for a form of influenza, by their serological reactions.

Paramyxoviruses are related to the myxoviruses but are larger, and the group includes the parainfluenza and mumps viruses; on the basis of morphology and haemagglutinating properties the measles and respiratory syncytial viruses have been provisionally allocated to this group.

Rhabdoviruses have one important member that is pathogenic for man, the rabies virus. All warm-blooded animals are susceptible to infection, the virus having a predilection for mucus-secreting glandular tissue and the central nervous system.

Fowl leukosis viruses include the Rous sarcoma virus, which in 1911 was shown to induce tumour formation in hens (p. 18.112).

Mouse tumour viruses are oncogenic agents and one member is described on p. 18.113.

Adenoviruses were first isolated from apparently healthy tonsils, but many different types of both human and animal origin are now recognized. All share a common cross-reacting antigen and are stable within wide ranges of pH and temperature. The human viruses can be recovered from the respiratory and alimentary tracts, but not all types have been shown to be associated with disease. Recently, much interest has been shown in the adenoviruses because of their ability to induce malignant tumours in hamsters (p. 18.110).

Papovaviruses contain the viruses of **pa**pilloma and **po**lyoma and the **va**cuolating agents. They are oncogenic and include the human wart virus (plate 18.3b). The vacuolating agents produce their effects in tissue culture cells *in vitro*. They can cause latent infections in monkeys and as a result they may contaminate tissue cultures produced from such animals. Simian virus 40 (SV40) can be detected readily in tissue culture of monkey kidney; it may interfere with the growth and detection of other viruses (p. 18.110), and it may contaminate stocks of virus prepared for use as vaccines.

Herpesviruses form a large group including a number of human pathogens which have a similar distinctive structure. Herpes (Greek, *herpein*, to creep) was applied to describe the lesions of the herpes simplex virus in skin.

Poxviruses are the largest of the true viruses, being just within the limits of resolution of the light microscope. The characteristic skin lesion or pox (old English for pustule) gives the name to the group which includes the viruses responsible for variola (smallpox), vaccinia and molluscum contagiosum. Members of the group also cause disease in a wide range of vertebrates and the animal pathogens include the viruses of cowpox, rabbit myxoma, and rabbit and squirrel fibroma (plate 18.3a, facing p. 18.96).

THE PHYSICAL AND CHEMICAL PROPERTIES OF VIRUSES

Size of viruses

The size of a virus particle was formerly estimated from its ability to pass through graded filters of known pore diameter, but the electron microscope (EM) now permits more precise measurements. Untreated virus particles are not readily visualized in the EM, but their electron density can be increased by one of the following methods.

In **shadow-casting**, the virus specimen is suitably mounted and subjected to a stream of vaporized heavy metal such as gold. The vapour condenses on the side of the virus nearer the source of the metal and the particles appear dark on the EM screen. If the metal vapour is directed at an angle, metal is deposited on the virus particle and part of the supporting film is shielded. This shadow area lacks any metallic deposit and so appears bright. The size of the shadow allows the height of the particle to be calculated. The particles, however, appear dense and detail of their structure is not seen.

In thin sections, viruses may be revealed by **positive staining** due to interaction of a heavy metal with protein. Virus suspensions are usually **negatively stained** with phosphotungstic acid (PTA) at neutral pH. Here the electron-dense stain surrounds the particles and penetrates surface hollows. The substructure is then visible in the EM and this technique is of use in grouping viruses of similar structure and in estimating the number of virus particles in a suspension. Enumeration usually involves mixing the virus with a suspension of latex spheres of known concentration. After staining, the proportion of virus to latex particles is counted and the concentration of the virus suspension calculated.

PTA STAINING AND INFECTIVITY
Individual virus particles vary in appearance after PTA staining. In some, the centre of the capsid is not penetrated by PTA and is unstained, whereas others are penetrated and appear dark. The unstained centres in some particles are due to a nucleic acid core which excludes the stain; these particles are potentially infective. A differential count of stained and unstained centres indicates the proportion of particles that contain nucleic acid in a suspension and this may then be related to the infectivity of the preparation as measured biologically. In plant viruses, infectivity is low and often only 0.1 per cent of

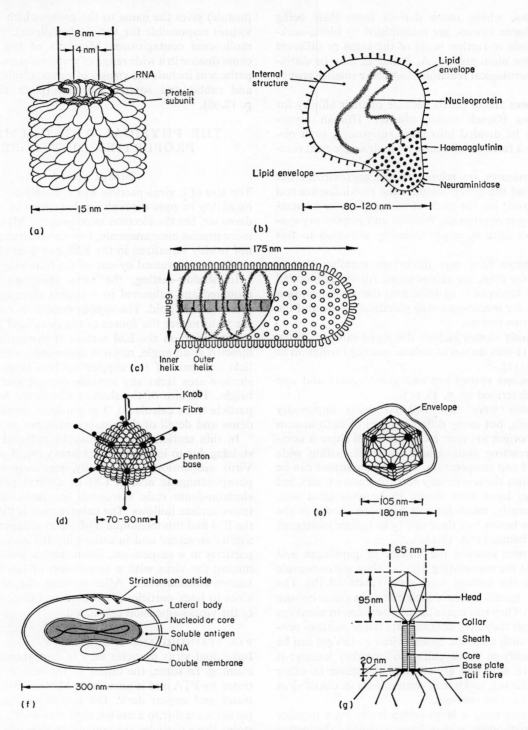

FIG. 18.41. Examples of the three recognized types of viral structure. Tobacco mosaic virus (a), influenza virus (b) and rabies virus (c) are helical. Adenovirus (d) and herpesvirus (e) are isometric viruses. Vaccinia (f) and the bacteriophage T4 (g) are complex viruses. (a) and (d) after Cohen, (e) after Fenner and (g) after Hayes.

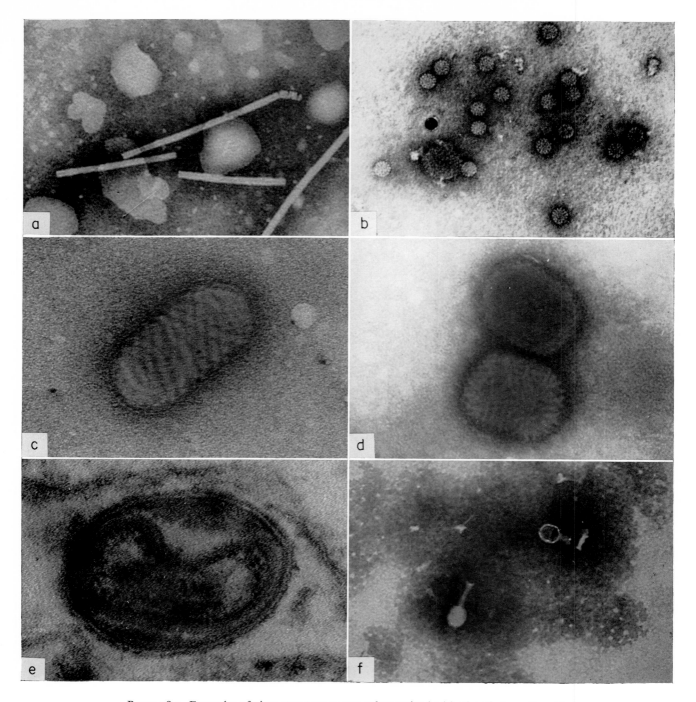

PLATE 18.3. Examples of virus structure as seen when stained with phosphotungstic acid.

(a) A helical virus, tobacco mosaic virus ($\times$ 131,600); (b) an isometric virus, human wart virus ($\times$ 75,200); (c), (d) and (e) are examples of complex animal viruses of the pox group; (c) orf virus from a human case ($\times$ 131,600), (d) viruses of molluscum contagiosum with one empty particle, note the difference in protein substructure ($\times$ 131,600), (e) the internal structure of cowpox virus showing an outer double membrane containing a double-membraned core ($\times$ 203,000); (f) *Escherichia coli* T4 bacteriophage preparation: the particle on the left contains its nucleic acid, whereas the other has an empty head and a contracted tail sheath ($\times$ 56,800).

Preparation (e) by A.G.E. Dunn.

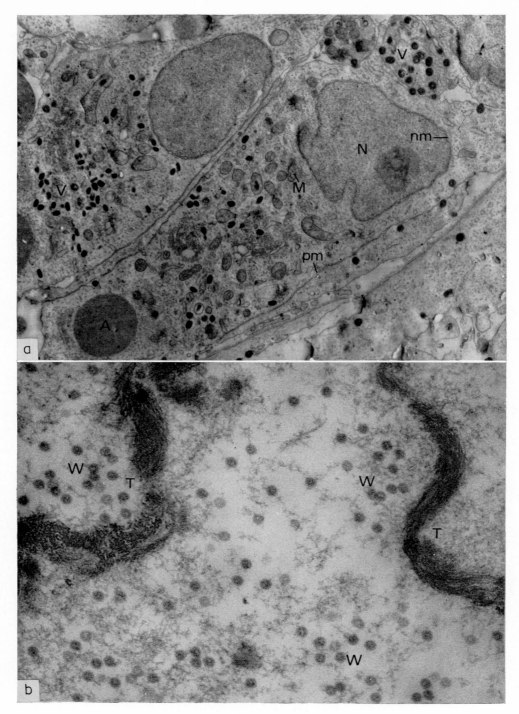

PLATE 18.4. Virus particles in tissue sections.

(a) Low power EM view of a section of a chorioallantoic membrane of a hen's egg infected with cowpox virus. In the cell, the nucleus (N), nuclear membrane (nm), plasma membrane (pm) and mitochondria (M) are seen. The developing virus particles (V) and a type-A inclusion (A) are also noted (×6000).

(b) High power EM view of a section of a stratum granulosum cell showing wart virus particles (W) and tonofibrils (T) in the cytoplasm (×60,000).

Preparations by A.G.E. Dunn.

the particles are infective. In animal viruses, the number of infective particles may be 1–10 per cent, whereas with bacteriophages almost every particle observed is infective.

Non-infective particles, devoid of nucleic acid, are less heavy than infective ones and so can be separated in a caesium chloride density gradient. The more buoyant non-infective particles equilibrate at a higher level in the tube and are accordingly termed the 'top component'.

Nucleic acid

This may be either DNA or RNA but never both. The **genome** may be a single strand of RNA (picorna-viruses), a double strand of RNA (reoviruses), a single strand of DNA (bacteriophage Φx174), or a double strand of DNA (poxviruses). The double-stranded DNA of the papovaviruses is unusual in being circular or super-coiled. The mol. wt. of the nucleic acid in a virus may range from about 1.7×10^6 up to 160×10^6. The size of the strand controls the number of polypeptides that can be coded for or specified by a virus. Thus, a polyoma virus which has relatively little nucleic acid (mol. wt. 3.5×10^6) can specify only ten polypeptides and has a simple protein capsid. In contrast, the T phages of *Esch. coli* with much more nucleic acid (mol. wt. 120×10^6) can specify almost 400 polypeptides and so provide the basis for much more complex external structures.

Structure

The EM shows three types of virus structure, helical, isometric and complex (fig. 18.41, & plate 18.4).

HELICAL VIRUSES

Tobacco mosaic virus (TMV) is a cylinder 300 nm long and 15–17 nm in diameter with a central hole 4 nm in diameter. The protein coat is formed from 2130 identical polypeptide chains, each composed of 158 amino acids and interconnected by hydrophobic bonds; in addition there are noncovalent bonds between the protein subunits and the coil of single-stranded RNA which lies in a groove 4 nm from the centre of the helical virus (fig. 18.41a). X-ray analysis shows that forty-nine protein subunits are required for three full turns of the helix, which has a pitch of 2.3 nm. TMV is a rigid structure and of constant length when fully infective but, in common with other viruses, the protein subunits can assemble in the absence of the nucleic acid and there is then a great variation in the length and stability of the particle.

The helical structure of the myxo-, paramyxo- and rhabdoviruses is not at first evident and in the EM the two former appear pleomorphic and the latter is bullet-shaped (figs 18.41b & c). Treatment with ether ruptures their outer structure and releases the internal helical nucleoprotein. As the nucleoprotein helix of the myxo-viruses is 600–1000 nm long and is confined in a sphere of

80–120 nm diameter, it must be flexible. The mode of packing of the nucleoprotein in the outer, ether-sensitive structure is still unknown.

Phages also show helical symmetry. The filamentous phages of *Esch. coli* (coliphages) are 800–850 nm × 6.5 nm. The single-stranded DNA is thought to be in the form of a closed circle pulled taut so that the two strands lie parallel, surrounded by protein. The structure has been likened to a phage tail. The filamentous phages of *Pseudo-monas* bacteria are longer (1600 nm × 7.5 nm) and are flexible like the helices of the myxoviruses. This flexibility allows the development of rope-like structures which can be seen in EM preparations.

ISOMETRIC VIRUSES

A spherical virus, when examined by X-ray diffraction, shows 5:3:2 symmetry, i.e. it is an icosahedron (figs. 18.42 & 44). EM studies confirmed the presence of this

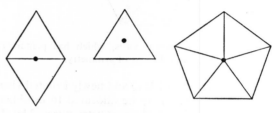

FIG. 18.42. The 2-, 3- and 5-fold axes of symmetry seen in icosahedral viral structure.

configuration in spherical viruses from many plant and animal sources, and it is the accepted fundamental structure of isometric viruses. A sphere can be formed from sixty identical or very similar subunits, but as no virus has yet been shown in the EM to have sixty morphological units, the actual substructure of a virus capsid was unresolved until attention was drawn to the architectural system exploited in the modern construction of geodesic domes. This involves the triangulation of a sphere into quasi-equivalent triangles grouped in fives and sixes. Isometric viruses could likewise be subdivided by triangulation of the twenty equilateral triangles to produce an icosadeltahedron defined by its triangulation number T; this is the number of equilateral triangles contained in the area defined by the three adjacent five-fold axes of symmetry (fig. 18.43b).

If each of the smaller equilateral triangles is composed of three asymmetric subunits, the total number of sub-units in the icosadeltahedron would be $20 \times T \times 3 = 60T$; when $T = 16$, the total number would be 960. These sub-units can be grouped in dimers, trimers or hexamers (fig. 18.43); at the vertices they occur in pentamers (fig. 18.44).

These morphological units or **capsomeres** are responsible for the substructure seen in PTA-stained preparations. The substructural arrangement of adenovirus ($T = 25$) and herpesvirus ($T = 16$) has been established

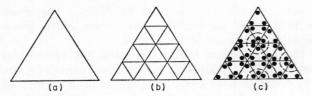

FIG. 18.43. One face of an isometric virus is shown (a), subdivided into sixteen equilateral triangles (b) when T=16. Each of the small triangles is defined by three subunits (●) grouped in hexamers on the faces and at contiguous edges of large triangles (c).

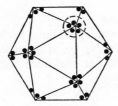

FIG. 18.44. An icosahedral virus, which has pentamer groupings at each five-fold axis of symmetry.

beyond doubt (fig. 18.41d & e) and newly isolated viruses from unrelated sources may be allocated to established groups on the basis of their substructure. The EM interpretation of the structure of the smaller viruses is difficult and the number of capsomeres has not yet been established with certainty (table 18.5). When T=7, enantiomorphism occurs, the right- or left-handedness of the structure must be stated. Human wart virus is therefore defined as 7D (dextro) while rabbit papilloma, its

mirror image, is 7L (laevo). In contrast to the protein subunits of TMV, which are identical and in which the sequence of amino acids is known, the composition of the subunits of isometric viruses is not known and it is not certain that all 60T subunits are identical.

Plant viruses, e.g. turnip yellow mosaic virus (T=3) also exhibit 5:3:2 symmetry. Phages show 5:3:2 or 4:3:2 symmetry.

The structural relationship of the nucleic acid to the capsid in the isometric viruses is not yet established, but there is evidence from the adenovirus group that the DNA may be sandwiched between an inner icosahedral protein structure and the capsid. In turnip yellow mosaic virus the RNA penetrates into the thirty-two capsomeres.

COMPLEX VIRUSES

Poxviruses may appear to be brick-shaped when dried and examined as shadow-cast preparations in the EM, but PTA-staining reveals their external structure. When they are cut in sections (fig. 18.41f), there is an outer double membrane which is virus-specific, an inner elongated core containing DNA and two lateral bodies of unknown significance.

Some *Esch. coli* phages have a very complex structure; there is an isometric head containing the DNA and internal protein. The tail is made up of a core with a sheath composed of twenty-four rings, and in addition, there are six tail fibres and a base plate with six spikes (fig. 18.41g).

ADDITIONAL STRUCTURES

Lipoprotein envelopes occur in myxo-, paramyxo-, leuko-, rhabdo- and herpesviruses. In the first four cases, the outer

TABLE 18.5. The properties and structural characteristics of some viruses.

Virus	Nucleic acid	Stranded-ness	mol. wt. of NA × 10^6	Size of virus (nm)	Nucleo-capsid	Length of helix or number of capsomeres	Proportion of the bases in NA					
							A	T	U	G	C	HMC
PLANT												
TMV	RNA	S	2	300 × 15	H		30	—	26	25	19	—
PHAGE												
T-even	DNA	D	120	200 × 65	Complex	—	32·5	32·5	—	18	—	17
Φx174	DNA	S/C	1·7	25	I	12	25	33	—	23	19	—
f2	RNA	S	ca 1	20–25	I	?92	22	—	25	26	27	—
ANIMAL												
Influenza	RNA	S	2	80–120	H	600–1000 nm	22–25	—	30–33	18–20	24	—
Reo	RNA	D	10	75	I	92 or 180	28	—	28	22	22	—
Polyoma	DNA	D/C	3·5	30–45	I	42 or 72	26	26		24	24	—
Herpes	DNA	D	70	180	I	162	14	13	—	38	35	—
Adeno	DNA	D	23	70–90	I	252	22	21	—	27	29	—
Vaccinia	DNA	D	160	250 × 300	Complex		31·5	31·5	—	18	19	—

NA, nucleic acid; A, adenine; T, thymine; U, uracil; G, guanine; C, cytosine; HMC, hydroxymethylcytosine; S, single; D, double; S/C, single, circular; D/C, double, circular; I, isometric; H. helical.

lipoprotein coat is formed from part of the plasma membrane of the infected cell. In contrast, herpesvirus derives its envelope from the nuclear membrane of its host cell.

Protein appendages are found on the surface of the myxoviruses and paramyxoviruses; these are haemagglutinin spikes which enable the viruses to combine with their specific receptors on the surface of red blood cells and on epithelial cells. The spikes are 8–10 nm long and are distributed over the lipoprotein membrane (fig. 18.41b). Rhabdoviruses have similar projections (fig. 18.41c).

Adenoviruses have fibres with terminal knobs that protrude from the pentamers under certain conditions. These structures are functional, as they correspond to the C antigen which are responsible for the specific haemagglutinating and cytotoxic properties of the adenovirus. The fibre, knob and pentamer are sometimes referred to as the penton (fig. 18.41d).

VIRAL ENZYMES

Very few viruses possess enzymes. Myxo- and paramyxoviruses have a neuraminidase which is possibly located near the base of the haemagglutinin spikes. Neuraminidase releases sialic acid (neuraminic acid) from glycoprotein substrates that occur at the surface of erythrocytes and are also present in many mucous secretions in the respiratory and intestinal tracts. The enzyme is very active and is responsible for the elution of the virus from red blood cells *in vitro*. Its ability to break down mucoproteins containing sialic acid probably facilitates viral contact with epithelial cells of mucous membranes *in vivo* and may be involved in release of virus from infected cells. The neuraminidase is strain specific and not related to the haemagglutinin.

The paramyxoviruses can also lyse red blood cells *in vitro* but the mechanism is not yet known.

The presence of ATPase has been reported in avian myeloblastosis virus, herpes virus, murine leukaemia virus and Newcastle disease virus. The envelope of each of these viruses is derived from the host cell and the occurrence of ATPase in the virus seems to be dependent on its initial presence in the host cell. In these four viruses, therefore, the ATPase is thought to be derived from the cell and not virus-specified.

ATPase and ATP have also been detected in the tails of coliphages that have contractile sheaths. The enzyme and its substrate may be a built-in store of energy, required for contraction of the sheath, but this is speculative.

Phages are known to contain a muramidase (lysozyme) with which they cleave the linkages of *N*-acetyl muramic acid with *N*-acetyl glucosamine in the bacterial cell wall.

Recently a DNA-dependent RNA polymerase (vol. 1, p. 12.9) has been detected on the surface of the core of vaccinia virus (a poxvirus) and this plays a part in uncoating of the virus within host cells.

THE PROPAGATION, DETECTION AND ENUMERATION OF VIRUSES

Viruses can be grown in appropriate host cells that supply the enzymes necessary for their energy production. Usually the presence of the virus is declared by the destruction of the cell, but sometimes there are more subtle alterations in the host cell and special tests may be necessary to detect the virus.

Animal viruses

CULTURE IN ANIMALS

At first, animal viruses were cultivated in whole animals but this had many limitations. If the host animal has already a latent viral infection, the second virus may trigger this off or the virus may be unable to replicate because of interference from the resident virus. Moreover, adult animals may have developed an immunity to various viruses. The only viruses now cultivated routinely in animals are the Coxsackie A viruses and the arboviruses. In both these cases suckling mice are used and this avoids the problem of the test animal having an established immunity to the challenge virus. Coxsackie A virus causes a flaccid paralysis and myositis in the mice whereas the arboviruses are lethal to the animals.

CULTURE IN EGGS

In the early 1930s, fertilized hen's eggs were introduced to grow viruses. Eggs are known to be free from any antibody response and were thought to be devoid of latent viruses, though it is now known that they may carry viruses of the leukosis group. Embryonated eggs are still used to propagate some viruses.

Ten to twelve day-old chick embryos are used for the growth of poxviruses and herpes simplex virus; the virus is introduced on to the surface of the chorioallantoic membrane which has been separated artificially from the shell membrane to form a new air space (fig. 18.45). After incubation for 48–72 hours, necrotic areas or **pocks** develop on the membrane. These pocks are characteristic

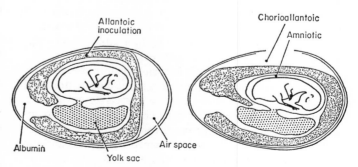

FIG. 18.45. Routes of inoculation used for the implantation of viruses in embryonated eggs.

for the virus; with variola and herpes simplex they are small, white and discrete, with vaccinia they are larger, cream-coloured and less clearly defined, and with cowpox, haemorrhagic. Not only can the type of pock be used to distinguish different viruses, but pocks can be counted and, as one infective virus particle can produce one pock, the number of pock-forming units (PoFU) per ml is a measure of the number of infective particles in a virus suspension.

The myxo- and paramyxoviruses normally have no visible effect on the eggs, but can agglutinate red blood cells and they can be detected by the haemagglutination reaction. The myxovirus is introduced into the amniotic cavity of a 12-day-old chick embryo. At this stage the embryo has begun to swallow, so the influenza virus gains access to the developing lung buds where it is able to replicate, and the virus is shed into the amniotic cavity. After incubation for 72 hours at 35°C, the amniotic fluid is harvested and examined for haemagglutinin. If influenza A virus is present, it agglutinates guinea-pig and human red blood cells, but not those of the fowl. After a few passages in the amniotic cavity, the original virus, O, becomes adapted to eggs and, when introduced into the allantoic sac, it replicates in the cells that line the cavity. There is then a good yield of derived virus, D, and this method is used in the production of influenza virus vaccine. In addition, when influenza A virus is grown in the cells of the chorioallantoic membrane it develops the ability to agglutinate fowl cells. This is known as the O–D variation.

CELL CULTURE

If cells from disaggregated mammalian or avian tissues are incubated aseptically in a suitable nutrient medium, the cells grow and divide within a few days. The advent of antibiotics greatly facilitated the handling of such cells *in vitro*. Tissues commonly used include monkey kidney, human amnion and chick embryo. Trypsin is usually employed to disperse the cells.

A sample of the dispersed cells is stained with a vital stain and the viable cells counted under the microscope. A suitable dilution is made in nutrient fluid to give 5×10^5 cells/ml and the cell suspension is then distributed into glass or plastic containers. The cells settle on the surface and grow during incubation to form a continuous sheet or monolayer. This is a **primary cell culture.**

The primary monolayer is in turn trypsinized to remove it from the vessel surface, diluted in tissue culture fluid and seeded into two or more culture vessels to produce a **secondary cell culture.** Such cells continue to grow exponentially, if given proper care, for up to forty to sixty cell divisions. The cultures are termed **cell strains** and the individual cells resemble the cells of the parent tissue in their morphological and other characteristics.

After 50 ± 10 divisions, the cells in a cell strain begin

to decline, despite provision of fresh nutrient and the correct environmental factors such as pH, temperature and atmosphere. The cells apparently grow old and die (p. 36.6).

Sometimes a cell strain begins to accelerate its growth rate. This reflects a spontaneous change; the cells no longer have a finite life and they are called a **cell line.** Other associated changes are evident in these cells and they include morphological changes to an epithelioid form, the development of heteroploidy, loss of their sex chromatin and of the Coxsackie A9 virus receptors; the cells support the growth of a wider range of viruses than that sustained by the parent cells. This step is the first on the gradient of transformation (p. 18.109). Unchanged cells (cell strains) do not produce a tumour when they are inoculated into hamsters. Cells that have undergone the change to cell lines produce tumours in hamsters and may be regarded as malignant.

TISSUE CULTURE

In contrast to the use of monolayers of tissue culture cells, it is sometimes advantageous to use a tissue explant to study the growth of a virus. The original method for the growth of tissue was to anchor it to the glass surface by means of clotted fowl plasma. The plasma had a double function, in that it held the tissue in place and protected it from deleterious changes in the environment. Fibroblasts migrate out from the tissue and these can be used as a source of cell monolayers.

Plasma clots are not widely used now, but organized cells are being employed for the cultivation of viruses. Respiratory viruses are known to attack nasal and tracheal epithelium; they can be grown on small pieces of trachea that have been excised and placed on the roughened surface of plastic Petri dishes. The tissue adheres to the rough surface and plasma is not needed to anchor the cells. The cilia on the epithelial surface are therefore not covered and ciliary movement can be observed with the microscope. Respiratory secretions are deposited on to these tissue fragments and viral growth stops the cilia beating before they stop in control preparations. The infected tissue fragments are then examined histologically and in the EM for evidence of the presence of viruses. By this means it has been possible to increase the number of respiratory viruses isolated.

In a diagnostic laboratory it is usual to employ a primary or early secondary cell strain and a cell line. Examples of cell strains are monkey kidney tissue culture cells used for the isolation of enteroviruses, and strains developed from human foetal material for the growth of a range of viruses including that of chickenpox. HEp–2 cells derived from a human carcinoma are a typical cell line and are used, for example, to grow adenoviruses. As HEp–2 cells began as malignant cells, they probably could never be properly classified as a cell strain. HeLa cells are another commonly used cell line which was derived from a patient (Helen Lane) with carcinoma of the uterine cervix.

DETECTION OF VIRUS IN TISSUE CULTURE

The introduction of a virus into a tissue culture may give rise to a recognizable change in the cells, called a **cytopathic effect** (CPE). The form of this varies; thus adenoviruses cause cells to swell and form cytoplasmic processes; wild strains of herpesvirus and poliovirus produce a rounding of the cells; measles and laboratory strains of herpes produce syncytia, and Coxsackie B and echoviruses shrivel the cells. The CPE spreads gradually from the infected cells throughout the cell sheet which is completely destroyed but it is possible to confine the effect by incorporating specific antiserum, agar or methylcellulose in the medium. In this way the foci of infection are restricted to their original positions and, as one virion may give rise to one focus of infection or **plaque**, the infectivity of a viral suspension can be determined and expressed in plaque-forming units (PFU)/ml.

The growth of some viruses may not be associated with a CPE. This is the case when influenza viruses are grown in monkey kidney (MK) cells but, as they produce a haemagglutinin, their presence can be detected by mixing a suitable suspension of erythrocytes with a sample of the culture fluid and demonstrating **haemagglutination**. If erythrocytes are added directly to the infected MK cells, they adhere to the tissue culture cells and are not removed by washing with saline. If a suitably diluted virus inoculum is used, this **haemadsorption** test makes it possible to count the foci of infection. The haemadsorption effect presumably depends upon the assembly of haemagglutinin for progeny virus at the surface of the MK cells which then become adhesive for the erythrocytes.

Rubella virus causes neither an obvious CPE nor haemadsorption but can be detected by an **interference phenomenon**. For this, the virus is inoculated into African green monkey kidney (AGMK) cells and, after incubation for a few days, it is challenged with a virus that normally produces a CPE in AGMK cells. If the rubella virus has replicated in the cells, it interferes with the multiplication of the challenge virus and no CPE results. Controls are necessary to ensure that the challenge virus produces a definite CPE.

Another method of detection of virus growth depends on the fact that tissue culture cells produce CO_2 during growth. In the **metabolic inhibition test** the growth medium contains an indicator that shows the gradual fall in pH during the normal growth of the cells; if a virus is introduced, the cells cease to respire and the pH of the medium is unchanged. This test is useful in the study of the neutralization of enteroviruses by antisera. Addition of specific antiserum neutralizes the challenge virus and the tissue culture cells into which the virus–serum mixture is introduced continue to grow. The medium therefore becomes acid in contrast to the virus-infected controls.

Cell fusion

A virus existing in a cell (A) in which it cannot complete its replication cycle may be recovered or recalled by fusing a different cell (B) on to cell A. The process of cell fusion is initiated by adding a suspension of inactivated paramyxovirus (e.g. Sendai virus) to the mixed cells and this induces them to adhere. The viral nucleic acid can then pass from the non-productive to the productive cell and new virions are produced. This promises to be of importance in the study of animal viruses.

Bacterial viruses

When a bacteriophage infects a sensitive bacterium, it can either replicate and lyse the host cells (visible like the CPE of animal viruses) or it may be incorporated in the host genome in a state of lysogeny. A **lytic response** is manifested when a liquid culture of the host bacterium clears or when areas of clearing (plaques) develop after a suitably diluted suspension of virus is sown on a 'lawn' of sensitive bacteria growing on a plate of culture medium (fig. 18.46). These plaques may be small or large, with

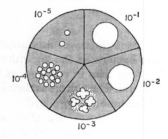

FIG. 18.46. The patterns of lysis produced when drops of graded dilutions of a phage suspension are applied to a lawn of a sensitive bacterium. Confluent lysis has been produced by the 10^{-1} and 10^{-2} dilutions, semi-confluent lysis by the 10^{-3} dilution and discrete plaques have been produced by the 10^{-4} and 10^{-5} dilutions.

clearly defined or diffuse edges; such features are stable characters and are useful in genetic analysis. **Lysogenic bacteria** carry the phage genome (prophage) integrated with the bacterial DNA. Occasionally the prophage expresses itself and then replicates and lyses the cell. This can be induced artificially by ultraviolet light or by mutagens such as nitrogen mustard (p. 29.4), hydrogen peroxide or mitomycin C (p. 20.14). The prophage is normally inhibited from replication in the lysogenic state by the presence of virus-specified repressor substance that controls the operon for the structural genes (vol. 1, p. 38.3). Ultraviolet light destroys the repressor substance and thus allows the phage to replicate. The presence of prophage and its repressor endows the host bacterium with immunity to similar phages; although the second phage may enter the cell, it cannot replicate because the repressor substance produced in response to the prophage is in control (fig. 18.47).

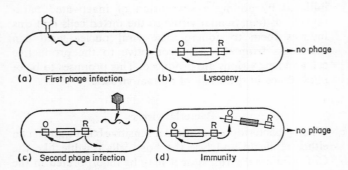

FIG. 18.47. Immunity conferred by lysogeny. Phage DNA is injected into the host bacterium (a). If the lysogenic state is established (b), a substance produced by the repressor (R) acts on the operon (O) within the phage DNA and represses the production of new infective phage. When a second related phage attacks the lysogenized cell (c), its DNA is injected but is immediately repressed (d) by the existing repressor substance.

To grow a lytic bacteriophage, it is usual to employ a culture of sensitive bacteria in the logarithmic phase and to introduce phage particles in numbers at least equal to the number of bacteria. The culture is then incubated and aerated for 90 min, time for two cycles of replication. A few drops of chloroform are then added to kill any residual bacteria and release any phage retained in intact cells. The suspension can be lightly centrifuged to remove the cellular debris and the resultant supernate containing the phage is tested for its infectivity. If the phage is required for phage typing, the routine test dilution (RTD) is determined by placing drops of tenfold dilutions of the phage suspension on a lawn of sensitive bacteria. The highest dilution that causes confluent lysis is taken as the RTD. In the example shown in fig. 18.46 the 10^{-2} dilution would be used in subsequent phage-typing experiments. The number of plaques can be counted at the 10^{-4} dilution and so the actual number of infective phage particles can be ascertained.

The infectivity of a virus preparation can be measured by either the **focal** or **quantal response**. When the focal response is the index, the numbers of foci of infection are counted and by calculation based on the volume and dilution of the inoculum, the infectivity of the original suspension is expressed in pock- or plaque-forming units/

ml. In the quantal or all-or-none response, the lethal dose of the virus required to kill 50 per cent of the animals (LD50) or to destroy 50 per cent of the tissue cultures (TCD50) is calculated (p. 3.6 and p. 20.3).

ANIMAL VIRUS AND HOST INTERACTIONS

There are three stages in the course of most virus infections. First, the virus starts to replicate in a tissue at a particular site in the host. Second, the virus spreads from this site, usually into the blood stream, and third, sites of viral replication are established in target organs such as susceptible cells in the CNS or skin.

Poliomyelitis in man provides a good illustration of these three stages. Infection is usually initiated by the ingestion of the virus, followed by replication in the tissues of the pharynx or alimentary tract. From these local sites the virus reaches the blood and may then attack and destroy nerve cells in the ventral horn of the spinal cord to produce paralysis. Specific and non-specific defence mechanisms may act at any of these stages to limit replication. The pre-existing immunity of the host plays an important part in determining the result of infection. The presence of humoral antibody is usually an effective means of blocking invasion, hence the value of immunization against virus diseases such as poliomyelitis and smallpox. Specific antibody acts on the virion only, and therefore may afford marked protection during the dissemination of the virus via the blood. However, IgA antibody can be detected in normal secretions and may act directly at the first stage of initiation of infection. Excess antibody may block adsorption of virus to a specific receptor on the host cell. In low concentrations, antibody may yet prevent penetration of virus into a cell, even after attachment of the virus to the cell surface, and antibody at the surface of the virion within the cell may interfere with the uncoating mechanisms.

IgE antibody (p. 22.11) mediates the type I hypersensitivity reaction (p. 22.19) and so may enhance defence mechanisms. The resulting local inflammation and exudation of serum antibody may increase concentrations of humoral antibody reaching the site of virus attack. Various nonimmunological mechanisms may also be enhanced in this way. Local acidity and reduced oxygen pressure at the site of inflammation may have an antiviral effect. A rise of local temperature of as little of 2°C may be critical for the growth of some viruses, e.g. variola.

Once the invading virus is established within target cells, antibody is usually not effective, although it may limit the further spread of infection. In some instances, e.g. with herpes simplex virus, virus may spread directly to adjacent cells without losing the protection of the host cell membrane.

During a primary virus infection, the role of antibody in determining the outcome of infection is debatable. Individuals with hypogammaglobulinaemia (p. 23.12) produce little or no detectable circulating antibody and are vulnerable to bacterial invasion, but are not so susceptible to viral infection. Interferon production (p. 18.108) may play an important part in recovery from virus infection. In the whole animal, interferon may have local and distant actions. Locally, interferon produced in the cells that are initially infected is available to adjacent cells in high concentration. These conditions are ideally suited to limit the spread of local infection. In addition, following the release of interferon from locally involved cells, it may protect target cells before the virus reaches them. Some of the claims made for the protective effects of interferon should nevertheless be reviewed in the light of recent evidence on the rapidity with which a protective degree of immunity develops at the cell level by immunological mechanisms that do not involve interferon.

Drugs that interfere with the normal host defences may render an individual unduly susceptible to virus invasion, or may activate latent viruses within the host. Patients with leukaemia, especially if they have been treated with X-rays, corticosteroids and other immunosuppressive agents (p. 24.6), may develop disseminated or severe infections with cytomegalovirus and other viruses (p. 18.116).

The replication of viruses

When a bacterial culture in the logarithmic phase of growth is infected with sufficient phage to give more than one phage particle per host bacterium, the initially turbid culture becomes translucent within about 30 min due to the replication of the phage and lysis of the host cell. If the culture is sampled for its phage content at regular intervals during this period the results may be expressed graphically as in fig. 18.48.

This represents a **one step growth curve** which is achieved when all the host cells are infected with phage simultaneously and the culture is examined for the presence of phage without artificial lysis of the host cell. As the cells have not been artificially lysed, the number of infective phage particles per infected cell does not appear to vary during the first 20 min; each unlysed bacterium is equivalent to one **infective centre**, no matter how many phage particles it contains (see below). The time represented by this part of the graph is known as the **latent period**. An animal virus–host cell system gives comparable results when the experiment is carried out under similar conditions, but the time scale would be in hours rather than in minutes.

If the same experiments are carried out with either the phage–bacterium or animal virus–mammalian cell sys-

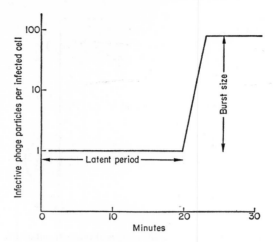

FIG. 18.48. The one-step growth curve of a phage.

tem, and the host cells are lysed before the amount of virus is estimated, the results are different. Fig. 18.49 shows three stages (a) adsorption and penetration, (b) eclipse,

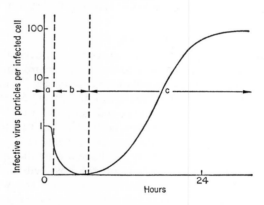

FIG. 18.49. Stages in the multiplication of virus particles during growth *in vitro*. After (a) adsorption and penetration (b) there is an eclipse phase followed by (c) maturation and release of virus.

and (c) maturation and release. With the phage, stage (a) is extremely short and the eclipse phase ends about 10 min after infection. New infective virus can be detected earlier in cells artificially lysed than in unlysed cells, because no matter whether each infected host cell contains one or 100 infective virus particles it will give rise to only one infective centre if its virus content is not artificially liberated.

For quantitative measurements on virus-infected cells, it is necessary to find out the number of infective centres in a culture and this can be done by plaque production with unlysed cells (fig. 18.50). Alternatively in the phage–bacterium system, the number of infected bacteria can be calculated by estimating the number of uninfected bacteria (after adsorption of the phage) and subtracting this number from the initial viable count

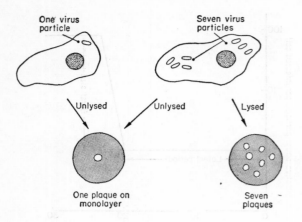

FIG. 18.50. The effect of artificial lysis of the host cell on the demonstrable number of infective virus particles.

of the bacterial culture employed. When the number of infected host cells is known it is possible to calculate the **burst size**, i.e. average number of infective virus particles produced per infected cell (see fig. 18.48).

ADSORPTION AND PENETRATION

The successful attachment of viruses to cells depends on the collision rate. In some virus-host cell systems specific receptor sites on the host cell are necessary; for example, T3, T4 and T7 phages of *Esch. coli* are attached specifically to the middle layer of the cell wall, and T2 and T6 phages to the outer lipoprotein layer. The T2, T4 and T6 coliphages have contractile sheaths; in some cases their tail fibres are activated by tryptophane during the operation that brings them to bear on the host cell surface. The phage then excretes muramidase (p. 18.99) which produces small holes in the cell wall. These can be repaired quickly, but if many phages attach to the host cell, the cell wall may become sieve-like, the cytoplasmic membrane loses its support and the bacterium is destroyed. This is termed **lysis from without**. In the normal course of events, the phage particle injects its DNA and internal head protein into the bacterial cell through the small hole that is subsequently repaired; host cell DNA synthesis is inhibited and phage replication commences. The T-even phages of *Esch. coli* have contractile sheaths which pump their DNA into the host cell, but it is not known how phages with non-contractile tails introduce their DNA into bacteria. After the phage DNA has entered the host cell, its outer protein coat is no longer required and can be removed from the cell with no detrimental effect on phage replication. The RNA phages have specific sites for adsorption on the pili of male bacteria (p. 18.56); by some unknown means they inject their nucleic acid into the pili and from there it travels into the soma of the cell.

Specific receptors are known to exist for only three groups of animal viruses. Myxoviruses and paramyxoviruses attach to the mucopolymers on the surface of the cells of the respiratory tract by means of their haemagglutinin spikes. Enteroviruses require specific lipoprotein receptor sites.

The animal virus–mammalian host cell relationship is very different from the phage–bacterium association on account of the structural differences between the bacterial cell wall and the plasma membrane of animal cells. The plasma membrane of the eucaryotic cell is not rigid (vol. 1, p. 13.6) and viruses can be engulfed by pinocytosis. The whole virus particle is taken into the host cell where the protein capsid is removed, leaving the nucleic acid ready to initiate replication. The adsorption, penetration and uncoating of the virus has been studied in detail in the case of vaccinia virus. Initially the virus is adsorbed by the host cell and appears in a vesicle. In this vesicle, the outer double membrane (fig. 18.41b) is removed by a nonspecific host cell reaction. The resulting core is then released into the cytoplasm by enzymic or mechanical rupture of the vesicle. The DNA remains within the core and cannot initiate replication until the core has been removed. However, on the surface of the core is a DNA-dependent RNA polymerase capable of producing the RNA for the specification of the proteolytic enzyme that effects the necessary break. Thus the first uncoating of vaccinia virus is a nonspecific host reaction, whereas the second is a virus-specified reaction. The events are summarized in fig. 18.51.

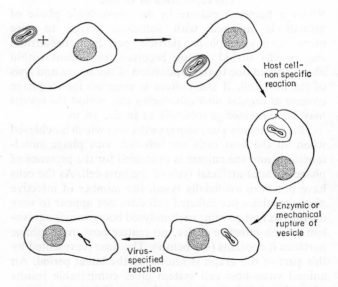

FIG. 18.51. The steps involved in the adsorption, penetration and uncoating processes of a poxvirus infection. The outer membrane of the virus is removed nonspecifically by the host cell, but the viral DNA is released from the core by a virus-specified reaction.

ECLIPSE PHASE

Comparison of figs. 18.49 and 18.50 shows that during the first 20 mins of a phage infection, or a longer latent period in the case of an infection with an animal virus, there is no increase in the number of infective centres. If the host bacteria are lysed by chloroform, or the host animal cells disrupted by physical means, titration of the resulting suspensions on suitable systems shows a fall in the number of infective particles. This is because early in infection the viral genome in the disintegrated cell is subjected to the nucleases present in the cell which destroy the viral nucleic acid; this leads to the fall in the titre of the virus. The critical period when infectious virus cannot be detected in artificially lysed cells is referred to as the **eclipse phase** which continues until progeny virus appears. At that point the titre of infectious virus begins to rise and then exceeds the number of infective centres.

If the cells are lysed artificially, new progeny virus is detectable as soon as it is assembled. The eclipse phase is therefore necessarily shorter than the latent period, which extends from time zero until the natural release of virus from the host cell. If only unlysed cells are examined, the number of infective centres does not show an increase, although some host cells may contain more than one virus particle.

Despite its name, the eclipse phase is a very active period in the replication cycle when the virus particle specifies the enzymes, nucleic acid and structural proteins necessary for its progeny. Much information about this phase comes from study of the T-even phages. The

NH_2

Hydroxymethylcytosine (HMC)

nucleic acid of these phages differs from that of the host DNA in that the cytosine is replaced by hydroxymethylcytosine (HMC). As it is possible to detect HMC chromatographically, its production can be studied by running chromatographs of infected host cell lysates at timed intervals. As the bacterium does not produce HMC normally, new enzymes are required for its production from the free cytosine in the cell and these are specified by the phage. If protein synthesis is inhibited by adding chloramphenicol to a phage-infected culture of *Esch. coli* at time zero (fig. 18.52) no phage nucleic acid or bacterial nucleic acid is produced. In the absence of chloramphenicol, there is only a small increase of DNA in uninfected host cells compared with the large increase in DNA of phage-infected cells. If the chloramphenicol is added at varying times after the infection of the bacterium with phage, the production of phage DNA increases in pro-

portion to the time interval between the infection and the addition (fig 18.53); this indicates that the necessary enzymes are produced early and, once they are synthesized, they assist with DNA replication.

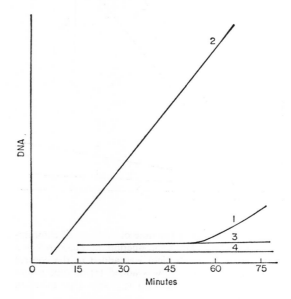

FIG. 18.52. The production of DNA by normal (1) and phage-infected bacteria (2) is inhibited when chloramphenicol is added at time O (3 and 4).

Esch. coli assembles its DNA from the four bases, adenine (A), thymine (T), guanine (G) and cytosine (C); deoxyribose (d) and phosphorylation gives the monophosphate (MP) nucleotides dAMP, dTMP, dCMP and dGMP which are phosphorylated to the respective nucleotide triphosphates before their incorporation into the bacterial DNA is mediated by bacterial DNA polymerase and a bacterial DNA template. In a metabolizing host bacterium there is therefore a pool of nucleotides and nucleotide triphosphates from which a phage can manufacture most of its glycosylated DNA.

The unique feature of the DNA of T-even phages is that HMC takes the place of C. The phage specifies a deoxycytidylate hydroxymethylase that converts dCMP from the bacterial pool into dHMCMP and further phosphorylates this to dHMCTP in preparation for its glycosylation and incorporation into the phage DNA.

In addition, the phage specifies a deoxycytidine pyrophosphatase that converts dCTP into dCMP. Two other phage-specified enzymes then convert this to the uridine and thymidine monophosphates, dUMP and dTMP, which are further phosphorylated by kinases, glycosylated and incorporated into phage DNA.

As the hydroxymethylase interferes with the normal phosphorylation of bacterial dCMP, and as the pyrophosphatase degrades bacterial dCTP, these two enzymes

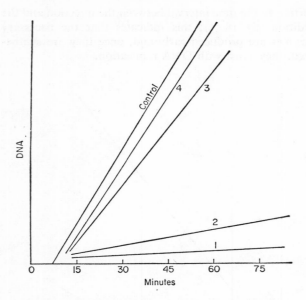

FIG. 18.53. The effect of the time of addition of chloramphenicol on phage DNA production in phage-infected bacteria. No chloramphenicol was added to the control suspension. The antibiotic was added (1) at time o and (2) at 4 min, (3) at 8 min and (4) at 12 min after infection (from Stent).

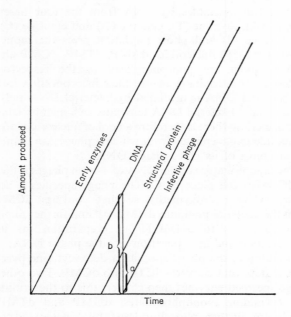

FIG. 18.54. An outline of the sequence of macromolecular synthesis in the production of infective phage. Production of 10–20 equivalents of structural protein (a) and 40–80 equivalents of DNA (b) is necessary before the first infective phage particle is detected.

may be regarded as the proteins that switch off bacterial DNA synthesis.

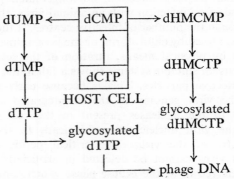

During the eclipse phase, structural phage proteins are also produced and the EM indicates that these are formed after the nucleic acid. The nucleic acid can be seen as coils that develop 8 min after infection with phage; 2 min later the tailless heads are seen, and phage particles, completely assembled, are evident at 12 min. The production of structural proteins can also be traced immunologically since these are antigenic. Fig. 18.54 illustrates the sequence of events. First the early enzymes are produced, next the DNA, then the structural proteins and lastly the infective phage. When the first infective phage particles are produced, there are 10–20 equivalents of structural protein and 40–80 equivalents of nucleic acid. These are still present at the end of the replication cycle and this excess implies that phage replication is an uneconomic exercise.

Animal virus infections

In these there is no convenient unusual nucleotide with which to monitor the production of nucleic acid, but in some cases there is definite evidence of the production of new enzymes that are virus-specified. The nucleic acid of herpes simplex virus contains a high proportion of guanine and cytosine (68 per cent) compared with its host cell (43 per cent). The virus produces an identical DNA polymerase in cells of three different species (human, rabbit and hamster) and so it may be concluded that this enzyme is virus-specified.

The production of arginyl transferase is another virus-specified function present in herpes-infected cells. It is known that arginine is required for the production of the virus and that the codons for arginine are AGA, ACG, CGU, CGA, CGC and CGG. Four of these codons have CG as the first two nucleotides of the triplet and, as herpes simplex virus has a much higher G+C content than its host cell, it is probable that the virus uses at least one of the CG codons to specify arginine. The codons used by the host cell for the specification of arginine may well be AGA or ACG and, if this is so, the cell may lack arginyl transferase(s) for the CG arginine codon(s). The virus would therefore have to specify its own arginyl transferase(s) for the CG codon(s). This appears to be the case, as one new arginyl transferase, distinct from that of the host cell, has been detected in herpes-infected cells.

As with bacterial viruses, animal virus replication is an uneconomic process. The various building blocks are produced in a similar time sequence, but the components of the new virus particle are not all produced at the same site in the host cell. In the eucaryotic cell, the nucleus is membrane-bound, so it is possible for the virions to produce their nucleic acid in either the nucleus or the cytoplasm; the protein capsid and other protein components are produced usually in the cytoplasm. Vaccinia virus is an example of a DNA virus that produces its nucleic acid in the cytoplasm, while both herpesvirus and adenovirus produce their DNA in the nucleus. Influenza viruses produce their RNA in the cell nucleus but paramyxoviruses in the cytoplasm only.

Control of production of virus-specified enzymes
Despite the uneconomic aspect of virus production, there is evidence of control in the sequential production of virus-specified enzymes. In the case of herpes simplex virus, the DNA polymerase (an early enzyme) is produced 2–4 hours after infection, but is followed at 6 hours by a viral DNAase (a late enzyme) which destroys at least some of the excess viral nucleic acid.

With vaccinia signs of regulation are also evident. Two peaks of incorporation of ^{14}C-uridine into RNA are

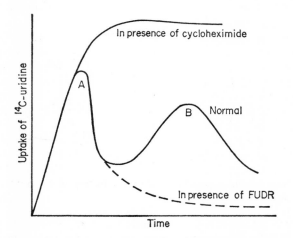

FIG. 18.55. The uptake of ^{14}C-uridine by tissue culture cells infected with vaccinia virus is normally biphasic (see A and B). Peak A represents RNA synthesis specified by the parent (input) virus whereas peak B is due to RNA synthesis specified by progeny virus. Cycloheximide interferes with translation of the RNA so that it accumulates. FUDR inhibits the production of progeny virus DNA so that a template for B is not provided. After Woodson B. (1967). *Biochem. biophys. Res. Commun.*, **27**, 169.

observed (fig. 18.55). Peak A may be due to the transcription of the parental DNA and peak B to the transcription of the progeny DNA. This explanation is acceptable because when cycloheximide, which inhibits translation of m-RNA, is added to the system, the incorporation of ^{14}C-uridine increases. The accumulation of m-RNA results because it is stable for some hours. Moreover if 5-fluoro-2-deoxyuridine (FUDR) is added instead of cycloheximide, the translation of the m-RNA does not cease but the incorporation of ^{14}C-uridine decreases as in the ordinary infection. This is because FUDR inhibits the production of new DNA, so there is no new DNA template for transcription of the second peak of RNA.

Double-stranded viral DNA replicates in the same manner as cellular DNA. The single-stranded viral DNA, such as in the phage Φx174, produces a second strand of DNA on initiation of the replication cycle, and this newly formed double-stranded DNA is sometimes called the replicative form (RF).

RNA viruses
The viruses that contain genetic material in the form of RNA are unique in the biological world and their replication is the subject of much research. Most present knowledge stems from a study of the RNA phages and the reoviruses and enteroviruses. Reovirus is a double-stranded RNA virus that apparently replicates without the aid of DNA. It seems to produce its new nucleic acid in a manner comparable to that of double-stranded DNA. The progeny are similar to the parent, and single-stranded RNA is found in association with the polyribosomes, presumably involved in the production of protein.

The single-stranded RNA viruses are more difficult to comprehend. There is evidence that DNA is required for viral replication in the avian leukosis group but not in some phages and the enteroviruses. On the contrary, there is evidence that a double-stranded replicative form of RNA is produced. Shortly after infection, a new RNA more resistant to RNAase is detected, which may be a double-stranded nucleic acid composed of the (+) input strand and a complementary (−) strand. As the virus replication proceeds, an excess of new (+) strands accumulates in the culture and replicative forms with one or more varying lengths of new (+) strands attached to them are also detected (fig. 18.56). These latter replicative forms with their attached (+) strands are known as replicative intermediates (RI). Tracer studies show that the input virus does not appear in the progeny, so the current theory is that the production of the new (+) strands of RNA involves a conservative mechanism employing only the (−) strand of the RF as template. The new (+) strand is incorporated into the protein capsid which is specified by the (+) strand in conjunction with the polyribosomes.

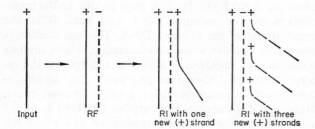

Input RF RI with one new (+) strand RI with three new (+) strands

FIG. 18.56. An outline of the stages involved in the conservative replication of single-stranded RNA in the synthesis of single-stranded RNA viruses. The input (+) strand provides a template for a complementary (−) strand and this complex is the replicative form (RF). The complementary component (−) of the RF then becomes the template for all further RNA synthesis and is called the replicative intermediate (RI).

MATURATION AND RELEASE

When all the macromolecules have been produced, the progeny viruses are assembled and released from the host cell by either bursting or leaking. The T-even phages are examples of bursters with their own mechanism of release. About halfway through the eclipse phase the production of lysozyme starts and when it reaches a critical level **lysis from within** occurs, with release of phage particles. Poliovirus also has an explosive mechanism which results in rupture of the cell and dissemination of the virus.

Many of the animal viruses do not rupture their host cell; instead they leak out over a period of time, and in the process may remove part of the cell membrane. Herpes simplex virus, which is assembled in the nucleus, has a protein capsid 105 nm in diameter, but on passing through the nuclear membrane it acquires an envelope that increases its diameter to 180 nm. The ribonucleoprotein helix (S antigen) of the influenza virus is produced in the nucleus. The haemagglutinin (V antigen) and neuraminidase are produced in the cytoplasm, and there is concurrent alteration of the plasma membrane of the cell. The actual method of assembly and release is uncertain, but the S antigen collects an outer envelope composed of altered plasma membrane with haemagglutinin and neuraminidase incorporated. The virus particle may be extruded from the cell by a process of budding. There is some evidence that the neuraminidase is involved in the release mechanism (p. 18.99).

Interference, exclusion and resistance

The replication of a virus in a host cell can be inhibited by other viruses under certain conditions. A simultaneous infection of a cell by two related types of virus may result in the production of progeny particles similar to the infecting viruses, although some particles may show recombination and phenotypic mixing. However, if the viruses are inoculated at different times, the second may not replicate. This is known as **interference**.

When a bacterium infected with coliphages T2, T4 or T6 is further challenged by a closely related phage, the second phage may attach itself to the infected bacterium and proceed to eject its own DNA. It seems that the initial infection alters the cell wall of the host to make it more resistant to subsequent phage action. The DNA of the second challenge phage fails to penetrate and is vulnerable to extracellular DNAase which degrades it. This is the phenomenon of **exclusion**.

Failure of phage replication in the presence of a normally sensitive bacterial cell may be attributable to two other factors. One is the lysogenic state (p. 18.101). The other applies when a mutation in the host bacterium results in a change in the cell wall that deletes the phage receptors so that the infective process cannot begin. This latter factor is known as host cell **resistance**.

Interferon

This protein is formed in infected cells and interferes with the growth of animal viruses. It has a mol. wt. of about 30,000 and is readily released from the infected cells. Almost all viruses, irrespective of whether they contain DNA or RNA, can induce interferon synthesis, and this has been detected both in tissue cultures and in intact animals, including man. The mechanism may be an important defence against viral infections.

Interferon production is a function of the host cell. Both transcription of host cell DNA and subsequent protein synthesis are necessary for its production (fig. 18.57). This is shown by the inhibitory effects of actino-

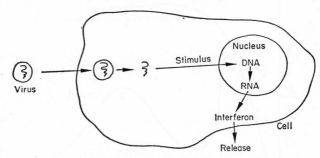

Virus Stimulus Nucleus DNA RNA Interferon Cell Release

FIG. 18.57. A possible mode of induction of interferon synthesis.

mycin D on DNA transcription and of puromycin on m-RNA translation. However, interferon-producing cells do not require to synthesize DNA for this purpose; the DNA inhibitor, FUDR (p. 18.107), has no effect on its production. Interferon can be assayed by its ability to reduce the number of plaques produced by a susceptible virus, and this allows the kinetics of its production to be followed in tissue culture. Interferon is detected soon after the production of infective virus; its concentration rises with that of the virus and falls when the cells show the effects of viral growth. Virulent and freshly isolated viruses, in general, induce less interferon than do laboratory or attenuated strains, as is well illustrated by the poliovirus. This may be due to a direct inhibition by the virulent viruses of host cell function. Inactivated viruses can also induce interferon, as may a number of organisms other than viruses, e.g. *Bedsonia* and *Rickettsia*, some bacteria and some extracts of *Penicillium* moulds. This suggests that interferon production may be a general cellular response to a foreign nucleic acid. Indeed, extracted viral nucleic acids and synthetic double-stranded polynucleotides induce interferon effectively. In the intact animal, endotoxins from Gram-negative bacteria can cause the appearance of interferon in the blood.

The mechanism of interferon induction has not been elucidated. It may occur in a manner similar to derepression (vol. 1, p. 38.2) and the incoming virus may act as a key unlocking the mechanism leading to synthesis of m-RNA and protein.

Interferon is species-specific. Thus a chick cell preparation is active in chick cells but much less effective in mouse cells. Thus it is difficult to manufacture potent interferon preparations for therapeutic trials in man.

Possible mode of action
Any explanation of the action of interferon must account for its activity against both DNA and RNA viruses. It is most effective if applied to cells before the virus, but activity can be demonstrated if it is introduced at the same time as the virus. Interferon acts early in viral replication, probably by interfering with the translation of viral m-RNA (fig. 18.58). In this way it may prevent the combination of the

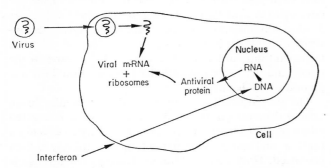

FIG. 18.58. The possible mode of action of interferon in preventing virus replication.

viral m-RNA with the cell ribosomes and thus abort the formation of functioning polyribosomes. As a result, production of early viral enzymes may not occur. The fact that prior treatment of cells with interferon is the most effective means of obtaining inhibition may indicate

that interferon is not the direct inhibitor of viral replication. As the action of interferon may be blocked by actinomycin D and puromycin, it may owe its antiviral activity to induction of the synthesis of an inhibitory protein.

Experimentally, the administration of interferon to animals before challenge with a lethal dose of virus can be protective. In man, if interferon is given intradermally before vaccination at that site, the vaccinia lesion does not develop. Interferon has many of the properties of an ideal antiviral agent but its present clinical applications are limited by difficulties associated with the production of large quantities of purified human interferon and the assessment of its activity in man.

ONCOGENIC AND DEFECTIVE VIRUSES

A brief account of viruses in relation to the causes of cancer in man is given on p. 28.10. It indicates that one or two neoplasms may be attributed to the effect of a virus, but that in the great majority of patients with cancer there is no evidence that a virus is responsible. What follows is an account of some of the properties of several oncogenic viruses; these have opened up a new and fascinating branch of biology. It is safe to say that this has no application to medicine in 1970; whether this will still be true in 1980 or 1990 any of us can guess.

Of the twelve recognized groups of animal viruses, three of the four DNA groups (papovavirus, adenovirus and poxvirus) and two of the eight RNA groups (avian leukosis and mouse tumour virus) have members that can cause tumours *in vivo* or are capable of transforming cells *in vitro*. Most oncogenic DNA viruses differ from RNA viruses in two ways. First, viruses are not detected in cells transformed (see below) by DNA viruses, but are present in those transformed by RNA viruses; second, most oncogenic DNA viruses do not produce tumours in their natural hosts, whereas most RNA viruses do.

Transformation
Tissue culture cells may transform spontaneously when the cell strains become cell lines (p. 18.100) but transformation can be induced by a number of factors that include carcinogenic agents and X-rays; in addition, polyoma virus, adenovirus and some RNA viruses transform certain cells. Cells after transformation have lost their property of **contact inhibition.** When cells are growing normally, they divide and then may glide over each other so that they lie in an orderly monolayer with no overlapping (fig. 18.59). Stoker has postulated that contact inhibition is due to emission and reception of signals between cells. Once a cell has been transformed, it no longer glides over its neighbours; it tends to lie on top of them and this lack of orientation results in a pile-up

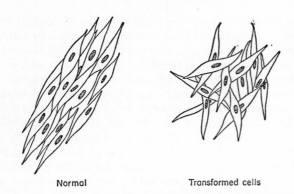

Fig. 18.59. A comparison of the different patterns of growth of normal and transformed fibroblasts *in vitro*.

of cells and a very different type of growth (fig. 18.59). Because transformed cells no longer emit signals, contact inhibition is lost. They still appear to receive signals however, because they can be confined by normal, untransformed cells. Virus-transformed cells gain the ability to grow out and form colonies in agar and this is exploited in studies of transformation. In addition, heteroploidy develops and their character is altered (p. 18.100). New antigens are expressed and this important change is discussed below.

Oncogenic DNA viruses

Polyoma virus, isolated from leukaemic mouse tissue but not the cause of the leukaemia, can replicate in mouse tissue *in vitro* and produce a CPE in the cells. Subsequent inoculation of the virus into normal suckling mice induces various types of tumour. If the virus is introduced into kidney cells of baby hamsters *in vitro*, little if any infective virus is produced but a number of the cells are transformed and no longer grow in an orderly fashion.

The proportion of cells transformed by polyoma virus (1–2 per cent) is only one-tenth of that transformed by Rous sarcoma virus, RSV (p. 18.95 and p. 28.10), but nevertheless the polyoma–hamster kidney cell system has proved a useful laboratory tool in the investigation of oncogenic viruses. The nucleic acid content of polyoma virus with a mol. wt. of $3 \cdot 5 \times 10^6$ can specify ten polypeptides; most of their functions have now been recognized although the actual part of the nucleic acid responsible for their specification has not yet been identified. Yet polyoma virus, unlike RSV, cannot be detected in the transformed cells and it cannot be induced by any of the methods used for the recall of lysogenic phage (p. 18.101). However, new antigens, known as a T or tumour antigen, and a transplantation antigen are also developed. The latter term is derived from the rejection of transformed cells transplanted into normal animals.

The evidence that at least part of the genome of the polyoma virus is present in the transformed cells is as follows:

(1) T antigen reacts with serum from an animal with a polyoma tumour, but not with serum from an uninfected animal, and is therefore thought to be virus-specified;

(2) a virus-specified m-RNA, which hybridizes with polyoma DNA but not with cellular DNA, has been detected in transformed cells.

Only part of the viral nucleic acid is necessary for transformation of baby hamster kidney cells. If polyoma virus is exposed to ultraviolet light, it can no longer produce new virus in mouse tissue culture cells but can still transform hamster kidney tissue culture cells. Just how this part of the polyoma genome is carried by the transformed cells is not understood.

Although adenovirus and SV40 (p. 18.95) produce tumours in suckling hamsters, they do not usually produce tumours when inoculated into adult animals. These viruses readily transform cells *in vitro*, and such cells also develop T antigen which reacts specifically with serum from animals carrying tumours induced by the same type of virus; e.g. cells transformed with adenovirus type 12 develop a T antigen that reacts only with serum from an animal bearing a tumour induced by cells transformed by type 12 virus. The T antigens do not correspond to the capsid antigen or protein, and do not require the replication of all the viral genome for their production. This can be illustrated by inhibition studies. If either FUDR or cytosine arabinoside is added to the virus infected cells, virtually no DNA is produced, but T antigen can be detected. The production of T antigen however depends on protein production since it is inhibited by actinomycin D.

The T antigens can be detected by complement-fixation tests with sera from tumour-bearing animals. They are developed in cells that have been transformed *in vitro* or *in vivo*. Fluorescent antibody procedures have demonstrated T antigen in the nuclei of transformed cells and transplantation antigen at the surface. It is clear that the oncogenic virus specifies both the T antigen and the transplantation antigen.

The development of transplantation immunity in an animal depends on its age. When SV40 virus is injected into a newborn hamster, the animal is likely to develop a tumour, and complement-fixing tumour antibody is then produced. However, no tumour develops when SV40 is injected into a young adult hamster; moreover, the adult animal thereafter rejects an inoculum of cells transformed by SV40 which would induce tumours and complement-fixing T antibody in an adult hamster not previously exposed to SV40. Thus, experience of SV40 before challenge with SV40-transformed cells results in transplantation immunity. Fluorescent antibody studies indicate that the antibody responsible for transplantation immunity acts at the surface of the cells. The relationship between the T antigen and the transplantation antigen is not clear. T-antigens produced in cells of different species are indistinguishable immunologically and this also holds for the corresponding transplantation antigens.

COMPLEMENTATION IN DNA VIRUSES

A number of years ago, attempts were made to adapt an adenovirus to monkey cells so that it might be used as a vaccine. The virus grew in the cells and produced T antigen, but SV40 antigen was also produced. When SV40 and monkey-kidney-adapted adenovirus were added simultaneously to simian cells, the number of adenovirus particles observed in EM sections of the cells was greatly in excess of the number obtained when the adapted adenovirus was added alone. The adenovirus vaccine was examined in more detail and shown to be contaminated with the SV40 genome; a salutary lesson for the producer of virus vaccines.

In human cells, adenovirus carries out its replication cycle of adsorption, penetration, uncoating of nucleic acid, production of T antigen in the nucleus, replication of DNA with transcription and migration of m-RNA for capsid protein into the cytoplasm, translation of the m-RNA to give capsid protein, migration of capsid

protein back into the nucleus, maturation and finally release of the new virus particles (fig. 18.60). In simian cells, however, the adenovirus cycle of replication is incomplete. The T antigen and viral DNA can be detected but no capsid antigen is produced. There is evidence that adenovirus m-RNA is present in the cytoplasm of the infected simian cells, so that the cycle seems to be blocked at the stage of translation of the m-RNA. Addition of SV40 to this system allows the adenovirus to complete its replication cycle but the presence of adenovirus does not influence the yield of SV 40. This is an example of **non-reciprocal complementation**, since the adenovirus requires assistance from SV40, but the SV40 itself is quite capable of replicating on its own. The action of the SV40 is either to supply the necessary mechanism for the translation of the adenovirus m-RNA or to repress some enzyme in the simian cell that is interfering with the translation. SV40 is not the only simian virus that can supply this function.

Further studies of the simian-adapted adenovirus vaccine show that it is a mixture of two different virus particles. One is the adenovirus and the other is composed of an adenovirus capsid with nucleic acid from both the SV40 and the adenovirus. This latter particle has been named PARA, i.e. **p**article **a**iding or aided by the **r**eplication of **a**denovirus. This is an example of **reciprocal complementation** since the adenovirus cannot replicate in simian cells in the absence of PARA, and PARA cannot replicate in simian cells in the absence of adenovirus. The dependence of PARA on adenovirus for capsid development can be demonstrated by transcapsidation. In this a PARA with an adenovirus type 7 capsid is mixed with an adenovirus type 2 in simian cells. The result is a mixture of PARA with an adenovirus type 2 capsid and adenovirus type 2. All evidence of the type 7 virus has disappeared (fig. 18.61).

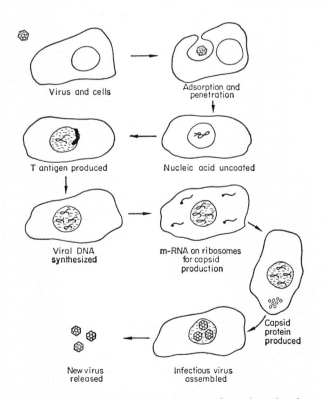

FIG. 18.60. The steps in the replication of an adenovirus in its host cell.

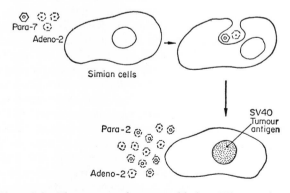

FIG. 18.61. The process of transcapsidation. When a mixture of PARA-7 virus and adenovirus type 2 is added to simian cells, SV40 tumour antigen is produced in the nuclei. The resultant progeny is a mixture of PARA-2 virus and adenovirus type 2.

Oncogenic RNA viruses

When Rous sarcoma virus (RSV) (p. 28.10) is inoculated into a culture of chick embryo fibroblasts, the virus multiplies, some of the cells are transformed and infectious virus can be detected (fig. 18.62). The transformed cells are recognized by the alteration in their

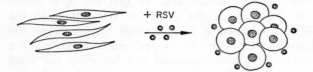

Chick embryo fibroblasts   Transformed cells and RSV

FIG. 18.62. The transformation of chick embryo fibroblasts by Rous sarcoma virus.

shape; they become round, do not exhibit contact inhibition and pile up in disorientated masses. In addition, their generation time is shorter than that of normal cells, which they eventually overgrow.

Under certain conditions, some strains of RSV cannot complete their replicative cycle unless an additional factor is present, and are known as **defective viruses.** An example is the Bryan high titre strain (BH–RSV). If this is added in high concentration to chick embryo fibroblasts, the cells are transformed and virus is produced in the usual way; but if the dose inoculated is reduced by dilution, no transformation occurs and the virus found in the culture medium is incapable of causing transformation. In fact, BH–RSV is a mixture of a transforming factor and a virus that is able to replicate in the chick cells but cannot itself transform them. It does, however, cause erythroblastosis in chickens and has been named the Rous associated virus (RAV). As BH–RSV contains more RAV than transforming factor, the component viruses can be separated by introducing a small dose of BH–RSV, probably containing about ten to twenty RAV and one to two transforming factors, into chick fibroblasts in tissue culture. The spread of RAV is limited by incorporating antiserum to RAV in the medium. After suitable incubation the cells are examined for any foci of transformation. Such cells are removed, trypsinized and reseeded on normal chick cells *in vitro*. The transformed cells grow more quickly than the normal cells and soon foci of transformation are observed but no infective virus can be detected. However, on addition of RAV to the culture, RSV and RAV can both be detected (fig. 18.63). It is concluded that the transforming factor is the RSV genome carried by the transformed cells but that it is incapable of completing its replicative cycle in them. BH–RSV is therefore termed defective RSV. Since the discovery of the original RAV, at least fifty such viruses have been isolated and designated RAV 1–50.

RSV and RAV cannot be distinguished antigenically and the RSV genome appears to be incapable of specifying its own protein coat, being dependent on RAV for this function. The RAV is known as the helper virus and the resultant protein coat of the RSV depends on the antigenic type of RAV used as helper. Thus, if the transformed, nonproducing cells are challenged with RAV-1, the resultant RSV will have an RAV-1 antigenic determinant, whereas if RAV-2 is used the resultant RSV has an RAV-2 protein coat.

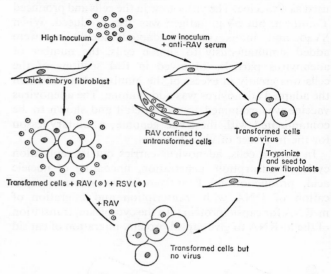

FIG. 18.63. The effect of BH-RSV on chick embryo fibroblasts. BH-RSV is a mixture of RAV and a small proportion of RSV. Introduction of a high inoculum into chick embryo fibroblasts results in transformation of the cells and production of both viruses. A low inoculum added with anti-RAV serum to fresh chick cells results in transformation, but no new virus can be detected in the medium. Virus can be recalled only by adding new RAV to the transformed cells.

The BH–RSV strain is the only one that has been shown to be defective in tests with chicken cells. The Schmidt-Ruppin strain (SR-RSV) is not defective in chicken cells *in vitro* but its yield is increased if RAV is added to the fowl cell–virus system. In mammalian cells, however, SR-RSV is apparently defective. It is capable of transforming mammalian cells but does not produce infective virus. These transformed cells nevertheless carry the SR-RSV genome; if they are mixed with chick cells in the presence of an ultraviolet-treated paramyxovirus (Sendai), the transformed mammalian cells and the chick cells become joined by cytoplasmic bridges. This technique is known as cell fusion (p. 18.101) or heterokaryon formation. After fusion, SR-RSV can be detected and it is thought that the SR-RSV genome which is unable to produce virus particles in the mammalian cell migrates via the cytoplasmic bridges to the chick cell where it is able to complete its replicative cycle. The species of host cell is therefore important in the study of cellular transformation *in vitro*, and the fusion technique may well lead to the detection of viral genomes in cancerous tissue if the correct second species of cell can be found (fig. 18.64).

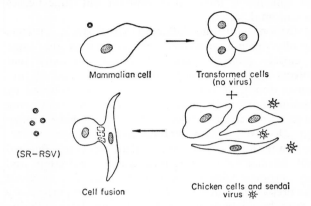

FIG. 18.64. The effect of Schmidt-Ruppin Rous sarcoma virus (SR-RSV) on mammalian cells. The cells are transformed but no virus can be detected unless chicken cells are fused to the transformed mammalian cells by the action of Sendai virus.

MOUSE TUMOUR VIRUS

This virus causes mammary cancer but the genetic strain, sex and hormonal state of the mice influence its development. Inbred females of the CH3 strain of mice have a high incidence of spontaneous cancer of this type which also develops in castrated males treated with oestrogens; this suggests that the female sex hormone is important in the development of the cancer. The foetus of the CH3 mouse is not normally infected *in utero* but infant mice may be infected by their mother's milk (p. 28.10).

CONCLUSION

In the search for a possible causal virus in human cancer, the models described in the previous pages should be borne in mind. In addition to assessing physiological and genetic factors concerning the host, it may be necessary to consider methods used in the recall of viruses unable to complete their replication cycle in the cell that they parasitize. Thus, cell fusion experiments and complementation studies provide approaches to further investigations which may prove of great value to medicine.

ANIMAL VIRUSES OF MEDICAL INTEREST

Picornaviruses

POLIOVIRUSES

At the beginning of the century, infection with poliovirus was widespread among children under 5 years of age, but only an occasional patient developed the typical infantile paralysis. With improvements in sanitation and environmental conditions, fewer young children were involved and the pattern of infection changed; **poliomyelitis** began to occur in epidemics of increasing severity and to affect older age groups. The increasing numbers of young adults affected was serious as both the incidence of paralysis and the mortality rate increase with age.

Poliovirus is worldwide and spreads either directly or indirectly from infected cases or convalescent carriers with no intermediate host. The virus usually gains access by ingestion, and multiplication occurs first in the tonsils, pharynx or small gut, probably in lymphoid follicles. Thereafter it may be recovered from the regional lymph nodes and may then reach the blood. A minor illness may develop at this time, with fever, headache, sore throat and vomiting. However, 90–95 per cent of infections are unnoticed by the patient and inapparent clinically. In a small minority of cases a major illness results from invasion of the central nervous system, probably due to spread by the blood or perhaps along nerve fibres; the illness takes the form of a meningitis (non-paralytic poliomyelitis) or of frank paralysis.

Killed and attenuated vaccines have been developed to combat the virus. As all three antigenic types of poliovirus cause paralytic disease, vaccines must include strains of each. Initially, a formalin-inactivated vaccine (Salk) was produced and reduced the incidence of paralytic disease by 80–90 per cent. Subsequently, attenuated (Sabin) strains of low virulence were developed for each of the three antigenic types, and vaccines incorporating the Sabin strains have now been used successfully on a wide scale (p. 22.22). Attentuated vaccines have advantages over inactivated preparations in ease of administration and in the degree and duration of the immunity that they confer.

OTHER ENTEROVIRUSES

Some strains of Coxsackie and Echoviruses have been associated with paralytic disease. More commonly, infection of the central nervous system with these viruses presents as aseptic meningitis. Coxsackie B viruses are responsible for **Bornholm disease** (pleurodynia, epidemic myalgia); this causes paroxysmal attacks of acute pain in the chest, which is associated with irregular fever and general malaise. The viruses may also cause pericarditis and myocarditis. Echoviruses are also responsible for short febrile illnesses which may be accompanied by a rash.

RHINOVIRUSES

These multiply mainly in the cells lining the nasal cavity and are a frequent cause of the **common cold**. In contrast to the polioviruses, many antigenic types have been recognized and this makes the development of suitable vaccines impracticable.

Arboviruses

Members of this group produce viraemia in a susceptible vertebrate host and are transmitted by blood-sucking arthropods, in whom the virus replicates. A member of this group is responsible for **yellow fever**, which has occurred in epidemics for hundreds of years. Two epidemiological patterns exist and the virus is transmitted from man to man, or from monkeys to man, by mosquitoes of the genus *Aedes* (p. 19.50).

Immunity in man is conferred by vaccination with attenuated strains of the virus. The 17D strain was attenuated by passage in tissue culture and is now grown in the developing chick embryo, and the immunity produced by this vaccine is of long duration. The use of such a vaccine is important not only in controlling the disease in the enzootic areas, but also in protecting travellers to such areas.

Arboviruses which cause **encephalitis** in man are transmitted by mosquitoes or ticks and give rise to recognized diseases in various parts of the world (p. 19.50). The only arbovirus known to be indigenous in the United Kingdom is that of louping-ill. This tick-borne disease of sheep may be occasionally transmitted to shepherds or laboratory workers, some of whom develop meningitis.

Myxoviruses

Influenza arises from infection with influenza A, B or C virus. It presents as a short illness of abrupt onset, with fever, headache, generalized aches and pains and cough. Infection is acquired by inhalation of virus in droplets from the respiratory tract of infected cases. Mortality associated with this condition is usually due to secondary bacterial invasion of the respiratory tract, and this is more likely to occur if there is pre-existing chronic disease of the lungs; a coagulase-positive staphylococcus is most commonly responsible, but *Haemophilus influenzae* may be involved also (p. 18.73).

Strains of the A virus show a marked degree of antigenic variation, and are placed in groups designated influenza A_0, A_1 or A_2. The appearance of a significantly different antigenic variant is attended with major outbreaks of the disease, because of the low level of general immunity to the new variant. In such epidemics, the disease is seen most commonly in patients aged 5–14 years and 25–34 years. Over a period of about 10 years, successive outbreaks produce widespread immunity to a particular family of strains, and this limits their ability to spread. At this stage, a new variant may appear and the previously prevalent strain disappears. Pandemics with influenza A viruses arose in 1918–19 and in 1957. The A_2 strain responsible for the 1957 pandemic was first encountered in China in 1956–57 and spread to Hong Kong early in 1957. Within a few months, it had reached most countries, initially producing local epidemics, often in military camps, schools or hospitals from which the virus spread to the rest of the population.

In contrast to the A virus, influenza B strains show less antigenic variation and, as a result, infection occurs in outbreaks at longer intervals, and these may coincide with influenza A epidemics. Serological studies indicate that influenza C infection is common, but clinical cases are seldom detected.

Infection with one influenza virus strain protects partially against subsequent challenge with the same or closely related viruses. A broad immunity that protects against the reappearance and spread of previously dominant antigenic types may be conferred by immunization with inactivated vaccines containing antigens of strains associated with epidemic infection. However, a new strain has to be incorporated, or administered as a monovalent vaccine. Purified viral haemagglutinin vaccines confer protection and may produce fewer local and systemic reactions than preparations of the whole virus. Patients particularly at risk should be immunized, including those suffering from chronic pulmonary, cardiovascular, renal or metabolic disease and also people in certain occupations, e.g. medicine, education, transport, whose absence from work may disrupt services in the community.

Paramyxoviruses

Infections with the parainfluenza viruses occur usually in children and cause **rhinitis, pharyngitis** and **bronchitis; bronchopneumonia** may also develop. They are also called **haemadsorption viruses** because they confer on infected cells in tissue cultures the ability to adsorb guinea-pig erythrocytes. Each antigenic type is stable and infection is often endemic in large populations. Occasionally epidemics with a single serological type arise. Immunity following infection is not complete and reinfections are usually less severe than the primary infection.

Infection with the **mumps virus** is common in children in all parts of the world and produces painful swelling of the salivary glands; the parotids are usually involved, hence the name epidemic parotitis. Subclinical infection is common and in older patients the testes, ovaries and pancreas may be affected. **Meningoencephalitis** occurs and affects males more often than females. Attenuated vaccines can be produced from strains by serial passage in the chick embryo but are not in regular use.

Measles virus causes a highly infectious disease of children, endemic throughout the world, but epidemics tend to occur every other year in the UK and USA. The characteristic features consist of rhinitis, conjunctivitis and bronchitis with cough and a maculopapular rash. In a child whose food supply is barely adequate, the infection may precipitate a severe state of malnutrition. In this way, measles is responsible for large numbers of deaths in many countries. Secondary bacterial invasion may result in otitis media and broncho-pneumonia. Severe encephalomyelitis and subacute sclerosing panencephalitis (p. 18.117) are very rare complications.

Both killed and attenuated virus vaccines have been produced; the general use of the attenuated virus vaccine is still debatable (p. 22.23).

Respiratory syncytial virus, so called because of its association with respiratory illness and its ability to produce syncytial cytopathic effects in tissue culture, is an important cause of **pharyngitis, bronchitis** and **pneumonia** in young children aged less than 5 years. Annual epidemics of infection in the winter months occur in urban areas in many parts of the world. The virus is unstable during slow freezing and this must be avoided in submitting specimens for virus isolation.

Rubella virus cannot as yet be assigned to any virus group but it is convenient to include it here. It is an RNA virus, sensitive to ether, with a particle diameter of 222 nm and it is capable of agglutinating erythrocytes of some species. **German measles** resulting from infection is mild, with lymphadenopathy and a transient macular rash. The disease assumes importance in pregnancy, especially during the first 4 months, when abortion, stillbirth or congenital defects may be produced. Virus invasion of the foetus occurs via the placenta. The rubella syndrome seen at birth includes anomalies of the eye, ear, heart and CNS. Immune tolerance to this virus does not occur, and the affected infants possess specific neutralizing antibodies. However, despite antibody production, the virus may persist in involved organs for many months after birth and this may reflect a defective cellular immune response, so that the virus is not cleared efficiently by the host. Attenuated rubella virus vaccines are being tested at present.

Rhabdoviruses

These include the causative virus of **rabies**, primarily a disease of carnivores, such as jackals, foxes, wolves and dogs, but a latent infection may occur in bats. The virus is excreted in the saliva, and the bite of a rabid animal can infect any mammal, including man. The disease was formerly widespread and still causes over 20,000 deaths each year in India. It remains endemic in the USA and Europe where national boundaries do not prevent its spread; the relative freedom from this disease in Britain depends on strict enforcement of quarantine laws.

The virus travels from the site of the bite to the brain via the peripheral nerves. The incubation period may vary from 7 days after a bite on the face to 60 days after a bite on the foot. Hydrophobia is often the first symptom, but is quickly followed by painful muscle spasms, delirium and coma. Death follows inevitably.

The virus can be detected in the brain where it produces in neurones a characteristic eosinophilic cytoplasmic inclusion body, the **Negri body**, especially in the hippocampus (p. 25.39). These inclusions are of diagnostic value. In an effort to combat the disease, Pasteur produced one of the earliest examples of a laboratory-prepared vaccine by passaging the 'street' virus in rabbits until he produced a 'fixed' virus; after drying and phenol treatment, it was used as an active immunizing agent to treat possible rabies infections. Even with modern preparations, the course of injections is long and adverse effects are produced. A killed vaccine prepared in duck embryos is a less potent antigen, but produces fewer reactions. Attenuated vaccine strains are also available and may be used in both man and animals.

Adenoviruses

Adenoviruses are responsible for mild respiratory tract infections, **viral pneumonia, pharyngoconjunctival fever,** acute **conjunctivitis,** and epidemic **keratoconjunctivitis** (shipyard eye).

Herpesviruses

HERPES SIMPLEX VIRUS
This may infect man in a number of ways. A vesicular eruption is produced by this virus which has a predilection for skin, mucous membranes and nerve tissue. The appearance of the eruption may be modified in different sites. Primary infection is seen most often as herpetic **gingivostomatitis** in children. Here the vesicular stage of the eruption is short and the lesions observed are usually shallow ulcers on the tongue or mucous membranes of the cheek and lips. During the primary infection antibody is produced, but the virus is not eliminated and it becomes latent within the tissues of the host, perhaps in nerve fibres. Despite the presence of circulating antibody, the virus may be reactivated; this leads usually to a cold sore at the mucocutaneous junction of the lip (**herpes labialis**) or the skin around the mouth and nose may be involved (**herpes facialis**). Many different precipitating factors have been held responsible for this reactivation including sunlight, menstruation, respiratory tract infection and febrile illness.

Apart from the mouth and face, primary and recurrent lesions may be seen elsewhere on the skin, in the eye and in the genital tract. The 'herpetic whitlow' may be encountered on the fingers of nurses and dentists. A severe form of infection of the skin, **eczema herpeticum,** may occur in eczematous children. Primary infection may also present as **aseptic meningitis** or **encephalitis**. Strains of herpes simplex virus can be divided into two serological types. Type 2 strains are associated with genital infections. The cervix uteri may be involved and the virus has been demonstrated in a proportion of biopsy specimens from cases of cervical carcinoma.

The virus is spread by direct contact with a primary or recurrent case. Poor hygiene and overcrowding spread the infection. Thus, although primary infection is frequent in young children, many escape infection at this age, especially if from a good home, and may acquire an infection at an older age. Primary herpetic stomatitis is not uncommon in teenagers and young adults.

VARICELLA-ZOSTER VIRUS

Primary infection is seen usually in children as **chickenpox (varicella)**. The disease presents as a widespread vesicular eruption, occurring in successive crops typically on the trunk, then on the back and face, and proximal parts of the limbs. After recovery, the virus may become latent in the nervous tissue of the host and remain so for many years. **Zoster** (shingles) probably results from reactivation of such latent infection in a partially immune host. It presents as a vesicular eruption, limited to one side of the body and usually to one or two dermatomes. Round cell infiltration and nerve cell destruction occur in the related dorsal root ganglion which is presumably the site of latent infection. The lesions are usually on the trunk, but the fifth cranial nerve may be involved. Varicella may be contracted from other cases of the disease, and epidemics occur. However, it may be acquired also from cases of shingles. Zoster on the other hand occurs sporadically and is not associated with contact with other cases of zoster or varicella.

CYTOMEGALOVIRUSES

These are found in various animal species and all have an affinity for salivary gland tissue. Human infection is widespread although seldom apparent. A severe form of infection occurs in the newborn, who contract the disease *in utero* and show involvement of most organs with the presence of typical inclusion-bearing cells. Infection at this stage may be fatal, although recovery can occur, and virus may be isolated from the throat and urine of such cases for many months, despite the presence of antibody. Evidence of disseminated cytomegalovirus infection may be found in patients with malignant disease of the reticuloendothelial system treated with corticosteroids and radiotherapy. Patients on immunosuppressive therapy may show widespread infection leading to prolonged fever. In these conditions the infection may represent a reactivation of a latent infection and the mechanism may be similar to that involved in herpes zoster infections.

INFECTIOUS MONONUCLEOSIS (glandular fever)

This is a disease of children and young adults and it presents with fever, headache, sore throat and cervical adenitis. Atypical mononuclear cells occur in the peripheral blood and liver function is frequently impaired. In some cases, a heterophile antibody capable of agglutinating sheep erythrocytes appears (**Paul–Bunnell antibody**). The serum of such patients has been found to react also with antigens of a virus which is probably a member of the herpesvirus group. This is the **Epstein–Barr (EB) virus** found in some cell lines derived from tumours of patients with Burkitt's lymphoma (p. 28.10). Thus, the classical form of infectious mononucleosis is associated with a positive Paul–Bunnell reaction and a possible EB virus aetiology. On the other hand, some patients with the infectious mononucleosis syndrome, usually with a negative heterophile antibody test, show evidence of infection with cytomegalovirus. A similar syndrome may occur in patients who have been transfused with whole fresh blood or who have undergone cardiopulmonary bypass procedures during cardiac surgery; these patients also show evidence of infection with cytomegalovirus.

Poxviruses

Smallpox (variola) has been recognized for centuries and was the first infectious disease against which active immunization was developed in man (p. 22.1). The disease is still endemic in India, Pakistan, South-East Asia and parts of Africa and South America, with a consequent risk of infected cases carrying the disease to Western countries. Smallpox usually presents as a febrile illness with severe prostration, headache, backache, and limb pains, appearing 12–13 days after contact with a case. Three to four days after the onset, a facial and peripheral rash appears and develops over some days through macular, papular, vesicular and pustular stages. The mortality from variola major may be up to 25 per cent. Infection with variola minor (alastrim) virus is less severe and has a much lower death rate.

Patients are infectious from the time of appearance of the rash. Infection is primarily by inhalation and may be acquired by contact with a patient or with fomites such as clothing or bed linen, the virus being stable and resistant to drying. An important source of spread is the unrecognized infection that may occur in a partially immune individual.

Active immunity is conferred by vaccination with a living related virus now known as **vaccinia** (p. 22.23).

Control of the disease follows a rigorous vaccination programme, but regular revaccination is necessary. In epidemics strict isolation of patients and contacts is necessary; methisazone (p. 20.36) during the incubation period is helpful.

Other members of the poxvirus group may cause local infections. **Cowpox** may develop after contact with infected animals, usually on the hand where it resembles a vaccinia reaction. Another local infection is produced by the virus of **orf** (contagious pustular dermatitis) acquired from infected sheep. In contrast, **molluscum contagiosum** is contracted only from human cases. The skin lesions in this case are nodular and may persist for several months.

Acute infectious hepatitis and homologous serum jaundice
These closely related conditions are presumed to be of virus aetiology although no virus has been isolated. Clinically, the diseases are similar, but may be distinguished by the features listed in table 18.6.

TABLE 18.6. Distinguishing features of infectious hepatitis and homologous serum jaundice.

	Infectious hepatitis	Homologous serum jaundice
Incubation period	15–40 days	40–160 days
Age group usually affected	Children and young adults	All age groups, mainly adults
Carrier state:		
blood infective	Up to 8 months	? lifelong
faeces infective	Up to 16 months	Faeces not infective
Routes of transmission	Usually by ingestion	Parenteral, ? other
Prophylactic value of γ globulin	Good	Limited, not generally practical

Infectious hepatitis is usually spread by faecal contamination from a patient or convalescent carrier of the disease. A single dose of γ-globulin confers passive protection to contacts and to travellers visiting countries in which the disease is common. The protection is highly effective and lasts about 6 months.

The relation between the agents responsible for these two diseases is unknown. Serum jaundice is transmitted by human blood or serum, usually introduced by transfusion or by the use of improperly sterilized instruments. The **Australia antigen** (Au) has been detected serologically in plasma of patients with serum hepatitus (SH). Particles of 20 nm diameter have been demonstrated in the blood of Au–positive patients, but it seems that these particles are not true viruses and may be protein complexes.

Slow virus infections
These are progressive conditions with incubation periods extending from months to years and apparently associated with a causative virus.

The best example is **subacute sclerosing panencephalitis** which seems to be caused by a myxovirus agent, morphologically and serologically indistinguishable from measles virus. Patients have high titres of antibody to measles virus in blood and CSF. There is a very variable latent period between a recorded attack of measles and the onset of the panencephalitis which may represent an aberrant adaptation of the virus to nervous tissue. The virus may be retained in a defective form in the CNS of those who develop the disease.

Kuru is a progressive and fatal form of subacute cerebellar degeneration that affects the Eastern Highlanders of New Guinea. The women are involved predominantly

and the practice of cannibalism, recently banned, in which brain and other offal was eaten primarily by the females, may account for the distribution of the disease. There appears also to be a genetic predisposition to kuru. The agent is transmissible from brain and visceral organs to chimpanzees and there is an incubation period of 2 years. Thereafter, the disease can be passed in chimpanzees with an incubation period of 1 year.

Kuru in man resembles scrapie and related slowly progressive neuromyopathies of sheep and other animals. The scrapie agent is remarkably resistant to deleterious agents. It is thermostable at 80°C, resists ultraviolet irradiation, is stable over a wide pH range, is highly resistant to formalin, and resistant to enzymes that range from proteinases to phospholipases. The scrapie agent therefore lacks the characteristics of recognized virus particles and some evidence suggests that it has a major carbohydrate component. It is transmissible and passes through filters of less than 100 nm pore diameter. Work in this field is at the crossroads of conventional virology, genetics, biochemistry and experimental pathology. The clinical and pathological features of these diseases resemble in some respects chronic degenerative diseases of the nervous system in man, such as multiple sclerosis and amyotrophic lateral sclerosis.

Waterson has pointed out that slow virus infections of the CNS share with models of viral oncogenesis:
(1) a common requirement for access to a susceptible host at a critically early age and
(2) a prolonged phase of latency. There are sound reasons for regarding the lysogenic state in bacteria (p. 18.101) as a basis for further investigations in these important areas.

Diagnostic methods for viral infections
The three approaches to the laboratory diagnosis of viral infections are:
(1) the isolation and identification of a virus known to be associated with the presenting clinical disease,
(2) the demonstration of virus particles or characteristic histopathological changes in affected tissues or material from the patient, and
(3) the demonstration of a serological response to a particular virus or virus antigen.

VIRUS ISOLATION
As in diagnostic bacteriology, the collection of the proper specimens at the appropriate time greatly influences the likelihood of success. The correct methods of transport for specimens and prompt delivery are important. In general, dry swabs should not be used. To avoid desiccation in transport, swabs or scrapings should be placed in medium, such as Hanks' balanced salt solution (BSS), and kept refrigerated until collected. The medium may be supplemented with a protective agent

such as gelatin or bovine serum albumin. Samples of tissues, exudates, blood, vesicle fluid and CSF should be sent without placing in transport media. A brief clinical history, indicating the date of onset of illness and, if possible the suspected causative virus, helps the laboratory staff to select the most useful tests.

In the laboratory, specimens are usually treated with penicillin, streptomycin and an antifungal agent to suppress contaminants. An account of the treatment of a specimen of faeces outlines these points. A 10–20 per cent suspension of the sample is made in Hanks' BSS, centrifuged to remove the debris, treated with antibiotics and allowed to stand for 2–3 hours; it is then inoculated into the appropriate culture systems. CSF is inoculated directly and not treated with antibiotics. If inoculation cannot be performed immediately, specimens are held at a very low temperature such as −30°C or −70°C.

To cultivate a virus it must be inoculated into a suitable cell system. This may be a tissue culture preparation, chosen from a number of primary cell strains or continuous cell lines, or embryonated hen's eggs, or a susceptible animal. Historically, viruses were first grown in animals and then chick embryos were used. The development of antibiotics made the use of tissue culture methods practical, and these are now the mainstay of diagnostic virology.

No single cell system is ideal for routine testing and it is common practice to inoculate several cell types. Primary cell strains such as monkey kidney, human amnion or human embryo lung and human cell lines such as HEp-2 or HeLa may be used; the choice depends on the availability of the appropriate systems and the likely causative agent. It is here that the clinical information can be of great importance as a guide.

After inoculation, cultures are incubated at 35°C and examined microscopically for several weeks for signs of virus growth. Observation of the type of CPE that develops may, in the light of the source and clinical data, indicate the identity of the causative virus, but the diagnosis may not be straightforward. It may be necessary to harvest the fluids from the tissue culture system first seeded, and pass them to fresh culture cells before a CPE becomes apparent. False positive results may arise from the reactivation of latent viruses in the animals from which the cell culture was prepared, e.g. SV40 (p. 18.111). A toxic substance in the original specimen may give a false CPE, e.g. drugs present in faecal specimens. Such a false CPE is not maintained in serial passage. Final identification of the virus isolated usually depends on serological procedures (see opposite).

A number of viruses are still isolated readily in the developing chick embryo or its membranes. These include influenza A, mumps, variola and vaccinia viruses.

Members of the poxvirus group and herpes simplex virus can be grown on the surface of the chorioallantoic membrane, where they produce characteristic pocks. The appearance of the pocks is often virtually diagnostic but the identity of the virus may be confirmed by the suppression of pock formation by specific antiserum. To distinguish between variola major and variola minor, incubation of inoculated eggs is carried out at different temperatures, since variola minor does not produce pocks at or above 38·3°C.

Although *Bedsonia* are not true viruses they may be isolated in eggs by inoculation into the yolk sac. Growth may be demonstrated in stained smears of the yolk sac membrane. If *Bedsonia* is the suspected cause of the patient's illness, this should be clearly indicated, because pretreatment of the specimen with certain antibiotics prevents growth.

Animal inoculation still has a place in diagnostic virology for the isolation of Coxsackie A viruses and arboviruses. For the isolation of the former suckling mice within 24–48 hours of birth are infected by the intracerebral, intraperitoneal or subcutaneous routes, and are observed over a period of several weeks for signs of infection, paralysis or death.

HISTOLOGICAL TECHNIQUES

Post mortem examination of stained sections of tissues may show cellular changes characteristic of infection with certain viruses. Similar changes may be seen in biopsy specimens, exfoliated cells, or scrapings from lesions. Variola and vaccinia virus infections produce intracytoplasmic inclusions, called Guarnieri bodies, and rabies virus produces Negri bodies. Intranuclear inclusions and giant cells may be found in infections with herpes simplex and the varicella-zoster viruses. Fluorescent antibody staining may also be used to demonstrate virus antigens within cells.

With members of the poxvirus group, direct visualization of virus particles is possible with light microscopy. Stained scrapings from lesions of smallpox may show not only Guarnieri bodies but also individual virus particles. In the EM, PTA-stained vesicle fluid may reveal the characteristically shaped poxvirus particles and this provides a rapid screening technique for identifying smallpox virus. The icosahedral shape of herpes particles may also be demonstrated in vesicle fluid.

SEROLOGICAL TECHNIQUES

Type-specific antisera are used to identify viruses isolated from specimens for diagnosis. In the case of entero- and adenoviruses, of which many serotypes are known, identification is facilitated by using pools of several antisera to test for neutralization of CPE or other effects of the virus on cells.

Serological reactions can also be used to identify virus-specific antigens within infected tissues or exudates. Complement-fixing or precipitating antigens can be detected in fluids obtained from vesicles of variola or vaccinia. Fluorescent antibody staining techniques can also be applied to clinical specimens, either directly or after growth in tissue culture. In the latter case, sufficient virus replication may occur during a short incubation period to allow a rapid diagnosis. The indirect staining technique is employed, utilizing a number of type-specific antisera and a fluorescein-conjugated antiglobulin. A rapid provisional diagnosis may be possible by these techniques, but the method is limited by the degree of specificity of the available antisera and the degree of non-specific staining.

Serum specimens from patients can be examined by a variety of techniques with the aim of demonstrating a significant antibody response during the course of an illness. It is advisable to examine at least two serum specimens, the first collected as early as possible in the acute phase of illness and a second collected 2–3 weeks later in the convalescent phase. Most viral serological methods employ a serial doubling dilution procedure and a significant response implies a four-fold or greater rise in titre between acute and convalescent sera. If serum is not withdrawn at the times indicated, it may not be possible to demonstrate a rise in titre. If only a single convalescent sample is available, a presumptive diagnosis may be made occasionally, if the titre is significantly high.

Serological diagnosis alone is feasible with certain groups of viruses, but as the number of recognized viruses has grown, it has become less practicable to screen serum for all the viruses that might be responsible for a particular syndrome. Knowledge of the clinical history and a provisional diagnosis are of great importance as they allow selection of the best range of antigens.

A number of methods are available for estimating the antibody content of serum.

Neutralization is the inhibition of virus infectivity, and may be demonstrated in animals, eggs or tissue culture. To assay neutralizing antibody, serial dilutions of the patient's serum are mixed with a standard, small infective dose of virus. The highest dilution of the serum that inhibits the virus infectivity is taken as the antibody titre. As the neutralizing response is highly specific, the application of the technique is limited to either demonstrating a serological response to a particular virus, or screening sera against a limited number of virus serotypes, for example the Coxsackie B viruses in suspected cases of Bornholm disease (p. 18.113).

Haemagglutination inhibition is used to detect antibodies against viruses that produce a haemagglutinin. Dilutions of serum are mixed with a standard haemagglutinating dose of virus, and the highest dilution of serum capable of inhibiting haemagglutination is determined. Before testing, all sera are treated to remove non-specific inhibitors and the treatment varies with the nature of these. For example, before testing for inhibition of influenza virus haemagglutinin, sera are treated with neuraminidase obtained from *Vibrio cholerae* or with periodate. These treatments destroy inhibitory mucoproteins in the serum that compete with the erythrocyte receptors for the viral haemagglutinin. Haemagglutination-inhibition is an extremely sensitive technique.

Haemadsorption-inhibition is used to detect antibodies to viruses that produce haemadsorption. This is of value with some influenza A, B and parainfluenza viruses.

Fluorescent staining by fluorescein-conjugated anti-human globulin can be used to detect the binding of human antibody by antigens present in cell preparations infected with specific viruses.

Complement fixation (p. 22.16) does not require any of the specialized facilities necessary for most methods of viral diagnosis. The procedure can be used to diagnose some infections caused by a specific virus, e.g. the mumps virus. In addition, it is useful for screening sera against a number of antigens in cases where no virus has been isolated, especially as infection with any member of some groups of viruses can be diagnosed by testing with a single antigen. For example, all influenza A strains possess a common complement-fixing ribonucleoprotein (S antigen).

INTERPRETATION OF LABORATORY FINDINGS
The isolation of a virus from a patient does not necessarily mean that it is the cause of the presenting illness. The probability is greater if a virus has been isolated from blood, CSF, effusions, vesicle fluid or biopsy specimens, than if one has been isolated from upper respiratory tract secretions or faeces. A virus isolated from the latter sites may be present as a result of a mild or unrecognized infection and may be unrelated to the current illness. More significance can be attached to isolation if the virus has been previously shown to be associated with a similar clinical syndrome. For example, the regular isolation of echoviruses from patients with meningitic symptoms has indicated the association of some members of this group with aseptic meningitis.

The demonstration of a rising titre of antibody response increases the probability that a virus isolated from a patient is responsible for his illness. Difficulties arise in serological diagnosis when cross-reactions occur among related viruses.

FURTHER READING

BURNET F.M. (1962) *Natural History of Infectious Disease*, 3rd Edition. London: Cambridge University Press.
CRUICKSHANK R. (1965) *Medical Microbiology*, 11th Edition. Edinburgh: Livingstone.
DAVIS B.D., DULBECCO R., EISEN H.N., GINSBERG H.S. & WOOD W.B. Jnr. (1968) *Principles of Microbiology and Immunology*. New York: Harper.

FENNER F. (1968) *The Biology of Animal Viruses*, vols. I and II. New York: Academic Press.

GILLIES R.R. & DODDS T.C. (1968) *Bacteriology Illustrated*, 2nd Edition. Edinburgh: Livingstone.

HAYES W. (1968) *The Genetics of Bacteria and their Viruses*, 2nd Edition. Oxford: Blackwell Scientific Publications.

HORSFALL F.L. & TAMM I. (1965) *Viral and Rickettsial Infections of Man*, 4th Edition. London: Pitman.

LURIA S.E. & DARNELL J.E. Jnr. (1967) *General Virology*, 2nd Edition. New York: Wiley.

MANDELSTAM J. & McQUILLEN K. (1968) *Biochemistry of Bacterial Growth*. Oxford: Blackwell Scientific Publications.

RIDDELL R.W. & STEWART G.T. (1958) *Fungous Diseases and their Treatment*. London: Butterworth.

SWAIN R.H.A. & DODDS T.C. (1967) *Clinical Virology*. Edinburgh: Livingstone.

WILLIS A.T. (1964) *Anaerobic Bacteriology in Clinical Medicine*, 2nd Edition. London: Butterworth.

WILSON G.S. & MILES A.A. (1964) *Topley and Wilson's Principles of Bacteriology and Immunity*, vols. I and II, 5th Edition. London: Arnold.

Chapter 19
Medical zoology

PROTOZOOLOGY

Protozoa are abundant in the animal kingdom, but owing to their minute size, their existence is not evident. Like bacteria, they can be defined as unicellular micro-organisms, but in their structural organization the two groups differ fundamentally. The organization of the protozoan cell is similar to that of multicellular animals and plants. Within the plasma membrane are a nucleus, mitochondria and the other structures which are characteristic of a mammalian cell (vol. 1, p. 13.1). The nucleus contains DNA combined with protein to form the chromosomes and it divides in a manner essentially similar to mitosis in higher animals and plants. Protozoan mitochondria resemble those of higher animals in structure and function. Whereas enzymic activity of bacteria occurs largely at the surface of the cell, in protozoa it is intracellular. Most protozoa ingest food in particulate form and digestion takes place within the cell in food vacuoles. Like other animals, protozoa are not affected by antibiotics in concentrations that are lethal to bacteria. In assessing the status of protozoa in relation to bacteria and mammals, these few but important differences make it reasonable to rank them nearer to the mammals.

As agents of disease, protozoa are similar in many respects to bacteria and viruses. They inhabit various sites in the host, e.g. the lumen of the alimentary and genital tracts, the tissues either as extracellular or intracellular parasites, the blood and other body fluids. Protozoa may gain entry to a host by ingestion in food or water, by inhalation, by the bites of bloodsucking arthropods, at coitus and across the placenta. Protozoa can multiply intensively in a host. They are antigenic and evoke the formation of specific antibodies. A species is not physiologically or antigenically homogeneous but is comprised of different strains, so that resistance developed to one strain may not protect against a second strain of the same species. The immunity developed by a host to protozoan infections is sometimes strong and long lasting, but more often it is of short duration. So far it has not been possible to immunize hosts by injection of killed protozoa; neither has passive immunization proved successful. Unlike bacteria, many parasitic protozoa have complex life cycles, different morphological and physiological forms of the organism developing in sequence. In this respect, protozoa resemble parasitic helminths.

Characters of protozoa

MOTILITY
Protozoa are motile but this is sometimes difficult to observe since they dart so rapidly across the field of the microscope; such protozoa bear **flagella** or **cilia**. Electron microscopy (EM) has shown that cilia and flagella have the same structural organization, the extended plasma membrane enclosing nine peripheral and two central tubular fibrils (vol. 1, p. 13.13), whether they occur on ciliated epithelia of multicellular animals, on protozoa or as the tails of sperm. The flagella of bacteria have a different structure. Flagellated protozoa have a small number, one to eight, of these motile processes; ciliated protozoa usually have many. How movement is effected in other protozoa is not so obvious. In amoebae the cell surface is mobile and cytoplasm streams into variously shaped protuberances, called pseudopodia. The mechanics of **amoeboid movement** are not fully understood. Some parasitic protozoa move by bending and twisting. In these cells the EM shows fibrils running longitudinally beneath the plasma membrane. If these are contractile and the pellicle elastic, such movements can be explained.

FEEDING
Most protozoa ingest particulate food, which may be of bacterial, plant or animal origin. A few feed exclusively by absorption of nutrients through the cell surface. Particulate food is taken into food vacuoles, which are pockets nipped off from the cell surface. Here digestion proceeds and undigested residue is ejected, often at a particular spot, the cell anus. Some protozoa have a conspicuous water-regulating system. A contractile vacuole appears and disappears rhythmically as fluid collects and is pumped out.

REPRODUCTION
This is by simple or **binary fission** in which the

nucleus divides by mitosis, followed by cytoplasmic fission and the formation of two daughter cells. Another mode of fission, common among certain parasitic protozoa, is known as multiple fission or **schizogony**. As the cell grows, the nucleus divides repeatedly, but cytoplasmic fission is delayed and the cell becomes multinucleate. When growth stops, segmentation occurs and numerous, small uninucleate products, **merozoites**, are formed. Protozoa grow at various rates. Under optimum conditions, the large *Amoeba proteus* requires 24 hours to complete a growth cycle, but the ciliate *Tetrahymena pyriformis* needs only 2 hours, and its growth capacity is of the same order as many bacteria. Sexual reproduction is not universal among the protozoa, but it is a necessary part of the life cycle in certain parasitic species, such as the malarial parasite. Gametes are formed from macrogametocytes, each of which produces one large, nonmotile macrogamete, and from microgametocytes which produce several small, motile microgametes. Such gametes do not survive unless two of opposite type or 'sex' fuse to give the zygote.

GROWTH CYCLES

When food is plentiful, cycles of growth and reproduction take place; the active feeding stage is known as a **trophozoite**. Change in environmental conditions may lead to the formation of inactive **cysts**. In encystation, a cell stops feeding, becomes spherical or oval, cilia or flagella are resorbed, and an outer covering or cyst wall is secreted. Metabolism is greatly reduced, and this allows the cysts of some protozoa to remain viable for many months. In a suitable environment the cell may become active again and re-assumes the characteristic form of the trophozoite.

Protozoa are found in any moist environment, fresh water, the sea, soil, decaying vegetation and as parasites in all the diverse groups of the animal and plant kingdoms. About thirty species of parasitic protozoa have been recorded from man, but about half of these are harmless parasites and exist as commensals.

Protozoa of the alimentary and genital tracts

Some fifteen species of protozoa have been recorded from the alimentary tract of man. By far the most important of these is *Entamoeba histolytica* (fig. 19.1) which causes amoebic dysentery and amoebiasis.

AMOEBIASIS

E. histolytica is small, measuring from 10–40 μm. On a warm stage, the cells are constantly active; pseudopodia containing hyaline cytoplasm erupt from the surface, first in one direction then in another. In locomotion, the cell elongates, the central core of cytoplasm streams towards the moving tip and then turns back in two counter streams along the periphery. In living cells, it is

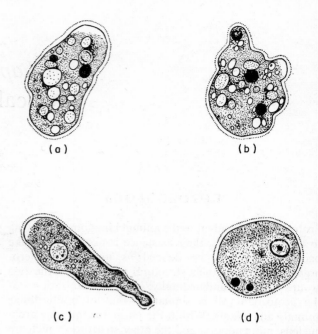

FIG. 19.1. *Entamoeba histolytica;* (a) and (b) trophozoites with ingested erythrocytes; (c) elongate trophozoite in locomotion; (d) stained trophozoite to show nuclear characters.

not easy to see the nucleus or indeed any other cytological detail. In amoebae which have been passed in the faeces from a case of acute dysentery, ingested red blood cells are usually conspicuous in the cytoplasm, and this feature is diagnostic. The cytology of the nucleus is used to distinguish species of parasitic amoebae. In stained specimens of *E. histolytica*, a small, deeply-stained granule, the **karyosome**, is seen in the centre of the nucleus and a ring of granules round the inner face of the nuclear membrane (fig. 19.1).

Life cycle

The primary site of development is the lumen of the large intestine, where the amoebae may thrive, feeding on bacteria and reproducing by binary fission. Often and for reasons unknown, the amoebae penetrate the epithelium and multiply in the gut wall causing ulceration and necrosis. Thence they may spread to other tissues such as liver, lung and brain; infection of the liver with abscess formation is common, but abscesses in other sites are relatively rare. In unfavourable conditions amoebae encyst. Living cysts look like air bubbles or oil droplets in a microscopic preparation. Sometimes small, refractile rods can be distinguished within the cysts. These are the **chromatoid bodies**, which stain intensely with basic dyes and are thought to be aggregations of ribosomes. They occur in the cysts of all species of the genus *Entamoeba*. The mature cyst contains four nuclei. Cysts pass out in the faeces and may remain viable and infective for several weeks outside the host. When cysts are ingested in water or food, they pass unaltered through the stomach and become activated in the small intestine. The cytoplasm starts to stream and the amoeba squeezes through a small hole in the cyst wall and escapes. Now each nucleus divides once, followed by cell division so that eight small amoebae are produced from each cyst. The survival of the organism outside the host depends on external conditions. Trophozoites may survive for two or three days in stools at 5°C, but they are not infective since they are destroyed in the stomach. Cysts are considerably more resistant and may remain viable for several weeks in stools or in water at 5°C but are rapidly killed at 50°C, and by drying. Cysts may be found readily in one sample of faeces, but may be scarce or absent in a succeeding sample. *E. histolytica* normally grows surrounded by bacteria, but some strains can be cultured without associated bacteria or any other living cells. Cysts do not form in such cultures unless bacteria are added. Furthermore, cysts have never been detected amongst amoebae which are growing in the host's tissues. To complete the life cycle, conditions must be favourable both for growth and for cyst formation.

Hosts

Amoebiasis is of world wide distribution and the infection in man is nearly always contracted from a human source. *E. histolytica* is a common parasite of monkeys and apes, but seldom invades the tissues of these hosts and so is not pathogenic. It can be established in laboratory animals such as rats, guinea-pigs, rabbits and golden hamsters, if introduced artificially by laparotomy.

Amoebic dysentery occurs wherever sanitation is unsatisfactory. The cysts enter the body in the drinking water or in food contaminated by flies. In places where night soil is used to manure vegetable gardens, this is another source of infection. The disease occurs also amongst those whose personal hygiene is poor, and there have been many outbreaks in mental institutions.

Differential diagnosis

Besides *E. histolytica* other species of amoeba, which are nonpathogenic, may inhabit the alimentary tract of man, so it is necessary to be able to distinguish it from these. Only *E. histolytica* engulfs red blood corpuscles and this often makes diagnosis easy. Otherwise it is difficult, even for the specialist, to distinguish one species of living trophozite from another, since little cytological detail can be seen, and all are similar in size and in the way they move. Differences between species are more easily discerned in the cyst forms (fig. 19.2 and table 19.1) Staining with iodine reveals the differential characters; the cytoplasm stains yellow, glycogen red-brown and the nuclei become demarcated.

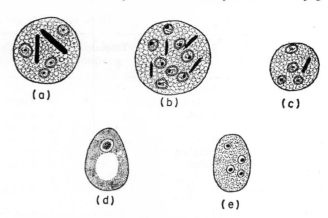

FIG. 19.2. Cysts of intestinal amoebae. (a) *E. histolytica;* (b) *E. coli;* (c) *E. hartmanni;* (d) *Iodamoeba butschlii;* (e) *Endolimax nana.*

Pathogenicity

E. histolytica may live in the lumen of the gut of a man for long periods without invading the tissues. Such people may pass typical cysts of *E. histolytica* without any signs of intestinal disturbance. They are known as cyst passers or carriers. Careful study has shown that there are two distinct populations of amoebae that produce cysts with four nuclei. People passing cysts which have a diameter of less than 10 μm (average 7 μm) never show the clinical symptoms of amoebiasis. These small amoebae are now assigned to a separate species, *E. hartmanni*, which is regarded as nonpathogenic. Amoebae producing cysts with a diameter greater than 10 μm (average 12 μm) may be associated with dysentery. However, not all people harbouring the larger amoebae have symptoms of dysentery. This may be because some strains of *E. histolytica* lack the invasive properties. Alternatively the behaviour of the amoebae may depend on the environment, such as the bacterial flora and the chemical nature of the contents of the large intestine, which vary from person to person. One environment may favour tissue invasion, another repress it. *E. histolytica* must always be regarded as a potential pathogen and in many tropical countries a very important one. Nevertheless, detection of this amoeba in a patient does not necessarily mean that the cause of the clinical condition has been ascertained.

TERRAMOEBIASIS

There is mounting evidence that free-living amoebae may occasionally cause rapidly fatal meningoencephalitis in man, and for this condition the term terramoebiasis has been proposed. A small number of patients presenting with similar symptoms and histories have been described from Australia, the USA and Czechoslovakia. All had a recent history of bathing in fresh water pools or lakes and in several, numerous amoebae, resembling free-living

TABLE 19.1. Differential characters of amoebae.

Species	Location in host	Trophozoite size (μm)	Cyst size and shape (μm)	No. of nuclei in cyst	Appearance of stained nuclei
E. histolytica	Large intestine	18–40	7–16 Round	4	Small, central karyosome, fine peripheral granules
E. hartmanni	Large intestine	5–12	4–10 Round	4	Small, central karyosome, fine peripheral granules
E. coli	Large intestine	20–30	10–30 Round	8	Small, acentric karyosome, coarse peripheral granules
E. gingivalis	Mouth	10–20	No cysts	–	Small, central karyosome, fine peripheral granules
Endolimax nana	Large intestine	6–12	6–9 × 5–7 Oval	4	Large, irregular karyosome
Iodamoeba butschlii	Large intestine	5–20	9–15 Round, oval, pear-shaped. Conspicuous glycogen vacuole	1	Large karyosome, scattered granules
Dientamoeba fragilis	Large intestine	7–12 binucleate	No cysts	–	Large, granular karyosome

species, were found in the brain at autopsy. In one case, the cerebrospinal fluid before death contained active amoebae and these were cultured successfully. Mice died within 10 days of rhinencephalitis following nasal instillation of 100–1000 amoebae.

There is also evidence that amoebae are associated with respiratory disease in children. Amoebae, which are normally free-living in soil or ponds, have been detected in several laboratories as contaminants of mammalian cell or tissue cultures. Some of these cell cultures had been seeded with nasal or pharyngeal swabs from man or

animals. It has been shown that some of these tissue culture amoebae infect and kill mice when introduced intranasally, or monkeys when introduced intracerebrally. However, since soil amoebae form cysts which are resistant to desiccation, the amoebae which develop in tissue culture could have originated from airborne cysts lodged in the respiratory passages, and not from an active infection.

The free-living amoebae found capable of infecting animals and man belong to two genera, *Acanthamoeba* and *Naegleria*. In both genera the nucleus, with its large,

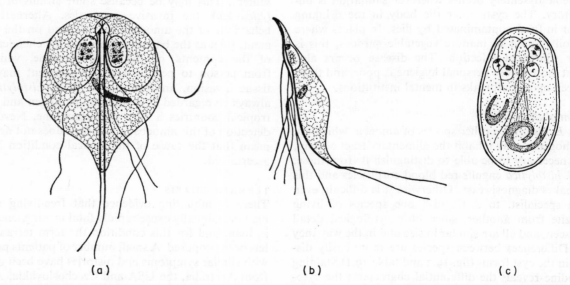

FIG. 19.3. *Giardia intestinalis*; (a) trophozoite, ventral view showing paired nuclei and four pairs of flagella; (b) lateral view; (c) cyst showing four nuclei and flagellar apparatus.

central nucleolus, is easily seen in the living cells and in histological preparations.

GIARDIASIS

Giardia intestinalis is a flagellate which is most abundant in the duodenum but may extend along the small intestine and into the bile duct. It may cause enteritis and diarrhoea, especially in children. The organism is flattened dorsoventrally and bears four pairs of flagella (fig. 19.3). It looks like a saucer with a stubby handle and the cells roll over and over tracing a wobbly path. If once seen alive and active, they are easily recognized again. In the host, the cells adhere to the mucosa, the concave ventral surface acting as a sucker. The organism has no cell mouth, but obtains nutrients from the semi-digested food which bathes it. It reproduces by binary fission and forms cysts. Normally only cysts are found in the faeces, and iodine-stained cysts can be recognized by their oval shape, rather thick wall, and the dark streaks in the centre, which represent the flagellar apparatus. Giardia occurs in many species of mammal and organisms from different hosts look very alike. The necessary cross-infection experiments have not been done to determine whether it is the same or different species of Giardia which occurs in the various hosts.

BALANTIDIAL DYSENTERY

Balantidium coli is a ciliated protozoon and is the only species of ciliate which parasitizes man. Like most protozoan parasites of the alimentary tract, *B. coli* inhabits the lumen of the large intestine, where it feeds on and digests bacteria. It reproduces by binary fission and forms cysts.

Balantidium coli is a large protozoon measuring from 40 to 200 μm in length (fig. 19.4). It is pear shaped and densely covered with short cilia arranged in closely set, longitudinal parallel rows. A depression at the anterior end leads to the cell mouth or cytostome, which is lined with longer cilia. A conspicuous structure in all ciliated protozoa is the large macronucleus, which stains uniformly and intensely; in *B. coli* it is kidney shaped. A much smaller micronucleus is also present. It is unlikely that *B. coli* would be confused with any other protozoa inhabiting the alimentary tract of man.

B. coli has been isolated from many species of mammals and is a common parasite of domestic pigs. In the pig, the organism is usually restricted to the lumen of the gut, but invasion of the mucosa sometimes occurs. Balantidial dysentery is rare in man but humans may harbour this species without suffering from dysentery. If *B. coli* from the pig established itself readily in man, cases of balantidial dysentery would be expected to occur more frequently. Perhaps the human and porcine parasites are different species; the prevalence of *B. coli* in pigs and its rarity in man support this view.

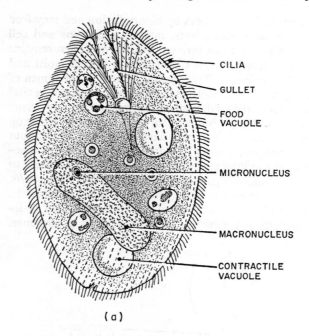

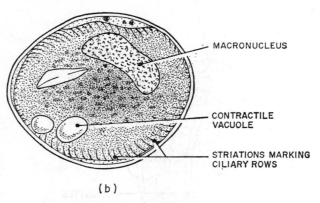

FIG. 19.4. *Balantidium coli*; (a) trophozoite; (b) cyst.

TRICHOMONIASIS

Flagellated protozoa of the genus *Trichomonas* are common parasites of a wide variety of animal hosts, including insects, birds and mammals. Most species inhabit the gut and are generally harmless. The species *T. vaginalis* inhabits the human genital tract and may be associated with vaginitis in the female or urethritis in the male. *T. vaginalis* is an oval-shaped cell, about 15 μm long, with a tuft of four flagella projecting from the anterior end of the cell (fig. 19.5). A fifth flagellum is directed posteriorly and extends about half-way down the cell forming a flange or undulating membrane. A small, spine-like process projects from the posterior end of the cell. In fresh preparations little else is seen, but the anterior free flagella, the short undulating membrane and the posterior spine permit identification.

T. vaginalis reproduces by binary fission and may feed on other micro-organisms, mucous secretions and cell debris. Cysts are not formed, but the organism remains viable outside a host for several days if kept moist and cool. In the female, *T. vaginalis* is found in the lumen of the vagina; in the male, it may travel along the genital duct as far as the epididymis. Transmission usually occurs at coitus, but organisms can survive on drops of water on lavatory seats. Women may harbour *T. vaginalis* without any symptoms, although frequently its presence is associated with inflammation of the vagina. Since it is usual to find other micro-organisms in the vagina with *T. vaginalis*, it has been argued that the protozoon is not responsible. A more likely explanation of the variable effects of infection with *T. vaginalis* is that strains differ in virulence.

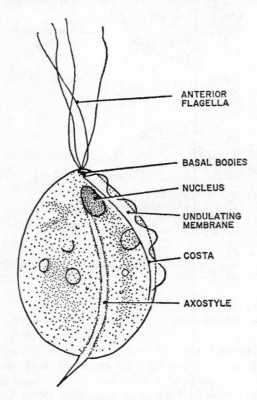

ANTERIOR
FLAGELLA

BASAL BODIES

NUCLEUS

UNDULATING
MEMBRANE

COSTA

AXOSTYLE

FIG. 19.5. *Trichomonas vaginalis.*

Protozoa of the blood and tissues

The flagellated protozoa which parasitize the blood and tissues of man belong to the family Trypanosomatidae. The family contains many species which parasitize such widely different hosts as insects, fish, birds and even plants. The species of medical importance belong to the genus *Trypanosoma* and *Leishmania*. They cause African trypanosomiasis or sleeping sickness, South American trypanosomiasis or Chagas disease and leishmaniasis or kala azar and oriental sore.

SLEEPING SICKNESS OR AFRICAN TRYPANOSOMIASIS

Sleeping sickness is caused by *T. gambiense* and *T. rhodesiense* and is transmitted from man to man or from animals to man by tsetse flies (*Glossina*). In the mammalian host the organisms inhabit the blood but may penetrate other organs where they occur in intercellular spaces. In a drop of blood, the trypanosomes appear as minute, wriggling objects, which jostle the erythrocytes as they push their way amongst them. In stained films, the trypanosomes are seen to be long, slender cells, about 26×3 μm, with a single flagellum which originates at the posterior end of the cell, runs forwards over the surface and extends freely at the anterior end (fig. 19.6). Where the flagellum is in contact with the cell, it forms a wavy flange, called the undulating membrane. In well-stained preparations, the nucleus can be seen lying about the centre of the cell, and the **kinetoplast**, situated a short distance from the posterior end. With one of the Romanowsky stains both these structures stain bright red in contrast to the bluish colour of the cytoplasm. The kinetoplast, an organelle peculiar to the *Trypanosomatidae*, has been shown by EM to be a specialized part of a single tubular mitochondrion and DNA accounts for its affinity for nuclear stains. Trypanosomes reproduce by longitudinal, binary fission, the nucleus and kinetoplast divide first, a second flagellum develops and finally the cell cleaves into two.

Development in Glossina

When a tsetse fly feeds, its toothed proboscis tears the skin causing a small haemorrhage to form. If trypanosomes are present, they are sucked into the gut of the fly with the blood drawn up from this pool. Fig. 19.6 shows the various forms that the trypanosomes assume during their development in the intermediate host. For the first few days after an infective feed, the trypanosomes are found in the midgut. Then some travel forwards to the proventriculus. For development to be successful, some must pass right forwards to near the tip of the proboscis where the opening of the salivary duct is located. They must then pass up the duct to the salivary glands where forms develop which are infective to the mammal. These are called metacyclic trypanosomes because they appear at the end of the developmental cycle. Reproduction takes place at all sites in the fly. The time required for this remarkable cycle is 2–3 weeks or even longer. Not only do the trypanosomes alter in morphology in the insect host, but they differ physiologically from the blood stream forms; the insect forms consume less O_2 and oxidize carbohydrates more completely than do the blood forms. Trypanosomes can be cultured but only as insect forms. The lack of suitable methods for culturing the mammalian forms has handicapped the search for chemotherapeutic agents.

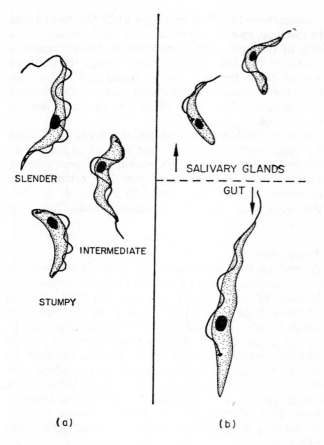

FIG. 19.6. Forms seen in the life cycle of *Trypanosoma gambiense* and *T. rhodesiense*; (a) in blood of mammal; (b) in tsetse fly.

Development in man

If a tsetse fly harbouring a mature infection bites man, metacyclic trypanosomes may be injected along with saliva. In the early stages of an infection the parasites may be found in the blood. A characteristic feature is that the number of trypanosomes builds up to a peak and then declines, and these cycles are repeated. During the increase most of the trypanosomes are long and slender, but as the number declines, short and stumpy forms appear. The trypanosomes stimulate the host to produce antibody which agglutinates and lyzes the organisms. Some of the trypanosomes become resistant to antibody and so a new population develops of different antigenic type; these flourish until specific antibody is again formed to destroy them. It is possible that the antibody causes the change from slender to stumpy forms, and that it is only the stumpy forms which can establish them-themselves in the vector. At later stages of the infection the trypanosomes become scarce or absent from the blood but invade the central nervous system to cause sleeping sickness.

Distribution

Sleeping sickness in man occurs only where tsetse flies are present and these insects are restricted to the hot and humid parts of Central and Southern Africa. But sleeping sickness in West Africa differs clinically and epidemiologically from the condition in East Africa. In the West, the disease generally runs a chronic course, in the East it is acute. In the West, man acquires infection from a tsetse fly which has fed previously on another infected human, whereas in the East man may acquire infection from a fly which has fed previously on a wild or domestic animal host. This permits the clinician to recognize the Western or Gambian form of the disease caused by *T. gambiense*, as opposed to the Eastern or Rhodesian form caused by *T. rhodesiense*. It must be stressed that the two species are identical morphologically and in their developmental cycles, and that there is yet a third species, *T. brucei*, with the same characteristics. *T. brucei* occurs in both East and West but is not infective to man.

Trypanosomes can establish and develop in a wide range of mammalian species, and have been isolated from many species of African game animals. In these hosts the association seems to be a benign one and the mammal remains in good health. But the same trypanosomes in man or in man's domestic animals are highly pathogenic. Trypanosomiasis of domestic animals is an urgent problem in large areas of Africa where stock cannot be reared because of the presence of tsetse flies and game animals.

Transmission

Probably at least 100 metacyclic trypanosomes are required to initiate an infection in man. By inducing flies to feed through a membrane on a small volume of blood, it has been shown that several hundred metacyclic trypanosomes are commonly ejected at each feed. Tsetse flies feed exclusively on blood and take meals every one or two days. A fly takes on average twenty feeds a month. It may require 2–4 weeks for *T. gambiense* and *T. rhodesiense* to develop to maturity in the vector, but once a mature infection has been established, the fly probably remains infective for the rest of its life, about 1–2 months. Hence one fly may transmit trypanosomes to at least twenty hosts. Some of the fly's meals may be taken on non-susceptible hosts such as crocodiles. However, identification of blood meals has shown that tsetse flies feed mostly on animals which are suitable hosts for the trypanosomes. That infection in man is not much more prevalent can be explained by the finding that *T. gambiense* and *T. rhodesiense* establish only with difficulty in *Glossina*. Rarely do more than 1 per cent of flies caught in the wild have mature infections, and even under laboratory conditions it is difficult to infect more than 10 per cent.

CHAGAS DISEASE OR AMERICAN TRYPANOSOMIASIS

Chagas disease is caused by *T. cruzi* and occurs in Central and South America. It is transmitted by blood-sucking bugs of the family Triatomidae.

Development in man

The parasite soon leaves the blood and settles in tissues, most frequently in cardiac, striated or smooth muscle. Here they lose their flagella and round up. They now start to multiply and clusters of several hundred cells may be formed, displacing muscle fibres. After a time, the colony starts to disperse; the cells elongate, each develops a flagellum and the new trypanosomes enter the circulation. Each is about 20 μm long, and is curved or sickle-shaped with a large kinetoplast lying near the pointed posterior end of the cell (fig. 19.7). When seen alive in a

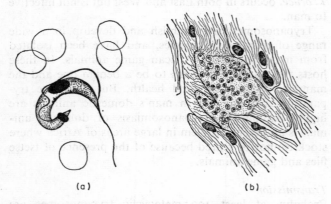

(a)   (b)

FIG. 19.7. *Trypanosoma cruzi*; (a) in blood film; (b) in heart muscle.

drop of blood the trypanosome twists and untwists into figures-of-eight. The trypanosomes remain in the circulation for several days and then again disappear into the tissues to undergo another reproductive cycle. In chronic infections the tissue phase predominates, since the blood forms can rarely be detected.

Development in the bug

If a bug sucks blood containing trypanosomes these become established first in the midgut. Here they multiply rapidly and within a few days some pass into the hindgut and infective forms begin to appear in the faeces. In contrast to the African trypanosomes, where the infective forms are situated anteriorly in the vector and are introduced into man by inoculation, the infective forms of *T. cruzi* are located at the posterior end of the vector's gut and infection is by contamination. Triatomid bugs ingest a large amount of blood relative to their body weight and the ingested blood

is concentrated by fluid excretion while the insect feeds. In this way, infective trypanosomes are deposited on the skin of the host. The trypanosomes cannot penetrate unbroken skin but may gain entry through the puncture wound. Since the bugs are nocturnal and feed on the face, the trypanosomes are more commonly smeared into eyes, mouth or nose where they penetrate mucous membranes.

T. cruzi develops in several species of bugs, all of which are good hosts. If ten bugs were allowed to feed on an infected person, all ten would probably become infected. Laboratory reared or 'clean' bugs are often used in diagnosis; it may be simpler to rear and maintain the bugs than to prepare culture media for diagnosis.

Distribution

T. cruzi has been found in many species of wild animals and in reduviid bugs in Central and South America and in some of the Southern states of the USA. Human infection in the USA is rare, but in parts of Central and South America the incidence of infection in man may be as high as 20 per cent. It has been established that some 35 million people are at risk to the infection. The infection may be spread from man to man or from animals to man. Domestic dogs and cats are reservoirs in urban areas. Drugs which are effective against the African trypanosomes have no action on human infections with *T. cruzi*; no curative drugs have yet been discovered against this parasite.

LEISHMANIASIS

Leishmania donovani causes **kala azar** or visceral leishmaniasis in man and animals, and the disease occurs in certain parts of all continents except Australia. It is transmitted by blood-sucking flies of the genus *Phlebotomus*, commonly known as sandflies.

Development in man

Leishmania is an intracellular parasite about 2 × 4 μm in size (fig. 19.8). In stained smears of infected tissue, clusters of parasites, called **Leishman–Donovan** or **LD bodies**, are seen in the cytoplasm of macrophages or lying free; host cells often rupture when the preparation is made. The organism may be recognized by the characteristic association of nucleus and kinetoplast; with Romanowsky stains the nucleus is round and stains pink, the kinetoplast is smaller, rodshaped and stains deep red. Whether they are phagocytosed or enter cells by their own activity is not certain. EM has shown that a small flagellum is present and in tissue cultures jerky movements of the cells can be observed. Once inside a suitable host cell, the parasites reproduce by binary fission until the cytoplasm becomes

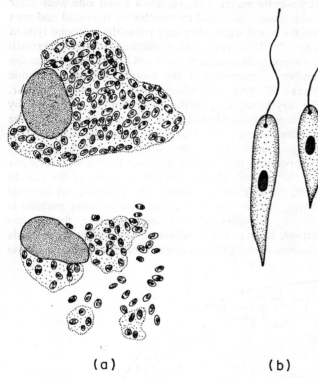

FIG. 19.8. *Leishmania donovani*; (a) parasites within macrophage cell and some lying free; (b) promastigate forms.

packed. It is presumed that the host cell then disintegrates and the freed parasites spread to other cells. The leishmanial parasites first develop locally at the site of the insect's bite, but later they spread by blood or lymph and become widely dispersed in the body.

Development in the sandfly

While feeding, sandflies ingest, in addition to blood, cells lying in the dermis outside the circulation. If cells containing LD bodies are ingested, the parasites are liberated in the midgut as the host cells disintegrate. The freed parasites elongate and a flagellum develops from the anterior end of each cell. These slender, active promastigotes reproduce rapidly so that within a few days hundreds may be found in the midgut of the insect and, as the numbers increase, they tend to move forward into the foregut. A fly is infective, however, only if some flagellates have moved into the tip of the proboscis, so that when this is inserted into the skin, the parasites escape into the tissues. The forward progression of promastigotes in the sandfly's gut is characteristic of leishmanias which infect man or other mammals.

Distribution

Leishmanial parasites are widely distributed throughout the warmer parts of the world, but the clinical and epidemiological aspects of the infection vary from place to place. **Cutaneous leishmaniasis** or **oriental sore** is caused by *L. tropica*. These parasites remain localized where they are introduced by the vector and give rise to an ulcerating sore. *L. donovani* and *L. tropica* are identical morphologically and in their developmental cycles, and may be transmitted by the same species of *Phlebotomus*. The markedly different behaviour in the human host justifies separation into two species. Furthermore, the two organisms differ antigenically; a person who has recovered from kala azar is fully susceptible to oriental sore and vice versa.

Cutaneous leishmaniasis, as it occurs in the American continents, is much more complex and some believe that five species should be recognized. *L. brasiliensis* causes espundia or **mucocutaneous leishmaniasis**. In this form the parasites spread, sooner or later, from the local lesion to involve the nasopharynx. In Mexico and British Honduras, cutaneous leishmaniasis is known as 'bay-sore' or **Chiclero's ulcer**, caused by *L. mexicana*, and is characterized by a single lesion, often on the ear. This infection is seen only in men who go into the forests, the chicle or gum gatherers and mahogany workers.

Leishmanial parasites can establish themselves in many species of mammals and man often acquires infection from a sandfly which has previously fed on an infected animal. The infection of humans from animal sources is termed a zoonosis, Chiclero's ulcer being a good example. Three species of forest rodents have been shown to harbour *L. mexicana*. In the Mediterranean basin, the domestic dog is the main reservoir host and destruction of dogs significantly reduces the incidence of kala azar in humans. It has been shown that in dogs the parasites are present in the skin as well as in the viscera. Sandflies feeding on dogs readily become infected, whereas it is difficult to infect the flies from a human host. In other parts of the world, jackals, foxes and various species of rodents may be the reservoir hosts of visceral or cutaneous leishmanial parasites. The Indian sub-continent is the only area where no animal reservoir of *L. donovani* has been found. But sandflies feeding on kala azar patients are readily infected.

Leishmanial parasites can be easily cultured in the insect or promastigate form, and culture of blood or tissues often reveals the presence of parasites which could not be detected microscopically. The golden hamster is a highly susceptible host and has been much used in the laboratory for studying the organisms and in diagnosis.

MALARIA

Malarial parasites belong to the genus *Plasmodium*. This genus contains many species which parasitize reptiles, birds and mammals. Man may be infected by four species, which are transmitted by mosquitoes of the genus *Anopheles*. Simian rodent and avian malarial parasites can be easily maintained in the laboratory and their study has contributed to the development of antimalarial drugs.

Development in man

The infective form, known as the **sporozoite**, is introduced by mosquito bites. It is a slender, spindle-shaped cell with a single nucleus (fig. 19.9). Sporozoites can remain in the blood for up to 1 hour. To survive and establish infection, sporozoites must reach and penetrate parenchymal cells of the liver. No other host cell is suitable and all efforts to find them in other tissues cells have failed. Most intracellular protozoan parasites are similarly specialized so that they survive and grow only in one type of host cell. Within the liver cell the first cycle of growth and reproduction takes place (the pre-

erythrocytic cycle). This occupies about one week after which several thousand **merozoites** are liberated and pass into the blood where they may parasitize a second type of host cell, the erythrocyte. Continuing cycles of growth and reproduction take place in red blood cells, and as the number of parasites in the blood increases, rhythmic attacks of fever and other clinical symptoms appear. The erythrocytic growth cycle can be followed by examining stained blood films. On entering a red cell, the parasite assumes a ring form with a central vacuole. This persists for about 6 hours, when the vacuole gradually disappears as the parasite increases in size until it nearly fills the red cell. During the last 12 hours of the growth cycle, nuclear fission occurs from which, on average sixteen merozoites are formed. The growing parasite is termed a **trophozoite** and, after nuclear fission has started, it is called a **schizont**. The erythrocytic cycle occupies about 48 hours (except for *Plasmodium malariae*

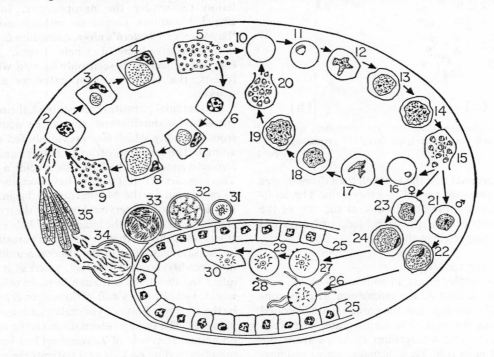

FIG. 19.9. Life cycle of malaria parasite; 1, sporozoites from salivary glands of mosquito enter liver cells; 2, liver cell containing early stages of primary exoerythrocytic parasite; 3 and 4, stages in development of the primary exoerythrocytic schizont in liver cells; 5, fully developed primary exoerythrocytic schizont rupturing and releasing merozoites; 6, liver cell containing merozoite of a secondary exoerythrocytic cycle of schizogony; 7–9, remaining stages in exoerythrocytic schizogony ending in second generation of merozoites; 10, red cell of circulating blood; 11–14, stages in erythrocytic schizogony in circulating blood; 15, fully developed erythrocytic schizont rupturing and releasing erythrocytic merozoites and gametocytes; 16–20, repetition of erythrocytic schizogony; 21 and 22, development of male gametocyte or microgametocyte in circulating blood; 23 and 24, development of female gametocyte or macrogametocyte in circulating blood; 25, wall of stomach of mosquito; 26, exflagellating microgametocyte producing microgametes in stomach of mosquito; 27, macrogamete; 28, microgamete free in stomach of mosquito and seeking macrogamete; 29, zygote, formed by fertilization of macrogamate by a single microgamete; 30, ookinete, or travelling vermicule formed by elongation of zygote; it is about to penetrate epithelial lining of stomach; 31, oocyst, formed by ookinete after penetration of stomach wall of mosquito; it lies under elastic membrane on outer surface of stomach; 32 and 33, stages in development of oocyst with production of sporozoites; 34, rupture of mature oocyst with dispersion of sporozoites most of which enter salivary glands of mosquito; 35, salivary gland of mosquito containing mature sporozoites. From Garnham P.C.C. (1966) *Malaria Parasites and other Haemosporidia*. Oxford: Blackwell Scientific Publications.

which has a 72-hour growth cycle) and attacks of fever coincide with the liberation of the merozoites into the plasma. Merozoites penetrate fresh red cells rapidly and are rarely seen free in the blood. How they get into cells is not known. It has long been known that the malaria parasite feeds on haemoglobin, utilizing the protein portion of the molecule but leaving the haem portion, which accumulates to form the familiar malarial pigment. EM has shown that the parasite feeds by phagocytosis, engulfing chunks of red cell cytoplasm; digestion takes place in food vacuoles, where the pigment accumulates until it is released into the plasma when the host cell ruptures and the merozoites escape. Shortly after the parasite has started reproducing in the blood, the sexual forms or gametocytes begin to appear in the red cells. Gametocytes may survive for several days in the mammalian host, but cannot develop further unless they are ingested by a suitable mosquito host. The single nucleus of the gametocyte distinguishes it from the fully grown asexual forms.

Development in the mosquito
The proboscis of the mosquito is composed of a number of fine stylets which are under muscular and sensory control. One of the stylets contains the duct from the salivary glands, which lie in the anterior part of the thorax of the insect. Saliva is pumped into the dermis during feeding and may contain agglutinins and an anticoagulant, but its nature varies with the species of mosquito. Salivary protein and/or carbohydrate are thought to cause the skin reactions of mosquito bites. In biting, the proboscis is thrust through the epidermis, then random probing movements can be observed. When a capillary is pierced blood is immediately drawn up the tube and, by means of a series of pumps and valves, is sucked and pushed into the distensible midgut or stomach. If the meal is taken from a person infected with malaria, the asexual forms of the parasite are destroyed in the stomach, but the gametocytes escape from the erythrocytes and in the microgametocyte three nuclear divisions take place, and eight whip-like microgametes break away from the body of the cell and lash around in the stomach. This process, aptly described as ex-flagellation, can be watched in a drop of blood on a microscope slide, and may be completed within 20 min of withdrawing blood. A single microgamete fuses with the larger macrogamete to produce the zygote, which soon pushes through the gut epithelium and comes to rest on the outside of the stomach. At this site, the final stage of the development cycle, **sporogony**, occurs. It is essentially another schizogony cycle in which a few thousand sporozoites are formed and takes 1–2 weeks for completion. On the stomach wall, the parasite assumes a spherical shape and is called an **oocyst**. The stomach of a heavily infected mosquito looks knobbly due to the many, rounded oocysts protruding from its surface. When mature, the oocyst ruptures and the sporozoites pass into the body cavity. They are motile and travel forwards to reach and penetrate the salivary glands. This takes place rapidly since, when oocysts are known to be maturing, the salivary glands contain sporozoites. Sporozoites can be obtained by culturing oocysts on mosquito stomachs. As these are infective, salivary secretion is not required for maturation of the sporozoites. However, under natural conditions, sporozoites must reach the salivary glands to allow a new cycle to start and so ensure the survival of the parasite.

Differential diagnosis
In suspected cases of malaria, diagnosis is made by examination of stained blood films (vol. 1, p. 26.2). For proper treatment it is important that the species should be identified. The chief differential characters of the four human species of *Plasmodium* are shown in table 19.2 and plate 19.1, facing p. 19.12. *P. falciparum* differs in several important respects from the other species.
  (1) It is the most pathogenic species.
  (2) Para-erythrocytic forms (see below) are absent.
  (3) Normally, only the early growth stages of the erythrocytic schizont are seen in peripheral blood because the parasitized red cells tend to clump and adhere to the capillary walls.
  (4) The gametocytes are crescent shaped and may persist in the blood for up to 4 weeks after drug treatment has removed the asexual forms. Thus a cured case can still infect mosquitoes.
    The other three species cause relapsing malaria. Relapse is caused by renewed invasion of the blood by merozoites produced from schizonts persisting in the liver (**exo-erythrocytic parasites**). It is convenient to divide these into two types, the pre-erythrocytic and the para-erythrocytic, which develop at the same time as the blood forms and persist after the blood infection has ended. What triggers the re-invasion of the blood by the para-erythrocytic merozoites is not known. Waning of the immune mechanism would seem an obvious explanation but it does not fit all the facts. For example, in some strains of *P. vivax* from temperate Europe, primary invasion of the blood may not occur until 6 months or so after infection from a mosquito bite. This seems to be a pretty adaptation on the part of the parasite to climates where mosquitoes hibernate during the cold season and are not available for transmission. It is important to appreciate that the various morphological forms also differ physiologically, so that a drug which is effective in killing the erythrocytic schizonts may have no action on the exo-erythrocytic forms nor on the gametocytes (p. 20.19). To effect clinical cure, a drug which destroys the asexual erythrocytic forms must be given, but in relapsing species the parasites may persist in the liver; consequently

TABLE 19.2. Differential diagnosis of human species of plasmodium.

Species Disease	*P. falciparum* Malignant tertian	*P. vivax* Benign tertian	*P. malariae* Quartan	*P. ovale* Oval tertian
Pre-erythrocytic forms	Mature 5–6 days 40,000 merozoites	Mature 8–9 days 15,000 merozoites	Mature 15 days 2,000 merozoites	Mature 8–9 days 15,000 merozoites
Para-erythrocytic forms	Absent	Present, about 3 yrs	Present, many years	Present, usually short-lived
Erythrocytic forms (a) Ring	0·15–0·5 diameter of RBC, cytoplasm fine in young rings, thick, older rings, marginal forms and multiple infections common	0·3–0·5 diameter of RBC, cytoplasm circle thin, faintly staining	0·3–0·5 diameter of RBC, cytoplasm circle thick, densely staining	0·3 diameter of RBC, cytoplasm circle thick, densely staining
(b) Trophozoites	Parasite compact, not usually seen	Irregular, sprawling, vacuolated	Compact, rounded, bandform	Compact, rounded
(c) Schizonts	Compact, about 0·6 of diameter of RBC, 8–24 merozoites, pigment black, clumped, not usually seen	Nearly fills RBC, 12–24 merozoites, pigment light brown, loose clump	Compact, 8 merozoites, sometimes in rosette form, pigment dark brown, clumped	Round, compact, nearly fills RBC, usually 8 merozoites, pigment dark brown, clumped
Gametocytes	Crescent-shaped, distorting RBC	Round, fills RBC	Round, fills RBC	Round, nearly fills RBC
Effect on RBC	Not enlarged, sometimes coarse stippling, Maurer's clefts	Enlarged, fine stippling, Schuffner's dots, often in reticulocytes	Not enlarged, sometimes Zieman's stippling	Slightly enlarged often oval, fine stippling, Schuffner's dots appear early, in rings

after a longer or shorter interval, the patient may suffer from a further attack of fever.

Transmission
A mosquito may ingest more than its own weight of blood at one feed and a normal meal may be 4 mm³, so that about 20 million red cells are ingested. This is a far larger number than it is practical to scan microscopically. Although few or no gametocytes may be detected in blood films, mosquitoes feeding on that host and dissected later may show many oocysts on the stomach. Sometimes several hundred oocysts may be found in one mosquito, which nevertheless appears healthy. It is thought that a few hundred sporozoites are required to initiate an infection in man and, since a single oocyst produces several thousand sporozoites, even lightly parasitized mosquitoes are infective. The number of sporozoites introduced into the host affects the initial severity of the malarial attack. Climatic factors may influence the development of malarial parasites in the vector, e.g. at low temperatures the developmental cycle takes longer than at higher temperatures. The gametocyte

is a vital stage in the parasite's life cycle, since it is the form which is established in the vector, thereby making possible spread to another host (p. 19.52).

Distribution
In the early 1950s about half the world's population lived in areas where malaria was endemic and were at risk to infection (fig. 19.10). At this time so much information about the malarial parasite and its vectors had been accumulated, that it became feasible for the World Health Organization (WHO) to launch a malaria eradication programme. Briefly, this novel aim, the eradication of a disease agent, was a practical proposition because:

(1) potent insecticides had been discovered which could be applied as sprays to human dwellings and which retained their insecticidal action for about one year,

(2) effective drugs were available which would eliminate the parasite from the human host, and

(3) there was no known reservoir of infection in hosts other than man.

Although it has since been discovered that some species

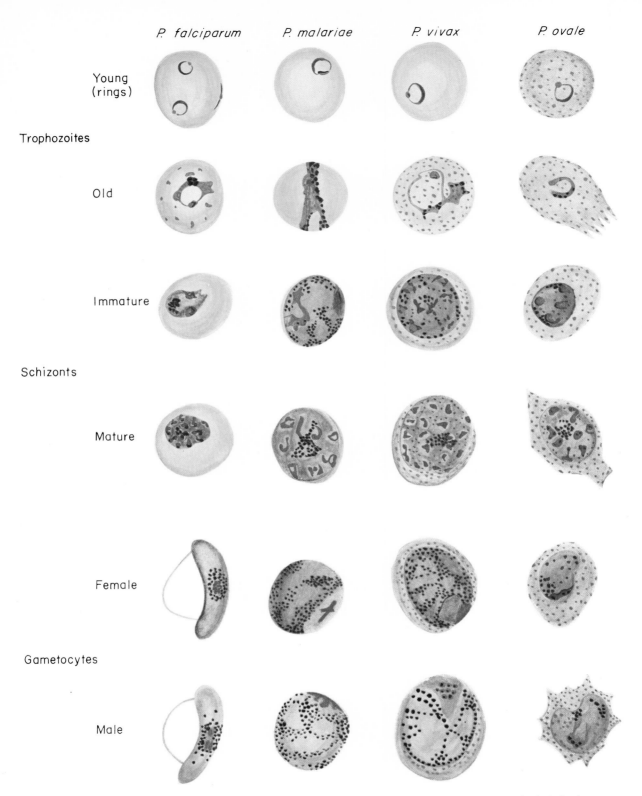

PLATE 19.1. Differential diagnosis of the species of human malaria. From Hoare C.A. (1960) *Handbook of Medical Protozoology*. London: Baillière, Tindall & Cassell.

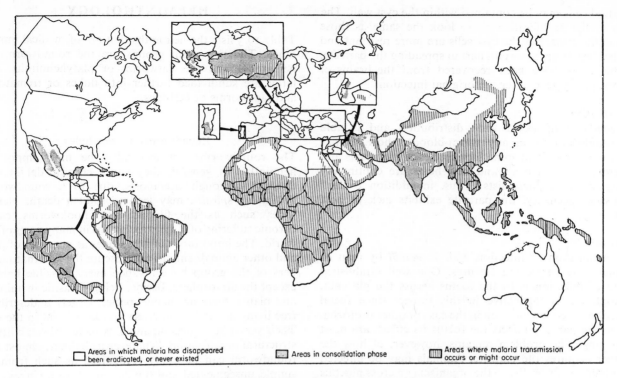

FIG. 19.10. World distribution of malaria in 1965. After WHO.

Areas in which malaria has disappeared been eradicated, or never existed

Areas in consolidation phase

Areas where malaria transmission occurs or might occur

of monkey malarial parasites are transmissible to man, it is unlikely that these species are a source of infection to man. The success of the malaria eradication programme may be judged by quoting from the 1966 WHO report: 'The population of areas now freed from the risk of malaria now amounts to 57 per cent of the population in the originally malarious areas of the world for which information is available'.

TOXOPLASMOSIS

The causative organism, *Toxoplasma gondii*, was first described in the gondi, a North African rodent, in 1908, but it was not until 1939 that it was recognized as a human infection.

Development

T. gondii is a small protozoon measuring about 2×5 μm. The cells are slightly curved, with one end broader than the other (fig. 19.11). The single nucleus lies near the centre of the cell. Reproduction is by a form of budding in which two daughter cells develop within the parent cell. *T. gondii* is an intracellular parasite, which, unlike most intracellular protozoa, can invade and multiply in any type of host cell except the non-nucleated erythrocyte. The organism is probably established first in cells near the site of entry, but after multiplication it is released and may be carried by blood or lymph to other sites,

including the brain and spinal cord. Usually there is a short period of rapid multiplication and spread (the proliferative phase) which is soon checked by the host response. Subsequently the parasites are restricted and their rate of multiplication greatly reduced. In this phase they are described as cysts, since they are

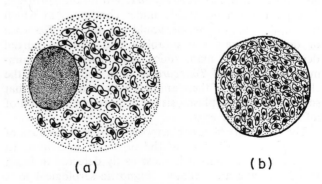

(a)   (b)

FIG. 19.11. *Toxoplasma gondii*; (a) proliferating form in a host cell; (b) cyst form.

enclosed within a clearly defined membrane and appear to be extracellular. The term cyst is misleading since the organisms reproduce within the enclosing membrane and the cyst grows. Young cysts may contain twenty to thirty parasite cells, but after a month or so several hundred cells may be contained within the cyst wall. The cells of the proliferative phase look the same as those within the cysts, but the cyst cells are more resistant and probably play an important part in spreading the parasite. Viable cysts have been recovered from the brains of guinea-pigs 5 years after the original infection.

Distribution

T. gondii is of world wide distribution and is able to establish itself in any warm-blooded host. It has been recovered from some fifty species of mammals and seventy species of birds and new hosts are continually being added to these lists. Thus, in addition to lack of tissue specificity, the parasite exhibits lack of host specificity.

Transmission

The acquisition of infection with *T. gondii* by man or animals has perplexing features. One well established route of infection is to the foetus across the placenta. Toxoplasma is distinctive in this respect since foetal infection is very uncommon in the case of other protozoa. When the parasite infects the foetus its effects are most damaging. The problem remains, however, of how the mother acquires the parasite. Animals may be infected by inhalation or orally, so the organism can cross mucous membranes. Toxoplasma may also be excreted in milk, urine and faeces and be found in secretions from the respiratory tract and in raw eggs. Cysts kept at 3°C for 1 month have been proved to be viable, although they are killed quickly at 50°C and by drying. There is no evidence that blood-sucking arthropods are involved in transmission.

Toxoplasma may be transmitted in the eggs of the nematode worm, *Toxocara mystax*. Within the worm egg, Toxoplasma remain viable under conditions in which the unprotected organisms would not survive. *Toxocara* of dogs and cats can establish and undergo partial development in man, mice and fowls. The common occurrence of *Toxocara* in dogs and cats and the close association of these animals with man suggests that some cases of toxoplasmosis are acquired by ingestion of infected *Toxocara* eggs.

The diagnosis of toxoplasmosis is difficult because of the diverse distribution of the organism in a host. In experimental animals it is most easily detected in brain tissue. Specific and reliable diagnostic serological tests have been developed. Serological tests have been used to determine the incidence of *Toxoplasma gondii* in man and animals. A survey of dogs from the London area showed an incidence of 45 per cent, and the incidence in human populations of different countries has varied from 0 to 68 per cent. These figures indicate that *T. gondii* is a common parasite of man, but the infection is usually cryptic and benign.

HELMINTHOLOGY

Table 19.3 lists the helminths that are of medical importance. The two main groups are the roundworms or nematodes and the flatworms or platyhelminths. The latter are subdivided further into flukes or trematodes and tapeworms or cestodes.

Roundworms or nematodes

The roundworms are medically the most important helminths. In general, they cause chronic debilitating diseases, although trichinosis, due to a roundworm, *Trichinella spiralis*, may lead to sudden death. Nematodes such as the filariae and hookworms cause chronic suffering of large populations in many parts of the world. The importance of nematodes as parasites of man and other animals should not obscure the fact that members of the group have invaded every possible habitat except the atmosphere. Besides being parasitic in animals and plants, there are many species, largely undescribed, free living in the soil, in rivers and lakes, and in the sea. Their versatility is accompanied by incredible stability in structural organization. Whatever its habitat, almost any roundworm can be easily recognized as such from its simple, unsegmented and tubular structure, an inner tube or gut, being surrounded by an outer one, the body wall. Between the two tubes is a cavity filled with fluid, the pseudocoelom (figs. 19.12 & 19.13).

It has been suggested that the structural conservatism of nematodes has been dictated by the peculiar mechanical principles involved in their locomotion, the basic oddity being the hydrostatic skeleton. The components of this system are an external cuticle containing a basket-work of inextensible criss-crossed fibres (fig. 19.14) and the pseudocoelomic fluid under very high pressure. The pressure is opposed by longitudinal muscles in the body wall (fig. 19.13) the contraction of which shortens the worm and tends to decrease its volume; the volume changes are the simple consequences of the geometry of the system. Muscle relaxation automatically lengthens the worm due to the force exerted by the pressure on the cuticular basketwork. Differential contraction of dorsal and ventral muscle-blocks accounts for the wave-like swimming action of most nematodes. The arrangement is unique in requiring muscles operating in one direction only, but it would be mechanically impossible without pressures much greater than are found in other worm-like creatures. Some of the secondary features of roundworm structure, such as the very muscular oesophagus (sometimes called the pharynx), the anal sphincter and the solid tissue surrounding the excretory ducts (the lateral lines) can be considered as special adaptations to combat the otherwise detrimental effects of such high internal pressures.

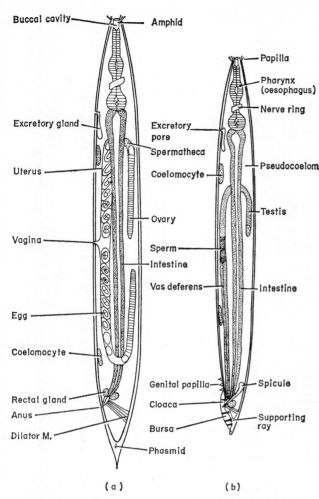

FIG. 19.12. Diagrammatic structure of adult female (a) and male (b) nematode, lateral views. From Lee D.L. (1965) *The Physiology of Nematodes*. Edinburgh: Oliver & Boyd.

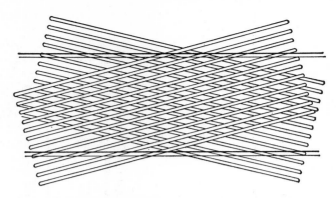

FIG. 19.14. Diagram of a small portion of the basketwork of fibres in the cuticle of *Ascaris suum*. The two heavy lines represent transverse annulations, approximately 20 μm apart, on the outside of the cuticle. From Lee D.L. (1965) *The Physiology of Nematodes*. Edinburgh: Oliver & Boyd.

The structure and chemical properties of the nematode cuticle are relevant to some immunological host–parasite relationships, and also to chemotherapy. The cuticular layers are almost completely protein in composition and cuticular proteins may be antigenic; but the intact cuticle is probably more inert in this respect than other constituents of roundworms, such as the pseudocoelomic fluid and their excretions and secretions. Thus the cuticle serves as a barrier between the parasitic nematode and the immunological attack of its host. It obviously serves as a barrier also to attack by anthelminthics if the compounds employed are unable to pass through, and the worms keep their mouths shut. Despite the fact that water together with many inorganic ions and other hydrophilic materials, such as amino acids and sugars, are able to penetrate the cuticle, most of the data on anthelminthic permeation can be explained on the basis of selectivity on the part of its thin outer layer of lipid. Thus the more hydrophobic drugs are able to penetrate with greater speed and are potentially the better nematocides.

As has been said, energy sources such as glucose are able to pass through the cuticle, but their rate of entry is too slow to be of nutritional value. Only glucose imbibed through the mouth is actively polymerized into glycogen. This contrasts with the parasitic flatworms where 'cuticular' feeding accounts for all nutritional uptake in tapeworms, and some of it in trematodes.

The structural uniformity of roundworms is matched by a comparable uniformity in the basic pattern of development. In the large number of species investigated the life cycle consists of six stages, i.e. an egg, four larval stages, and an adult (fig. 19.15). It is customary to refer to stages apart from the egg by number, starting with the 'first stage larva' and ending with the 'fifth stage', or adult. The sexes are separate in most species, differentiation of

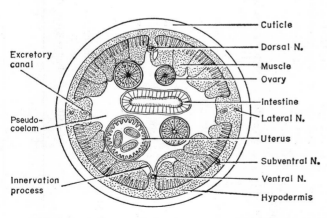

FIG. 19.13. Cross-section through a female nematode. From Lee D.L. (1965) *The Physiology of Nematodes*. Edinburgh: Oliver & Boyd.

TABLE 19.3. A summary of important helminths which infect man, giving the mode of infection, the resulting disorder and its distribution throughout the world: D, definitive host; I, intermediate host.

Parasite	Stages in man	Infection by	Major hosts in life cycle other than man	Condition caused	Distribution
NEMATODES (roundworms)					
RHABDIASOIDEA:					
Strongyloides stercoralis	3rd→5th	Skin penetrating larva	—	Enteritis	Tropical
STRONGYLOIDEA:					
Ancylostoma duodenale	3rd→5th	Skin penetrating larva	—	Enteritis: 'hookworm anaemia'	Tropical, subtropical
Necator americanus	3rd→5th	Skin penetrating larva	—	Enteritis: 'hookworm anaemia'	Tropical, subtropical
Ancylostoma braziliense *A. caninum* *Uncinaria stenocephala*	3rd	Skin penetrating larva	Dog, cat	Cutaneous larva migrans	Tropical, subtropical
OXYUROIDEA:					
Enterobius vermicularis	3rd→5th	Egg eaten in dust etc,	—	Enterobiasis: *pruritus ani*	Cosmopolitan
ASCAROIDEA:					
Ascaris lumbricoides	2nd→5th	Egg eaten in human faeces etc.	—	Enteritis; parasitic pneumonia	Cosmopolitan
Toxocara canis	2nd	Egg eaten in dog faeces	Dog (D), mice etc. (I)	Visceral larva migrans	Cosmopolitan
T. mystax	2nd	Egg eaten in cat faeces	Cat (D), mice, insects (I)	Visceral larva migrans	Cosmopolitan
DRACUNCULOIDEA:					
Dracunculus medinensis	3rd→5th	Intermediate host swallowed in drinking water	Copepod (freshwater) crustacean (I)	Cutaneous sores: allergic response	Tropical
FILARIOIDEA:					
Wuchereria bancrofti	1st, 3rd, 4th, 5th	Insect bites	Mosquitoes (I)	Elephantiasis	Tropical
Brugia malayi	1st, 3rd 4th, 5th	Insect bites	Mosquitoes	Elephantiasis	S. Asia, Far East
Loa loa	1st, 3rd, 4th, 5th	Insect bites	*Chrysops* (I)	'Fugitive swellings'— eye particularly	Tropical
Onchocerca volvulus	1st, 3rd, 4th, 5th	Insect bites	Blackfly (I)	Onchocerciasis 'river blindness,'	Tropical Africa Central America
TRICHINELLOIDEA:					
Trichinella spiralis	All stages	Undercooked meat, particularly pork	Pig and many other mammals	Trichinosis	Cosmopolitan
Trichuris trichiura	1st→5th	Egg eaten in human faeces	—	Enteritis	Cosmopolitan

PLATYHELMINTHS (flatworms)
TREMATODES (flukes)
FASCIOLIDAE

	Stage	Source of infection	Hosts	Disease	Distribution
Fasciolopsis buski	Adult	Vegetable food	Pig (D), snail (I)	Enteritis	Far East
Fasciola hepatica	Adult	Grass, watercress	Ruminants (D), snail (I)	Parasitic hepatitis	Cosmopolitan
OPISTHORCHIIDAE:					
Clonorchis sinensis	Adult	Undercooked fish	Snail (I), fish (I), cat (D)	Parasitic hepatitis	Far East
Opisthorchis felineus	Adult	Undercooked fish	Snail (I), fish (I), cat (D)	Parasitic hepatitis	Europe
HETEROPHYIDAE:					
Heterophyes heterophyes	Adult	Undercooked fish	Snail (I), fish (I)	Enteritis	N. Africa, Far East
TROGLOTREMATIDAE:					
Paragonimus westermanii	Adult	Undercooked crab	Snail (I), crab (I)	Pulmonary cysts	Far East
PARAMPHISTOMATIDAE:					
Gastrodiscoides hominis	Adult	?	Snail (?)	Enteritis	S. Asia
SCHISTOSOMATIDAE:					
Schistosoma japonicum	Adult	Skin penetrating larva	Snail	Enteric schistosomiasis	Far East
S. mansoni	Adult	Skin penetrating larva	Snail	Enteric schistosomiasis	Africa
S. haematobium	Adult	Skin penetrating larva	Snail	Vesical schistosomiasis	Africa
CESTODES (tapeworms)					
CYCLOPHYLLIDEA:					
Taenia solium	Adult (cyst rare)	Undercooked pork	Pig (I)	Enteritis (cysticercosis rare)	Cosmopolitan
T. saginata	Adult	Undercooked beef	Ox (I)	Enteritis	Cosmopolitan
Echinococcus granulosus	Cyst	Eating eggs in dog faeces	Sheep (I), dog (D)	Hepatic and pulmonary hydatid	Cosmopolitan
E. multilocularis	Cyst	Eating eggs in fox or wolf faeces	Vole (I), fox (D), wolf (D), dog (D)	Alveolar hydatid	Europe and N. America
Hymenolepis nana	Adult cyst	Eating eggs in human faeces	Mouse (D), rat (D), though strain differences	Enteritis	Cosmopolitan
PSEUDOPHYLLIDEA:					
Diphyllobothrium latum	Adult	Undercooked fish	Copepod crustacean (I), freshwater fish (I),	Enteritis, vit. B_{12} deficiency(?)	Europe, N. America
Diphyllobothrium spp.	Larva	Flesh of lower vertebrates and swallowing freshwater copepods	Copepods, (I), fish, (I), amphibia, reptiles (transport hosts)	Sparganosis	Cosmopolitan

male from female usually becoming morphologically obvious in the fourth stage. The completion of each stage from one to four is marked by a moult, or shedding of the cuticle, with the formation of new cuticle underneath.

The nematode larva differs from the larvae of other groups (e.g. insects) in that its structure is essentially the same as that of the adult, except for differences in size and in the degree of development of the gonads. For this reason the use of the term larva to describe the immature nematode may be questioned, but it is firmly entrenched.

When moults occur in mammalian tissues, there is a temporary increase in the flow of antigenic information from parasite to host, largely in the form of moulting fluid. This in turn has led to the theory that protective immunity to nematode infections results from the forma-tion of anti-moulting fluid antibodies, and that the moulting phases of the parasite are thus the immunogenic stages (but see p. 19.19). This is an extension of an old idea that protective antibodies are often anti-enzyme in character since moulting fluid is thought to contain enzymes which hydrolyse components of the cuticle.

The pattern of development persists even though a given stage in the life cycle may become adapted to very different habitats in different species. Some tele-scoping of the life cycle has occurred in highly evolved parasites, such as *Ascaris* and *Wuchereria*, which are isolated from the outside environment at all stages of development. Less well-adapted forms, such as the hookworms, pursue a free-living existence as far as the third stage. Some nematodes, such as the *Strongyloides*

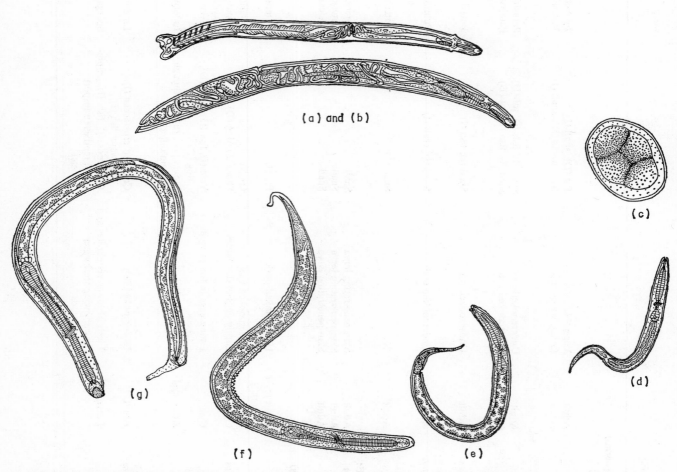

FIG. 19.15. A complete nematode life cycle; *Ancylostoma duodenale*; (a) adult male, (b) adult female, (c) egg, (d) first stage larva, (e) second stage larva, (f) third stage infective larva, (g) fourth stage. Compared with (a) and (b), (c) is drawn on a scale ×500, (d), (e) and (f) ×20 and (g) ×7; the adult female is 10–13 mm long.

species, have the luxury of a parasitic life for their fourth and fifth stages for some of the time, but may return to the outside world for a completely free-living existence.

It has been suggested that nematodes, because of the resistant third stage larva which is found in many members of the group, including free-living forms, were preadapted to a parasitic existence. It has also been proposed that heavy immunological selection has been brought to bear on the struggling parasitic nematode, and that such selection has been more rigorous than that operating on most viruses and bacteria and that it leads to a different end point. Bacterial parasites usually reproduce in the host's body and are released within the period of the primary immunological response. Selection of antigen mutations, or 'immunological drift', is thus random in the sense that any different antigen is unrecognized by a host immunized by an earlier infection, and so is advantageous to the parasite. In the case of nematodes and other metazoan parasites the stages destined to pass on the infection are rarely, if ever, developed or released until after the primary response is fully developed. In fact an immune state will have supervened whilst the parasites are reproducing and disseminating their transmission stages. This is likely to select against parasitic antigens which elicit a protective immune response in the host at the very first encounter. Thus parasites of this type may evolve antigens like those of the host, since most random variation would be disadvantageous. Such a process is called **molecular mimicry**. Combative evolutionary trends in the host can be expected while any degree of pathogenicity exists, and may take the form of a balanced genetic polymorphism in the host population with regard to the relevant antigens. The genetics and distribution of the human blood groups have been explained by arguments along similar lines.

The various stages of nematodes may be found in many regions of the host's body. The larvae of most of the human parasites, such as *Trichinella spiralis*, *Ascaris lumbricoides*, the hookworms, and *Strongyloides stercoralis* travel via blood and/or connective tissue for some of their parasitic existence. Adult filarioids, e.g. *Wuchereria bancrofti* and *Loa loa*, as well as larvae, are tissue dwellers, having escaped completely from the site of most adult parasitic nematodes, the gut. On the theory that tissue stages are predominant in eliciting an immune response, most of the nematodes infecting man are likely to be immunogenic at some stage of their invasion. Is it valid to assume, however, that their noninvasive stages are not immunogenic, or that the complete development of parasites like *Enterobius*, which live in the lumen of the gut and have no invasive stage, are spared the onslaught of the host's specific defences? Experimental

evidence is against such assumptions; transplantation of adults of the nematode *Nippostrongylus brasiliensis*, for example, from one rat's intestine to another elicits good protective immunity in the recipient even though the invasive stages of the life cycle have been omitted. This particular result also shows that moulting is not a crucial immunogenic stage, as some believe (p. 19.18).

The current position is clear to the extent that the ideas of the 1920s, that metazoan parasites were inaccessible to immunological mechanisms for one reason or another, have been refuted. However, the precise nature of the protective reaction against nematode invasion seems to be related to other poorly understood immunological phenomena, such as immediate (p. 22.19) and delayed hypersensitivity (p. 22.20). Although specific γ-globulins appear in the serum as a result of nematode infections, they have at best an indirect role in protection. In many host-parasite systems the mass of worms behaves like a homograft between genetically similar, though not identical, members of the same species. In particular, there often appears to be a threshold level in the size of infection below which the parasitic 'graft' is tolerated and above which rejection occurs. This is circumstantial evidence for a partial antigenic similarity between host and parasite and supports the evolutionary arguments for the development of molecular mimicry.

The immunological differences between microbial infections and metazoan parasitism may also result from the fact that the helminths are self-limiting in any individual host (providing, of course, reinfection does not occur), whereas bacteria and viruses multiply inside the host until it either dies or mobilizes an effective defence system.

In the foregoing account, the morphological and developmental uniformity of nematodes has been emphasized. When one considers the many roles a roundworm may play, it would be surprising if they were as physiologically inflexible. Indeed, even the rudimentary knowledge we possess makes it plain that within this group there is a wealth of biochemical and physiological diversity awaiting analysis.

Flatworms or platyhelminths

In general, parasitic flatworms are medically less important than the nematodes, with one or two notable exceptions. Among the exceptions are the three species of *Schistosoma*, causative agents of major human diseases in Africa, South America and the Far East. Hydatidosis of man, due to the cyst of *Echinococcus granulosus*, is important in sheep-rearing areas such as Australasia. With these, and the possible addition of fasciolopsiasis and clonorchiasis in the Far East, the catalogue of really significant platyhelminth diseases is complete. However, in developed countries, where devastating disease is largely under control, it is natural that attention is paid to the eradication of minor clinical entities such as taeniasis and diphyllobothriasis.

All flatworms have a few common features although much less uniform in structure and development than the nematodes. Nearly all are hermaphrodite (the schistosomes are exceptions), all have flame cells in their osmoregulatory–excretory systems (fig. 19.16), and their internal organs are cushioned in a loosely packed cellular

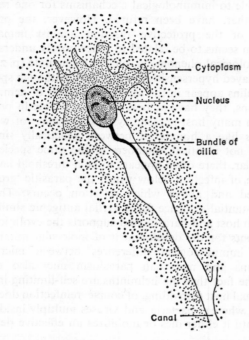

FIG. 19.16. A flame cell typical of all flatworm osmoregulatory–excretory systems. From Borrowdale L.A. *et al.* (1963) *The Invertebrates*, 4th Edition. London: Cambridge University Press.

parenchyma and not in any kind of body cavity. The basic structure of the gonads is a fairly constant feature, particularly that part of it concerned with assembling the various components of the egg, the so-called shell gland or Mehlis' gland (fig. 19.17).

FLUKES OR TREMATODES

The digenetic flukes have typically two hosts in the life cycle, sometimes more but never less. The definitive host, i.e. the one harbouring the sexually mature parasite, is always a vertebrate; the intermediate hosts are invertebrates. The first intermediate host is some kind of mollusc, generally an aquatic or amphibious snail. A high degree of host specificity is shown in this phase of the life cycle in contrast to others, such as the adult phase which, for a particular fluke, can occur in a number of species. Low specificity is shown too, in the choice of second intermediate hosts where these are utilized, so

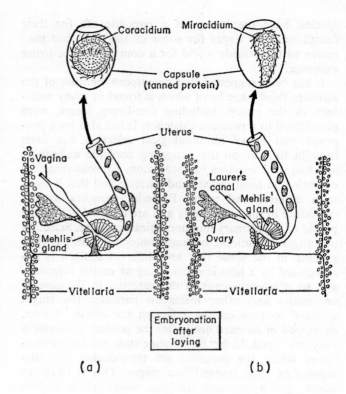

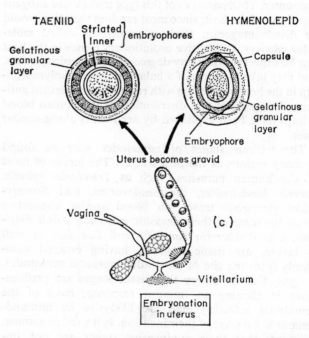

FIG. 19.17. Diagrammatic comparison between the female reproductive organs and eggs of pseudophyllidean cestodes (a), digenetic trematodes (b) and cyclophyllidean cestodes (c). From Smyth J.D. (1962) *Introduction to Animal Parasitology*. London: English University Press.

that control of fluke parasites is best concentrated on the mollusc host.

Morphologically, the typical adult digenetic fluke is represented by *Clonorchis sinensis* (fig. 19.18). Different

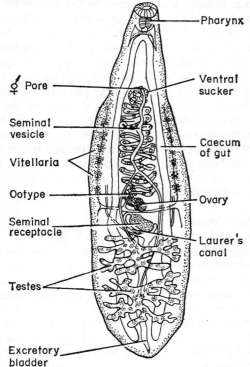

FIG. 19.18. Adult *Clonorchis sinensis* showing the structures visible after fixing and staining. From Smyth J.D. (1962) *Introduction to Animal Parasitology*. London: English Universities Press.

species differ in shape, although the contours of the body may be modified by the organism's movements, in the position of the oral and ventral suckers, the presence of spines or scales on the cuticle, the position of the gonads in the body, the extent to which the vitellaria (the site of synthesis of the shell and yolk material) fill the lateral margins of the fluke, the form taken by the gut caeca, and so on. Unless fixed and stained, however, the fluke reveals little of its internal structure and, in life, appears as a flat, leaf-like, cream-coloured object, in most cases visible to the naked eye.

Digenetic flukes are often parasites of the gut of vertebrate hosts, though they may be found in the liver. or the lungs, or in cysts in other parts of the body. Particularly important in man are those flukes which live in the blood, i.e. members of the family Schistosomatidae.

Life cycle

In cases where the adult lives in the gut or an associated organ, the eggs it lays pass in the faeces. The egg is usually

operculate (fig. 19.19), and requires development outside the host to the first larva, a ciliated **miracidium** (fig. 19.19b). This motile stage, having hatched, is very short lived and must find the correct species of snail in a matter of hours; it then burrows into the snail's tissues and sheds its cilia to become the next stage in the life-cycle, the **sporocyst.** The sporocyst typically produces, by internal budding from its wall, the next larval stage, or **redia.** A varying number of these, depending on the species of fluke, are produced for each sporocyst. The rediae may produce further generations of rediae, or they may produce directly the last stage to develop in the snail, the **cercaria.** This is a tailed motile stage which emerges from the snail, and usually turns into a **metacercaria** by losing its tail and secreting a tough

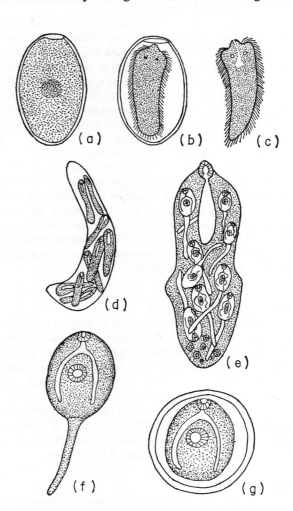

FIG. 19.19. The development stages of a digenetic trematode; (a) egg when laid, (b) egg with miracidium developed, (c) hatched miracidium, (d) sporocyst, (e) redia containing cercariae, (f) cercaria, (g) metacercaria. From Hackett C.J. (1954) *Manual of Medical Helminthology*. London: Cassell.

protective wall. A metacercaria is essentially a very young fluke; it has the oral and ventral suckers of the adult and a small gut with the two lateral caeca (fig. 19.19g), but the gonads are absent. It may form shortly after release from the snail, encysting on herbage as in the case of two-host flukes like *Fasciolopsis*. In three-host flukes such as *Clonorchis*, the metacercaria is formed in the second intermediate host (a fish in *C. sinensis*) after active penetration by the cercaria. Alternatively, no metacercariae may be formed at all; a condition found in schistosomes.

In some fluke life cycles one or other larval stage may be omitted or curtailed; the absence of a metacercaria in schistosomes is an example. The schistosomes also lack a redial stage, multiplication inside the snail being restricted to sporocysts.

If a metacercaria of an intestinal fluke is swallowed, it excysts in the gut and then grows to the adult worm, attaching itself to the gut wall. In the life cycles of flukes which live in the liver or the lungs or other tissues, migration must take place, and this is usually through the peritoneal cavity to the liver, or further, through the diaphragm to the lungs and other organs. The schistosome cercariae penetrate the skin and find their way into the blood via the lymphatic system.

The extensive migrations of these young flukes through the tissues suggests that immune responses may follow their invasion, and certainly antigen–antibody reactions can be detected. However, there is little evidence of a protective immunity against the trematodes of man though there is a vast serology related to the schistosomes. The sera of patients suspected of harbouring schistosomes may be tested against various antigens derived from schistosome eggs and cercariae.

TAPEWORMS OR CESTODES

Many features of the cestodes reflect structures which are found in the trematodes. The form of the adult reproductive organs, the type of parenchymatous tissue, and the structure of the tegument or cuticle have many similarities; the cestodes, however, have no internal gut, and there is the characteristic feature, certainly in all the human tapeworms, of the repetition of identical units, the **proglottids**, forming a segmented structure. The means of attachment, the holdfast (also called the head or scolex), is another unique feature of the group.

Life cycle

The adult tapeworm is restricted almost exclusively to the gut of the definitive host, and this applies to all species in man. The life cycle is very different from that of trematodes, though members of the Pseudophyllidea have some superficial resemblances. Except in one species there are at least two hosts; *Hymenolepis nana*, the dwarf tapeworm of man, although often using two, can dispense with its intermediate host.

The definitive host is always a vertebrate. The intermediate host may be a vertebrate or an invertebrate and this stage is some kind of cyst. In the vertebrate intermediate host this is a bladder worm, a fluid-filled sac containing one or more heads which ultimately become adult tapeworms. In invertebrate intermediate hosts the cyst, a **cysterceroid**, is smaller and is simply the head of a tapeworm surrounded by parenchymatous tissue, often bearing a small tail-like structure. The intermediate host must become infected by eating the egg or the larva which emerges from the egg. This larva is known as a **hexacanth embryo**, i.e. a small sphere with three pairs of characteristic hooks. Muscles are attached to the hooks within the body of the larva (figs. 19.24c, j & l), and these are instrumental in its migrations through the tissues of the intermediate host.

Immunity reactions

Experimental immunology of adult tapeworm infections suggests that a protective immunity may be developed, though this has been studied only in rat tapeworms of the genus *Hymenolepis*. Immune responses of mammals to larval tapeworm infections have also been studied in model laboratory systems, and, as one might expect for such predominantly tissue dwellers, an immunity is elicited. In a number of experimental situations in which acquired protective immunity to platyhelminth infections can be demonstrated, it seems that somatic antigens are important in eliciting the protective antibody response, unlike the situation in nematodes, where excretion–secretion antigens (plate 19.2) are the functional ones in this respect. The difference is interesting when one examines the character of the integument of the two types of parasite. In the case of the nematode, it appears to be an inert structure, in other words, a true cuticle. Electron microscopy and biochemical studies show that the cuticle of the parasitic platyhelminths is far from inanimate, and that it has many metabolic functions. It is therefore unlikely to be the same kind of immunological or chemotherapeutic barrier as is the case in nematodes. It is possible that the greater significance of somatic antigens in immune reactions to flatworm infections compared with nematodiases is to some extent related to these differences in cuticular structure. To emphasize these differences the term 'tegument' may be preferable to 'cuticle' when referring to the outside of a platyhelminth. In particular, in cestodes, the tegument must perform the function of a gut; it has to take in nutrient material, and specific biochemical transport mechanisms have been demonstrated which selectively take up amino acids and monosaccharides. Indeed the rate of uptake of glucose may control the number of worms in the host's gut. If the popula-

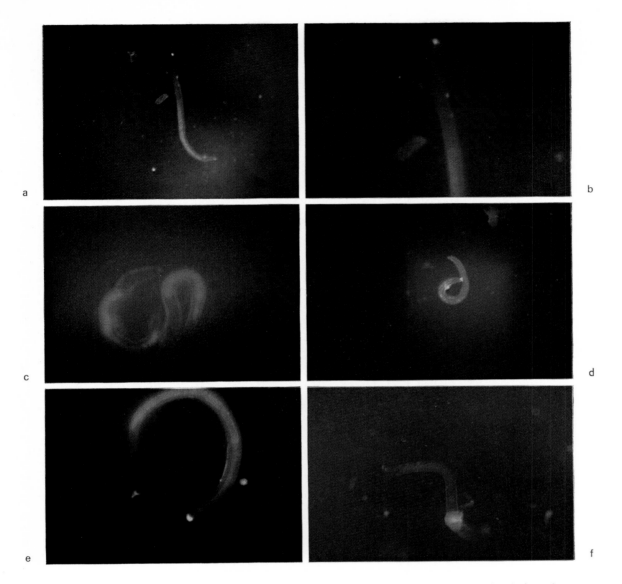

a

b

c

d

e

f

PLATE 19.2. Use of near ultraviolet fluorescence microscopy in the immunodiagnosis of visceral larva migrans (VLM).

Larvae of *Toxocara canis* placed in fluorescein isothyocyanate-labelled globulin from the sera of experimental rabbits (a, b, c & d) and known human cases of VLM due to *T. canis* (e & f). Labelled globulin from uninfected rabbits (c) shows the autofluorescence of the larval intestine only. The bright yellow fluorescence identifies specific antibody from one globulin fraction of infected rabbits (a & b) and human subjects (e & f) conjugating with excretion–secretion (ES) antigens produced at the mouth, excretory pore and anus of the larva. Another globulin fraction shows less specific labelling of antigens scattered at random over the surface of the larva (d). The specific fraction from sera of people infected with, or allergic to, roundworms other than *Toxocara* spp. gives no reaction with *T. canis* larvae.

From Hogarth Scott R.S. (1966) Visceral larva migrans. *Immunology*, **10**, 217. By kind permission of the author and the H.E. Durham Fund of King's College, Cambridge which has borne the cost of the plate.

tion of parasites is sufficiently large, competition for sugar is a growth-limiting factor. In the gut the tapeworm has to compete with the host's intestinal epithelium for a supply of sugars, which is always limited by rapid absorption.

There are few tapeworm parasites of man and in most he is the definitive host. These are of minor clinical importance. There are, however, two genera in which the cyst is found in man; one of these, *Echinococcus*, producing hydatid or alveolar cyst, can be very dangerous. The other is the genus *Taenia*, which normally infects man in the adult stage, but the species *T. solium* can occasionally give rise to cysticercosis, i.e. the cystic stage may develop as a result of autoinfection from a patient's own faeces containing the tapeworm's eggs. This, although comparatively rare, can give rise to serious disease, particularly if the cyst migrates into the central nervous system.

Helminth parasites of man

The following summary has been arranged, not according to zoological classification, but according to the manner in which man becomes infected.

INFECTION BY EATING UNDERCOOKED MEAT

Undercooked pork is commonly the carrier of infections of the important nematode parasite, *Trichinella spiralis* (fig. 19.20) which causes **trichinosis**. This in many ways is an atypical nematode; the adults are short-lived in the gut and, though they may cause temporary inconvenience, they are not the primary cause of the illness.

The females lay larvae which invade the mucosa of the gut and migrate to skeletal muscle in various parts of the body, particularly the diaphragm, intercostal muscles, larynx, tongue and masseter muscles. In these positions they become enclosed in lemon-shaped cysts of reactive tissue formed by the host, taking a number of weeks for complete development. The disease results from damage to the muscles, its exact form depending on the site and number of larvae. Particularly dangerous is invasion of the intercostals and muscles of the larynx, which may lead to fatal hypoxia. Unless calcified by host reaction, larvae stay dormant in the muscle and infective for another host eating such meat. The cysts are digested out of the tissues by the new host's enzymes; the larvae emerge, moult to the adults, and the life cycle is completed.

Although discovered as long ago as 1835 by an enterprising medical student during dissection, *T. spiralis* is still the subject of controversy. For instance, the traditionally accepted vascular route of larvae to the muscles has been challenged recently. It may turn out that they travel via the peritoneal cavity and connective tissue, a suggestion that agrees well with their final distribution in the body.

Epidemiologically the picture is complicated because, unlike most nematodes, *T. spiralis* has a wide host range.

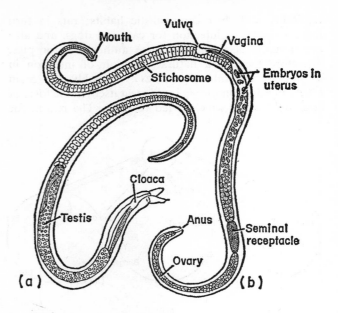

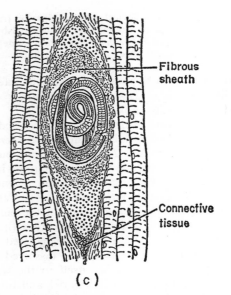

FIG. 19.20. *Trichinella spiralis*; male (a), female (b) and infective larva encysted in skeletal muscle (c). From Smyth J.D. (1962) *Introduction to Animal Parasitology*. London: English Universities Press.

As well as pigs and man, most carnivorous or omnivorous animals can be infected, and this includes other sources of food for man. In the Arctic for instance, bear meat is a source of infection. The wide host range means also that the epidemiological cycle involves animals other than man and pig even where pig is the only carrier of human infection. Wild rats carry an endemic infection of *Trichinella* because of their susceptibility and their cannibalistic habits; rats in turn form a source of infection for cats and dogs, and also occasionally, according to some authorities, for pigs. Therefore there is a natural reservoir of infection in livestock and game (fig. 19.21). Probably the main source of infection for pig is pig meat itself, in the form of household waste which is fed to them. The reason for

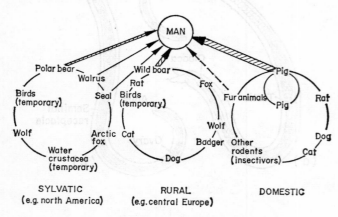

FIG. 19.21. Epidemiological relationships for trichinosis in different types of community. From Soulsby E.J.L. (1965) *Textbook of Veterinary Clinical Parasitology*, vol. I. Helminths. Oxford: Blackwell Scientific Publications.

considering this to be so is that *Trichinella* infections are virtually absent in areas where pigs are fed garbage which has been rigorously cooked.

Another parasite which may be acquired through eating undercooked pork is the tapeworm *Taenia solium*. It is not as dangerous as *Trichinella spiralis*, but it merits serious consideration due to rare variations in the life-cycle affecting man. Usually infection of man results from eating the cysts (*Cysticercus cellulosae*) of the tapeworm which may be found in any of the pig's skeletal muscles. The cyst is a typical cysticercus (fig. 19.22c), i.e. a bladderworm with a single invaginated proscolex.

When eaten by man the cyst is dissolved away, the head evaginates and attaches itself to the wall of the small intestine by means of its hooks and four circular suckers. The neck of the tapeworm just behind the head then starts to proliferate proglottids, reaching chain lengths of up to 70 cm. The segments, which have successively become mature (fig. 19.25b) and then gravid (fig. 19.22), are shed at the end of the chain. Thus packets of eggs are passed in the faeces for infection of the intermediate host, i.e. the pig. The tapeworm is specific in both phases of its life cycle; it is found only in the adult stage in man, and in the cysticercus stage in the pig. Man may act artificially as the 'intermediate host' by becoming infected with the eggs (p. 19.23), a condition known as **cysticercosis**. When eaten by the pig, the egg of the tapeworm containing the hexacanth embryo passes

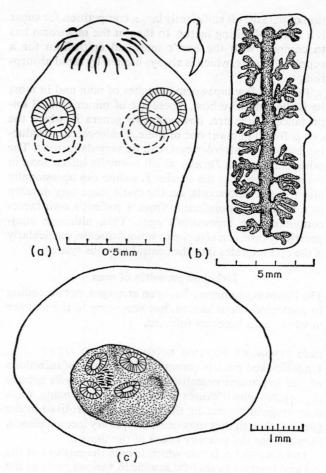

FIG. 19.22. *Taenia solium*; (a) holdfast, (b) gravid segment, (c) *Cysticercus cellulosae*. From Hackett C.J. (1954) *Manual of Medical Helminthology*. London: Cassell.

down into the small intestine; the embryo hatches and burrows into the gut wall, enters the portal blood and is carried through the liver into the heart, the pulmonary circulation, back through the heart, and finally into the systemic circulation leading to the peripheral capillaries and body musculature. In this position the hexacanth embryo develops into the cysticercus by growth and the formation of the typical bladderworm having the invaginated holdfast with its hooks and suckers. The cysticercus in the muscle, surrounded by an adventitious connective tissue coat, is infective for man and may survive for a considerable time, though ultimately the calcification reactions of the host's defence mechanisms kill it.

The beef tapeworm, *Taenia saginata*, is as host specific as *T. solium* and has a life cycle which is very similar, with the ox as the intermediate host. Slight morphological differences, such as the absence of hooks on the scolex of *T. saginata* and details of the gravid segments, provide means to distinguish the two worms. Unlike those of *T. solium*, the gravid segments of the beef tapeworm often migrate out of faeces, distributing eggs as they break up. They may even migrate out of the anus from inside the host; a patient may discover the infection when a gravid segment is found wandering in his clothing. *T. saginata* is less important than *T. solium* because it has never been incriminated in cases of human cysticercosis, but it is the only one of the two which occurs in Britain due possibly to the suggested epidemiological picture outlined in fig. 19.23.

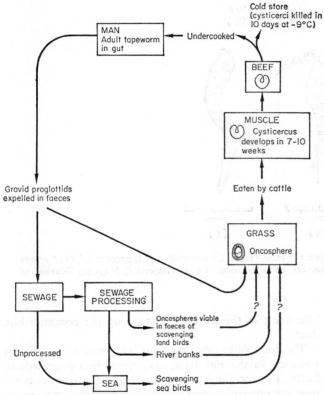

FIG. 19.23. *Taenia saginata*; suggested epidemiological cycle in the United Kingdom.

Control measures
Thorough cooking of meat prevents the infection of man with parasites of this type. Meat inspection is effective against tapeworms, debatably so against *Trichinella*. In the USA, where serious local epidemics of trichinosis are not infrequent, the inspection of pork for *Trichinella* cysts has been discontinued. The reason for this is that the cyst is small, and its detection requires microscopic examination of meat using an apparatus called a compressorium (two pieces of glass sheet between which the suspected meat can be squashed). These procedures are inefficient and lead to a false sense of security. Another way of controlling such diseases is to prevent

infection of food animals. Methods to achieve this differ depending upon whether taeniasis or trichinosis is involved. The source of *Trichinella* infection for pigs is primarily household waste containing infected pig meat. In the case of the pork and beef tapeworms, pigs and cattle become infected by eating human faeces, and therefore a different regime must be adopted for their control. The existence of many reservoir hosts for *Trichinella* must also be taken into account in any control programme (fig. 19.21).

INFECTIONS FROM EATING UNDERCOOKED FISH AND CRUSTACEA
Throughout the world many species of freshwater fish carry infection of the broad tapeworm of man, *Diphyllobothrium latum*. As in other pseudophyllideans, the head is inserted into the wall of the small intestine and expanded to grip laterally. The spatulate muscular holdfast with two longitudinal grooves (fig. 19.24a) is clearly adapted for this function and does not need the hooks and suckers typical of cyclophyllideans (fig. 19.22a). Differences in the segments of the two types of tapeworm can be seen in fig. 19.25a and b.

The operculate eggs of *Diphyllobothrium* are laid through the uterine pores of mature segments, pass out in the faeces and develop to the hexacanth embryo outside the host. The embryo inside the egg is surrounded by a ciliated coat which enables it to swim about once it has hatched. The eggs must reach ponds or streams before the larvae or coracidia hatch, for it is in such habitats that the intermediate hosts are to be found. Various species of freshwater copepod crustacea are the first intermediate hosts, becoming infected when they eat the larvae. Once the copepod, often a species of *Cyclops* (fig. 19.24e), has eaten a larva, the hooks of the hexacanth embryo are used to burrow from the gut into the body cavity, where the procercoid develops. This still contains the three pairs of hooks of the hexacanth embryo, as well as a main body with penetration glands at one end (fig. 19.24d). Continuance of the life cycle requires the infected copepod to be eaten by a small freshwater fish, whose tissues become invaded by the procercoid. Growth and morphogenetic processes produce the next stage, the plerocercoid (fig. 19.24f), within the fish, which is a true second intermediate host potentially capable of carrying the infection to the definitive host. However, it is common for the infected stickleback, or similar fish, to be eaten in turn by a larger predator fish such as a pike. When this happens the plerocercoid is able to invade the body cavity of the predator and still remain infective for a definitive host. A pike playing such a role is classed as a transport host for the reason that no development or reproduction of the parasite takes place. Man is only one of a number of fish-eating mammals in which the adult tapeworm may develop. Salmon and trout,

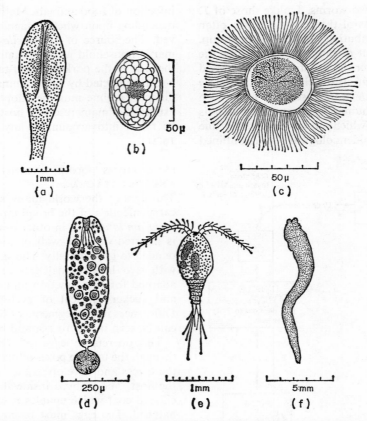

FIG. 19.24. *Diphyllobothrium latum*; (a) holdfast, (b) egg as it appears in fresh faeces, (c) coracidium, (d) procercoid, (e) *Cyclops* containing procercoids, (f) plerocercoid. Note the different scale for each drawing. From Hackett C.J. (1954) *Manual of Medical Helminthology*. London: Cassell.

perch, pike, eel, and other species can act as transport hosts.

In addition to the broad tapeworm, three kinds of fluke may be transmitted to man by eating undercooked fresh-water fish. An important species in the Far East is *Clonorchis sinensis* (fig. 19.18), which lives in the bile ducts of its hosts. The molluscan phase is unusual in that the mollusc must eat the egg containing the fully developed miracidium, a case of curtailment in the life cycle. Cercariae, which emerge from the snail, burrow into the muscles of the freshwater fish, and the metacercariae which are formed are infective for man and other fish-eating mammals (fig. 19.26). A similar life cycle is undergone by the minute, heterophyid gut flukes, the commonest being the North African species, *Heterophyes heterophyes*. The second intermediate hosts of this species, as in *C. sinensis*, are freshwater food fish. In Europe a species of fluke very closely related to *C. sinensis*, *Opisthorchis felineus*, is sometimes found in man, though it is more frequently a parasite of cats. The *Clonorchis* and *Opisthorchis* species do not migrate through the tissues of the mammal's body; they enter the bile ducts in the liver by passage up the common bile duct.

The lung fluke, *Paragonimus westermani*, (fig. 19.27) common in the Far East, also needs two intermediate hosts. The second intermediate hosts in this case, however, are crustacea; man becomes infected by eating crabs and crayfish, either raw or pickled in vinegar or wine.

Control measures
These helminth infections occur in areas where raw fish and crustacea are particular delicacies. The recommendation to cook food of this type is therefore unlikely to have much effect. Refrigeration, salting or drying, are not effective in killing the infective stages. To control all these diseases, one must aim at the removal of the sources of infection for the fish. This is a difficult problem because wild and domestic fish-eating mammals are often infected though *Diphyllobothrium* infections in man primarily arise from human sources and other reservoirs are insignificant. In the trematodiases, however, nonhuman reservoirs are important, and certainly in some areas of China, clonorchiasis would not exist

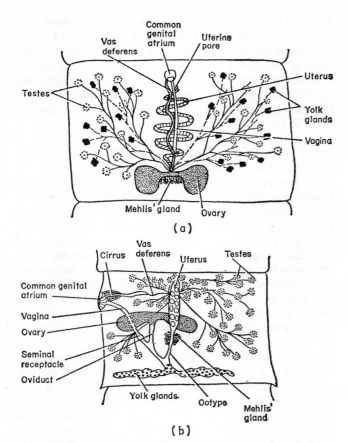

FIG. 19.25. Comparison of mature segments of a pseudo-phyllidean (*Diphyllobothrium latum*) (a) and a cyclo-phyllidean (*Taenia spp.*) tapeworm (b). From Hackett C.J. (1954) *Manual of Medical Helminthology.* London: Cassell.

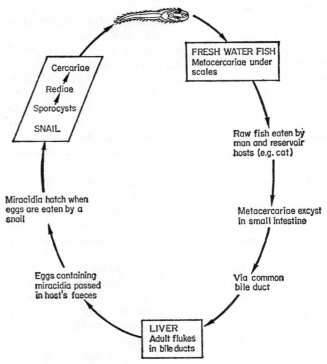

FIG. 19.26. Life cycle of *Clonorchis sinensis.*

were it not for infections in domestic animals. For the control of *Diphyllobothrium*, therefore, the life cycle can be effectively broken by preventing human faeces from entering the environment of the intermediate hosts. This is less likely to be successful in dealing with the fluke diseases originating from aquatic food and really the only protection for man is to be sure that the fish he eats is cooked adequately.

INFECTION FROM VEGETABLE FOOD

The gut fluke, *Fasciolopsis buski*, is acquired by man through eating raw vegetables, usually two plants extensively cultivated in the Far East, the water chestnut and water caltrop. There is a close ecological relationship between man, the food crop, and the intermediate host snail. Pigs, as well as man, can be infected with *F. buski*. The morphology of the fluke and its life cycle resemble closely those of *Fasciola hepatica*, the common liver fluke of sheep. The latter occasionally infects man, and recent outbreaks of human **fascioliasis** have been reported in England, South America, France and North Africa.

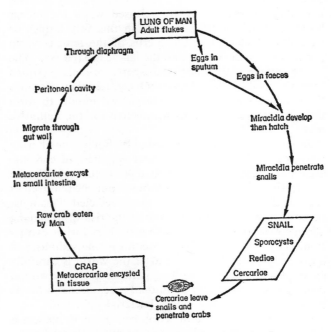

FIG. 19.27. Life cycle of *Paragonimus westermani.*

Control measures

If human or pig faeces containing *Fasciolopsis* eggs were not used as fertilizer, then the primary cause of human epidemics would be removed. Meanwhile entry of the metacercariae into the human host could be prevented by scalding vegetables before they are peeled; alternatively, cooking would solve the problem, but the material is generally eaten raw. Human infection with *Fasciola* can be prevented by avoiding ingestion of the metacercariae; grass should not be eaten, nor watercress grown, in areas where sheep or cattle are commonly grazed.

Under some circumstances *Ascaris lumbricoides* may be transmitted to man by vegetables which have been fertilized with human faeces. Ascariasis is more commonly a direct result of low standards of public and personal hygiene, however, and is discussed below.

INFECTIONS FROM DRINKING WATER

A parasite acquired through the drinking of unclean water is the 'fiery serpent' or Guinea worm, *Dracunculus medinensis* (plate 19.3a) common in parts of Asia and Africa. The infection is carried by a small freshwater copepod, often a species of *Cyclops* (fig. 19.24e). The *Cyclops'* intermediate host harbours the third stage infective larva and this, once swallowed by man, burrows into the wall of his gut. It passes into the peritoneal connective tissue, where it lives for some time. After several months and two moults, the adult female migrates to subcutaneous tissues in the limbs, where a blister forms just over the site of the worm. The female, by this time, is fully gravid, and contains many hatched first stage larvae which are released when the blister bursts. When a patient infected in this way bathes or wets the infected area, the uterus of the female worm prolapses into the water, and the larvae are released. The larvae mingle with other microscopic organisms which form the food of the copepods. Once eaten they pass into the copepod's haemocoel, undergo two moults to form the third stage, and are then infective for the definitive host.

Dracunculiasis can be prevented by boiling or filtering water or the use of tapped water supplies. In endemic areas treatment of infected individuals reduces the chance of infection of other people. Worms should be removed as soon as the characteristic blisters are detected. This must be done rather carefully because of the risk of damaging allergic reactions if the parasite is broken during extraction. The generally adopted procedure is long, tedious, and apparently primitive. The head of the worm is carefully externalized and then the long parasite is slowly wound onto a small stick with additional precautions as far as possible to prevent secondary bacterial infection.

Another water borne infection can occur in man as a result of tapeworms related to *Diphyllobothrium latum*.

This is the condition called **sparganosis**. Plerocercoids, or spargana, may be found wandering in the tissues of many animals, including man. One of a number of ways of becoming infected with such parasites is by accidental ingestion of a copepod intermediate host containing the tapeworm's procercoid larva (fig. 19.24d), which traverses the gut wall and develops to the plerocercoid, or sparganum, in the tissues.

INFECTION RESULTING FROM SUBSTANDARD PUBLIC AND PERSONAL HYGIENE

Roundworm and cestode infections may result from the ingestion of the parasites' infective stages due to inadequate sanitation or poor personal hygiene. The most important is **hydatidosis**, due to cysts of taeniid tapeworms of the genus *Echinococcus*. *E. granulosus* is responsible for 'hydatid' proper and *E. multilocularis* associated with 'alveolar hydatid'. Hydatidosis granulosus occurs in sheep farming areas, human infection being accidental. The natural cycle stems from the domestic dog, which becomes infected by eating sheep offal containing hydatid cysts. The adult tapeworms (fig. 19.28a) develop in the small intestine of the dog from the numerous proscolices of the cyst, and shed gravid segments in the same way as other cyclophyllidean tapeworms. Faeces carrying tapeworm segments adhere to the dog's fur and generally contaminate the animal and its environment. Normally the intermediate host is the sheep, and the life cycle is completed when a sheep eats the eggs or the gravid segments. The hexacanth embryo burrows into the wall of the sheep's small intestine, enters the portal system and, in most cases, becomes arrested in the hepatic capillary beds where the slow growing cyst begins to develop. Other embryos may pass on in the circulation to the lungs and through these to the systemic circulation. The sites where cysts may form in man are similar, most in the liver, some in the lung, and a few, approximately 5 per cent, in other regions such as the central nervous system or the muscles. The danger for man is that the hydatid never ceases to grow. Other tapeworm cysts have a limit to their size, and disentegration does not set up metastases in other sites. In the case of hydatid, the individual cyst grows continually and, if broken, the germinal epithelium or the contents of the cyst may be carried to other parts of the body where new foci of infection are set up. Thus, there is the danger of damage to particular organs as a result of enlargement of a cyst, or because of the invasion of a vital area by metastasizing daughter cysts. The detailed structure of a hydatid is shown in fig. 19.28b.

Alveolar hydatid cysts infiltrate the tissues in a very different manner; they are naked protoplasts invading tissues of all kinds, including even the Haversian system. The natural cycle of *E. multilocularis* involves foxes and wolves as definitive hosts and small rodents, such

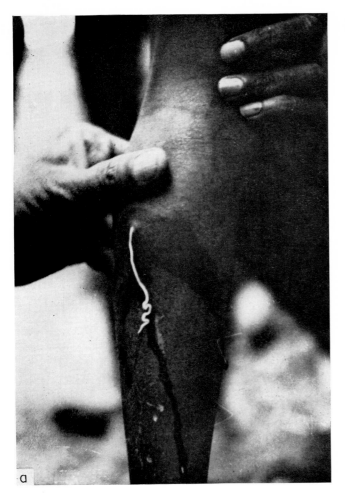

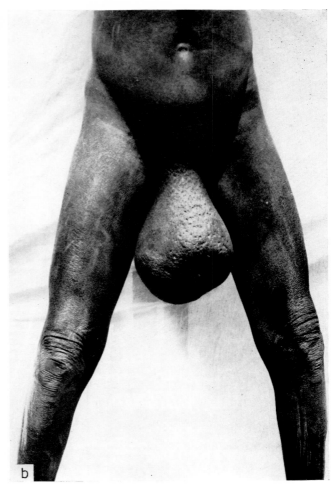

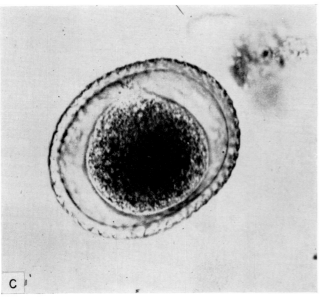

PLATE 19.3.

(a) Female *Dracunculus medinensis* partially extracted from the leg. Courtesy of the Wellcome Museum of Medical Science.

(b) Elephantiasis of the scrotum due to *Wuchereria bancrofti*. Courtesy of the Wellcome Museum of Medical Science.

(c) Egg of *Toxocara canis*. From Soulsby E.J.L. (1965) *Textbook of Veterinary Clinical Parasitology*, vol. I, Helminths. Oxford: Blackwell Scientific Publications.

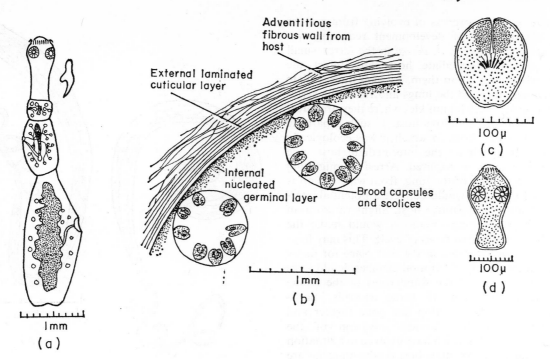

FIG. 19.28. *Echinococcus granulosus*; (a) adult tapeworm, (b) portion of hydatid cyst, (c) invaginated proscolex removed from cyst, (d) evaginated proscolex. From Hackett C.J. (1954) *Manual of Medical Helminthology*. London: Cassell.

as voles and field mice, which act as their prey. Man becomes infected accidentally as a result of contact with wolf or, in special circumstances, dog faeces.

E. granulosus is not uncommon in the United Kingdom, but *E. multilocularis* has been reported only once in the recent past. Many measures contribute to the control of hydatid disease, including those to prevent infection of domestic dogs. The faeces of these animals should be examined routinely in endemic areas and tapeworm infections thus diagnosed treated with anthelminthics. Raw sheep offal must not be fed to dogs and material known to be infected with hydatid should be destroyed. To guard against human infection, particularly of children, care in handling dogs and then food must be scrupulous. Official New Zealand policy advises that children in some sheep farming areas should be forbidden to handle dogs. The domestic dog may be infected with *E. multilocularis*, and this is commonly the case in the Arctic where sledge dogs are sometimes a source of infection for man.

Hymenolepis nana, the dwarf tapeworm of man, is included in this section because ingestion of human faeces is the main mode of infection. It is the only tapeworm known to be able to dispense with its intermediate host if necessary; all stages of development from hexacanth through cysticercoid to adult occur in man's small intestine. It is of small clinical importance even though it is not uncommon in many parts of the world.

The roundworms whose success can be attributed to poor hygienic habits are the ascaris of man, *Ascaris lumbricoides*, and two roundworms common in children, the pinworm, *Enterobius vermicularis*, and the whipworm, *Trichuris trichiura*. All these species are cosmopolitan, though **ascariasis** and **trichuriasis** are probably less common in Britain than they used to be.

On first acquaintance the life cycle of *Ascaris lumbricoides* seems eccentric, to say the least. The larvae which emerge from the infective eggs after they have been swallowed by man burrow into the intestinal mucosa, and pursue extensive and apparently purposeful migrations in the blood stream, being carried through the liver into the heart, pulmonary circulation and lung capillaries. Here they moult to the third stage, and after a short while burst into the alveolar sacs and undergo a further moult. These larvae, now in the fourth stage, migrate up the bronchial tree and, aided by the cilia of the trachea, reach the back of the throat where they are carried down into the digestive tract when the host swallows. In the small intestine once more, they perform the final moult to become adult. Thus the parasite comes full circle; it migrates round the body from the small intestine back to the same site, an apparently pointless sequence of events unless there is some evolutionary explanation. The explanation which has been offered is that *A. lumbricoides*, having, as it does, only one host in the life cycle, is in the process of evolving from a more primitive ascarid type of development requiring two hosts. In some species, e.g. *A. devosi* in the ferret, small mammals act as intermediate hosts and infect the carnivores which prey upon them. In such intermediate hosts larvae pass through the lungs and reach the systemic circulation and skeletal muscles where they are infective for the carnivore definitive host. If such a parasite were to invade a new host, in which it was ecologically advantageous to eliminate the intermediate host, one simple change would be required. Arrest of migrating larvae in the capillaries of the lung, from which there is direct access to the gut, would convert a potential intermediate host into the definitive host. Slight variation in larval growth rate during migration would make the difference between the two types of cycle. This may have been how selection operated in the first place for many more physiological and behavioural changes would have been necessary to curtail the wanderings of the larvae at the time of hatching. In some ascarids, particularly those of birds, selection has gone further and virtually eliminated such 'useless' invasion of the host's tissues. Life cycles which have evolved in a situation where a facultative intermediate host is advantageous are those of the dog and cat ascarids, and these are relevant to the dangerous condition in man, visceral larva migrans (p. 19.34).

The eggs produced by the adult female *A. lumbricoides* (fig. 19.36i), living in man's small intestine, are robust and live for a long time after they have passed out in the faeces and developed to the infective stage. They survive disposal in advanced sewage systems, and withstand desiccation and low temperature. Similarly resistant are the eggs of the pinworm (fig. 19.36n), *E. vermicularis*, commonly found in children. Its route of infection is the same though there is no tissue migration, the life cycle being very much simpler. Second stage larvae which hatch from infective eggs in the duodenum moult, then migrate to the caecum, moult twice more and grow to maturity. The gravid female pinworms migrate from the caecum, reach the anus, and deposit their eggs on the perianal skin, often bursting in the process. Eggs adhere to the skin, where they develop to the infective stage. Reinfection, as well as transmission to others, usually results from hand contamination. This is made more likely by scratching of the anal region in attempts to allay the extreme pruritus which accompanies the parasite's activities. Eggs may also drop off the skin and become generally distributed in the environment of infected individuals. Although children in the family setting may become infected, the condition is typically found in the institutionalized young; the eggs become disseminated throughout the dust and on the door knobs, etc., of communal dwellings, and are able to survive long periods of desiccation. Communal living, infrequent bathing and

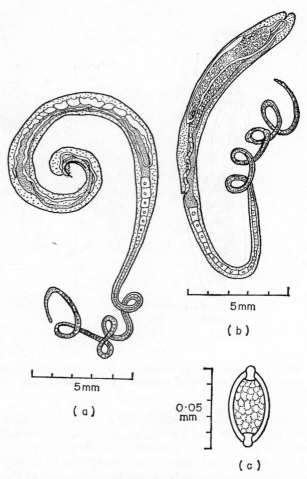

FIG. 19.29. *Trichuris trichiura*; (a) male, (b) female, (c) egg. From Hackett C.J. (1954) *Manual of Medical Helminthology*. London: Cassell.

contaminated clothing combine to produce epidemics of **enterobiasis**.

Whipworm infection often coexists with ascariasis, the epidemiology of the two conditions being very similar, though *Trichuris* eggs (fig. 19.29c) are less robust than those of *Ascaris*. Like *Enterobius*, *Trichuris* adults (fig. 19.29a & b) are found in the caecum where their long, thin anterior ends are embedded in the tissue of the gut wall. Eggs are laid in the caecum, pass in the faeces and develop to infective first stage larvae which lie dormant inside their shells until eaten by man. Development of the adult worms takes place without tissue migration.

Control of these three roundworms is straightforward since they are host specific, man being the sole source of infection for himself. Where high standards of hygiene prevail the problem is insignificant.

The extreme robustness of the infective stages of these parasites excludes the possibility of breaking the cycle by killing them, though interim measures to prevent their ingestion by man should be obligatory. However, the adult parasites are not too difficult to remove from the host by chemotherapy, and therefore a check on infection rates, particularly in institutionalized children, should be maintained, with ensuing treatment of detected cases. *Ascaris* and *Trichuris* eggs are found by microscopic examination of the faeces, and those of *Enterobius* by similar examination of a Scotch tape smear taken from the perianal skin. Many of the precautions to be taken against infection with pinworm apply to *Hymenolepis nana*, since again, human sources of infection are epidemiologically the important ones, and children are the most likely subjects.

Cysticercosis in man resulting from infection with the tapeworm *Taenia solium* is relevant to the present discussion. Reference to p. 19.24 indicates how infection is brought about, and why it should now be mentioned in dealing with inadequate personal hygiene, since cysticercosis must have its origin in human faeces.

INFECTION BY SKIN PENETRATION

Infection of man through the skin occurs in the important human helminth parasites, the schistosome blood flukes and hookworms. *Strongyloides stercoralis*, although very common in tropical areas, is of minor clinical importance.

Three species of schistosome occur in man and are responsible for the chronic disease **schistosomiasis** (bilharziasis). *Schistosoma mansoni* is found in South America and Africa; throughout Africa, particularly in Egypt, the common species is *S. haematobium*; the third, *S. japonicum*, is confined to the Far East. These flukes live in the vascular system associated with the gut (*S. mansoni* and *S. japonicum*) or with the bladder (*S. haematobium*). Infection is caused by the skin-penetrating fork-tailed cercariae (fig. 19.30) which in endemic foci abound in waters where men bathe. The cercaria sheds its tail on entering the skin and invades the lymphatic system, reaching the blood stream by this means. After extensive migration the parasites settle in veins and venules which the particular species tends to frequent, *S. mansoni* and *S. japonicum* in the portal system of the gut wall, *S. haematobium* in the bladder venules. In these sites the males and females develop together, almost always being found in copula (fig. 19.31), and the female lays eggs in the distal extremities of the venules. The nonoperculate eggs have spines on them, the position of the spine depending on the species (figs. 19.36b, c, f). The spines anchor the eggs in the small blood vessels initially, and then assist them in their slow passage through the tissue into the lumen of the gut or bladder. During their stay in the tissue the miracidia develop and are ready to hatch once the eggs are passed in the faeces or urine. Hatching is triggered by light and also by dilution of the medium. The mira-

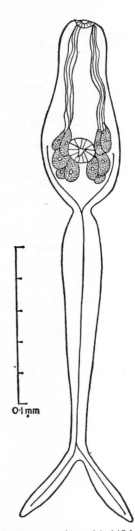

FIG. 19.30. Furcocercous, i.e. with bifid tail, cercaria of *Schistosoma* spp. Note penetration glands with their ducts opening anteriorly. From Hackett C.J. (1954) *Manual of Medical Helminthology*. London: Cassell.

cidia of all digenetic flukes enter the appropriate snail intermediate host to multiply and produce the free-swimming cercariae (fig. 19.33).

The 'New World Hookworm', *Necator americanus*, occurs, as one might expect, in North and South America; it belies its name, however, by being endemic also in large areas of Africa, India and South-East Asia. The 'Old World Hookworm', *Ancylostoma duodenale* is also misnamed to the extent that it is also found in North America. It has occurred in hot damp mines in northern Europe where conditions are favourable for transmission. The life cycles of the two species are similar. The adult worms live in the small intestine. The females lay thin-shelled eggs which pass out in the faeces of the host; the

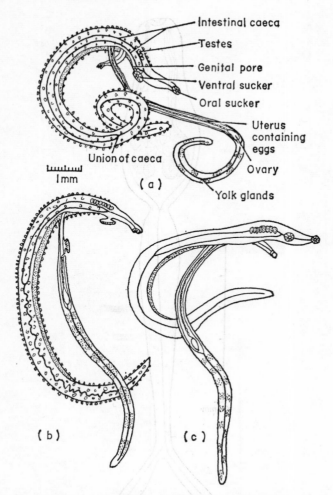

FIG. 19.31. Male and female schistosomes showing the females gripped in the gynaecophoral grooves of the males; (a) *Schistosoma haematobium*, (b) *S. mansoni*, (c) *S. japonicum*. From Hackett C.J. (1954) *Manual of Medical Helminthology*. London: Cassell.

first stage larvae develop in the eggs and hatch, feed on bacteria in the faeces, and grow and moult to the second stage. The process is repeated, though at the second moult, the cuticle is loosened and retained as a sheath around the body of the larva. This nonfeeding third stage contains food stores, mainly in the form of lipid, and, depending on the environmental conditions, may be able to survive for a month or so. It enters a new host by penetrating the skin, an event made much more likely by walking barefoot. Immediately on penetration and shedding of the sheath, larvae enter the bloodstream and are carried through the venae cavae to the heart and then to the pulmonary capillary network, where they are arrested. The third moult occurs after the worms have burst into the alveoli; it may happen during their passage up the bronchial tree to the rear of the throat, or it may

not occur until the larvae have been swallowed and have arrived in the small intestine, which is the final site. Here they moult to the fifth stage, completing the cycle (fig. 19.15). The adult worms have large mouths with heavily cuticularized teeth and lancets, by which they attach themselves to the mucosa of the small intestine and cause incisions in it which enable them to suck blood. Much of the pathology of hookworm infection is due to anaemia.

Another skin-penetrating nematode, *Strongyloides stercoralis*, is typical of the rhabdiasoid roundworms in that its development involves what is called 'alternation of generations', i.e. a parasitic generation is followed by one in which all stages of the life cycle are capable of development outside the host. The parasitic phase (fig. 19.32) involves a developmental sequence very like that of hookworms, though the adult worm in the small intestine does not suck blood and is a female-like organism which reproduces parthenogenetically. The other phase of the life cycle, the completely free-living one, involves fourth stage larvae and bisexual adults morphologically different from the parasitic ones and very similar to many nematodes found in soil. Identification of the stages of the free living cycle is therefore very specialized.

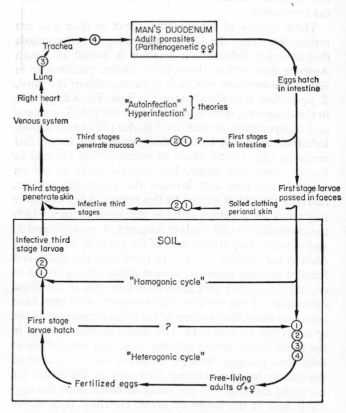

FIG. 19.32. Life cycle of *Strongyloides stercoralis*. Numbers in circles indicate moults.

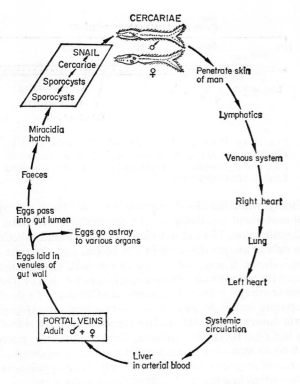

CERCARIAE

SNAIL
Cercariae
Sporocysts
Sporocysts

Miracidia
hatch

Faeces

Eggs pass
into gut lumen

Eggs go astray
to various organs

Eggs laid in
venules of
gut wall

PORTAL VEINS
Adult ♂ + ♀

Liver
in arterial blood

Penetrate skin
of man

Lymphatics

Venous system

Right heart

Lung

Left heart

Systemic
circulation

FIG. 19.33. Life cycle of *Schistosoma mansoni.*

Control measures

The exact methods used to combat the skin-penetrating helminths depend on the type of parasite. Schistosomiasis can be minimized if people at risk avoid contact with infected waters. Long term eradication requires the introduction in endemic areas of adequate sewerage which eliminates contamination of slow flowing freshwater canals and streams (the preferred habitats of the intermediate hosts) with untreated human faeces and urine. The control of hookworm disease is again dependent on the adequate disposal of human faeces, though in this case the object is to remove the source of infection from man's immediate vicinity and to place the hookworm's stages in an environment in which they will not survive.

Most of the skin-penetrating helminths are potentially simple to control in theory since their epidemiology is related to human sources of infection only. Schistosomiasis eradication programmes should include an assault on the intermediate host. This is best done by attempting to change the ecological conditions of areas which are likely to be contaminated by human faeces. There are ways of killing the snails, but these are probably not to be preferred in the long run because of other damaging ecological consequences of such treatment. A powerful lesson learnt over the years in Egypt is that irrigation schemes may well extend the range of the

16

intermediate host and with it the endemicity of human infection. In practice control has proved extremely difficult and expensive.

S. mansoni infects mammals other than man and the house mouse is an amenable host providing a means for the laboratory study of schistosomiasis.

INFECTIONS CARRIED BY BITING ARTHROPODS

The human filarial worms, including *Wuchereria bancrofti*, *Brugia malayi* (causes of elephantiasis); *Loa loa* (the eye worm); *Onchocerca volvulus* (cause of human onchocercosis), and a number of other species, are all transmitted by biting insects belonging to the order Diptera. Probably the most important are *W. bancrofti* and *B. malayi*, the former being very widely distributed in tropical areas. *B. malayi*, is more restricted, being found in Southern Asia and the Far East.

The adults of *W. bancrofti* live in the lymphatic system where the females lay first stage larvae enclosed in an elongated egg shell. The larvae, or 'microfilariae' (*Mf*) migrate via the lymphatic system to the blood stream where they are available to the mosquito intermediate host. Many species of mosquito, both anopheline and culicine may transmit Bancroft's filariasis, the cycle in the insect resulting in the concentration of third stage infective larvae in the haemocoele of the labium. When the mosquito bites, larvae emerge and enter the wound. The infection is not actively pumped into the definitive host by the mosquito's hypodermic mouthparts as in the case of malaria. Having entered the body, the parasite completes development, moulting twice and undergoing prolonged migration through the tissues before reaching adulthood and producing microfilariae approximately one year after infection. Commonly the lymph vessels draining the extremities or the pelvic region are affected, and their blockage as a result of interactions between parasite and host leads over many years to **elephantiasis** (plate 19.3b, facing p. 19.28). *Brugia malayi* has a life cycle similar to that of *Wuchereria*, though it is possibly less frequently implicated in elephantiasis. **Onchocercosis** in Africa and Central America results in subcutaneous lesions where the adults are found. The microfilariae of *Onchocerca volvulus* do not enter the blood stream, but remain in subcutaneous tissue in the vicinity of the nodule formed by the adult worms. Species of *Simulium* (blackflies) are the intermediate hosts. *Loa loa* is a form in which the adult worms migrate frequently and may be found infecting the eye. The intermediate host in this case is the fly, *Chrysops*. A controversial feature of the biology of many of the filarial worms is the cyclic appearance of their microfilariae in the peripheral blood of the host. These variations are related to a 24-hour rhythm, peak numbers occurring either during the day (*Loa loa*) or during the night (*W. bancrofti*). That this periodicity is in some way influenced by the host's circadian rhythms seems beyond doubt; it is clear also that it correlates with the behaviour of the intermediate hosts, for *Loa loa* uses a day biting insect and *W. bancrofti* a crepuscular one (table 19.4). One view of the more fundamental mechanisms at work, and the adaptive significance of periodicity, has been put forward in vol. 1, p. 44.7. Two important elements of this view are (1) the attribution of endogenous (circadian) rhythms to the larvae and (2) the phasing of larval behaviour specifically by the host's temperature cycle. The adaptive significance is, by implication, self-evident; periodicity correlates with the behaviour of the vector, therefore it is of survival value to the parasite.

Sceptics claim that evidence for endogenous larval rhythmicity is lacking, and that experiments purporting to demonstrate specific temperature effects are unrealistic. In regard to benefits to the parasite, periodicity may well be essential for survival simply because it is such a common phenomenon, but it is far from obvious why it is so crucial. When they are not swept passively into the peripheral blood, larvae must strive to stay in the pulmonary circulation and so expend energy in 'escaping' from the most favourable place. It would seem more logical for them to conserve their efforts and remain in the peripheral blood continuously.

Since the adult worms are usually in the depths of the body, they are not commonly available for diagnostic purposes, and the diagnosis is based on the characters of the microfilariae. A number of criteria may be used.

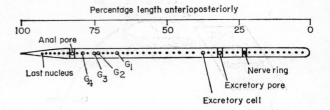

FIG. 19.35. Diagram of microfilarial 'landmarks' used in identification; G1–4 are genital rudiments. From Smyth J.D. (1962) *Introduction to Animal Parasitology*. London: English Universities Press.

Firstly, while the blood preparation is still fresh, the type of movement that living larval worms exhibit is of value in identification. The site in which larvae are found, whether in subcutaneous tissue or in the blood, and the type of periodicity, if any, are obviously relevant. Criteria used once the worms have been stained in a blood film or tissue smear are specialized. The presence or absence of a sheath separate some species from others; for instance, *Microfilaria bancrofti* and *Mf. malayi* are sheathed, *Mf. volvulus* is not (fig. 19.34). In addition, the structure of a microfilaria as seen after haematoxylin staining is made up of a series of so-called 'landmarks', deeply staining points and clear areas in a less well defined column along the central rachis of the worm (fig. 19.35). Careful measurements of the total length of the worm and the relationship of each of the landmarks to the total length provide a complex formula for the specimen which can be related to reference data for the different species of microfilaria.

The epidemiology and control of the arthropod-borne helminthiases are intimately bound up with the behaviour, breeding habits, physiology and ecology of the intermediate hosts. These aspects are examined in the section on medical entomology.

VISCERAL LARVA MIGRANS, CUTANEOUS LARVA MIGRANS AND MISCELLANEOUS TISSUE MIGRATING FORMS

Visceral and cutaneous larva migrans are conditions which typically arise in man from helminths truly specific to other hosts, but which can invade human tissues and there pursue an abortive existence of varying duration. In medical parasitology visceral larva migrans is the condition specifically arising from infection with the eggs of the dog and cat ascarid nematodes, *Toxocara canis* (plate 19.3c, facing p. 19.28) and *T. mystax*. The second stage larvae which emerge from the eggs after they have been accidentally eaten by the human host migrate to many parts of the body. The larvae are dangerous when they enter the CNS, and in a number of cases have caused blindness of children. Currently there are attempts to perfect an immunological method to detect visceral larva migrans (plate 19.2, facing p. 19.22). Infection

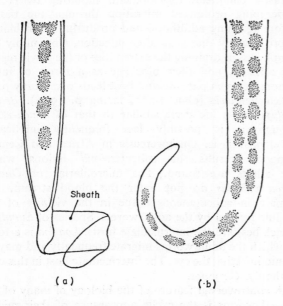

FIG. 19.34. Rear end of sheathed and unsheathed microfilaria after staining in blood film; (a) *W. bancrofti*, (b) *O. volvulus*. From Smyth J.D. (1962) *Introduction to Animal Parasitology*. London: English Universities Press.

occurs in man, as in hydatidosis, when handling dogs or when dust or soil contaminated with dog or cat faeces is ingested. Therefore parents of children are well advised to have their dogs and cats checked for infection by faecal examination and treated if necessary. Anthelmin-

thics (p. 20.22) are very effective against the roundworm of these animals.

The third stage infective larvae of the three dog hookworms, *Ancylostoma caninum*, *A. braziliense* and *Uncinaria stenocephala*, although they cannot complete development in man, may invade his skin and undergo considerable migration in the subcutaneous tissue, leaving visible, irritating lesions in their wake. Another human dermatitis may result from bathing in water contaminated with the cercariae of schistosomes which develop to maturity in birds or mammals other than man. These may infect both marine and freshwater habitats, the marine or freshwater molluscan intermediate hosts being the immediate cause of the water contamination. The condition is commonly called 'swimmer's itch'.

ARTHROPODS

The numerically dominant animals of our age are the insects. There are nearly a million known species and some of them are represented by astronomical numbers of individuals. Out of such numbers, it is not surprising that some species challenge man's economy and assume the role of pests. Pests have a place in the earliest literature and in the book of Exodus lice, flies and locusts appear as three of the ten plagues of Egypt. Although systematic studies of insects began in the eighteenth century, interest in the diversity of their structure and biology, and a close study of insects as pests began only in the middle of the nineteenth century. Applied entomology then developed rapidly, first in the agricultural field and later in medicine.

Medical entomology began in 1879 when, in South China, Manson discovered that mosquitoes play a part in the life cycle of the worm which causes one form of human filariasis. Manson suspected mosquitoes of playing a similar role in the transmission of malaria and encouraged Ross in India to undertake his fruitful researches. The end of the nineteenth century saw the successful studies by Walter Reed and his co-workers in Cuba on yellow fever. These three medical men, each turned entomologist, implicated mosquitoes in the natural history and transmission to man of three major diseases caused by distinct types of infective organism, a nematode worm in filariasis, a protozoan in malaria and a virus in yellow fever.

It was at once clear that attack on the insects might control the diseases themselves. Although yellow fever was soon almost eliminated from towns by attacks on its mosquito vector, it was recognized that more expertise was needed to attack successfully other insect-borne diseases. Hence medical entomology expanded its scope and much of the work had interests which were no longer primarily medical. On this account, of the three branches of medical zoology, entomology

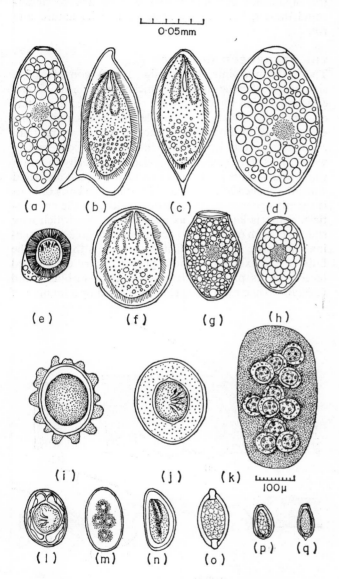

FIG. 19.36. Eggs of helminths affecting man; (a) *Gastrodiscoides hominis*, (b) *Schistosoma mansoni*, (c) *Schistosoma haematobium*, (d) *Fasciolopsis buski*, (e) *Taenia* spp., (f) *Schistosoma japonicum*, (g) *Paragonimus westermani*, (h) *Diphyllobothrium latum*, (i) *Ascaris lumbricoides*, (j) *Hymenolepis diminuta*, (k) Egg 'nest' of *Dipylidium caninum*, a tapeworm of dogs occasionally found in man. (l) *Hymenolepis nana*, (m) *hookworm*, (n) *Enterobius vermicularis*, (o) *Trichuris trichiura*, (p) heterophyid fluke, (q) *Clonorchis sinensis* or *Opisthorchis felineus*. From Hackett C.J. (1954) *Manual of Medical Helminthology*. London: Cassell.

might appear to have the least claim today to a part in the medical training. A doctor clearly needs to recognize and identify the helminthic and protozoal agents of disease before he can reach a definitive diagnosis, whereas knowledge of their insect vectors is diagnostically irrelevant. For progress in epidemiology, on the other hand, knowledge of the vectors is a *sine qua non*. Malaria, typhus and plague, all insect-borne diseases, have been counted the three greatest killers. Although each is now much diminished, they are far from being eradicated and great epidemics can again break out.

Lice, fleas, tsetse flies and sandflies soon followed mosquitoes in being assigned a medical role. But before any insect had been shown to transmit disease in man, Theobald Smith proved that *Babesia bigemina*, the protozoan agent of the cattle disease Texas Fever was transmitted by the tick, *Boophilis annulatus*. In this century ticks and mites have been convicted of spreading human diseases. Medical entomology is, therefore, no longer concerned exclusively with insects.

General characteristics of arthropods

Insects, ticks and mites belong to the phylum *Arthropoda* whose members are characterized by the following features.

(1) The body is invested with an inelastic cuticle secreted by the epidermal cells which, among other things, functions as an exoskeleton (fig. 19.37). This prevents increase in size and hence postembryonic growth proceeds by a series of **ecdyses** or **moults** when the cuticle is shed and replaced. In addition to increase in size the successive **instars** or **stages** involve changes in form and structure and so growth is accompanied by metamorphosis.

(2) Embryonic development reveals segmental structure and some features of this are retained up to the adult instar. There are segmentally arranged paired appendages provided with articulations which permit movements; hence the name of the phylum. The appendages are structurally modified at different positions along the body length to serve the functions of feeding (mouthparts), locomotion (legs) and reproduction (gonopods) (fig. 19.38).

(3) The circulation is an open system in which the heart is a long muscular tube running along the back and opening in front. This propels haemolymph (blood) forwards into the **general body cavity**, or **haemocoel**, where it flows backwards to re-enter the heart through a series of laterally placed openings termed **ostia**.

(4) The central nervous system contains a series of paired ganglia disposed segmentally along a ventral nerve cord. This ends anteriorly in a **cephalic ganglion** to which it is joined by a pair of circumoesophageal commissures.

The taxonomy or naming of arthropods is based mainly upon their external cuticular structures. Insects preserved on pins in a museum are no more than cuticles within which the soft structures have dried and shrivelled. In life the cuticle has a profound modifying influence on the organism's physiology and biology and to understand these it is necessary to appreciate its nature and role.

THE ARTHROPOD CUTICLE

The arthropod integument (fig. 19.37) consists of a single layer of epidermal cells which secrete the inanimate cuticle in which three zones are recognizable; the outer-epicuticle overlays an exocuticle and endocuticle. The **epicuticle** is multilayered, although rarely more than 2 μm thick. It is lipoprotein in nature but covered by waxes. This layer gives the organism its capacity to retain water and survive in air. The **exocuticle** is hard and rigid while the **endocuticle** is soft and flexible. The basis of both is the nitrogenous polysaccharide, **chitin**. In the endocuticle, chitin is laid down as parallel lamellae which may slide over each other and so permit some degree of stretching and hence flexibility. Chitin forms less than half the bulk of the exocuticle whose properties are determined largely by its protein, **sclerotin**, which is insoluble and resistant to chemicals. Sclerotin is formed by a tanning of

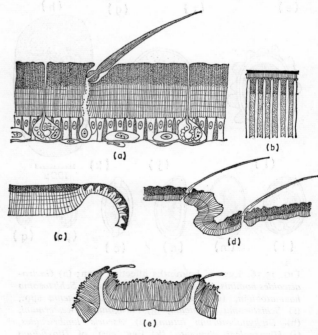

FIG. 19.37. Sections of insect cuticle; (a) epidermis and dermal glands with overlying endo- and exocuticles; (b) epicuticle and pore canals at greater magnification; (c, d & e) sections at various sites showing how rigidity and flexibility are achieved by different arrangements of the exocuticle.

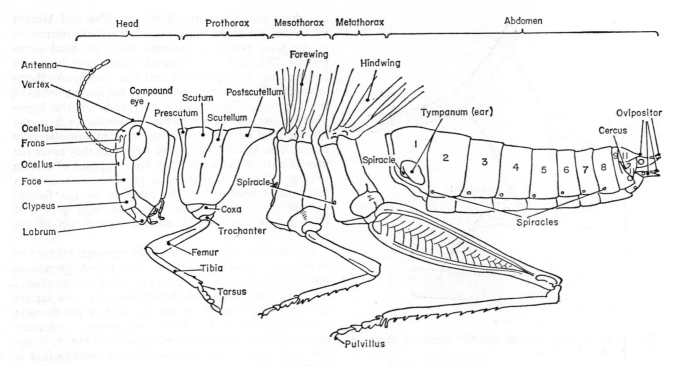

FIG. 19.38. External anatomy of the locust.

the original exocuticular protein. The endo- and exo-cuticles are crossed by pore canals through which cytoplasmic extensions of the epidermal cells can control events in the distant structures. The arthropod cuticle thus recalls the structure of vertebrate bone or dentine.

In the newly moulted insect the cuticle is pale, soft and distensible, but after a few hours exposure to the atmosphere it hardens and darkens. This tanning is due to quinone substances formed in newly exposed cuticle by the action of polyphenol oxidase on derivatives of tyrosine. Also derived from tyrosine is the pigment, melanin, to which much of the darkening is due.

Sclerotized areas or **sclerites** are hard plates of fixed form and disposition, interrupted where flexibility or articulation is required. Their fixity within and variation between species recall the bones of vertebrates. In regions of flexibility the exocuticle is often broken up into small discrete blocks (fig. 19.37).

The cuticle is continued internally to line the surfaces of all ectodermal structures, such as the anterior and posterior gut, the distal parts of the gonoducts and the respiratory system. The midgut in insects is often protected by a loosely applied fine chitinous membrane, the peritrophic membrane. Respiration in insects and acarina is mediated by a system of finely branching tubes lined by cuticle in which the sclerotization is arranged spirally. This pattern, while preserving patency, permits flexibility. The tubes or **tracheae** open to the exterior through

spiracles, whose aperture is controllable. Their finest branches or tracheoles end in intimate contact with all the cells of the body and here the gaseous exchange takes place (fig. 19.39). The tracheal system with its fine ramifications around and within the internal organs provides an important support mechanism and incidentally imposes a barrier to fine dissection. The events which occur at ecdysis are as follows.

(1) The chitin is dissolved by a chitinase and resorbed.

(2) The epidermis, now isolated from the cuticle, lays down first the epicuticle, then the exocuticle and finally the endocuticle.

(3) The internal pressure is increased by consumption of air (or of water in aquatic forms) until the old cuticle fractures along predetermined lines.

(4) The organism then emerges and the new cuticle undergoes tanning; thus a new complement of rigid structures of increased dimensions is acquired. These processes are under a complex hormonal control.

Classification

The phylum is divisible into classes of which the most familiar are:

(1) *Crustacea* including crabs, lobsters, shrimps, water fleas, etc.,

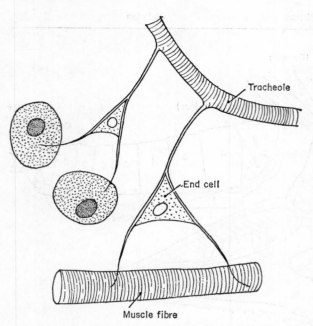

FIG. 19.39. A tracheole with end-cells supplying tissue cells and a muscle fibre.

(2) *Chilopoda* or centipedes,
(3) *Diplopoda* or millipedes,
(4) *Arachnida* e.g. spiders, scorpions, ticks and mites,
(5) *Insecta*.

The crustacea, whose significance in the transmission of certain helminth infections has already been discussed (p. 19.25), are mainly aquatic at all stages in their life history whereas the other four classes are mainly terrestrial at least in their adult stage. Medical interest in the arthropods is virtually confined to the last two classes (table 19.4). Further, out of some dozen orders of *Arachnida*, only one, the *Acarina*, need concern us and out of some two dozen orders of Insecta, only four, *Hemiptera* (bugs), *Siphunculata* (blood-sucking lice), *Siphonaptera* (fleas) and *Diptera* (two-winged flies). These five orders include species which have some degree of parasitic dependence on man, either occasional or regular, through which they contribute to the range of human infective disease.

General morphology

INSECTS

The insect body is divided into three regions of head, thorax and abdomen (fig. 19.38). The head, a strongly sclerotized rigid structure bears the mouth and contains the cephalic ganglion. Anterior to the oral region there is a pair of sensory appendages, the antennae, which are primitively multisegmented filiform structures but subject to great modification in different types of insect. Behind are the mouthparts, mandibles, maxillae and labrum which are the structurally modified paired appendages of the three post-oral segments which the head incorporates. The anterior and posterior margins of the mouth (labrum and hypopharynx) and the mouthparts themselves are all structurally adapted to the feeding habits of the organism. The salivary duct ends on the hypopharynx but the paired glands lie further back in the thorax. The eyes are normally situated dorsolaterally but in some insects they are so large that they cover the greater part of the head. They are composed of a large number of optical units, each provided with its own lens and retinal organ. In addition to the faceted or compound eyes, many insects have a group of three simple eyes (ocelli) situated on the top of the head.

The thorax comprises three body segments referred to as pro- meso- and metathoracic. Their paired appendages are well-developed walking legs of which insects always have six. The meso- and metathoraces in most insects each bear a pair of wings and the bulk of the thoracic space is occupied by flight musculature. Primitive apterous insects are of no medical concern but the wingless state as a secondary evolutionary modification is found in lice, fleas and the bed-bugs. Flies of the order Diptera have only one pair of wings developed for flight, the anterior or mesothoracic; their metathoracic wings are modified to form a pair of small knobbed stalks, the halters or balancers (fig. 19.40). Insect wings are essentially integumental sacs from which the epidermis is lost and the haemocoelic cavity obliterated by the close application of the dorsal and ventral cuticles. The tracheal branches, which were functional during development of the wing, persist as a skeletal framework supporting the cuticular membrane and are revealed as the wing venation. The pattern of the wing venation is often sufficiently characteristic for a particular group as to afford a basis for its recognition (fig. 19.41).

The abdomen, which contains the reproductive system and the bulk of the gut, has an obviously segmental structure, each segment bearing separate sclerites both dorsally and ventrally. In embryological life there are some twelve abdominal segments but terminal modifications reduce the evident number in the mature insect to from four to eight according to the species. Except for the terminal segments, which retain appendages modified for copulation and oviposition (genitalia), the abdomen is devoid of appendages.

ARACHNIDS

In the Arachnida the head is never differentiated and at most the body shows a division into cephalothorax and abdomen. In the Acarina, the only order of major medical interest, even this separation is lacking (fig. 19.45). The most anterior appendages, the chelicerae, lie

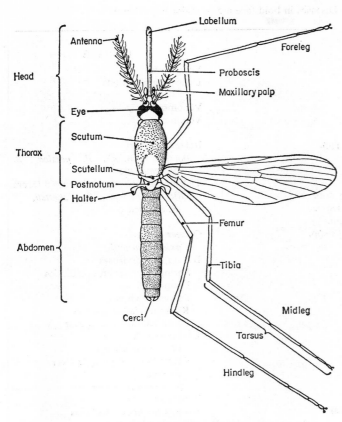

FIG. 19.40. A mosquito.

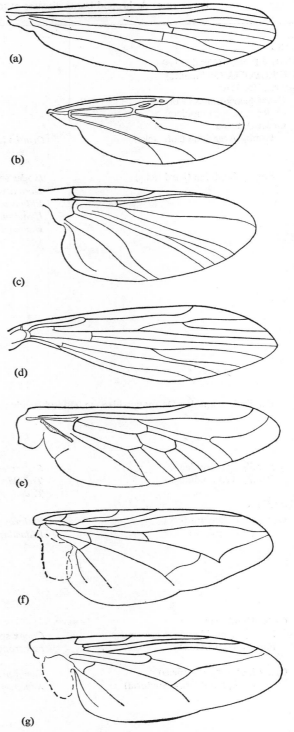

FIG. 19.41. Wing venation of Dipterous insects; (a) *Culicidae*, mosquitoes; (b) *Ceratopogonidae*, midges; (c) *Simulidae*, black flies; (d) *Psychodidae*, sandflies; (e) *Tabaniade*, clegs or horseflies; (f) *Calliphoridae*, blowflies; (g) *Glossina*, tsetse flies.

anterior to the mouth; they display a wide range of modifications but their primary function is in feeding. Behind them lie the pedipalps, also subject to a wide range of modifications. Four pairs of walking legs complete the complement of arachnid appendages. Arachnida lack both antennae and compound eyes but ocelli are not uncommon. The tracheal system of the Acarina communicates with the atmosphere through a single pair of spiracles whereas in insects spiracular openings are numerous, the thorax having two pairs and the abdomen one pair for each of its developed segments. Small Acarina lack spiracles, and in them respiration is cutaneous.

DEVELOPMENT OF INSECTS AND ARACHNIDS
Most insects and arachnids are oviparous. Embryonic development is unremarkable but postembryonic development merits discussion since it has a controlling influence on the ecology of the organism. In the hemimetabola (figs. 19.43, 44, 50 & 51), metamorphosis is gradual, and in holometabola (figs. 19.46–49) it is radical and abrupt.

The **hemimetabola** include the Acarina, bugs and lice which emerge from the egg similar to the adult in general

TABLE 19.4. Arthropod borne diseases of man. Diseases in bold face are of major importance.

CLASS		DISEASE
CHILOPODA (Centipedes)		Venomous
DIPLOPODA (Millipedes)		Urticating secretions
ARACHNIDA		
Order Scorpionida (scorpions)		Venomous
Order Araneida (spiders)		Venomous
Order Acarina		
Family Argasidae (soft ticks)	*Ornithodoros* spp.	**Relapsing fevers**
		Borrelia duttonii, B. persica, B. hispanica etc.
Family Ixodidae (hard ticks)	*Ixodes* spp.	Tick-borne typhuses and spotted fevers
	Dermacentor spp.	*Rickettsia conori, R. rickettsii,*
	Rhipicephalus spp.	*R. siberica*
	Hyalomma spp.	
	Haemaphysalis spp.	**Q fever**
		Coxiella burnetii
		B group arboviruses
		Spring–summer encephalitides
		Louping-ill
		Powassan virus
		Kyasanur forest disease
		Omsk haemorrhagic fever
		Unclassified Viruses
		Colorado tick fever
		Crimean haemorrhagic fever
		Tularaemia
		Pasteurella tularense
		Tick paralysis
Family Laelaptidae Dermanyssidae etc. (Blood sucking mites)		Korean nephroso-nephritis
		Murine typhus
		Rickettsia mooseri
		Rickettsial pox
		Rickettsia akari
Family Sarcoptidae	*Sarcoptes scabiei*	**Scabies**
Family Trombidiidae	*Trombicula akamushi*	**Japanese river fever**, scrub typhus
	T. deliensis	*Rickettsia tsutsugamushi*
INSECTA		
Order Siphunculata (lice)	*Phthirus pubis*	Pubic phthiriasis
(=Anoplura)	*Pediculus humanus*	Head and body phthiriasis
		Epidemic typhus
		Rickettsia prowazekii
		Trench fever
		Rickettsia quintana
		Epidemic relapsing fever
		Borrelia recurrentis
Order Hemiptera		
Family Cimicidae	*Cimex* spp. (bedbugs)	Noxious
Family Triatomidae	*Panstrongylus megistus* etc.	**Trypanosomiasis (Chagas's disease)**
		T. cruzi
Order Siphonaptera (fleas)	*Tunga penetrans* jigger fleas	Ulceration
(=Aphaniptera=Suctoria)	*Xenopsylla* spp. etc.	**Bubonic plague**
		Pasteurella pestis
		Murine typhus
		Rickettsia mooseri
		Tapeworms
		Dipylidium caninum
		Hymenolepis diminuta

TABLE 19.4. (*continued*)

Order Lepidoptera (moths and butterflies)		Urticating hairs
		Scholechiasis
Order Coleoptera (beetles) Cantharidae		Canthariasis
Order Diptera		
Family Culicidae (mosquitoes)		
Tribe Anophelini	*Anopheles* spp.	**Malaria**
		Plasmodium vivax, P. falciparum, P. malariae, P. ovale
		Filariasis Brugian and Bancroftian
Tribe Culicini	Especially important *inter alia Aëdes aegypti and Culex pipiens fatigans*	**Filariasis** Brugian and Bancroftian
		A group arboviruses
		Eastern, Western and Venzuelan Equine Encephalomylitides
		B group arboviruses
		Yellow fever
		Dengue fevers
		St Louis encephalitis
		Japanese B encephalitis
		? Murray Valley fever
		West Nile fever
		Unclassified arboviruses
		Rift Valley fever
Family Ceratopogonidae	*Culicoides* spp.	Filarioid infections
(midges, punkies etc.)	*Leptoconops* spp.	*D. perstans*
	Lasiohelea spp.	*M. ozzardi*
Family Simuliidae (black flies)	*Simulium* spp.	Hypersensitivity
		Onchocerciasis—River blindness
		Onchocerca volvulus
Family Psychodidae (sandflies)	*Phlebotomus* spp.	**Leishmaniases**
		Kala azar oriental sore, muco-cutaneous leishmaniasis, infantile leishmaniasis
		Leishmania spp.
		Sandfly fever (Arbovirus)
		Oroya fever, verruga peruana
Family Tabanidae (horseflies and clegs)	*Chrysops silacea and C. dimidiata*	Loaiasis (Calabar swellings)
		Loa loa
	Chrysops spp.	Tularaemia
	Tabanus spp.	*Pasteurella tularense*
	Haematopota spp.	
Family Muscidae. Non-blood sucking	*Musca* group	Enteric infections (mechanically)
Blood sucking group.	*Glossina* spp. Tsetse flies	**Trypanosomiasis**
		T. gambiense, T. rhodesiense
Family Calliphoridae	*Calliphora* spp.	
	Chrysomyia spp.	
	Callitroga spp.	Ulcerative and wound myiasis
	Wohlfartia spp.	
	Sarcophaga spp.	
	Cordylobia anthropophaga	African furuncular myiasis
Family Tachinidae	*Dermatobia hominis*	American furuncular myiasis
	Oestrus spp. (nasal flies)	Orbital myiasis
	Rhinoestrus spp.	
	Hypoderma spp. (warble flies)	Creeping myiasis
Family Gasterophilidae	*Gasterophilus* spp. (bot-flies)	Creeping myiasis
Miscellaneous families		Intestinal myiasis

appearance and are adapted for life in the same environment. At each successive ecdysis there is a slight change in appearance until full adult form is achieved at the final ecdysis. The immature instars of hemimetabola are termed nymphs. Wings are not functionally developed until the adult instar is reached. In the first instar of acarina, the fourth pair of legs and the spiracles are lacking but they are present and fully developed in the second instar (fig. 19.51).

The **holometabola** include the fleas and dipterous flies. The immature stages (larvae) of these insects are entirely different from their parents in appearance, environment and feeding habits. After a series of ecdyses when the larva increases in size and may change in appearance, although not towards the adult form, it reaches its full growth. At the next ecdysis it becomes a pupa when its form resembles neither larva nor adult. Feeding stops and, after disintegration of many larval organs and tissue, a complete structural reorganization takes place. Finally the pupa moults and the adult insect emerges. Viviparity is occasional among the holometabola in some of which, such as Sarcophagine blowflies, numbers of first stage larvae are deposited. Tsetse flies (fig. 19.49) deposit fully developed larvae singly after a gestation period of some 10–14 days. During this time the larva grows from the nourishment it receives *in utero* and after deposition it pupates forthwith.

Venoms

Among the terrestrial arthropods there are predatory forms which incapacitate or kill their victims by injection of venom. The composition of venoms varies but as they rapidly paralyse small animals, it is presumed that most contain neurotoxins. Man is not infrequently injured by centipedes, spiders, and scorpions (fig. 19.42) and by ants, bees and wasps whose poison claws or stings can penetrate human skin. The effects of venoms vary according to the species. Some stings cause little more than local pain and oedema which subsides rapidly. More potent venoms produce severe pain which may persist for hours or days and produce local necrosis. The most powerful venoms, found in some scorpions and spiders, may produce general syndromes and may be fatal to children. Spiders of the genus *Latrodectus* which are widely dispersed in warm regions are among the most venomous of the arthropods; the best known is the American black widow, *Latrodectus mactans*. The folklore which has grown around the Mediterranean tarantula, *Lycosa tarantula*, greatly exaggerates its effects. Scorpion stings may be mild or severe, but there is little

correlation between the size of a species and the severity of its sting. Antisera can be prepared against most arthropod venoms.

Irritating fluids, whose role is presumably protective, occur in the caterpillars of some Lepidoptera, moths and butterflies, and in some Coleoptera or beetles. The best known among these is the beetle *Lytta vesicatoria*, the Spanish fly from which cantharidin is prepared. When taken orally this may cause nausea and vomiting, but when excreted in the urine induces priapism. For this reason it gained a reputation as an aphrodisiac among the early Greeks and Romans. It is potentially dangerous and may cause death.

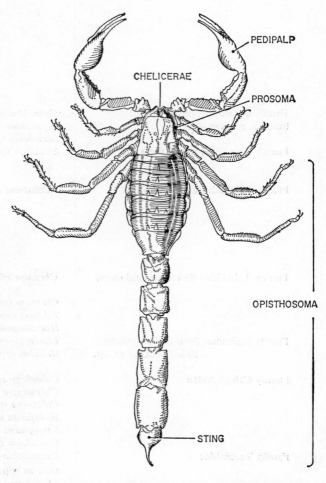

FIG. 19.42. A scorpion. Size varies in different species, from 2 up to 20 cm in length.

Permanent parasites

On the human host, permanent parasites are few and only the lice and the scabies mite merit notice.

LICE

Rather more than two hundred species of blood-sucking lice have been described, but only two infest man.

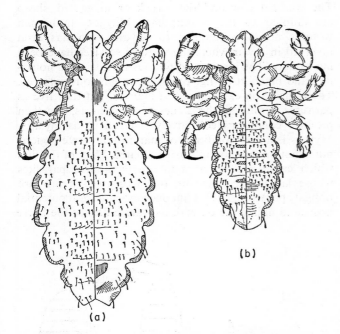

FIG. 19.43. Body or head-louse (*Pediculus humanus*) × 20; (a) female left-dorsum, right-venter; (b) male left-dorsum, right-venter.

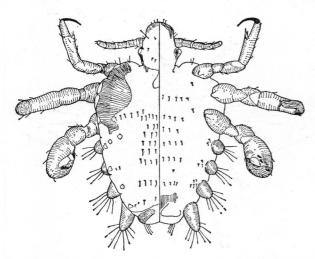

FIG. 19.44. Crab louse (*Phthirus pubis*); right-venter, left-dorsum, × 40.

These are *Pediculus humanus* (fig. 19.43), which occurs in two forms: the head louse and the body louse, and *Phthirus pubis* (fig. 19.44) the crab louse. They can live and breed only on man and survive only a few hours away from the host. Hence infestations can be acquired only from human sources and they are spread mainly by personal contact. Fugitive infestations by lice of other mammals and birds can follow close contact with their hosts but are of no importance since such lice cannot survive and breed on man. *P. pubis* establishes itself readily in pubic hair and is spread mainly by sexual contact; it lives in axillary and beard hair but not in scalp hair which is too fine and closely packed. It can establish itself in children only in the eyelashes and eyebrows. *Pediculus humanus* lives either in the scalp hair or underclothing. In well washed communities it is seldom found except as a scalp infestation in neglected children. Infestations are common in cold weather amongst persons who seldom change their underclothes.

Lice that infest man feed only by piercing the skin with their modified mouth parts to draw blood. They attach their eggs, **nits**, to hairs or clothing and the nymphs live and feed in the same manner as their parents. Their claw structure enables them to grasp and hold hairs among which they move easily but their progress is limited on plane surfaces. Louse infestations (**pediculosis** or **phthiriasis**) irritate and induce scratching which leads to secondary infections; when infestation is prolonged the skin becomes thickened and pigmented. Their importance as disease vectors, however, overshadows their physical and aesthetic disadvantages. *P. humanus* transmits *Rickettsia prowazekii* and *Borrelia recurrentis*, the agents of epidemic typhus and epidemic relapsing fever respectively (pp. 18.86 and 84).

SCABIES

The scabies mite which infests man, *Sarcoptes scabiei* (fig. 19.45) is morphologically indistinguishable from the sarcoptic mange-mites common on domestic animals especially pigs and dogs in Britain. Strains show some specificity for their particular host but cross infestation can occur. Man can contract infestations from animals but these are transient and their effects mild. Infestation by human strains is persistent and its effects are progressive and may be severe. Like lice these mites are obligate parasites throughout their life cycle; their survival away from the host is brief and their transmission mainly through direct contact. The mites, easily seen with a hand lens, live within the keratinized layers of the epidermis. The female burrows within the skin and lays her eggs at intervals as she progresses. Up to thirty eggs may be laid during the three week life of the female. The eggs hatch within three to four days and by the tenth day development, comprising one larval and one nymphal instar, is

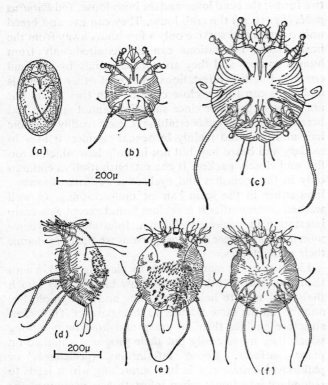

FIG. 19.45. Itch mite (*Sarcoptes scabiei*); (a) egg; (b) larva; (c) male; (d, e & f) female.

complete. Diagnosis is made by recognition of the mites in skin scrapings. The mites are found most frequently in the web and sides of the fingers, the fronts of the wrists, nipples, umbilicus and genitals, the fronts of the knees and tops of the feet. In extensively affected cases the whole anterior aspect of the body may be involved but infestation rarely extends to the back, face and scalp. The typical lesion is the galleried skin in which the burrows appear as sinuous lines from 1 to 10 mm in length. Skin sensitization causes pruritus, and scratching causes secondary infection which may obscure the characteristic burrows. Pediculosis may coexist with scabies when the more conspicuous lice may distract attention and obscure the diagnosis of scabies.

Acariasis due to quite different types of mite is occasionally seen as an occupational hazard. Normally free living mites infest flour, sugar and other foodstuffs, and sometimes become temporary cutaneous parasites of man. They produce a dermatitis popularly termed grocer's itch or miller's itch. These conditions, which are not readily contagious, are differentiated from scabies by circumstantial evidence and entomological identification of the agents confirms diagnosis.

Part free living parasites

Though few arthropods are wholly parasitic on man, there are numbers of species whose life cycles contain alternate free living and parasitic phases, the latter involving either myiasis or haematophagy.

Myiasis

The warbled cow and the struck or maggoted sheep are familiar to the countryman. Maggots in human wounds are also familiar to anyone who has been involved in a war where the medical services have been inadequate. The larvae of dipterous flies, such as houseflies and bluebottles (fig. 19.46) are acephalous maggots. These thrive on carrion and in manure, but they live as parasites feeding on the tissues of living hosts, and then produce conditions collectively referred to as myiasis. Myiasis is a rare condition of man in temperate regions but is not uncommon in warm climates. Most of the flies which cause myiasis in man are facultative parasites whose larvae are normally free living but a few are obligate parasites. Man is but one among several potential hosts and unlike the ox with its warble flies or the horse

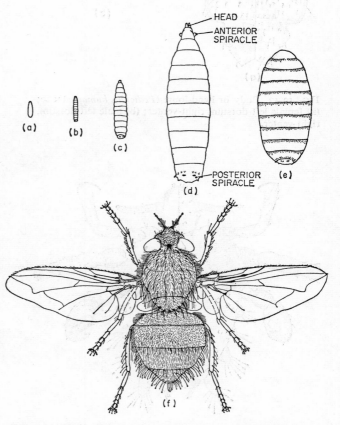

FIG. 19.46. Life cycle of a blue bottle (*Calliphora sp.*); ×4; (a) egg; (b-d) larval instars 1–3; (e) pupa; (f) adult.

with its bot-flies, he is not the unique host for any species of myiasis fly.

Open wounds or noisome discharges from natural orifices attract gravid females of many species and induce oviposition. Myiasis may occur in extensive ulcerative lesions in the skin and subcutaneous tissues or in the nose, mouth and orbit. About one week is required for larvae to complete their growth before they drop off to pupate. The lesions have an enhanced attractiveness to gravid flies and hence repeated reinfestation may occur, especially among uncared for infants, physically handicapped persons and mental defectives and other neglected cases. The principal agents of infestation are species of greenbottle genera, *Callitroga* and *Chrysomia*, and black and white larviparous *Wohlfartia* spp. Larvae of the former are known in America as screwworms as the rows of small spines resemble the thread of a screw. *Chrysomyia bezziana*, the most important myiasis fly of the Old World is an obligate parasite which attacks many species of host. In Africa it is important as a parasite of cattle, but man is rarely attacked except in India. *Callitroga americana* has been exterminated from parts of the American continent by a method which was pioneered in the Dutch Caribbean island of Curaçao. This utilizes the fact that females of this species mate only once. Measured irradiation of pupae produces infertile but sexually competent males. Natural populations can be reduced to extinction point by release of sterile males bred *in vitro*. The method is now exploited commercially.

Furuncular myiasis is caused by the tumbu or mango fly, in Africa and by the 'human warble', in tropical America. Larvae penetrate deeply into the subcutaneous tissues and, either singly or in small numbers, produce painful swellings topped by breathing holes. The eggs of the African fly are laid and hatch on the ground and the larvae are acquired by passing rats, dogs and humans. Children are infected directly but adults more often from clothing laid on the ground in laundering. The American fly attaches its eggs to insects such as mosquitoes which serve as transport agents. Hatching, emergence and skin penetration take place on the host (horses, cattle and man) on whose blood the transport insect feeds. Larval development is completed in about three weeks for *C. anthropophaga* but in *D. hominis* is delayed for some three months.

Very rarely **intestinal myiasis** may follow ingestion of fly eggs or larvae in food and water and is manifest where such are present in the vomit or faeces.

Creeping myiasis due to larvae beneath the skin may be produced by the cattle warbles, *Hypoderma* spp. and the horse bot-flies, *Gasterophilus* spp. In their normal hosts these larvae penetrate the skin or mucosa and enter a preliminary migratory phase before settling down in their development sites. The nasal fly of sheep, *Oestrus ovis*, and the pharyngeal fly of horses, *Rhinoestrus purpureus*, have been recorded in cases of human orbital and nasopharyngeal myiasis but in man they cannot complete development and migrate further.

HAEMATOPHAGY

In general, the holometabolous blood suckers, e.g. fleas and dipterous flies, require blood only in their adult life before breeding. Their pre-adult development and growth is nourished by a wide range of food materials including algae and other micro-organisms. For example, mosquitoes (fig. 19.52) and blackflies (fig. 19.47) may feed on algae and other micro-organisms; midges, clegs and horseflies on organically enriched soil; fleas and sandflies (fig. 19.48) on organic debris and stableflies on dung. Some are predatory in their larval stages, for example some mosquitoes and tabanids.

The bloodsuckers with a hemimetabolous life cycle are, in contrast, wholly dependent upon blood. Among these are the soft and hard ticks (fig. 19.50), mites, true bugs and blood-sucking lice and bed bugs (fig. 19.51). The holometabolous tsetse flies (*Glossina* spp.) are exceptional in that the larva feeds *in utero* and hence these species, like the hemimetabola, are entirely dependent upon blood.

Blood is not a wholly adequate diet for arthropod existence and is supplemented by the activity of symbiotic intracellular micro-organisms, which are transmitted from one generation to the next.

Blood sucking arthropods can cause great pain, panic and sheer misery. This is an economically significant aspect of their activities. Biting flies, where their numbers are great, impede agricultural, sylvicultural and fishing operations and inhibit tourism in potentially attractive areas, as visitors to the West Highlands of Scotland or the beaches of the Caribbean can confirm. The direct effects of attack include irritation of the skin, especially of the face, pain following the injection of saliva and loss of blood. Irritation from insects on the skin and the sense of helplessness in face of large numbers contribute to the distress. The variety of mouth structures lead to very variable amounts of pain. Some mosquitoes and many hard ticks have such exquisitely refined cutting structures that their bites may pass unnoticed at first. On the other hand the coarse stylets of the tabanid flies or clegs produce wounds which are acutely painful at once. Notoriously painful also are the bites of triatomid bugs, which are colloquially known as kissing bugs from their propensity to bite the face of sleeping subjects, and soft ticks.

Blood loss is probably the least important result of attacks by biting fly. Humans rarely sustain the weight of attack which would be required to produce marked effects. Death through exsanguination is, however, not uncommon among domestic animals in the tropics

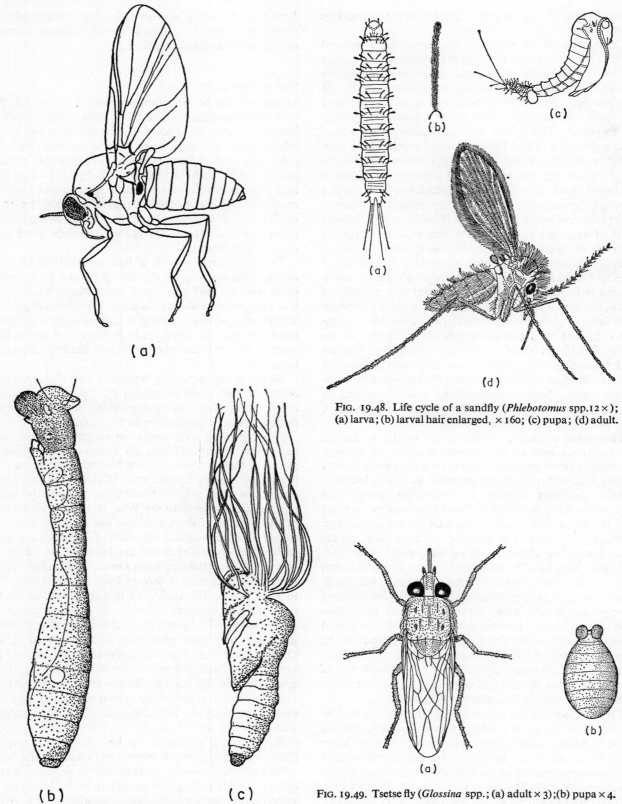

(a)

(b)   (c)

FIG. 19.47. Life cycle of a black fly (*Simulium* spp.);
(a) adult × 12; (b) larva × 10; (c) pupa × 10.

(a)   (b)   (c)

(d)

FIG. 19.48. Life cycle of a sandfly (*Phlebotomus* spp.12×);
(a) larva; (b) larval hair enlarged, × 160; (c) pupa; (d) adult.

(a)   (b)

FIG. 19.49. Tsetse fly (*Glossina* spp.; (a) adult × 3);(b) pupa × 4.

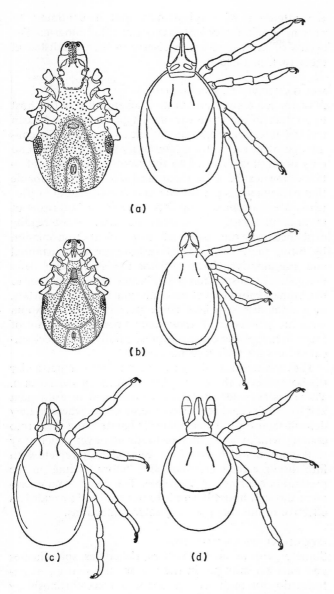

FIG. 19.50. A hemimetabolous life-cycle, the palaeartic hard tick (*Ixodes ricinus*); (a) female, venter-left, dorsum-right × 15; (b) male, venter-left, dorsum-right × 15; (c) nymph × 25; (d) larva × 40.

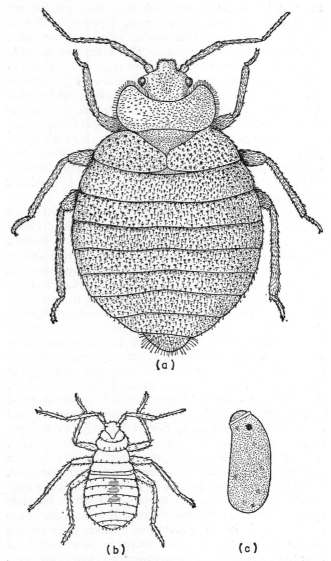

FIG. 19.51. A hemimetabolous life-cycle, the bedbug (*Cimex lectularius*); (a) adult, × 20; (b) nymph, × 20; (c) egg, × 30.

especially when they are the victims of uncontrolled infestation by ticks. Anaemia has been reported in travellers and residents of swamp areas infested with gnathobdellid leeches which are haematophagous annelid worms of widespread tropical distribution. Leech bites are painless and their anticoagulant secretions leave free-bleeding wounds after detachment. *Hirudo medicinalis* held an important place in medical practice until bleeding ceased to be fashionable.

Salivary secretions, which often contain anticoagulants and haemolysins, produce markedly different symptoms in different individuals, ranging from little more than red spots in some to extensive oedema, itching or pain in others. Scratching aggravates the symptoms. Saliva is antigenic in many cases and subjects who react slightly at first may become sensitized later. Direct and delayed reactions may then appear in which there is severe local pain and often general malaise. Hypersensitivity is particularly evident where simuliids (black-flies) are involved. During the first few days of a fishing trip in areas where simuliids are abundant (e.g. Eastern Canada) the angler may complain of the attacks he sustains, but in his second week he is incapacitated and obliged to discontinue his sport. Hypersensitivity in animals unable to avoid further exposure sometimes results in calamitous losses. The abundant simuliid faunas of the North Saskatchewan river, the Mississippi and the Danube have caused losses counted in tens of thousands of cattle in some years. Following the period of sensitization further exposure can produce desensitization and a relative immunity. This is probably the reason for the indentured African labourer carrying with him a private supply of the domestic soft tick, *Ornithodoros moubata*, which maintains his immune status and so allows him to avoid the discomfort a return home might otherwise entail.

Some individuals of certain species of hard tick, such as *Dermacentor andersoni* in Western Canada, *Ixodes rubicundus* in South Africa and *I. holocyclus* in Eastern Australia cause a particularly serious condition known as **tick paralysis**. Although animals (cattle and sheep in Canada, sheep in South Africa and dogs in Australia) are affected more frequently than humans, it is sufficiently common, especially among children, for local medical practitioners to be continuously alert during seasons of tick activity. Understanding of the ascending paralysis is incomplete. Female ticks are principally responsible and one alone can produce the condition; symptoms appear only after the tick has been attached for several days. Although the course of the syndrome is progressive and may terminate fatally if uninterrupted, discovery and removal of the offending tick is followed by a rapid regression of symptoms and ultimate complete recovery. It is presumed that paralysis, which results from a failure of release of acetylcholine at motor nerve endings, is caused by a toxin present in the saliva of some individual ticks. Antisera can be prepared which alleviate symptoms in severely affected cases. The incidence of the paralysis toxin in tick populations appears to be subject to wide variation and this is reflected in the geographical distribution of cases. *Dermacentor andersoni* is an interesting example. Although this tick is widespread in Southern Alberta and British Columbia in Canada and in the American states of Idaho, Montana, Wyoming and Colorado, nearly all the numerous records of paralysis due to it are from North of 49°N and West of the Rockies in British Columbia.

Vectors in Disease

A **vector** is any organism which acts as intermediary agent in the transfer of a parasite from one host to another. In the course of its transmission a parasite may or may not undergo developmental and or multiplicative processes and hence vectors play either a purely mechanical or a biological (cyclical) role.

The role of haematophagous arthropods as disease vectors was the aspect of their activity that first engaged the attention of medical men and it continues to present a major problem to medical entomologists. The agents of arthropod-borne disease in man are listed in table 19.4, p. 19.40.

MECHANICAL TRANSMISSION

A vector can convey organisms unchanged from one host to another in the same way as a hypodermic needle can transfer infection from one patient to another. The contamination of the vector is temporary and superficial, and only organisms adhering to the mouthparts cause infection of the next host. On theoretical grounds it is probable that parasitaemias in man due to viruses, bacteria or protozoa are transmissible in this way; some outbreaks of anthrax in South Indian populations are most readily explained on the basis of mechanical transmission by biting flies. The evidence is, however, circumstantial and presumptive. Indeed, there are some who deny mechanical transmission a significant role in relation to the human subject; it is certainly much more important in animal disease where some parasites, e.g. myxoma virus in rabbits or *Trypanosoma evansi*, the agent of Surra in horses and camels, depend wholly upon mechanical vectors for their transmission.

The non-haematophagous muscid flies, in particular the houseflies of the genus *Musca*, present a special case. These insects undergo larval development in excrement and the adults feed readily on the substrata whereon they deposit their eggs. Their domestic habits bring them into contact with exposed human foodstuffs over which they walk and on which they feed. Flies already replete with filth disgorge their crop contents before feeding on the preferable offerings of the table. The route from excrement through housefly vomit to human food provides an effective means for spreading enteric infections.

CYCLICAL TRANSMISSION

Some organisms such as viruses, rickettsias, spirochaetes and bacteria multiply in the vector; the filaroid nematodes do not multiply but undergo metamorphosis by moulting from a first stage larva (microfilaria) to a third stage or infective larva; and the haemoflagellate and haemosporidian protozoa both develop and multiply in the vector. Depending upon the location of the cyclical process there are various ways in which the infection is transmitted.

The simplest situation is found when the louse, *Pediculus humanus*, ingests blood containing *Rickettsia quintana* (trench fever). The organism remains in the gut lumen where it multiplies and from which it passes out in the faeces. However, *R. prowazekii* (epidemic typhus) enters the epithelial cells of the midgut, where it multiplies before being passed in the faeces. *Trypanosoma cruzi* (p. 19.8) metamorphose and multiply in the mid-gut and hindgut of triatomid bugs before the infective form gains the exterior in the dejecta. Infection follows entry through scratches, sometimes through mucous membranes (*T. cruzi*) and possibly by inhalation (*R. prowazekii*). It follows that personal infestation by lice is not required for an individual to contract epidemic typhus and doctors and nurses in attendance upon patients may develop louse-borne typhus in this way.

Inoculative infection with leishmania and trypansomes follows developments in the gut of sandflies and tsetse flies respectively. Leishmania in the anterior gut lumen migrate forwards to the mouthparts where the infective stage is reached. The trypanosomes follow a complex route in the midgut around and through the peritrophic membrane and thence forwards to the opening of the common salivary duct on the hypopharynx. They reach the lumina of the salivary glands after migration up the ducts and the metacyclic forms are injected into the host with the saliva of the insect.

A peculiar method of transmission applies to *Pasteurella pestis* (bubonic plague) after multiplication in fleas (especially the rat fleas, *Xenopsylla cheopis* and *X. brasiliensis*). Multiplication in the foregut produces a compact bacterial mass. When the blocked flea, as it is termed, attempts to feed, the pharyngeal pump directs blood into the foregut but its further passage into the midgut is prevented by the bacterial occlusion. When the pharyngeal muscles relax the blood surges forward again as the distended walls of the foregut contract. Regurgitation of contaminated blood into the wound produces a new case of plague. Inability to satisfy hunger leads the blocked flea to frequent attempts to feed and so enhances transmission.

In some instances there is deeper invasion of the vector organism. The malaria sporozoites migrate from the gut wall through the haemocoel to penetrate and accumulate in the salivary glands from which they are transferred to a new host when the mosquito feeds. *Borrelia duttonii*, the agent of African tick borne relapsing fever, multiplies in house infesting soft ticks of the group *Ornithodoros moubata*. Related species responsible for relapsing fevers in America, Asia and North Africa utilize other ticks. *Borrelia recurrentis*, which causes epidemic relapsing fever, undergoes cyclical development in *Pediculus humanus*. All these spirochaetes penetrate the gut wall to enter the haemocoel of the vector where they multiply. The tick-borne species invade several of the organs of the vector and are transmissible by the saliva, by the secretions of the coxal glands (which regulate salt and water balance after the tick has fed) or by the eggs of the next generation of ticks.

The arboviruses invade successively the gut epidermis, the haemolymph and various organs in whose cells they multiply. In all cases transmission is by saliva and in the tick borne also by eggs. *Rickettsia rickettsii*, which is transmitted by *Dermacentor andersoni* and other

hard ticks, has similar invasive properties, as have the other tick borne rickettsias (table 19.4). Infection acquired at one feed is retained during the moult and transmitted by salivary inoculation at the feed of the next instar, or may be passed through the egg to be transmitted at the first feed of the next generation. *R. tsutsumagushi*, the agent of scrub typhus is transmitted by trombidiid mites. Stage to stage transmission is impossible here since the vectors are parasitic once only during their life-time. Infection acquired in the parasitic larval stage is retained through the two moults to nymphal and adult stages and then passes through the egg to be transmitted by the larva of the next generation.

Filarioid larvae penetrate the gut wall to undergo growth and moulting in the muscles and other organs of the appropriate vector. Development completed, they migrate forwards in the haemolymph to the labrum. When the vector feeds they emerge actively through the arthropod integument and then penetrate the skin of the vertebrate host.

The profuse multiplication which sometimes occurs in the arthropod host can be utilized for diagnostic purposes. It is often very difficult to demonstrate the trypanosome parasites in suspected cases of Chagas's disease. Clean triatomid bugs are fed on suspected cases and, after an appropriate interval, infection can be confirmed by the abundant trypanosomes, readily recognized in the arthropod gut (xenodiagnosis).

Infestation of the flight muscles by filarioid nematodes impedes flight in the vector hosts and heavy infestations impair their life expectancy. Similarly the life span of lice infected with *R. prowazekii* is greatly reduced since the louse has no mechanism for the replacement of damaged gut cells. Apart from these examples it is remarkable how little effect most of the above organisms have on the vigour or life expectancy of infected arthropods. Mosquitoes or ticks with high arbovirus titres, malarious mosquitoes, trypanosome-infected tsetse flies, soft ticks carrying spirochaetes, etc., appear as healthy as their uninfected fellows.

Epidemiological considerations

FEATURES OF CYCLICAL TRANSMISSION

The **extrinsic incubation period** is the time required for the development cycle of the pathogen in the vector. Development is rapid when the temperature is high, slow when the temperature falls and stops when a threshold is reached. The temperature threshold is characteristic for the organism. Many organisms can survive prolonged exposure to low temperatures (e.g. arboviruses) and can resume growth when temperatures become favourable. This is obviously important in hibernating arthropods. When an anopheline mosquito feeds upon a malarial patient with a gametocytaemia, a developmental cycle (p. 19.10) has to be completed before the mosquito can inflict an infective bite. This takes time. Indeed, the infected mosquito takes three or four more blood meals before it begins to transmit malaria. For *Plasmodium falciparum* the extrinsic cycle requires over two weeks at 25°C, over three weeks at 20°C and below 17°C development ceases. The comparable figures for *P. vivax* are rather less than two weeks at 25°C, two and a half weeks at 20°C, and development is not arrested until temperatures of 15°C and less are reached. These figures alone explain why benign tertian malaria may be widespread in temperature regions where malignant tertian disease is unknown. The absence of malaria of all types from cool temperate regions despite abundant anopheline mosquitoes is also explained.

It is generally true, although filarioid nematodes are an obvious exception, that once infective, a cyclical vector remains infective throughout its life. The culicine mosquito, *Aëdes aegypti*, transmits yellow fever for a period of three months until it dies, and many ticks and mites can pass infections (virus, rickettsia or spirochaete) to their progeny.

Cyclical transmission of any particular organism is restricted to a limited range of vectors. Plasmodia infective to man can complete their development in anopheline mosquitoes only, whereas species infective to birds often fail to develop in anophelines but produce sporozoites freely in culicine mosquitoes.

FEATURES OF MECHANICAL TRANSMISSION

There is no latent period and the infected vector immediately acquires infectivity which is transient and declines exponentially over a period rarely exceeding 24 hours. Temperature, except as it affects arthropod biting activity, has no effect on the process.

Transmission is not limited to a particular vector. Myxomatosis in rabbits, for example, can be spread by fleas, lice, mosquitoes and other biting flies. However, the probability of mechanical transmission depends on the number of parasites in the host, whereas a cyclical vector can transmit from patients in whom parasites cannot be found directly (e.g. in *Trypanosoma cruzi* infections). It is important to realize, however, that the quantum of infection taken up has a critical importance also for cyclical vectors. This is particularly evident in relation to arbovirus transmission. For the examples which follow virus concentrations are expressed as median lethal doses for mice per 0·03 ml of intracerebral inoculum, i.e. LD50.

The virus of Rift Valley fever is noninfective to the mosquito *A. aegypti* at a concentration of $10^{7\cdot0}$ but at $10^{8\cdot0}$ a large proportion of the mosquitoes becomes infected. Similarly, no individuals of the mosquito *Orthopodomyia signifera* can be infected by blood containing $10^{6\cdot5}$ eastern equine encephalitis virus but

most are susceptible when the concentration is $10^{7\cdot7}$. Thus there is an **infection threshold**, definable within precise limits for each mosquito species. For any one virus this threshold is of great epidemiological importance.

There is the complementary phenomenon of host-characteristic viraemic levels in different vertebrate species. Western equine encephalitis, a disease of man and horses in the USA, was long regarded on circumstantial grounds as mosquito borne. The discovery of frequently infected *C. tarsalis* confirmed this suspicion, although attempts to infect mosquitoes experimentally from viraemic patients were unsuccessful. These mosquitoes normally feed on birds. Surveys showed that in birds, infection produces high levels of viraemia, although unaccompanied by the morbidity seen in man and horse. Hence man and horse, in which viraemia rarely exceeds the infection threshold of the vector, are not part of the natural life cycle of the virus. Similar factors are responsible for the spread of Murray valley encephalitis in Australia.

Man is in a similar position in relation to the tick borne viral encephalitides and haemorrhagic fevers. Human infection is tangential to a wild animal cycle. The multiplication phase of arboviruses in the vertebrate host is very short and hence their long term interepidemic maintenance has to be in the arthropod vector. Hard ticks, which feed three times in their life cycle at intervals as long as twelve months apart, can obviously serve as maintenance hosts. Their efficiency is often enhanced by ovarian transmission and congenital infection. In mosquitoes, on the other hand, there is no evidence of ovarian transmission and hence virus maintenance is limited to the term of their adult life. For many mosquito borne viruses the problem of interepidemic maintenance remains unsolved.

YELLOW FEVER TRANSMISSION

Yellow fever occurred in epidemic form throughout the warm seaboard areas on both sides of the Atlantic, until its urban transmission by the domestic mosquito, *A. aegypti*, was understood and measures were adopted for its control. In tropical regions, where breeding of *A. aegypti* was continuous and uninterrupted, human epidemics ran a full course to decline and disappear as the numbers of susceptible people decreased. In sub-tropical and temperate places, where mosquito breeding is interrupted by the dry or cold season, epidemics were terminated abruptly by the disappearance of adult mosquitoes. *A. aegypti* passes adverse seasons as dormant eggs and can thus play no part in virus maintenance. Yellow fever, therefore, was explicable as a man–mosquito–man cycle maintained by humans travelling from one centre to another. When yellow fever was found to affect other primates, it was realized that a sylvatic monkey–mosquito–monkey cycle would support the urban one. Monkeys in the vast equatorial forest were thus an additional reservoir, from which infection could spread. Other possibilities, however, have been identified. Yellow fever crossed the Panama Canal in 1948 and began a northward advance into the then unaffected monkey populations of Central America. It affected principally the forest populations among which transmission was mediated by *Haemagogus spegazzini*. This mosquito is adult and active in the wet seasons but in the dry it aestivates in the egg. Yellow fever advanced north each wet season but neither monkeys nor *H. spegazzini* could maintain the virus in the dry seasons. The maintenance host was found to be another mosquito, *Sabethes chloropterus*, unimportant during epidemic periods but important between epidemics because it aestivates in the adult stage. Before the inactive period, mated females of this species take a blood meal and, instead of maturing eggs, they develop a fat body (gonadotrophic dissociation) on which they subsist during the dry season. Virus survives in infected individuals and it is transmitted when activity is resumed in the next wet season. Today, human epidemics in Africa and America derive intermittently from the jungle cycle by the introduction of virus into domestic mosquito populations either when workers return after being infected in the forest or when infected monkeys make forays against agricultural settlements.

THE SPREAD OF TYPHUS

The role of vectors in the epidemiology is well illustrated by the human rickettsioses. Louse borne typhus due to *Rickettsia prowazekii* has been recorded from most parts of the world. Its earliest recognizable presence in Europe was in Spain at the siege of Granada in 1489 and its greatest outbreak involved thirty million cases in Russia between 1918 and 1922. Persistent endemic foci of greater or lesser geographical extent have long been recognized in which hyperendemics periodically occur and from which epidemics can develop. These occur usually in winter time, associated with increased incidence of lice and the cycle man–louse–man is entirely responsible for the epidemic spread. This was seen in the Naples outbreak of 1944, where lack of soap and the life in air raid shelters favoured multiplication and dissemination of lice. Louse control on patients and their close contacts rapidly stopped the typhus epidemic. The problem of the inter-epidemic maintenance of typhus appears to have been largely solved by the finding that the usually mild febrile illness, Brill–Zinsser disease, was a recrudescent form of typhus, occurring in the absence of lice. *R. prowazeki* can persist in such latent human infections for as long as twenty years and thus man himself can act as the reservoir. This simple view, however, may not be

the whole story since *R. prowazeki* was isolated in 1955 in Ethiopia from domestic animals and their hard ticks.

The transmission of murine typhus (*R. mooseri*) by the rat louse (*Polyplax* spp.) presents an analogy with classical typhus in man. This organism, however, multiplies freely in the gut of rat fleas (*Xenopsylla* spp. etc.) and these insects readily attack man to produce human infections. The human disease is world wide, but essentially sporadic and local in its incidence. It is most likely to occur in those who come in contact with rat infestations by working in granaries and food stores. Murine typhus is not lethal to rats and hence is not accompanied by deviation of rat fleas to man on the scale found in murine bubonic plague. This probably accounts for the lack of any tendency for this disease to become epidemic for man while it remains flea borne. It is not normally transmissible by human lice but there is evidence that murine typhus has produced strains adapted to the human louse with consequent epidemic tendencies and it has been suggested that epidemic typhus, which is antigenically related to murine typhus, has evolved in this way. Where murine typhus shows varying seasonal prevalence its peak incidence in man is in summer (Near East) or autumn (USA) as is to be expected for a flea-borne infection and not, as in classical louse-borne typhus, in winter.

Scrub typhus (*R. tsutsumagushi*) which has a wide distribution in the Far East is another mainly murine infection in which the vectors are the tromidiid mites *Trombicula akamushi* in Japan and *T. deliensis* in Burma. The cycle, rodent–mite–egg–mite–rodent, flourishes in conditions of secondary scrub adjacent to cultivation. The scrub favours mite survival and the nearby activities of man favour rodent populations. The incidence of scrub typhus in man depends upon the degree of his contact with the 'typhus islands' and its seasonal variation is determined by changes in the population of larval mites which is maximal during the monsoon.

The epidemiology of the tick-borne rickettsioses is a complex problem currently engaging the attention of workers in many parts of the world. All can develop in a range of ticks, in most of which transstadial and transovarian passage are regular features. Ticks can, therefore provide long term reservoirs for each rickettsia species. Infections of a range of mammal and bird hosts allow circulation and dispersal. The picture in man has always been confused by the occurrence within each rickettsial species of antigenically indistinguishable strains of greatly differing virulence. Since the development of effective antibiotics, it has become harder to record the true incidence in man and this makes the study of the epidemiology more difficult.

Rickettsia rickettsii is widely distributed in the American continents where it is known by many local names of which the best known is Rocky Mountain spotted fever (RMSF). Man is affected in varying degrees according to local faunal and ecological patterns although mainly in sporadic fashion. RMSF occurs either when man enters the feral environment to be bitten by wild ticks or when human environments encroach upon the domain of or are invaded by feral hosts and become infested by their associated ticks. In the western States, where *Dermacentor andersoni* is the principal vector, infection is observed mainly in adult male field and forest workers. In the eastern States, surburban development encloses tick populations among which *D. variabilis* readily transfers to domestic dog hosts. In these circumstances RMSF may occur among women and children. These are but minor details, however, in an epidemiological complex which in the United States, involves at least eighteen species of birds, thirty-one species of mammals and some dozen species of ticks. *R. sibirica* (Siberian tick typhus) shows many similarities with that of *R. rickettsii*. Recent work on *R. conori*, the agent of Boutonneuse, Marseilles or Mediterranean tick fever which had a wide distribution in southern Europe, Africa and southern Asia, shows that this too has an epidemiology of comparable complexity. The close association between *R. conori*, domestic dogs and the kennel tick, *Rhipicephalus sanguineus*, suggested by earlier work in North Africa has been confirmed in Bulgaria but in France several other species of tick (*Ixodes* spp., and *Dermacentor* spp.) also play a role. It is probably more than coincidence that a significant decline in the incidence of boutonneuse fever in man has followed the reduction of rabbit populations in Europe by myxomatosis.

Further examples are not needed to show that, although the phenomena of pathogen transmission by vectors can be analysed and interpreted on the basis of a few simple concepts, the epidemiological issues of practical significance are often ascertainable only after close study of the vectors and their ecological relationships. Where the disease is a zoonosis the interrelationships of man, reservoirs, vectors and pathogen may be of such complexity that rationally devised control measures can be applied only in an atmosphere of expectancy. Even the strict anthroponoses of malaria have resisted half a century of effort because until recently their ecology was only imperfectly understood. A full understanding of the vector and its ecology are essential. Progress in this field has contributed substantially to the planning of control measures where the probability of success is calculable before control is initiated and where modifications can be devised rationally when required during its course. Malaria is the most instructive example of this.

Malaria transmission

Human malaria affects all parts of the world except the cool regions of high latitude and high altitude where the extrinsic developmental cycle fails, and some Pacific islands from which anopheline mosquitoes are absent. It is transmissible by anopheline mosquitoes only and for all practical purposes schizogony cycles can take place only in man. Around 250 species have been described in the genus *Anopheles* and they fall into some four or five taxonomically distinct groups or sub-genera. Many species have been experimentally tested for their susceptibility to infection by human *Plasmodium* spp. and of these only a very small proportion have proved wholly refractory. Nevertheless, although the potential range of vectors is great, field evidence implicates little more than one dozen species as major vectors and it is notable that between them they represent all the anopheline subgenera. Clearly it is not systematic relationships but individual characteristics which determine the vector role of a particular species. Many anophelines have specialized breeding requirements which restrict their distribution and limit their numbers. A species which requires dense equatorial forest, for example, can never have more than a marginal and local importance. The major vectors are found among species which are tolerant of a range of environments or whose preferred conditions are widely available. They are species which co-exist with human populations and human activities such as agriculture, mining and civil engineering provide breeding conditions by intentional or accidental impounding of water. Though the prerequisite of contact between human and anopheline populations may be satisfied, many anopheline species remain unimportant because they do not have a good life expectancy in the adult instar or do not feed readily on man. The north Indian *Anopheles subpictus* fails because it rarely survives long enough to complete the extrinsic cycle, while the European *A. messeae* is unimportant because of its preference for cattle.

A MATHEMATICAL MODEL

Malaria transmission can be represented by a mathematical model in which the terms for mosquito longevity and anthropophily (human-biting tendency) are important components. A hypothetical numerical example illustrates the weight these items contribute. Assume that all the mosquitoes in a given locality bite human subjects and the population size is such that a patient infected with *Plasmodium vivax* supplies 100 blood meals during the gametocytaemic phase. If the probability P of any mosquito surviving one day is 0·9, i.e. assuming mortality is randomly distributed in the mosquito population and the daily mortality 10 per cent, some 116 new cases would become infected from the original case provided the mean temperature remained above 25°C. A drop in temperature to 20°C would prolong the extrinsic incubation period and reduce the frequency of mosquito feeding so that the number of

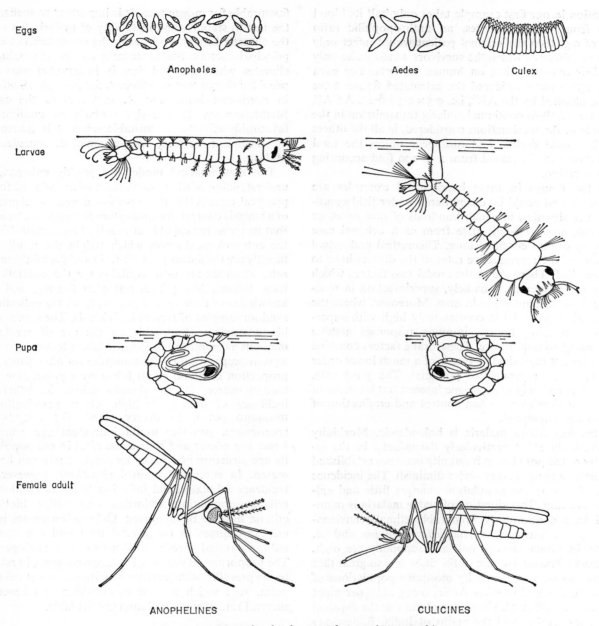

Eggs

Anopheles   Aedes   Culex

Larvae

Pupa

Female adult

ANOPHELINES   CULICINES

FIG. 19.52. Mosquito developmental stages (not to scale).

new cases would be reduced to about fifty-four. If in the same situations the probability of mosquito survival were 0·8, a daily mortality of 20 per cent, the numbers of new cases would be down to ten at the higher temperature and five at the lower. In all these situations the incidence of malaria would increase since each case produces an increased number of new cases. With a mosquito survival reduced to 0·7, however, a single new case from each original one would merely permit the maintenance of the disease at the higher temperature, but at the lower

temperature well under one new case would be produced and malaria would decline in the population. In this last situation malaria maintenance would be restored only if the total mosquito population were to undergo a two- to three-fold increase.

Consider now the more normal experience where mosquitoes take their blood meals from many hosts. From the point of view of malaria it is immaterial what other hosts are attacked and it is the probable rate of human attack that matters. If we assume that the mosquito population in our first example takes only half its blood meals from human sources, an anthropophilic ratio (AR) of 0·5, then the original patient would infect only fifty mosquitoes of which the survivors would make only half their infective bites on human subjects. For each of the situations considered the calculated figures have to be multiplied by the AR^2, i.e. $0·5 \times 0·5 = 0·25$. An AR of 0·1 would allow continued malaria transmission in the first only of the six situations considered, in all the others malaria would decline and disappear unless the total population were increased from 2 to 200 fold according to the situation.

All the figures in these hypothetical examples are reasonable and could be encountered under field conditions. The situation in which hundreds of new cases, or thousands when $P > 0·9$, arise from each original case obviously cannot continue long. Theoretical and actual estimates of the reproductive rates of the disease have to be reconciled. There are in the model two factors which reduce the discrepancy, namely, superinfection in mosquitoes and superinfection in man. Moreover, where the transmission potential is continuously high with superinfection in man, human immune responses assume epidemiological importance. These brake factors combine so that the net reproductive rate is of a much lower order than the gross reproductive potential. The gross rate, however, is not only of academic interest but becomes of paramount significance when control and eradication of malaria are attempted.

In tropical Africa malaria is holendemic. Morbidity and mortality affect particularly the infants. In the remainder of the population immunity becomes established with increasing age and episodes diminish. The incidence of the disease in the population changes little and epidemics are rare. This situation of **stable malaria** is maintained in a continuously favourable climatic environment by the mosquitoes *Anopheles gambiae* and *A. funestus* in which survival and anthropophily are high. The gross reproductive rate of the disease is so great that malaria can be maintained by mosquito populations of very small size and in West Africa 0·025 bites per night per person is sufficient. **Unstable malaria** was the classical pattern for Ceylon and the plains of India. Endemicity was low and immunity in the population negligible. The vector, *A. culicifacies*, has a low anthropophilic ratio and a poor survival rate and hence to maintain malaria its population size requires to be large; for example, ten bites per night at least are needed to maintain malaria in Madras. The monsoon climate of India causes mosquito populations to undergo vast numerical fluctuations. The alternation of humid and arid seasons also profoundly affects mosquito survival. Consequently, malaria transmission in India is seasonal and in the past disastrous epidemics involving all sections of the population have occurred in those years when conditions were particularly

favourable for mosquitoes. It is important to realize that the key to stability and instability of malaria lies not in the climatic background but in the characteristics of the principal vectors. Stable malaria can be maintained in climates where transmission is interrupted seasonally provided the vectors are efficient, for example *A. minimus* in north-east India and *A. sacharovi* in the eastern Mediterranean. Conversely, malaria in continuously favourable climates is unstable when it is transmitted by inefficient vectors, for example *A. maculatus* in Malaya.

The mathematical model has greatly enhanced the understanding of the epidemiology of malaria. Its further practical value is that it can provide a measure of progress of a malaria control. Its application presupposes, however, that its terms are capable of practical estimation. Two of the entomological terms which weight the result significantly are the anthropophilic ratio and the adult survival rate. Methods are now available for the estimation of these factors. Mosquitoes rest after feeding, and local knowledge of their resting places allows the collection of random samples of replete individuals. The source of its blood meal is identifiable by the use of serological methods as employed in forensic laboratories, on a dried squash preparation of the mosquito on filter paper. The proportion of blood meals taken by a population from human sources is thus directly calculable. Where the incidence of malaria is high, direct examination of mosquito gut and salivary glands for oöcysts and sporozoites, provides useful individual age estimates. From the oöcyst and sporozoite rates in the population its age structure and hence its survival rate can be estimated. In successful control situations, however, the incidence of plasmodial infection becomes too low for reliable population estimates and other biological criteria have to be employed. Oviposition causes recognizable changes in the genital tract and consequently nulliparous and parous individuals can be distinguished. The proportion of parous to nulliparous gives, in relation to the prevailing temperature conditions, an age reference point from which the age composition and hence the survival rate of the population is calculable.

Vector control
The aim of medical entomology is the elimination of arthropod-borne disease. Immunoprophylaxis has contributed greatly to this end in the control of such diseases as yellow fever, and chemoprophylaxis among those fortunate enough to be able to afford it limits the incidence of malaria. A more radical approach by attacking their vectors offers the possibility of insulating human populations from feral sources of pathogens and of eradicating pathogens involved in human disease. Arthropod populations are reducible by altering the environment to deprive them of the conditions which

favour their survival. They are also susceptible to chemical attack. In either case knowledge of the ecological relationships is a prerequisite for success. Environmental control is too complex a subject for consideration within the present limits. It is of particular importance, however, where urban development and mining or engineering enterprises in the tropics are under consideration since it is precisely these activities which in the past have created many of the environments favourable to noxious arthropods.

Chemical control of arthropods is a major industry which has developed since the introduction of **dicophane** (DDT). This event was as far reaching for insect control as was the introduction of penicillin for microbiology. The term DDT is derived from the chemical name **d**ichloro**d**iphenyl**t**richlorethane, the chemical formula of which is given on p. 6.14. Surprisingly, DDT is as toxic to mammals, when given intravenously, as it is to insects; the susceptibility of arthropods is due to the fact that the compound easily penetrates the exoskeleton. It then kills the arthropods by rendering the axonal membranes unstable. The key to the DDT revolution lies not in its potency, in which its advantages over earlier agents are unremarkable, but in its physical inertness and chemical stability. Its residual properties considerably exceed those of any of its predecessors. The first major success of DDT in the medical field was in 1944 when treatment of victims and their close contacts arrested the typhus epidemic in Naples, the first occasion when typhus was effectively controlled during winter. No less notable has been its impact on malaria control. Before the advent of DDT the reduction of mosquito populations through the use of chemicals was practicable only through attacking their aquatic stages when they are most readily accessible. Indeed, this method scored many successes of which the most remarkable was the eradication of *A. gambiae* from Brazil, whither it had been accidentally introduced from Africa in the early thirties of this century. Such results, however, were vastly expensive to achieve since they depended upon rigorous and close supervision by a large personnel. Moreover, as we have seen, the effect *vis-à-vis* malaria transmission of total reduction of mosquito populations depends upon their efficiency as vectors. Success in an area of unstable malaria such as Madras could be achieved with comparatively inefficient methods of larval destruction. Success in areas like West Africa where the vectors are highly efficient demanded larval mortalities which are beyond practical achievement. Residual insecticides have introduced a new dimension to insect control in so far as they provide a means of attacking adult insects. This has a twofold result, it reduces the population but more appropriately it reduces the life expectancy of adults. The addition of diminished survival to a reduced biting rate has made malaria eradication a practicable possibility.

Insecticide resistance is the new problem which places an obstacle before the ultimate goal, and this is analogous to the problem of drug resistance which complicates the employment of antibiotics and chemotherapeutic agents. Insecticide resistance is usually a preadaptive genetic character. Where it appears, it can only be overcome by variation of insecticidal agents, which, fortunately the available range is steadily increasing. These include the organophosphorus compounds, e.g. **parathion, malathion** and **dichlorvos** (DDVP), carbamide insecticides, e.g. **carbaryl** and **aprocarb** which have been widely used as residual sprays, and other chlorinated hydrocarbons such as **dieldrin**. Possible hazards to man from the use of insecticides are discussed on p. 32.6.

Zoology and medicine

It is sad that, although most of man's animal parasites had been described and their mode of transmissions known by the early years of this century, they continue to cause an enormous morbidity and mortality. The reason is not neglect of their study, because medical zoology has attracted the attention of many parasitologists and entomologists, many of the most distinguished of whom have been medically qualified. Unhappily, the application of knowledge is hindered by social and economic problems. The industrialized communities of the West may fail to appreciate the importance of parasitic diseases, since by chance, rather than by design, they have become isolated from the wild environment. Yet the modern cities of the Pacific seaboard of the USA are still only islands in a countryside where bubonic plague is endemic in feral rodents.

Interest in protozoal and metazoal parasites also flags as rapid expansion of new branches of the biological sciences tends to crowd them out of medical and zoological curricula. Such exclusion would be unfortunate, especially for the medical profession who pioneered the development of medical zoology and whose continuing leadership in this field is required. The incorporation of serious study of animal parasites in medical training contributes substantially in terms of potential aid to countries with large numbers of poor rural communities, and to preparedness for the occasional episodes caused by the return of the parasite to prosperous areas in developed countries. The intrinsic interests of the field also provide an impelling reason for its study. The multiplicity of interrelationships between the animal parasites and their human and other hosts provide a background for understanding of the natural history of diseases and their quantitative definition. The research problems which arise offer, as malariology alone can show, as full an intellectual challenge as any field of biology.

FURTHER READING

ADLER S. (1964) Leishmania, in *Advances in Parasitology*, vol. 2. New York: Academic Press

ARTHUR D.R. (1962) *Ticks and Disease*. Oxford: Pergamon.

BUSVINE J.R. (1966) *Insects and Hygiene*, 2nd Edition. London: Methuen.

BUXTON P. (1950) *The Louse*. London: Arnold.

FAUST E.C. (1960) The multiple facets of *Entamoeba histolytica* infection, in *International Review of Tropical Medicine*, vol. 2. New York: Academic Press.

FAUST E.C. & RUSSELL P.F. (1964) *Clinical Parasitology*, 7th Edition. London: Kimpton.

GARNHAM P.C.C. (1966) *Malaria Parasites and other Haemosporidia*. Oxford: Blackwell Scientific Publications.

GORDON R.M. & LAVOIPIERRE M.M.J. (1961) *Entomology for Students of Medicine*. Oxford: Blackwell Scientific Publications.

JACOBS L. (1967) Toxoplasma and toxoplasmosis, in *Advances in Parasitology*, vol. 5. New York: Academic Press.

LEE D.L. (1965) *The Physiology of Nematodes*. Edinburgh: Oliver & Boyd.

MACDONALD G. (1957) *The Epidemiology and Control of Malaria*. London: Oxford University Press.

NEAL R.A. (1966) Experimental Studies on *Entamoeba* with reference to speciation, in *Advances in Parasitology*, vol. 4. New York: Academic Press

SMART J. (1965) *A Handbook for the Identification of Insects of Medical Importance*, 4th Edition. London: British Museum.

SMYTH J.D. (1962) *Introduction to Animal Parasitology*. London: English Universities Press.

WOLSTENHOLME G.E.W. & O'CONNOR M. eds. (1962) *Bilharziasis*, CIBA Foundation Symposium. London: Churchill.

Chapter 20
Principles of chemotherapy

Chemotherapy means curing by chemicals but, as this definition would include all drug treatment, the word is restricted to the use of a chemical compound in a patient to kill an infective organism or neoplastic cell. Since most compounds which poison micro-organisms may also poison man, it is necessary to select those which are as toxic as possible for the micro-organisms but which exert minimal injury on the host. Although modern compounds are often remarkably successful in this respect, they are not in themselves beneficial to the patient. Compounds which kill micro-organisms outside the patient are called disinfectants or antiseptics and are described on p. 18.39.

History of chemotherapy

Most major advances in science depend on developments in other branches of knowledge and occur in a social and economic environment which offers rewards for successful solutions to urgent problems. This is illustrated by the history of modern chemotherapy which began in the early years of the present century. On the one hand, the organisms responsible for most infections had been recently discovered and were available for study in the laboratory. On the other, organic chemists were synthesizing large numbers of new compounds, the structure and properties of which could be subjected to endless modification; chemical factories were being set up to make new dyes for the textile industry and so new compounds became available for medical investigation. An additional economic stimulus was provided by the development of Africa and other parts of the tropics to European enterprise; new and often fatal infectious diseases which required new remedies were encountered. Finally, the genius to exploit these circumstances was Paul Ehrlich, one of the greatest of medical scientists, who made outstanding contributions to immunology, haematology and cancer research. The science of chemotherapy was invented and founded largely by him and his disciples in Germany.

SALVARSAN AND ARSENICAL COMPOUNDS
At the end of the nineteenth century a fatal infection of

horses and cattle in Africa, carried by tsetse flies, prevented the use of draught animals in exploring and developing central Africa. Later, a similar infection was found to occur in man, causing the fatal disease called sleeping sickness. Both infections were due to protozoa in the blood called trypanosomes (p. 19.6), which could be transmitted from mouse to mouse by syringe and which killed the mice in a few days. Ehrlich was already studying dyes such as trypan red, which could cure mice of these infections, when in 1905 Thomas, in Liverpool, discovered that infected animals and later man, could be cured by an organic compound of arsenic called **atoxyl**. This observation was quickly followed up by Ehrlich and his associates who discovered its formula. This structure is

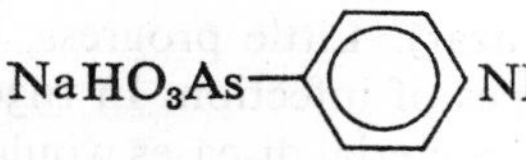

$$NaHO_3As-\langle\bigcirc\rangle-NH_2$$

Atoxyl

particularly favourable to chemical modification since innumerable side chains can be joined to the benzene ring and to the —NH₂ group. Ehrlich made and tested large numbers of such compounds, seeking chemical modifications which made them less poisonous to the mouse and more curative against the trypanosomiasis. In this process, many of the fundamental conceptions about chemotherapeutic agents, which are described below, were developed. Eventually in 1910, the 606th compound to be tested was found to be particularly effective, not only in curing trypanosomiasis in mice, but also in curing syphilis in man. This compound was named **salvarsan** (salve + arsenic + aniline), or **arsphenamine**, and it rapidly became the standard treatment for

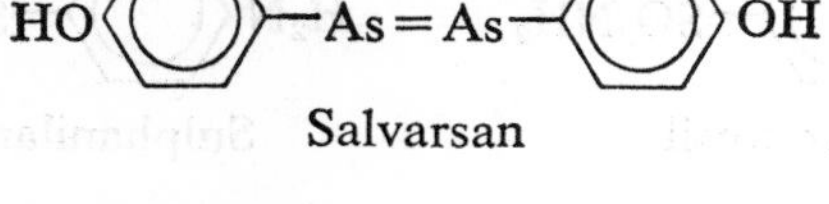

$$H_2N \quad\quad\quad\quad NH_2$$
$$HO\langle\bigcirc\rangle-As=As-\langle\bigcirc\rangle OH$$

Salvarsan

syphilis. Its discovery is one of the landmarks of medical science, since it provided the first example of an infection

20.1

being cured by a chemical compound specially invented for the purpose. Salvarsan tended to be toxic and was soon replaced by a less toxic compound called **neosalvarsan,** which was universally employed until it was superseded by penicillin in 1945. The discovery of salvarsan also caused a revolution in medical therapeutics from the economic and sociological viewpoint. Large commercial organizations engaged originally in manufacturing dyes now set out to discover new remedies which they could sell at a profit, and they were prepared to invest money on a hitherto undreamed of scale for this purpose. This state of affairs has continued up to the present and the pharmaceutical industry has become increasingly large and complex. At first, the field was dominated by large German firms such as Farben, Bayer and Hoechst; this dominance continued until 1939, when British and American firms and those in other countries began to take an interest in the subject. Since the war, particularly with the great developments in antibiotics, the major investments and discoveries have come from the United States, although important contributions have been made in other countries.

SULPHONAMIDES

The success of salvarsan stimulated similar work on other infections and new cures were found for protozoal infections such as malaria, amoebic dysentery and leishmaniasis (kala azar). Little progress, however, was made with other types of infection. In 1930, the opinion was widely held that bacterial diseases would not be cured by chemical means; many substances could be found which killed the bacteria in the test tube, but none of these was sufficiently harmless to give to patients. A team of workers in Germany, including Domagk, Mietsch and Klarer, persisted in testing drugs against streptococcal infections of mice; eventually between 1933 and 1935 they found that these infections could be cured by a red dye named **prontosil** which had been synthesized in 1920; it also cured streptococcal infections in patients, though it was inactive *in vitro*. This major advance led to increased research in many other countries. It was soon found that the active part of the dye liberated in the body was a substance called **sulphanilamide.**

Prontosil   Sulphanilamide

This substance interfered with the uptake by the bacteria of *p*-aminobenzoic acid (PABA) which is a constituent of folic acid and which the bacteria, but not the patient or animals, required for folic acid

p-Aminobenzoic acid

synthesis and their growth. Woods and Fildes subsequently showed that PABA, when present in excess, inhibited the antibacterial effect of sulphanilamide, since both compete for the same enzyme receptor site. It has also been shown that sulphanilamide competitively inhibits folic acid synthetase purified from *Esch. coli*; this enzyme condenses PABA in the formation of folic acid. Folic acid is capable of overcoming the inhibition of bacterial cell growth exerted by sulphanilamide, since it is the compound which is produced by the reaction which sulphanilamide inhibits. The selective action of sulphanilamide on some microorganisms, in contrast to the cells of human tissue, appears to be dependent on the fact that unlike man most bacteria cannot use the preformed exogenous folic acid present in body fluids.

Sulphanilamide was soon subjected to countless modifications of its molecule to yield the class of compounds known as **sulphonamides**. With these substances it soon became possible to cure infections due to streptococci, meningococci, pneumococci, gonococci and dysentery bacilli. Later sulphonamides were used to treat leprosy and they may also be valuable in the treatment of malaria. The sulphonamides led to a new development in the theory of chemotherapy, i.e. drug action by antimetabolites.

ANTIBIOTICS

The next great discovery was that of penicillin and the antibiotics, which have a different and chequered history. As early as 1877, Pasteur and Joubert had observed that 'common bacteria' prevented the growth of anthrax bacilli in urine and had suggested that this might be used clinically. Other workers made preliminary investigations but obtained no practical success. In 1899, Emmerich and Löw prepared a substance, pyocyanase, from *Ps. pyocyanea*, which was used as a throat spray for diphtheria and other infections of the throat until 1914, but it was never widely accepted or developed. In 1929, Fleming in London found that colonies of a penicillium mould prevented the growth of staphylococci in their neighbourhood. He made an extract of this mould, called it penicillin and used it therapeutically as a local application. As it was difficult to prepare and unstable, it was not developed further at this time. However, in 1938, Florey, Chain and their colleagues began an academic study of various antibacterial substances produced by micro-organisms, including the active substance in Fleming's extracts. When the product, still very impure, was tested on mice infected with haemolytic streptococci, the results were so promising that the material was given to a patient at Oxford with spectacular results. Large scale investigations followed with results that are now common knowledge. The success of this first antibiotic led to a search for other similar substances and a long series of compounds has become available, e.g. streptomycin, tetracyclines, chloramphenicol and many others.

A recent development has been the addition of suitable side chains *in vitro* to the nucleus of the penicillin molecule, made by the mould *in vivo*, by the techniques of synthetic chemistry (p. 20.12). This represents a combination of the new technique of obtaining an active antibiotic from fungal growth and the old techniques of chemical modification to obtain more favourable properties. In this way a new range of penicillin derivatives has been obtained, e.g. phenethicillin, cloxacillin and ampicillin. Thus the distinction which the term 'antibiotic' makes between the naturally occurring and synthetic antimicrobial or chemotherapeutic substances is not of fundamental significance.

General theory

As already stated, the aim of chemotherapeutic research is to find a compound which interferes with the growth and survival of the infective organism without poisoning the patient. For this purpose it is desirable to reproduce a similar infection in some small animal. The mouse is ideal for this since it is cheap, easy to handle, available in large numbers and is readily standardized. The compound under trial is given to a series of mice in graded doses, and its effect upon the mice and upon the course of infection is watched. Higher doses often kill the mice, i.e. they are toxic. The lower doses, if the compound is active, may show a curative action by suppressing the infection or by prolonging the life of the mice compared with the untreated controls. In this way, it is possible to find the maximum dose which is tolerated by the animal without causing death, i.e. the maximum tolerated dose (MTD), and the minimum dose which cures the infection (MCD). The ratio between these two doses was named by Ehrlich, the **chemotherapeutic index.**

Chemotherapeutic index (CI) $= \dfrac{\text{maximum tolerated dose}}{\text{minimum curative dose}}$

This provides a rough measure of the probable therapeutic value of a compound, and the first objective of experimental research in a chemotherapeutic laboratory is to prepare compounds with as large a chemotherapeutic index as possible. Unfortunately, however, experience soon showed that these quantities were not so

easy to measure accurately as had first been supposed. Mice vary a great deal among themselves, no matter how carefully they are standardized, and both the MTD and MCD are only statistical approximations which refer to groups of animals. Unless the group is inconveniently large, the accuracy of the approximation is low. Consequently attention was shifted from the MTD to the dose which kills 50 per cent of the animals (lethal dose LD 50), which is more sharply defined statistically, and similarly from the MCD to the dose which cures 50 per cent (CD 50). So the chemotherapeutic index became:

$$CI = \frac{LD\ 50}{CD\ 50}$$

With compounds which have a steep dose–response curve, where a small increase in the dose produces a great increase in the percentage of animals killed or cured, this index is satisfactory for its laboratory purpose. But with compounds with a flat dose–response curve, where a large change of the dose is required to produce a small change in the percentage killed or cured, it is better to base the index on the ratio:

$$CI = \frac{LD\ 20\ (\text{dose which kills 20 per cent})}{CD\ 80\ (\text{dose which cures 80 per cent})}$$

Each laboratory chooses its definition of the index to suit its own particular purposes.

Two further qualifications are needed. Men do not always or even commonly react exactly as mice do, and the compound which is most active in curing a mouse is not necessarily the same as the one most active in curing man. All the same, the power to cure infection in mice is a valuable indication as to which compounds should be investigated for their curative power in man. Secondly, the criteria of toxicity are usually not the same in the two cases. In mice the investigator measures chiefly the maximum dose which can be given without killing the animal, i.e. without fatally damaging its liver, kidney, brain or heart. In man, the clinician is limited by the amount which can be tolerated without producing symptoms such as vomiting, headache, skin rashes, etc. In spite of these qualifications the concept of the chemotherapeutic index still plays a fundamental part in modern chemotherapy.

Procedures for finding chemotherapeutic drugs

FINDING AN ACTIVE CHEMICAL

The practical procedure for discovering and developing a chemotherapeutic drug may be illustrated by a description of the development of antimalarial drugs, which has received much attention during the past 40 years. The first step is to devise a suitable animal infection that can be used for screening, i.e. carrying out a simple standard test to see whether a compound is likely to have activity against malarial parasites. In the case of many infectious agents, e.g. trypanosomes, streptococci or tubercle bacilli, the human pathogens may infect laboratory animals. The human malarial parasites, however, do not grow outside man, so that related parasites which produce malaria in birds or animals must be used. In the past, different organisms have been employed, e.g. *Plasmodium relictum* in canaries, *P. lophurae* in ducklings and *P. gallinaceum* in chicks; nowadays *P. berghei* in mice is mainly used. Each of these has its own pecularities, and none is exactly similar in its drug-sensitivity to the human parasites. Much preliminary study is therefore necessary to work out a convenient and reliable procedure and to determine its limitations. The next step is to administer chemical compounds to the infected animals in an arbitrary scale of doses, e.g. 1 mg, 0·3 mg, 0·1 mg per mouse. The compounds chosen for this testing must be selected in various ways. The simplest is to test practically all the compounds which the laboratory or pharmaceutical firm can lay hands on. Although this may seem unimaginative and wasteful of effort, activity has often been found in chemical compounds that would never have been suspected on theoretical grounds. A more scientific, but not necessarily more productive method, is to start with compounds which have some resemblance to a substance known to be active, e.g. quinine, or to make compounds on some hopeful hypothesis, e.g. that compounds of the pyrimidine type may interfere with the synthesis of a nucleic acid and the formation of the cell nucleus. Such a hypothesis has the advantage of stimulating and encouraging the synthetic chemist through what is usually a long series of disappointments. But many of the active compounds thus discovered have been found ultimately to have been based on the wrong hypothesis. Once a compound has been found to be active, the proud discoverer, often assisted by hindsight, can usually explain the logical steps by which he was led to synthesize that particular compound. Unfortunately, he is not able to predict reliably what the next type of active compound will be! Whichever method of selecting compounds is used, it is generally found that 99 out of 100 substances tested are disappointing. Many are inactive on both animal and parasite except in big doses; many are toxic to the animal but not to the parasite; only rarely is one found which suppresses the parasite, when given in doses which the host can tolerate. This may be regarded as the first step on the long road to producing a practical drug.

The next stage is to modify the compound by introducing side chains in different parts of the molecule, in the hope of improving the antimalarial activity or diminishing the toxicity or both. Several hundred derivatives may be made in this way and tested by the standard procedure to see which has the highest chemotherapeutic index. Often the index can be greatly improved by this procedure. Eventually two or three compounds of the series

are chosen as being the most hopeful for further development. The most important criterion is of course the ratio between activity and toxicity (CI) but ease of synthesis, cheapness and stability must also be considered.

FINDING A NEW ANTIBIOTIC
The early development of new antibiotics follows a different course. The starting point is often a sample of earth from a homely or exotic location. A ground aqueous suspension of soil in high dilution is spread on agar plates seeded with some test organism, e.g. *Staphylococcus aureus*. Colonies develop from various organisms in the soil suspension, and round some of these there will be a clear halo where the growth of the underlying staphylococci has been inhibited. These colonies are picked off and cultures are made from them. Extracts of the cultures are tested for antibacterial action against a wide variety of micro-organisms. Promising cultures are then grown on a much larger scale; further investigations are made to improve the growth of the organism and to encourage a good yield of the active principle. When sufficient material is obtained, preliminary chemical investigations must be made to see how it can be extracted from the bulk of the organism, how it can be kept stable during handling and storage and to discover its type of chemical structure. Preliminary tests are made of its actions on infections in mice and of its toxicity. The latter tests are always difficult to evaluate in the case of an impure preparation, for until a relatively pure compound is obtained, it is impossible to say how much of the toxicity is due to the antibiotic itself and how much to an impurity. Only after much preliminary study can one be certain of avoiding two pitfalls, first that the active compound itself is too toxic for therapeutic use and secondly that the substance has already been isolated and described in some other laboratory. Many compounds are discarded at each stage of their development. Those antibiotics which survive this preliminary assessment are subsequently developed in the same way as other chemotherapeutic compounds.

PILOT CLINICAL TRIALS
The next step is to make careful toxicity trials on larger animals to make sure that the compound can be given safely to man. Hitherto, toxicity has been measured only as the dose which just fails to kill half the mice or birds. Now it is necessary to find out the action of the compound on the main systems of the body, e.g. liver, kidney, bone marrow, heart and nervous system, of several species of animals, preferably including dogs and monkeys. Preliminary investigations are made also on the absorption of the compound from the alimentary canal or subcutaneous tissues, the concentration in the blood and the rates of excretion and degradation. It is not necessary to show that the compound cannot be toxic for

man; almost all active compounds are toxic if given in sufficiently high doses. Rather it is necessary to know how the compound may be toxic and what doses may be given safely without the risk of producing adverse effects. For ethical reasons, these investigations must be completed before the compound can be given to a single human patient, and are legally enforced in many countries. The recent public alarm about the possible dangerous effects of new drugs, the legal requirement in the United States and the obligations placed on manufacturers in Britain may present a serious obstacle to further progress.

The next step is to carry out a pilot trial on a small number of human patients. This is always an anxious moment for the investigator. No matter how carefully the animal toxicity tests have been made, there is always the possibility that the human organism will react differently and that a dose which is safe for an animal may produce a dangerous or fatal reaction in man. Compounds which are active on the animal parasite may often be quite inactive on the human ones. Usually, however, tests on ten or fewer patients show whether the compound is likely to be active in man, useless or dangerous. If the compound surmounts this hurdle, the question of its development begins again at a new level.

LARGE SCALE DEVELOPMENT

Manufacture, which up to this stage has been conducted at a bench level, must be developed on a pilot-plant scale, and this usually involves many new technical difficulties. Larger clinical trials must be planned and conducted in accord with all the administrative checks and precautions now enforced by the British, American and other governments. Comparison must be made with other similar drugs to ensure not only that the new compound is therapeutically effective, but that it has some clear advantage, e.g. greater activity, less toxicity or comparative cheapness, over existing remedies. When all these are completed, regrettably sometimes earlier, a publicity campaign is started to make the compound known to the medical profession and to official bodies likely to use the compound on a large scale. After this, the fate of successful new compounds tends to follow a common pattern. For several years, there is a flood of published papers reporting great successes. After a time, critical papers begin to appear, reporting failures of the compound to cure or describing adverse reactions to it. These papers become more numerous until soon it seems that the only reports which people feel are worth publishing are bad reports. Finally, a more or less balanced evaluation of the new compound is reached, in which it is realized that it is not quite as effective or as safe as was first claimed, but that it is still a valuable new addition to our therapeutic armamentarium. At this point, of course, the compound

may be superseded by the appearance of some other remedy and the whole process starts again. Somewhere during this long history, usually about the time when it is first established that the new compound is definitely a valuable remedy, investigations are made into its mode of action; these often reveal new biological facts, e.g. the role of muramic acid in the building up of the walls of bacterial cells, which had previously been unsuspected (p. 20.10).

From a commercial point of view, all the above developments constitute a long, expensive and hazardous procedure. At any stage, even after having been put on the market, the compound may fail to surmount some hurdle and have to be discarded; the ultimate product, although miraculous in its cures, may be unpatentable, like isoniazid used in the treatment of tuberculosis, because its chemical constitution, but not its therapeutic action, had long been known; or the compound, although constituting a big advance, may be speedily superseded by a new competitor. Most of the compounds which are developed fail in this way and the pharmaceutical company must pay the losses. It is only the rare product, which survives and begins to earn a profit, that pays for the previous failures and primes the pump for new developments.

Relations of the compound to the infective organism

The action of chemotherapeutic compounds and antibiotics may be considered from two aspects, that of the infective organism and that of the patient.

LETHAL ACTION ON THE ORGANISM

The action of a chemotherapeutic compound on an organism is to kill it (**bactericidal action**) or to prevent its growth (**bacteristatic action**). The distinction between bactericidal and bacteristatic compounds can be readily made *in vitro*. In the case of bactericidal agents, micro-organisms exposed to the drug die even if they are transferred to a fresh drug-free medium. Bacteristatic compounds inhibit growth, but this begins again after transfer to a fresh medium. The distinction is less clear when these compounds are employed clinically since their antibacterial effect is modified by cellular and humoral defences and is influenced by their concentration in body fluids. Table 20.1 indicates commonly used bactericidal and bacteristatic antimicrobial substances.

Killing may be the result of some lethal action, e.g. phenyl arsenoxides combine with enzymes containing SH groups and so kill trypanosomes quickly; most of the compounds acting on malaria parasites and other protozoa produce their effects in this way. Alternatively the compound may interfere with the utilization of some essential nutrient; thus sulphanilamide blocks the uptake of the similarly shaped molecule of PABA essential for the

TABLE 20.1. Action of antimicrobial agents.

Bactericidal antibiotics	Bacteristatic antibiotics
Penicillins	Sulphonamides
Streptomycin	Tetracyclines
Neomycin	Chloramphenicol
Kanamycin	Novobiocin
Polymyxins	Erythromycin
Cephalosporins	

multiplication of many bacteria. This antimetabolite type of action is common to the sulphonamides and antifolic acid agents, e.g. pyrimethamine and mercaptopurine. Antibiotics act in a variety of ways. The compound may upset the formation of mucopeptides, necessary for the bacterial cell wall, as is the case with penicillin. Penicillin has no antibacterial action on resting bacteria and it does not destroy them until they begin to divide and to require new cell walls. Alternatively, it may exert a direct effect on the cell membrane, e.g. the polymyxins, or interfere with protein synthesis within the bacterial cell, e.g. tetracyclines. Finally, the compound may have an opsonin type of action, as is the case with diethylcarbamazine and microfilariae. This compound is quite harmless to the microfilariae *in vitro* but, when it is given to an infected man or animal, it somehow alters the microfilariae so that they become attractive to the large macrophages in the liver which seize and destroy them. In many cases the action of compounds on organisms is not yet understood, and it usually involves detailed knowledge of intracellular biology and biochemistry. The biochemical basis of the action of the more important antibiotics is given on pp. 20.9 to 17.

SYNERGISM

It appears theoretically probable that many compounds may inhibit some metabolic pathway in a micro-organism, perhaps by blocking one particular enzyme. Cells, however, are versatile and it is occasionally possible for the micro-organism to switch the reaction to some other, possibly less efficient, pathway and so circumvent the blocking action of the compound. If however, a second compound can be applied which blocks the second pathway, the combined action of the two compounds may be much more difficult for the micro-organism to withstand than that of either alone. In practice, this occurs in a limited number of cases. Thus, sulphonamides interfere with the early stage of the anabolism and utilization of folic acid, and pyrimethamine interferes with some of the later stages. When given to animals infected with malarial parasites or toxoplasma, the two compounds reinforce

one another, small doses of the two together being as effective as much larger doses of either alone. This is known as **synergism** or **potentiation**. There is a variety of other reasons which have been advocated for using antibiotics or chemotherapeutic substances in combination. Some of these are clinical and arise from the need to treat mixed bacterial infections. *In vitro* studies have shown that in some cases, i.e. when an organism is exposed to two antibiotics simultaneously, development of resistance to each drug is delayed. This has been shown to be of particular importance in the case of tuberculosis and is discussed on p. 20.31. However, the clinical value of combinations of synergistic drugs is limited.

DRUG RESISTANCE

If all the organisms are not killed by their first contact with the compound, some of the survivors are found to be resistant to the further action and this resistance is found in their descendants, so that the whole population becomes resistant. This phenomenon was first seen by Ehrlich and his colleagues in trypanosomes exposed to dyes or arsenicals; it has since been observed in other protozoa, in bacteria, viruses, cancer cells, insects and rats. Its consequences are particularly unfortunate when staphylococci are resistant to penicillin and other antibiotics, when tubercle bacilli are resistant to isoniazid and streptomycin, and when malarial parasites develop resistance to chloroquine and other antimalarials. Some organisms, e.g. *Entamoeba histolytica* and most parasitic worms, have not shown drug resistance. Some chemicals, e.g. arsenic trioxide, emetine and quinine have never produced it.

The change which takes place when an organism becomes resistant to a drug depends on the organism and the drug. Apparently resistance may be achieved through different mechanisms. Trypanosomes, which are resistant to phenyl arsenical compounds, show diminished absorption of the compound. Increased destruction of the drug, e.g. by penicillinase-producing staphylococci and to a lesser degree by other enzymes which destroy cephalosporins, tetracyclines, sulphonamides and streptomycin, is responsible for resistance in some instances as well as is the development of an altered receptor mechanism. The development of resistance to sulphonamides sometimes depends upon increased production by the micro-organism of PABA or alteration in its metabolism so that the organisms cease to be dependent on it. In most cases, however, the mechanism of resistance is not fully understood. The resistant organism is often slightly less efficient at multiplication or survival than the normal organism, even in the absence of the drug. Sometimes it may be less pathogenic and show morphological changes. Further, if a mixture of sensitive and resistant organisms is free to multiply *in vivo* or *in vitro* in the absence of the drug, the sensitive organisms tend to outgrow the resistant ones and so resistance is gradually lost. On the other hand, therapeutic selection favours the spread of resistant organisms, when sensitive strains are eliminated by the prolonged use of a single chemotherapeutic substance or antibiotic. Thus, while penicillinase-secreting staphylococci existed in very small numbers prior to the discovery of penicillin, the widespread use of this antibiotic over the last 15 years has led to a vast increase in the numbers of resistant organisms especially in the hospital environment. Similar therapeutic selection appears to be responsible for the increased number of sulphonamide resistant gonococcal strains which have appeared in recent years.

In most cases drug-resistance is probably due to the spontaneous appearance of mutants independent of exposure to the drug during the process of cell division, some of which may be more resistant to drug action than the normal strain. Resistance may thus develop to a maximum by a series of discontinuous steps, each step corresponding to a discontinuous change in the genetic material, but marked resistance may be achieved by a single step as with streptomycin. For many years mutations which resulted in the development of resistance to antimicrobial agents were regarded by many to represent adaptive changes provoked by the presence of the agent in the bacterial environment. Experimental evidence indicates that this view is incorrect and may, for example, be demonstrated by the technique of **replica plating**. A thick layer of bacteria is seeded on a master culture plate and is recultured on two other plates, one containing a suitable antibiotic, e.g. streptomycin, in a concentration sufficient to inhibit the growth of the organisms. When resistant organisms appear on the plate containing the antibiotic, a sample of cells is taken from the corresponding position on the antibiotic-free master plates and inoculated on to a second antibiotic-free plate. Colonies are again removed from this and grown on yet another streptomycin-containing medium to determine their resistance. When this sequence is repeated, the proportion of resistant strains increases at each cycle. The results show that mutations which convey resistance occur in cells which have never been exposed to the antibiotic and that the change is spontaneous rather than adaptive.

Once drug resistance has developed in a bacterial population, it can be transferred to other bacteria of the same species by the genetic mechanisms of transduction or conjugation. The pathway varies with the organism. In some bacterial species, e.g. *Staph. aureus*, genetic DNA elements independent of the bacterial chromosome which resemble plasmids are responsible for transferring resistance to penicillin (p. 18.59). In others the **resistance transfer factor** (RTF) mediates the conjugation and transfer of DNA material between the cells and is a genetic element containing a number of drug resistant loci (p. 18.57).

Transfer of multiple drug resistance was first observed in Japan in 1959 during the treatment of bacillary dysentery. Pathogenic strains of *Shigella* resistant to four unrelated drugs, sulphonamides, streptomycin, chloramphenicol and tetracyclines, suddenly appeared and resistance was also conveyed to harmless strains of *Esch. coli*. Since mutations can account only for the development of one resistance at a time, it was suggested and subsequently established that transfer of patterns of resistance could also occur. The resistance is acquired extremely rapidly and has earned the description infectious. In addition to the drugs already mentioned, infectious resistance occurs for kanamycin, neomycin and penicillinase-sensitive penicillins. Concern over the potential danger of these mechanisms for the future has been emphasized by the spread of infectious resistance among intestinal organisms of farm animals fed antibiotics, which have then spread to man. It is likely, however, that the widespread use of antibiotics in the treatment of human disease is mainly responsible for the spread of resistance of this type.

To reduce the incidence of resistant strains, therapeutic practices which favour the development of drug resistance should be avoided whenever possible. Thus, chemotherapeutic compounds should be administered in full doses from the start, aiming to kill 100 per cent of the organisms and to leave no survivors which might develop resistance. In general the course of treatment should be kept short when possible, e.g. less than 10 days, to avoid long continued contact between compound and organism. Indiscriminate use of small doses of a compound over long periods, without proof that sensitive organisms are present and are causing harm, is bad practice and leads to drug-resistance in the organism and possibly to drug-sensitization in the patient (p. 23.10).

Another procedure, particularly useful in the treatment of tuberculosis, is to administer a mixture of two or even three of the standard remedies, streptomycin, isoniazid and *p*-aminosalicylic acid. This is based on the theory that if the chance of the appearance of a mutant resistant to any one of the three drugs is $1:10^9$, the chance of the appearance of a mutant simultaneously resistant to two of the drugs is the square of this, $1:10^{18}$; and the chance of one resistant to all three is the cube, $1:10^{27}$. This theory has been borne out by practice and the use of a combination of two or three compounds in the treatment of tuberculosis has diminished the number of resistant strains of the tubercle bacillus which have developed.

Relations of the compound to the patient
ABSORPTION, DISTRIBUTION AND EXCRETION
Some compounds, like sulphanilamide, are rapidly absorbed from the alimentary canal and can be given by mouth. Others are destroyed by the acid in the stomach

(penicillin G) or are not absorbed from the intestine (streptomycin) or cause vomiting; these must be given by injection. Some compounds, e.g. penicillin and streptomycin, are not irritant and can be given by intramuscular injection; others, e.g. neoarsphenamine, are highly irritant and have to be given slowly by intravenous injection. If immediate action is required, as in severe malaria or pneumonia, a compound may be injected intravenously. If a slower action is desired, extending over hours, days or weeks, the compound may be mixed with an insoluble base and injected intramuscularly, so that a depot of the drug is formed.

After the compound has been introduced into the patient, the question of its distribution must be considered. Some compounds, like sulphanilamide, are distributed quickly and evenly over most parts of the body. Others are concentrated particularly in one organ, e.g. chloroquine in the liver. Many compounds, e.g. penicillin and streptomycin, are unable to pass the blood–brain barrier and thus to enter the central nervous system, and this is important in the treatment of brain infections or meningitis. Even among the constituents of the blood, distribution may be uneven; some compounds do not enter the red blood cells in appreciable amounts, e.g. sulphadimethoxine; others, like mepacrine, are particularly concentrated in the white blood cells. Some compounds, e.g. suramin and many long-acting sulphonamides are tightly bound to the blood proteins; although they may be detected in large concentration in the blood by chemical measurements, only a small amount is free and exerts a therapeutic action.

Much information about the absorption and excretion of a compound may be obtained from a graph showing the blood concentration and urinary excretion at various intervals of time up to 24 hours after a single dose. In order to interpret such graphs, information about the concentration in various organs, especially the liver and kidneys, may also be necessary. In the case of some compounds, e.g. sulphonamides acting on bacteria, a relatively low concentration of drug maintained over a long period is most effective. With other compounds, e.g. arsenicals acting on trypanosomes and treponemata and most antimalarial compounds, a very high concentration, which may last only a short time, gives the best results.

Excretion of a compound often occurs through the kidneys into the urine, in which the concentration is commonly many times higher than it is in the blood. Antibacterial compounds which are excreted in high concentration in the urine, e.g. sulphonamides, cyloserine or ampicillin, are valuable in the treatment of infections in the urinary tract. The compound may be found also in the intestinal contents and faeces; part of this may represent drug which has been taken by mouth but not completely absorbed and part may represent compound which has been absorbed into the body and then excreted again via the bile or other secretions back into the intestine. Small amounts may be excreted in the milk (which may be important for breast-fed babies), tears, vomit, sweat etc. Clearance follows a decay curve and with most compounds the greater part is eliminated in 12–48 hours.

METABOLISM

Most compounds undergo chemical change in the body. Sometimes, this leads to the liberation of a more active compound, e.g. active trivalent arsenical compounds formed from inactive non-toxic pentavalent ones like tryparsamide, or the active metabolite formed from the inactive antimalarial compound, proguanil. More often the chemical changes lead to loss of activity from breaking up of the specific structure of the compound into less active fragments. Often the compound is combined with detoxifying radicles, e.g. acetyl derivatives, glucuronates, etc., which make a compound less active. The sulphonamides tend to be combined with the acetyl radical (p. 2.11) but as the resulting derivatives are often relatively insoluble, crystals of them may form in the kidney tubules and ureters and lead to blockage. Details of the steps by which some compounds are metabolized are given on pp. 20.17 to 33.

ADVERSE EFFECTS

Although all chemotherapeutic substances are poisons and have been selected for medicinal use because they poison the micro-organisms more than the patient, they may exert significant adverse effects on the patient. Thus streptomycin tends to poison the auditory nerve as well as the tubercle bacillus, so that it may produce deafness as well as cure; many compounds may produce nausea, vomiting, and headache. In addition to these effects, which are usually proportional to the dose, other severe reactions may be produced in a few specially susceptible patients by relatively small doses. These include haemolytic anaemia, depression of the bone marrow leading to aplastic anaemia or agranulocytosis, skin sensitization and exfoliative dermatitis, necrosis of the liver or thrombocytopenia with fatal haemorrhage into the brain.

These reactions arise in two ways. There may be a congenital absence or relative lack of some enzyme in the body, e.g. glucose-6-phosphate dehydrogenase, so that 8-aminoquinoline antimalarial compounds cause acute haemolysis. The mechanisms involved in this reaction are described on p. 31.10. More seriously, the patient may have become immunologically sensitized to the compound, or to a combination of compound plus protein (hapten) as a result of previous exposure. This occurs especially with penicillin so that a later injection of penicillin may cause immediate anaphylactic shock or death. The mechanisms involved here are discussed on p. 23.1. Alternatively the hypersensitivity reaction does not come

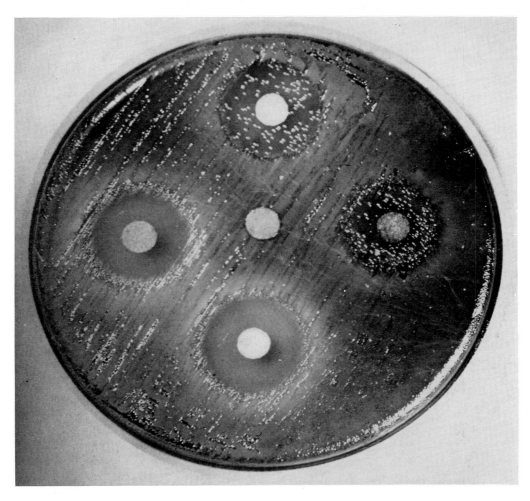

PLATE 20.1. Disc test showing different degrees of sensitivity to various antibiotics. Susceptibility of the test organism is indicated by clear zones around two antibiotic-impregnated discs. The organism is resistant to the antibiotic in the central disc. Resistant variants have produced colonies within the zones of general sensitivity in the other two instances.

on for some days after the first dose. Such reactions are particularly liable to happen after arsenicals but they also occur with sulphonamides and many other compounds (p. 23.10). Adverse effects of individual compounds are described in the section on therapeutically useful compounds (p. 20.17).

GENERAL SCOPE OF CHEMOTHERAPY

Chemotherapeutic agents are now available for most of the infections with the exception of those caused by viruses. The majority of bacterial infections can be cured, usually by antibiotics, but as already indicated spontaneous or acquired resistance to different individual antibiotics may occur. The sensitivity of the strain may be tested by methods in which the organism is exposed, usually on a solid culture medium, to which is added a standard amount of antibiotic. The latter is incorporated either in the medium or in a disc of blotting paper applied to its surface. Another method is to punch out a hole in the medium which is then filled with antibiotic solution. The antibiotic diffuses into the medium and inhibits growth of the organism over an area which under standard conditions depends on its **sensitivity**. Although these methods do not allow the minimum inhibitory concentration (MIC) of the antibiotic to be determined, they are rapid and sufficiently accurate for routine purposes to indicate whether an individual bacterial species or strain is sensitive, moderately sensitive or resistant to usual doses (plate 20.1). Chemotherapeutic substances, which kill or inhibit one or a limited number of microbial species, are described as **narrow spectrum** and those which affect a large number are said to possess a **broad spectrum**. Nystatin for example is active only against certain fungi and is a narrow spectrum compound, while tetracyclines and ampicillin are broad spectrum antibiotics. Accurate estimates of MIC can be obtained using serial dilutions of pure antibiotics to which are added standard inocula of organisms. Subsequent subcultures are made on appropriate solid media to determine whether the organism has been killed or inhibited. Assay of the concentration of antibiotic in blood or other body fluids can be performed using similar methods. In this way, it is possible to determine whether the dose of antibiotic is sufficient to meet the sensitivity characteristics of the particular organism under investigation.

Protozoal infections, e.g. malaria, sleeping sickness etc., can all be cured, with the exception of Chagas' disease due to *Trypanosoma cruzi* in South America; the acute attacks can be cut short with one of the 8-aminoquinolines but the infective organism cannot be eradicated.

Helminthic infections can mostly be cured. Those of the alimentary canal present little difficulty. Filariasis due to *Wuchereria bancrofti* and to *Loa loa* can be cured with diethylcarbamazine, but the treatment of onchocerciasis is still unsatisfactory. However, the chief problem among the worm infections is schistosomiasis (bilharziasis), which is a common and important trematode infection in many parts of the tropics where irrigation is practised and water snails become abundant. It was found in 1915 that it could be cured with difficulty by a long course of injections of sodium or potassium antimony tartrate or tartar emetic; in spite of an immense amount of research since 1945, tartar emetic treatment has not yet been definitely surpassed, at least for certain species (p. 20.18).

Rickettsial infections, e.g. typhus, respond well to chloramphenicol and to tetracyclines.

Virus diseases cannot yet be treated effectively in practice by means of chemotherapy although a few encouraging results have been obtained in limited fields, e.g. idoxuridine (p. 20.36) cures or ameliorates herpes simplex keratitis and methisazone (*N*-methylisatin-β-thiosemicarbazone) is prophylactic against smallpox (p. 20.36).

The conditions in virus infections are in general unfavourable to chemotherapeutic treatment, since when clinical symptoms first appear the virus has already firmly established itself inside the body cells and has begun to cause damage there. Many animal cells prepare interferon, which inhibits virus infection and this may be one of the body's defence mechanisms against such infections. Interferon appears to be a protein; it has not yet been possible to develop it sufficiently for general clinical use (p. 18.106).

Mycoplasmas, which include the organisms causing atypical pneumonia, respond to tetracyclines, streptomycin and some other antibiotics.

Systemic fungal infections, such as *Candida albicans*, are often made more virulent by the administration of tetracyclines and they sometimes form an unwelcome complication of tetracycline therapy. They respond to some extent to the polyene antibiotics, e.g. nystatin and amphotericin B, but their treatment is still unsatisfactory. Dermatophytic infections, e.g. ringworm due to *Trichophyton rubrum*, respond to the antibiotic griseofulvin, which is given by mouth. An account of the more important therapeutic compounds is given on p. 20.17. Their use in the treatment of individual diseases is discussed in vol. 3.

Cancer has been the subject of extensive chemotherapeutic research, and the subject is described in chap. 29.

THE BIOCHEMICAL BASIS OF ANTIBIOTIC ACTION

It has already been emphasized that all antibiotic substances depend for their effect on an ability to inhibit a biochemical process or disrupt a vital cell structure in an

17

invading organism without having a significant effect on the host. The best antibiotics approach this ideal behaviour closely, and many of the therapeutically useful compounds inhibit biochemical reactions, or disrupt the formation or function of cell structures, which do not occur in the host cells at all. For example, the penicillins and cephalosporins inhibit bacterial cell wall synthesis, and mammalian cells contain no equivalent structure. Similarly, polymyxin disrupts the structural integrity or biosynthesis of the bacterial cytoplasmic membrane, and this structure also seems to differ in significant respects from the membranes found in mammalian cells.

In many cases, however, an antibiotic relies for its action on having a greater effect on some biochemical reaction in the invader than in the host. Such differential effects can arise in a number of different ways; in some cases the relevant enzyme in the host has a lower affinity for the inhibitor and thus is less sensitive at low concentrations. Sometimes the enzyme is present in much larger amounts in the host and therefore less sensitive to complete inhibition; but in other cases the host enzyme is relatively inaccessible to the inhibitor because of the intervention of one or more permeability barriers. Another type of differential sensitivity, which is less commonly met with in the action of antibiotics than in the action of chemotherapeutic agents, is caused by the ability of the host, but not the invader, to satisfy its requirement for a given metabolite by using a collateral biosynthetic pathway. In this case, addition of the inhibitor blocks the target enzyme in both host and invader, but the essential product of the inhibited reaction is provided by the alternative route in the host cell alone.

Whatever the biochemical basis of these differential effects, and some are extremely subtle in operation, such a differential between host and invader is an inescapable necessity for successful antibiotic action. In this section, the action of some important antibiotics is examined to identify the biochemical processes which are inhibited and to describe the basis of the differential inhibitory action. The antibiotics have been chosen either because they are important clinically or because they have proved useful in biochemical investigations.

Antibiotics which interfere with bacterial cell wall synthesis

In order to appreciate the action of antibiotics that interfere with bacterial cell wall synthesis, it is important to consider the chemical structure of the wall and its biosynthetic origin.

BACTERIAL MUCOPEPTIDE STRUCTURE AND SYNTHESIS

The walls of most bacterial species are complex structures containing a number of types of macromolecule but in most cases, and particularly in Gram-positive organisms, the structural rigidity is imparted by the mucopeptide component. In Gram-negative organisms the mucopeptide is frequently intimately interlayered with protein and lipid components.

Although the exact details of the chemical structure of the mucopeptide complex varies from species to species, in all cases it seems to adhere to the basic chemical pattern shown in fig. 20.1. Species differences seem chiefly to involve the lysine position and the nature of the cross bridge from the lysine to the terminal D-alanine, for lysine can be replaced by other diamino acids, such as diaminopimelic acid, ornithine and α,γ-diaminobutyric acid, and the cross-linking bridge may contain additional amino acids, such as glycine or serine.

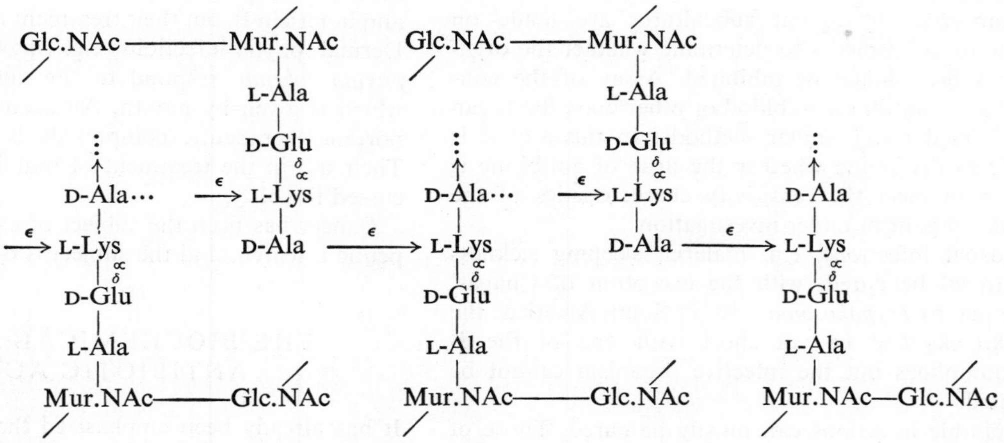

FIG. 20.1. General structure for the mucopeptide part of bacterial cell wall; peptide bond, —CO→NH—; Mur, muramic acid; Glc, glucosamine; NAc, *N*-acetyl—.

Mucopeptide is essentially an enormous sack-like molecule made up of a network of molecular chains. One type of chain is a mucopolysaccharide polymer of alternating units of *N*-acetyl glucosamine and *N*-acetyl muramic acid, whereas the other can be considered as a polypeptide chain containing certain linkages, such as ε-linked lysine and δ-linked glutamic acid, which are not found in proteins. Furthermore, certain of the amino acids, unlike protein amino acids, are in the D-configuration. The whole structure is held together by a system of cross links as shown diagrammatically in fig. 20.1.

The synthesis of this sack-like structure is an extremely complicated process which is incompletely understood, but at least thirty enzymes and perhaps a good many more, seem to be involved. The early steps that build a pentapeptide side-chain on the *N*-acetyl muramic acid are summarized as follows:

(1) Uridine diphosphate-*N*-acetyl-muramic acid
(UDPMurNAc)+L-Ala → UDPMurNAc.Ala

(2) UDPMurNAc.Ala+D-Glu → UDPMurNAc.Ala.Glu

(3) UDPMurNAc.Ala.Glu+L-Lys →
UDPMurNAc.Ala.Glu.Lys

(4) UDPMurNAc.Ala.Glu.Lys+D-Ala.D-Ala →
UDPMurNAc.Ala.Glu.Lys.Ala.Ala

Note that the two terminal D-alanines are inserted together as D-Ala.D-Ala. This dipeptide is synthesized from D-alanine by a separate enzyme, D-alanyl-D-alanine synthetase.

The next step in the synthesis of mucopeptide consists of the condensation of the uridine diphosphate-*N*-acetyl muramyl pentapeptide formed by reaction 4 with uridine diphosphate-*N*-acetyl glucosamine, thus:

(5) UDPMurNAc.Ala.Glu.Lys.Ala.Ala
+
Uridine diphosphate-*N*-acetylglucosamine (UDPGlcNAc)

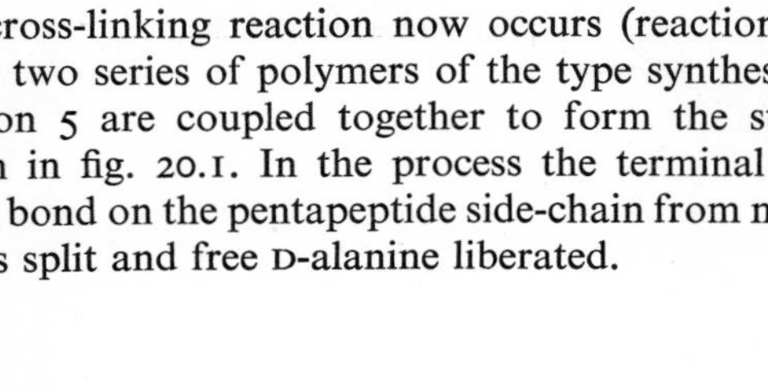

↓

—MurNAc—GlcNAc—MurNAc—GlcNAc—
| |
L-Ala L-Ala
| |
D-Glu D-Glu
|δ |δ
|α |α
L-Lys L-Lys
| |
D-Ala D-Ala
| |
D-Ala D-Ala

A cross-linking reaction now occurs (reaction 6a) in which two series of polymers of the type synthesized by reaction 5 are coupled together to form the structure shown in fig. 20.1. In the process the terminal D-Ala. D-Ala bond on the pentapeptide side-chain from muramic acid is split and free D-alanine liberated.

These reactions can be summarized:

(6a) GlcNAc.MurNAc.L-Ala.D-Glu.L-Lys.D-Ala.D-Ala
+
GlcNAc.MurNAc.L-Ala.D-Glu.L-Lys.D-Ala.D-Ala

↓

(6b) GlcNAc.MurNAc.L-Ala.D-Glu.L-Lys.D-Ala
| +D-Ala
GlcNAc.MurNAc.L-Ala.D-Glu.L-Lys.D-Ala.D-Ala

↓

GlcNAc.MurNAc.L-Ala.D-Glu.L-Lys.D-Ala
| +D-Ala
GlcNAc.MurNAc.L-Ala.D-Glu.L-Lys.D-Ala

The enzyme in reaction 6a is called glycopeptide transpeptidase and that in 6b is D-alanine carboxypeptidase.

ANTIBIOTICS WHICH INHIBIT MUCOPEPTIDE SYNTHESIS

D-cycloserine is a structural analogue of D-alanine and as such, is an effective inhibitor of the formation of the dipeptide D-alanyl-D-alanine from D-alanine. This dipeptide is essential for reaction 4 in the above sequence and

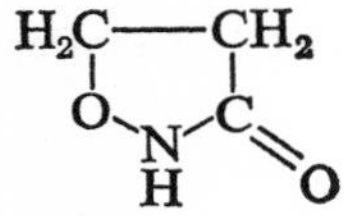

$$H_2C——CH_2$$

Cycloserine

without it mucopeptide synthesis ceases and the products of reaction 3 accumulate within the bacterial cells. In addition to this reaction, however, D-cycloserine (and probably the L-isomer as well) inhibits the interconversion of D- and L-alanine by the bacterial enzyme alanine racemase, and this action helps to augment the inhibitory effect of the antibiotic. In this case the differential effect of the antibiotic arises from the fact that mammalian cells contain no structure analogous to the bacterial cell wall, and that D-alanine does not seem to be required for mammalian cell metabolism. The clinical use of this antibiotic is described on p. 20.30.

The **penicillins** and **cephalosporins** (figs. 20.2 & 4b) are closely related groups of antibiotics produced by various species of moulds of the genera *Penicillium* and *Cephalosporium*. A number of naturally occurring antibiotics of this group are known, all of which differ in the nature of the substituents inserted into the penicillin and cephalosporin nucleus. The penicillins and the cephalosporins inhibit both reaction 6a and 6b in the above series,

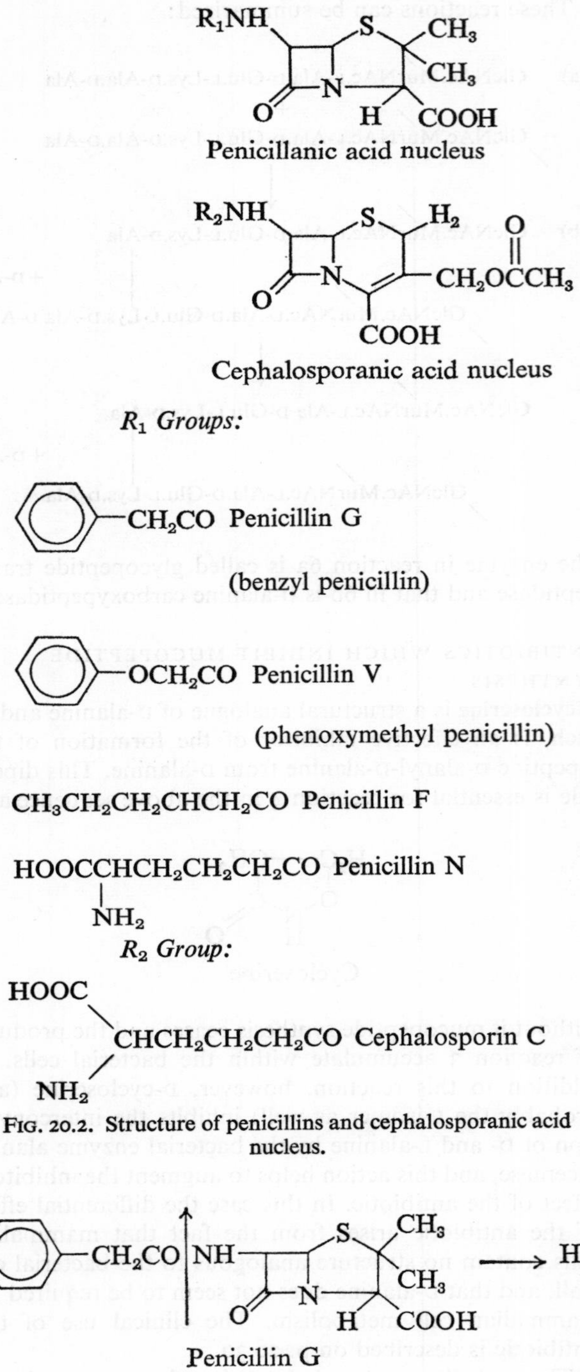

Penicillanic acid nucleus

Cephalosporanic acid nucleus

R_1 *Groups:*

CH₂CO   Penicillin G

(benzyl penicillin)

OCH₂CO   Penicillin V

(phenoxymethyl penicillin)

$CH_3CH_2CH_2CHCH_2CO$ Penicillin F

$HOOCCHCH_2CH_2CH_2CO$ Penicillin N
$\quad\quad\;\;|$
$\quad\quad NH_2$

R_2 *Group:*

$\begin{array}{c} HOOC \\ \qquad CHCH_2CH_2CH_2CO \\ \quad\; NH_2 \end{array}$ Cephalosporin C

FIG. 20.2.   Structure of penicillins and cephalosporanic acid nucleus.

and by this means block the cross linking reaction in mucopeptide synthesis. As with cycloserine, the penicillins and cephalosporins may cause the accumulation of mucopeptide precursors, although in this case it is the product of reaction 4 that accumulates to the greatest extent.

The bacterial cell normally relies on the rigid mucopeptide component of its cell wall to contain the high osmotic pressure of the cell contents, and any weakening of this wall leads to death of the cell by bursting. Since the penicillins and cephalosporins only inhibit mucopeptide synthesis, they have little effect on non-growing cells as these have an adequate amount of mucopeptide to give the wall sufficient rigidity. It is only when growth of the cell leads to an increase in cell contents that the reduced mucopeptide synthesis cannot contain the cell contents, and the organisms burst. The detailed biochemical action of the penicillins and cephalosporins therefore provides an explanation at the molecular level of the repeatedly observed phenomenon that penicillin is only active against growing bacteria.

Although all bacteria probably contain mucopeptide, it accounts for a much smaller part of the cell walls of Gram-negative bacteria than is the case with the Gram-positives. And this observation is possibly connected with the fact that, in general, Gram-negative bacteria are less sensitive to penicillin action than the Gram-positive. Furthermore, the more complex cell wall of the Gram-negative organisms probably hinders penicillin from reaching the site of mucopeptide synthesis.

At first the only penicillins available were the compounds which could be obtained from the mould *Penicillium chrysogenum* under fermentation conditions (fig. 20.2). Now, however, a method has been devised to use these natural penicillins as a source of a new range of compounds which can be made by chemical synthesis in the laboratory, the **new** or **semi-synthetic penicillins**. The synthetic route to these new penicillins is as follows: penicillin G is hydrolysed by an enzyme preparation to give 6-amino penicillanic acid (fig. 20.3a). This product

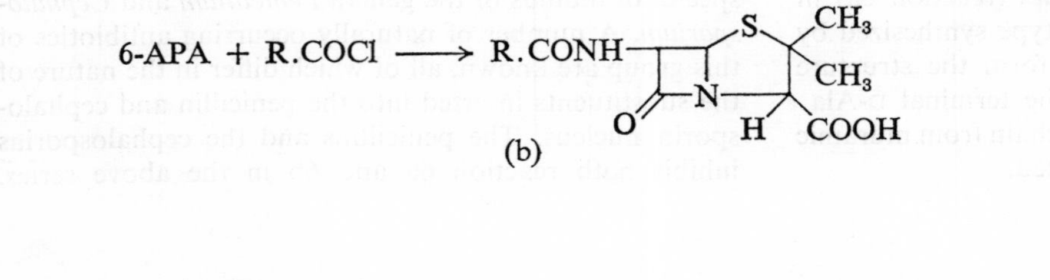

Penicillin G   →   6-Amino penicillanic acid (6-APA)

(a)

6-APA + R.COCl ⟶ R.CONH—

(b)

FIG. 20.3. Synthetic route to the new penicillins. (a) Splitting penicillin G to give 6-amino penicillanic acid (6-APA). (b) Coupling 6-APA to give a new penicillin with side chain R.

Methicillin

Oxacillin

Cloxacillin

Ampicillin

Carbenicillin

(a)

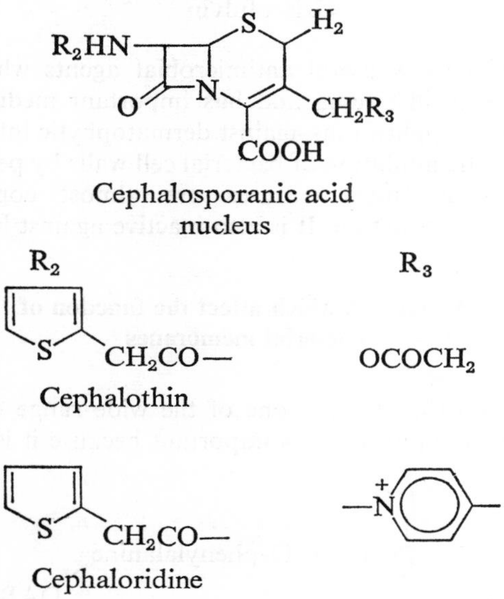

mucopeptide synthesis, by inhibiting reaction 5 in the mucopeptide biosynthetic sequence. As with the penicillins and cycloserine, the inhibition of mucopeptide synthesis by these compounds leads to the accumulation of the biosynthetic intermediates of mucopeptide synthesis, in this case mainly uridine diphosphate-N-acetyl-muramic acid pentapeptide. Uridine diphosphate-N-acetyl glucosamine does not accumulate, presumably because it can be used as a substrate in reactions not inhibited by these antibiotics.

Summary of antibiotics which inhibit bacterial cell wall synthesis
Of the antibacterial antibiotic substances whose action

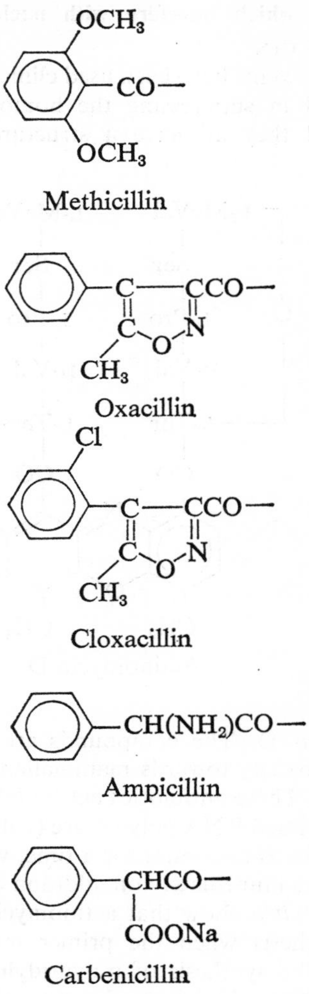

Cephalosporanic acid nucleus

Cephalothin

Cephaloridine

(b)

FIG. 20.4. (a) Side chains of the new penicillins. (b) Cephalosporanic nucleus and cephalosporins (p. 20.28).

can then be reacted chemically with a variety of acyl chlorides to give a new range of penicillins (fig. 20.3b).

These semi-synthetic penicillins have a range of novel properties which make them a major addition to the armoury of antibacterial agents. Although all of them act by inhibiting bacterial cell wall synthesis, one group, methicillin, oxacillin, and cloxacillin (fig. 20.4a), has the advantage that they are not destroyed significantly by staphylococcal pencillinase, an enzyme which renders many staphylococcal cultures resistant to penicillin action (p. 20.26). Another of the new penicillins, ampicillin (fig. 20.4), is able to reach the site of mucopeptide synthesis in Gram-negative bacteria and is consequently a more potent inhibitor of these organisms than old penicillins such as benzyl or phenoxymethyl penicillin.

The structure of neither **ristocetin** nor **vancomycin** is yet completely worked out. They both inhibit bacterial

has been elucidated so far, penicillin, cephalosporins, cycloserine, vancomycin and ristocetin act by inhibiting mucopeptide synthesis. Bacitracin may also act this way, but in this case the precise mode of action is unknown. The fact that bacterial mucopeptide synthesis is so often the target for antibacterial compounds presumably reflects the main requirement for a successful antibiotic which was mentioned above, namely that the compound must inhibit a bacterial enzyme system without affecting the organism that produces the antibiotic. Since mucopeptide synthesis is a biosynthetic process confined to bacteria it is an eminently suitable target for antibacterial agents.

GRISEOFULVIN
The cell walls of fungi do not contain mucopeptide but often rely on chitin or a chitin-like polymer for their

rigidity. Chitin is more widely distributed in nature than mucopeptide and is frequently found in the shells of crustacea. The biosynthesis of the polymer in fungi can be inhibited by certain antibiotics, such as griseofulvin, which is produced by mycelia of *P. griseofulvum*. It is

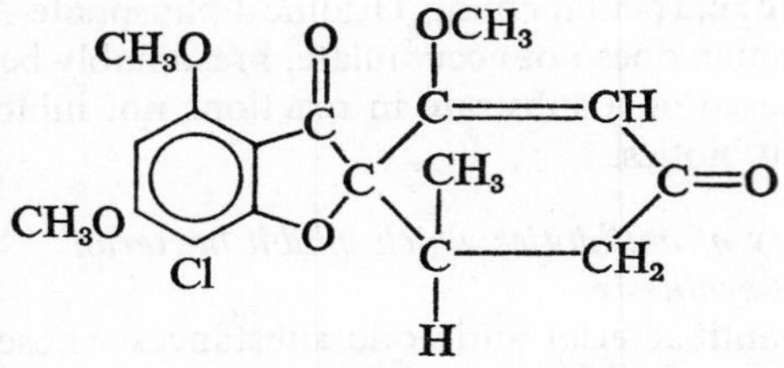

Griseofulvin

one of the few useful antimicrobial agents which are effective against fungi and has important medical and veterinary applications against dermatophytic infections. As with the inhibition of bacterial cell walls by penicillin, nongrowing fungal cultures are almost completely resistant to its action. It is also inactive against bacteria.

Antibiotics which affect the function of bacterial membranes

POLYMYXIN

Polymyxin (fig. 20.5) is one of the wide range of polypeptide antibiotics and is important because it is one of

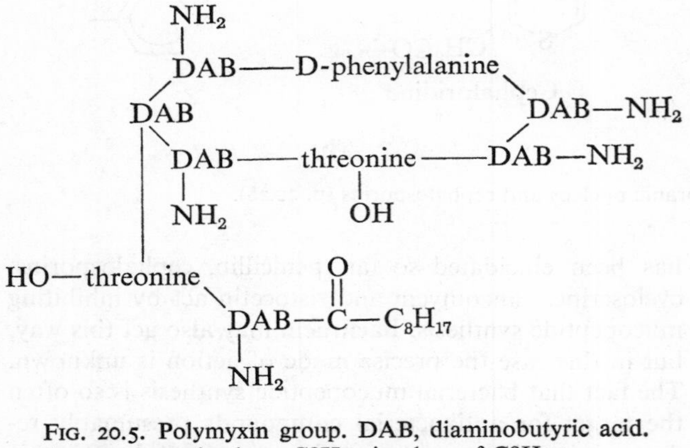

FIG. 20.5. Polymyxin group. DAB, diaminobutyric acid. Some polymyxins have C_8H_{15} in place of C_8H_{17}.

the few antibiotic substances which are active against bacteria of the genus *Pseudomonas*, which is an increasing cause of postoperative infections of wounds.

Polymyxin is bound specifically to the bacterial cytoplasmic membrane where it damages the permeability properties of the structure. Thus bacteria treated with polymyxin rapidly liberate all the small molecular weight components normally concentrated within the membrane into the culture medium.

Antibiotics which interfere with nucleic acid synthesis

ACTINOMYCIN

The actinomycins have been used clinically as antitumour agents and in suppressing the homograft reaction (p. 29.12) and they all have a structure very similar to

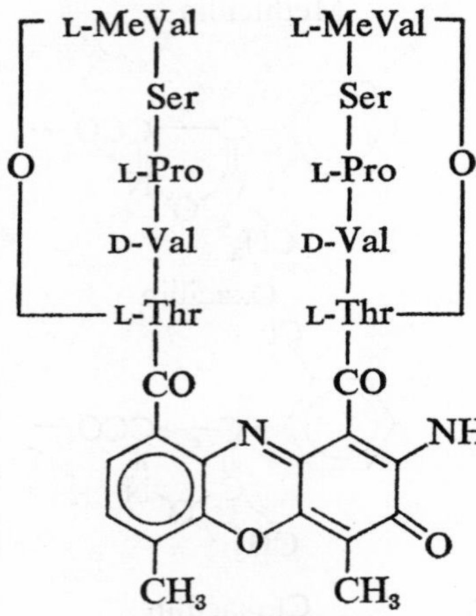

Actinomycin D

actinomycin D. The compounds are also bacteristatic but their toxicity towards mammalian cells makes them dangerous. These antibiotics act by inhibiting the action of DNA primed RNA polymerase (vol. 1, p. 12.9) so that DNA synthesis continues for a time, whereas RNA synthesis ceases immediately on addition of the antibiotic.

Tests *in vitro* show that actinomycin D only inhibits RNA synthesis when the primer molecule is rich in guanine. The synthesis of polyuridylic acid on a polydeoxyadenylic acid primer, for example, is insensitive to actinomycin D, whereas the synthesis of polycytidylic acid on polydeoxyguanylic acid is completely inhibited. As mammalian DNA contains about 20 per cent of guanine spread randomly through the strands, the synthesis of RNA by the action of DNA primed RNA polymerase is rather sensitive to actinomycin inhibition.

A number of molecular models have been suggested to explain the action of actinomycin. The most plausible suggests that the actinomycin molecule is drawn into the minor groove of the DNA by formation of specific intermolecular hydrogen bonds to the guanines of the DNA polydeoxyribonucleic acid chains and that this complex is inactive thereafter as a primer for the RNA polymerase enzyme.

MITOMYCIN C AND NALIDIXIC ACID

Mitomycin is an antibiotic that is rarely used in medicine because of its extreme toxicity. It acts by inhibiting the DNA-primed DNA polymerase, thus causing inhibition of DNA synthesis.

Nalidixic acid also acts by inhibiting DNA polymerase and has a spectrum of activity very similar to that of mitomycin C.

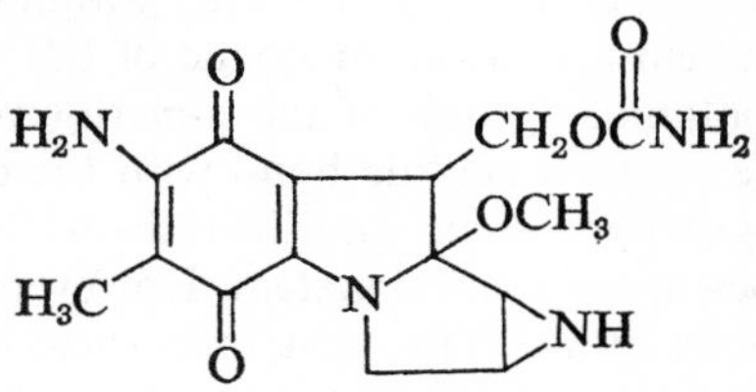

Mitomycin C

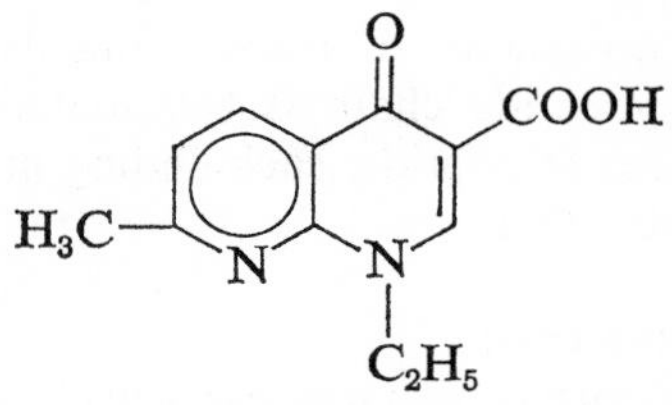

Nalidixic acid

Antibiotics which interfere with protein synthesis

STREPTOMYCIN

Streptomycin is used widely in clinical medicine and has been invaluable in the treatment of tuberculosis. The antibiotic has many effects on bacterial cells but probably the most significant is the inhibition of protein synthesis. The antibiotic is bound to ribosomes, particularly that part of the ribosomal structure that adsorbs the transfer-RNAs. One theory suggests that any messenger RNA

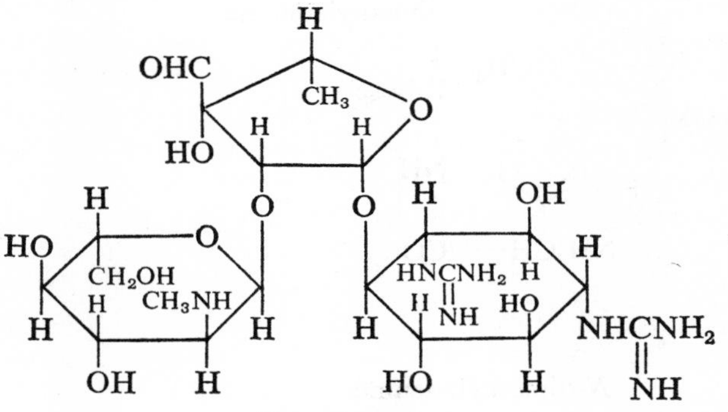

Streptomycin

molecules which reach ribosomes with streptomycin bound on them are 'misread' in the course of protein synthesis (vol. 1, p. 12.4). Thus the cause of bacterial death is the widespread synthesis of proteins which are so different from the correct versions, because of misreading, that they cannot adequately carry on the metabolism of the cell. Some support for this hypothesis comes from the fact that streptomycin dependent bacteria can be isolated. These bacteria need streptomycin for growth and this

bizarre finding can be explained if the streptomycin dependent cells carry a mutation which itself leads to a degree of misreading of messenger RNA. In these mutants the essential role of streptomycin could be to correct by 're-misreading' the errors introduced by the mutation. Although this hypothesis of phenotypic modification by streptomycin is superficially attractive, it is doubtful whether it explains all the facets of streptomycin action.

KANAMYCIN AND NEOMYCIN

Two other antibiotics, kanamycin and neomycin, have a structure broadly similar to streptomycin and one of them, kanamycin, has been shown to cause misreading of the messenger in a manner analogous to streptomycin. The

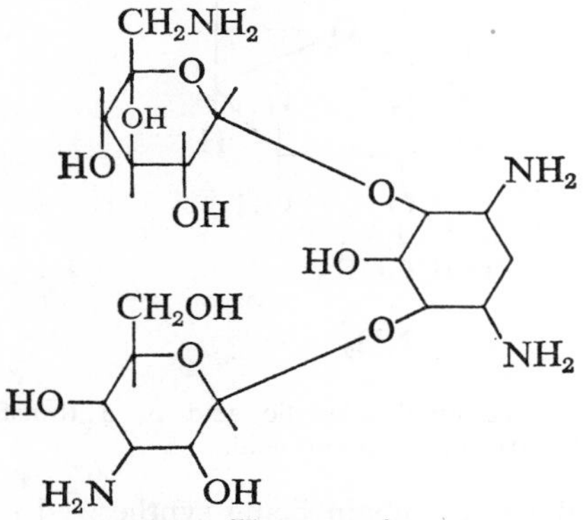

Kanamycin

therapeutic value of kanamycin centres around the experimental finding that streptomycin resistant strains are frequently kanamycin sensitive. This presumably reflects a slightly different binding site on the ribosome for the two antibiotics.

PUROMYCIN

Puromycin is not used widely for clinical purposes, but it is the one antibiotic whose mode of action is known precisely and it has been used extensively in biochemical studies on the mechanism of protein synthesis. The antibiotic acts as a structural analogue of the terminal adenine

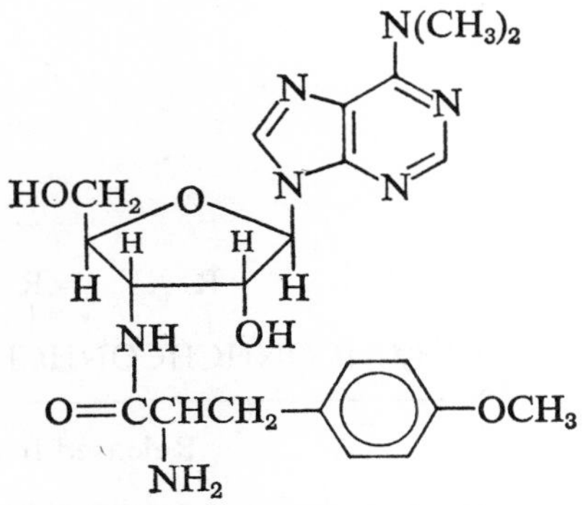

Puromycin

residue of a transfer RNA molecule when that molecule is loaded with an amino acid (fig. 20.6). The inhibitor acts to cause premature termination of the polypeptide chain during its biosynthesis and its liberation from the ribosome. In the course of this process, the carboxyl end of the polypeptide chain is substituted with a puromycin molecule. The exact sequence of reactions is shown in fig. 20.7 and should be compared with the action of t-RNA shown in vol. 1, p. 12.9.

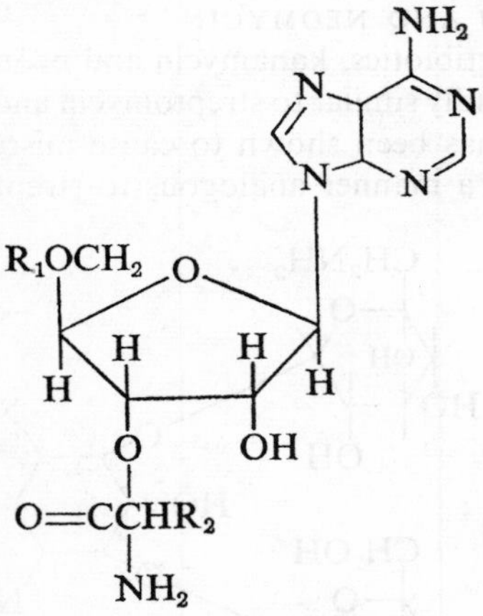

FIG. 20.6. Terminal adenylic acid of a transfer-RNA molecule carrying an amino acid.

In a polypeptide chain being synthesized on the surface of a ribosome (vol. 1, chap. 12) the carboxyl end of the chain is bound to t-RNA$_1$. The next step in the synthesis is the approach of t-RNA$_2$ already carrying its

appropriate amino acid. Normally the amino group of the amino acid on t-RNA$_2$ forms a peptide bond with the carboxyl group at the end of the growing chain, thus displacing t-RNA$_1$ which is liberated without its amino acid. Puromycin acts as an analogue of t-RNA$_2$ in this scheme. The amino group of the *p*-methoxy-phenylalanine residue forms a peptide bond with the carboxyl of the growing peptide chain and liberates t-RNA$_1$ just as t-RNA$_2$ does in the normal system. However, unlike the normal process in which the next amino acid is added via t-RNA$_3$ (fig. 20.7 and vol. 1, p. 12.9), the substitution of the growing chain with a puromycin residue detaches the nascent polypeptide chain from the ribosome so that t-RNA$_3$ has no chance of transferring its amino acid. Thus the polypeptide chain is terminated prematurely and short pieces of peptide, each ending in a puromycin residue, are liberated.

CHLORAMPHENICOL

Chloramphenicol has been used extensively against Gramnegative infections such as typhoid. It seems likely that this antibiotic interferes in some way with the binding of messenger RNA to the ribosomes, since RNA accumulates in chloramphenicol treated cells and a large proportion of this RNA has messenger-like properties. Whatever the precise mode of action, however, the net effect of chloramphenicol action is to inhibit polypeptide synthesis by blocking the formation of new peptide bonds.

The antibiotic relies for its effectiveness on the fact that, in the intact organisms at least, only bacterial protein synthesis is sensitive to the antibiotic. Why protein

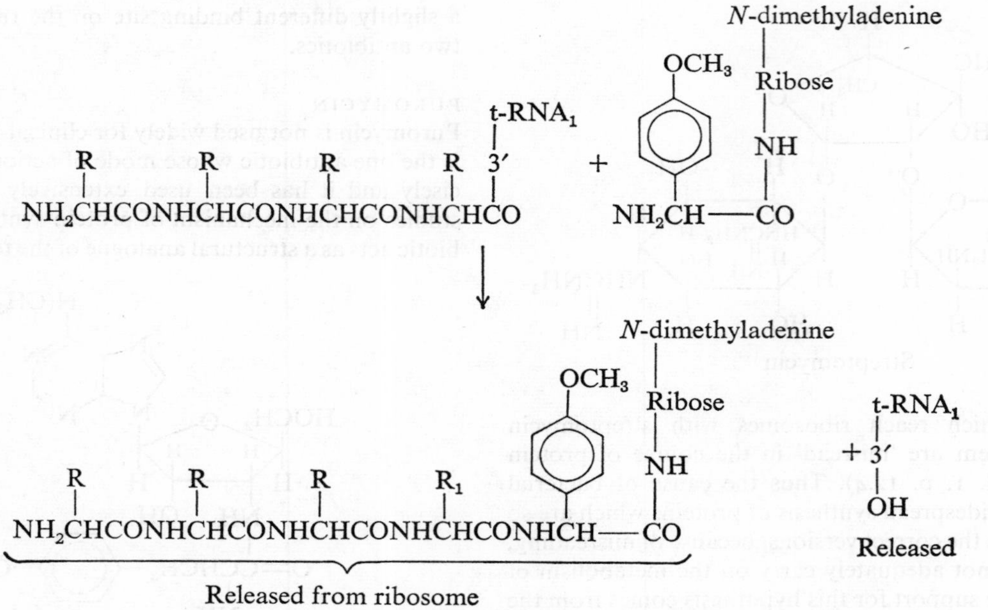

FIG. 20.7. Action of puromycin to terminate the synthesis of a peptide chain prematurely (compare with step 1, vol. 1, p. 12.9).

synthesis in mammals is insensitive to chloramphenicol is not known; possibly mammalian ribosomes are different

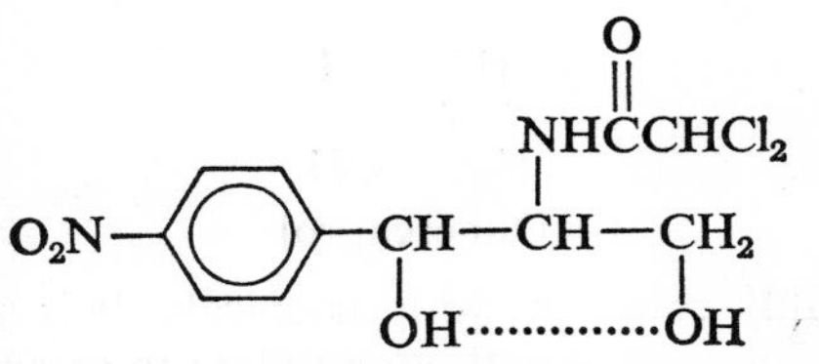

Chloramphenicol

from their bacterial counterparts or chloramphenicol cannot reach its target in mammalian cells because of a permeability barrier not present in bacteria.

TETRACYCLINES

Three tetracyclines, **tetracycline** itself, **chlortetracycline** and **oxytetracycline** are used commonly in medicine and probably all act in the same way. As with streptomycin, the antibiotics have many effects on bacterial cells but their action in interfering with protein synthesis is probably crucial. The precise step in the process which is inhibited is not known but the activation of amino acids and the transfer of the activated residue to the t-RNA are

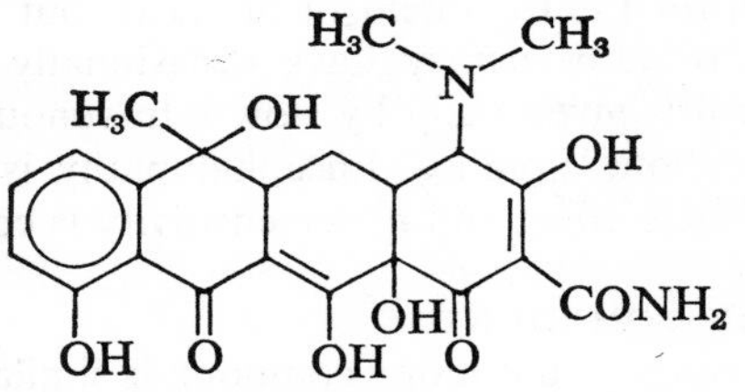

Tetracycline

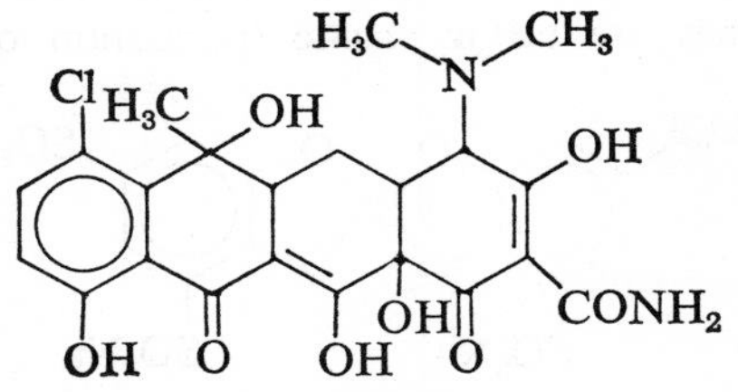

Chlortetracycline

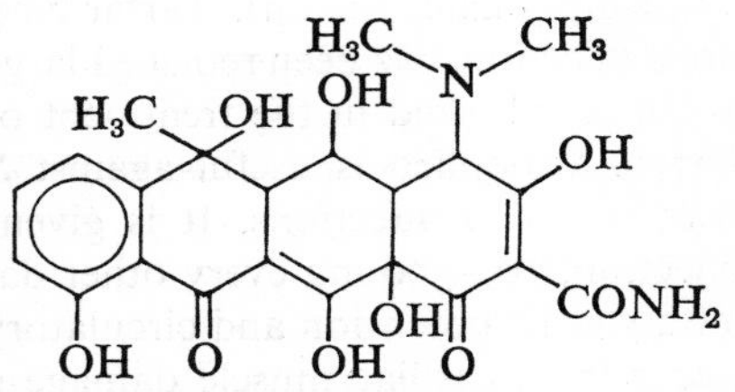

Oxytetracycline

certainly normal. The antibiotic seems to block either the attachment of the t-RNA-amino acid complex to the ribosome or the transfer of the activated amino acid to the growing peptide chain. The accumulation of RNA which occurs during tetracycline treatment argues, however, that neither messenger RNA synthesis nor ribosomal RNA synthesis is inhibited by these antibiotics.

THE MACROLIDE ANTIBIOTICS: ERYTHROMYCIN, SPIRAMYCIN AND OLEANDOMYCIN

This group of antibiotics, of which erythromycin is the most commonly used, are effective antibacterial com-

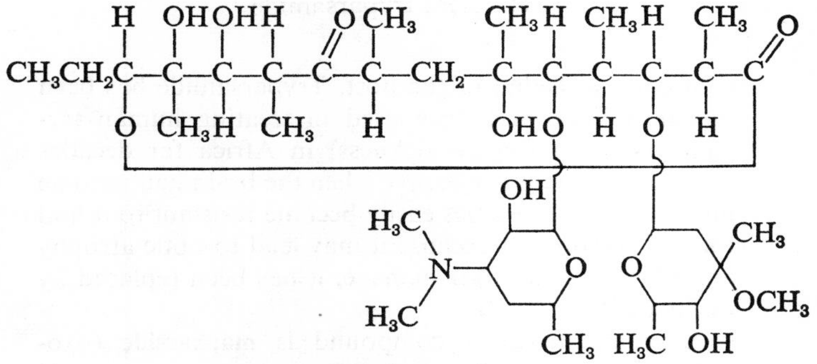

Erythromycin

pounds. They act by inhibiting bacterial protein synthesis but their exact mode of action is unknown.

MAIN THERAPEUTIC COMPOUNDS

During the last 60 years great numbers of therapeutic compounds have been introduced; the present list illustrates the main types which have been found valuable clinically. The compounds are grouped according to the nature of the organism against which they are used. The details of their use in clinical medicine are given in vol. 3. For historical reasons one may begin with trypanosomes and arsenical compounds.

Compounds active against trypanosomes, leishmaniae and spirochaetes

The earliest and most important compounds were the phenyl arsenicals. These consisted of a benzene ring joined to a suitable side chain on the one hand and, on the other, to an arsenic atom which might be quinquevalent or trivalent, thereby greatly altering the biological action.

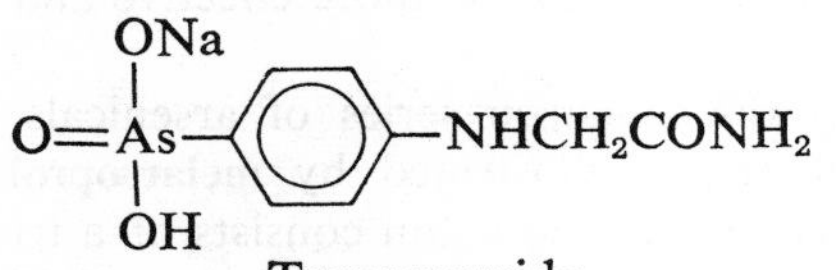

Tryparsamide

A typical quinquevalent compound is **tryparsamide**. This drug is of low toxicity. It diffuses throughout the body and and readily penetrates the CSF and nervous system. It is inactive until reduced in the body to the trivalent form which actively kills trypanosomes and spirochaetes but which is also fairly toxic. It is likely that arsenical compounds combine with SH dependent enzymes, e.g. hexokinase. The selective action of arsenicals may then be due to the relatively high rate of metabolism

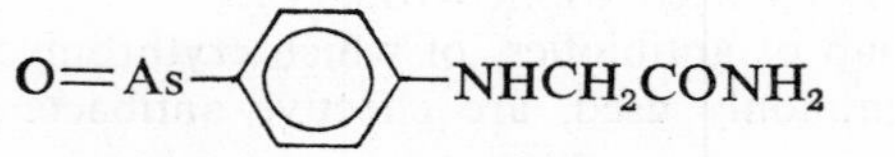

Trivalent tryparsamide

compared with that of the host. Tryparsamide has been the most important drug used in treating human trypanosomiasis (sleeping sickness) in Africa for decades and was particularly effective when the brain had become infected. Trypanosomes easily become resistant to it and for this reason and because it may lead to optic atrophy and blindness and liver damage, it has been replaced by melarsopol.

A typical trivalent compound is **mapharside** (oxophenarsine) which is active against trypanosomes and

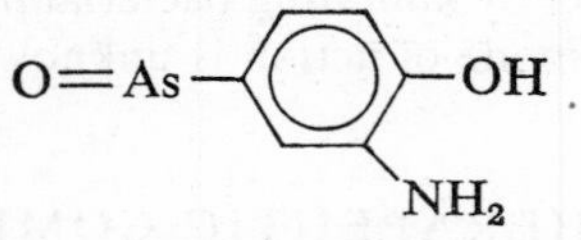

Mapharside

spirochaetes but is also toxic. It was used to treat syphilis until supplanted by penicillin.

The arsenobenzol series is also represented by **neoarsphenamine** (neosalvarsan). In this, the arsenic atom is still further reduced. This compound is highly effective

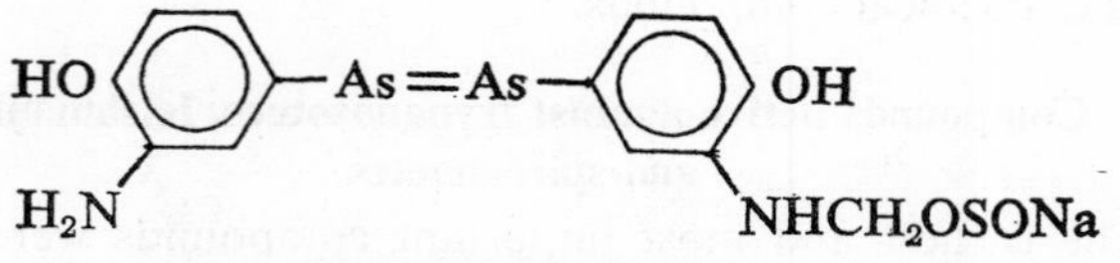

Neoarsphenamine

against syphilis and is less toxic than mapharside. It was the main treatment for syphilis for 30 years until it was also superseded by the more effective and less toxic penicillin.

Recently the melarsen series of arsenicals has been introduced and is illustrated by **melarsoprol** (Mel B, arsobal). Here the side chain consists of a triazine ring which acts as an antimetabolite to folic acid. The arsenic

acid is trivalent, but it is partly blocked by a molecule of **dimercaprol**.

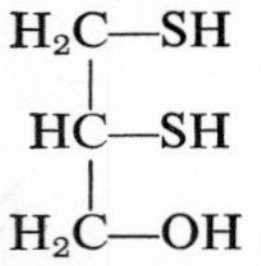

Dimercaprol

which readily combines with arsenicals. It is surprising that this combination with an antidote to arsenic should result in an active drug. Although toxicity is reduced, the

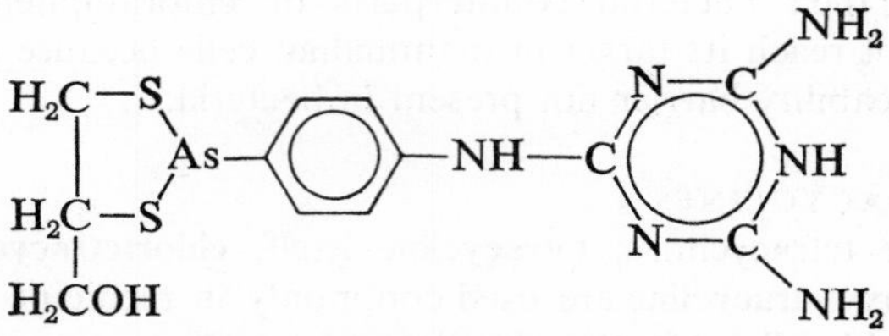

Melarsoprol

compound remains highly active against trypanosomes including those resistant to tryparsamide and is able to penetrate into the CSF and cure infections of the nervous system. A water-soluble modification, **melarsonyl potassium** (Mel W), which can be given intramuscularly, is under trial for the treatment of filariasis, but fatal reactions due to idiosyncrasy have occasionally occurred. Melarsoprol is given daily by slow intravenous infusion in a dose about 3 mg/kg. Encephalopathy is the most serious adverse effect and hypersensitivity is common.

ANTIMONY COMPOUNDS

There is a range of antimony compounds similar to those of arsenic. Both quinquevalent and trivalent forms occur. They are used chiefly for the treatment of leishmaniasis, e.g. kala azar, and for schistosomiasis. The most important ones are **tartar emetic** (potassium or sodium

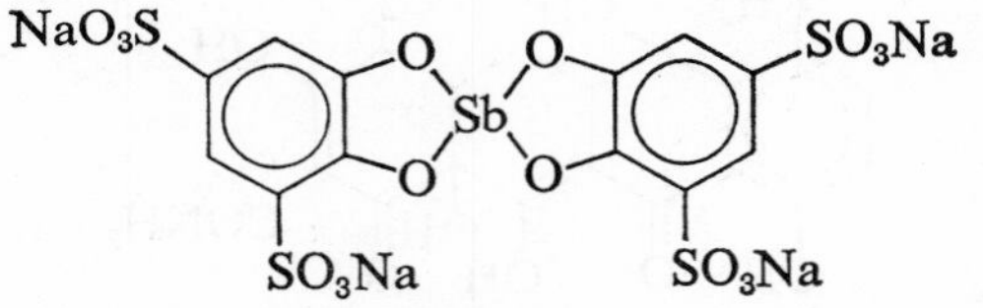

Stibophen

antimonyl tartrate), and **stibophen** (sodium antimony bis-catechol-3:5-disulphonate, fuadin). Tartar emetic, given by intravenous injection, has been replaced largely by less toxic drugs but is still used in the treatment of *Schistosoma japonicum*. Stibophen is useful against *S. haematobium* and *S. mansonii* infections. It is given by intramuscular injection, 100–300 mg every other day up to a total dose of 2.5 g. Hypotension and circulatory collapse may also occur from cardiac muscle damage and overdosage may be treated with dimercaprol.

OTHER TRYPANOCIDAL COMPOUNDS

These include the aromatic diamidine compounds, particularly **pentamidine** and **stilbamidine**, which have been

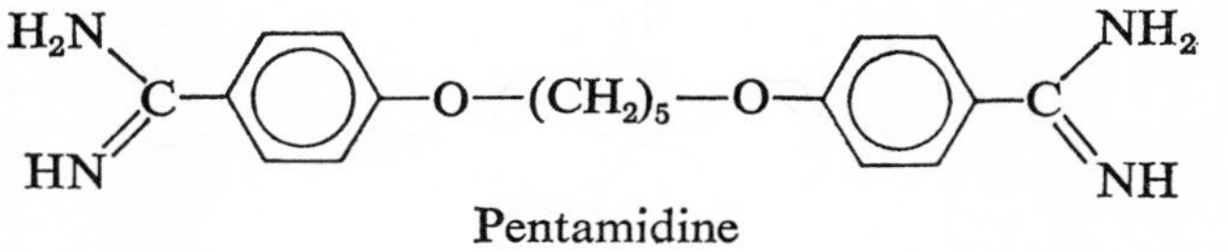

Pentamidine

used widely for the prophylaxis of sleeping sickness in Africa; one intramuscular injection protects against infection for six months. Discovery of the chemotherapeutic activity of this group of drugs was accidental. Trypanosomes have long been known to die on culture in the absence of glucose. One of the diguanides (p. 6.00) was tested for trypanocidal activity and it was found to be active even *in vivo*. This led ultimately to the synthesis of the diamidines which are particularly effective against organisms with a high aerobic glycolysis. Given by intramuscular or intravenous injection in doses of 300 mg/day for 10 days, the drug induces occasional hypersensitivity reactions and a drop in blood pressure. Occasionally numbness and paraesthesia over the distribution of the trigeminal nerve occur.

Suramin (antrypol, germanin, Bayer 205) has a complex structure of benzene rings, joined by urea bridges and has been valuable against sleeping sickness and also against onchocerciasis. The mechanism of the trypanocidal action is unknown. Very firm binding occurs with proteins and this may be partly responsible for its effect. Given intravenously by a single injection (1–2 g) the compound is detectable in the blood for up to 3 months and is used in this way prophylactically. Access to cell fluid and CSF is limited. A variety of adverse effects include proteinuria, nausea, vomiting, conjunctivitis and dermatitis, and fall in blood pressure.

Antimalarial compounds

The oldest of these is **quinine**, obtained from the bark of the South American cinchona tree and discovered several centuries ago. Quinine itself has been almost entirely

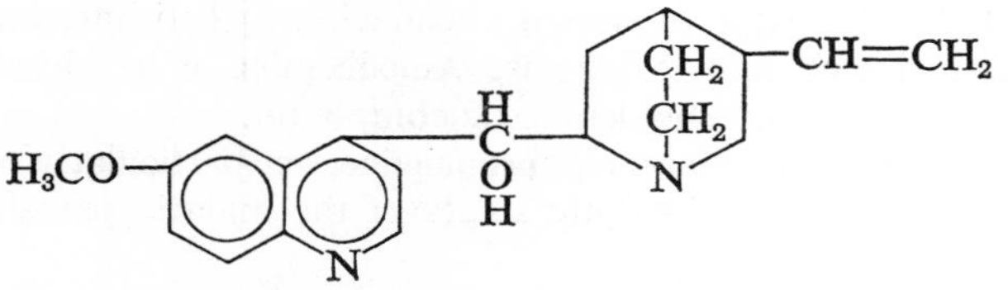

Quinoline group   Quinuclidine group
Quinine

replaced by more active and less toxic compounds derived from its quinoline group although it is still recommended by some for the treatment of cerebral malaria.

4-Aminoquinolines, e.g. **chloroquine**, are the most

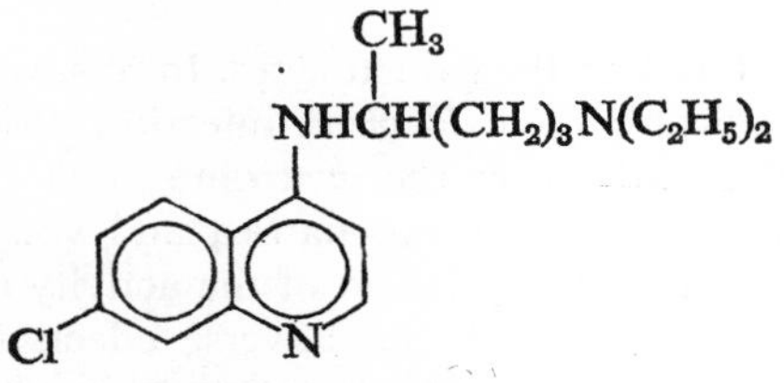

Chloroquine

widely used compounds for the treatment, prevention and suppression of malaria. Chloroquine kills all stages of the malaria parasite in the red blood corpuscles. It is therefore an effective suppressive drug of all types of malarial parasites. Because it has little effect on the exoerythrocyte stage of *P. vivax* infection, relapses may occur. Strains of *P. falciparum* resistant to chloroquine have become a serious problem in some parts of the world.

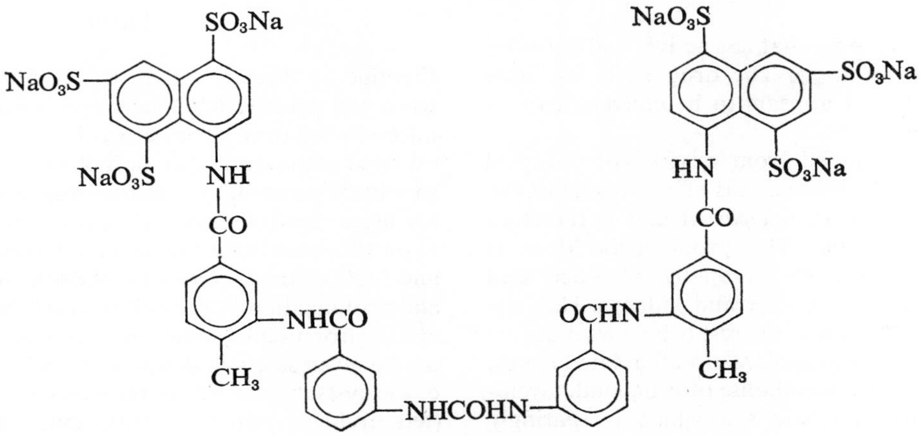

Suramin

It is rapidly absorbed from the gastrointestinal tract and is concentrated in the liver. This fact suggested its usefulness against amoebic infections of the liver (p. 20.21). For control of an acute attack of malaria 0·5–1 g chloroquine is given for 3 days. Toxicity is low but includes blurring of vision, headaches, gastrointestinal disturbance and psychosis. **Amodiaquine** is a closely related and possibly less toxic compound.

8-Aminoquinolines, e.g. **primaquine**, act particularly on the early exoerythrocytic stages of the malaria parasite

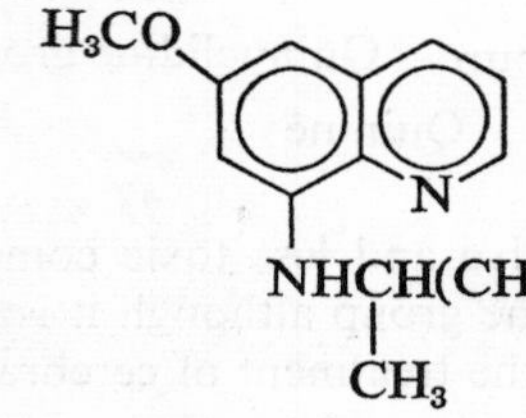

Primaquine

in the liver and on the gametocytes. In this way they produce a radical cure of *P. vivax* infection. Primaquine is absorbed rapidly from the gastrointestinal tract and is rapidly excreted. Anorexia, nausea and vomiting occasionally occur but depression of the activity of the bone marrow is the most serious adverse effect. Haemolytic anaemia occurs in individuals and races in whom there is a deficiency of glucose-6-PO_4 dehydrogenase (p. 31.10). The usual dose is 15 mg/day for 14 days.

Proguanil (paludrine) acts on the malaria parasite both in the blood and in the liver, probably by interfering with the reduction of folic acid. Although less toxic

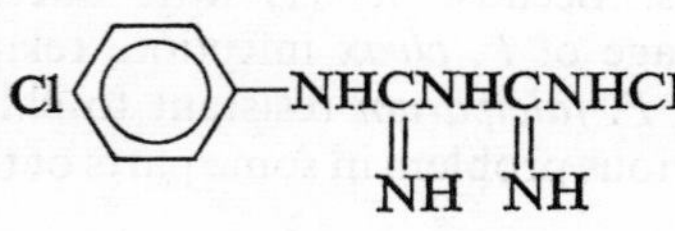

Proguanil

than chloroquine it is somewhat less active, and parasites may become resistant to it. The drug itself has little antimalarial activity but appears to be converted to an active derivative by the host.

Proguanil was developed from a series of chemical modifications to sulphadiazine. It is effective against the pre-erythrocyte stage of *P. falciparum* and is therefore useful as a prophylactic. The prophylactic dose is 100 mg/day by mouth. It is rapidly absorbed and distributed especially to the liver and kidneys. Half the drug is excreted in the urine, the rest being metabolized. **Chlorproguanil** and **cycloguanil** are closely related drugs, the latter being an active metabolite of proguanil. Cycloguanil given as an embonate salt which is sparingly soluble is being assessed as a long term prophylactic

against malaria.

Pyrimethamine (daraprim) is a remarkably active substance which, like proguanil, is effective by interfering

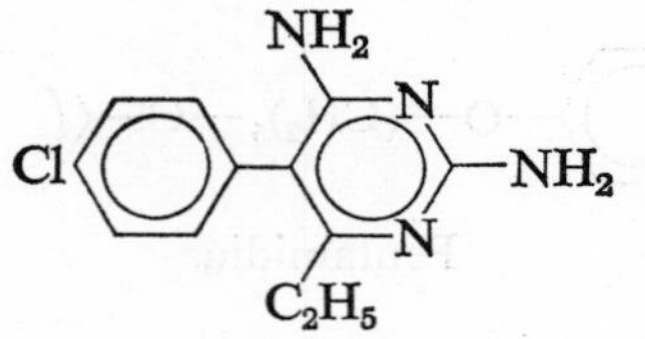

Pyrimethamine

with the formation of N^5-formyl tetrahydrofolic acid (folinic acid) from folic acid. It can be used both for treatment and for prophylaxis, but parasites may also become resistant to it. Pyrimethamine is given by mouth in doses of 25–50 mg once weekly. Larger doses cause megaloblastic anaemia and convulsions.

In recent years interest has grown in the use of sulphonamides in the treatment of malaria. They appear to potentiate the effect of pyrimethamine probably also by interfering with the synthesis of folic acid.

Compounds active against Entamoeba histolytica
The chief compound is **emetine** which was isolated from the root of *Cephaelis ipecacuanha* by Pelletier, the French chemist who discovered quinine, and which has a complicated structure.

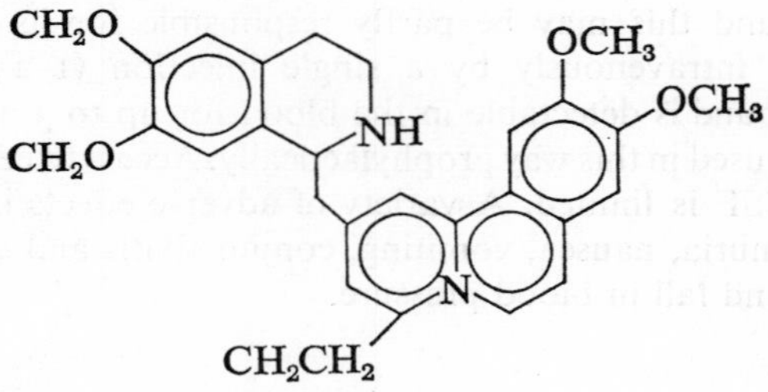

Emetine

Emetine is directly lethal to *E. histolytica* especially when the parasite is in the trophozoite stage. Given by injection the drug accumulates in the liver and is slowly excreted in the urine. No more than 1 mg/kg body weight should be given daily and the drug should not be given for more than 10 days. The most important toxic effect is on the heart with fall in blood pressure, tachycardia and ECG changes consisting of depression of the T-wave and prolongation of the P-R interval. Nausea is common and neuromuscular symptoms also occur. Emetine cannot be given safely in doses which will ensure eradication of the cysts in man. Other remedies, including antibiotics (tetracyclines, paromomycin), quinolines, phenanthrolines, etc. are less toxic and unpleasant to take, but are less reliable than emetine in destroying the amoeba. **Dehydro-emetine** appears to be as active as emetine and is also less toxic.

ARSENICAL DRUGS
Carbasone is an organic arsenical compound originally synthesized by Ehrlich and has been used for many years.

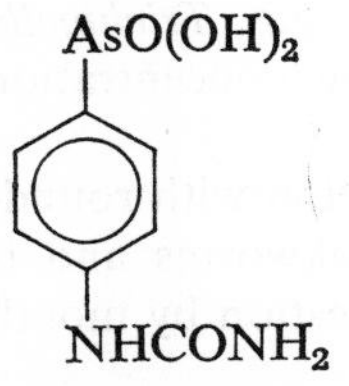

AsO(OH)$_2$

NHCONH$_2$
Carbasone

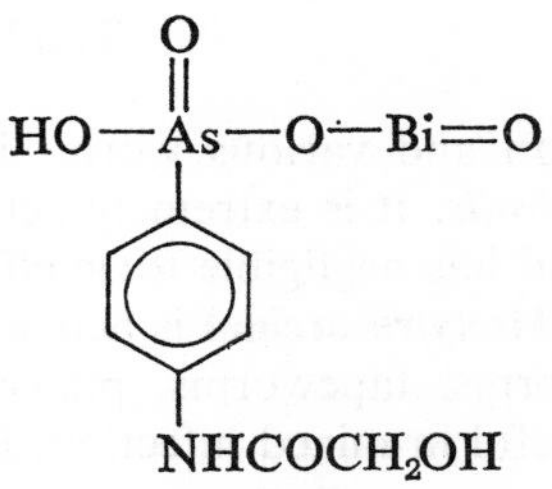

$$HO-\overset{\overset{O}{\|}}{As}-O-Bi=O$$

NHCOCH$_2$OH
Bismuth glycolylarsanilate

It is directly amoebicidal, destroys the trophozoites and, like emetine, is not active on the cysts. It is not effective in the treatment of liver infection. When given by mouth in adults for 10 days, the drug accumulates and is comparatively nontoxic; overdosage results in arsenic poisoning with blindness, skin rashes, encephalopathy and liver necrosis may result. Carbasone is best given in conjunction with other drugs in doses of 0·25–0·5 g daily.

Glycobarsol (bismuth glycolylarsanilate) is a similar compound which contains both arsenic and bismuth. Although not well absorbed from the gut, it is useful in intestinal infections.

Quinolines, e.g. **chloroquine** described on p. 20.19 is of value in the treatment of amoebic hepatitis because it is absorbed from the gut and is concentrated in the liver. A variety of iodinated quinolines which are given by mouth are also useful for intestinal forms of the disease. These include **diodoquin**, **chiniofon** and **vioform**. They are relatively nontoxic.

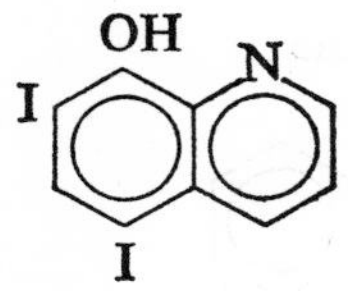

Diodoquin

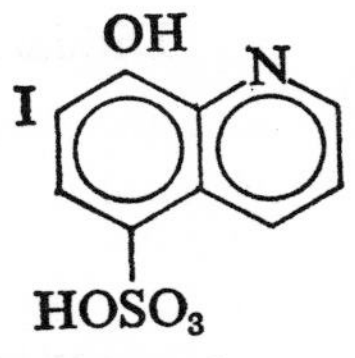

Chiniofon

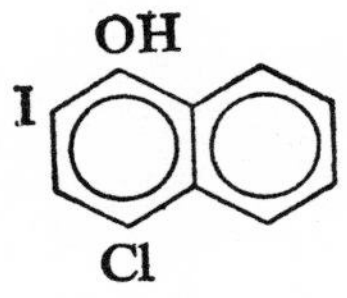

Vioform

Recently it has been found that amoebic infections respond well to **metronidazole** (see below) given by mouth as 2–4 g daily for 10 days, which is a much bigger dose than those used against *Trichomonas*. This treatment is effective and nontoxic, and metronidazole is now the best compound for amoebiasis.

Compounds active against Trichomonas vaginalis
The chief compound now in use is **metronidazole** (flagyl), which is very effective in the treatment of vaginitis or of

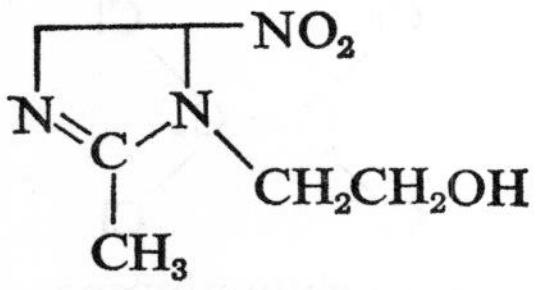

Metronidazole

male infections with *Trichomonas*. It is given by mouth in doses of 750 mg/day for 10 days. Toxic effects are uncommon but it may produce leucopenia.

Compounds active against worms (anthelminthics)
These are of great importance as helminthiasis is worldwide. Many traditional herbal remedies, such as santonin and extract of *Filix mas* are effective against worms in the alimentary canal, but have been abandoned because of toxicity and the discovery of more effective remedies. The following is a list of the more important drugs now in use.

Mepacrine (atebrin, quinacrine) is a powerful antimalarial drug which was synthesized in Britain just in

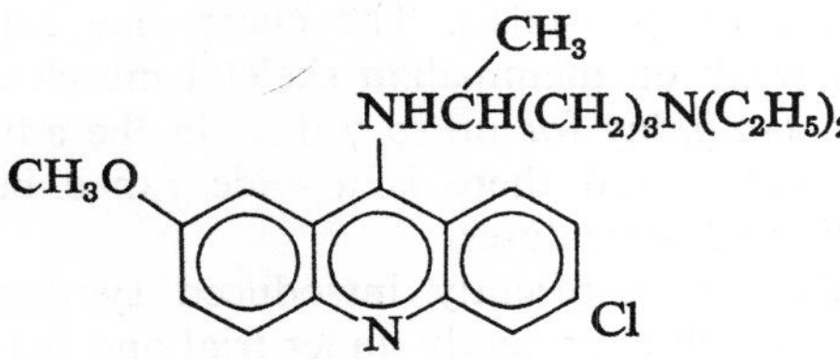

Mepacrine

time to replace the supply of quinine lost when the Japanese captured Indonesia in World War II. Without mepacrine it is doubtful if India could have been defended successfully. However, it is now discarded in favour of chloroquine, but has found a new use as a remover of tapeworms. Adverse reactions are rare, but include nausea, vomiting and dizziness. Yellow colouration of the skin is common, but harmless.

Dichlorophen is also useful against large tapeworms in man and animals. A single oral dose of 6–9 g for adults

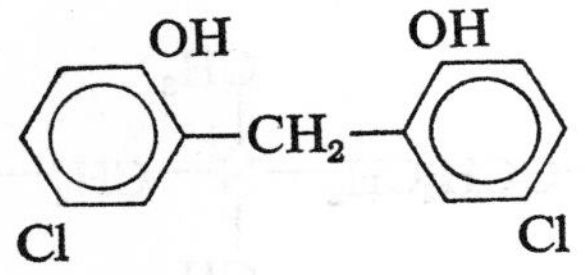

Dichlorophen

is effective in a large number of cases. It also causes nausea and intestinal colic.

Tetrachlorethylene has entirely replaced carbon tetrachloride (CCl_4) as an effective treatment against hook-

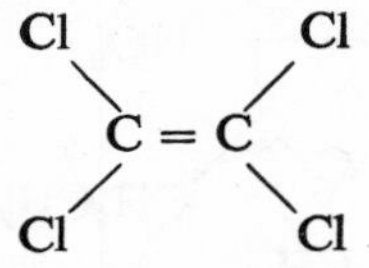

Tetrachlorethylene

worms due to *Necator americanus*. Although poisonous to the liver if damaged by severe anaemia or virus hepatitis, it is cheap for mass therapy, and many millions of people have been successfully treated. Given by mouth on an empty stomach it is absorbed only in small amounts. A suitable dose is 0·1 ml/kg up to a total dose of 5 ml.

Piperazine hydrate is effective against *Ascaris lumbacoides* (round worm) and *Enterobius vermicularis* (threadworm), and acts by paralysing the worms by curare-like

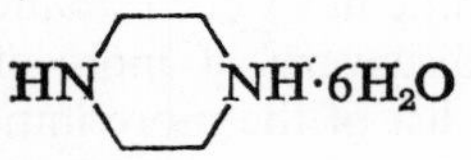

Piperazine hydrate

action at the myoneural junction so that they are expelled alive by peristalsis. The curare-like activity is extremely weak on mammalian skeletal muscles. Given by mouth 1–2 g/day for up to 7 days in the adult, it is partly absorbed and there is a wide range betweeen therapeutic and toxic doses.

Tetramisole is a recently introduced synthetic anthelminthic which is presently under trial and may prove

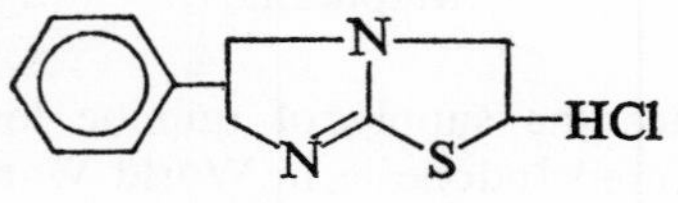

Tetramisole

useful in the treatment of ascariasis when given with piperazine. It inhibits the formation of succinate but appears to have no effect on the response of ascaris to acetylcholine. The adult dose is 200–400 mg/day.

Bephenium hydroxynaphthoate is active against hookworms and roundworms. Given orally it is nontoxic but somewhat expensive. A suitable single dose is 5 g.

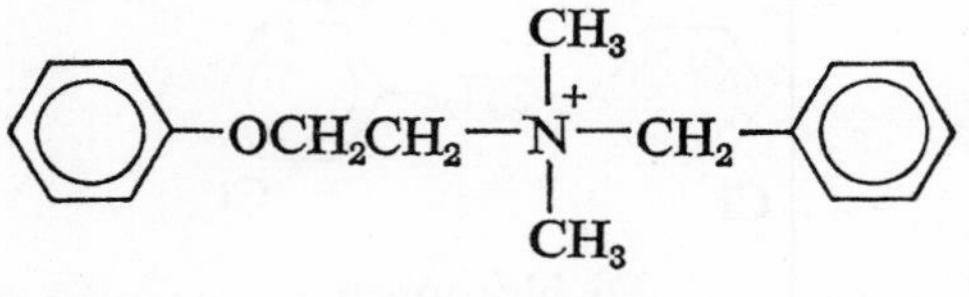

Bephenium

Thiabendazole is a new compound introduced for veterinary use but also active against *Strongyloides* in

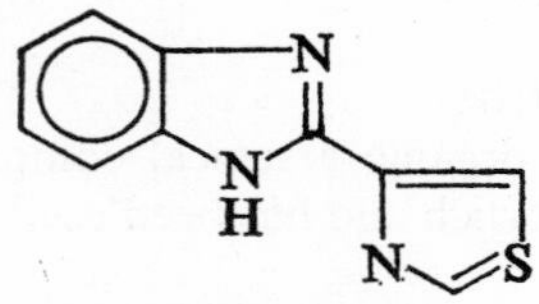

Thiabendazole

man and various worms in the tissues, e.g. *Trichinella spiralis*. It is extremely active at very low concentration and has negligible toxic effects in man.

Hexylresorcinol is active against infection with roundworms, tapeworms, pinworms and hookworms and is useful in mixed infection. Following ingestion by mouth

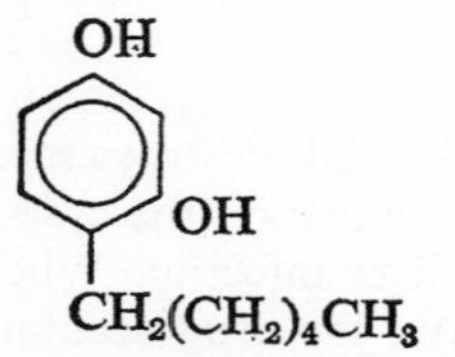

Hexylresorcinol

the drug partially paralyses the worms and because it is only partly absorbed its toxicity is low. It is irritating to mucous membranes and is often given in gelatine coated capsules. The adult dose is 1 g. Repeated doses may cause necrosis of the mucous membrane of the intestine.

Two compounds developed from a study of the anthelminthic activity of cyanine dyes are **dithiazanine** and **viprynium**. The former, given as the iodide salt, is

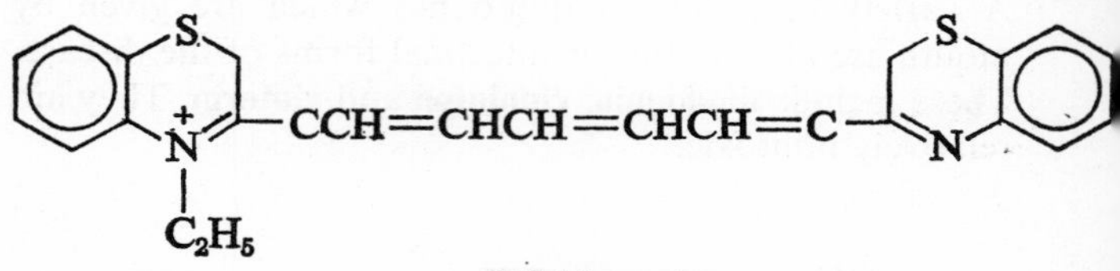

Dithiazanine

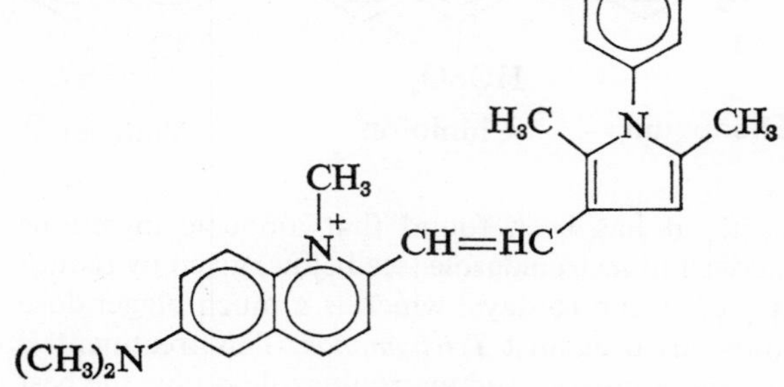

Viprynium

used against enterobiasis, ascariasis, trichuriasis and strongyloidiasis. Viprynium, given as the embonate salt, is active against enterobiasis and strongyloidiasis. The dose is 5 mg/kg. Cyanines appear to inhibit the O_2 uptake of the parasites, but have no effect on mammalian cytochromes. Both compounds are given by mouth, are not absorbed to any appreciable extent and colour the stools. Dithiazanine causes gastrointestinal symptoms and deaths have been reported from its use. Viprynium is relatively free from adverse effects.

Diethylcarbamazine (hetrazan, banocide) is a piperazine derivative remarkably active against filariasis due

Diethylcarbamazine

to *W. bancrofti*, *Loa loa* and *Onchocerca volvulus* and is nontoxic. It is inactive *in vitro* and seems to act like an opsonin, causing the microfilariae in the blood to be devoured by the fixed macrophages of the liver. It is given by mouth (6 mg/kg/day) and is readily absorbed.

Schistosomiasis is an important infection in the tropics, and search for an effective remedy has been made on an enormous scale during the last 20 years. Nevertheless no really satisfactory compound has yet been found. The commonest treatment is some form of antimony compound, e.g. **stibophen**, a trivalent antimony compound or antimony lithium thiomalate (anthiomaline) or **astiban** (TW Sb). **Lucanthone** (Miracil D) is a thiaxan-

Lucanthone

thone and is effective against *S. haematobium* and *S. mansonii* but ineffective against *S. japonicum*. The mechanism of action is unknown. It may interfere with egg laying. Its main disadvantage is its liability to produce gastrointestinal upsets, tremors, vertigo, headache and insomnia. It is absorbed rapidly from the gut and is largely destroyed in the body. A suitable dose is 10–20 mg/kg daily for 5–10 days.

A new and promising derivative, called **hycanthone** has recently been introduced for the treatment of *S. mansoni* infections; it is given by intramuscular injection in doses of 3 mg/kg/day every 3 days for three doses.

The best current compound for the schistosomiasis is

probably **niridazole** (ambilhar) which was introduced in 1965. This compound is given by mouth in twice daily

Niridazole

doses of 12·5 mg/kg for 5–7 days. It is very effective against *S. haematobium*, quite effective against *S. mansoni* and moderately effective against *S. japonicum*. It is well tolerated except that in older patients, particularly if the liver is impaired; it may occasionally produce convulsions or psychosis. Another promising compound for the treatment of *S. haematobium* infections is **metriphonate**.

Compounds active against bacteria
SULPHONAMIDES

A list of the more important sulphonamides is given in fig. 20.8. These may be regarded as derivatives of the basic compound, sulphanilamide. The para-amino group (*) is essential for antibacterial activity. Its substitution yields compounds such as succinylsulphathiazole and pthalylsulphathiazole in which the substituent group is slowly released in the intestine after oral administration and these are used in the treatment of intestinal infections. Substitution of the amide group (**) yields compounds of variable potency of which the most widely used is sulphadiazine and sulphadimidine.

Apart from the compounds specially designed to treat intestinal infections, sulphonamides are absorbed rapidly when given by mouth. All compounds are bound to a varying extent to plasma proteins. The degree of binding greatly influences their pharmacological behaviour and is partly responsible for the differences between the compounds. Acetylation at the para-amino position is the most important pathway of degradation and the acetylated metabolites are bound to proteins to a greater degree than their parent compounds. The degree of acetylation varies with the different compounds and the conjugated compounds which are bacteriologically inactive are sometimes more insoluble and more toxic. Sulphonamides and their acetylated derivatives are largely excreted in the urine, though the rate of elimination varies considerably and part of a dose is oxidized in the body. The protein free moiety of the drug is filtered at the glomerulus and the drug is reabsorbed by the renal tubules to a varying degree.

Sulphadiazine is distributed throughout total body water and is able to penetrate the cerebrospinal fluid, pleural, synovial and other fluids and also to the foetus. If given as a single dose of 4 g to an adult, sulphadiazine

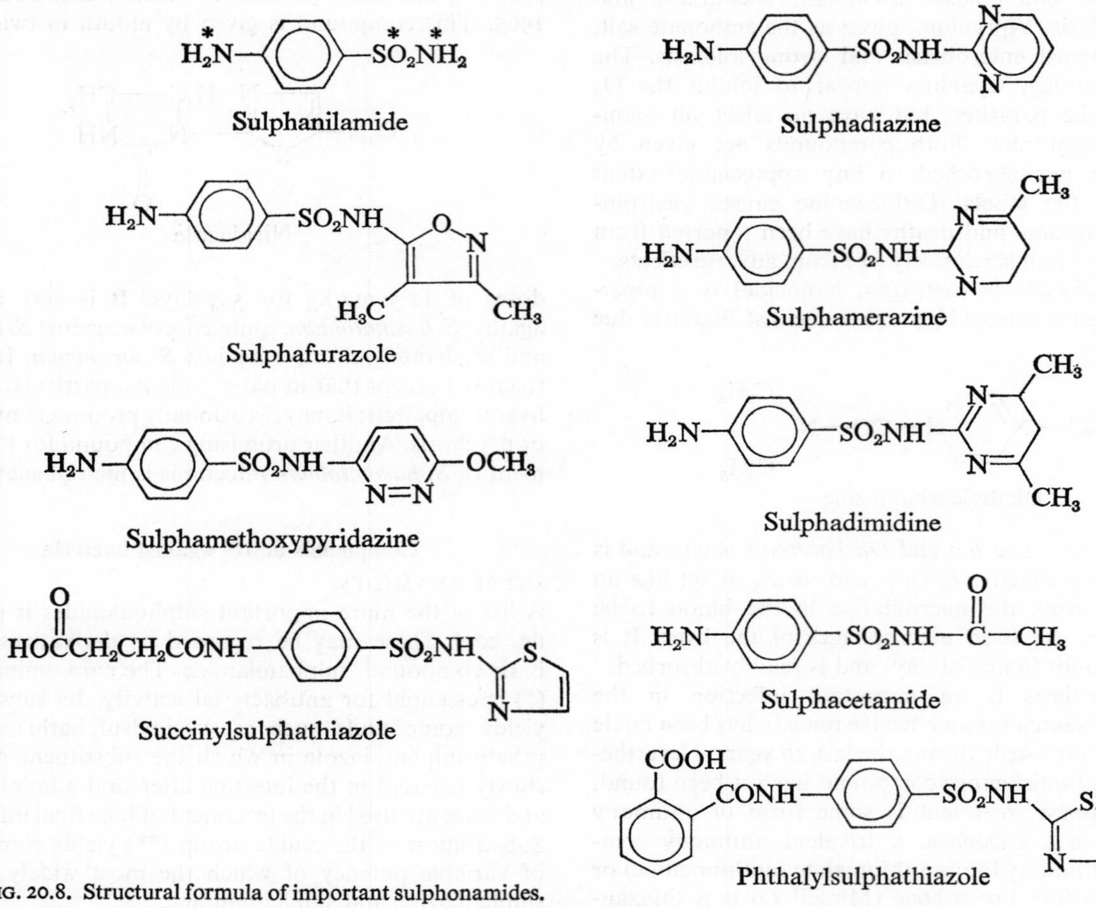

FIG. 20.8. Structural formula of important sulphonamides.

reaches a maximum blood concentration of about 10–15 mg/100 ml in 3–4 hours. More than half of the drug is eliminated from the body in 24 hours and the rest within 48 hours. At normal therapeutic blood levels, 25–50 per cent of the drug is bound to proteins. **Sulphamerazine** and **sulphadimidine** are two methylated derivatives of sulphadiazine. They are absorbed slightly more quickly from the gut than their parent compound and are bound to plasma proteins to a greater extent. This, together with the fact that over 80 per cent of both substances are reabsorbed by the renal tubules, renders them more slowly excreted; their therapeutic dose is therefore smaller than that of sulphadiazine and they need to be given less frequently in the course of the day. They also penetrate the CSF to a smaller degree. **Sulphafurazole** (sulphisoxazole) is one of the most soluble of the sulphonamides and this is also true of its acetylated metabolite. Its volume of distribution within the body however is much less than that of sulphadiazine and its derivatives, and amounts to little more than that of the extracellular fluids. On average, the concentration in the CSF is only about one-third of that of the blood. **Sulphamethoxazole** is closely

related to sulphafurazole and has similar properties. **Sulphacetamide** is also a more soluble compound, being about 100 times more soluble than sulphadiazine. Very high concentrations of sodium sulphacetamide are non-irritating to tissues and this has led to its local use in eye infections in concentrations of up to 30 per cent.

In contrast to these sulphonamides which are rapidly eliminated from the body, **sulphamethoxypyridazine** is absorbed readily from the gastrointestinal tract and over 90 per cent is bound to plasma proteins. For this reason only a small amount of the drug is available for glomerular filtration and, after a single dose, the drug may be detected in the urine after 4 days. For the same reason, the concentration in the CSF is low. The closely related compound, **sulphadimethoxine**, resembles sulphamethoxypyridazine in its rapid absorption and relatively slow rate of excretion in the urine. This, however, is due to the fact that the drug is reabsorbed by the renal tubules after filtration to a considerable degree rather than to binding to plasma proteins which, paradoxically, is quite low. Long-acting sulphonamides have been recommended for long-term suppressive treatment of recurrent urinary tract infections and recurrent throat infections but their use for these purposes is controversial.

Succinylsulphathiazole and **pthalylsulphathiazole** are both poorly absorbed from the gastrointestinal tract and have been advocated for the treatment of intestinal infections and for prophylactic use in elective operations on the colon. They are hydrolysed in the intestine liberating the chemotherapeutically active compound which may reach concentrations of several hundred mg/100 ml within the gut with less risk of systemic toxicity and with minimal blood concentrations.

Trimethoprim, a diaminopyrimidine is a recently synthesized compound which resembles part of the folic acid molecule. In contrast to aminopterine (p. 29.7) the substance has a high affinity for the bacterial enzyme and

Trimethoprim

little affinity for mammalian cells. Thus, it acts as an antimetabolite for the synthesis of N^5 formyl THF in bacteria and in protozoa. Acting alone it is a bacteristatic compound of limited potency but it strongly potentiates sulphonamides. It is readily absorbed when taken by mouth and 50 per cent of a single dose is excreted in the urine in 24 hours. In combination with a sulphonamide, e.g. sulphamethoxazole (septrin, bactrim), the adult dose is 0·5 g/day and so far adverse effects have been few.

Spectrum of activity and resistance
Sulphonamides are not specific in their action on bacterial species, differences in potency being quantitative. Relative potencies may be determined by estimating the minimum concentrations needed to inhibit growth in an artificial medium or by measuring the ability of the sulphonamide to counteract the antibacteristatic action of *p*-aminobenzoic acid. Most strains of β-haemolytic streptococci causing human infection are highly susceptible. Pneumococci and meningococci are the most sulphonamide sensitive of all pathogenic bacteria. Many strains of gonococci are susceptible but increasing numbers of insensitive strains are developing. Staphylococci are insensitive or only moderately sensitive. The presence of pus associated with staphylococcal infection, by virtue of its high concentration of PABA, renders sulphonamides unsuitable for treatment in these cases. Pathogenic bacilli vary considerably in their vulnerability. This is particularly true of *Esch. coli*, *Proteus* and *K. aerogenes*. Many strains of *Shigella* are inhibited

and *K. pneumoniae* and *Vibrio cholerae* are also sensitive. Actinomyces and the agents of lymphogranuloma venereum, and trachoma are also susceptible (p. 18.86).

Bacteria, initially sensitive to sulphonamides, may develop resistance to the action of the drug. As already described, resistant strains are likely to be due to random mutations which are then favoured in the presence of the drug. The biological basis of drug-induced resistance is unknown. The most common change is probably the ability of some bacteria to synthesize increased amounts of PABA to counteract the action of the drug. This is not a constant finding however, and other mechanisms are probably responsible (p. 20.6).

Adverse reactions
All sulphonamides are potentially toxic drugs. Untoward effects are numerous and varied and may involve almost every organ system. Slight effects occur in 5–10 per cent of patients. A few reactions are severe and may occasionally be fatal. In the early days of sulphonamide therapy, injury to the urinary tract due to the formation and deposition of crystals within the renal tubules and in the ureters was common. Sulphonamides now in use are more soluble and urinary complications are less common. The solubility of nearly all sulphonamides is increased by alkalinization of the urine and dangers of precipitation can be avoided by ensuring a good fluid intake. This is of special importance in the case of sulphadiazine, sulphamerazine and sulphamethazine. Disorders of the haemopoietic system were also among the more serious adverse effects of sulphanilamide and other early compounds. However, acute haemolytic anaemia, agranulocytosis and thrombocytopenia are now comparatively uncommon. The majority of adverse reactions are due to hypersensitivity reactions. These consist of skin reactions which include urticaria, erythematous and petechial rashes, exfoliative dermatitis and photosensitivity. Fever, malaise, arthralgia and bronchospasm may also occur. A rare hypersensitivity reaction which is a variety of erythema multiforme, the Stevens–Johnson syndrome, is usually fatal. Jaundice due to focal or diffuse hepatic cell necrosis may develop. If given to pregnant women or neonates they may aggravate kernicterus (p. 12.18) by competing with bilirubin for binding with serum albumin. Drowsiness, fatigue, depression and peripheral neuritis are rare. Anorexia, nausea and vomiting and headache develop in some patients. Occasionally, cyanosis due to the formation of methaemoglobin or sulphaemoglobin occurs but is relatively harmless. Teratogenic activity has been reported in experimental animals but no evidence of this has been found in man.

Dosage and administration
Sulphonamides are nearly always given by mouth. Rapidly absorbed and rapidly excreted sulphonamides

used for the treatment of systemic infection, e.g. urinary tract infection, meningitis, etc., are given in an initial dose of 3–6 g/day for an adult in divided doses throughout the day. Thereafter between one-half and two-thirds of this dose is given for up to 10 days. In severely ill patients sodium sulphadiazine (0·1 g/kg body weight) can be given slowly intravenously. Rapidly absorbed and slowly excreted sulphonamides such as sulpha-methoxypyridazine may be given in a dose of 1–2 g/day in the adult and continued as suppressive doses of 0·5 g/day for some weeks. Poorly absorbed sulphona-mides such as succinylsulphathiazole and pthalylsulpha-thiazole are given in a dose of 5–10 g/day in divided doses.

PENICILLINS
The chemical structure of the naturally occurring semi-synthetic penicillins and their mode of action are given on p. 20.12 & 13. Their pharmacological properties and anti-bacterial spectrum differ considerably and are described individually.

Penicillin G (benzylpenicillin) was one of the first of the naturally occurring penicillins to be discovered and has proved to be the most effective clinically. Absorption from the gastrointestinal tract is limited and the antibiotic is destroyed rapidly by acid gastric juice. Apart from the duodenum where absorption is rapid, penicillin G is not absorbed by the other parts of the small intestine. Under favourable conditions only about one-third of an oral dose is absorbed, so this route of administration is generally inadvisable. When given by subcutaneous or in-tramuscular injection, absorption into the blood is rapid. After a single injection, the maximum blood concentration is reached within 30 min and falls to very low levels within 3–4 hours. This rapid elimination from the blood led to the development of complexes of penicillin G which are more insoluble and from which the active compound is slowly released. The most commonly used of these are **procaine penicillin G** and **benzathine penicillin G** suspensions. A single injection of procaine penicillin produces a maximal blood concentration within three hours and a therapeutically effective concentration may persist for 24 hours. Benzathine penicillin G is more slowly absorbed from the site of injection and a single injection yields detectable levels after several days.

Penicillin G is distributed unevenly throughout the body. It penetrates the CSF only to a slight extent and only small amounts enter synovial fluid, pleural or peri-cardial cavities and ocular fluids. The restricted volume of distribution is largely due to the fact that over 20 per cent is bound to plasma proteins. This limitation has led to the use of intrathecal injections in the treatment of intra-cranial infection. In the presence of normal renal function, over 50 per cent of a single dose of penicillin G is excreted in the urine within 1–2 hours. Renal excretion is achieved largely by tubular secretion and may be greatly reduced by the use of a competitive inhibitor such as pro-benecid and by other organic acids (p. 11.10). A small percentage of administered penicillin G is excreted in bile where it is concentrated. The moiety of penicillin, not excreted, is destroyed in body tissues by mechanisms which are unknown. These characteristics lead to marked fluctuations in blood level when penicillin G is given intermittently, and frequently daily injections are needed if satisfactory blood levels are to be maintained throughout the 24 hours.

Antibacterial spectrum and resistance
In adequate concentration, penicillin G kills a wide range of bacteria including Gram-negative and positive cocci. Pathogenic strains of *Strep. pyogenes* are highly suscep-tible. When first employed this was true of the majority of strains of staphylococci. Today, however, the incidence of resistance varies with the population studied but may be as high as 90 per cent of hospital patients. With minor exceptions, gonococci are vulnerable but meningococci are not so susceptible to penicillin G as they are to sul-phonamides. No significant resistance of pneumococci to the antibiotic has been reported. Some strains of *Esch. coli*, *Salmonella* and *Shigella* are sensitive to penicillin G. *Treponema pallidum* is extremely vulnerable but *Leptospira* are inhibited less readily. Clostridia are also vulnerable. *Pseudomonas*, *Klebsiella*, *Proteus*, *Vibrio*, *Brucella*, mycobacteria, rickettsiae, fungi, yeasts and viruses are resistant to penicillin.

Bacteria may commonly be naturally resistant to the action of penicillin G or acquire resistance only after exposure to the drug. Some pathogenic organisms, how-ever, notably pneumococci and pyogenic streptococci, do not possess natural resistance and never appear to acquire it. Naturally occurring resistance to penicillin and resistance that develops during treatment are due to the production of the enzyme penicillinase by the organism and are genetically determined. This substance hydrolyses penicillin to inactive penicilloic acid and by opening the β-lactam ring renders the drug ineffec-tive. By a process of natural selection, i.e. the elimination of sensitive strains, penicillinase-producing and penicillin resistant staphylococci accumulate in closed populations such as hospital communities. In general these organisms are highly pathogenic (p. 18.70).

Dosage and administration
Naturally occurring penicillins, such as penicillin G, are standardized on the basis of their potency against test organisms. One mg of penicillin G equals 1667 Inter-national Units, so that 1 unit is the pencillin activity in 0·6 μg of the master standard. Organisms inhibited by less than 0·1 unit/ml are considered highly susceptible, where-as those inhibited by less than 1 unit penicillin/ml are only moderately so. Blood levels of up to 5 units/ml are easily

achieved by therapeutic doses. Penicillin G is generally given in doses of up to 100,000 units 3–6 times a day, procaine penicillin in doses of 300,000 units twice daily, and benzthazine penicillin in doses of 600,000 units twice daily. Much larger doses may be required in special cases.

Phenoxymethyl penicillin (penicillin V) is closely related to penicillin G and differs pharmacologically only in that it is more resistant to acid and is therefore more stable if taken by mouth. After administration it is absorbed in the duodenum and upper intestinal tract and its fate in the body is similar to penicillin G. It is given in doses of 250 mg once or twice daily. **Phenoxyethyl penicillin** is for all practical purposes similar to phenoxymethyl penicillin and is also given orally in similar doses.

Methicillin is a semisynthetic penicillin, the importance of which lies in the fact that it is highly resistant to the action of penicillinase and is therefore valuable in the treatment of penicillin G resistant *Staph. aureus*. This resistance is probably due to the effect of the *O*-methoxy groups adjacent to the site of attack by the enzyme. Methicillin is destroyed by acid gastric juice and is poorly absorbed from the gastrointestinal tract; it is therefore given parenterally. After an intramuscular injection of 1 g to an adult, therapeutically effective concentrations are present in the body for up to 6 hours, so that four to six injections per day are generally required for effective blood levels to be sustained. It is bound to plasma proteins to about 20 per cent and does not readily penetrate the CSF. It is excreted in the urine in a way similar to penicillin G. *Staph. aureus* may rarely become resistant to methicillin by mechanisms which do not involve the production of penicillinase. It has no activity against Gram-negative organisms and possesses weak effects against pneumococci or streptococci. The adult dose is 2–4 g/day but 8–12 g is required in some cases.

Oxacillin and **cloxacillin** are semisynthetic penicillins and share some of the pharmacological properties of methicillin and phenoxymethyl penicillin. They may be given orally as they are not destroyed by gastric acid and are absorbed by the gastrointestinal tract to the extent of about 50–60 per cent. Cloxacillin is superior to oxacillin in this respect. They are unaffected by penicillinase and are therefore effective against penicillinase secreting staphylococci. Because they can be given by mouth they are very useful in the treatment of staphylococcal infections and are replacing methicillin for this purpose. The usual daily adult dose is 2–4 g.

Ampicillin is a semisynthetic penicillin which is acid stable but susceptible to the action of penicillinase. It differs from all other penicillins in possessing a very wide bacteriological spectrum, being effective against many Gram-negative and positive organisms. These include *Haemophilus influenzae*, *Esch. coli*, certain strains of *Proteus*, *Salmonella* and *Shigella*. Although its adsorption from the gastrointestinal tract is variable, it is usually given orally. It resembles penicillin G in its distribution and excretion in the urine and bile. An average adult dose is 2–4 g/day.

Hetacillin is a derivative of 6-amino penicillanic acid which undergoes hydrolysis to ampicillin in aqueous solution and in the body. It seems likely that it has no antibacterial activity itself and is merely another way of giving ampicillin.

Carbenicillin is one of the newer semisynthetic penicillins which possesses an even wider range of activity against Gram-negative bacteria than ampicillin. It is the first of the penicillins to be effective against some strains of *Ps. pyocyanea* but only in high concentrations. Carbenicillin is given parenterally in doses up to 30 g/day. Table 20.2 summarizes some of the pharmacological properties of the penicillins.

TABLE 20.2. Resistance of penicillins to acid and penicillinase.

	Acid	Penicillinase	% Protein binding
Penicillin G	+	o	25–50
Penicillin V	+ +	o	50–60
Methicillin	o	+ + +	15–20
Oxacillin	+ +	+ + +	80–85
Cloxacillin	+ + +	+ + +	80–85
Ampicillin	+ + +	o	20–25
Carbenicillin	+ + +	+ + +	45–50

Adverse effects

Penicillins are virtually nontoxic and doses far in excess of those normally used may be given without ill effect. With usual therapeutic doses, blood levels far in excess of the usual concentration are achieved in patients with renal failure without untoward reactions. Very high concentrations which may be reached in some cases of renal failure are, however, toxic to the central nervous system and may cause convulsions. Irritation at the site of injection develops occasionally and an inflammatory response may follow intrathecal injection or if penicillin is injected in error into the sciatic nerve.

By far the most serious reactions are due to hypersensitivity and penicillin is one of the most common causes of drug allergy. The mechanism of these reactions is uncertain. The penicillins or their transformation products can react with the ε-amino groups of polypeptides and proteins to form stable co-valently linked hapten protein conjugates, e.g. penicilloyl protein which promote the production of specific antibodies. Another view is that a highly reactive preformed antigen exists in penicillin preparations derived from products used in their preparation. There appears to be no reliable practical method of detecting sensitivity to penicillin but inquiry concerning reactions to previous administrations should always be made. Patients who suffer from sensitivities to other agents are more liable to react adversely to penicillin and sensitivity induced by one penicillin may lead to similar reactions to others. Reactions are usually more severe when the drug is given parenterally, but may be fatal even after oral administration. The incidence varies from 1–5 per cent but may be as high as 15 per cent in the case of ampicillin.

Reactions include skin rashes of all types, fever, arthralgia, lymphadenopathy, stomatitis and glossitis. Acute anaphylactic reactions with shock, bronchospasm, prostration, cardiac arrest and death may occur.

CEPHALOSPORINS

Cephalosporin C was first isolated from a cephalosporium mould from the sea near a sewage disposal area off Sardinia. It was thought that this might be an ecologically promising area for a micro-organism which might destroy typhoid bacilli. Its formula is given on p. 20.12 and is similar to the penicillins. The antibiotics available, **cephalothin**, **cephaloridine** and **cephalexin**, are semisynthetic derivatives. The first two are not absorbed from the gastrointestinal tract but are readily absorbed from an intramuscular site and may be given intravenously. Cephalexin is given orally. They are distributed widely in the body, including the CSF and are bound to plasma proteins to about 20–60 per cent. They rapidly excreted in the urine largely unchanged within 6–8 hours after a single dose.

The semisynthetic cephalosporins are effective against a large number of Gram-negative and Gram-positive bacteria. Cephaloridine is less effective than cephalothin in treating infection due to penicillinase-secreting staphylococci but both drugs are active against *Strept. pyogenes*, pneumococcus, *Cl. welchii*, meningococcus, actinomyces, many strains of *Salmonella*, *Esch. coli*, *H. influenzae* and *Shigella*. *Proteus* and *Pseudomonas* are insensitive. The usual daily dose is 2–4 g in the adult and should be given in one-sixth of this dose every 4 hours.

Hypersensitivity reactions similar to those seen with penicillin occur occasionally, but cross-reactions with the penicillins are uncommon. The wide bacterial spectrum of these antibiotics occasionally leads to infection with insensitive organisms such as *Pseudomonas*. High doses may give rise to proteinuria and transient neutropenia.

CHLORAMPHENICOL

The formula of **chloramphenicol** is shown on p. 20.17. It is unique among naturally occurring substances in containing a nitrobenzene group. It possesses a wide spectrum of activity and readily inhibits the growth of *Esch. coli*, *K. pneumoniae*, *H. influenzae*, *Bord. pertussis*, *Pasteurella*, *Actinomyces*, *Salmonella* species, some strains of *Proteus*, *Brucella*, *Vibrio*, *Shigella* and *N.*

gonorrhoea, *Rickettsiae*, psittacosis, lymphogranuloma–venereum group and mycoplasma.

Chloramphenicol is water soluble and rapidly absorbed from the gut. It is conjugated by the liver with glucuronic acid and hydrolysed, and the metabolites are excreted in the urine. A small proportion of the active drug is also eliminated in this way. The drug is widely distributed in the body and enters the CSF, bile and milk and readily passes the placenta. The drug is usually given by mouth, in doses of 1–2 g/day for adults. A usual dose for children is 50 mg/kg. It may also be given intramuscularly or intravenously.

By far the most important adverse effect of chloramphenicol is leucopenia, thrombocytopenia and aplasia of the marrow which is related to its nitrobenzene radical. This effect is most likely to occur after prolonged dosage or after repeated courses of the drug but it may occur after a small or initial treatment and is almost invariably fatal. For this reason, chloramphenicol should be reserved for the treatment of serious infections not susceptible to other drugs, e.g. typhoid fever or severe whooping cough. Infants and neonates are particularly liable to develop serious side effects such as vomiting and circulatory collapse. This may be due to immaturity of the hepatic conjugating mechanism or to slow renal excretion (grey baby syndrome). Other adverse effects include fever, skin reactions and glossitis. As in the case of other broad spectrum antibiotics, superinfection with resistant organisms may develop and changes in the bacterial flora in the gut may be responsible for a fall in prothrombin activity.

TETRACYCLINES

The tetracyclines were the outcome of research into the antibiotic producing potentialities of soil organisms following the discovery of penicillin. **Tetracycline**, **chlortetracycline** and **oxytetracycline** are close derivatives of a single polycyclic compound (p. 20.17), and for all practical purposes they are identical in their pharmacological and antibacterial properties. **Dimethylchlortetracycline** also resembles these compounds but is twice as potent.

The tetracyclines possess a wide range of activity against both Gram-negative and positive bacteriae. They also inhibit amoebae, *Mycoplasma*, *Rickettsiae*, *Coxiella*, and the agents of lymphogranuloma venereum, psitticosis and trachoma. They are not active against viruses. The bacteria against which these compounds act as bacteristatic agents include some strains of streptococci, pneumococci, gonococci, *Clostridium*, *Brucella*, *Klebsiella*, *H. pertussis* and *H. influenzae*, menincogocci, some strains of *Esch. coli*, *Salmonella* and *Shigella* organisms and anthrax bacillus. *Ps. pyocyanea* and *Pr. vulgaris* are unaffected.

Tetracyclines are only partially absorbed from the

gastrointestinal tract but satisfactory blood levels may be obtained when taken orally. They are bound to plasma proteins to different degrees (chlortetracycline > dimethyl chlortetracycline > tetracycline > oxytetracycline); they are also widely dispersed throughout body water. They are concentrated in the bile and excreted by the liver into the gut where they undergo an enterohepatic circulation. Penetration into the CSF is slow, but they readily pass the placental barrier. The drugs are excreted mainly in the urine but also in the faeces.

All tetracyclines may cause hypersensitive reactions and cross sensitivity is almost invariable. These reactions include fever, skin rashes, glossitis, angioneurotic oedema. Anaphylaxis may also occur.

Gastrointestinal irritation by tetracycline results in heartburn, nausea, vomiting and diarrhoea, and these symptoms are more severe when higher doses are given. Very occasionally severe diarrhoea may also occur from superinfection with resistant organisms such as *Staph. aureus*, *Cl. albicans*, *Proteus* and *Pseudomonas*, sometimes with fatal results. This complication may follow oral or parenteral administration, presumably in the latter case due to its excretion into the gut in the bile. Leucopenia and thrombocytopenia may follow long term use. Sensitivity of the skin to light occasionally develops and after large doses hepatic necrosis has been noted. With the exception of chlortetracycline, the drugs are excreted freely in the urine and high blood level may occur in renal failure. Tetracyclines are chelating agents and bind bivalent metal ions, e.g. Ca^{++}. They are therefore taken up in the growing bones and teeth of the foetus, neonates and children. Hypoplasia of dental enamel occurs and yellow discoloration of the teeth may be permanent if the drugs are given under 7 years of age. Chelation takes place with calcium and a complex is formed at these sites. Even short exposure to the drug in pregnancy damages the first dentition: serious deformity of permanent teeth or bones following use in pregnancy has not so far been reported but cannot be excluded as a possibility. Tetracyclines which have been exposed to air for several months slowly become degraded chemically and may induce renal tubular damage with aminoaciduria, reduced ability to secrete $[H^+]$, glycosuria and proteinuria.

Tetracyclines have widespread metabolic effects and in large doses they may reduce protein synthesis in the body. The rate of urea formation also rises and, in patients with renal failure, uraemia is aggravated. Increased urinary excretion of riboflavine, folic acid and nicotinamide also occurs and many doctors prescribe Vitamin B preparations when tetracyclines are given for long periods of time. This has not been shown to be necessary.

The usual oral dose of tetracyclines is 1–3 g/day in the adult. Dimethylchlortetracycline is more completely absorbed and more slowly excreted in the urine and a dose of 300 mg twice daily is usually sufficient. Intra-venous infusion of tetracyclines in a dose of 1 g/day in one or two doses is often used but may cause thrombophlebitis.

MACROLIDES

This group, so called because of the large lactone ring in their molecule, includes erythromycin, oleoandomycin, spiramycin, magnamycin and leucomycin. In general these are similar to penicillin G in their range of activity but they readily induce resistant organisms.

Prior to the availability of the newer penicillins, **erythromycin** (p. 20.17) was used widely to treat infections with penicillin-resistant staphylococci. Exposure to the drug, however, often leads to resistance and the antibiotic is now reserved for streptococcal, pneumococcal or staphylococcal infections in individuals who are allergic to the semi-synthetic penicillins. When given in the form of a stearate salt (erythromycin estolate) absorption from the gastrointestinal tract is rapid and acid destruction in the stomach is small. Diffusion occurs rapidly throughout the body fluids except those of the brain, but penetration into the CSF is greater in meningeal inflammation. Excretion takes place largely by way of the bile, urinary loss being very low. Hypersensitivity reactions occasionally occur of which the most important is jaundice, due to inflammation around the intrahepatic biliary canaliculi similar to that occasionally induced by chlorpromazine. This complication is more liable to develop during prolonged treatment or after repeated courses. The usual dose is 250 mg given four times daily for an adult with appropriate reduction for children.

Oleoandomycin, triacetyloleoandomycin and **spiramycin** closely resemble erythromycin in their spectrum of bacterial sensitivity and general pharmacological properties. There is a limited degree of bacterial cross resistance within the group.

POLYMYXINS

Polymyxins are polypeptides (fig. 20.14) derived from certain strains of *B. polymyxa* which are soil organisms. Five polymyxins have been identified and those commercially available are **polymyxin B (polymyxin)** and **E (colistin)**. Their importance lies in the fact that they are effective against *Pseudomonas* organisms which are resistant to all other antibiotics except gentamycin (p. 20.31) and carbenicillin (p. 20.27). The reason for this is unknown. They are also active against many other Gram-negative bacilli but have no action on *Proteus* or Gram-positive organisms. Being polypeptides they are not absorbed by mouth and are best given intravenously or intramuscularly in the treatment of systemic infections; occasionally polymyxin B is applied topically. Since pure preparations are not readily available, their dosage is given in terms of units, 1 mg of pure polymyxin B being equivalent to 10,000 units and 1 mg colistin to 30,000 units. The parenteral dose of polymyxin B is 1–2 mega units/day and is given in three or four divided doses. Adverse reactions include allergic skin reactions and fever, flushing of the face, circumoral and glove and stocking parasthesia, ataxia and respiratory depression. Renal damage with proteinuria and renal failure may also occur. As the drug is largely excreted in the urine, the dose should be reduced in the presence of renal failure.

Colistin is given intramuscularly in doses of 9–18 mega units/day in divided doses when renal function is normal. Adverse effects are similar to those induced with polymyxin B but, in addition, include leucopenia and deafness.

Both compounds are supplied as the polymyxin sulphate but some or all of the amino groups of the polymyxins can be replaced by sulphomethyl radicals. Sulphomethyl polymyxin B (thiosporin) and sulphomethyl polymyxin E (colomycin) are less toxic, and more rapidly excreted than their parent compounds.

Bacitracin is not a polymixin but a polypeptide antibiotic active against many Gram-positive bacteria and *Neisseriae*. It is used now only locally for skin infections.

NEOMYCIN AND KANAMYCIN
Some bacilli of the streptomyces group produce antibiotics which resemble streptomycin in their antibacterial activity. The most important are neomycin and kanamycin.

Neomycin is a paired compound in which a deaminohexose linked to D-ribose is joined to a deaminohexose and deoxystreptomycin. **Kanamycin** has some structural similarity to streptomycin and neomycin. Both compounds have wide antibacterial activity, like streptomycin, but differ in that bacterial resistance is slow to develop. Neither are absorbed by mouth and neomycin is too toxic to be given parenterally. It is useful for topical treatment and it is also given orally in the treatment of gastrointestinal infections, especially due to *Esch. coli* (2–4 g/day). Kanamycin may be given parenterally (1 g/day) and is valuable in *Esch. coli* septicaemia and *Proteus* infections resistant to other compounds. Kanamycin is toxic to the kidneys and the vestibular apparatus. Hypersensitivity reactions also occur. It is mostly excreted in the urine and its dose should be reduced in renal failure. Neomycin and kanamycin reduce ventilation during general anaesthesia by a neuromuscular blocking action (p. 5.69).

NOVOBIOCIN
Novobiacin is a dibasic acid with the empirical formula $C_{31}H_{36}N_2O_4$ with unusual antibacterial properties which most closely resemble penicillin. It is active against *Staph. aureus*, pneumococcus, *H. influenzae* and gonococcus; curiously, streptococci are relatively resistant. Some strains of proteus are sensitive. It is also inactive against *Pseudomonas*, *Salmonella* and *Esch. coli*. Its mode of action is unknown but it has been suggested that it damages the cell wall by binding magnesium ions. It is absorbed from the gut; only a small amount is excreted in the urine, the great bulk of a given dose being excreted in the bile where it is conjugated with glucuronic acid. Its use in neonates should be avoided for the same reason as that given for chloramphenicol. It does not readily penetrate the CSF. Hypersensitivity reactions are common and other toxic effects include diarrhoea and vomiting and alopecia. Indications for the use of novobiacin are now uncommon.

CYCLOSERINE
Cycloserine (p. 20.11), a compound structurally related to the amino acid D-alanine, was originally used in the treatment of tuberculosis, but it has wide antibacterial activity particularly against *Esch. coli* and organisms of the psittacosis–lymphogranuloma group. It is rapidly absorbed from the stomach and small intestine. It readily diffuses throughout total body water and the greater part is excreted in the urine in high concentration. A suitable therapeutic blood level is 20–30 μg/ml; in view of toxicity which occurs with levels above 50 μg/ml, determinations of the concentration in the blood are commonly required. Adverse reactions involve the CNS and include headache, confusion, tremor, psychotic reactions and convulsions; they rapidly disappear if the drug is stopped and the blood level falls. Because it is excreted largely in the urine, patients with renal failure are particularly susceptible to toxic effects. The usual daily dose is 1–2 g/day.

LINCOMYCIN
Lincomycin is chemically distinct from other antibiotics and is a derivative of propylhygrinic acid. It probably acts by depressing DNA and protein synthesis and has a similar antibacterial spectrum to erythromycin against some strains of *Staph. aureus*, streptococci, pneumococci and anthrax bacilli; it is ineffective against most Gram-negative bacilli. Its greatest value lies in the treatment of deep-seated pyogenic infections, including those in bone (osteomyelitis), but resistance to its action is common and relatively easily induced. It is almost free from toxic effects though occasionally produces diarrhoea. It is readily absorbed when given by mouth. The average adult dose is 1–2 g/day. It is absorbed rapidly from the upper gut and is excreted largely into the lower gut. Adverse reactions include gastrointestinal disturbance, jaundice and pruritus. The usual adult daily dose is 1·5–2 g.

SODIUM FUCIDINATE (FUCIDIN)
Fucidin has a basic steroid structure similar to that of naturally occurring adrenocorticoids but is free from hormonal effects. Penicillinase-secreting staphylococci are sensitive to it. It is absorbed from the gastrointestinal

tract and is excreted largely in the bile and eliminated from the body in 24–48 hours after a single dose. Adverse reactions are few but include gastrointestinal disturbances The usual adult dose is 1·5 g/day given in divided doses.

GENTAMYCIN

Gentamycin is a recently discovered compound the structure of which is not fully known. Produced from *Micromonospora*, an actinomycete, it consists of two related substances which are oligosaccharides related to streptomycin. It has a wide range of activity; most strains of staphylococci, *Esch. coli* and *Pseudomonas* and some strains of *Proteus* are sensitive. Resistance develops slowly. When given by intramuscular injection it is absorbed rapidly; after a single dose most of it is excreted in the urine in 12 hours. As in the case of streptomycin, vestibular damage may occur if gentamycin is given in excessive dose or for longer than 7 days especially if renal failure is present. The usual adult dose is 40 mg 8 hourly.

NALIDIXIC ACID

Unrelated chemically to other antibacterial agents nalidixic acid is a naphthyridine derivative (p. 20.15). It is active against Gram-negative organisms, particularly *Esch. coli*, *Proteus*, *Salmonella* and *Shigella*. Absorbed rapidly from the gut it is excreted almost entirely in the urine in free and conjugated forms within 24 hours. Effective blood levels are obtained in adults with 3–4 g/day, and there is evidence to indicate the drug is concentrated in renal tissue. Nausea, vomiting, dizziness and drowsiness, itching and skin rashes may occur. Subjective visual abnormalities also may develop. It is used mainly for urinary tract infections.

NITROFURANTOIN

Nitrofurantoin is a substituted furan derivative. It is mainly active against Gram-negative organisms but most strains of *Ps. pyocyanea* are resistant to it. Its antibacterial mechanism is not known; the compound is used exclusively in the treatment of urinary tract infections.

Nitrofurantoin

It is rapidly absorbed from the gastrointestinal tract and about 50 per cent of the drug is excreted in the urine. Nausea and vomiting are common and peripheral neuritis also occurs. The usual daily dose for an adult is 300–600 mg.

VANCOMYCIN

The formula of vancomycin is unknown. It is an amphoteric compound of mol. wt. about 780. Vancomycin is not absorbed from the gastrointestinal tract and is always given intravenously. It is effective only against Grampositive organisms; consequently the discovery of the newer penicillins, cephalosporins and erythromycin has greatly reduced its use but occasionally staphylococci may be sensitive only to it. It is largely excreted in the urine within 6–8 hours after a single injection. It does not readily penetrate the CSF, synovial or pleural fluids. The dose is 30 mg/kg given in two or three divided doses. Hypersensitivity reactions of any degree of severity may occur. Deafness and renal damage with transient rise in the concentration of blood urea occasionally develop; severe renal failure has been reported and the drug should either be avoided in renal failure or given in reduced dosage. Ristocetin, a compound with similar properties to vancomycin, is no longer used clinically.

RIFAMIDE (RIFAMYCIN)

Rifamycins are extracted from *Streptomyces mediterranei* and have a novel chemical structure with a long aliphatic ridge spanning an aromatic system. They act by inhibiting RNA polymerase as do the actinomycins. They are specially active against Gram-positive organisms and tubercle bacilli. Given intramuscularly 150 mg daily, the drug is rapidly excreted in the urine. Rifamide is also highly concentrated in the bile. Although Gramnegative organisms, which are mainly responsible for infection in the biliary tract, are relatively resistant, its concentration in the bile is so high that it may prove useful in this condition.

Compounds active against mycobacteria

The discovery of drugs which might be useful in the treatment of tuberculosis or leprosy has been influenced by certain features peculiar to these organisms. *Mycobacterium leprae* does not grow on artificial media and *Mycobacterium tuberculosis* does so with difficulty after lengthy periods of incubation. Furthermore, the susceptibility of animals to experimental tuberculosis and leprosy varies greatly between species so that conclusions of the effect of potentially useful drugs are difficult in man where the disease is frequently chronic and unpredictable in its behaviour.

ANTITUBERCULOSIS DRUGS

Streptomycin (p. 20.15) was discovered in 1944 as a metabolite of soil micro-organisms, streptomycetes, and after penicillin was the next important antibiotic to be isolated. Dihydrostreptomycin was produced 3 years later by catalytic hydrogenation of streptomycin, but it is now rarely used because it is more likely than streptomycin to damage the cochlear nerve and produce deafness.

Streptomycin was the first antibiotic to cure experimental tuberculous infections in guinea-pigs, to inhibit the multiplication of the organisms in culture and to cure tuberculous meningitis, formerly a fatal disease.

Streptomycin is not absorbed after oral administration but is absorbed rapidly into the blood after injection. About 30 per cent of the drug is bound to plasma proteins and it does not readily penetrate the CSF unless the meninges are inflamed. Distribution throughout the ECF is rapid and includes the pericardial, pleural and especially the peritoneal spaces. It also passes the placental barrier; the concentration in the liver and kidney is high. Over 50 per cent of the drug is excreted unchanged in the urine within 24 hours, largely by glomerular filtration, and toxic blood levels are reached if normal doses are given in the presence of renal failure. After a single dose, maximum concentrations of streptomycin occur in the blood in 1–2 hours and fall rapidly to low levels in 6–12 hours. Apart from tubercle bacilli, other organisms usually sensitive to the antibiotic include *Brucella, Esch. coli, H. influenzae* and pneumococcus, *Pasteurella pestis* and *P. tulerense*, and *Shigella*. The antibacterial action of streptomycin is also pH dependent, the drug being more effective in an alkaline medium. Unfortunately streptomycin induces bacterial resistance more readily than any other antibiotic and this may occur after exposure of only a few hours. The development *in vivo* of resistance to streptomycin is an important factor in the use of the drug for tuberculosis. It increases with the duration of use and is due to the occurrence of resistant mutant strains. The simultaneous use of other antituberculous agents hinders the emergence of such strains and, accordingly, in the treatment of tuberculosis, streptomycin should always be combined with other drugs.

The most serious adverse effects of streptomycin affect the central and peripheral nervous system. In particular, damage to the vestibular component of the eighth cranial nerve occurs with acute dizziness, headache and nausea; ataxia may develop in a few weeks and may persist for many months or years. Some diminution of auditory acuity progressing to severe deafness may also occur, preceded by warning tinnitus. These complications are particularly likely to develop in old people and are due to overdosage. Other less common reactions include encephalopathy with nystagmus, nausea, somnolence, slow respirations, fever, delirium and peripheral neuritis. Hypersensitivity reactions include skin rashes, blood dyscrasies, stomatis, anaphylactic shock, pruritus and lymphadenopathy. Respiratory arrest has followed peritoneal instillation and is due to neuromuscular blockade; this is particularly liable to occur if skeletal muscle relaxants have been given (p. 5.69). Transient proteinuria is occasionally seen.

The usual dose of streptomycin is 1–2 g/day by intramuscular injection. Details of dose schedules for tuberculosis and other infections are given in vol. 3.

The discovery of antituberculous effect of **sodium (or calcium) p-amino salicylic acid (PAS)** followed the

$$H_2N-\!\!\!\bigcirc\!\!\!\overset{\text{OH}}{-}\!\!\!COOH$$

p-Amino salicylic acid

demonstration that salicylic acid increases the O_2 consumption of tubercle bacilli and suppresses multiplication and growth. The precise mechanisms of action are unknown though the effect is antagonized competitively by *p*-aminobenzoic acid. This suggests that the inhibition may be similar to the antibacterial action of sulphonamides although the latter are ineffective against tuberculosis. PAS does not possess any of the analgesic or antipyretic properties of salicylic acid. Given by itself to experimental animals, PAS has a beneficial if slight antituberculous effect but its greatest importance lies in the fact that when given with streptomycin or isoniazid the emergence of drug resistant strains is greatly delayed.

PAS is rapidly absorbed from the gastrointestinal tract, is dispersed throughout the total body water and penetrates into chronic fibrocaseous areas of tuberculous infection. Almost all of a given dose of PAS is excreted by tubular secretion in the urine within 12 hours; about 50 per cent of it is acetylated and is relatively insoluble.

Anorexia, nausea, epigastric pain and vomiting are the most troublesome adverse effects. Occasionally gastric ulceration develops. A wide range of sensitivity reactions may occur and include fever, joint pains, hepatic necrosis, sore throat, lymphadenopathy, blood dyscrasias, encephalopathy and others. The drug reduces prothrombin formation by the liver and long continued treatment induces enlargement of the thyroid gland with hypothyroidism by preventing the formation of thyroxine.

The usual dose in antituberculous therapy is 8–12 g/day. It is usually given in cachets which also contain isoniazid.

Isoniazid (isonicotinic acid hydrazine INH) is the most powerful and effective antituberculous drug. Its discovery was a development from the finding that nicotinamide had antituberculous activity. Its mode of action is unknown. DNA formation is suppressed but bacterial wall

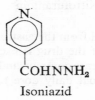

COHNNH₂
Isoniazid

synthesis is unaffected. Tubercle bacilli exposed to isoniazid lose their properties of acid-fastness. The drug is absorbed rapidly from the gastrointestinal tract and is freely distributed through body water, including the CSF and milk. About 75 per cent is excreted in the urine within 24 hours in the form of free isoniazid, acetylisoniazid and isonicotinic acid conjugates. The extent of acetylation is relatively constant for any given individual but certain persons acetylate the drug slowly and excrete large amounts of free compound instead. The ability to acetylate is genetically determined and, when it is slow, peripheral neuritis is more likely to develop as a toxic effect (p. 31.11).

Hypersensitivity reactions similar to those for other antibacterial agents and drugs occur. Peripheral neuritis is common with high doses but may be prevented by giving pyridoxine. This effect may be due to the fact that isoniazid competes with pyridoxal phosphate. Other untoward effects include optic neuritis, muscle twitching, euphoria, memory loss, psychotic reactions, convulsions and intolerance of alcohol. A more serious development has been the discovery that isoniazid is carcinogenic in albino mice. The implications of this on the use of the drug in man are not so far clear, but the compound has now been used on great numbers of patients for many years without clinical evidence of carcinogenesis. The usual daily dose is 200–300 mg.

Other less commonly used antituberculous drugs are **cycloserine** (p. 20.11); **viomycin**, a polypeptide antibiotic; **pyrazinamide**, a pyrazine analog of nicotinamide; **thiacetazone**, a semicarbazone and **ethionamide**, a pyridine derivative like isoniazid and **ethambutol** (ethylene diaminobutanol). These drugs are potentially toxic and are reserved for patients who are intolerant to streptomycin, PAS or isoniazid, or when the infecting organisms are resistant to them. Rifamide (p. 20.31) is also occasionally used.

ANTILEPROTIC DRUGS
Soon after the discovery of the sulphonamides a class of compound, the sulphones, was investigated for antistreptococcal activity. These were found to be effective but were believed to be too toxic for clinical use. They were then found to have antituberculous effects but here too they were rapidly superseded by streptomycin and other compounds. Nevertheless, a favourable effect on leprosy was observed and today they remain the most important drugs in the treatment of this disease.

All sulphones of clinical value are derived from

$$H_2N - \bigcirc - SO_2 - \bigcirc - NH_2$$

Dapsone

dapsone (diaminodiphenylsulphone). Other effective sulphones include **sulphoxone, sulphetrone** and **thiazolsulphone** (promizole). These compounds may depend on their effect by the liberation of dapsone in the body which remains the most effective agent clinically. The mechanism of action against *Myco. leprae* is believed to be similar to that of other sulphonamides, as *p*-aminobenzoic acid inhibits the bactericidal activity of the drugs. Failure of the leprosy bacillus to grow in culture renders it impossible to test this hypothesis and so it is not known why they are specially effective against leprosy bacilli.

Dapsone is slowly absorbed from the gastrointestinal tract and persists in the blood for 1–2 weeks. It is distributed widely in the body and undergoes excretion in the bile with subsequent reabsorption, an enterohepatic circulation which greatly prolongs its half life in the body. These peculiarities influence the pattern of therapy and dapsone is often given in slowly rising doses starting with 25 mg rising to 300 mg twice weekly. The most common adverse effect is anaemia due to hypersensitive reactions; the drug may be given safely over 5 years and eventually cure most cases. It is an inexpensive drug, an important consideration, since great numbers of people have to be treated in poor countries.

Other antileprotic drugs include **thiambutosine** a derivative of thiourea (p. 6.7), which is given by mouth and to which the organisms frequently become resistant, and **thiacetazone**.

Drugs effective against fungi
Antibiotics are comparatively ineffective against fungal infection which, however, is sometimes a serious complication of antibacterial antibiotic treatment.

Nystatin, named after the New York State Department of Health, is a conjugated double bonded polyene with a large molecular weight and its precise structure is unknown. It is most effective when applied directly on to fungal infected surfaces, e.g. the mouth, vagina or throat. It is not absorbed when given by mouth and has no systemic effect. *Candida albicans*, cryptococcus, histoplasma and other fungi are usually sensitive. It is given for fungal infections of the mouth or gastrointestinal tract in doses of 1–2 million units/day.

Griseofulvin was originally derived from a penicillium mould and inhibits the growth of epidermophyton, tricophyton and microsporum which cause athlete's foot, ringworm and tinea. The structural formula of griseofulvin is shown on p. 20.14. Chemically it resembles that of colchicine and like this compound is beneficial in gout. Given by mouth it is partially absorbed and is incorporated into the keratin of skin, nails and hair, particularly in areas which are affected by the organisms. Gastrointestinal symptoms occasionally occur but are rarely severe. Hypersensitivity may also develop. The adult dose is 250 mg four times/day.

Amphotericin B, like nystatin, is also a polyene of large molecular weight and its structural formula is unknown. It is the most effective available agent for systemic fungal infection due to histoplasma, cryptococcus, coccidiodes, blastomyces and *Candida* species. It is given only intravenously (or by intrathecal injection in meningeal infection) in progressively increasing dosage. The initial dose is 1–2 mg/day gradually increasing to 50 mg/day. It is irritant and toxic. Severe reactions, e.g. chills, fever and vomiting are common, and so are hypersensitivity reactions. Liver damage and renal failure may occur. Nevertheless the compound is valuable since it is effective in a number of formerly fatal infections.

VIRAL CHEMOTHERAPY

In contrast to the number of antimicrobial compounds available for the treatment of bacterial, fungal and other parasitic infections relatively few are useful in viral chemotherapy. The reason for this difference is easily understood. While bacteria possess their own structural, metabolic and genetic apparatus, viruses become integrated with specific host cells, the metabolic machinery of which synthesizes new viral material under the direction of viral DNA or RNA. For this reason, many inhibitors of specific cell functions interrupt similar processes involved in viral replication, e.g. actinomycin D and rifamycins inhibit viral DNA-dependent RNA polymerase, and puromycin, which inhibits protein synthesis in cells, also prevents viral protein synthesis. Although it is not easy to interrupt viral nucleic acid and protein synthesis without affecting the host cell, a variety of chemicals are known that either distinguish between virus and host cell or between infected and noninfected cells.

Antiviral substances can be classified on the basis of the stage of the cycle of virus replication at which they act. They may produce an effect,
(1) on free extracellular virus,
(2) at the adsorption, penetration or uncoating stage,
(3) at the stage of macromolecular synthesis, or
(4) at the stage of assembly and release of new virus.

ACTION ON FREE VIRUS
At the free virus stage, specific antibody is the most effective antiviral agent and some of its actions are discussed on p. 22.17. The administration of purified globulin preparations in human viral infections, however, has not invariably proved of value; for example, the prevention of rubella in this way is not always effective; on the other hand, contacts of cases of viral hepatitis have been reliably protected by doses of 0·5–1 g given intramuscularly.

Isoquinoline derivatives (fig. 20.9) affect free virus directly. These compounds are antineuraminidases and inactivate some members of the myxovirus and paramy-xovirus groups, perhaps by combining with the neuraminidase present on the outer envelope of the virus. Both infectivity and haemagglutinating ability may be reduced after a period of direct contact with the drug. Apart from this action which has been noted against influenza A, B and C strains, parainfluenza and measles virus, a possible inhibitory action of isoquinolines during the intracellular replication of some enteroviruses and rhinoviruses has also been noted. In human volunteers, prior treatment with these drugs confers some protection against infection with influenza B virus.

ACTION AT STAGE OF ADSORPTION OR PENETRATION
Amantadine is the L-amino derivative of adamantane, a tricyclic saturated hydrocarbon. It does not act against free virus but at the level of penetration and uncoating of the infecting virus. It is effective against some influenza A and C viruses and rubella virus in tissue culture, but the results of studies in small animals and men challenged with a drug-sensitive virus have not shown that amantadine produces definite protection *in vivo*. Adverse psychic and neurological effects have been reported in man at the recommended dose of 200 mg/day.

INHIBITION OF INTRACELLULAR VIRAL REPLICATION
2-(α-hydroxybenzyl)-benzimidazole (HBB) and **guanidine** inhibit the replication of some members of the enterovirus group by preventing viral RNA synthesis as a result of blocking the formation of a functional virus-induced RNA polymerase. In animals, no definite protective effect can be demonstrated because drug resistant mutants arise rapidly. Cross resistance between the two drugs is not complete, although they appear to act at the same level. Many derivatives of HBB have been studied, and some have been found to be more effective inhibitors than the parent substance. In infant mice challenged with low doses of **Coxsackie A9** virus, the L-propyl derivative has been reported to protect the mice or to delay the time of death.

The halogenated derivatives of deoxyuridine have been shown to interfere with the synthesis of both host cell DNA and viral DNA. The substitution of the halogen is at the 5 position of uracil, and the resulting deoxynucleosides are 5-fluorodeoxyuridine (FUDR), 5-bromodeoxyuridine (BUDR), and 5-iododeoxyuridine (IUDR) or **idoxuridine**. Within cells these compounds are phosphorylated by thymidine kinase yielding the 5-monophosphates. The mode of action of FUDR differs from that of BUDR and IUDR in that it inhibits thymidylic synthetase, thus preventing the incorporation of thymidine into DNA. BUDR and IUDR interfere with enzymes synthesizing DNA but can be converted to the triphosphates

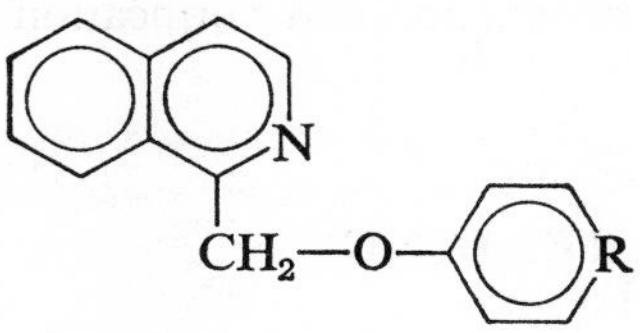

Isoquinolines
R = −OCH₃
= −Cl

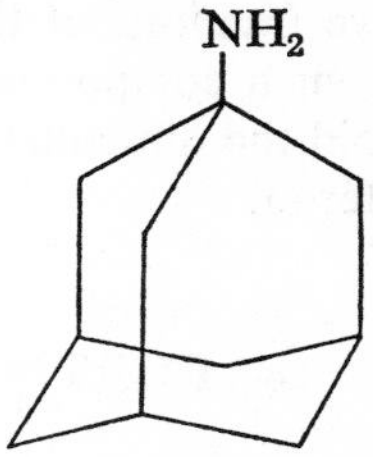

1-Adamantanamine

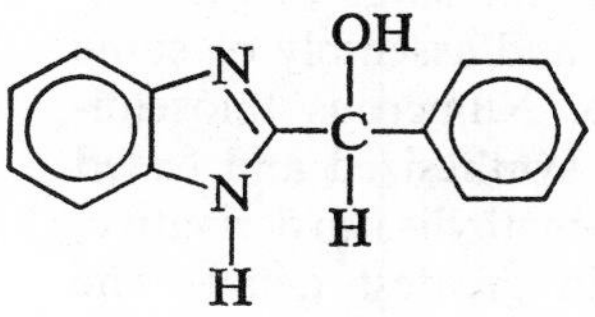

2-(α-Hydroxybenzyl)
-benzimidazole

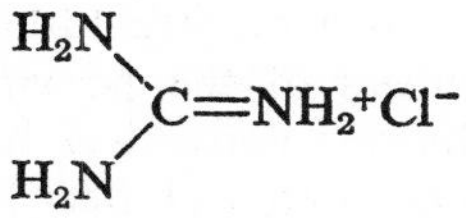

Guanidine hydrochloride

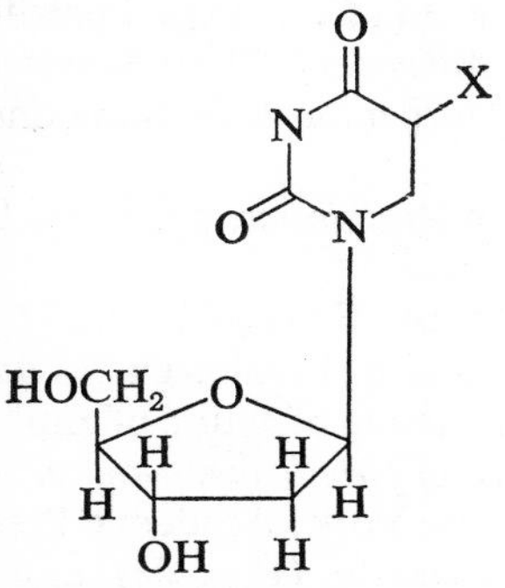

5-Substituted deoxyuridines
X = CH₃ : Thymidine
= F : 5-Fluorodeoxyuridine
= Br : 5-Bromodeoxyuridine
= I : 5-Iododeoxyuridine

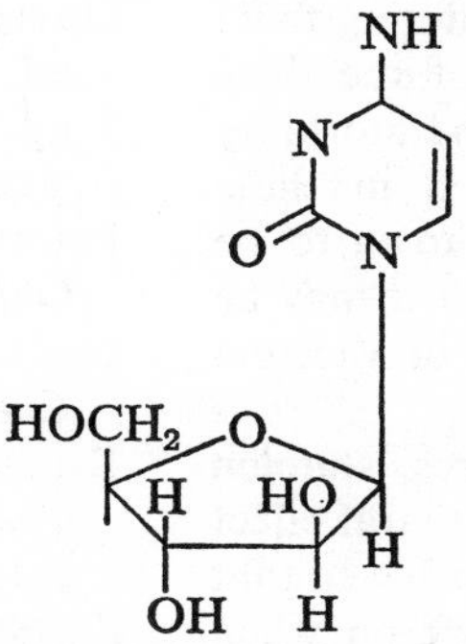

Cytosine arabinoside

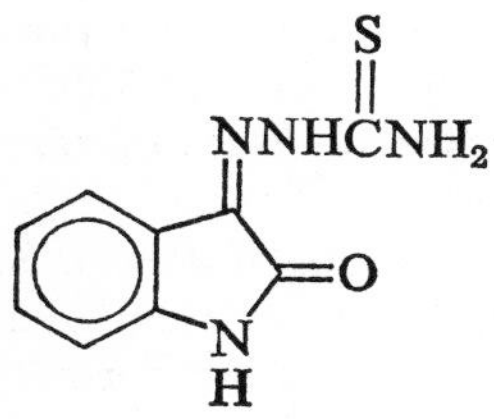

Isatin β-thiosemicarbazone

FIG. 20.9. Some antiviral agents.

and incorporated into DNA. The resulting fraudulent DNA may replicate but gives rise to nonfunctional proteins and virus maturation is accordingly prevented. Since the synthesis of both host cell DNA and viral DNA involves similar mechanisms it is necessary to give some explanation for the apparently selective action of these compounds on viral replication.

Infection with vaccinia and herpes simplex viruses results in the appearance of a thymidine kinase that is probably specified by the virus. The presence of this enzyme in infected cells brings about the phosphorylation of the halogenated deoxyuridines that is a necessary prerequisite for their action; the discriminating effect may be more marked in animals than in tissue cells, as in the whole animal at any point in time many cells are not synthesizing DNA and hence are resistant to the inhibitory action of these chemicals. However, the chemicals affect some of the host cells and substituted deoxyuridines (especially IUDR) have consequently been investigated and used mainly in surface infections with DNA viruses such as those of vaccinia and herpes simplex. Infection of the cornea by herpes simplex virus can be treated successfully with idoxuridine when dendritic ulcers with or without stromal keratitis are present, or

when there is extensive corneal involvement, especially if steroids have been applied to the eye. The administration of IUDR allows the use of corticosteroids in the presence of herpes simplex virus in the treatment of deep keratitis. Some reduction in the duration of the symptoms of herpetic skin infection has been claimed when IUDR is used, but penetration of the drug to the site of viral replication is inadequate. Systemic use of IUDR has been confined to potentially lethal disorders such as encephalitis caused by herpes simplex virus. It seems likely that the drug may be incorporated in DNA of normal cells and might result in late complications such as neoplasm or other genetic damage. Leucopenia, thrombocytopenia and hepatic necrosis have been noted. Apart from their possible clinical use, the three analogues of IUDR have been widely used in studying the replication of DNA viruses and host–virus interaction. Their inhibitory effect is reversible by the addition of thymidine.

Inhibition of DNA synthesis can also be demonstrated with the compound **cytosine arabinoside**. This blocks the conversion of cytidilic acid to deoxycytidilic acid. Little or no selective antiviral action is found perhaps because no virus-specific enzyme is involved in the phosphorylation step.

ACTION AT STAGE OF ASSEMBLY OR RELEASE
Isatin-β-thiosemicarbazone acts at the stage of the synthesis of viral structural proteins and assembly of some members of the poxvirus group. Numerous thiosemicarbazone derivatives have been synthesized and tested for their antiviral effect, and the *N*-methylisatin derivative, **methisazone**, has been studied in greatest detail. The inhibitory action is not on viral DNA or RNA synthesis, but apparently on late viral messenger RNA, preventing the formation of polyribosomes that synthesize late structural proteins.

In man, methisazone has been shown to be effective in preventing disease in contacts of patients suffering from smallpox. In contacts, two doses of 3 g of the drug reduce both the number of infections and the mortality but vaccination should also be undertaken in these circumstances. Methisazone has not been shown to be effective in treating established infections, but it may be useful in some cases of eczema vaccinatum or vaccinia gangrenosa.

Two extracts of *Penicillium* mould cultures, **statolon** and **helenine**, have been found to have an antiviral effect similar to that of interferon (p. 18.109). It is believed that these products induce the synthesis of interferon when administered to the whole animal. This induction may be brought about by virus-like particles or RNA present in

the active fractions of these preparations. The development of such compounds and synthetic polynucleotides may avoid the difficulties of production and purification of interferon.

FURTHER READING

BUSCH H. & LANE M. (1967). *Chemotherapy. An Introductory Text*. Chicago: Year Book Medical Publishers.
DATTA N. (1965). Infectious drug resistance. *Brit. med. Bull.* **22**, 254.
DOYLE F.P. & NAYLER J.H.C. (1964). Penicillins and related structures, in *Advances in Drug Research*, vol. 1, pp. 1–69, ed. N.S. Harper & A.B. Simmonds. New York: Academic Press.
FLOREY H.W. (1949). In *Antibiotics*, pp. 1–73. London: Oxford University Press.
GARROD L.P. & O'GRADY F. (1968). *Antibiotics and Chemotherapy*, 2nd Edition. Edinburgh: Livingstone.
ROGERS H.J. (1968). The mode of action of antibiotics, in *The Biological Basis of Medicine*, vol. 2, ed. E.E. Bittar & N. Bittar. New York: Academic Press.
SCHNITZER R.J. & HAWKING F. (1963–64). *Experimental Chemotherapy*, vols. 1–3. New York: Academic Press.

Chapter 21
Inflammation

By inflammation is meant the defensive reactions of the body's tissues to injury of any kind. Such reactions follow a broad general pattern but vary in detail according to the nature of the injurious agent and the site and severity of the injury. The many types of injurious agents which give rise to an inflammatory response may be summarized as follows:

(1) bacteria and their toxins, viruses, rickettsiae, fungi, protozoa and helminths;

(2) trauma, which may be mechanical, thermal, electrical or chemical; ionizing irradiation, no less damaging because it is invisible, is also a form of trauma;

(3) death (necrosis) of tissue arising as a result of loss of blood supply or from any other cause (p. 25.4);

(4) an immune reaction, i.e. the interaction of an antigen and a specific antibody; this is equally true whether the antibody is directed against a foreign protein or against the body's own tissues, i.e. autoimmunity (p. 23.7), and

(5) most malignant neoplasms.

Inflammation may be divided broadly into two types, acute and chronic. In **acute inflammation** a succession of changes takes place within a short period, which may be anything from a few minutes to a few days; it is brought to an end either by a return of the tissue to normal (resolution) by fibrosis (p. 21.14) or by conversion to a chronic form. **Chronic inflammation** is of longer duration and may last months or years; during this time the inflammatory reaction may fluctuate in severity but retains essentially the same character throughout. Chronic inflammation differs from acute inflammation in several other important respects. Subacute inflammation is a term occasionally used to describe an inflammatory reaction intermediate between acute and chronic and partaking of the characters of both. In any individual case the type of inflammatory response present may not fall precisely into any one category.

The morphological changes in inflammatory conditions are made up of the direct effects of the causative factor and the defensive responses of the body to the injury. These components are closely intermingled and cannot always be readily disentangled from one another.

The gross signs of acute inflammation were recognized and accurately described a very long time ago, though only within the last hundred years has it been appreciated that the process represents nonspecific defensive reactions to many different kinds of injury and does not constitute a specific disease. In the first century A.D. Celsus described the four cardinal signs of acute inflammation as **tumor** (swelling), **rubor** (redness), **calor** (heat) and **dolor** (pain). Galen, in the second century, added a further sign, **functio laesa** (loss or impairment of function). Thus acute inflammation, if it occurs in an easily observed site, can be recognized as a swollen, red, hot, painful lesion which interferes with the function of the affected part.

Not until the advent of the microscope and the acceptance of the cellular basis of pathology was it possible to understand the events which give rise to the cardinal signs. In the middle of the nineteenth century early observations were made on transparent membranes such as the mesentery or the webbed foot of the frog, where the sequence of events could be readily observed under the microscope. Cohnheim's celebrated lectures, published in 1882, give an account of the morphological changes which to this day can scarcely be bettered; he demonstrated the essential part played by the vascular system and the leucocytes of the blood in the acute inflammatory process, while Metchnikoff in the following decade focused attention on the phenomenon of phagocytosis.

The acute inflammatory process is highly complex, comprising different sequences of events which occur almost simultaneously, so that it is scarcely possible to give an account of the changes in strict chronological order. There are, as it were, so many subsidiary plots that it would be necessary, as in a Shakespearean drama, to keep interrupting the main story in order to discover what the lesser characters were doing. Moreover, the details of the inflammatory process vary so much according to the nature and severity of the initiating stimulus and according to the structure of the affected organ or tissue that no single description is applicable to all examples of inflammation.

The inflammatory response

It is common knowledge that if a hand is scalded with hot water the skin becomes reddened. The response lasts for a variable period of time, and if the scald is severe the area remains red for some days. Compared with the surrounding skin, the inflamed part is warm to the touch and may be swollen; it is also painful. When the scald is on the arm or the leg, the whole limb is kept still, for movement is restricted by swelling and pain. The skin has responded to this heat injury by a succession of changes; similar inflammatory changes occur when the skin is injured or irritated in other ways and may follow trauma, i.e. mechanical injury by scratching, pinching or direct blows, and also injury caused by chemical reagents such as acids, alkalis and a host of organic and inorganic irritants. Many people, especially those with fair skins, are familiar with the redness and pain which follows exposure to bright sunlight; in this case, the ultraviolet radiation produces the inflammatory response. Moreover, similar reactions of the skin occur when bacteria or other parasites multiply in cutaneous or subcutaneous tissues.

It is apparent that the skin reacts to a variety of injuries by a common pattern of response and the sequence of changes is the **acute inflammatory response**. This occurs also when other tissues are injured, for instance the peritoneum, bronchi or synovial sheaths. The suffix -itis, as in peritonitis, bronchitis, or synovitis, indicates inflammation in the part named.

If the injury to a part is severe enough, there is death (necrosis) of cells (p. 25.28). A bad scald or burn may kill the whole thickness of the skin, both epidermis and dermis. The dead skin obviously cannot show inflammatory changes; however, around the central necrotic area the tissues that have been injured but not killed become inflamed. Burdon Sanderson defined inflammation as 'the changes which occur in a living tissue when it is injured, provided that the injury is not of such a degree as at once to destroy its structure and vitality'. In the case of a severe heat injury the necrotic area may separate from the still living, inflamed tissues and be rejected as a scab or **slough**, leaving behind a raw area or ulcer. This may become infected with pathogenic organisms; in this event inflammatory changes produced by the bacteria are added to those produced by the burn. From the surface of the infected ulcer there exudes protein-containing fluid derived from blood plasma; this fluid may be clear, or it may be thick, and coloured in varying shades of yellow and green, a **purulent exudate** or **pus**, or it may be blood stained or **haemorrhagic**. Purulent exudates contain liquefied dead tissue, polymorphs, dead and alive, which have emigrated into the area from the small blood vessels, and plasma or serum, as well as invading or contaminating micro-organisms.

Similar changes occur in the inflammatory reaction of tissues or organs deep to the skin. If the site of inflammation lies on a surface of a body cavity, the protein-containing exudate is discharged into that cavity.

An inflammatory exudate in a serous cavity or in a loose body tissue may be abundant and watery; this is sometimes referred to as a **serous exudate**. However, in many cases of acute inflammation of the serous sacs, i.e. in pericarditis, pleurisy or peritonitis, the extravasated fluid contains a large quantity of fibrin, and is less abundant but thicker; this is called a **fibrinous exudate** (plate 21.1a). An exudate in a serous sac may also be purulent. If the inflammatory area is not on a surface, and the inflammatory process is severe, death of tissue occurs and pus is formed. A collection of pus in a solid organ or tissue is called an **abscess** (plate 21.1b); its wall often becomes well defined and in time consists of fibrous tissue. An abscess may, sooner or later, discharge on to a surface, e.g. the skin or the peritoneum or, in the lung, a bronchus. It does this by tracking through and breaking down the intervening tissues to form a discharging channel or **sinus**. The sequence of such an inflammatory response is seen on a small scale when a hair follicle becomes infected with *Staph. aureus*. There is an initial inflammatory reaction with redness, pain and swelling, giving rise to a small abscess, usually called a boil, which discharges its purulent contents on to the skin surface.

An **ulcer** is the name given to a lesion of an epithelial surface in which the epithelium is destroyed, exposing the underlying tissues, and in most cases this is accompanied by inflammation of the surface so that a layer of polymorphs, fibrin and necrotic tissue lies on the ulcer floor. In an acute ulcer, healing, with regeneration of the epithelium, may occur rapidly, but in a chronic ulcer, with much tissue damage, fibrous tissue develops in the floor (p. 21.14) and epithelial regeneration may be delayed or may never occur (plate 21.1c).

Resolution of an acute inflammatory process consists of recession of the signs of inflammation, with return of the tissue to its normal state. If tissue has been destroyed by the inflammatory process this is restored by means of **repair** and **regeneration**. In tissues capable of being stimulated to cell division, as for example the epidermis, replacement may occur at least in part by the tissue cells themselves, but in other tissue, such as cardiac muscle, in which the highly differentiated cells can no longer divide, replacement is by scar or fibrous connective tissue which develops through the process known as **organization**.

Sometimes a balance is struck between the extension of the inflammatory response and the processes of resolution and repair, and then the tissue becomes chronically inflamed.

In many circumstances, second or subsequent exposures to pathogenic bacteria or foreign proteins produce inflammatory reactions which differ from those of the first exposure. This constitutes an altered tissue reactivity or hypersensitivity and is shown specifically to that particular foreign material and not to others (p. 22.18).

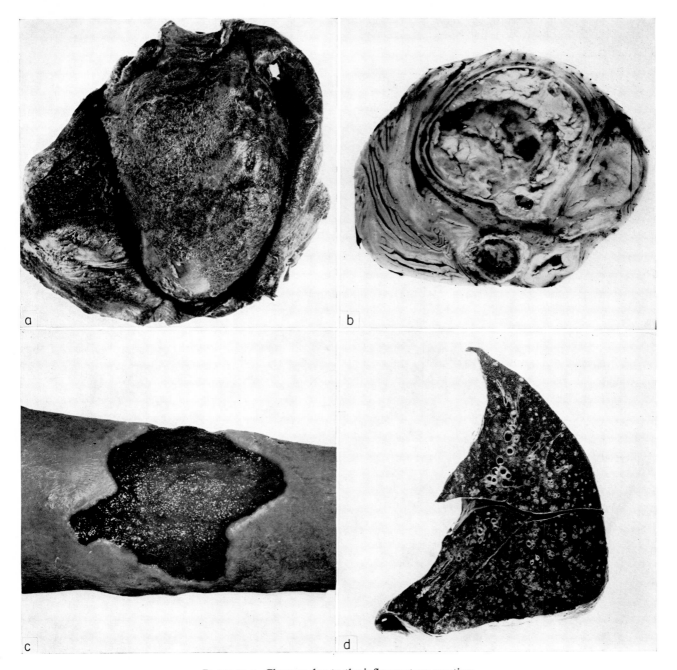

PLATE 21.1. Changes due to the inflammatory reaction.

(a) The pericardial sac has been opened to show the fibrinous exudate on the opposing surfaces in this case of fibrinous pericarditis. The strands of fibrin are clearly seen.

(b) Several chronic abscesses are seen in this section of cerebellum, each containing thick purulent material and enclosed by a well-defined wall.

(c) This chronic gravitational ulcer of the leg failed to heal, partly because of infection and partly because of impaired circulation due to varicose veins.

(d) On the cut surface of the lung, miliary tubercles are seen as discrete, pale foci, each only a few millimetres in diameter.

The basic components of the inflammatory response are now considered under the following heads:

(1) changes in the microcirculation,

(2) alteration of permeability of the vessel walls, and

(3) emigration of leucocytes, chemotaxis and phagocytosis.

Changes in the microcirculation during the acute inflammatory response

THE TRIPLE RESPONSE

The naked-eye appearance of an inflammatory reaction in the skin has already been described. The redness is due to an increased volume of blood flowing through the inflamed area. Because of this the temperature of the inflamed skin rises and approaches that of the blood in the central regions of the body, i.e. deep body temperature. The part, therefore, feels hot to the patient and to the observer.

Some of the vascular reactions of inflammation can be seen if a firm line is drawn with a blunt point over a suitable area of skin, for instance over the anterior surface of the forearm. As Sir Thomas Lewis pointed out in 1927, there is first a transitory white line which is, after a few seconds, succeeded by a **red line**; vasoconstriction and emptying of the vessels of the microcirculation is followed by vasodilation. A **weal**, or area of local oedema, begins to appear in association with this red line and surrounding both of these there is an irregular area of redness that spreads out 1 cm or so on either side of the red line; this is called a **flare**. The role of histamine in the triple response is discussed on p. 14.4, and the nervous mechanism is illustrated in fig. 21.1.

EXPERIMENTAL TECHNIQUES FOR OBSERVING THE MICROCIRCULATION

Observations are most satisfactorily made on thin sheets of tissue in the living animal. The light used for transillumination should not damage the tissue by heat or UV radiation; the cold light reflected down a quartz or 'Perspex' rod is very suitable. Observations by Leeuwenhoek early in the 1700's were made on the transparent tails of fish and tadpoles, and they became favourite objects of study; a nineteenth century gentleman's microscope was supplied with tubes to contain eels for such purposes. Later Waller and Cohnheim made accurate and detailed observations on the circulation of the frog in the thin web of tissue between the toes and in the pinned-out tongue. These observations have been extended to mammals by using the web of a bat's wing or an everted hamster cheek pouch. The mesenteries of many species are also thin enough, but this tissue must be kept moist and obviously the experiment has to be made on anaesthetized animals; both procedures may influence the inflammatory response. An ingenious preparation for

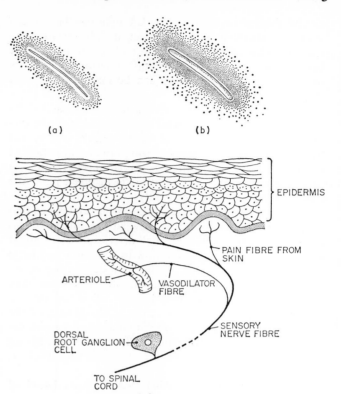

FIG. 21.1 Thomas Lewis' triple response.

(a) Soon after the skin has been stroked firmly by the marker, a red line appears surrounded by a diffuse reddening.

(b) Three to five minutes later this diffuse red area, the flare, becomes more sharply defined. The stroke is now oedematous and is raised slightly, making the weal. The weal is still present 30 min later, but the oedema fluid spreads out and the weal therefore becomes flattened and has less sharp edges.

The red line is due to dilation of the vessels of the microcirculation at the site of injury; the flare is produced by vasodilation brought about by the so-called axon reflex illustrated in (c).

(c) When the sensory nerve endings subserving pain are stimulated, afferent impulses travel up the sensory nerve fibre; branches from the sensory fibre pass to the nearby arterioles and produce vasodilation. If the main sensory trunk is cut, the axon reflex can be elicited for a few days but disappears as the separated proximal fibres degenerate.

accurate observation is the rabbit ear chamber. At a sterile operation, a hole is punched in a rabbit's ear and a chamber inserted so that the defect is filled by two cover glasses, a few millimetres apart. Blood fills the space between the two glasses but soon becomes organized, i.e. replaced by vascularized connective tissue. In a few weeks, when the tissue reaction has settled down, the microcirculation can be observed in the connective tissue in the ear chamber of a rabbit which has been trained to remain motionless in a quiet, darkened room. Injuries can be inflicted on the tissue by UV light or a laser beam without disturbing the chamber at all. Modifications in the technique allow the insertion of a few pathogenic bacteria in order to study inflammation caused by organisms. Similar chambers can be made in the loose skin in the flank of mice.

Other microcirculations which have been studied include that of the thin sheet of skeletal muscle of the cremaster in the young rat. The retinal vessels can be seen with a binocular microscope through the cornea without disturbing the eye. If fluorescein is injected into the carotid artery and observation made in green light, the retinal vessels show up brilliantly.

Using any of the above preparations it can be seen that in normal circumstances the flow in the larger vessels is laminar; in the veins and small arteries it has a rate of up to 150 mm/sec, while the flow in the aorta and large arteries may be as much as 800 mm/sec. As the blood passes from the larger to the minute vessels the flow falls to 0·5–1 mm/sec. The velocity of blood flow is inversely proportional to the cross sectional area of the vessel. Since the total cross-sectional area of the circulation increases markedly as the smaller arteries divide into arterioles, the flow diminishes at these sites (vol. 1, p. 28.26).

As the red cells pass in laminar flow, they are deformed into drop-like shapes and they may be deformed again as they pass through the narrowest capillaries, some of which may be only 2 μm in diameter, whereas erythrocytes are normally about 8 μm. Krogh estimated that there were in a section of skeletal muscle some 2000 capillaries/mm². The other vessels of the microcirculation and their internal diameters are as follows; the smallest arteries 250–30 μm, the arterioles 30–20 μm, the postcapillary venules 20–50 μm and the small veins 50–250 μm. Vessels larger than 300 μm are visible to the naked eye and are not considered part of the microcirculation. The geographical organization of the capillary bed has been described in great detail for the mesentery, the cremaster muscle, the rabbit's ear chamber and other systems. In some circulations, e.g. the hamster cheek pouch, there is an arch-like arrangement of small arteries and veins with a net of capillaries filling in the arch. In others, e.g. the mesentery, the capillary bed is in parallel with by-pass vessels, and in this case smooth muscle sphincters around the precapillary vessels can divert the blood either into the bed or through the by-pass vessel. These muscle sphincters can be seen to contract and relax rhythmically at intervals of from one second to many minutes, a process called **vasomotion**. Sometimes, as in the cremaster muscle, there is a ladder-like arrangement parallel to the muscle fibres, with horizontal vessels forming cross connections. In other capillary beds, there appears to be a less highly organized arrangement of vessels.

OBSERVATIONS ON THE MICROCIRCULATION DURING INFLAMMATION

During and after injuries of various kinds the changes are those that would be expected from naked eye observations of the triple response. There is often an initial vasoconstriction, but after a few minutes this gives place to arteriolar dilation. About 30 min after an acute injury the whole capillary bed is suffused with blood at an increased pressure. Capillaries which were closed open up and those already patent dilate. The venules participate in the dilation, and there is an increased flow of blood in the draining veins. The flow continues to be rapid in all vessels for a while, but as the reaction develops the blood in the widely dilated capillaries and venules begins to slow and in many vessels may stop completely, i.e., **stasis**, or oscillate to and fro. Slowing and stasis may occur centrally in the lesion while rapid flow continues more peripherally. However, a secondary extension of stasis may develop after a few hours and involve peripheral areas as well.

The phase of rapid flow through a widely dilated microcirculation results from vasodilation of the arterioles and of such specialized structures as the precapillary sphincters. The succeeding phase of stasis is more difficult to explain. The pressure in the capillaries increases as stasis develops so there must be an associated increase in resistance to outflow. The pressure in the small veins may be increased by a rise in pressure in the interstitial fluid due to oedema, and there may be some venomotor activity; there is also increased viscosity of the blood due to exudation of fluid from the minute vessels with consequent concentration of the remaining cells. Clumping of erythrocytes intravascularly produces a characteristic appearance in the living circulation when seen under the microscope; the cells appear aggregated into an amorphous jelly-like material, a process which has been called **sludging**. However, if the circulation in the vessel starts again, the red blood cells separate once more.

Alterations in permeability of the vessel wall

From the very earliest stages of inflammation, the vessel walls of the microcirculation become much more permeable to plasma proteins. This may be shown by a simple experiment on rats. The dye, Evans blue, injected intravenously, becomes attached to plasma albumin. The shaved skin of such rats has only a slightly bluish tinge. An area of inflamed skin can then be produced in an anaesthetized rat by pressing a disk, heated to 45°C, for a few minutes to the shaved part. The disk-shaped area shows the classical signs of inflammation, and it gradually becomes deep blue. Increased amounts of albumin, labelled in this case with dye, leak out of the microcirculation. The tissue fluids of the inflamed area contain an abnormally high concentration of protein, about the same as the plasma. Acute inflammation due to other injuries, including invasion by pathogenic micro-organisms, similarly produces excess tissue fluids with a high protein content. The lymph flow draining in-flamed areas is increased and the protein content is, naturally, high. The lymphatics are kept open by their fibrous attachments to the surrounding tissue but little is known about the permeability of the lymphatics and their role in areas in which the tissue tension is raised by inflammatory oedema. This tissue oedema leads to swelling of the affected part though it is recognized per-haps more easily macroscopically than microscopically. In tissue sections separation of the fibres and cells of the connective tissue, with clear spaces between them, is seen. Similar separation may occur, but to a much less degree, between the cells of a compact epithelial organ.

The factors which predispose to the formation of excess extravascular fluid include a fall in intravascular colloid osmotic pressure due to the increased permeability of the small vessels, and an increase in pressure within the small vessels of the inflamed area. This increase of pressure, which has been measured directly, is due to arteriolar dilation and to obstruction of outflow, in part caused by packing of erythrocytes, leucocytes and platelets on the venous side. The pressure within the capillaries and venules is raised even when there is vascular stasis.

Three questions now arise.

(1) Which vessels become more permeable to protein in an inflamed area?

(2) What changes occur in the blood vessel wall to allow more protein to escape?

(3) What is the mechanism by which many types of noxious agent produce a common pattern of response?

It has for long been assumed that the vessels which show increased permeability in inflammation are the capillaries. It is now known that in the microcirculation of muscle the venules are the vessels most commonly affected (fig. 21.2). What happens to the vessel walls may be seen in electron micrographs. Changes in permeability may be studied by injecting into the circulation electron-dense particles in colloidal suspension; mercuric sulphide (HgS) can be used or the iron-containing protein, ferritin. In normal vessels of muscle, the endothelial cells abut on one another with less than 2 nm separation between the plasma membrane of one cell and that of the next. Junctions between cells known as maculae adhaerentes or desmosomes (vol. 1, p. 13.11) may help to seal the two cells together though, as we shall see, cells can be pulled apart at these junctions. Outside the endo-thelial cells there is normally an intact basement mem-brane which splits to enclose the phagocytic peri-cytes (fig. 21.3). In the minute vessels of the liver, how-ever, which normally leak much plasma protein, there are gaps between the cells. In inflamed muscle, a similar, but in this case abnormal, separation of the endothelial cells occurs in the venules. Gaps as much as 800 nm

18

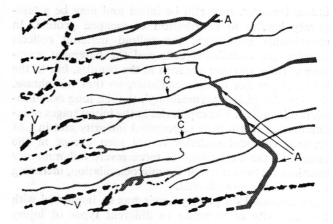

FIG. 21.2. The microcirculation of the cremaster muscle of the rat after a local injection of histamine. The animal has received systemic injection of colloidal HgS. The leaking vessels have been labelled by these particles.

There is deposition of the tracer particles particularly on the venous side. The arterioles and considerable lengths of the finest capillary segments are spared.

A = arteriole; C = capillary; V = venule

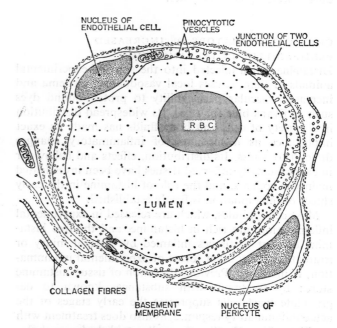

FIG. 21.3. The EM appearance of a section through a small venule or capillary. Two endothelial cells are sectioned; in one the section has not passed through the nucleus. The basement membrane is split and encloses a pericyte.

appear within a few minutes and injected colloidal material can be seen, on EM photographs, lying in the gaps between the endothelial cells. The basement membrane, however, may still be intact and may be a temporary barrier to distribution of escaped protein. In experiments with HgS, the colloid material collects between the endothelial cells and the basement membrane. These changes are seen in the venules, but in the initial stages not in the capillaries, so that the phrase, 'increased capillary permeability', though long established, is misleading. The capillaries in the initial stages of inflammation retain their endothelial integrity and in EM sections colloidal material is not seen except in the lumen. In the later stages of more severe inflammatory reactions all the vessels of the microcirculation, including the capillaries, are affected.

As discussed on p. 14.5 Lewis was so impressed with the similarity of response to different types of injury that he suggested these changes were brought about by a common mediator which he called the H-substance or histamine-like substance. Since Lewis' day, other vasoactive substances have been shown to be liberated from damaged tissue and from platelets; these include 5-HT, ATP and ADP, kinins such as the nonapeptide bradykinin and many others. The problem is now to find out which of the many vasoactive substances discovered have roles in the inflammatory response and during which phases they act.

CHEMICAL MEDIATORS OF INCREASED
PERMEABILITY IN INFLAMMATION

Histamine, when injected into the skin of experimental animals or man, causes local vasodilation, oedema and increased vascular permeability to protein-bound dyes such as Evans blue (p. 14.4). Its widespread distribution in a variety of cells and body fluids has made its exact importance as a mediator of inflammatory changes difficult to assess. Its distribution, effects and behaviour in experimentally inflamed tissues have been investigated mainly in rodents, and the role of histamine in the early stages of inflammation is firmly established.

Mast cell granules, which are released in experimental inflammation, are rich in histamine, and the free histamine content of tissues inflamed by thermal injury or irradiation or by other forms of experimental inflammation, is increased. Previous depletion of tissue histamine stores by treatment with substances known to degranulate mast cells suppresses the early stages of the acute inflammatory response, as also does treatment with antihistamines. Finally, the well established morphological change resulting from the action of histamine, i.e. the separation of endothelial cell junctions in venules, is consistent with the observed increase in vascular permeability to plasma proteins.

Whether or not histamine has a continuing role in the inflammatory process beyond the first half hour or so is less certain. Depletion of measurable tissue histamine and treatment with antihistamines do not affect this later phase of inflammation and there is a strong presumption that some other mediator takes over, although it has been argued that the widespread distribution of histidine decarboxylase, the enzyme involved in histamine production, means that the local production and action of histamine may continue. The question of exactly how histamine causes the opening up of endothelial gaps is still unsolved. Contraction of smooth muscle in small veins, causing passive congestion in the smaller venules, is one possibility, while another is that it affects a contractile mechanism in the endothelial cells.

5-Hydroxytryptamine (5-HT) in low concentration produces vascular effects similar to those of histamine in some species. Since this amine is also widely distributed, particularly in rat mast cells and human platelets, a function as a mediator of inflammation has been suggested for it, but the evidence for this is not as strong as is that for histamine. In any event, as with histamine, any action it may have is likely to occur in the initial stages only.

Peptides resulting from the partial hydrolysis of several different proteins have been found to have vasodilator and permeability-increasing effects. These are known collectively as kinins, and those about which most is known are bradykinin and kallidin, as found in various body fluids (p. 17.3). These have clear cut actions consistent with roles as mediators of inflammation. Kinins are relatively quickly destroyed by kininases, which makes their investigation difficult *in vivo*, but, being produced from a precursor abundant in plasma and tissue fluid, these peptides are strong candidates for the mediators of the acute inflammatory response beyond the first half hour.

Other substances with possible roles in inflammation of various types are currently under investigation and include RNA and its breakdown products, and a high molecular weight factor isolated from lymph node cells which may be concerned with the inflammatory changes in delayed hypersensitivity reactions. This substance, the **lymph node permeability factor** (LNPF), has been purified from guinea-pig lymph nodes after ultrasonic disintegration. The local concentration of LNPF parallels the severity of the inflammatory response in the tuberculin reaction. The factor is a potent leucotactic substance and may also increase vascular permeability.

LNPF is of interest in that it has vasodilator and permeability-increasing actions, but, unlike the other mediators, no histamine-like action on smooth muscle, nor does it lower blood pressure (p. 14.16).

Some of the mediators described above may also affect leucocyte emigration or may cause pain in inflamed tissues, but the evidence is insufficiently strong to label any one of them the chemotactic or pain-producing agent.

Emigration of leucocytes and phagocytosis

NEUTROPHIL POLYMORPHS

The polymorphs have an obvious role in the reactions of the tissues to invasion by bacteria such as *Staph. aureus.* If not killed first, polymorphs may eat up the disease-producing bacteria. Normal tissues contain few extra-vascular polymorphs; in inflammation, however, these cells, formed in the bone marrow and released into the circulating blood, escape from the microcirculation through the vessel wall. In this way an easily mobilizable reserve of short-lived cells is provided by dispersed manufacturing centres, for use in any infected part of the body.

What is the mechanism by which polymorphs leave vessels only in inflamed tissues? Observations of the microcirculation in preparations such as the ear chamber show that immediately following any injury the blood polymorphs stick momentarily to the endothelium; they roll along the inside surface of the vessel wall, slower than the axial stream of red cells, adhering briefly before they are once more swept off into the circulation. After a few minutes, more and more adhere so firmly that they are not dislodged by the blood flow. The endothelium comes in this way to have a lining of adhering polymorphs, by a process sometimes called **margination** (fig. 21.4 and plate 21.4a, facing p. 21.10). Other leucocytes, platelets and red cells may also stick to the endothelial cell surface. There is most probably some change in the properties of the endothelial cell membrane, but the change is beyond the limits of resolution of the present-day EM. Vaso-active substances such as bradykinin cause leucocytes to stick to the vessel wall; it has also been suggested that proteolytic enzymes from lysosomes may be partly responsible.

The marginated polymorph leaves its intravascular site by its own efforts; this is called **emigration** or **diapedesis** (walking through, plate 21.4b, facing p. 21.10). No chemotactic stimulus has been demonstrated to emigration

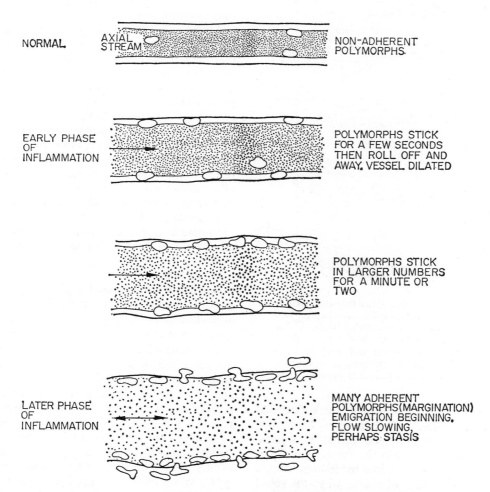

FIG. 21.4. Adhesion of polymorphs to a venule wall in an inflamed area. After Clark E.R. & Clark E.L. (1935) *Amer. J. Anat.* **57,** 385.

which seems to follow inevitably from adhesion to the endothelial wall. The cell moves by the spread of pseudopodia, and this is sometimes referred to as amoeboid movement. From a polymorph adhering to the vessel wall in an inflamed area, a pseudopodium insinuates itself between the endothelial cells, apparently not impeded by the tight junctions. The bulk of the cell, including the nucleus, passes through the intercellular space and comes to lie outside the endothelial cell. It has still to pass the basement membrane, which forms a definite barrier to penetration, as is seen in the EM. The manner in which the polymorphs pass through this barrier is not known, but no gaps visible by EM are left behind. All this takes time, but within 60 min from their adhesion to the vessel wall, polymorphs are moving through the interstitium of the tissues (figs. 21.5 & 6 and plates 21.2 & 3).

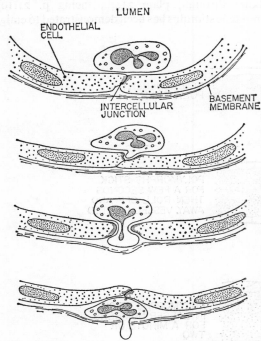

FIG. 21.5. The migration of a polymorph through a venule in acute inflammation. Using a rabbit's ear chamber and making direct observations in the living state, it has been shown that the time taken for migration is about 5–10 min. Once through the vessel wall and its basement membrane, the polymorph can move at 20 μm/min. After Marchesi V.T. & Gowans J.L. (1964). *Proc. roy. Soc. B.* **159**, 283.

Sometimes erythrocytes pass through the endothelial wall in the wake of emigrating polymorphs. Moreover, weakening of the vessel wall by endothelial cell separation, with a high pressure within the vessel, sometimes allows small leaks of erythrocytes into the tissues. Minute haemorrhages may take place, of course, when the vessel walls are involved in tissue destruction caused by bac-

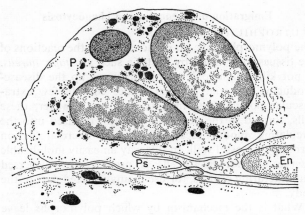

FIG. 21.6. A polymorph (P) adherent to the endothelium of an inflamed vessel of a rat's mesentery. A pseudopod (Ps) is extending into the endothelium (En) and is apparently separating the intercellular junctions; ahead of the advancing pseudopod the junction looks morphologically intact. After Marchesi V.T. (1961) *Quart. J. exp. Physiol.* **46**, 115.

teria. Haemorrhagic exudates often denote a serious inflammatory process.

After emigration, are polymorphs then guided by chemotaxis (chemical attraction) or do they move at random? If by chemotaxis, do the chemotactic agents come from bacteria or from the damaged tissues? These questions have not been answered by direct *in vivo* experiments, but *in vitro* observations on isolated polymorphs in culture media have shown that bacteria, alive or dead, can exert a chemotactic effect. A chemotactic stimulus is produced also after antigen–antibody complexing (p. 22.13); this involves two or more steps and results in the production, from one of the plasma proteins, of a chemotactic agent. No satisfactory evidence exists that dead tissues themselves, autolysed or not, attract polymorphs. It has been suggested, however, that the chemotactic substance is produced by a reaction between an enzyme in the serum and a component of damaged tissues.

In an inflamed site, the polymorph in its wanderings through the tissues comes into the chemotactic orbit of bacteria or of the plasma factor, produced by a bacterial antigen–antibody complex. The cell must now move up the concentration gradient of the chemotactic stimulus to the bacteria in an approximately straight line. Here the cytotoxic products of the bacteria may kill the cell. If it stays alive, however, contact between bacterium and cell surface results in adhesion followed by ingestion of the organisms by the cell. This is, of course, **phagocytosis** (vol. 1, p. 13.11). If isolated bacteria and suspensions of polymorphs are brought into contact randomly by being rotated together in a tube, ingestion of the bacteria occurs almost equally well at room temperature as at 37°C. When clumps of organisms or tissue debris are ingested, the cytoplasm of the polymorph flows around

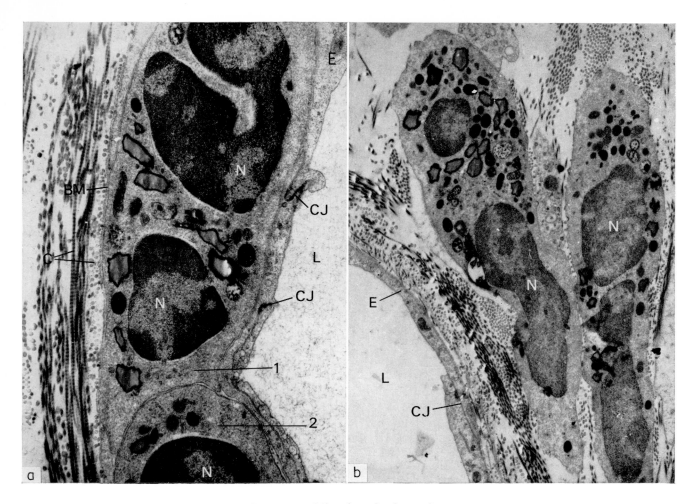

PLATE 21.2. Migration of polymorphs.

(a) Section through a small vessel of a rabbit's ear inflamed by ultraviolet radiation. Two polymorphs (1 and 2) have migrated through the endothelium (E) and are lying in a subendothelial position. There are two intact cell junctions (CJ) in the endothelium, and the basement membrane (BM) of the endothelial cells is seen; this has been stripped away from the cells by the leucocytes. Bundles of collagen fibres (C) in the perivascular sheath run at right angles to one another, those near the basement membrane being cut transversely and those further away longitudinally; N, nucleus; L, lumen; (× 17,000). From Florey H.W. & Grant L.H. (1961) *J. Path. Bact.* **82**, 13. By courtesy of Lady Florey.

(b) In this section, two polymorphs are shown free in the connective tissue surrounding a small blood vessel; they have passed through the basement membrane. Lumen (L) of the vessel; E, endothelium; CJ, cell junction; N, nucleus; (× 15,300). From Florey H.W. & Grant L.H. (1961) *J. Path. Bact.* **82**, 13. By courtesy of Lady Florey.

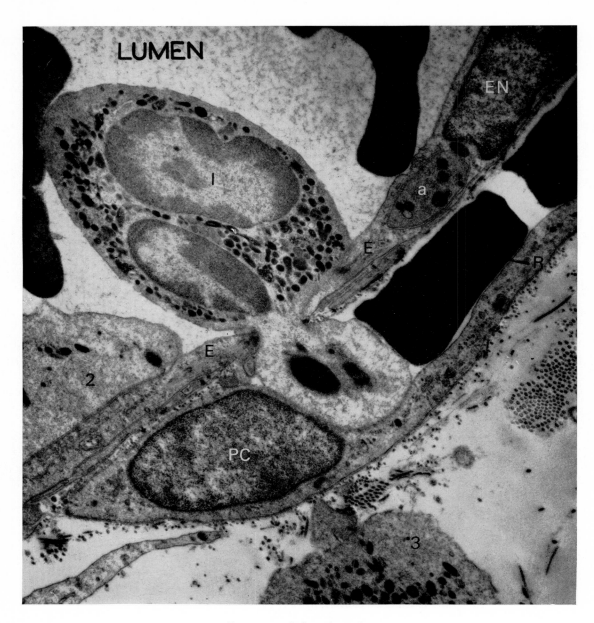

PLATE 21.3. Inflamed venule.

Cell 1 is a polymorph passing through the endothelium (E). Its advancing process is seen in contact with a periendothelial cell (PC). Two red cells (R) are in the periendothelial space. An object (a), which might be a platelet or the tip of a polymorph, can be seen pushing into the endothelial cytoplasm. Cell 2 is a polymorph adherent to the endothelium, and cell 3 is a polymorph in the perivascular connective tissue; (×15,500). From Marchesi V.T. & Florey H.W. (1960) *Quart. J. exp. Physiol.* **45**, 343.

the particle which is eventually included, if small enough, in a large, membrane-bounded vesicle within the cell.

Using isolated cells it can be shown that the ingestion of bacteria and other particles is greatly enhanced by the presence of antibodies. These phagocytosis-promoting Ig-globulins which coat the bacterium or other foreign body are called **opsonins** (fig. 21.7 and p. 22.14).

Once the bacterium has been ingested it is often killed and digested by the lysosomes of the polymorph; these contain proteolytic and other hydrolysing enzymes which are discharged into the vesicle containing the organisms. Whether it has eaten and digested bacteria or not, the cell undergoes degenerative changes after a day or so. The nucleus is rounded up and the cell comes to resemble the small round cell of the tissues surrounding a focus of subacute or chronic inflammation (p. 21.10). In some circumstances, ingested bacteria may continue to multiply and the cell may burst open releasing infective micro-organisms into the tissues. Some micro-organisms are indeed adapted to intracellular life, e.g. *Neisseria*.

We have considered emigration and phagocytosis by polymorphs in relation to the inflammation caused by micro-organisms. There are disastrous consequences when the bone marrow fails to produce polymorphs. This may happen after radiation damage, or as a feared reaction to treatment with drugs such as chloramphenicol, or in leukaemia. Death in these cases results from bacteria multiplying unchecked in the tissues.

A typical sequence of responses resulting in massive emigration of polymorphs can occur in inflammation due to nonbacterial causes, for instance after the injection of turpentine.

EOSINOPHILS

The eosinophil polymorphs emigrate in small numbers from blood vessels in inflamed areas. They have, *in vitro*, an ability to move, to be attracted chemotactically and to phagocytose similar to that of the neutrophil polymorph. However, they are inconspicuous in most inflammatory responses but larger numbers are present in hypersensitivity reactions and in helminth infections.

MONOCYTES

The polymorphs are not the only cells to leave the microcirculation during inflammation. Blood monocytes also can be seen to stick to the endothelial cells. Proportionately fewer monocytes than polymorphs adhere; there are, of course, in the blood usually six times as many polymorphs. The adhering monocytes emigrate by their active movements through intercellular gaps just as the polymorphs do, and accumulate in an area of tissue damage or at a bacterial focus. Chemotactic responses can be shown *in vitro* but how important these are in inflammation is not known. In a day or so after

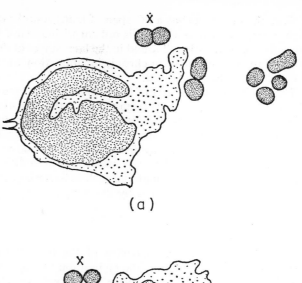

(a)

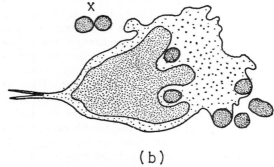

(b)

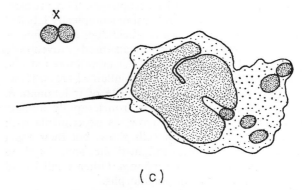

(c)

Fig. 21.7. Phagocytosis. Successive traces taken at 2 min intervals of a leucocyte as it ingests pneumococci in the presence of a specific antibody (opsonin). In this *in vitro* preparation, the leucocyte is moving across the field from left to right. There are eight cocci in the field; two, labelled x, do not touch the cell, but the remainder are ingested. After Wood W.B., Smith M.R. & Watson V. (1946) *J. exp. Med.* **84**, 387.

emigration, monocytes become indistinguishable in both appearance and function from tissue macrophages; they are actively phagocytic, eating tissue debris and bacteria. They can, on occasion, be seen to engulf polymorphs.

Since the monocyte has a life span of many months or even years, rather than days, it is not surprising that it is often the characteristic cell found in the later stages of the inflammatory response or in chronic inflammation when emigration has largely ceased.

These cells constitute part of the population of macrophages. Another part comes from the local tissue histiocytes. Macrophages engulf bacteria, dead polymorphs, and particulate material; some of this is digested by their lysosomal enzymes. They are instrumental in removing the debris to the regional lymph nodes and in addition they may process antigenic material such as bacteria prior to the formation of antibodies by the lymphocyte series of cells.

LYMPHOCYTES

What happens to the lymphocytes of the blood? Do they take part in margination and emigration? Relatively few circulating lymphocytes adhere to inflamed vessels, and consequently few are seen penetrating the inter-endothelial gap. In this context the surface properties and behaviour of lymphocytes differ from those of polymorphs and monocytes, for they do not adhere to glass or move towards any known chemotactic stimulus. Yet lymphocytes have a special affinity for the endothelial surface of the venules of the lymph nodes; they penetrate the actual cells of these vessels during their normal recirculation between blood and lymph.

It has been suggested that the small round cells in and near an inflammatory lesion are lymphocytes and that these differentiate into macrophages. This problem can be investigated in the rat, using isotopically labelled small lymphocytes from the thoracic duct or thymus or lymph nodes. When such cells are transfused intravenously to another but untreated rat of the same inbred strain, the labelled cells do not appear in inflamed areas. However, there are round cells at the site of inflammation. These appear to be derived in part from a rapidly dividing line of cells in the bone marrow, as experiments with transfused labelled marrow cells show, but their exact nature is unknown. In an inflamed site, some of these cells differentiate into macrophages. Other small round cells may be derived from polymorphs.

In an acute inflammatory focus, therefore, there are living, dying and dead polymorphs, all of which have crawled out of the nearby dilated vessels of the microcirculation, principally the venules. Some of the degenerating polymorphs are seen as small round cells in fixed and stained preparations. Present in smaller numbers are emigrated monocytes and tissue macrophages; after a day or so these two cell types are indistinguishable. In addition other cells, morphologically small round cells, which have come out of the circulation are present; these are not part of the population of re-circulating lymphocytes, but have been formed in the marrow during the previous 24 hours. They can mature into macrophages. Plasma cells are also present in relatively small numbers at this stage, and varying amounts of fibrin can be seen in fixed and stained sections (plate 21.2c). As described on p. 21.2, an acute inflammatory exudate on a serous membrane is often mainly fibrinous in character (plate 21.1a, facing p. 21.2).

Inflammatory responses can spread and involve more tissue. Cell death and pus formation can lead to a further progression of the lesion or, if a well defined wall develops around a localized collection of pus, to abscess formation. Dead polymorphs accumulate at the inflammatory focus and liberate digestive enzymes which cause liquefaction of dead tissue cells. The liquefied mass becomes visible to the naked eye as thick yellow pus; the process by which the pus is formed is called **suppuration**, and the exudate is referred to as **suppurative** or **purulent**. Pus consists of dead and living polymorphs, macrophages, the remains of necrotic tissue cells and microorganisms. The wall of an acute abscess consists of fibrin and polymorphs. During the process of suppuration and abscess formation the marrow increases production of polymorphs and the blood contains a number of young cells with a smaller number of lobes in the nuclei (a reduced Arneth count).

If the acute inflammatory process subsides and the condition becomes chronic, the cardinal signs of Celsus disappear.

Chronic inflammation

A chronic inflammatory state may persist for months or years but a state where the destructive and healing processes are nicely balanced is infrequent. Usually periods of repair are interrupted by further acute inflammatory changes with exudation, emigration, etc., to be followed by a further period of regression and repair.

Chronic inflammation differs from the acute in two important ways. Firstly, the cellular exudate becomes more varied, but is made up mostly of mononuclear cells. Secondly, chronic inflammation is attended by proliferation of the connective tissues of the affected area; because of the formation of new tissue, the process is described as **formative** or **productive**, in contrast to the **exudative** nature of acute inflammation, where exudation of fluid and plasma proteins plays such an important part.

The mononuclear cells are lymphocytes, plasma cells and macrophages (plate 21.4d). Of these, only the macrophages are under chemotactic influence and capable of phagocytosis. The plasma cells and lymphocytes provide a more subtle and enduring defence by means of antibody formation. There is no clear understanding of how lymphocytes and plasma cells differ in function, or of why one cell type sometimes greatly outnumbers the

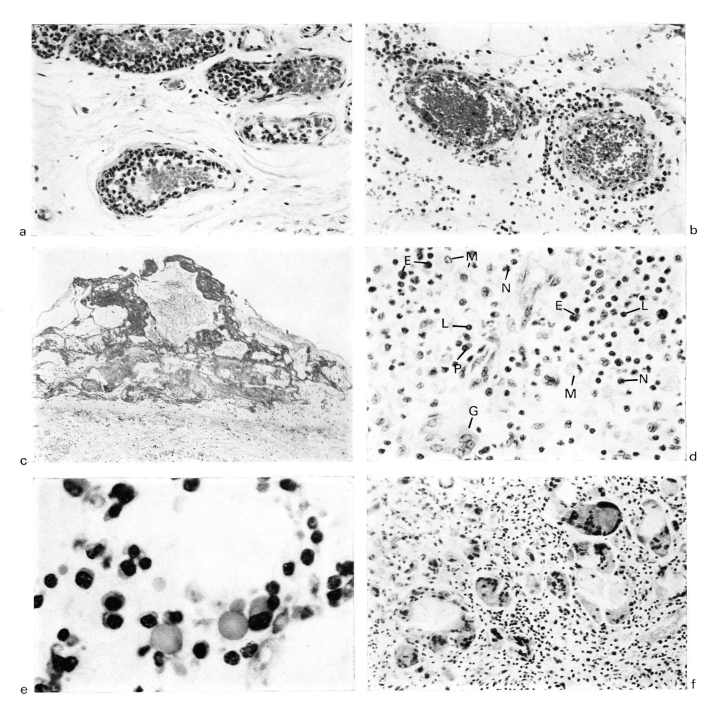

PLATE 21.4. Histology of inflammation.

(a) In the early stage of acute inflammation, polymorphs aggregate at the periphery of the blood stream, along the inner margin of the vascular walls, prior to passage through the walls. This is known as margination. Haem. & eosin (× 240).

(c) In this field from a specimen of fibrinous pericarditis, eosinophilic, structureless strands of fibrin are seen covering the surface; a little myocardium is demonstrable deep to the exudate. Haem. & eosin (× 50).

(e) The rounded, hyaline eosinophilic masses are Russell bodies; they are derived from plasma cells actively synthesizing antibody, and may be found intracellularly or extracellularly. Haem. & eosin (× 650).

(b) While margination of polymorphs is still seen, many are now passing or have passed through the vessel wall (emigration); they are infiltrating the surrounding tissue. Haem. & eosin (× 180).

(d) This field is taken from a focus of chronic inflammation. In addition to neutrophil polymorphs (N), there are lymphocytes (L), plasma cells (P), macrophages (M), and a few eosinophils (E) and giant cells (G). Haem. & eosin (× 370).

(f) Multinucleated foreign-body giant cells are aggregated around faintly-staining foreign material; other inflammatory cells are also present. The giant cells show different patterns of nuclei, including peripheral arrangement. Haem. & eosin (× 160).

other. Round hyaline masses, about the size of a plasma cell but without a nucleus, are occasionally seen in long-standing chronic inflammatory lesions. They are known as **Russell bodies**, and are thought to be derived by extrusion from the cytoplasm of plasma cells (plate 21.4e & vol. 1, p. 27.12).

Other inflammatory cells occur less constantly. Some neutrophil polymorphs may persist when an acute inflammatory process becomes chronic; in a chronic pyogenic abscess, polymorphs persist in the suppurative centre while the picture of chronic inflammation develops at the periphery.

Eosinophils are peculiarly unpredictable in their occurrence. They tend to be most numerous in chronic inflammation involving the skin, the lungs and the intestinal tract, and are conspicuous in inflammatory processes of allergic or parasitic origin. They occur, however, in other reactive lesions without demonstrable cause, though not during the acute phase, so that their presence may be an indication of chronicity, or perhaps of healing. Their function is obscure. Though phagocytic, they seem to have little or no part to play in the defence against bacteria. Their life span is thought to be much longer than that of neutrophils. It is possible that they are concerned with absorption of the products of an antigen–antibody reaction, and another action may be as an antagonist to histamine.

Macrophages assume distinctive forms in certain circumstances. In the presence of necrotic fat, their cytoplasm develops a foamy vacuolated appearance, and they may then be called **lipophages**. In lesions where there has been much haemorrhage, phagocytosis of iron pigment results in a pigmented stippling of the cytoplasm, and such cells are termed **siderophages**.

Macrophages may fuse to form **multinucleate cells**, in which several nuclei are contained within one cytoplasmic mass; another possible mechanism of formation is by nuclear division without division of cytoplasm, but this seems unlikely. Multinucleate cells may reach a very large size, up to 10–12 times the size of a mononuclear macrophage, and are then called **giant cells** (fig. 21.8).

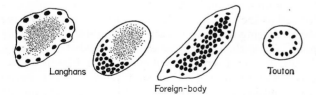

Langhans   Foreign-body   Touton

FIG. 21.8. Tuberculous, or Langhans, giant cells typically have nuclei around the periphery or aggregated at one pole; in foreign-body giant cells they tend to be scattered throughout the cytoplasm, and Touton cells, associated with phagocytosis of fat, possess a ring of nuclei. These features, however, are not rigidly exclusive, and any of the types may be seen in any one condition.

These have large numbers of nuclei, and since the diameter of the cell greatly exceeds the thickness of an ordinary histological section, the number of nuclei must be much greater than appears in the two-dimensional view under the microscope. Giant cells form around particles which are too large to be engulfed by mononuclear phagocytes, such as foreign bodies of extraneous origin, unabsorbable surgical suture material or the cholesterol deposits which occur in sites of old necrosis or haemorrhage. They may then form clusters or elongated syncytial masses around the foreign body (plate 21.4f). A distinctive type of giant cell is more rounded and has its nuclei arranged in a complete or incomplete peripheral ring; this is the **Langhans giant cell**, most often associated with tuberculosis. Another type is the **Touton giant cell**, seen in conditions which involve phagocytosis of lipid; the cytoplasm is foamy, as in the mononuclear lipophage, while the ring of nuclei is not peripheral but is separated from the cell boundary by a zone of cytoplasm. Giant cells occur also in measles and other viral infections.

Repair and Regeneration

When an inflammatory lesion subsides completely, vascular dilation diminishes and oedema disappears as the fluid exudate is reabsorbed by the lymphatics. Polymorphs which have perished in the battle are phagocytosed and destroyed by macrophages or are carried to the lymph nodes and meet a similar fate there. It is remarkable how completely all trace of the inflammatory process can be removed. Even fibrinous exudate can be digested by enzymic action and the products absorbed.

Repair and regeneration do not await the completion of the inflammatory process; the reparative phase begins before the inflammatory phase is complete, and the one merges imperceptibly with the other.

The simplest form of the repair process occurs in a surgical wound, where destruction of tissue is minimal, the margins of the wound are closely apposed, and with proper precautions bacterial infection can be excluded. In this form of healing, called 'primary union' or 'healing by first intention', the essential elements of the process are proliferation of fibroblasts, which ultimately form collagen, and formation of new capillary vessels.

In many inflammatory and traumatic lesions, however, there may be substantial loss or displacement of tissue, or destruction of tissue by necrosis or haemorrhage. In these circumstances, and especially if there is also bacterial infection, the healing process is necessarily slower and more complex, since it involves absorption of the inflammatory exudate and of the dead tissue, as well as replacement of tissue which has been lost or destroyed. This is called secondary union, or healing 'by granulation' or 'by secondary intention'.

The process of repair is described in relation to a heat

injury, since this has been used as a model for acute inflammation, although of course the processes described are common to the repair of any inflammatory or traumatic lesion. Let us assume that the injury is such that, over a central area of a few square centimetres, the cells of the epidermis and of the dermis have been killed by heat (a third degree burn). Around the central necrotic area there is an intermediate zone where epidermis but not dermis is largely destroyed; further out, the skin is severely inflamed and shows vascular stasis, oedema and leucocyte emigration. At the periphery of the lesion, say 10 or 15 cm from the necrotic centre, little more than the vascular flare of a triple response occurs.

Healing is delayed if pathogenic organisms gain access to the scalded area and multiply there; in these circumstances the area of inflammation and tissue injury extends. It is therefore of great importance clinically to keep pathogens away by sterile dressings and careful aseptic nursing technique. If this is done, the inflammatory response subsides gradually in the outer zone of the inflamed area. In the tissues where there is much exudation and emigration of leucocytes, multiplication of fibroblasts and laying down of collagen occurs. In this way, an interstitial inflammatory exudate is replaced by firm fibrous material; the area becomes hard to the touch and is said to be indurated.

Repair in the more central areas presents further problems. For the purpose of analysis we may separate,

(1) healing where the epithelial cells of the surface alone have been killed (a second degree burn), and

(2) healing in the central areas where epidermis and dermis have been destroyed (a third degree burn).

EPITHELIAL REPAIR

The epithelial cells at the margins of the ulcer begin to spread across the dermal surface denuded of epithelium. At a cellular level, at least three processes are involved, more or less simultaneously. The adhesive properties of the cells at the edge change so that they are no longer tightly bound together but slide on one another. Within a few hours of injury the cells leave the margins of the lesion to cover the edges of the bare surface with a layer of cells; they are no longer attached to each other by the normal intercellular adhesions. Secondly, the cells of the basal and spinous layers of the epithelium multiply faster. The highest rates occur not at the very edge of the ulcer but a millimetre or so out from this. Cell division occurs also in the cells that have moved in from the margins of the lesion. Thirdly, by a process sometimes called dedifferentiation, the morphological characteristics of the epithelial cells of the margins change. The cells that move across the surface, for instance, are more flattened than normal basal squamous epithelial cells and their nuclei have a looser texture. Similar changes take place in the repair of all wounds

and discontinuities involving epithelia; the repair of a surgical incision through the skin, or of an acute gastric ulcer or a bladder incision is associated with diminution of cell adhesiveness, increased mitotic rates and dedifferentiation of nearby epithelial cells.

In spite of years of work, it is not yet possible to define precisely the way in which these changes are brought about. Perhaps we shall have to discover first the method by which a normal epithelium so regulates its cell division, adhesive properties and differentiation that continuity is maintained but overgrowth prevented. Does interruption of continuity by a burn or an incision or ulcer remove factors inhibiting multiplication and separation of cells, or alternatively, does injury to tissue produce humoral substances, wound hormones, that stimulate division and separation? There is indirect support for both views. For instance, normal cells when plated out in tissue culture as a dense suspension of single cells move short distances over the surface until they come into contact with other cells; their movement is then inhibited because the cell surfaces in contact stay at rest. Cells derived from invading neoplasms show little or no contact inhibition. In tissue culture explants of normal cells, the margin of growth is directed outwards, because of contact inhibition; if a sheet of cells is allowed to grow in tissue culture, the rate of division is greatest at the periphery. In addition, a small area of the growth in a tissue culture may be punched out at a distance from the advancing edge, where there is little growth or movement. Repair is then effected by directional movement of cells, freed from contact inhibition, while cells around the defect will be stimulated to divide. Other experiments with tissue culture may indicate the role of humoral factors and some of these are discussed on p. 27.2.

In the injury we are considering, a second degree burn of the skin, the cells that have formed the epithelial covering have been destroyed. The area is re-covered by living cells moving and growing in at the edge of the lesion. Often small epithelial islands may develop in the middle of the denuded area; these originate from invaginations of the original epidermis associated with hairs, and sweat and sebaceous glands. These cells, embedded as they are in the depths of the dermis, may have escaped being destroyed. Very useful additional growing points for epithelial replacement are provided in this way. A surgeon may create artificially such islands of regeneration by taking epithelial fragments (skin grafts) from another part of the skin and laying them on the burnt area, but only autografts can be used (vol. 1, p. 27.13).

CONNECTIVE TISSUE REPAIR

We now have to consider healing in the central areas where the whole thickness of the skin, epidermis and dermis, has been destroyed, with perhaps death of some underlying tissues. In this case there is loss, not only of epithelium, but also of connective tissue, blood vessels, lymphatics, nerves, both sensory and vasomotor, sweat and sebaceous glands and a number of other cell types. The ulcerated area exudes a protein-containing fluid closely resembling blood plasma, mixed with emigrated white cells and a variable number of erythrocytes. Fibrinogen escapes with the other plasma proteins and this forms fibrin strands in the exudate. Whether the exposed area continues to 'weep' in this way depends, of course, on whether the lesion remains free of pathogenic bacteria, and also on how the lesion is dressed, on the extent of tissue destruction and on environmental conditions. A crust consisting of dried exudate may form over the necrotic area. This occurs readily if the lesion is exposed to a hot and dry atmosphere. Such a crust may be beneficial by preventing further loss of fluid and at the same time access to the living tissue by pathogens. In Baghdad, where the temperature is often 40°C and the humidity less than 10 per cent, severely burnt or scalded people have been successfully treated by being nursed naked and without dressing to the lesions, to encourage the formation of protective crusts.

How does repair occur in such lesions? The overall response when there is not a great deal of tissue damage is the replacement of the exudate by a highly vascularized loose connective or granulation tissue that is gradually covered by epithelium from the margins of the crater. The vascularity then becomes less and the connective tissue fibres shorten until a white scarred area is formed.

The whole process from the first ingrowth of cells to the final white scar may take many months, but the first parts of the response are quite rapid. Within a few hours of the burn, macrophages from nearby living tissue at the base of the lesion wander into the exudate amongst the fibrin strands and the remnants of white and red cells. The macrophages are actively phagocytic, eating up tissue debris and helping to liquefy the more or less solid exudate. If there is much dead tissue, the macrophages are unable to cope with it, and a necrotic slough separates with encrusted exudate from the living tissue, leaving an exuding ulcer behind.

The macrophages are not the only cells to enter the exudate from the underlying tissue. After two or three days, buds of vascular endothelial cells sprout from existing capillaries by cell migration and cell division, processes we have already seen in the skin epithelium at the edge of wounds. The solid cores of endothelial cells push up into the exudate at the rate of about 0·25 mm/day. Very soon lumina appear and lining endothelial cells become recognizable in the vascular buds; blood can now enter from the parent capillary. Nearby capillary buds join up, and in this way loops of capillaries are

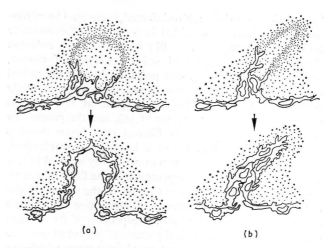

FIG. 21.9. Growth of capillary sprouts during repair. A chemical burn has been made in the cornea; capillaries are sprouting into the tissue debris of the lesion. (a) The loosened endothelial cells divide and migrate into the area of tissue weakness. (b) Cross connections form between two adjacent sprouts. After Schoefl G.I. (1964) *Ann. N.Y. Acad. Sci.* **116**, 789.

formed, projecting into the exudate. Blood flows freely through the loops (fig. 21.9).

The density of new capillaries is at first very high. In a few days the surface of the crater becomes a carpet of capillary loops; these are very easily damaged and the base is prone to bleed when touched. The new vessels are, moreover, quite permeable to protein and even intermittently to red blood cells. The capillary loops often seem to grow into areas softened by the action of a preceding advancing line of macrophages.

About three days after injury, at the same time as capillary endothelium is sprouting, the fibroblasts of the living tissue start to move into the exudate and into the material between the capillaries. The fibroblasts appear as elongated cells in the light microscope; in EM sections they can be seen to have a well developed endoplasmic reticulum with an abundance of attached ribosomes; they are cells making protein for export. At first little collagen is laid down in the organizing exudate; by about the fifth or sixth day, however, fibres which have the characteristic EM appearance of collagen are seen. From this time on, more and more collagen is deposited, and the reaction gradually becomes less vascular and more fibrotic. The fibroblasts and the fibres they produce are orientated in directions determined by the mechanical stresses within the area. The fibroblasts arise from fibrocytes of the surrounding tissue which have a high rate of mitosis; fibroblasts in the repair tissue itself also divide freely. There is no convincing evidence that fibroblasts can arise by differentiation from macrophages.

At this stage, about a week after the initial injury, the

base of the central area, if uninfected, is covered by newly-formed capillaries embedded in a growth of connective tissue containing active fibroblasts, some collagen fibres, intercellular ground substance and, of course, macrophages and emigrated polymorphs. To the naked eye the base of the lesion is red, and appears finely nodular or granular. The repair tissue at this stage is called **granulation tissue** (plate 21.5a), and the process by which it and subsequently fibrous scar tissue develop from an inflammatory lesion is known as organization. The term granulation tissue was originally applied in this way to the macroscopic appearance in the floor of a healing ulcer, but it is now used to refer to the characteristic light microscopic appearance of reparative fibroblastic and endothelial proliferation, irrespective of its site and cause. The same histological pattern of granulation tissue is seen, for example, around an abscess from which the pus has been released, or at the margins of a healing myocardial infarct, although in these sites it does not form macroscopic 'granules'. Sometimes an excessive amount of granulation tissue is produced, and it protrudes from the surface of an ulcer making re-epithelialization difficult. Granulation tissue once formed is remarkably resistant to infection and pathogenic bacteria will not gain a foothold in such highly vascularized tissue containing numerous leucocytes and a high concentration of antibodies. It is in the first few days, before granulation tissue has formed, that wounds may easily become infected.

The lesion is now well on the way to complete repair. During the next week or two, epithelium gradually extends over the granulation tissue. Some of the newly-formed vessels differentiate into arterioles, venules, arteries and veins by acquiring smooth muscle and fibrous coats. The smooth muscle tissue probably derives from existing undamaged cells which divide and move along the growing vessel wall. There is no good evidence that fibroblasts can differentiate into smooth muscle cells. Not all the capillaries remain or develop into larger vessels; some regress.

There is a parallel development of lymphatic vessels; as with blood vessels, endothelial cells are loosened, multiply and slide apart to form masses of cells that eventually become canalized. The new overgrowth of lymphatics into granulation tissue and the surrounding areas may be well seen if injections are made into the tissue in the vicinity of the healing wound (fig. 21.10).

Peripheral nerve fibres, including those of the autonomic nervous system, are capable of regeneration, and they grow into repair tissue from the nearest viable nerves. They establish connection with the muscle coats of new large vessels and with the newly formed sub-epithelial tissue. Specialized skin receptors are not reformed at nerve endings.

At the same time as the vascular bed is developing in

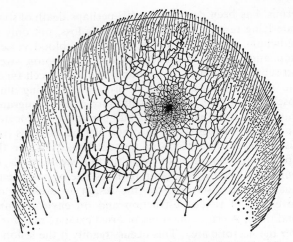

FIG. 21.10. Lymphatics of a mouse's ear injected with a suspension of carbon particles. Twenty-one days previously an abscess was produced by injecting a small quantity of turpentine; a small perforation occurred as a result of the abscess. The growth of lymphatics around the lesion is well shown. After Pullinger B.D. & Florey H.W. (1937) *J. Path. Bact.* **45**, 157.

the repair tissue, more collagen is being formed and the fibres already laid down by the fibroblasts are shortening. This draws the edges of the wound together and reduces the surface which has to be epithelialized. After two weeks or so, collagen shortening is marked and the contracting wound may pucker the surrounding skin. Thus a scar, or **cicatrix**, is formed (plate 21.5b). If tissue damage is extensive, scar contraction may severely limit movement and so incapacitate the patient.

Since the amount of scar tissue is increased when the lesion is infected, it is very important to keep pathogens away from such lesions, particularly of the hand or face.

The repair of the skin lesion that we have been considering is now nearing completion, and the pace of the response slows down once the granulation tissue has been covered with epithelium. Fibrosis is now the predominant reaction as the vascularity decreases. The bright red, recently healed wound becomes slowly an avascular white scar. The newly formed epidermis is at first very thin, but it will become over the weeks as keratinized as the surrounding skin.

When there are large masses of dead tissue this sloughs off and the spatial defect is filled first by blood clot and then by highly vascularized granulation tissue and finally by scar tissue.

Fibrosis is an essential part of the healing process, but may itself produce harmful effects when it develops in certain anatomical sites. Cicatricial contraction occurring in a hollow organ, for example, may narrow and even obstruct the lumen. Again, a fibrinous exudate occurring on a serous surface such as the pleura may not be absorbed, becoming converted into fibrous tissue; the result-

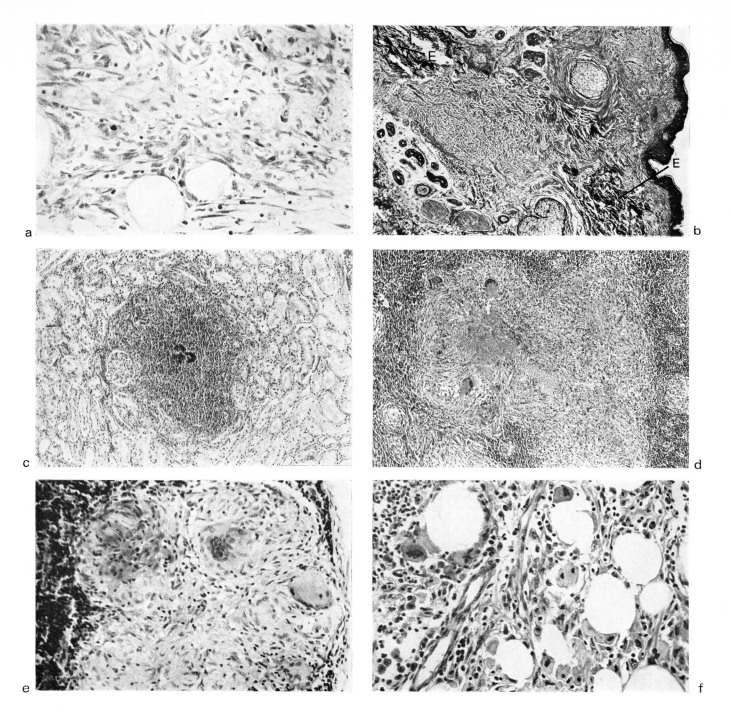

PLATE 21.5. Histology of inflammation.

(a) Granulation tissue showing fibroblasts, which are the long fusiform cells, collagen fibres and newly formed capillaries. The large empty spaces represent adipose tissue and some inflammatory cells are present. Haem. & eosin (×220).

(c) Pyaemic abscess in kidney. In the centre of the mass of polymorphs is a clump of bacteria. Haem. & eosin (×65).

(e) This sarcoid follicle, like the tubercle, is made up of epithelioid and giant cells, but lacks the central zone of caseation. Haem. & eosin (×220).

(b) Scar from a surgical incision. A narrow zone of (red) collagen fibres extends through the dermis. Sebaceous and sweat glands, present on either side, are absent from the scar, and the black elastic fibres (E) have failed to regenerate. The epidermis is complete. Elastic–van Gieson (×50).

(d) This tuberculous follicle is made up of pale epithelioid cells, with several giant cells. The central caseous zone is pink and homogeneous and the follicle is surrounded by lymphocytes. Haem. & eosin (×55).

(f) Fat necrosis. Macrophages with foamy cytoplasm, some of them multinucleate, surround spaces from which fat has been dissolved during preparation of the section. Other types of inflammatory cell are present. Haem. & eosin (×180).

ing adhesions between the parietal and visceral layers of the serous membrane may interfere with the function of the lung. Similar adhesions in the peritoneal sac can cause intestinal obstruction. Fibrosis takes place in the wall of an abscess cavity, if healing and reabsorption have not occurred. This thick and relatively avascular wall hinders the access of antibiotics to micro-organisms in the centre.

Fig. 21.11 shows the relative size of the cells involved in inflammation and repair.

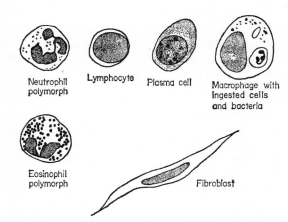

FIG. 21.11. The cells of acute and chronic inflammation and repair as seen in stained preparations and drawn approximately to scale.

Spread of infection

If the defensive reactions fail to overcome and destroy invading micro-organisms the inflammation can spread, especially by lymphatic and blood vessels, to involve other organs and eventually become generalized throughout the body.

The infecting micro-organisms may gain entrance to the lymphatics and pass to the regional lymph nodes where the events of acute inflammation are enacted anew, and the cardinal signs are observed again. For example, if spread of infection occurs from an initial site in the finger, involvement of the lymphatics is manifested by a thin, painful, red line extending up the arm, i.e. acute lymphangitis, while its arrival at the lymph nodes is signalled by a painful swelling in the axilla, acute lymphadenitis. Before the discovery of antibiotics, the onset of acute lymphangitis and lymphadenitis was a sign of grave import, indicating that the invading micro-organisms were overcoming the body's defensive reactions and possibly heralding a generalized infection which often proved fatal. Nowadays, prompt treatment at this stage usually reverses the trend to generalized spread.

More serious still is entry of the multiplying micro-organisms, such as streptococci, into the blood stream, i.e. septicaemia (p. 18.29). This may occur directly at the site of initial infection, or indirectly via the lymphatics. The micro-organisms are rarely so numerous that they can be identified microscopically in the blood, but their presence can be verified bacteriologically by blood culture.

Septicaemia, if untreated, may itself be fatal but if not, foci of acute inflammation may be set up in different organs remote from the original site. Sometimes, perhaps as a result of small infected thrombi being disseminated in the blood stream, these distant inflammatory foci take the form of multiple small abscesses; these are especially liable to occur in the brain, lungs and kidneys (plate 21.5c). The condition is now referred to as pyaemia, and the abscesses in distant organs as pyaemic abscesses.

If inflammation, especially of a suppurative type, spreads extensively and rapidly along natural tissue spaces, the condition is called, inappropriately, **cellulitis**. This is seen particularly in subcutaneous tissues. A similar condition in the skin is **erysipelas**. Certain micro-organisms particularly prone to cause suppuration are known as the pyogenic cocci (p. 18.67).

Spread of a deep-seated abscess may allow it to reach and ulcerate an epidermal or mucosal surface, forming a channel through which the inflammatory exudate may continue to discharge for a long period. Such a channel is called a sinus. It may be formed also as a result of eruption of an acute abscess on to an epithelial surface.

When such a communication is formed in this way between an internal hollow organ and the skin, or between two internal hollow organs, the resulting channel is called a **fistula**. For example, a faecal fistula occurs when chronic inflammation causes the intestinal tract to open on to the anterior abdominal skin, and a bronchopleural fistula when destruction of lung tissue brings about a communication between a bronchus and the pleural sac.

THE INFLAMMATORY RESPONSE TO SPECIFIC INFECTIONS

Certain forms of chronic inflammation by reason of their distinctive morphology need separate consideration.

Prime among these are **infective granulomata**, of which the principal examples in temperate climates are tuberculosis and syphilis. These infections, though differing in their aetiology, share a common characteristic, in that the inflammatory lesions take a nodular or tumour-like form. The term granuloma, though firmly established, is misleading. It implies a neoplasm of granulation tissue, but the tumour is simply a swelling, while the granulation tissue is strikingly different from that of ordinary non-specific inflammation. Leprosy, lymphogranuloma venereum, brucellosis and actinomycosis are other examples of infections which may give rise to a granuloma.

Tuberculosis

The initial infection by tubercle bacilli occurs most frequently by way of the respiratory tract, but the disease may spread to almost every organ or tissue in the body. Irrespective of the site, the basic lesion is a small nodule of inflammatory nature, the **tuberculous follicle** or **tubercle**, from which the disease derives its name (plate 21.5d, facing p. 21.14). Formation of the tubercle begins after a transient acute inflammatory response, with polymorph infiltration. The tubercle has a highly characteristic microscopic appearance and is recognized by the presence of epithelioid cells, giant cells, caseation, lymphocytes and sometimes tubercle bacilli.

The **epithelioid cell** is an elongated cell, with ill defined margins. The nucleus is oval or spindle-shaped, poorly-staining, but with a definite nuclear membrane, while the cytoplasm is eosinophilic and faintly granular. In a developing tuberculous follicle, the epithelioid cells form a fairly well circumscribed mass or nest; they possess cytoplasmic processes which merge imperceptibly with one another. Epithelioid cells belie their name, since their appearance does not in any way suggest an epithelial origin; indeed they are sometimes referred to as endo-thelioid cells, a synonym which is less inappropriate since they have at least some resemblance to the endothelial cells which line blood vessels. Unlike other inflammatory cells, they are not a normal constituent of the blood or reticuloendothelial system, but occur only under patho-logical conditions. They are probably derived from macro-phages and assume their epithelioid form after ingestion of the lipid material which is a component of the tu-bercle bacillus.

At first sight they may seem rather featureless cells, and it is unfortunate that the cells which provide an essential clue to the diagnosis of tuberculosis should be so lacking in character. Yet they are like none other, and can with practice be recognized both by their morphology and by their characteristic follicular grouping.

Langhans giant cells (p. 21.11) have the same faintly granular eosinophilic cytoplasm as epithelioid cells, from which they are derived. The nuclei are arranged in a peri-pheral ring or crescent, or become clustered at one pole of the cell, an arrangement which distinguishes this type of giant cell from the many others. The Langhans giant cell occurs occasionally in other granulomatous condi-tions, so that its presence is not absolutely diagnostic of tuberculosis. Equally important, giant cells are not essential for the diagnosis of tuberculosis, and they are often absent in the more acute and rapidly spreading forms of the disease. When present in a tubercle, they are usually in small numbers, and commonly occur around the periphery.

Caseation, or caseous necrosis, develops in the centre of the follicle. The necrotic tissue is unlike that of a pyo-genic abscess, but has something of the character of cream cheese, as implied by the term 'caseation'. Microscopi-cally, necrosis of the central epithelioid cells results in almost total loss of cellular outline and of nuclear staining, and all that remains within the enclosing ring of surviving epithelioid cells is a central mass of very finely granular eosinophilic material. Caseation, like the formation of epithelioid and giant cells, may owe its peculiar character to the high lipid content of the organism, and when present it is one of the most typical features of the tubercle follicle, serving to distinguish tuberculosis from other granulomatous lesions. Its cause is still obscure; it has been thought to be due to ischaemia in the centre of the tubercle, because of involvement of small vessels in the disease process and diminution of their lumina, but this is unproven. From its time of onset, it appears likely to be the result of the development of hypersensitivity to the bacteria.

The morphological picture of the tubercle is com-pleted by the presence in some cases of numbers of lymphocytes around the epithelioid cell mass.

The tubercle is just visible to the naked eye, being initially only about a millimetre in diameter. It grows by formation of epithelioid cells at the periphery, balanced by continuing necrosis in the inner zone, so that the caseous centre steadily expands while the enclosing zone of epithelioid cells remains of about the same thickness. It may grow in this manner to a large size, always re-taining at its margins a layer of epithelioid cells, enclosing an area of caseation and surrounded by a zone of lympho-cytes. Commonly, several tubercles coalesce to form a single lesion. A large lesion has a necrotic centre as in a pyogenic abscess, but lacks the macroscopic as well as the microscopic features of pyogenic inflammation and is sometimes known as a **cold abscess**.

The presence of tubercle bacilli within the follicle is the most certain demonstration of its tuberculous nature, and using the Ziehl–Neelsen method, or fluo-rescent techniques, these organisms can be demonstrated in tissue sections. Enormous numbers of bacilli can some-times be seen, especially in the more acute forms of the disease; they are present both in the caseous areas and among the epithelioid cells. Very often, however, they are scanty, and in very chronic lesions may be so sparse that only one or two are found after a painstaking search of several sections. They may be especially difficult to find if the patient is receiving antituberculous drugs. Culture on the appropriate media or inoculation of infected material into a guinea-pig sometimes serves to identify the organisms in cases where they cannot be found in tissue sections.

THE KOCH PHENOMENON

In 1891, Robert Koch inoculated a guinea-pig locally under the skin with tubercle bacilli, and found little observable reaction for 7–10 days, after which a nodule appeared at the site, breaking through the skin to produce an ulcer, which showed no healing tendency. From this primary site the organisms spread to the regional lymph nodes, then to the blood stream and eventually the animal died of disseminated tuberculosis. If an animal was reinoculated with the bacteria a week or two after the first infection, a local nodule appeared within a few days, ulcerated much more rapidly than the first, but healed without involving the regional lymph nodes.

This Koch phenomenon is a specific example of a cell-mediated immune response described in general terms in vol. 1, p. 27.2. It is also a type IV hypersensitivity or allergic reaction and its relation to immunity and other types of hypersensitivity is described on p. 22.18.

In an individual who has not been in contact with them before, tubercle bacilli excite an initial reaction which is quite different from that developing subsequently or following a second exposure. In the primary exposure, the inflammatory process is relatively slow, and not very severe. After a short-lived infiltration of the tissues with polymorphs, thought to be due to the presence of the polysaccharide fraction of the bacteria, mononuclear cells accumulate around the organisms and this continues for about 10 days. During this time the individual develops hypersensitivity to the organism, and this has two main results in regard to tissue reaction. First, the proliferative response, i.e. the infiltration by mononuclear inflammatory cells, is greatly accelerated; these cells become transformed into the epithelioid cells described already, and giant cells begin to form. Secondly, caseous necrosis begins in the centre of the cellular mass and extends. Sensitization of the tissues is exhibited when a second exogenous or endogenous infection occurs after healing of a previous primary infection. This allergic phenomenon is the basis of the tuberculin skin testing techniques, such as the Mantoux test, which are used clinically to discover whether or not a person has previously suffered from a tuberculous infection (p. 22.18).

Altered sensitivity is a cellular phenomenon, and cannot be passed on from one experimental animal to another by injecting serum from the sensitized to the nonsensitized animal. The cells involved in the sensitizing process are lymphocytes.

The speeding up and increase in severity of the local inflammatory process in a sensitized animal is in time associated with a fibroblastic tissue response, so that the lesion becomes walled off by a fibrous tissue barrier; this tends to hinder the spread of organisms.

The allergic state is apparently produced by the protein fraction of the organism. It seems, however, that for the protein fraction to act in this way it must be contained within the mycobacteria; if tuberculoprotein only is injected into an animal, it does not induce the hyper-sensitivity state, although it is capable of causing the response once the animal has become sensitized.

SPECIFIC IMMUNITY

This develops together with cell-mediated hypersensitivity, but appears to be distinct from it. The tissues of an individual possessing such immunity to tubercle bacilli kill the organisms much more effectively and rapidly than those of the nonimmune patient, and for this reason the local lesion heals. The increased ability to kill the bacteria appears to be due to a change in the macrophage reaction; these cells not only infiltrate the tissues more rapidly, but also become more capable of destroying the organisms which they engulf. In the nonimmune individual, i.e., in a first infection, the macrophages (epithelioid cells) take the organism into their cytoplasm, but as a result the cells rather than the micro-organisms are likely to be destroyed. Later in the clinical disease and also on subsequent infections, some change takes place which enables these mononuclear cells to kill the organisms. Again, therefore, the phenomenon is cell-mediated and is not accompanied by circulating antibodies in the serum.

It seems likely that hypersensitivity and immunity, although related, are not in fact the same phenomenon. If guinea-pigs which have been sensitized to tuberculoprotein are desensitized by a series of injections of this material, a stage is reached where they are no longer hypersensitive, but still exhibit specific immunity.

The practical result of this reaction is the destruction of mycobacteria with subsequent tendency to healing of the lesions. It has already been pointed out that hypersensitivity leads to the development of fibrosis around the tuberculous lesion, and this is of benefit to the patient, being complementary to the immune response.

PRIMARY AND SECONDARY TUBERCULOSIS

A first infection occurs probably most commonly in childhood, and in countries where tuberculous infection of milk has been eliminated the usual route is by the respiratory tract. Little or no reaction is seen in the bronchial mucous membrane at the site of entry of the organisms, and the first detectable lesion is a subpleural patch of tuberculous consolidation, commonly at the base of one of the upper lobes of the lung, known as the **Ghon focus**. From this focus the bacteria rapidly spread by the lymphatics to the lymph nodes at the hilum of the lung, where they set up a further focus of caseous tuberculosis. The Ghon focus and the lesions in the hilar lymph nodes together constitute the **primary complex**. In most instances complete healing of the primary complex occurs, and all that remains in the adult lung to mark the site of the Ghon focus is a tiny subpleural nodule of fibrosis or calcification.

If the primary focus is initiated by the swallowing of

infected milk, the lesion is in the small intestine, with secondary involvement of mesenteric lymph nodes. The intestinal lesion itself may disappear completely and quite rapidly, leaving only caseous or calcified lymph nodes.

Secondary infection may be either exogenous, due to further inhalation of significant numbers of mycobacteria, or endogenous, due to spread from some existing tuberculous lesion within the body. The lesions are more chronic than those of primary infection and tend to remain localized at the site of infection, with less tendency to involve the regional lymph nodes. If in the lung, the lesions, again unlike those of the primary complex, are most commonly situated at or just below the apex of an upper lobe.

HEALING OF TUBERCULOUS LESIONS
Healing of tuberculous lesions, like that of nonspecific inflammation, occurs by fibrosis. Fibroblasts proliferate around the lesions, forming new fibrous tissue which ultimately replaces the tuberculous granulation tissue. The smaller lesions may thus undergo total fibrosis. Substantial foci of caseation, however, are not readily replaced. They may, like pyogenic abscesses, erupt on to an epithelial or serous surface, or be evacuated by surgical intervention. Eruption on to the skin, such as may occur from caseous tuberculosis of the cervical lymph nodes, results in a tuberculous ulcer, with necrotic base and characteristically undermined edges; this, if untreated, is very slow to heal.

Large caseous lesions which cannot discharge their contents become enclosed by a zone of fibrous tissue. The caseous centre may calcify, and the final irreversible lesion is a hard, craggy calcareous mass, a lesion which is easily demonstrated by a radiograph during life.

A large caseous lesion, while developing a fibrous or calcified capsule, may retain its caseous centre indefinitely. In such lesions there is little or no epithelioid cell reaction between the caseous mass and the capsule, yet a few organisms may persist within the caseous material and remain a potential source of re-infection should the patient's resistance to tuberculosis later become diminished.

In the lung, a large caseous mass of this type may erupt into a bronchus and the necrotic material be coughed up, leaving a tuberculous cavity.

Healing of tuberculosis is delayed in lesions which have become secondarily infected by pyogenic organisms.

SPREAD OF TUBERCULOSIS
Spread of the disease may occur in other ways than by expansion and coalescence of established tubercles. When the patient's resistance is insufficient to overcome or localize the infection, the defensive reactions themselves may paradoxically favour disseminaton of the bacteria.

Those organisms that survive ingestion by phagocytes are carried within these motile cells along tissue spaces to other parts of the affected organ, where they set up new foci of infection. Similarly, the organisms, or phagocytes containing viable organisms, may enter the lymphatics and so spread from one part of the lung to another or to the regional lymph nodes. When infection reaches the pleura, pericardium or peritoneum, where there are no physical barriers to its progress, it may spread with great rapidity throughout the serous sac, the membrane becoming studded with tiny tubercles. Such spread does not necessarily involve the entire serous sac, as the development of adhesions may provide barriers which are lacking in the healthy state.

Another mode of spread is along the lumen of a hollow viscus. This is most prone to occur in the respiratory tract, where infected sputum may carry infection from one bronchus to another, and into associated alveoli (tuberculous bronchopneumonia), or to the larynx or to the intestine if the sputum is swallowed. Similarly, infection may be transmitted from one site in the intestinal tract to another more distal, or from the kidney to the bladder, or from the uterine tube to the endometrium.

Another route of spread is by the blood stream. The avascular nature of the tuberculous follicle provides some protection against organisms escaping into the circulation. However, bacteria may reach the blood stream by way of the lymphatic system and the thoracic duct, or more directly by eruption of a caseous lesion into a vein. Tuberculous foci, single or multiple, may then be produced in any organ. This is the means by which foci of tuberculosis arise in organs such as kidney, bone, brain or adrenal; these lesions may be initiated in childhood at the time of the primary infection, lie dormant for many years, and eventually either heal completely or break down at a later time to produce clinical tuberculosis of the organ involved.

Massive infection of the blood stream by erosion of a blood vessel may result in generalized **miliary tuberculosis**, a condition in which countless tiny tubercles form almost simultaneously throughout the viscera; the condition is called 'miliary' because the lesions in their size and their profusion supposedly resemble millet seeds. Macroscopically, the miliary tubercles appear as greyish-white specks, best seen on the cut surface of the liver, spleen, lung and kidney (plate 21.1d, facing p. 21.2). Microscopically, they have the usual characters of tuberculous follicles, with caseous centres. The original lesion is often in the lung, and the bacteria enter the pulmonary venous system so that they are spread through the body viscera. Should the infection enter the blood stream by a systemic rather than a pulmonary vein, the mycobacteria pass through the right side of the heart into the pulmonary arteries, and miliary tuberculosis may then be almost confined to the lungs.

The lesions of miliary tuberculosis, pulmonary or generalized, are not necessarily of uniform size, since the earlier lesions continue to grow and coalesce while successive waves of infection give rise to further crops of fresh miliary tubercles. Miliary tuberculosis was rapidly fatal before the introduction of chemotherapy and antibiotics (p. 20.31).

Of all the results of blood-borne tuberculosis, the most feared is tuberculous meningitis. Infection of the meninges may occur in the course of generalized miliary tuberculosis, especially in children, although it probably arises more commonly as a result of eruption of tuberculous lesions of the brain into the ventricles or on to the surface of the brain. The lack of anatomical barriers in the subarachnoid space allows rapid dissemination of the infection and the lesion therefore assumes a more diffuse and cellular form than in other organs. Tubercles may be so poorly formed that they cannot be readily observed macroscopically; even microscopically the epithelioid cells may not form classical follicles, and giant cells may be absent, while caseation tends to be diffuse rather than confined to the centre of follicles. The condition was always lethal prior to the discovery of antituberculous drugs.

Syphilis

Syphilis is one of the major infective granulomata and the most important venereal disease (p. 18.84). Like the tubercle bacillus, the causal organism, the *Treponema pallidum* is invisible in tissue sections stained by the ordinary methods, so that one must depend on recognition of the inflammatory response for the first suspicion in histological diagnosis.

LESIONS

As described on p. 18.84 the disease usually unfolds in three stages. The **primary chancre** presents as a hard, painless papule which gradually enlarges and then ulcerates the skin or mucous membrane. Although the ulcer may reach a diameter of several centimetres, as it is painless it may pass unnoticed in some sites, e.g. the uterine cervix.

The microscopic appearance of the chancre is that of a chronic inflammation, and is characteristic but not diagnostic of syphilis. The tissue is very heavily infiltrated by lymphocytes, plasma cells and macrophages, the density of the infiltration accounting for the characteristic hardness. Plasma cells are often predominant, as they may be in any stage of syphilis. Polymorphs play relatively little part; they are present in the floor of the ulcer and become much more numerous if secondary pyogenic infection occurs.

There is a conspicuous proliferation of small vessels and fibroblasts, the highly vascular picture contrasting sharply with the avascular lesions of tuberculosis. Two changes concerning the vessels are particularly striking. One is the tendency for chronic inflammatory cells to become aggregated around the small vessels; such **periarteritis** or **perivascular cuffing** is best seen in the deep margin of the lesion, where the diffuse inflammatory infiltration is less intense. The other is an intimal proliferation in the small arteries, which narrows the lumen and is known as **endarteritis**. Neither periarteritis nor endarteritis is diagnostic of syphilis, since both occur in other chronic inflammatory states, but they are specially marked in syphilitic lesions.

Unless there has been much superimposed pyogenic infection, healing of the chancre occurs with remarkably little fibrosis, and the scar may be almost invisible.

The lesions of **secondary syphilis** occur on the skin and all visible mucous membranes. The rash on the skin is symmetrical and commonly maculopapular (a macular rash is an area of skin differing in colour from normal; a papule is a small raised area in the skin). The mucous membrane lesions are most readily seen in the mouth; they take the form of raised white patches, which may ulcerate and produce irregular elongated lesions, aptly termed snail-track ulcers. On the mucocutaneous surfaces of the penis, vulva or anus, they appear as broad elevated lesions (condylomata or venereal warts). Lymph nodes are usually enlarged.

Microscopically, secondary syphilis has essentially the same characters as the primary chancre, but the cellular infiltration is less intense. Plasma cells are again prominent, as are periarteritis and endarteritis. The squamous mucous membranes, if not ulcerated, show hyperplasia and hyperkeratosis, especially in the condylomata.

The lesions of **tertiary syphilis** are strikingly different from those of the first two stages. They lack the symmetrical distribution of the secondary stage; they may be very few in number and are not accompanied by enlargement of lymph nodes. Most important of all, they involve extensive destruction of tissue and do not heal with the restoration of tissue that occurs in the earlier stages; on the contrary, healing is accompanied by such a degree of fibrosis as to cause serious permanent damage to the affected organ.

The lesions commonly take the form of a diffuse chronic interstitial inflammation, which microscopically has much the same characters as those of the earlier stages and is not in itself diagnostic of syphilis. The inflammatory process, however, is both more diffuse and more prolonged, leading to formation of syphilitic granulation tissue which is eventually succeeded by diffuse fibrosis. Periarteritis and endarteritis may again be present.

Less common but more characteristic of syphilis is the **gumma**, a nodular mass of syphilitic granulation tissue which bears some resemblance to the tuberculous follicle and is the lesion which entitles syphilis to its place among the infective granulomata. Like the tuberculous nodule, it ranges in size from a lesion scarcely visible to the naked eye to a tumour-like mass several centimetres in diameter, with a necrotic centre and an enclosing zone of epithelioid and other inflammatory cells. The necrotic centre does not undergo the softening so characteristic of tuberculous caseation, so that the gumma remains firm and rubbery. When it erodes the skin or a mucous membrane, the result is an ulcer of rounded or serpiginous outline; its straight edges give it a 'punched-out' appearance, contrasting with the undermined edge of a tuberculous ulcer.

Microscopically, the gumma differs from the tuberculous lesion in its vascularity, the more mixed character of its inflammatory infiltrate, its smaller and less numerous giant cells, and its greater degree of enclosing fibrosis. As well as epithelioid cells there are numerous plasma cells and lymphocytes, and as in all syphilitic lesions periarteritis and endarteritis are prominent. The necrotic centre is different too, often retaining definite cell outlines and even nuclear fragments.

Both the diffuse and the gummatous forms of tertiary syphilis may affect any organ in the body, but they have a special predilection for the skin and mucous membranes, the liver, the bones, the testes, and the cardiovascular and central nervous systems.

Congenital syphilis, in countries where medical services are good, does not carry its former menace to child life and health. The disease broadly follows the pattern of adult syphilis with conspicuous involvement of skin and mucous membranes. Some of the lesions are so characteristic as to deserve separate mention, e.g. fissures at the angles of the mouth and involvement of the upper respiratory tract ('snuffles'). Syphilitic infection of growing bones takes the form of epiphysitis and perichondritis; in particular, destruction of the bridge of the nose leads to a 'saddle' deformity and infection of the tibiae causes the bowing of 'sabre' tibia. Interstitial keratitis leads to opacity of the cornea. Interference with the developing enamel of the teeth causes a characteristic peg-shaped deformity, narrowing the apices of the teeth ('Hutchinson's teeth'). Diffuse involvement of the liver is very common, resulting in diffuse fibrosis or cirrhosis, and a similar diffuse fibrosis may occur in the lungs. In general, the lesions are much more of the diffuse inflammatory and fibrosing type, less often of the nodular or gummatous type.

Tuberculoid reactions

While the tuberculous follicle, complete with central caseation, in which mycobacteria can be specifically stained by the Ziehl–Neelsen or fluorescent methods, is diagnostic of tuberculosis, there are many other infective and noninfective inflammatory processes which simulate it in varying degree. Such tuberculoid reactions are characterized by focal aggregations of epithelioid macrophages with giant cells and in some instances central necrosis, but of course mycobacteria are not found. The infective granulomata (p. 21.15) constitute one group; in some of these conditions the formation of granulomatous follicles is not the sole or even the common form of the disease.

There remains a motley group of noninfective tuberculoid conditions which give rise to problems in clinical and histological differential diagnosis. The chief of these is sarcoidosis, while the others include Crohn's disease, berylliosis, rheumatoid disease, fat necrosis, and tuberculoid reaction to malignant neoplasms. Giant cell lesions unaccompanied by epithelioid cells, as in foreign-body reactions, are not correctly included among tuberculoid lesions, but are histologically similar and are described on p. 21.11.

Sarcoidosis is an uncommon disease of unknown origin, occurring usually in early or middle adult life, and characterized by the presence of tuberculoid granulomata in many different organs and tissues. The granulomatous foci are composed of epithelioid cells and Langhans giant cells, with a sparse lymphocytic infiltration around the periphery. The foci are more sharply circumscribed than is usual in tuberculosis. Caseation does not occur in their centres (plate 21.5e, facing p. 21.14). The lesions heal either by resolution or by progression to hyaline fibrosis. Inclusion bodies may be present in the giant cells and assist in the diagnosis though they are not pathognomonic of sarcoidosis.

Sarcoidosis has been reported to involve almost every organ in the body, but the commonest sites are the lymph nodes, the lungs, the bones, especially the small bones of the hands and feet, the liver and spleen, the skin and the eyes. Even if it appears clinically to be confined to one organ or system, microscopic examination usually shows the disease to be much more widespread.

Crohn's disease is an ulcerative disease of the intestinal tract, originally described as occurring in the terminal ileum but now known to affect any part of the small or large intestine. Its cause is unknown. Thickening and induration of the bowel wall occur in one or more sharply localized segments, narrowing the lumen. The microscopic features include small granulomatous foci, especially in the submucosa and subserosa. The foci do not caseate; they remain discrete and they might fairly be termed 'sarcoid-like' rather than tuberculoid.

Berylliosis or beryllium poisoning is an industrial disease affecting workers engaged in the manufacture of fluorescent lights. In the chronic form, noncaseating granulomata closely resembling those of sarcoidosis occur in the lungs and in the skin (p. 32.6).

Rheumatoid disease (p. 30.12) is best known by its involvement of joints, i.e. rheumatoid arthritis, but a nodular form of the condition may affect other organs and tissues. The nodules do not resemble tuberculosis very closely, since the centre is formed by a serpiginous zone of collagen necrosis unlike caseation, and the bordering zone of histiocytes or epithelioid cells has a characteristic parallel or palisaded arrangement; giant cells are not prominent. Histological differentiation can on occasion, however, be difficult.

Fat necrosis provokes a distinctive type of inflammatory response. It occurs in adipose tissue, the commonest sites being in the breast, where it is often attributable to trauma, and in the pancreas and neighbouring retroperitoneal fat, where it is due to escape of pancreatic fat-splitting enzymes from the system of glands and ducts to which they are normally confined.

The lesions form circumscribed firm patches, to which the deposition of fatty acids imparts an opaque white or yellow appearance. Microscopically, there is a mixed cellular infiltrate, made up of polymorphs, mononuclear cells and giant cells. Lipid-filled macrophages have a peculiar foamy appearance, because of their finely stippled and sometimes vacuolated cytoplasm, and can occasionally be mistaken for tuberculous epithelioid cells. In the giant cells which are derived from these lipophages the cytoplasm is similarly foamy. The inflammatory reaction is accompanied by fibroblastic proliferation, and the subsequent fibrosis forms a firm localized mass which may be mistaken clinically for a neoplasm or a tuberculous focus. Extensive lesions may ultimately become calcified (plate 21.5f., facing p. 21.14).

Noncaseous tuberculoid foci are occasionally seen in lymph nodes draining the site of a **malignant epithelial tumour** (carcinoma), while in primary malignant neoplasms of the reticuloendothelial system, such as **Hodgkin's disease**, similar foci may occur within the neoplastic tissue itself. The tuberculoid lesions are found in cases of malignant neoplasia where there is no suspicion of coincident tuberculosis or other granulomatous condition, and it must be assumed that they represent a variant of the chronic inflammatory response which usually accompanies malignant tumours (p. 28.14)

Reactions to the introduction of inorganic or nonliving material into the tissues often take a characteristic form. This is the presence of scattered groups of multinucleated giant cells, often seen to contain the foreign material, with few accompanying macrophages. These focal aggregations of cells, **foreign body granulomata**, are often associated eventually with marked fibrosis of the tissue. Such a reaction can be seen in relation to dust or dirt after trauma, cholesterol crystals following haemorrhage in a solid organ, or suture material left after an operation.

Fungus infections

Fungus infections affecting man are described briefly on p. 18.17. The lesions which they produce range from tuberculoid foci with or without central necrosis to abscess formation. In none of these conditions is the organism conspicuous, and indeed if suitable methods are not employed for the demonstration of fungi, the condition may be misdiagnosed as pyogenic infection or as a granuloma of unknown nature. Fungi, however, can also be secondary invaders, flourishing especially when bacterial infection has been suppressed by antibiotic therapy, and their presence may distract attention from the primary disease. In the lungs, for example, *Aspergillus fumigatus* more often represents a secondary than a primary invader.

Virus infections (p. 18.93)

Virus infections have no general identifying characteristic, either macroscopically or microscopically. They differ from other infections, however, in that the infecting agent is always intracellular, since a virus is capable of surviving and multiplying only in the living cell. In some infections inclusion bodies, thought to represent aggregates of viruses, can be seen microscopically within the cell. These are minute, rounded, basophilic or eosinophilic bodies, which may be present either in the nucleus, as in chickenpox, or in the cytoplasm, as in rabies. Particularly large and profuse intracytoplasmic inclusion bodies occur in molluscum contagiosum, a tumour-like virus infection of the skin. A very characteristic intranuclear inclusion body is seen in cytomegalic inclusion disease, in which the inclusion enlarges the nucleus and is separated from the nuclear membrane by a distinct halo ('owl's eye' appearance). In smallpox, inclusion bodies may occur both in the cytoplasm and in the nucleus (p. 18.116).

However, a cell infected by virus may appear histologically quite normal. In some cases the virus may cause cellular necrosis, or the cells may proliferate with or without subsequent necrosis, and in experimental animals certain viruses induce such cellular proliferation as to lead to the production of a tumour (p. 18.109). Affected cells may fuse to form multinucleated giant cells. Virus infections of certain organs may cause characteristic features in that organ, e.g. virus hepatitis. The effects on cells are further discussed on pp. 25.22 & 39 and 18.101.

Virus infections are usually accompanied by an inflammatory cell infiltration. The infiltrate has no distinguishing features, and may be lymphocytic as in virus pneumonia or of giant cell type as in measles. The infiltrate is usually mononuclear, but polymorphs may be present as in poliomyelitis. The inflammatory cells may be found particularly around small blood vessels. This perivascular cuffing is common in but not diagnostic of virus infections. It may be uncertain how far the inflammatory reaction is due to the virus infection itself, and how far to secondary bacterial infection.

Helminth infections (p. 19.14)

Inflammatory tissue reactions to larger parasites such as helminths vary in type with the organism concerned, with the duration of the infection and with the individual tissue involved. In the early stages the parasites in the tissues, e.g. trichinella, may be accompanied by a polymorph infiltration, associated with death of tissue cells, the lesion sometimes amounting to abscess formation. Commonly, e.g. with the filarial worms, the reaction is of a more chronic type, with infiltration by lymphocytes, plasma cells and macrophages. However, in virtually all such infections, infiltration of the tissues by eosinophils is a prominent feature, and the presence of significant numbers of these cells in an inflammatory exudate should always raise the suspicion of metazoan infection.

Several of the helminths excite a granulomatous reaction in the tissues; follicles consisting of epithelioid cells with a few giant cells and lymphocytes, may be formed, occasionally simulating a tuberculous lesion. A further change which may be seen in inflammatory reactions to such parasites is endothelial cell proliferation of smaller blood and lymph vessels, sometimes producing obstruction to blood flow and lymphatic drainage, as in elephantiasis. The later stages in most infections involve fibrosis and scarring; some parasites e.g. in hydatid disease, give rise to cyst formation, and old cysts may become calcified.

The effects of radiation

The inflammatory response to radiation possesses several special features which are discussed on p. 25.12, and p. 33.7.

FURTHER READING

FLOREY H.W. (1969) Inflammation, in *General Pathology* 4th Edition. London: Lloyd-Luke.

SPECTOR W.G. & WILLOUGHBY D.A. (1963) The inflammatory response. *Bact. Rev.* **27**, 117.

SPECTOR W.G. ed. (1964) The acute inflammatory response. *Ann. N. Y. Acad. Sci.* **116**, 747.

SPECTOR W.G. (1967) The cytokinetics of chronic inflammation, in *Scientific Basis of Medicine Annual Reviews*. London: Athlone Press.

WALTER J.B. & ISRAEL M.S. (1965) The inflammatory reaction; the body's response to infection; wound healing; chronic inflammation; tuberculosis, syphilis and actinomycosis, in *General Pathology*, 2nd edition. London: Churchill.

ZWEIFACH B.W., GRANT L. & McCLUSKEY R.T. eds. (1965) *The Inflammatory Response*. New York: Academic Press.

Chapter 22
Immunity

Immunity is an old word meaning exemption and was originally used to describe exemption from military service or from paying customs or taxes. In times of epidemics not everybody is affected and those who do not contract the disease are said to be immune. Immunology arose as the study of those biological processes that protected an organism against the attack of a living parasite. It soon became concerned with the reactions against other foreign substances which might enter the body, particularly if they were protein in nature. This aspect of immunology is now of considerable interest in relation to tissue grafts and transplantation reactions; it is the reactions in the tissues of the host, provoked by the presence of a foreign protein, that cause a graft or transplant to be rejected. Immunology is also concerned with the problems of how the tissues recognize a protein as foreign and distinguish it from a protein component of the body. A failure of such recognition may occur and result in inappropriate immune reactions which lead to a group of disorders known as autoimmune diseases (p. 23.7). All these mechanisms fall within the scope of immunology, which extends in modern biology and medicine far beyond the original problem of exemption from infectious diseases.

INFECTION AND RESISTANCE
Immunity to infectious disease is a graded phenomenon. The interaction between an infectious agent and host is such that in some instances the micro-organism, and in others the host, gains the upper hand. It is common knowledge that some species of animal are exempt from infection by particular micro-organisms whilst other species are readily infected. Man is readily infected by the common cold virus, while a dog is not. The dog can, on the other hand, be infected readily by distemper virus while man cannot. The absence of suitable receptors on the cytoplasmic membranes is the most important well recognized reason for the inability of viruses to infect cells. The study of immunity to micro-organisms involves an understanding of the host mechanisms which determine the end result of the interaction, whether it be complete **susceptibility** of an individual to infection, its converse complete **resistance** or somewhere between these two states. The characteristics of the infective agent, including the dose required to induce disease, its invasiveness, virulence and communicability have already been discussed (p. 18.29).

Susceptibility can be thought of as being determined by the effectiveness of the mechanisms or factors which deter an infective agent from becoming established in the body, either by hindering or preventing its access to the tissues or because the environment is unfavourable for its multiplication. In as much as these mechanisms do not arise directly as a response to the infective agent they may be said to be **passive**. Resistance on the other hand can be defined as an **active** response by the tissues to the presence of an infective agent and determines the result of the infection. Individuals may vary greatly in susceptibility and resistance to infection and immunology is concerned with both processes.

SCOPE OF IMMUNOLOGY
The science of immunology has developed in three overlapping phases:

(1) immunology in relation to infectious disease,

(2) immunochemistry of antigens and antibodies and their interaction, and

(3) autoimmunity and transplantation immunology.

The first phase arose from the recognition that those who survived an infectious disease were less likely to develop the disease again than those who had not previously been infected. Although prophylactic immunization made great strides after the development of the germ theory of disease by Louis Pasteur, empirical measures had already been in use in Britain for nearly 200 years. In 1717, Lady Mary Wortley Montagu, wife of the British Ambassador in Turkey, introduced variolation as a measure to combat smallpox. This procedure, which was probably first used in China where dried crusts of smallpox lesions were taken as snuff, involved pricking the skin through a drop of the exudate from a smallpox lesion in an active case. It carried considerable risk of actual infection rather than protection. Variolation was made illegal in Britain in 1840, and was succeeded by the less dangerous technique of **vaccination**, in which a virus related to the smallpox virus is used to produce a localized infection (vaccinia) in the skin, which immunizes against smallpox. This was developed by a physician, Edward Jenner, from the observation of Benjamin Jesty, a Dorsetshire farmer, who was responsible for the first successful vaccination. It is interesting that techniques similar to variolation were used in Edinburgh in the eighteenth century by Francis Home to protect children against measles.

With Louis Pasteur's discovery in the mid-nineteenth century that disease could be caused by micro-organisms, various successful attempts were made to induce immunity by using organisms of reduced virulence. Such attenuated organisms may be produced by growth under unfavourable conditions (p. 18.31). The immunity produced in an animal by the action of micro-organisms is an **active immunity**.

The next important advance came with the demonstration that the blood from an animal immunized against diphtheria had a neutralizing effect on diphtheria toxin. This discovery was made in the Koch Institute in Berlin by von Behring and Kitasato in 1890. The effect was due to a factor in the blood, called **antibody**, which acted on micro-organisms and their toxins. Serum containing antibodies, if given to another animal, could convey to that animal a **passive immunity**.

The role of the phagocytic cells of the body in taking up and destroying micro-organisms was elucidated at this time by Metchnikoff in Russia. Later, the helpful effect of antibody in the phagocytic process was established, the antibody coating the micro-organisms and making them more appetizing to the ingesting cells.

The specificity of antibody for the agent, i.e. the **antigen**, which induced its formation, led to a further important development in which antibody was used as a powerful analytic tool. The antigenic characters of bacterial and non-bacterial substances could be worked out, and Landsteiner was able to recognize and define the A, B and O blood groups on the basis of the antigenic differences in red cells. Thus immunochemistry, founded by Paul Ehrlich, was developed, and an understanding of antigenic specificity was obtained, using characterized chemical groupings attached to carriers of high mol. wt. as antigenic determinants. Precise and sensitive methods for measuring antigen–antibody reactions were established and concepts of chemical equilibria were applied to their interaction.

The extensive use of antisera in the treatment of infectious diseases soon led to the discovery that the immune response was sometimes a disadvantage to the individual. Serum, usually horse serum, given for purposes of passive immunization, itself acted as an antigen and induced the formation of antibody in the recipient. The combination of this antibody with the horse serum in subsequent injections resulted in severe shock and other clinical features, called **immediate hypersensitivity**. Sir Henry Dale in 1910 showed that this was due to the release into the circulation of pharmacologically active agents, notably histamine, stimulated by the combination of antibody and antigen (p. 14.14). Symptoms were severe if amounts of antibody and antigen were large. Immediate hypersensitivity is important as it arises not only as a result of reactions with antigens injected in the course of serum therapy, but also with antigens entering by other routes. Thus it is in large part responsible for the symptoms of asthma and hay fever following the inhalation of foreign substances which act as antigens. Many drugs and common foods also produce reactions after ingestion by susceptible individuals.

During the 1930's, a large amount of detailed information became available about antibodies and antigens and their interaction which led to the use of immunological techniques by chemists, geneticists and others in their own studies. The need also arose to provide a sound biological explanation covering the essential facts of immunity, why and how an immune response occurs following the introduction of foreign antigenic material, and why there is normally no response to the individual's own constituents.

In some human diseases a tissue antigen fails to be recognized as part of self, and therefore antibodies to it are produced by the body. This raises the whole question of the process of self-recognition, and how it might go wrong. The first attempt at an answer was made by Sir Macfarlane Burnet who proposed several ingenious theories to explain self-recognition, foremost being his clonal selection theory of antibody formation. These new developments in immunology led to an awakened interest in organ and tissue transplantation. The pioneer work of Medawar and his colleagues with skin grafts in mice confirmed Burnet's prediction that introduction of a foreign antigen in early life, before the immunological system was mature, could lead to the acceptance of the foreign material as part of self. Today there is great interest in possible methods of permitting an individual to accept foreign grafted material by modifying his normal immune response (p. 24.1).

Although antibodies have been thought of as protective agents against infective micro-organisms, and indeed the term immunity carries this connotation, it is now realized that antibodies may have many biological functions. The recognition that there are various classes of antibody, each with differing biological activities, encourages this attitude, and the possible role of antibody in the control of cell metabolism or in the clearing away of tissue breakdown products must be considered. It is even conceivable that the phenomenon of self-recognition lies behind the maintenance of the cellular integrity of different organs and tissues.

Innate immunity

In the absence of previous contact with a particular micro-organism the healthy individual is able to protect himself from infection by means of **innate immune mechanisms**. This non-specific first line of defence is of great importance in providing protection from the vast numbers of micro-organisms in any environment.

The main determinants of innate immunity are the species or strain and to a lesser extent the genetic make-up of the individual. Age, hormonal balance and sex play lesser roles. These factors are listed in table 22.1 where the mechanisms involved are also summarized.

TABLE 22.1. Innate immunity. The first line defences are of great importance in maintaining an individual free of infections. They cannot readily be enhanced by external interference.

Host determinants	Structural barriers	Active agents
Species and strain, Genetic make-up,	Skin, mucous membranes, Anatomical traps, e.g. nasal cavities	Antimicrobial secretions of skin and mucous membranes, e.g. tears, gastric juice, sweat and sebaceous secretions,
Age, Hormonal balance, Sex		Mechanical cleansing, e.g. cilia, Antimicrobial substances of tissue fluids, e.g. lysozyme, interferon and properdin, Cellular uptake and digestion of material, e.g. phagocytosis

SPECIES

Species react to micro-organisms in different ways; e.g. the rat is not at all susceptible to diphtheria whereas the guinea-pig and man are highly susceptible. The rabbit is peculiarly susceptible to myxomatosis and man to syphilis, leprosy and meningococcal meningitis.

STRAIN

Marked variations in resistance to infection between different strains of mice occur. In man, the habits and environment of a community affect its ability to resist particular infections by acquired immune mechanisms developing at an early age. This form of resistance is easily confused with innate immunity and makes the detection of differences in innate immunity difficult. It is accepted, however, that the American Indian and the Negro are more susceptible to tuberculosis than Caucasians. These differences can probably be accounted for by natural selection.

The term **herd immunity** refers to differences in susceptibility to infection of different groups. While this is sometimes innate, it may also be acquired. The extent to which a herd is immune influences the spread of epidemics (p. 22.21).

GENETIC FACTORS

The role of heredity in determining resistance to infection is illustrated in studies on tuberculous infection in twins. If one monozygotic twin develops tuberculosis, the other twin has a 3 to 1 chance of developing the disease, whereas the chances are reduced to 1 in 3 if the twins are dizygotic. Familial predisposition to other types of diseases involving immune reactions such as rheumatoid arthritis also occurs. Sometimes genetic abnormalities are an advantage to the individual in resisting infection, e.g. the protection against attack by malaria parasites provided by sickling (p. 31.13).

AGE

Infectious diseases are more severe at the extremes of life, although the reasons for this are not well understood. In the young animal, immaturity of the immunological mechanisms is likely to be important and chick embryos or newborn mice are frequently used to grow viruses. In the elderly, physical abnormalities are a common cause of increased susceptibility.

HORMONAL INFLUENCES

There is decreased resistance to infection in diseases such as diabetes mellitus, hypothyroidism and adrenal dysfunction. Cortisol in pharmacological doses diminishes the resistance to infection and its use may cause extension of the lung lesions in tuberculosis.

SEX

The sex of an individual does not usually affect the susceptibility to infectious disease to a marked degree. Both infectious hepatitis and whooping cough have a higher morbidity and mortality in females than in males, but the overall mortality from infectious disease is greater in the male than in the female in *homo sapiens* and in other species of mammals.

MECHANISMS OF INNATE IMMUNITY

The skin and mucous membranes and epithelial linings of the respiratory, alimentary and urinary tracts serve as physical barriers to the entry of micro-organisms. Furthermore, the nasal conchae reduce the inhalation of foreign particles into the lower respiratory passages, and the moist surface of the mucous membranes are also very efficient traps for inhaled material. The cilia of the respiratory tract sweep out foreign material.

The skin and mucous membranes also produce secretions which are active against many micro-organisms. The sebaceous secretions and sweat contain unsaturated fatty acids, and other substances which combine to produce a bactericidal effect. These mechanisms are rendered ineffective by prolonged exposure to moisture and it is therefore important that a skin dressing used to treat a wound should be permeable and allow evaporation of moisture.

The mucous secretions of the respiratory and genital tracts contain substances with bactericidal and viricidal properties, some of which, such as lysozyme, are present also in the tissue fluids. The high acidity of the stomach secretion is also an effective defence. In the lower intestinal tract the competitive effects of many types of micro-organisms prevent the exclusive establishment and growth of any particular species of organism.

ANTIMICROBIAL SUBSTANCES OF THE TISSUE FLUIDS

The tissues, which possess the basic ingredients for an excellent culture medium for micro-organisms, fortunately contain a variety of antimicrobial substances. Some of these have been characterized chemically but detailed information on their activities is not available. **Lysozyme,** described by Fleming in 1922, is the best known of them; it is a basic protein which functions as a mucolytic enzyme and splits mucopeptides of the bacterial cell wall, resulting in lysis of the bacterium. It is particularly effective against Gram-positive organisms and is present in many body fluids, being found in high concentration in the tears and in the cytoplasm of polymorphs. A number of other antimicrobial agents which are basic polypeptides are present in the tissues, but little information is available about their structure and mode of action.

The blood of healthy animals contains **normal antibodies** which occur in serum from early life and are believed to arise without prior antigenic stimulation. However, it is possible that these antibodies have developed as a result of subclinical infections by micro-organisms. In addition, similar antigens may be shared by many types of bacteria. **Properdin** is a protein (mol. wt. 1×10^6) which acts against Gram-negative organisms in conjunction with certain ions and a normal serum component called complement (p. 22.16). Some immunologists believe that properdin is not a separate entity but represents the combined activities of the normal antibodies.

INFLAMMATION AND CELLULAR MECHANISMS IN INNATE IMMUNITY

The entry of micro-organisms into the tissues leads to a degree of inflammation depending on the nature of the infective agent and the particular tissue involved. Inflammation is associated with vasodilation and increased permeability of vessels and leads to accumulation of fluid and phagocytic cells at the site of invasion. There is much argument as to whether this brings about more efficient localization of the micro-organisms and their destruction by the phagocytic cells or whether the massive infiltration of fluid leads to spread of organisms through the distended tissue spaces. It appears on balance that by mobilizing the phagocytic cells and bringing tissue fluids containing bactericidal substances to the site of infection, inflammation is a useful mechanism. Even if some organisms escape they are likely to be taken up into the lymphatic channels and to find themselves in the hostile environment of a lymph node (p. 21.15).

The phagocytic cells of the body, that is the polymorphonuclear leucocytes of the blood and macrophages present both in the blood and fixed in tissues, are extremely efficient at ridding the body of micro-organisms. Millions of organisms can be cleared from the blood within a matter of minutes. In fact, if free bacteria are found in the blood, one must suspect their continual release from some large focus such as an abscess.

After being engulfed by a phagocyte, a bacterium comes to lie in a vacuole within the cell cytoplasm. Then an adjacent lysosome discharges its contents of digestive enzymes into the vacuole and kills the organism. Many bacteria such as the pneumococci and *B. proteus* are killed within a few minutes after they have been engulfed. On the other hand, some organisms survive and even multiply inside phagocytic cells, e.g. *Myco. tuberculosis* and *Brucella*. The engulfment of a micro-organism by a phagocyte is aided by **opsonins** which make the organism more appetizing to the phagocyte by coating the surface of the former. This effect is probably brought about by altering the surface charge of the organism. Serum proteins readily perform this function and specific antibody is particularly effective.

Phagocytic cells provide the link between innate immunity and acquired immunity, for they pass on antigenic information to the antibody-forming cells, stimulating them to produce specific antibody.

Antigens

NATURE AND SPECIFICITY OF ANTIGENS

Antigens have been defined as substances capable of producing an immune response (vol. 1, p. 27.2). They are recognized as foreign substances by the immunologically competent lymphoid cells. Antigens are usually complex macromolecules containing protein, but antigenicity may depend on the presence of a simple foreign chemical group. A substance which acts as an antigen in one species of animal may not do so in another because it is represented in the tissues or fluids of the second species. For example, egg albumin is an excellent antigen in the rabbit, but of course fails to induce an immune response in a fowl. The more foreign a substance is to a particular species the more likely it is to be a powerful antigen. A good antigen need not contain different building blocks, e.g. amino acids of a protein, but their arrangement should be such that at least part of the surface of the molecule presents a configuration which is unfamiliar to the animal. Since macromolecules have a three dimensional structure, it is easy to visualize how they could become folded so as to present new and peculiar surface arrangements.

Alternatively, 'foreignness' can be a property which depends upon the presence in a molecule of chemical groupings which are entirely unfamiliar to an organism, e.g. when an arsonic acid group is introduced artificially by diazotization into a protein molecule. Such a group is known as a **hapten** and acts as the **determinant** of the **antigenic specificity** of a molecule. This means that the antibody which is formed in response to the antigen reacts specifically with the chemical determinant. Any change in the chemical determinant, even as minor as the removal of the AsO_3H_2 group from amino benzene arsonic acid, results in loss of ability to react with specific antibody (fig. 22.1). If the AsO_3H_2 group is replaced by

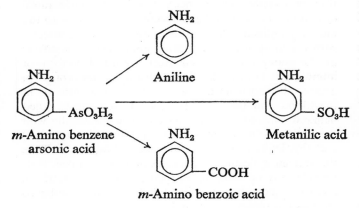

FIG. 22.1. Example of chemical group determinants of antigenic specificity.

another acidic group such as COOH or a SO_3H the ability of the antibody to the arsonic acid to react with the substituted substances is much reduced.

The influence of shape rather than removal or substitution of groups is shown by studies with stereoisomers of macromolecules containing tartaric acid where the antibody to L-tartaric acid fails to combine with D-tartaric acid.

Studies of this type carried out by Landsteiner in the early part of this century did much to establish the specificity of antibody for the antigen which induced its formation and illustrated the need for an extremely close fit between antibody and antigen before firm combination could take place. A slight variation in the shape of the antigen determinant prevents the antibody from forming a stable bond with the antigen. However even today immunologists are still far from understanding the chemical nature of the determinant groups in complex proteins and polysaccharides. Studies with synthetic poly-

peptides show that the surface arrangements of the amino acids in a branched polyamino acid structure are critical as determinants of antigenic specificity. Furthermore, when the three dimensional structure of a protein is changed by denaturation, it no longer reacts with antibody to the original material.

An essential requirement for a substance to be antigenic in its own right, i.e. without requiring to be attached like a hapten to a carrier protein, is that it has a sufficiently high molecular weight. Substances with mol. wt. below 5000 are not readily antigenic and have to be given combined with some other material, e.g. coated on carrier particles such as acrylic particles or red blood cells, or given with a material which acts as a nonspecific stimulus to the immune response, i.e. an adjuvant (p. 22.8).

Substances with a high mol. wt. on the other hand make good antigens, although the reasons for this are not clear. It is not simply a question of a large molecule having more and different antigenic determinant groups, or that larger molecules are excreted more slowly. The reasons may involve factors such as the physical state of the antigen, whether it is in a soluble or a particulate form, and how readily it is phagocytosed by macrophages. Thus if a solution of bovine serum albumin, which is highly antigenic, is filtered so as to remove the larger aggregates and the filtered material injected into a rabbit, antibody formation is largely prevented.

In the case of the polysaccharide dextran, a sample of mol. wt. 600,000 is antigenic, whereas one of mol. wt. 100,000 is not. There is no obvious reason for these differences, as the two materials are made up of identical building blocks and do not differ as far as the type of antigenic determinant is concerned.

In apparent contradiction to these findings is the observation that many quite simple chemical substances of low molecular weight such as picryl chloride, formaldehyde and drugs such as aspirin, penicillin and sulphonamide, can induce an immune response if injected, or in some cases even if applied to the skin. The reason for this is that these materials form complexes by means of covalent bonds with tissue proteins, and are then able to bring about an immune response, which can lead to the development of hypersensitivity states (p. 22.19).

HOST INFLUENCES

Whether or not a particular natural substance stimulates an immune response can be determined, as indicated above, by the phylogenetic relationship between the animal or micro-organism providing the antigen and the animal to be exposed to the antigen. When the two differ widely, e.g. bacterial antigens and mammals, the immune response is usually strong.

There appear to be genetic factors which determine whether an animal responds to some antigens. Thus two strains of mice differed markedly in their ability to produce antibody to a polymer of tyrosine and glutamic acid attached to a branched synthetic polypeptide carrier. When tested with a polymer in which the tyrosine had been replaced by histidine, the responsiveness was found to be reversed and the strain which responded poorly to the tyrosine antigen was found to respond well to the histidine antigen, and vice versa. Here the genetic controls determined the specific response, as the carrier for both antigens was the same. Different strains of rabbits may also vary in their ability to respond to certain antigens, but how important these genetic factors are in determining immune responses is not clear (p. 23.8).

ANTIGENS OF MICRO-ORGANISMS

Bacterial and viral antigens are in common use in medical practice as a means of inducing immunity to infectious diseases such as smallpox, diphtheria, measles, poliomyelitis, typhoid fever and many others. In general, there are four different types of antigen preparations or **vaccines.**

(1) **Toxoids** are the soluble exotoxins of bacteria, e.g. the diphtheria and tetanus bacilli, modified by the addition of formalin and by gentle heating. They are administered either in solution or precipitated on alum. Many years of useful immunity can be achieved by these procedures.

(2) **Killed vaccines** are cultured organisms killed by heat, usually 60°C for 1 hour, ultraviolet irradiation or chemicals such as phenol, alcohol and formalin. Protection against whooping cough, poliomyelitis and perhaps cholera can be achieved in this way.

(3) **Substances isolated from infectious agents**, e.g. the capsular polysaccharide of the pneumococci, a diffusible factor of *B. anthracis* and a cell wall antigen preparation of haemolytic streptococci have been shown to induce immunity, but such preparations are not in general use in medical practice.

(4) **Attenuated living vaccines** are made from strains of organisms which have lost their virulence by growth in culture or in animals where the conditions are not favourable for the growth and proliferation of the virulent strain. Strains develop which, whilst not able to produce disease, can induce immunity; such strains are known as attenuated organisms. The BCG vaccine (Bacille Calmette–Guerin) is the outstanding example of this type of vaccine, providing protection against tuberculosis. The oral administration of a strain of poliomyelitis virus induces a powerful immunity without producing the disease. This virus spreads from one individual to another and so is able to produce immunity in a community. An attenuated strain of yellow fever virus has been developed, obtained from the original virulent material by prolonged cultivation in tissue culture. Attenuated strains of measles virus are also used.

Living virulent organisms can also be used to induce immunity without the development of disease. This is achieved by introducing an organism, e.g. dog distemper virus, by a route different from that by which it normally gains access. The organism may also be combined with antibody and then injected, the neutralized organism being able to induce immunity but not infection.

Some practical aspects of immunization are described on p. 22.21.

Acquired immunity (fig. 22.2)

Pathogenic micro-organisms which overcome or circumvent innate immunity confront the host's second line of defence. This form of immunity, known as acquired immunity, is associated with the appearance in the blood of globulins known as antibodies or immunoglobulins. Its main characteristic is that it is specific for the particular micro-organism which calls it forth. Antibody formation is usually also associated with the appearance of lymphoid cells which are specifically sensitized to the inducing antigen. The sensitized cells can react directly with the antigen and may bring about cytotoxic effects on, for example, foreign cells from a graft. This form of immunity is known as **cell-mediated immunity** (vol. 1, p. 27.2) as distinct from that due to circulating antibody in the blood and tissue fluids which is sometimes called **humoral immunity**. Antibodies combine specifically with the antigen which stimulated their production (p. 22.8) and this leads to some remarkable consequences. Thus the antigen molecules or particles may be clumped, their toxicity may be neutralized, their uptake by phagocytes and subsequent digestion facilitated and cellular antigens such as red blood cells or bacteria may be lysed.

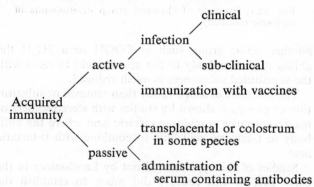

FIG. 22.2. Mechanisms of acquired immunity.

It is important to note that the formation of immunoglobulins is a physiological response to the introduction into the body of foreign material, irrespective of whether the material is harmful or not. Further, antibody may be directed at antigens of micro-organisms which have become inaccessible to the serum proteins and thus the antibody performs no protective role.

In all mammalian species, individuals vary greatly in their ability to produce antibodies, and also in the degree of resistance developed as a result of antibody formation.

ACTIVELY ACQUIRED IMMUNITY

This form of immunity may be induced by means of overt clinical infection or inapparent subclinical infection, and falls into two general categories. Some infections, such as diphtheria, whooping cough, smallpox and mumps, usually induce a lifelong immunity. Others such as the common cold, influenza and pneumococcal pneumonia, confer immunity for a shorter time, sometimes of only a few weeks' duration.

Failure of the second group of infections to induce lasting immunity is due to various factors, and particularly to the fact that different members or strains of the same species of organism may be involved and the acquisition of immunity to one strain does not prevent infection by another strain of the same organism.

Vaccination, whereby the individual is exposed to attenuated or killed organisms, is a widely practised method of inducing active acquired immunity.

PASSIVELY ACQUIRED IMMUNITY

This is the form of acquired immunity which is transferred to a non-immune individual by blood or other body fluids, or experimentally by cells from an actively immunized animal.

The human mother transfers antibodies to her infant via the placenta, and in some species, such as the rat and the dog, antibodies are also transmitted through the colostrum via the intestine. In other animals, notably the pig and the calf, transfer to the young occurs only by way of the colostrum.

Administration of specific immune sera is a therapeutic procedure in acute toxic diseases such as diphtheria, tetanus and gas gangrene. It is of temporary protective value for patients in danger of developing these infections, for travellers likely to be exposed to infective hepatitis, for very young children exposed to measles and for patients with hypogammaglobulinaemia (pp. 22.21 and 23.12).

Production of antibodies

The immune response resulting from exposure to antigenic substances has certain well defined characteristics. After the first exposure there is an interval of about two weeks before antibody can be found in the blood; the concentration then rises slowly to a low level and subsequently declines. This is known as the **primary response** (fig. 22.3). If a second dose of antigen is given at this stage, any remaining circulating antibody is rapidly mopped up by combination with the antigen; then after only a day or two a remarkable rise in the level of antibody begins and reaches within a few days a peak which can be from 10 to 50 times as high as the primary response.

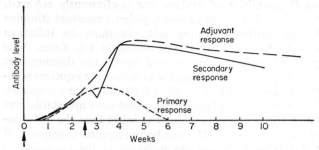

FIG. 22.3. Primary, secondary and adjuvant (p. 22.8) type responses. Second arrow shows time of injection for secondary response. Note small fall in antibody level due to combination of existing antibody with antigen.

This is the **secondary response**. Having reached its peak, the secondary response falls more slowly than the primary response and is boosted to even higher levels by further injection of antigen until a stage is reached when no further increase occurs.

For a maximum response the interval between the primary and secondary injection should not be less than about 10 days. Subsequent injections should be spaced out to weeks and then months; this allows time for the increase in numbers of antibody-forming cells which can be stimulated by subsequent injections. Even when the level of circulating antibody falls, the cells retain a memory of the antigen and are stimulated rapidly to form antibody anew by further contact with the antigen.

Some of the host determinants of acquired immunity have already been discussed. The nature of the antigen, the form in which it is presented and the dose given also have marked effects on the response.

PHYSICAL STATE OF THE ANTIGEN

It is common practice to enhance the ability of an antigen to stimulate antibody production, i.e. its antigenicity, by altering its physical state. A practical procedure is to adsorb the antigen on to mineral gels such as aluminium hydroxide or phosphate. The alum-precipated antigens are widely used as immunizing agents for humans. It seems that they are more readily antigenic than antigen given in soluble form, and this leads to a more efficient production of antibody. If all the particulate or aggregated material is removed from a solution of protein antigen by high speed centrifugation or by filtration, its ability to induce antibody formation is much reduced.

Other methods have been developed to enhance the antibody response, although at present they are used mainly in experimental work. The most important of these consists of the preparation of a water-in-oil emulsion; an aqueous solution of antigen is emulsified in a light mineral oil so that tiny droplets of the antigen solution are dispersed throughout the oil. The emulsion forms a depot of antigen in the subcutaneous tissues, from which small quantities of antigen are continuously released, sometimes for a year or more, giving a constant stimulus to the antibody-forming cells. In man, an influenza vaccine has been used successfully in this form. New possibilities have been opened up by the development of a multiple form of vaccine in which the aqueous solution is dispersed first in oil and the oil is then dispersed in a final water phase. These emulsions are stable and much less viscous and difficult to inject than the water-in-oil type. An even better antibody response is achieved if killed tubercle bacilli are included in the emulsion; a wax constituent of the bacterial wall is responsible for this effect. This method is used only for work in experimental animals. Water-in-oil emulsions are often called Freund's adjuvants.

The great advantage of these **adjuvant methods** is that both the primary and the secondary immune responses are achieved by only one injection of the antigen and that peak antibody level is maintained over a very long period by the small quantities of antigen released from the depot.

DOSE OF ANTIGEN
To induce a primary antibody response in which circulating antibody is found in the blood, a threshold dose of antigen is required, usually of the order of a few hundred μg for a protein antigen. Smaller doses, whilst not inducing detectable antibody formation, prime the antibody-forming cells so that a second injection gives a rapid secondary type of response.

The increase in the antibody response is small in proportion to the increase in the dose of antigen given and is proportional approximately to the square root of the increase in antigen administered. With some bacterial antigens the second injection of antigen should equal or preferably exceed the first dose if the best response is to be achieved. Excessive quantities of antigen inhibit rather than stimulate the antibody response and with some polysaccharide antigens, e.g. pneumococcal polysaccharide in mice, even quite small quantities are capable of doing this. This is possibly due to the absence in mice of enzyme systems capable of breaking down the polysaccharides which therefore persist in the tissues indefinitely and block the antibody-forming cells.

MATURATION OF TISSUES INVOLVED IN IMMUNE REACTIONS
Phylogeny
Lymphoid tissues are absent in invertebrates and the most primitive of the vertebrates, e.g. the hag fish. This system developed late in phylogeny, the first vestiges appearing in the lamprey where it is associated with a limited ability to produce an immune reaction. The complement system evolved some time later in evolution and is present in the jawed vertebrate, e.g. the paddle-

fish. With increasing structural complexity of animals the immune reaction became more diversified and effective.

Ontogeny
The immune system arises in the human embryo from gut-associated tissue. Lymphoid tissue first appears in the thymus at about 8 weeks of gestation (vol. 1, p. 27.5). Peyer's patches are distinguishable in the gut by the 5th month and immunoglobulin-containing cells appear in the spleen and lymph nodes at about 20 weeks. It has been shown that both IgG and IgM globulin (p. 22.12) are formed by the foetus from this period onwards, with IgM predominating. Maternal IgG is passed via the placenta, and at birth umbilical cord serum contains a concentration of IgG comparable to that of maternal serum. The newborn infant does not receive IgM antibodies from the mother and this probably accounts for the susceptibility to infection by Gram-negative organisms. However, the infant is able to respond to antigen of Gram-negative organisms producing antibodies of the IgM class. The infant is protected by the maternal IgG antibodies against Gram-positive bacteria and viruses. The neonatal human begins to synthesize IgM antibodies at an increasing rate soon after birth and at about 6 days the serum concentration rises sharply but reaches adult levels only by about 1 year of age.

IgA globulins are detectable from 13 days after birth, but adult levels are not reached until between the 6th and 7th years of life. IgG from the mother gradually disappears during the first 6–8 months of life and is replaced by an increased rate of synthesis by the infant itself, starting about 1 month of age and reaching adult levels at about the same time as IgA.

Cell-mediated immune reactions (vol. 1, p. 27.2) can be stimulated at birth but then are not as powerful as in the adult (e.g. homograft rejection).

TISSUES CONCERNED IN ANTIBODY PRODUCTION
The lymphoreticular organs (vol. 1, p. 27.2) are the site of antibody formation, but the method of immunization determines in which of these tissues the greater part of the antibody is formed. If an antigen is given intravenously, most of the antibody is produced in the spleen and some in the lung and bone marrow; on the other hand, if given subcutaneously or intradermally, the antigen travels via lymphatics to the local lymph nodes where antibody production is initiated. When antigen is given with adjuvants, there is a local accumulation of inflammatory cells, and antibody production occurs in the resulting granulomatous tissue.

The lymphoid tissues in the spleen and lymph nodes produce a greater quantity of antibody for a given weight of tissue than any other site of antibody production, although, because of its great bulk, the bone marrow contributes a higher proportion of the total antibody than other tissues.

CELLS CONCERNED IN ANTIBODY PRODUCTION

The lymphoid tissues responsible for humoral antibody production are associated developmentally with the gut and consist of lymphocytes and plasma cells in the lymph nodes and spleen. The lymphoid tissues responsible for cell-mediated immune reactivity are associated with the thymus. In the spleen and lymph nodes there are areas of thymus-dependent lymphoid tissue lying close to the central arterioles in the spleen and the post capillary venules in the medulla of the lymph node. It is in these areas that the cell-mediated immune processes are generated by contact with antigen caught by up the phagocytic cells in the lymphoid tissues (vol. 1, p. 27.12).

In the case of the humoral immune response, immunoglobulins are secreted into the blood by lymphoid cells, predominantly plasma cells fixed in the spleen and lymph nodes. The cell-mediated immune response is, on the other hand, brought about by migration of stimulated cells themselves from the lymphoid tissues via the efferent lymphatics to the blood stream; this they leave rapidly through the capillary endothelium and circulate in the tissue fluids; they are then ready to interact with foreign antigenic material, thus providing increased protection for those areas outside the blood circulating system.

The plasma cells have already been described and their role as the main producer of antibody indicated (vol. 1, p. 27.12). These oval cells (fig. 22.4) contain an abundant

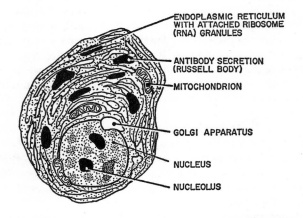

FIG. 22.4. Plasma cell showing cytoplasm containing antibody secretions (Russell bodies) produced by the ribosome granules of the endoplasmic reticulum.

endoplasmic reticulum, bearing ribosomes which make protein; this may aggregate to form Russell bodies (p. 21.10). The antibody nature of this protein can be shown quite clearly by immunofluorescent techniques

(vol. 1, p. 13.4) on sections of lymphoid tissue from an immunized animal. In animals making large amounts of antibody, antibody can be shown to be present also in large and medium-sized lymphocytes, although much less is seen than in the plasma cells.

MECHANISM OF STIMULATION OF ANTIBODY-PRODUCING CELLS

Isotope-labelled antigen injected into the subcutaneous tissues reaches the regional lymph nodes where it is localized by the reticuloendothelial cells. This localization would seem to depend upon the presence of small amounts of antibody at the surface of particular cells. The antigen can localize on two types of cell, macrophages and lymphocytes (fig. 22.5a, c). The surface of these

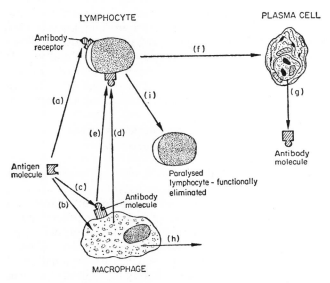

FIG. 22.5. Diagram of possible sequence of events in antibody formation. For explanation of letters, see text.

cells is coated with immunoglobulin, taken up passively by the macrophage and actively secreted by the lymphocyte. The specificity of the secreted immunoglobulin is thought to be determined by the genetic make-up of the lymphocyte, although some consider that antigen may have played a role by acting within the cell (p. 22.10). The function of antigen at the surface of the lymphocyte is to induce it to transform and proliferate into active antibody-producing cells (f, g). How this is brought about is not yet clear but certain antigens, e.g. bacterial flagella and haemocyanin, can bring it about readily and directly. Other antigens are less active and have to be taken into a macrophage and processed in such a way that they can influence the lymphocyte (b, d). The processing may involve the formation of a complex between antigen fragments and macrophage RNA. Some antigen appears to be retained on the surface of macrophages where it serves as a depot for the maintenance of the immune response, being passed on to lymphocytes over a long period of time (e). The macrophage also serves the purpose of catabolizing excess antigen (b,h). Another possible result of the interaction of certain types of antigen, e.g. aggregate-free serum protein antigens, with the surface of the lymphocyte is that the cell is prevented in some way from transforming for antibody production and is functionally eliminated from further participation in antibody production (i).

The lymphocyte population is a heterogeneous group of morphologically similar cells. Some of these depend on the thymus, are present in the blood, spleen and lymph nodes and involved in the cell-mediated immune reaction (vol. 1, p. 27.13). The cells concerned in the production of circulating antibody are probably derived from the bone marrow and are also present in the blood, spleen and lymph nodes. Some lymphocytes after transformation by antigen probably do not go on to become antibody-producing cells but remain dormant. It is possible that these cells retain a memory of the original contact with antigen. These 'memory' cells can then perhaps be reactivated on later contact with antigen.

Immunological learning processes

MOLECULAR PROCESSES INVOLVED IN ANTIBODY FORMATION

The ability of an individual to recognize a foreign antigen and to respond to it by producing antibody, retaining a memory which can be evoked on subsequent contact with the antigen, is an example of a learning process comparable to learning to ride a bicycle or to swim and involves the acquisition and evocation of specific skills.

There exists at present no satisfactory explanation of the cellular mechanism of antibody formation which can account for all the known characteristics of the immune response. This state of affairs is not due to lack of speculation and experimentation, and in the last few years much effort has been made to clarify this problem. Basically, the question concerns the external direction by antigen of the synthesis of protein (antibody) in the specialized cells of the lymphoid system (plasma cells).

Two main kinds of theory have evolved which are referred to as directive and selective theories. The **directive theory** was put forward by Haurowitz, Mudd and Alexander in the early 1930's and later modified by Pauling. The antigen is conceived of as a mould or template which can enter any globulin-producing cell and cause the pattern of amino acids laid down to be altered to fit the template, so that the globulin molecule is formed with a spatial configuration complementary to that of the antigen molecule. In order to account for the continued production of the antibody, it is assumed that the antigen, or part of it, remains in the cell as a template to direct future antibody production by the cell. Alternatively, it is proposed that the antigen modifies the genetic information in the DNA of the cell so that it and its daughter cells continue to produce the specific globulin.

The **selective theories**, on the other hand, propose that the antigen selects from the population of cells capable of making antibody only those few cells which already have the genetic ability to make such antibody. The antigen serves simply as a trigger to the globulin-producing process. The **clonal selection theory** of Sir Macfarlane Burnet is the best known of the selective theories and was formulated to take account of (1) the hitherto unexplained phenomenon of recognition by the normal individual of tissue antigens as part of self (tolerance to self) and (2) the human diseases where this recognition breaks down and antibodies are made against self antigens, the so-called autoimmune diseases (p. 23.7). The theory proposes that if antigenic material, either part of self or a foreign material, comes into contact with the cells of the antibody-forming system at the stage before the cells have reached maturity, i.e. in foetal life, the result is suppression rather than stimulation of antibody formation against the particular antigen concerned; this is referred to as immunological tolerance to the antigen. The antigen probably persists within the cell and blocks its ability to make antibody. The unblocking of a cell inherently capable of producing antibody against self antigens would explain autoantibody formation. It is for this aspect of immunity in particular that the clonal theory provides a more plausible explanation than the directive theory, which requires that all antibody-forming cells are blocked by self antigens rather than simply those cells destined to respond to the antigen concerned.

The other main characteristics of antibody formation, i.e. the specificity of antibody for antigen and the differences between the primary and secondary response, can be explained equally well by both the directive and selective theories. The clonal selection theory, however, is the most complete attempt so far to take into account all the known facts of antibody production.

Biological role of the immunoglobulins

Knowledge of the physical and chemical properties of the immunoglobulins is necessary to understand their behaviour. Unfortunately at present this provides only some hints as to how structure affects the activities of the immunoglobulin molecules.

Since the work of Tiselius and Kabat in 1936, using electrophoresis which identified antibody activity in the γ-globulin fraction of serum, it has been possible to show that the γ-globulins are a heterogeneous group of closely related proteins with overlapping physical and chemical properties (plate 22.1, opposite). Different types contain 1·5 to 10 per cent carbohydrate. Most of the molecules have a mol. wt. around 160,000, although some

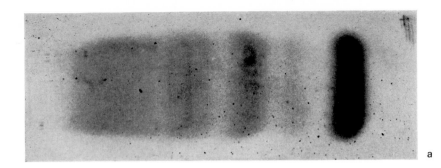

a

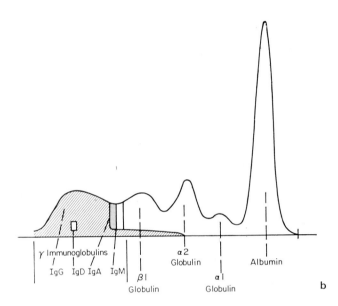

b

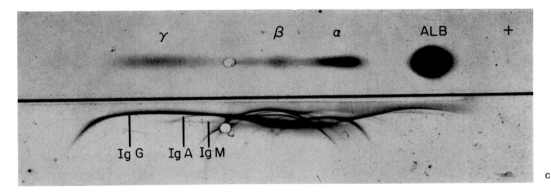

c

PLATE 22.1. Electrophoresis and immunoelectrophoresis.

(a) Electrophoresis of human serum.

(b) Tracing of protein peaks obtained from (a) showing diagrammatically the main classes of immunoglobulins.

(c) Immunoelectrophoresis technique. Top pattern shows serum protein distribution after electrophoresis in agar; serum components stained to render them visible. Lower pattern shows the precipitin bands which develop when antiserum is allowed to diffuse from a longitudinal trough towards the separated serum components: these components are not themselves visible as they have not been stained. In each case the whole serum was placed in small circular wells prior to electrophoresis.

may be as large as 1,000,000. The immunoglobulins are referred to as Ig or γ-globulins. On the basis of antigenic differences between the molecules it is possible to distinguish three main classes, G, M and A, using the technique of immunoelectrophoresis (plate 22.1). The first major group, IgG, has a molecular weight of 150,000 and is present in the serum in a concentration of 1200 mg/100 ml; the molecules have two combining sites for antigen, and play a major part in the common serological reactions (p. 22.13). The second class is known as the IgM and has a mol. wt. of 900,000–1,000,000, with about 10 per cent carbohydrate. They are present in serum in a concentration of 100 mg/100 ml and have five to ten antibody-combining sites. As a result they are most effective in agglutination reactions (p. 22.15). In addition, they are more effective than IgG immunoglobulins in bringing about lysis of cells by complement (p. 22.16).

The third main class, IgA, is present in the serum at a concentration of about 400 mg/100 ml. The IgA molecule is mainly made in plasma cells of the lamina propria and secreted into the mucous secretions as a dimer with an added secretory piece which prevents its digestion in the gut.

Two further classes known as the IgD and IgE globulins have recently been described, and the former appear to have some of the properties of the IgG globulins, although little is known of their serological and biological activities. IgE globulins on the other hand have been implicated in various forms of allergic reactions such as hay fever and asthma. They have the distinctive property of possessing an affinity for cell surfaces (p. 22.19).

STRUCTURE AND FUNCTION OF THE IMMUNOGLOBULINS

Porter in London made the discovery that the antibody molecule can be split by proteolytic enzymes into three parts, two of which contain the antibody-combining sites and the other the antigenic determinants.

New insight into the structure of the immunoglobulins and the relationships of the different classes has been obtained in the last few years by the discovery that these proteins are made up of distinct subunits held together in the whole molecule by disulphide (S–S) bonds. The bonds can be broken by reducing agents, so that the molecule falls apart into two pairs of polypeptide chains called light and heavy chains, individual light chains having a mol. wt. of 20,000 and the heavy chains of 52,000. Porter made a major advance when he developed methods of breaking the molecule into these chains and at the same time retaining the biological activity of the fragments (fig. 22.6).

The subunits are probably synthesized under independent genetic control since genetically inherited properties of the molecules can be shown to be associated

with different subunits; in the pathological condition of plasma cell myeloma in which plasma cells proliferate throughout the body, one of the subunits, very often of light chains, is made in excessive quantities and a dimer (i.e. two similar molecules attached together as a unit) of light chains may appear in the urine as Bence Jones protein (p. 28.4). Similar subunits have been found in the γ-globulins of species other than man, including the horse, guinea-pig and mouse.

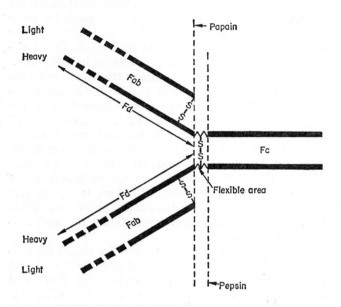

FIG. 22.6. Possible arrangement of the heavy and light chains and their fragments in the antibody molecule. Variable portions are shown by broken lines.

The common structural feature of all the immunoglobulins is the combination of light and heavy chains and it is tempting to suppose that the antibody-combining site involves this combination. Recent evidence indicates that the specificity of the antibody-combining site is carried by the heavy chain and that the light chain takes part through some nonspecific action, perhaps being responsible for maintaining the three-dimensional structure of the heavy chain. The part of the heavy chain (Fd fragment), together with the light chain, is called the Fab fragment and this is able to combine with antigen. The N-terminal end of the light chain has been shown to vary in amino acid sequence from one antibody to another whilst the C-terminal end is stable and it is thought likely that a similar pattern is exhibited by the heavy chain. The variation in amino acid sequence would be likely to account for the specificity of individual antibody molecules for their particular antigens. Two types of light chain exist, K and L. Individual Ig molecules have only one type. In IgG, 60 per cent are usually K and 30 per cent L type chains. The part of the heavy chain, the Fc fragment, carries a number of features which are responsible for the antigenic differences between the different classes of immunoglobulin and also the different biological functions of the immunoglobulins.

The activation or fixation of complement, a complex heat-labile substance present in the serum of humans and animals (p. 22.16), depends upon changes in configuration of immunoglobulin molecules when they are brought into close apposition during reaction with antigen, and it is the Fc fragment of the heavy chain which carries the predominant part of the molecule responsible for complement fixation. Both IgG and IgM molecules have the capacity to fix complement, but monomeric IgA molecules appear to be unable to do so whilst its dimer can.

IgM antibodies are more efficient than IgG antibodies in linking particulate antigens together for agglutination (p. 22.15), and rabbit IgM anti-salmonella antibodies have been shown to be twenty-two times as active as IgG antibodies in bacterial agglutination and 500–1000 times more efficient in the induction of phagocytosis of the organism. On the other hand, IgG antibodies are more efficient than IgM antibodies in the neutralization of diphtheria toxin and poliomyelitis virus. It appears that the Fc fragment is involved in neutralization, in addition to the part of the molecule containing the antibody-combining sites.

IgM antibodies are unable to sensitize tissues for anaphylactic reactions (p. 22.19) although IgG and IgA molecules, are able to do so. Recent work has shown that a new class of immunoglobulin, IgE, is a major factor in tissue sensitization. The transport of IgG globulin across the placenta is an active process depending upon an active site in the Fc fragment.

Transplantation of tissues and organs

The grafting of skin or other tissues from one normal individual to another results in most instances in a rapid rejection of the donor tissue (vol. 1, p. 27.13). The mechanism underlying the rejection is immunological, the recipient responding to foreign antigens in the donor tissue. Such antigens are thought to be mucopolysaccharides or lipopolysaccharides of the cell surface and are known as **transplantation antigens**. Two antigen systems are known to influence graft compatibility in man, the ABO erythrocyte and the leucocyte systems or HL-A antigens. Matching for ABO compatibility presents no difficulties, but because of the complexity of the HL-A antigens matching for these is not fully developed. Only when these antigens are exactly the same in the recipient and the donor are grafts accepted. This occurs only in the case of identical twins or in individuals from highly inbred strains of animals, such as mice, whose genetic constitution is identical. Animals of this type are called **isogenic**, whereas individuals of different genetic constitution are called **heterogenic**. Grafts between isogenic individuals are known as **isografts** and between heterogenic individuals as **homografts**. Skin homografts when applied for the first time, become vascularized and appear healthy for 3–14 days, depending upon the degree of genetic difference between the donor and recipient. The circulation then begins to fail, the graft becomes infiltrated with inflammatory mononuclear cells and later necrotizes and sloughs. If a second similar graft is now applied to the same recipient there is an accelerated and greatly increased inflammatory reaction with rapid necrosis; sloughing of the graft occurs within three or four days, indicative of the development at the first exposure of an active immunity to the antigens of the donor tissue. The blood of the recipient now contains antibodies against the donor cells, but such antibody alone cannot bring about rejection of a skin or organ graft, except in the case of grafts of isolated cells (marrow or tumour cells). However, lymph node or spleen cells from such animals does bring about graft rejection, and it is considered that the mechanism of skin homograft rejection is similar to that operating in delayed cellular hypersensitivity type reactions (p. 22.20) with the cell-mediated immune reaction as the predominant factor.

The main clinical problem in the field of transplantation of human tissues, apart from the selection of suitable donors, is the suppression of this immune response, and much effort is being expended in the search for acceptable methods of achieving this, involving the use of immunosuppressant drugs such as 6-mercaptopurine, or X-rays, and more recently the use of antilymphocytic serum. Such procedures carry the risk of permanently destroying the haemopoietic tissues and the ability of the patient to deal with infective micro-organisms (p. 24.1 and p. 32.4); thus, infection and sepsis are the commonest cause of transplant failure and death after renal grafts.

IMMUNOLOGICAL SURVEILLANCE

It appears possible that the homograft rejection mechanism serves an important physiological role in the normal individual in bringing about the elimination of spontaneously arising neoplastic cells which might represent a potential threat to the individual. In support of this possibility is the observation that the incidence of tumours is highest at the two extremes of life when the immunological mechanisms are at their least efficient. In animals whose immune systems have been deranged by thymectomy the incidence of tumours induced by chemical carcinogens and viruses is higher than in sham thymectomized controls.

This type of cell-mediated immune mechanism probably arose at an early stage in evolution with the development of multicellular organisms and would be effective also against exogenous parasites.

The ability of some tumours to initiate an immune

response can be clearly shown in pure strain mice who become immune to chemically induced tumour tissue from another mouse of the same strain; oncogenic viruses (p. 28.10) also induce new antigens in tumour cells.

The foetus as a homograft

Reference has been made in vol. 1, p. 27.19, to the immunological problem of viviparity. The foetus is genetically dissimilar from the mother and the uteroplacental interface is strictly analogous to the homograft situation. In the haemochorial human placenta, foetal tissues are bathed in maternal blood and there is the closest apposition of foetal trophoblast to maternal decidua, amounting even to cellular fusion. In human gestation this situation is tolerated for about 266 days, a period long exceeding the duration of normal graft tolerance, and yet there is no evidence of rejection. The mechanisms by which the mother tolerates her foetal homograft are still unknown, but several principles can be considered.

In order for rejection to occur, three conditions must be satisfied;

(1) the conceptus must make its antigenicity known to the mother;

(2) the pregnant recipient must be capable of normal immune response; and

(3) the mother must be able to communicate this response to the foetus.

The antigenicity of the embryo *per se* is not relevant in this context since the embryo does not come into direct contact with the mother. The only foetal tissue which is in contiguity with maternal tissues is trophoblast, with the possible exception of the transfer of foetal blood cells into the maternal circulation. There is strong evidence that trophoblast is an ineffective antigen and this must be a major factor in the mother's acceptance of foetal tissues. Trophoblast is potentially antigenic, as placental tissue from F_1 hybrid mice can be used to immunize the mother so as to cause rejection of paternal skin, but it seems likely that these antigens are masked by a fibrinoid layer (p. 30.3) which surrounds the trophoblast.

Experimental evidence has shown that skin homografts to pregnant rabbits survive for twice as long as in nonpregnant animals, and there is evidence for a similar effect in human but not in cattle and mouse gestations. This damping down of the immune response seems to be caused by corticosteroid hormones secreted in increased amounts during pregnancy. Thus, a pregnant woman may be relatively unresponsive to her husband's antigens, and this may be specific for her husband. Whether or not this is a function of insemination or conception is uncertain, as is its significance as a factor in the maintenance of pregnancy.

Several studies have shown that a foetus is protected against maternal immunity. For example, Woodruff immunized female rats and rabbits, prior to mating, with skin homografts from their male mates. About the 15th to 16th day after conception these immunized pregnant females received a graft of limb tissue from one of their own foetuses. These explanted limbs were rapidly rejected, yet the remaining foetuses escaped unharmed from the uterus at term. Lanman used the technique of ovum transplantation in rabbits so that there was no genetic relationship between mother and offspring, and he induced sensitization prior to pregnancy by homografts from both donor parents. In some cases he regrafted at the time of implantation or later in pregnancy. In none of these contrived situations could he demonstrate any change in the normal outcome of pregnancy. These experiments argue strongly that the foetus is usually protected against maternal immunological attack.

It is clear that the key to the immunological puzzle of pregnancy lies at the decidua–trophoblast interface. It is here that trophoblast confronts its potentially aggressive neighbour, and it has a critical pacifist role by virtue of its antigenic nonintervention and by its control of cellular traffic between mother and foetus.

Interaction of antibody with antigen

When molecules of antibody and antigen are brought together in solution, they interact with each other by the formation of a link between an antibody-combining site on the globulin molecule and an antigenic determinant group of the antigen molecule. The molecules are held together by intermolecular forces (van der Waals' forces) which are effective only when the two molecules are able to lie closely alongside. This means that the three-dimensional structure of the antibody-combining site must be complementary to that of the antigenic determinant group. It is considered that no more than ten to twenty amino acids out of the 1500 or so which make up the antibody molecule are present in the combining site. The combination of antibody with antigen is usually maximal at physiological pH and osmolality, and the strength of the union becomes more firm as immunization proceeds, indicating that the closeness of fit improves as the cells become more educated in making the antibody molecules.

The primary interaction of antibody with antigen is the first stage in a complicated series of events which may follow. These secondary phenomena vary according to the particular type of immunoglobulin which is taking part in the reaction and may be biologically advantageous, e.g. by killing micro-organisms or by neutralizing toxic substances derived from them. On the other hand, the secondary phenomena can act to the distinct disadvantage of the individual and lead to hypersensitivity reactions and damage to cells and tissues rather than protection.

The secondary phenomena can bring about several observable changes when carried out *in vitro* and these are used in tests to demonstrate the presence of antibody in the sera of patients suffering from infectious disease and to identify a particular antigen in the tissues or body fluids.

These reactions include **precipitation**, which occurs between antibody and antigen molecules in solution, **agglutination**, in which the antibodies are directed against surface antigens of particulate materials such as micro-organisms or erythrocytes and link them together in large clumps or aggregates, and **complement fixation**, in which antibody molecules, after reacting with antigen, fix the complex heat-labile constituent of the blood known as complement.

In addition to these classical serological phenomena a number of other effects of antibody–antigen interaction are of medical importance. These include neutralization of toxins by antibody, neutralization of viruses, precipitation of antibody and antigen in semi-solid media (gels), and phagocytosis of particulate antigen after exposure to antibody (**opsonization**). Antigen–antibody interaction is the basis of immunoassays for hormones (vol. 1, p. 25.5).

PRECIPITATION

Following combination of antibody and antigen molecules in solution, precipitation may occur, depending on the relative concentration of the two reactants. If a series of tubes (fig. 22.7) is set up, each containing a constant

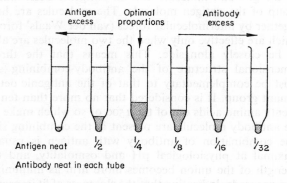

FIG. 22.7. Diagram illustrating the precipitin reaction.

amount of antiserum and decreasing amounts of antigen are added to the tubes, precipitation, appearing initially as a haziness and gradually increasing to clearly visible aggregates, can be seen to develop along the series, reaching a maximum and then falling off with the lower antigen concentrations. Dean and Webb in 1926 showed that the tubes in which most precipitate appears contain the **optimal proportions** of antigen and antibody for precipitation, and the proportions are constant for all dilutions of the same reagents. The composition of the precipitate varies with the original proportions of the antibody and antigen; if antigen is in excess the precipitate contains

relatively more of this component; similarly it contains more antibody if this is present in excess. As has been noted, on the antigen excess side of optimal proportions less precipitate appears, and this is due to the inability of the antigen–antibody complexes formed to link up to other complexes and so form a large aggregate of lattice which appears as a visible precipitate (tube 1 of fig. 22.8). Large aggregates of antibody and antigen form best under conditions of optimal proportions, which are such that, after initial combination of the molecules, free antibody-combining sites and antigen determinant groups remain, enabling the complexes to link up into a

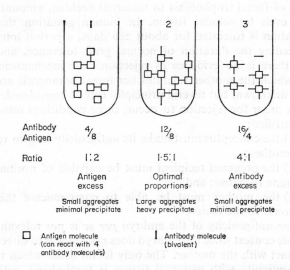

FIG. 22.8. Diagram of the effect of alteration of the ratio of antigen and antibody in the precipitin reaction.

large lattice formation (tube 2 of fig. 22.8). In antibody excess, all the free antigen determinants are soon used up by antibody so that very little further cross-linking can take place between the complexes (tube 3 of fig. 22.8).

The precipitin test can be carried out in a quantitative manner by estimating the protein content of the precipitate at optimal proportions. The qualitative test is of value in detecting and identifying antigens and is used in typing streptococci and pneumococci; when an extract of the organism is layered over antiserum, a ring of precipitate forms at the interface (the ring test). The technique is used also in forensic studies and in detecting adulteration of foodstuffs. A modification of the test, in which precipitation is allowed to occur in agar gel, is used widely for detecting the presence of antibody in serum or antigen in unknown preparations and is valuable for showing the identity of different antigen preparations (fig. 22.9). A variation of this method can be used to identify the individual antigens in multi-component systems such as serum. The components of serum are first separated by electrophoresis in agar gel,

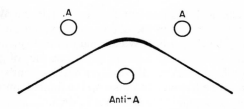

Reaction of identity; may be slightly skewed if different
concentrations in A wells

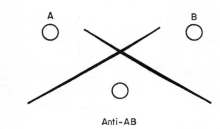

Reaction of non identity; pattern obtained when two
serologically different antigens are used with an antiserum
containing antibody to both

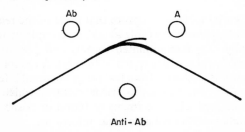

Reaction of partial identity 'spur' formation at junction of
of precipitin bands.

Fig. 22.9. Commonly observed patterns found in double
diffusion plates where two antigen solutions are compared
using antiserum as the analytic agent. From Cruickshank R.
(1968) Medical Microbiology, 11th edition. Edinburgh:
Livingstone.

and an antiserum prepared against the serum is allowed
to diffuse towards them forming precipitin bands (plate
22.2). This method, known as immunoelectrophoresis, is
valuable in showing the presence of abnormal globulin
constituents in the serum of patients with plasma cell
myeloma (p. 28.4).

AGGLUTINATION
In this reaction the antigen is part of the surface of particulate material such as a red blood cell, a bacterium or
perhaps an inorganic particle, e.g. polystyrene latex,
which has been coated with antigen. The addition of antibody to a suspension of such particles links them together to form visible aggregates or agglutinates. In
practice, an agglutination test is carried out in round-
bottomed test tubes, or perspex plates into which round-
bottomed wells have been moulded. A doubling dilution

19

series of the antiserum is made up in the tubes (neat,
$\frac{1}{2}$, $\frac{1}{4}$, $\frac{1}{8}$, etc.) and an equal quantity of the particulate
antigen added to each. After incubation at 37°C, agglu-
tination is seen in the bottom of the tubes, the last tube
showing clearly visible agglutination being taken as the
end point of the test. The dilution of the antiserum at the
end point, e.g. 1/256, the **titre** of the antiserum is used as
a measure of the number of antibody units per unit
volume of serum; e.g. if the end point occurs at a 1/256
dilution of the antiserum and if the test has been carried
out in 1 ml volumes, the titre of the serum is 256 units/ml
of serum. A practical difficulty of importance in agglutination tests is the occasional inhibition of agglutination in the first tubes of an antiserum dilution series,
agglutination occurring only in those tubes containing
more dilute antiserum. This is known as the **prozone
phenomenon** and is probably due to the stabilizing
effects of high protein concentration on the particles; the
protein coating increases the net charge of the particles
and brings about increased electrostatic repulsion between
individual particles, thus opposing the efforts of the antibody molecules to link them together. However, once the
protein concentration is reduced by dilution, the antibody
molecules can exert their effect and bring about agglutination. Agglutination has been shown to be dependent also
upon the presence of electrolytes, and is usually performed for this reason in isotonic saline.

One of the best-known applications of the agglutination test in diagnostic bacteriology is the Widal test used
in the investigation of the serum of patients suspected of
enteric fever for antibodies to the salmonella organisms.
Agglutination is used also in blood grouping (vol. 1,
p. 26.17). Red blood cells and inert particles such
as polystyrene latex can be coated with various antigens.
Thyroglobulin-coated red blood cells are used in a
diagnostic test for thyroid antibody (p. 23.3), and
IgG-coated cells or latex particles are used in the
detection of rheumatoid factor (p. 30.12). Hormone-
coated red blood cells or inert particles are used in many
hormone assay procedures which are based on the inhibition of the antibody (Ab)-induced agglutination of the
particles by hormone added to the sample under test.

Anti-hormone Ab + red cell coated with hormone →
Agglutination
Anti-hormone Ab + free hormone + red cell coated with
hormone → No agglutination.
Tests of this type are used for pregnancy diagnosis.

Certain viruses, e.g. the myxoviruses, influenza virus
and mumps virus, have the property of bringing about
agglutination of red blood cells. Inhibition of this
agglutination by antibody in patients' serum is used
widely as a diagnostic procedure. The presence of antibody in the patient's serum is detected by its ability to
link with the virus particles and prevent them from bringing about agglutination of the red blood cells.

IgM antibodies capable of agglutinating human red blood cells may be serologically active between 0°C and 4°C. Such substances are found in certain human diseases, including primary atypical pneumonia, malaria, trypanosomiasis and acquired haemolytic anaemia and they are often called **cold agglutinins**.

The presence of antibody globulin on red blood cells may not result in direct agglutination of the cells, for example, in some Rh negative mothers with Rh positive infants (vol. 1, p. 26.20) or in acquired haemolytic anaemia. It is, however, possible to show that the red blood cells are coated with antibody globulin by adding an anti-globulin serum (produced in the rabbit by injecting human globulin) which will bring about agglutination of the cells. This is called the antiglobulin test and is a very widely used serological procedure (p. 23.2, fig. 23.1).

COMPLEMENT FIXATION

The fact that antibody is able to activate the complement system, once it combines with antigen, is used as a method of demonstrating the presence of a particular antibody in a serum, e.g. the Wasserman antibody in syphilis, or of identifying an antigen such as a virus.

The complement system consists of a group of nine factors, globulins in nature, present in the serum of normal individuals. The complement of most species reacts with antibody derived from other species and guinea-pig serum is a common laboratory source of complement. Some of the components of complement are destroyed by heating at 58°C for 20–30 min. The individual components of the complement system are taken up by the antibody–antigen complex in a particular order and destruction of the heat-labile components, which are taken up early, prevents the remaining components from taking part.

For most antigens, the reaction of the complement system with the antigen–antibody complex causes in itself no visible effect and it is necessary to use an indicator system consisting of sheep red blood cells coated with anti-sheep red blood cell antibody to detect whether any free complement remains. Complement has the ability to lyse the antibody-coated cells, probably by virtue of the esterase activity of one of the components acting on the red cell membrane. In a test, the antibody, complement and antigen are first mixed together and after a period of incubation the indicator system, antibody-coated sheep red blood cells, is added. If the complement has been taken up during the incubation stage by the original antibody–antigen complex, it is not available to lyse the red cells. Thus a positive complement fixation test is indicated by absence of lysis of the red cells; in a negative test the unfixed complement is shown by lysis of the red cells (fig. 22.10).

The classical complement fixation test is the Wassermann reaction used in the diagnosis of syphilis, in which the test system consists of Wassermann antigen mixed with dilutions of the patient's serum in the presence of guinea-pig complement. After the antigen and patient's serum have had time to react and take up the limited amount of complement available in the system, the indicator system is added to show whether or not there is free complement.

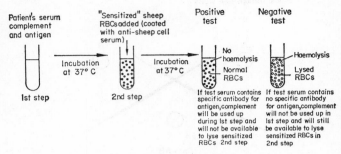

FIG. 22.10. The possible results of a complement fixation test. From Cruickshank R. (1968) Medical Microbiology, 11th Edition. Edinburgh: Livingstone.

Controls are included to ensure that none of the reagents are anti-complementary (able to take up complement non-specifically, e.g. contaminated serum) and positive and negative control sera are tested in parallel. A complement fixation test is also useful as a test for gonococcal infection and for detecting viruses in tissue cultures which have been inoculated with specimens of blood or tissue fluids from humans with probable virus infections.

ANTIGEN–ANTIBODY REÀCTIONS USING FLUORESCENT LABELS

The precise localization of tissue antigens or the antigens of infecting organisms in the body, of anti-tissue antibody and of antigen–antibody complexes was achieved by the introduction of the use of fluorochrome-labelled proteins by Coons and Kaplan in 1950. The absorption of ultraviolet light between 290 and 495 nm by fluorescein and its emission as green light (525 nm) makes protein, which has been labelled with the dye, visible. The technique is more sensitive than precipitation or complement fixation, and can detect protein at a concentration of the order of 1 μg/ml.

Applications

Some of the uses to which the technique has been put include the localization of the origin of a variety of serum protein components, for example immunoglobulin production by plasma cells and lymphoid cells. The demonstration and localization in the tissues of antibody globulin in a variety of autoimmune conditions has been achieved, including an antinuclear antibody in the serum of some patients with systemic lupus erythematosus and thyroid autoantibodies in the serum of patients with chronic thyroiditis (p. 23.7). In the diagnostic field human pathogens can be demonstrated by immunofluorescence and a tentative diagnosis may be given much sooner than by cultivation; however, the fluorescent method is at present used to supplement rather than to replace conventional methods.

Two main procedures are in use, the direct and indirect methods (fig. 22.11). The direct method consists of bring-

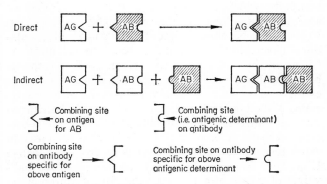

FIG. 22.11. The direct and indirect fluorescent antibody methods. Hatching represents fluorescein conjugated antibody. From Cruickshank R. (1968) Medical Microbiology, 11th Edition. Edinburgh: Livingstone.

ing antibodies to which fluorescein has been attached into contact with antigens fixed on a slide, e.g. in the form of a tissue section or a smear of organisms, allowing them to react, washing off excess antibody and examining under the fluorescent microscope. The site of union of the labelled antibody with its antigen can be seen by the apple-green fluorescent areas on the slide. The indirect method can be used both for detecting specific antibodies in sera or other body fluids and also for identifying antigens. This method differs from the direct method in the use of a non-labelled antiserum which is layered on the section or smear; whether or not this antiserum has reacted with the material on the slide is shown by means of a fluorescein-tagged antiglobulin serum, specific for the globulin of the serum applied first. Such an antiglobulin serum can be used to detect in sera antibody globulin to a variety of different antigens, which gives it a considerable advantage over the direct test; it is also more sensitive.

Role of antibody in protection against infective agents

The production of antibody, the primary interaction between antibody and antigens of an infective agent, and the secondary phenomena, which such union may induce, do not guarantee that the infective agent will be inactivated or eliminated from the body. Micro-organisms

have numerous ways of protecting themselves from, and side-tracking, the immune reaction of the host. For example, the pneumococcus produces large quantities of capsular polysaccharide which repels phagocytes and mops up the antibody produced, thus allowing the pneumococcus itself to proliferate unhindered. Trypanosomes can change their surface antigens from one generation to the next, so that the antibody made to the original organism is inactive against the ones which appear later. Some micro-organisms, particularly tubercle bacilli, brucella and many viruses, disappear inside tissue cells before sufficient antibody is produced to act against them. In short, a particular micro-organism is pathogenic because in some way it circumvents, at least initially, the immune response of the host. Luckily, however, the host immune response in most instances eventually comes out on top, and finally the infective agent is eliminated from the body.

How does the production of antibody and its reaction with antigen bring about these desirable consequences? First consider the effect of antibodies on the exotoxins produced by diphtheria, tetanus and gas gangrene organisms (antitoxins). For protection, antibodies must be present in sufficient quantity to neutralize toxin faster than it is produced. In this event the host is kept alive while the invading bacteria are eliminated by immune reactions directed at the bacteria themselves. An animal which has been previously actively immunized against the toxin has an immunological memory of the toxin; it can produce antibody rapidly and has an advantage over one which has had no previous experience of the antigen. The infected individual with no immunological memory may require to be given antibody prophylactically in order to tide him over the first stages of infection.

Where a micro-organism does not secrete exotoxins, the protection afforded by antibodies depends largely on the enhancement of phagocytosis of the micro-organism brought about by the antibody's action as an opsonin.

The effect of antibody on the bacterium is to change the cell surface and facilitate phagocytosis. In the case of pneumococci, as already mentioned, the capsular polysaccharide prevents this by mopping up antibody unless the infection is controlled before the organisms proliferate and produce the polysaccharide. The streptococcus contains material known as M protein which enables the organism to resist intracellular digestion. However, in the presence of antibodies against the M protein, the organism is not only phagocytosed more rapidly but can also be digested by the enzymes of the phagocyte.

In virus infections the efficacy of antibody depends largely on whether the virus passes through the blood stream in order to reach its target organ. The poliovirus, after crossing the intestinal wall, is carried in the blood stream to the spinal cord and brain where it proliferates.

Small amounts of antibody in the blood can neutralize the virus before it reaches the nervous tissue. Other viruses which pass through the blood stream to their target organ are those of measles, mumps, rubella and chickenpox. These infections are characterized by a prolonged incubation period, in contradistinction to viruses which have a short incubation period such as the influenza and common cold viruses, where the target organ is the site of primary infection, namely the respiratory mucous membranes. In this type of virus infection, although the blood antibody level may be high it is relatively ineffective against the infection, compared with its effect on blood-borne viruses. It seems likely that in these cases the effective immunoglobulins are those made locally in the mucous membranes, such as the IgA, which is present in higher concentration in such membranes than in the blood. Thus, in this type of virus infection, immunization by conventional methods is likely to be less effective than in the case of the blood-borne viruses.

A quite distinct type of resistance mechanism in virus infection is the production of **interferon**, which interferes with the synthesis of new virus by cells of the host. Interferon, unlike antibody, is not specific for the virus which may have induced its formation but is able to interfere with other quite different groups of virus. Interferon rather than antibody is probably responsible for cure in virus infection in the non-immune individual. It is worth noting that persons with hypogammaglobulinaemia, who have little resistance to infections where circulating antibodies are known to play an important part, can usually survive virus infection. This may be due in part to the interferon mechanism and also to an immunity induced in the actual infected cells, the kind of immune response which is exemplified by the delayed cell-mediated hypersensitivity reaction of the tuberculin type (p. 20.20).

CELL-MEDIATED IMMUNE RESPONSE

In the immunologically mature individual, contact with an antigen leads not only to the production of circulating antibody, but also to the development of a separate cell-mediated immune response. This is brought about by cells in the lymphoreticular system, as described in vol. 1, p. 27.2. The response may give rise to a variable degree of delayed hypersensitivity reaction (p. 22.20) and it is by means of this that cell-mediated immunity is recognized. These reactions characteristically follow the intradermal injection of antigen in a suitably sensitized individual and develop more slowly, as the name suggests, than the immediate type of reaction. After a few hours, slight redness may appear at the injection site, developing gradually over 18–48 hours into an indurated lump consisting mainly of perivascular masses of mononuclear cells (macrophages and lymphocytes); this contrasts with the immediate type of hypersensitivity

reaction where the cellular response is mainly of polymorphonuclear leucocytes.

Delayed hypersensitivity is characteristically induced by infectious agents which are predominantly intracellular in the infected host. This includes many virus infections (measles, smallpox, herpes) and some bacterial infections (tuberculosis, brucellosis, pertussis, syphilis). The micro-organisms responsible for these diseases are to a large extent protected from circulating antibody by their intracellular position, and it is likely that cell-mediated immunity which they induce is the primary defence against them. However, this is a highly controversial issue and has been the subject of much study and speculation. Tuberculous infection has been studied most exhaustively in this respect (p. 21.17). A skin response based on this type of reaction can be induced by various extracts of tubercle bacilli and is the basis of the **tuberculin** or **Mantoux test**, which is widely used in humans to discover whether the individual has been previously exposed to the tubercle bacillus; this test has been used in cattle to eliminate bovine tuberculosis from the British Isles. Thus an intradermal injection in a sensitized individual of 0·1 ml of a 1 in 1000 dilution of a protein extract of tubercle bacilli (purified protein derivative, PPD) induces an inflammatory indurated response appearing gradually over 18–48 hours.

The efficacy of BCG vaccination in preventing tuberculosis has been substantiated in the last few years by a large scale Medical Research Council trial. However, the mechanism of this immunity is not understood; circulating antibody is produced against various antigenic constituents of the tubercle bacillus, but transfer of such antibody to a second individual does not give protection from infection.

The inhibitory effect of monocytic cells from an immunized guinea-pig on the growth of tubercle bacilli has been shown both *in vivo* and *in vitro*. Furthermore, individuals with congenital hypogammaglobulinaemia can be successfully immunized with BCG vaccine, despite their inability to produce circulating antibodies. They produce positive tuberculin skin tests; in addition, after infection with measles, chickenpox and mumps, they are well known to develop resistance to further infection with these viruses and show positive delayed type skin tests to them. Although it is not possible to prove the role of cell-mediated immunity in resistance to infectious disease, these observations strongly suggest that it may play a valuable part.

Hypersensitivity

Early in the study of immunity it became apparent that the immune response to the antigens of micro-organisms sometimes failed to give protection, and might even produce harmful effects. These effects are known as **hypersensitivity reactions**, and are mainly due to tissue damage caused by pharmacologically active agents such as histamine which are formed following combination of antibody with antigen. It was soon found that hypersensitivity could be evoked also by intrinsically harmless substances such as foreign serum protein and even simple chemicals.

The term **allergy** was coined by von Pirquet at the beginning of the century to describe the altered reactivity of an animal after exposure to a foreign antigenic material. For him this included both protective and hypersensitivity reactions. However, over the years allergy has had a more restricted use and now refers only to hypersensitivity.

Fig. 22.12 summarizes the possible consequences of the development of immunity. The hypersensitivity states can be divided into two groups. The immediate, humoral

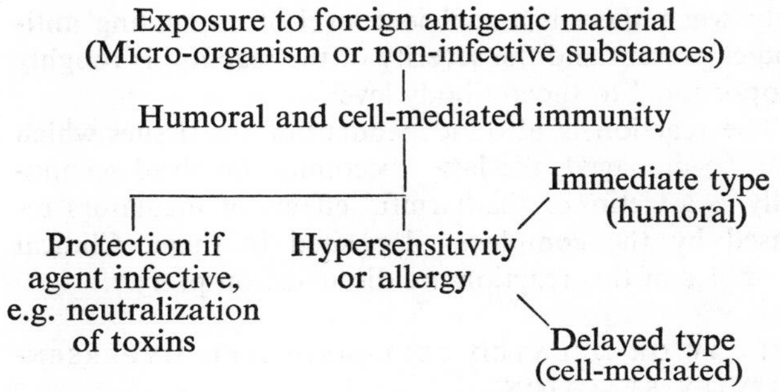

Exposure to foreign antigenic material
(Micro-organism or non-infective substances)

Humoral and cell-mediated immunity

Protection if agent infective, e.g. neutralization of toxins

Hypersensitivity or allergy

Immediate type (humoral)

Delayed type (cell-mediated)

FIG. 22.12. Consequences of the development of immunity.

type depends on the reaction of humoral antibody with antigen, and appears within minutes, but can occur up to several hours. It depends on the formation of pharmacologically active substances which affect vascular permeability and cause contraction of smooth muscle (p. 14.14) and is further subdivided into three types (table 22.2). The delayed, cell-mediated type (type IV, table 22.2) depends

TABLE 22.2. Hypersensitivity reactions

Type	Reaction
I	*Anaphylactic reaction* Systemic anaphylaxis Local anaphylaxis (hay fever, asthma, urticaria, food allergy)
II	*Cytolytic or Cytotoxic reaction* Transfusion reactions Haemolytic disease of newborn Autoimmune haemolytic anaemias Drug-induced haemolytic anaemia, purpura and agranulocytosis
III	*Toxic-complex reaction* Arthus reaction Serum sickness
IV	*Delayed cell-mediated hypersensitivity* Bacterial allergy (delayed skin reactions of tuberculin type) Contact dermatitis Autoimmune states

on the interaction of lymphoid cells with antigen and appears slowly. It involves the release of substances including that of a pharmacological mediator (lymph node permeability factor) which is distinct from those substances released by humoral antigen-antibody interaction (p. 14.16).

TYPE I OR ANAPHYLACTIC REACTION

This depends on a foreign antigen reacting with antibodies present in the tissues. An anaphylactic reaction can take place only in an individual who has been previously sensitized by contact with antigen. In most cases the directly observable effects can be attributed to the release of histamine from mast cells. Systemic anaphylaxis or anaphylactic shock was first described by Richet in 1902; he observed that dogs, after a single injection of an antigen, might die rapidly after a second injection a few days later. This increased susceptibility to a foreign substance he called anaphylaxis. Severe and fatal anaphylactic shock is associated with difficulty in breathing due to constriction of the bronchi and bronchioles, urticaria, pulmonary oedema and fall in blood pressure. It can be produced relatively easily in dogs, rabbits and guinea-pigs, but rats and other rodents are very difficult to sensitize; most monkeys can be sensitized only with difficulty. Severe anaphylactic shock occurs in man under a variety of conditions (p. 23.1), but it is not common and there are great variations in susceptibility.

Local anaphylaxis may occur when an antigen gains access locally to any surface of the body; it is especially prevalent in the respiratory mucous membranes, where it is responsible for the symptoms of hay fever and asthma. Urticaria and other skin reactions and a variety of gastrointestinal disturbances are also due to local anaphylaxis (p. 23.1). Colloquially, allergy usually refers to one or other of these manifestations of local anaphylaxis.

Mechanism of anaphylaxis

The nature of the immunoglobulin involved in anaphylaxis has posed a problem for many years. Known as the **reaginic antibody** it was found to be closely associated with IgA globulins. A new class of immunoglobulin, IgE, was first isolated and identified from the serum of patients suffering from plasma cell myeloma (p. 23.12) where it is often present in large excess. An immunoassay was developed and IgE can now be estimated in normal serum, where it is found in very small quantities. The amount of IgE in normal serum is 1/40,000 that of IgG and 1/5000 that of IgA. IgE certainly has reaginic activity, but doubt remains whether reaginic antibody is IgE in all cases.

The reaginic antibody appears to have a particular affinity for cell membranes and can remain fixed there for many weeks, e.g. to skin cells, thus rendering the tissue susceptible to antigen with the ensuing development of an anaphylactic response. If the antigen could be diverted from the tissue-fixed reaginic antibody, no anaphylaxis would take place. One method by which this can be brought about is by the antibody, freely circulating in the blood and tissue fluids, and not fixed to cells, mopping up the antigen. It is known that anaphylaxis occurs only when the level of freely circulating antibody is low, for example towards the end of an immune state, perhaps months or years after an immunizing injection, or in a poorly immunized animal. Guinea-pigs can be rendered susceptible to anaphylaxis by the injection of a small amount of serum from a well immunized (hyperimmune) animal whilst a larger quantity of serum fails to induce the anaphylactic state.

Desensitization can be brought about by raising the level of circulating antibody sufficiently to mop up antigen before it reaches tissue cells coated with reaginic antibody. How this may be effected in human anaphylactic states is discussed on p. 23.2.

The reaction between antigen and reaginic antibody on the cell surface releases histamine and other pharmacologically active substances which are discussed on p. 14.14.

TYPE II CYTOLYTIC OR CYTOTOXIC REACTION
These reactions are initiated by an antigenic component which is either part of a tissue cell or closely associated with a tissue cell, e.g. a drug attached to a cell wall. The antibodies, which are IgG or IgM in type, are directed against such a cell-associated antigen and bring about a cytotoxic or cytolytic effect, usually involving complement. Transfusion reactions due to the action of anti-red or white cell antibodies fall into this category, as does haemolytic disease of the newborn and certain forms of autoimmune disease (p. 23.2). Drug hypersensitivity can also be brought about by this mechanism, since drugs can form an antigenic complex with red cells, white cells or platelets. Sedormid thrombocytopenic purpura is a classical example of the result of complex formation between platelets and the drug sedormid, a carbamide analgesic which is no longer in use (p. 23.3).

TYPE III OR TOXIC-COMPLEX REACTION
Complexes between antigen and antibody may form in the blood stream and tissues in conditions where there is a relatively high level of circulating antibody. Mechanical blocking occurs when the complexes are precipitated in the small blood vessels and this can produce a variety of lesions. The classical example in experimental pathology is the **Arthus reaction**. In 1903, Arthus showed that when rabbits were inoculated at one site with repeated doses of horse serum, the initial injections were without effect. After a few injections, swelling and oedema occurred at the site of inoculation. These were at first transient and localized, but later firm, indurated swellings were formed which sometimes became necrotic. The intensity of these reactions was shown to vary directly with the level of precipitating antibody in the blood. Poorly vascularized tissues such as the cornea were less affected by contact with antigen.

These reactions can be explained as attributable to disturbances in nutrition following a failure of capillary function. The initial formation of the antigen–antibody complex attracts circulating leucocytes; these, together with platelets and fibrin, become lodged in a small vessel. This may lead to release of histamine and other chemical mediators and cytotoxic enzymes, and be followed by thrombosis, haemorrhage and necrosis. The intensity of these reactions in an animal can be reduced by decreasing the numbers of circulating platelets and leucocytes and by giving heparin. The toxic-complex reactions are distinguished from anaphylactic reactions in that they occur only when there is a sufficient level of circulating antibodies present and the severity of the reaction is roughly proportional to the antibody level.

The reaction is also independent of the tissues which may be damaged, the latter becoming involved secondarily as a victim of the harmful effects of mediators released by the complexes deposited in them. Clinical examples of this reaction are discussed on p. 23.7.

TYPE IV OR DELAYED CELL-MEDIATED HYPERSENSITIVITY REACTION
This is described on p. 22.18 as a specifically provoked, slowly evolving mixed cellular reaction involving particularly lymphocytes and macrophages, in no way dependent on circulating antibody. The classical example of this type of reaction is the tuberculin response.

These reactions, characteristically induced by intracellular infectious agents, can also occur by skin contact with a variety of simple chemical substances ranging from picryl chloride, paraphenylene diamine in hair dyes, and metals such as nickel, to drugs, including penicillin. These substances are not themselves antigenic and only become so by covalent binding to proteins in the skin. The clinical features induced in contact hypersensitivity reactions (contact dermatitis) include redness, swelling, vesicles, scaling and exudation of fluid (p. 23.7).

The nature of the mechanism whereby lymphoid cells react with these antigenic materials is not understood but is likely to involve antibody-like receptors on the surface of the lymphoid cells. The changes which occur following interaction of a sensitized cell with antigen probably depend on a pharmacologically active substance distinct from those responsible for the immediate type reaction. A material known as lymph node permeability factor (LNPF), as yet undefined, has been recovered from both normal and sensitized lymphoid cells (p. 14.16). Other factors including one with a cytotoxic effect have been found.

Active and passive immunization in clinical practice

Active and passive immunization have important applications in clinical practice. The chance of spread of an infection in a community is much reduced if 60–80 per cent of the population is immunized against it, and then the herd immunity is said to be favourable. In infections that are not acquired from case to case, e.g. tetanus, the state of the herd immunity does not influence an individual's chances of acquiring the disease although its incidence is likely to be lower the greater the number of the population who are immunized; nevertheless cases may continue to occur until 100 per cent immunization of the population is achieved.

SAFETY

A community will accept immunizing procedures only if the advantages clearly outweigh the disadvantages. The dangers in immunization arise mainly from adverse reactions due to hypersensitivity in individuals who are treated, errors in the preparation of the material and in its administration. Encephalitis or generalized vaccinia after smallpox vaccination, febrile convulsions after whooping cough vaccines and transverse myelitis after rabies vaccines are well known to immunologists; these and other similar reactions are exceedingly rare and the risk from them is, in general, much less than the risk of the patient contracting a serious form of the disease against which protection is required. Very rarely paralytic poliomyelitis occurs in an individual shortly after receiving a prophylactic inoculation for another disease, e.g. diphtheria, and the paralysis is usually restricted to the limb used for injection. This is known as provocation poliomyelitis and occurs during symptomless infection with the virus. The risk of a child developing provocation poliomyelitis as a result of receiving an immunizing agent has been reduced to negligible proportions by the development of poliomyelitis vaccines that are used early in childhood.

Vaccine preparations have been issued in which the immunizing agent has not been rendered avirulent or in which there has been contamination by other pathogenic organs. This can lead to disaster. However, the fingers of one hand probably suffice to count such disasters in over sixty years during which millions of batches of vaccine have been issued.

By far the greatest danger to the individual now arises from the introduction of infection at the time of administration of the vaccine. The greatest care must be taken to use a sterile technique. In a wealthy community, it should be normal practice to use a separate disposable syringe and needle for each patient. In the mass inoculation of large numbers of people in poor countries, this is obviously impossible. However, in all circumstances every effort should be made to ensure the sterility of the procedure. In particular the risk of transmitting jaundice must be borne in mind. Serum hepatitis is a dangerous disease, which has been responsible for many deaths.

ASSESSMENT OF ACTIVE IMMUNIZATION

There are difficulties in the standardization of a vaccine for human use and in assessing its possible ill effects. Laboratory techniques are available for assessing the potency of immunizing agents and often involve protection tests in animals; but there may be differences in the response of experimental animals and those of man. The most convincing evidence is afforded by properly controlled field trials and some vaccines have been assessed in this way. For example, the efficacy of BCG vaccine against tuberculosis has been established beyond doubt by several well-planned trials.

In some cases, a vaccine has established its merit in practice, as is illustrated by the record of diphtheria immunization in Britain. Notifications of diphtheria in Britain averaged about 70,000–80,000 annually until 1940 when mass immunization commenced. There were 60,514 notifications in 1940 and 61,834 in 1941. By 1947 the numbers had decreased to 6672, by 1951 to 798, and in 1967 there were just 6 cases notified in England.

Since 1941 most of the cases have occurred in non-immunized individuals, and no immunized person has died from diphtheria in Britain since 1948. Since 1955, with the exception of small localized outbreaks, diphtheria has been virtually eradicated from Britain and Canada, as well as several other countries.

PRIORITIES IN ARTIFICIAL ACTIVE AND PASSIVE IMMUNIZATION

The principles of artificial active and passive immunization are illustrated by reference to the problems involved in the prevention of tetanus. This is not a common disease in Britain, but it remains a major cause of morbidity and mortality in large areas of the world.

Tetanus toxin can be readily converted to a nontoxic toxoid, and a course of toxoid injections stimulates the production of protective antitoxin. Since the initial injection does not stimulate an adequately protective antibody response, active immunization requires at least two injections at about 6 weeks interval to ensure a secondary response. If the secondary response is boosted after a further interval of about 6 months, protection lasts for at least 5 years. The incorporation of an adjuvant (aluminium hydroxide) on which the toxoid is adsorbed, increases its antigenicity. As there is a delay in producing immunity, tetanus toxoid is of no immediate use in an emergency, but it produces a durable immunity and no adverse reactions.

When a person is injured and is considered to be at risk from tetanus, there is no time to wait for the development of active immunity and passive protection must be achieved. This is also the case when diphtheria is suspected. Under these circumstances, pre-formed antitoxin may be given to the patient. Antitoxin is usually produced by the injection of courses of antigen into horses so that large amounts of serum are available. Although the serum is subsequently refined, it is still liable to produce occasional reactions in man and passive immunization with antitoxin is associated with this accepted risk. The reactions range from negligible effects to dangerous and sometimes fatal anaphylactic responses. Thus, the immediate production of a protective level of antibody obtained by the injection of antiserum into a patient is achieved at the cost of a possible hypersensitivity reaction. Moreover, as the protein is foreign to the recipient, the antibody is fairly rapidly eliminated and the protection afforded is shortlived and may be sustained for only 2 or 3 weeks. Many of the problems associated with passive artificial immunization may be avoided if the antibody is developed in man and the use of homologous antiserum in human patients is likely to be extended in the future. Human γ-globulin is already used for the protection of patients at risk from various diseases. Although the protection afforded by homologous antiserum to patients is also transient, it is effective for periods varying from several weeks to a few months and it is unattended by the risks associated with the use of heterologous sera. There is nevertheless a place for the continued use of heterologous sera in special circumstances, for example in countries that cannot yet afford to produce stocks of homologous serum.

IMMUNIZATION SCHEDULES (table 22.3)
Immunization schedules may be considered with regard to protection of the child against diseases that are likely to present their challenge at predictable times in life. Thus, procedures currently practised in Britain differ from those that might be appropriate elsewhere and recommendations concerning active immunization should be made with local or national conditions in mind. Epidemiological and financial considerations frequently dictate the programme that can be made available. After primary courses of immunization have been given to a significant proportion of the population, periodic booster doses may be used to maintain the herd immunity and primary courses must continue to be given to succeeding generations. When an immunization campaign has been successfully prosecuted for a decade, there is a risk that apathy to the particular disease is engendered in the population and the numbers then submitted for primary courses begin to decrease. If this happens in Britain with regard to diphtheria, for example, it will not be long before the disease reminds the population of its lethal potential.

In Britain, a child is normally actively immunized during its first year of life with a vaccine that contains diphtheria and tetanus toxoid in combination with a killed suspension of whooping-cough (pertussis) organisms. The **triple vaccine** (dip-tet-pert) provides a strong antigenic stimulus, enhanced by the adjuvant action of the pertussis component. This vaccine is effective in early childhood; three doses are required, the first being given as early as 3 months, but the response is better if this is delayed until 6 months of age. Thereafter, the second dose is given 6–8 weeks later and the third dose after an interval of about 6 months. The injection of the triple vaccine may be combined with three oral doses of poliomyelitis vaccine so that, early in the second year of life, the child is protected against diphtheria, whooping cough and poliomyelitis and immunity against tetanus is also ensured. The vaccination against smallpox is given by applying one dose of living relatively avirulent vaccine into the skin during the second year of life, the complications of primary smallpox vaccination being least common in this age group. Measles vaccination may also be offered during the second year. Immunity to diphtheria, tetanus, poliomyelitis and smallpox is reinforced by booster doses of vaccine given at 5 years or at the age of school entry when the child is likely to be exposed to these diseases. Further vaccination against whooping cough is not usually undertaken, as the risk of serious complications of the disease is slight in older children. Booster doses of tetanus, poliomyelitis and smallpox vaccines are given at age 15–19. The living attenuated BCG vaccine, which confers immunity to tuberculosis, is given to children who have not acquired a natural immunity to the disease within their first ten years of life.

Travellers are exposed to infectious hazards in different countries. By international agreement, international certificates of vaccination against smallpox, cholera and yellow fever have been prescribed and one or more of these are essential documents for travellers between many countries. These seek to protect not only the individual but also the community to which he is going. The traveller is often well advised to seek immunization against other diseases that he may encounter and these include typhoid and paratyphoid fevers, plague, influenza and typhus fever. Adult travellers occasionally forget that poliomyelitis and diphtheria are significant risks in some countries. It is not yet possible to be artificially actively immunized against infective hepatitis, but effective passive protection against this disease can be acquired for a short period by accepting an injection of normal pooled human γ-globulin which contains the appropriate antibodies. Immunization against mumps, Q-fever and tularaemia may now be offered to laboratory workers and others at special risk. Vaccination has similarly been practised against brucellosis and leptospirosis in man, but the vaccines used are not generally available and their protective value against occupational hazards is not yet fully established.

TABLE 22.3. A schedule of vaccination and immunization procedures. After the Department of Health & Social Security (1969).

Age	Prophylactic	Interval	Notes
During the 1st year of life	Dip-tet-pert and oral polio vaccine (first dose)		The earliest age at which the first dose should be given is 3 months, but a better general immunological response can be expected if the first dose is delayed up to 6 months of age.
	Dip-tet-pert and oral polio vaccine (second dose)	Preferably after an interval of 6–8 weeks.	
	Dip-tet-pert and oral polio vaccine (third dose)	Preferably after an interval of 6 months.	
During the 2nd year of life	Measles vaccination	Not less than 3 weeks after a previous vaccine.	
	Smallpox vaccination	Not less than 3 weeks after a previous vaccine.	While the 2nd year is recommended for routine vaccination against smallpox, in individual cases and if special circumstances call for it, vaccination against smallpox may be carried out during the 1st year.
At 5 years of age or school entry	Dip-tet and oral polio vaccine or Dip-tet-polio vaccine Smallpox revaccination		With the exception of smallpox revaccination these may be given, if desired, at 3 years of age to children entering nursery schools, attending day nurseries or living in children's homes.
Between 10 & 13 years of age	BCG vaccine		For tuberculin-negative children.
At 15–19 years of age or on leaving school	Polio vaccine (oral or inactivated). Tetanus toxoid. Smallpox revaccination		

VACCINATION

Active immunity against smallpox is conferred by **vaccinia** virus; its origin is uncertain and it may be derived from variola or cowpox viruses (p. 18.116). The vaccine consists of lymph obtained from vesicles produced on the skin of calves or sheep by inoculating the scarified skin with the virus.

The vaccine lymph is supplied usually in glass capillary tubes; if it is stored frozen, its potency is maintained for about a year at −10°C and it may be kept in a domestic refrigerator for up to 2 weeks. It is inactivated at room temperatures and no vaccine should be used after more than 7 days from the date of dispatch, unless it has been kept in a refrigerator. The vaccine is administered intradermally, usually on the upper arm, and the multiple pressure procedure is recommended. A drop of vaccine lymph is spread over an area of skin about 0·5 cm in diameter. The skin must be clean, but no disinfectant should be used. Pressure is applied to the skin through the vaccine with a sterile large flat needle, held so that it is almost parallel to the surface. To introduce the vaccine into the epidermis, the needle is applied quickly, but not so vigorously as to draw blood. From 10 to 30 such 'pressures' are recommended, ten sufficing usually for a

'take' in primary vaccination. The dermojet, which is recommended when large numbers of vaccinations have to be done, is a small pistol-like injector which squirts a tiny stream of vaccine on to the skin at very high pressure.

After vaccination, excess lymph is wiped off with sterile cotton wool and the site allowed to dry. It is not necessary to apply a dressing at this stage. The patient should be advised to avoid wetting the site and a dry dressing should be applied if a pustule develops.

Three types of reaction may occur:

The **primary** reaction, seen in persons not previously vaccinated, consists of a red papule which appears in 3–4 days. A vesicle develops in 5–6 days, becoming pustular in 8 days. After 11 days a dry scab has usually formed, which falls off after about 21 days.

The **accelerated reaction**, occurring only in persons previously vaccinated successfully, is similar but more rapid. The vesicle is formed on the third day and becomes pustular next day and the scab is off within 8 days.

An **immediate reaction** consists of an erythematous papule appearing usually within 24 hours and reaching a maximum in 72 hours, when it fades rapidly without the formation of a vesicle. This occurs only in persons previously vaccinated and is a type IV hypersensitivity reaction. It does not necessarily indicate immunity, although often occurring in immune subjects.

A primary or accelerated reaction involves a sore arm during the vesicular and pustular stages. There is usually little or no general malaise, though small children may appear temporarily upset, but some restriction of activity is necessary and children should be forbidden vigorous games. The lesion is infectious at the pustular stage and patients should be advised accordingly.

Complications are very rare. Encephalitis and generalized vaccinia have already been mentioned. In persons with a history of dermatitis, the local reaction may be severe and constitute **eczema vaccinatum.** Necrosis of the skin may occur; this may be progressive in patients with hypogammaglobulinaemia or in patients receiving immunosuppressive drugs and is known as **vaccinia gangrenosa.**

Primary vaccination usually confers a good immunity for 5–10 years. Revaccination every 7 years has been the orthodox advice for a long time and this is sensible, but vaccination should have been carried out within 3 years if an assurance of protection is sought after there has been direct contact with a case of smallpox or during an epidemic. An international certificate of vaccination is needed for travel between most countries and this must be renewed every 3 years.

In countries such as Britain, in which smallpox is rarely seen, some responsible persons consider that the risk of death or disability as a result of smallpox is even less than the very small risk of developing one of the serious complications of vaccination. They therefore recommend that in such countries, primary vaccination should not be carried out except when there is an outbreak of smallpox. Others take the view that, since the risk of developing a serious complication is least when primary vaccination is performed in the early years of life, it is best to vaccinate children as a routine. It is difficult to compare these very small risks accurately, but most doctors who have had experience in treating smallpox get their own children vaccinated in the second year of life, as recommended above.

FURTHER READING

CRUICKSHANK R. & WEIR D.M. eds. (1967) *Modern Trends in Immunology—2.* London: Butterworths.

GELL P.G.H. & COOMBS R.R.A. (1968) *Clinical Aspects of Immunology,* 2nd Edition. Oxford: Blackwell Scientific Publications.

HOLBOROW E.J. (1968) *An ABC of Modern Immunology.* London: Lancet.

HUMPHREY J.H. & WHITE R.G. (1969) *Immunology for Students of Medicine,* 3rd Edition. Oxford: Blackwell Scientific Publications.

PARISH H.J. (1968) *Victory with Vaccines.* Edinburgh: Livingstone.

PORTER R.R. (1967) *The Structure of Antibodies.* Scientific American Offprint No. 1083. San Francisco: Freeman.

Chapter 23
Immunological mechanisms in the production of disease

The last chapter contains an account of the nature of hypersensitivity reactions. Here the concern is to discuss how these reactions cause disease in man. It is now more than fifty years since the role of anaphylaxis in diseases such as asthma, hay fever and food sensitivities was first discovered. Since then the immune mechanisms responsible for transfusion reactions, haemolytic disease of the newborn and other blood disorders have been elucidated. The discovery during the last fifteen years that aberrant immunological reactions are also the probable cause of many important diseases, previously labelled as idiopathic, has been one of the most exciting events in modern medicine. Immune reactions are implicated in the apparently spontaneous atrophy of various tissues such as the thyroid, parathyroid and adrenal glands and the gastric mucosa, either individually or collectively. They may also be involved in the progressive destruction of organs, such as the kidneys i.e., glomerulonephritis and in certain conditions of the liver. The changes produced in these tissues are basically inflammatory in nature and the conditions are therefore referred to as chronic thyroiditis, gastritis, etc. Other inflammatory diseases of these tissues, mainly of known infective aetiology are given the same general name, but are not relevant to the mechanisms discussed here.

The present chapter is based on the classification of hypersensitivity reactions given in table 22.2, p. 22.19. The major diseases that may arise from each of the four main types of hypersensitivity are considered in turn. Disorders of connective tissue in which aberrant immunological mechanisms may play an important role are described on p. 30.9.

The rare group of diseases which arise when one or more parts of the immunological system fail to develop is also described, together with some disorders in which immunoglobulins are present in the blood in excess. An account is also given of drug hypersensitivity.

Type I or anaphylactic reactions

Systemic anaphylaxis occurring in animals is described on p. 22.19. In man it may be induced by a foreign protein, e.g. antitetanus or antidiphtheria horse serum, some-times by drugs such as penicillin or local anaesthetics and very occasionally by streptomycin, PAS, iodine-containing contrast media used in radiography and insect stings. Anaphylactic shock is fortunately rare and it is often fatal. Within 30 min of receiving an injection of the offending serum or drug, the patient collapses with wheezing and a feeling of tightness over the chest; the blood pressure falls, urticaria, cyanosis and convulsions follow and death may occur from cardiac arrest in a few minutes.

More limited reactions, **local anaphylaxis**, caused by antigens gaining access to the tissues via the respiratory and gastrointestinal tracts, are much more frequent. Common allergens are present in strawberries, nuts, egg, fish, pollens, dandruff, milk and fragments of insects; aspirin has also been implicated.

Respiratory symptoms include hay fever, rhinitis and asthma arising from bronchiolar constriction. In the skin there may be urticaria (nettle rash or hives), oedema, purpura or eczema. Oedema sometimes involves the eyelids, lips, tongue and larynx, when it is called angioneurotic oedema. Common gastrointestinal symptoms are dyspepsia, vomiting and diarrhoea. In severe cases headache, fever, joint pains and circulatory collapse may develop.

Sudden death of babies in their cot is sometimes due to aspiration of cow's milk which induces a local anaphylactic response in the lungs followed by asphyxia due to pulmonary oedema. The severe oedema of the lung in lobar pneumonia due to the pneumococcus has also been ascribed to type I allergy; this may explain the severity of the reaction of the tissues to a bacteria from which no soluble toxic factor can be identified (p. 18.69).

A local reaction occurs in a person who is generally sensitized, and this would be revealed if sufficient of the antigen were absorbed. It is not known, however, why one person with general sensitization exposed to an antigen present in the inspired air experiences asthma, whereas another exposed to the same antigen develops only hay fever. This is hard to explain as a quantitative dosage effect, and there may be some as yet unknown local predisposing factors. IgE is raised in the blood in persons subject to anaphylactic reactions, sometimes as much as sixfold and it is possible that its concentration may be related to the severity of the reactions. Allergens which invoke IgE do so in extremely low concentrations of < 1 pg/ml.

Hypersensitivity reactions in any one patient may not be limited to any one type. Thus in patients with asthma associated with pulmonary *Aspergillus fumigatus* not only are reaginic antibodies present but other types of antibodies associated with type III reactions are also involved (p. 23.6).

One of the curious features about reagin is that its known actions are harmful and of no obvious benefit to the individual or the species. The concentration of IgE however has been found to be raised in Ethiopian children, especially those infested with *Ascaris lumbricoides*. It remains to be established whether this is responsible for effective protection against worms.

DESENSITIZATION
This is achieved by repeated small subcutaneous injections of the antigen to which the patient is hypersensitive over a period of a few months. The dose is slowly increased during the course, as the injection of a large quantity of antigen at the start would carry a risk of an anaphylactic reaction, particularly if accidentally given intravenously. The antibody which develops as a result of this treatment is sometimes referred to as 'blocking antibody' as it blocks antigen from contact with reaginic antibody coating tissue cells. The titre of blocking antibody can be readily followed in the serum by means of agglutination tests with red cells coated with the appropriate antigen (p. 22.15).

The main problem associated with this treatment, particularly in local anaphylaxis, e.g. hay fever and asthma, is that it is frequently difficult to be sure which of a number of possible antigens is responsible for the hypersensitivity. The patient is usually tested by an intradermal injection or prick through a drop of antigen on the skin, with a panel of different antigens; even if the panel contains an antigen to which the patient is sensitive, cross reactions frequently occur which make it difficult to arrive at a precise diagnosis. Furthermore, the precise chemical nature of the hypersensitivity-inducing antigens is not known, and the methods employed in making them for use in desensitization procedures are relatively crude, the end product inevitably containing contaminating material of no value in desensitization. When reproducible and precise *in vitro* methods of antigen assay are eventually developed, considerable advances in this field of therapy should be possible.

Drugs that are used to ameliorate the anaphylactic response are described on p. 24.4.

Type II cytolytic or cytotoxic reactions
In this type of hypersensitivity, antibody receptors combine with either an antigenic component of a tissue cell or

with an antigen or hapten which has become intimately attached to tissue cells. The antibody is usually of the classical IgG or IgM type. When they combine with antigens of invading micro-organisms they immobilize them.

Transfusion reactions involve the lysis of red cells by antibody and by complement. Following incompatible transfusion (vol. 1, p. 26.19) lysis may occur intravascularly or in the spleen where the sensitized cells are more readily destroyed with or without the participation of complement. Following blood transfusion, type I reactions, e.g. urticaria, oedema, bronchospasm, may also occur and are possibly due to traces of soluble foreign antigens in the donor's plasma reacting with reaginic antibody in that of the recipient or vice versa.

Haemolytic disease of the newborn occurs at birth or within the first two or three days of life and the rhesus (Rh) factor is the sensitizing antigen (vol. 1, p. 26.20).

Autoimmune haemolytic anaemias are a third example of a type II reaction; in these the red blood cell destruction is due to damage to the cells resulting from adsorption of autoantibodies arising spontaneously. The presence of adsorbed antibodies on the surface of the red cells can be demonstrated by the direct or indirect antiglobulin test (fig. 23.1). The removal of red blood cells

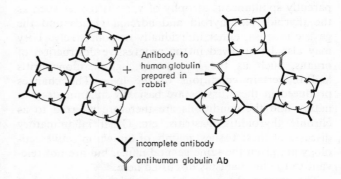

FIG. 23.1. The antiglobulin reaction (Coombs technique) is used to detect antibody adsorbed to the surface of the red blood cell (incomplete antibody). It can be carried out in two ways using either the patient's own red cells (direct test) or normal red cells previously mixed with the patient's serum (indirect test). Antihuman-globulin is added to the red blood cell suspension and causes agglutination of the cells when the incomplete antibody is present on their surface (vol. 1, p. 26.18).

from the circulation is probably brought about by the antibodies affecting their surface properties and by damage to the metabolism. The incomplete type of autoantibody causes their removal largely by the spleen; agglutinating and complement-fixing antibodies lead to removal by the reticuloendothelial system, the liver playing an important role by virtue of its size. An important factor in determining the filtering action of the spleen and liver is the intensity with which the antibody-affected cells undergo autoagglutination. In addition antibodies which are demonstrably lytic *in vitro* and present in sufficient titres may cause intravascular haemolysis. Erythrophagocytosis is important as a means of disposing of cells coated with complement-fixing antibody.

The study of blood disorders associated with **cytopenia** exemplifies another pathological immunological mechanism. Tissue cells may be rendered temporarily susceptible to the cytotoxic action of antibody and complement by adsorption of an antigen (e.g. a bacterial product) or a hapten (e.g. a drug) to their surface. Reaction of the bacterial antibody or antibody to the cell–drug complex then results in the destruction of the cell. Reference has been made to the generalized purpura due to thrombocytopenia which may develop following the administration of the drug apronal (sedormid, p. 22.20). Quinidine, aspirin, PAS, phenylbutazone, thiazides, stibophen, phenazones, tetracyclines, streptomycin, thiourea derivatives, troxidone, phenobarbitone, oestrogens, sulphonamides and other drugs may induce purpura in the same way, but do so much less frequently. A comparable disorder giving rise to **haemolytic anaemia** may follow the use of drugs showing an affinity for the red blood cells; these include stibophen, phenacetin, PAS, isoniazid, sulphasalazine, phenothiazines and penicillins. A similar mechanism involving the white cells may be the basis of one form of **drug-induced agranulocytosis**, e.g. phenothiazines, PAS, thiouracil, diuretic and antidiabetic sulphonamides and colchicine. Methyldopa also occasionally causes haemolytic anaemia; the antibody responsible appears to react with one of the Rh antigens on the patient's red blood cells which then become antigenic.

A group of disorders characterized by IgG antibodies in the serum, which show a high degree of organ specificity, include some forms of thyroid disease, i.e. **thyrotoxicosis, chronic thyroiditis** or Hashimoto's disease (plate 23.5a, facing p. 23.6) and **primary thyroid atrophy**, gastric atrophy (plate 23.5c) associated with pernicious anaemia and certain cases of adrenal atrophy (plate 23.5b), parathyroid atrophy and premature gonadal failure. Thus four different IgG antibodies that react with different components of thyroid cells or their secretions have been described; these are antibody to thyroglobulin (plate 23.1a, facing p. 23.4), antibody to an iodine-free component of thyroid colloid, complement fixing antibody reactive with the microsomal fraction of thyroid cells (plate 23.1b) and long acting thyroid stimulating substance. Gastric antibodies include those reacting with cytoplasm of oxyntic cells (plate 23.2a) and at least two reacting with different sites on intrinsic factor. Some patients with idiopathic adrenal atrophy have antibodies reactive with steroid-producing cells in the gonads (plate 23.2c) as well as those in the adrenal cortex. There is a clinical and even more pronounced immunological overlap between the diseases in this group. Thus 20–30

per cent of patients with thyroid autoimmune disease have gastric oxyntic cell antibodies in the serum as well as thyroid antibodies; over half of the patients with idiopathic primary adrenal atrophy have thyroid, gastric or parathyroid antibodies in the serum, the majority also having IgG antibodies specific for adrenocortical cells (plate 23.2b).

Although the presence of these specific IgG antibodies can be taken as evidence that the patient's immunological mechanisms are disturbed, it does not prove that they are responsible for any of the pathological features of the diseases. However, type II reactions may be important in this respect since thyroid microsomal antibodies, for example, are highly cytotoxic to human thyroid cells in tissue culture provided complement is present (plate 23.4a & b, facing p. 23.5). Nevertheless, thyroid disease has never been transferred successfully in experimental animals by means of this particular thyroid IgG antibody although this may be due to the antibody having difficulty in gaining access to the antigen *in vivo*. If, however, the animal's thyroid is previously damaged by irradiation, the infusion of thyroid microsomal antibodies may then augment thyroid damage. Likewise, although thyroid, gastric and adrenal antibodies are all capable of crossing the placenta into the foetal circulation, there is no evidence that, with the exception of LATS, this does the foetal organs any harm. As is described on p. 23.7, type IV reactions are also possibly concerned with the pathogenesis of autoimmune diseases.

THE LONG ACTING THYROID HORMONE (LATS) AND THYROTOXICOSIS

In 1957 Adams and Purves in New Zealand were studying a bioassay method for thyrotropic hormone (TSH) in mice. In this test (vol. 1, p. 25.4) TSH is injected into a suitably prepared animal, organically bound ^{131}I is released from the thyroid into the blood, and the increase in plasma radioactivity is recorded. The peak rise in blood ^{131}I occurs about three hours after the TSH is given (fig. 23.2). However, when the plasma of patients with thyrotoxicosis was injected, the time course for the plasma radioactivity was much more prolonged with the peak occurring in about 12 hours. The substance responsible for this late release was named long acting thyroid stimulator (LATS). Preparations of LATS were made from the glands of patients with thyrotoxicosis and on injection into rats these caused hyperplasia of the thyroid epithelial cells and also increased the uptake of ^{131}I by human thyroid cells in tissue culture. LATS was shown to be an immunoglobulin of the IgG type. In man the occurrence of LATS in the plasma correlates closely with thyrotoxicosis and seldom occurs in any patient who is not thyrotoxic or who has not been thyrotoxic in the past. Its transmission across the placenta correlates with thyrotoxicosis in the newborn. In the absence of associated

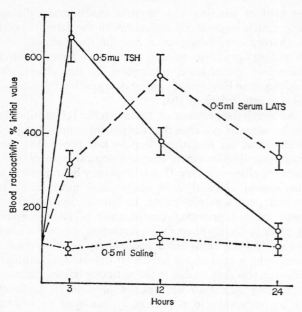

FIG. 23.2. Contrasting time courses of action of TSH and LATS in ^{131}I bioassay.

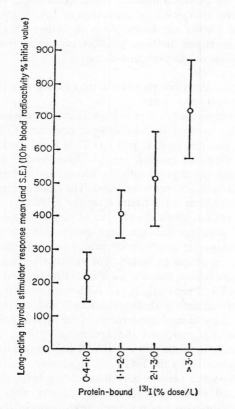

FIG. 23.3. Correlation between LATS level in serum and the turnover of ^{131}I in the thyroid gland in thyrotoxicosis. From Carneiro L. *et al.* (1966) *Lancet* **2**, 878.

thyrotoxicosis, LATS does not occur in chronic goitrous thyroiditis nor is it found in primary hypothyroidism, although both conditions are associated with a high incidence of other thyroid autoantibodies. Furthermore, in thyrotoxic patients before treatment has been initiated, there is a correlation between the level of LATS in the plasma and the severity of the thyroid overactivity (fig. 23.3). There was initial hesitancy in accepting LATS as an autoantibody due to the notion that antibodies must necessarily be damaging or inhibitory as implied by the terms cytotoxic and cytolytic.

Other examples of stimulation by antibodies as part of type II hypersensitivity reactions include the transformation of lymphocytes into lymphoblasts under the influence of antilymphocytic serum. This, however, is more immediately relevant to antigen recognition than to any specific disease process.

THE KIDNEY AND HYPERSENSITIVITY REACTIONS

There are two different and distinct mechanisms whereby the host's antibody response may cause glomerulonephritis, which may lead to progressive renal failure:

(1) the patient may produce antibodies capable of reacting with his own glomerular capillary basement membrane (GBM) antigen/s (a type II reaction), and

(2) the patient may produce antibodies capable of reacting with exogenous or nonglomerular endogenous antigens with the formation of circulating antigen–antibody complexes which may become trapped in the renal glomeruli (a type III reaction, p. 23.6).

Both of these processes serve to induce an antigen–antibody reaction in the glomeruli in which inflammation occurs. The degree of glomerular injury appears to be related directly to the quantity and quality of antibody and/or antigen involved. There is no evidence that delayed or cell-mediated hypersensitivity (type IV reaction) is important in the genesis of glomerulonephritis. Mononuclear cells, the hallmark of delayed sensitivity, are inconspicuous if indeed they participate at all.

These two mechanisms have distinctive immunohistochemical and morphological characteristics, making it possible to differentiate them in biopsy specimens. In lesions induced by anti-GBM antibody (type II reaction), antibody and complement are arranged in a uniform pattern along the inner aspect of the GBM and are readily detected by EM or immunofluorescence (plate 23.6a, facing p. 23.8). In type III reactions circulating nonglomerular antigen–antibody complexes, plus complement, accumulate in discrete irregular granules along the outer aspect of the GBM beneath the epithelial cells. These deposits are readily demonstrable by immunofluorescence or EM (plate 23.6b) and may even be visible in light microscopy.

Glomerulonephritis can be produced in animals by injecting heterologous, homologous or autologous GBM

Positive reactions in the indirect immunofluorescence test for autoantibodies to various antigens; the sera of patients with conditions referred to in the text have been used. The disease conditions shown in parenthesis are those in which the occurrence of the corresponding antibody in the serum is typical, but these antibodies may occur with a lesser incidence also in other related conditions and in control subjects.

In the indirect immunofluorescence test, unfixed air-dried sections are prepared from snap frozen tissue. The sections are treated with the test serum, washed and treated with antihuman γ-globulin (mono- or polyvalent) conjugated with fluorescein isothiocyanate. After further washing, the sections are examined by ultraviolet fluorescence microscopy.

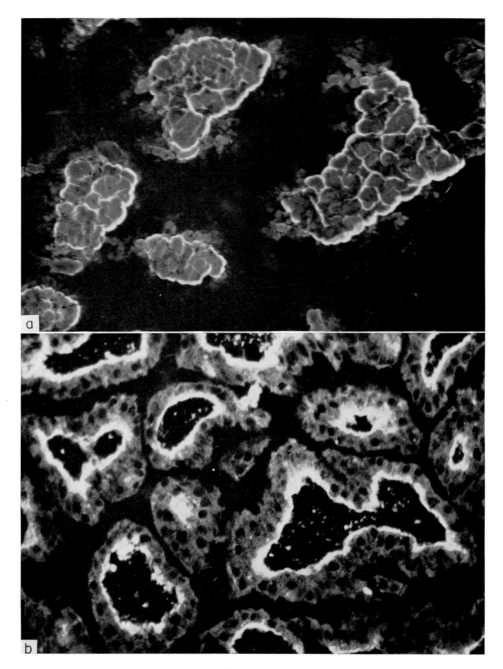

PLATE 23.1.

(a) Human thyroglobulin in the colloid of thyroid vesicles (× 210).

(b) Cytoplasm of human thyroid epithelial cells (× 210).
(Thyroid autoimmune diseases: thyrotoxicosis; chronic thyroiditis (Hashimoto's disease); primary atrophic hypothyroidism.)

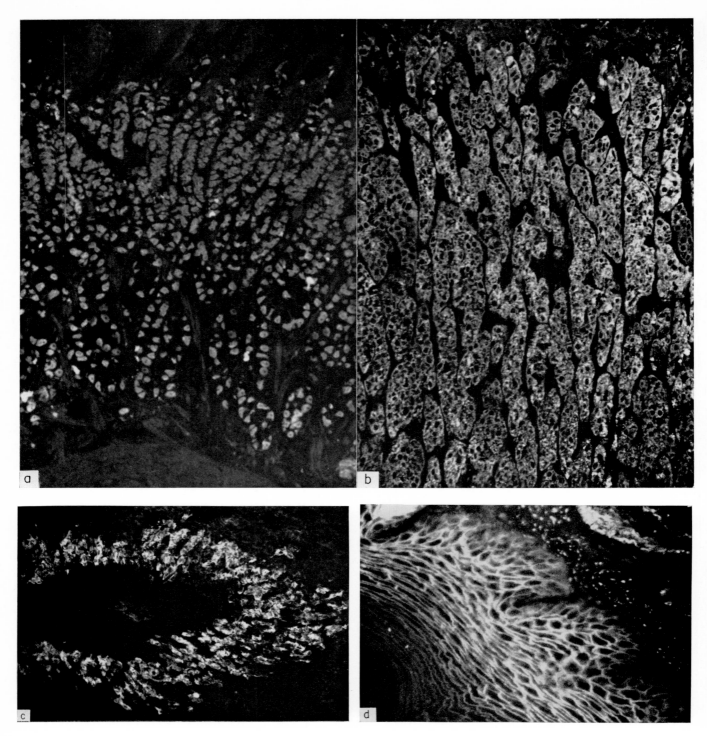

PLATE 23.2.

(a) Human gastric parietal cells ($\times$ 240). (Addisonian pernicious anaemia.)

(b) Cytoplasm of the secretory cells of human adrenal glands ($\times$ 220). (Idiopathic adrenal atrophy.)

(c) Theca cells of a Graafian follicle in human ovary ($\times$ 140). From Irvine W.J. *et al.* (1968) *Lancet* ii, 883. (Premature ovarian failure associated with idiopathic adrenal atrophy.)

(d) Stratified squamous epithelium of rabbit oesophagus ($\times$ 260). From Ablin R.J. and Beutner E.H. (1969) *Clin. exper. Immunol.* **4,** 283. (Pemphigus).

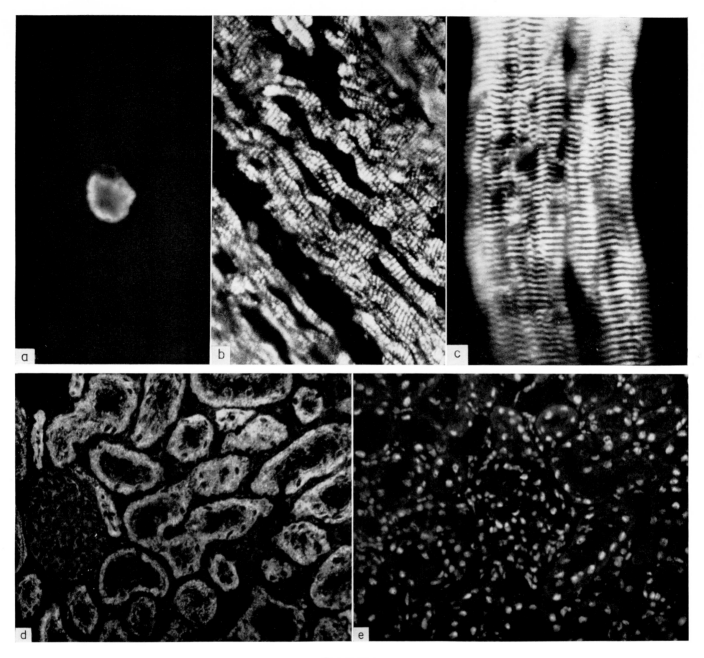

PLATE 23.3.

(a) Thymus myoid cells (p. 23.5) (×630).   (b) Heart muscle (×810).   (c) Skeletal muscle of calf (×810).
All three tissues possess a common antigen. (Myasthenia gravis.)

(d) Mitochondria in rat kidney tubules (×260). (Primary biliary   (e) Nuclei in rat kidney (×260). (Systemic lupus erythematosus.)
cirrhosis and active chronic hepatitis.)

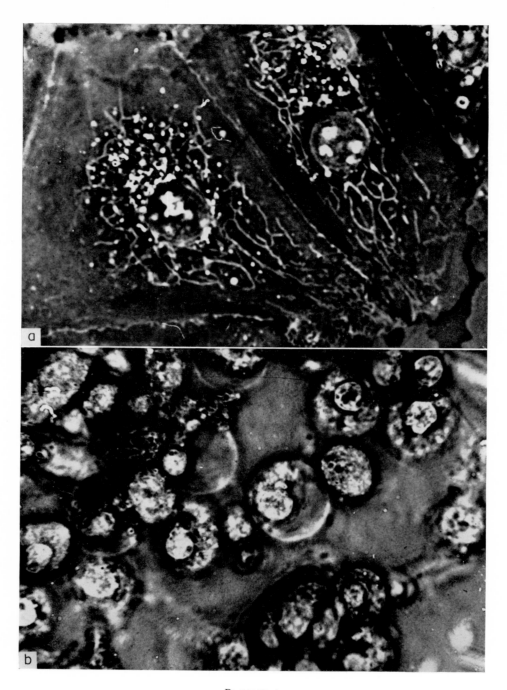

PLATE 23.4.

(a) Human thyroid cells trypsinized to get them into suspension and then cultured *in vitro* in 10 per cent normal human serum. The cells spread out as a monolayer on the coverslip (× 1100).

(b) Same as above but a few minutes after changing the culture medium to 10 per cent serum from a patient with chronic thyroiditis (Hashimoto's disease) (× 1100).

A comparable cytotoxic effect, specific for thyroid cells, has not been demonstrated with cells that have not been previously subjected to enzyme treatment. This illustrates that thyroid specific antibodies may be damaging to human thyroid cells provided they can gain access to the thyroid antigen which is in relation to the cell membranes.

From Irvine W.J. (1961) *Advances in Thyroid Research*. Ed. Pitt-Rivers, R. Oxford: Pergamon Press.

antigens. Antigens cross-reactive or identical with GBM antigens are present in the urine of all healthy mammals studied. These may be extracted from the urine of normal rabbits and used to induce nephritis similar to that produced by autologous, homologous and heterologous antigens. In such nephritic animals, little anti-GBM antibody can be found in the circulation, but if they are nephrectomized it accumulates in the serum, presumably as a result of the removal of the target antigen. Anti-GBM antibodies can also be readily eluted from the kidneys of these animals. Glomerulonephritis, induced by immunizing an animal with GBM, may be considered autoimmune in the sense that it is the host's antibody reacting with his own GBM which is the cause of the disease; the fact that the original immunizing antigen need not be autologous is irrelevant.

An important step in demonstrating the participation of anti-GBM antibodies in human renal disease was their isolation in 1967 from the serum and kidneys of patients with glomerulonephritis. Acid elution of homogenates of kidneys from such patients demonstrated not only the presence of anti-GBM antibodies but also their localization in the affected organ. In other patients anti-GBM antibodies were detected in the serum only after total nephrectomy undertaken prior to renal transplantation. The appearance of circulating antibodies after nephrectomy parallels the experimental observations in animals and indicates how efficiently the GBM, exposed to the circulation by the fenestrae, removes circulating anti-GBM antibodies. As little as 6 mg of globulin eluted from human kidneys with anti-GBM type nephritis when injected into monkeys cause immediately a severe, progressive glomerulonephritis.

In one patient, circulating anti-GBM antibodies which were demonstrated after nephrectomy fell in a linear manner and were no longer detectable one day after a renal transplant. An immediate and persistent glomerulonephritis developed in the transplanted kidney. These observations show not only that these antibodies are reactive *in vivo* but also that they can damage the renal glomerulus. It appears that patients forming anti-GBM antibodies may not be good candidates for renal transplantation since they are likely to reproduce in the transplant the same nephritic changes already suffered by their own kidneys. When patients with this form of glomerulonephritis require organ replacement, nephrectomy followed by a period of maintenance by haemodialysis and immunosuppression until the antibodies disappear from the circulation would seem to be a wise preliminary procedure.

MISCELLANEOUS OTHER CONDITIONS

Recent studies in **pemphigus**, a serious and fortunately uncommon disease of the skin characterized by bullous eruptions, show that autoimmunity is almost certainly concerned in its pathogenesis. The reaction of serum immunoglobulins with intercellular antigen peculiar to squamous epithelium can be demonstrated in frozen sections of skin obtained from man or laboratory animals. The titre of the antibody to the intercellular antigen is proportional to the severity of the disease. The antigen, a heat-labile water-insoluble substance, lies between squamous epithelial cells at a site corresponding to the lesion of the disease (plate 23.2d). The pathogenesis, however, cannot be attributed solely to autoimmunity; injection of serum from patients with pemphigus into the skin of monkeys produces intercellular fixation of antibody but not the fully developed disease. If the antibody is a cause rather than a result of the disease, additional features must be involved, such as increased tissue permeability allowing access of complement or other mediators of inflammation to the intercellular spaces of squamous epithelium.

In contrast to the diseases described above that are characterized by the occurrence of organ-specific antibodies, certain forms of liver disease, notably **primary biliary cirrhosis** (plate 23.5d, facing p. 23.6) and **active chronic hepatitis**, are associated with antibodies in the serum that are reactive with mitochrondria (plate 23.3d) and with smooth muscle. These antibodies are not specific for any particular organ and clearly their role in producing liver damage cannot be of great significance, although other immune mechanisms not so readily demonstrated may well be. Antinuclear antibodies, frequently called antinuclear factors (ANF), are reactive against components of tissue nuclei and their reactivity likewise does not show any precise organ specificity (plate 23.3e). The occurrence of ANFs in the serum is characteristic of systemic lupus erythematosus, with a lesser incidence in other connective tissue disorders (p. 30.12).

Myasthenia gravis, a disorder affecting neuromuscular function (p. 4.5) and commonly associated with enlargement of the thymus is also of particular interest. There is a high incidence of IgG antibodies in the serum which react with A or I bands of skeletal muscle (vol. I, p. 15.4) and which cross-react with cardiac muscle and certain cells in the medulla of the thymus that are derived from muscle cells present at an early stage in foetal development (plate 23.3a, b & c). The site of reactivity of the antibody with skeletal muscle cannot explain the block of neuromuscular transmission which is the characteristic functional abnormality in the disorder. In myasthenia the thymic medulla is frequently the site of germinal centre formation (plate 23.5e), which is abnormal, and recent studies have shown that a neuromuscular-blocking factor which is not immunological may be produced by the gland under these conditions. As described later under type IV reactions, the thymitis may be immunologically induced.

Antigens may be shared between an exogenous, e.g. bacterial, factor and a normal constituent of the body's tissues. The formation of antibodies to the exogenous factor would then result in these antibodies cross-reacting with the body constituent. Such a mechanism may be a factor, for example, in the pathogenesis of **rheumatic fever**, where there is evidence that antigen in the human cardiac myofibrils may be shared with components of certain streptococci (p. 30.10). A similar mechanism may occur in relation to **ulcerative colitis** where there is evidence that an antigen of a type of *Esch. coli* (i.e. 014) is shared with a constituent of the mucosal cells of human colon.

Type III or toxic complex reactions

Serum sickness, first described by Von Pirquet and Shick in 1905, is the classical example in man. The reaction may occur 8–12 days after a single injection of an antigen, which is usually horse serum, e.g. antitetanus. It consists of skin rashes, fever, joint pains and often swelling of the regional lymph nodes. The symptoms vary greatly, as do their duration. The illness is seldom serious, though it may give rise to much discomfort. Now that antitoxins and other horse serum preparations are much less used in medicine, serum sickness is not commonly seen. However, many drug reactions, especially those involving the penicillins and sulphonamides, are probably due to toxic complexes formed by drug haptens reacting with specific antibodies, formed in response to previous exposure to the drug.

As mentioned on p. 23.4, type III reaction has been implicated in some forms of glomerulonephritis in man. Further evidence for this comes from studies on a highly inbred strain of New Zealand black (NZB) mice. These animals frequently develop a characteristic glomerulonephritis and they are also infected chronically with one or more viruses. The glomerulonephritis is associated with the formation of antinuclear antibodies and complexes of these antibodies with nuclear antigens and complement can be demonstrated in the glomeruli. The primary abnormality in this experimental model, which closely resembles lupus erythematosus in man, may well be the presence of nuclear antigen, but whether this is derived from the infecting viruses or from abnormal catabolism of the host's own nuclear material, perhaps as a result of the infection, is uncertain. Thus the relation between the infection and the renal disease is not clear. This disorder, however, is a good example of glomeruli trapping an antigen–antibody complex with a consequent focal inflammatory reaction. The size and shape of the complex in relation to the local capillary circulation would seem to be at least one factor determining the probability of trapping.

In man, glomerular lesions arise in association with

systemic lupus erythematosus (SLE, p. 30.12), **streptococcal infections** (p. 18.69) and **quartan malaria**. In these conditions the presence of a focal antigen–antibody complex in the glomeruli can be demonstrated and the antigens involved in the complexes are identified or suspected (plate 23.6a, facing p. 23.8). In SLE, antinuclear antibodies have been found in high titres in affected kidneys, and complexes of nuclear antigens, host immunoglobulin and complement demonstrated in the glomeruli. During exacerbations of the renal disease, antinuclear antibodies have been found in the circulation, an event which is almost certain to lead to the formation of complexes. In poststreptococcal glomerulonephritis, host immunoglobulins and complement can readily be detected in deposits in the glomeruli. Evidence for the presence of streptococcal antigens is less strong, but suggestive. Similarly immunoglobulins and complement have been found in characteristic complexes in the glomeruli in cases of quartan malaria associated with glomerular inflammation. These complexes can be demonstrated also in the circulation and may be presumed to contain antigen derived from the malarial parasites.

In addition to these three entities in which the nature of the antigen is at least partly known, granular deposits containing host immunoglobulin and complement and resembling antigen–antibody complexes have been found along the basement membrane of the glomeruli in a number of cases of children and adults with acute and chronic renal disorders in which there is little hint as to the antigens involved. Endogenous or autoantigens and many infectious agents could result in the formation of such complexes. Immunological analysis of tissue obtained by percutaneous renal biopsy from a sufficient number of cases of glomerulonephritis may in the future provide estimates of the frequency with which different antigens cause the disease.

The source and supply of antigen is relevant to the course of any disease arising from a type III hypersensitivity reaction. If the antigen has been given in a single dose, as in serum sickness, the lesion should quickly regress. If, however, the antigen is given repeatedly, as in penicillin treatment, or is endogenous, as is the case in lupus erythematosus or intractable streptococcal infection, then the lesions persist or recur.

Reference has been made to the tendency for some individuals to produce reagins with the development of asthma when various antigens are inhaled (p. 23.1). However, under certain circumstances a type III response develops in the tissues around bronchi and alveoli on exposure to certain organic dusts. The spores of *Aspergillus fumigatus* are able to grow in the lungs and provide a persisting source of antigen. In some individuals, asthma is associated with a type I reaction, but in others, circulating antibodies are found and a type III reaction develops with extensive patchy involvement of the pulmonary

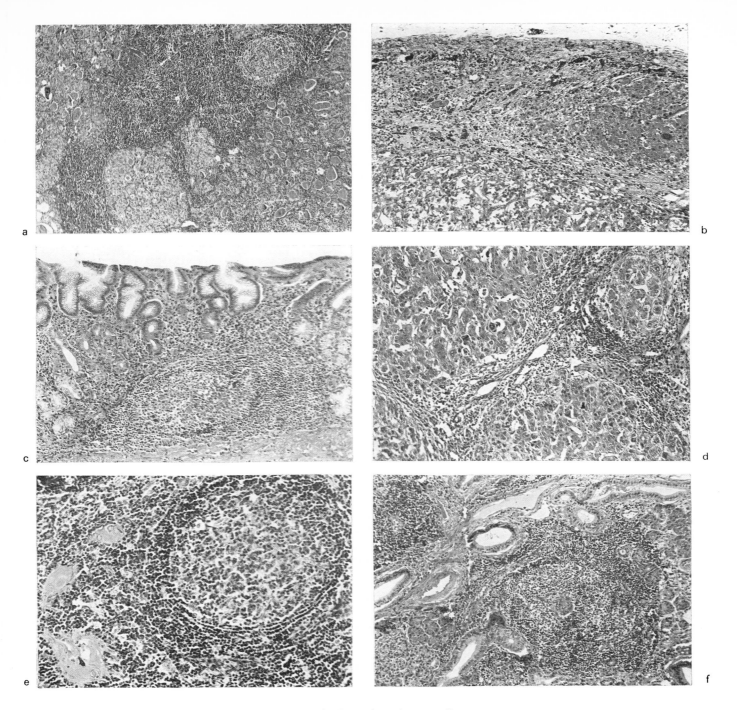

PLATE 23.5. Histology of autoimmune diseases.

(a) A field from the thyroid in a case of chronic thyroiditis (Hashimoto's disease). Atrophy of the parenchymal tissue is seen; the remaining thyroid follicles are small and lined by large cells with very eosinophilic cytoplasm (Askanazy cells). Much of the tissue is replaced by lymphoid follicles and aggregations of lymphocytes. Haem. & eosin ($\times 50$).

(c) Gastric mucosa from the body of the stomach in a case of atrophic gastritis. Note the absence of parietal and zymogenic cells, the paucity of glands and the increase of lymphoid tissue with infiltration of the lamina propria by small mononuclear cells. Haem. & eosin ($\times 100$).

(e) Chronic thymitis. Section of thymic medulla showing the presence of a lymphoid follicle together with three Hassall's corpuscles. Haem. & eosin ($\times 170$).

(b) An adrenal gland in primary adrenocortical atrophy; the upper half of the field shows a narrowed cortex with only a few groups of parenchymal cells; much of the tissue is fibrovascular connective tissue infiltrated by lymphocytes. The lower half consists of unaffected medulla. Haem. & eosin ($\times 85$).

(d) Primary biliary cirrhosis showing abnormal hepatic architecture; nodules of regenerating liver tissue, bands of fibrous tissue infiltrated by lymphocytes and plasma cells, and canaliculi distended with plugs of bile, indicating biliary obstruction, are seen. Haem. & eosin ($\times 95$).

(f) A field from a salivary gland in a case of Sjögren's disease. Several dilated ducts are seen; there is severe atrophy of the glandular tissue, with replacement by lymphoid tissue. Residual glands are present at the periphery of the field. Haem. & eosin ($\times 95$).

tissue analogous to an Arthus reaction. Similar reactions to the inhalation of certain species of actinomycetes from mouldy hay gives rise to a diffuse infiltrative pulmonary disease known as **Farmer's lung**; exposure to other antigens, e.g. dust from mushrooms or pigeon droppings, leads to similar allergic occupational hazards.

Type IV or delayed cell-mediated hypersensitivity reactions

MICROBIAL HYPERSENSITIVITY
The classical example is the tuberculin reaction which is described on p. 21.17 and p. 22.18. Similar inflammatory reactions occur in other chronic microbial infections in which the parasites may be intracellular, e.g. leprosy and brucellosis; they may be found also in fungal and viral infections, e.g. histoplasmosis, coccidiomycosis and psittacosis, and in helminthic infestation and Leishmaniasis. It is difficult to assess the significance of these reactions for the host although it is possible they represent a mild and delayed defence mechanism. On the other hand, unlike the more violent anaphylactic reactions, they do not constitute in themselves disease processes. Decreased delayed sensitivity is characteristic of sarcoidosis but the explanation for this is unknown (p. 21.20). Type IV reactions may also be responsible for the reaction of tissues to silica and beryllium (p. 21.20) in which granulomatous lesions are found in the lungs. Graft rejection also possesses features in common with type IV reactions, i.e. infiltration with mononuclear cells and failure of transfer by serum.

CONTACT DERMATITIS
This may occur in sensitized persons after exposure to a variety of substances, plants, household and industrial chemicals and drugs. These substances must be soluble and penetrate tissue. Primulas and, in America, poison ivy are two plants which have a bad reputation in this respect. As most of the chemicals which cause contact dermatitis are not themselves antigens, they must first form compounds with skin proteins, and these then cause the sensitization. The hypersensitivity of the skin is generalized and may be detected by the application of a small patch test containing the allergen anywhere on the body. The delayed reaction takes up to 48 hours to develop, and it is important to distinguish it from reactions due to direct irritation or toxicity. For many years it was believed that the allergy was confined to the cells of the skin, and that it spread over the body surface by continuity. This has been shown to be incorrect by experiments on guinea-pigs in which skin sensitization was tested after isolation of an area of skin from nervous lymphatic and vascular connections. Sensitization occurs only when lymph drainage to the regional lymph nodes is intact and the allergy is conveyed to the whole skin by immunologically competent cells in the blood stream.

Transfer of contact dermatitis has been achieved in animals and man with cells from the thoracic duct and spleen.

AUTOIMMUNE DISEASE
The evidence that type IV reactions are involved in some of the autoimmune diseases in man is largely indirect. In many of these conditions there is a marked accumulation of mononuclear cells in the thyroid, adrenal or parathyroid glands, gastric or colonic mucosa and liver or thymus (plates 23.5a–e) which is similar if not identical with that found in delayed hypersensitivity reactions. Provided adjuvants are used, comparable histological lesions, e.g. thyroiditis, gastritis, adrenalitis, orchitis, thymitis and encephalomyelitis, can be induced in experimental animals by the injection of suitable antigens and can be transferred from an affected to a normal animal by means of lymphocytes, though not by serum. The animals also develop positive skin tests for the antigen which are of the delayed hypersensitivity type. Furthermore the development of experimental thyroiditis or of allergic encephalomyelitis, can be prevented by prior treatment of the animal with antilymphocytic serum (p. 24.3).

An experimental model of myasthenia gravis can be produced in laboratory animals by immunizing with skeletal muscle extracts together with Freund's adjuvant. This produces an infiltration of lymphocytes in the thymic medulla and antibodies in the serum reactive with the A or I bands of skeletal muscle. The production of the block in neuromuscular transmission is dependent on the presence of the thymus although skeletal muscle antibodies may be produced with or without the thymus.

In man, the experimental opportunities are more limited. However, the lymphocytes from a patient with the autoimmune type of thyroiditis proliferate *in vitro* under the stimulus of thyroid antigen. Likewise, lymphocytes from a patient with autoimmune chronic inflammation of the adrenal glands give *in vitro* reactions indicating that they have been specifically sensitized for adrenal cortex. The leucocytes, but not the serum, from a proportion of patients with ulcerative colitis can exert a specific cytotoxic effect on colon cells *in vitro*, provided complement is present in the system.

It is not known whether type II reactions operate synergistically with type IV reactions in contributing to the origin or manifestations of autoimmune diseases. One of the difficulties is that techniques for study of humoral antibodies are far more advanced than those for the study of cell-mediated immunity.

Rheumatoid arthritis is another disorder about which there has been even more speculation on the role of autoimmune delayed hypersensitivity reactions. Rheumatoid factor (p. 30.12) is an IgM immunoglobulin and can be detected in moderate or high titres in the sera of the majority of patients with rheumatoid arthritis, while such titres do not occur in nonrheumatoid subjects. However, apart from its importance in drawing attention to the possible role of autoimmunity in the pathogenesis of rheumatoid arthritis, the rheumatoid factor has not yet been implicated in the pathogenesis of the disease. The development of typical rheumatoid lesions in subjects with congenital hypogammaglobulinaemia shows that neither circulating antibodies nor plasma cells, which give rise to them, can play a basic pathogenetic role. It has been suggested that the rheumatoid state might result from delayed hypersensitivity to one or more products of inflammation. The histopathology of the synovial membrane with its diffuse infiltration of plasma cells and the aggregations of lymphocytes with formation of germinal centres could then be interpreted as the immunological response to the local persistence of antigen. The nature of this antigen is not known and various claims for the implication of mycoplasma or other agents have not been adequately substantiated. Other indirect hints that delayed hypersensitivity may be important in the pathogenesis of rheumatoid arthritis include the demonstration that an arthritis virtually indistinguishable from rheumatoid arthritis can be induced in rabbits by the intra-articular injection of fibrin, if the animals have been previously made sensitive by intradermal injection of fibrin in Freund's adjuvant.

Sjogren's disease or syndrome is a chronic benign disorder which occurs in middle-aged females with involvement of the uveal tract and the salivary glands. In about one half of patients, this is associated with some form of connective tissue disease, usually rheumatoid arthritis or, less commonly, systemic lupus erythematosus. The lacrimal and salivary glands show extensive chronic inflammatory cell infiltration and acinar atrophy with failure of secretion (plate 23.5f). Antibodies to the salivary duct cell cytoplasm have been demonstrated in the sera of such patients. Rheumatoid factor and antinuclear factors are also commonly present in the serum. Although the lesion in the salivary glands produced by immunological techniques in animals do not exactly resemble those seen in the human disease, delayed hypersensitivity reactions are more probably involved in the pathogenesis than are type II reactions.

Why should these immune reactions occur?

Type I reactions occur in individuals who are so constitutionally disposed, and the nature of the reaction to the allergen depends largely on the immunological reactivity of the subject. This also appears to dictate whether a type I reaction, leading for example to asthma, or a type III reaction, leading to an allergic pulmonary disease, occurs. In the case of type I reactions the basic abnormality is the capacity to produce reagins and is

probably inherited, but at present it is impossible to fit any genetic hypothesis to the existing data. The genetic basis for an inherited disease may be either a single gene or it may be multifactorial. Individuals affected by type I reactions tend to develop the disorder in childhood if both parents are allergic subjects but do so at a much later age in the absence of a family history. Since only a small proportion of children in allergic families develop the disease, penetrance is clearly incomplete. Environmental influences may also be expected to contribute substantially. More accurate information on the inheritance of this type of hypersensitivity reaction is further complicated by the difficulties in diagnosis. All forms of bronchospasm are not allergic in origin and likewise there is clinical difficulty in defining allergic skin reactions, particularly in infants. The problem of inheritance and its role in human allergy is likely to be further advanced only when IgE reagin antibody is more readily detectable and the specificities of the antigens determined.

The formation of autoantibodies (type II and type IV reaction) must be considered in terms of the general theory of antibody formation and tolerance. It is reasonable to suppose that the consequences of antigenic stimulation depend on the same factors for autoantigens as for exogenous or foreign antigen, and it is not necessary to invoke any special mechanism whereby the animal or individual 'recognized' their own antigens as being part of 'self'.

Autoantigens may be considered in two groups:

(1) those to which tolerance is not normally fully established, and

(2) those in which antibody formation is a result of breakdown of a previously established tolerance.

Antigens in the first group, if suitably extracted and injected in the correct dosage, give rise to antibody formation in normal animals; antigens in the second group do not do this. The distinction between these two groups is not absolute and there are important genetic factors which determine the ease with which animals form antibodies to autoantigens; adjuvants also facilitate autoantibody formation. Furthermore, immunization with related or chemically modified antigens may cause autoantibody formation when the autologous antigen does not.

The clearest example of an autoantigen of the first type is one which has been sequestrated anatomically, i.e. it has never met the animal's reticuloendothelial system. Good examples of this are antigens in the anterior chamber of the eye which lacks lymphatic and vascular connections. Antigens in such special sites do not give rise to any immune response but will do so if injected parenterally. Thus, if the lens of the eye is damaged by trauma, leakage of antigen from the lens into the circulation may occur and antibodies are formed. This is probably the basis of **sympathetic ophthalmia** which may

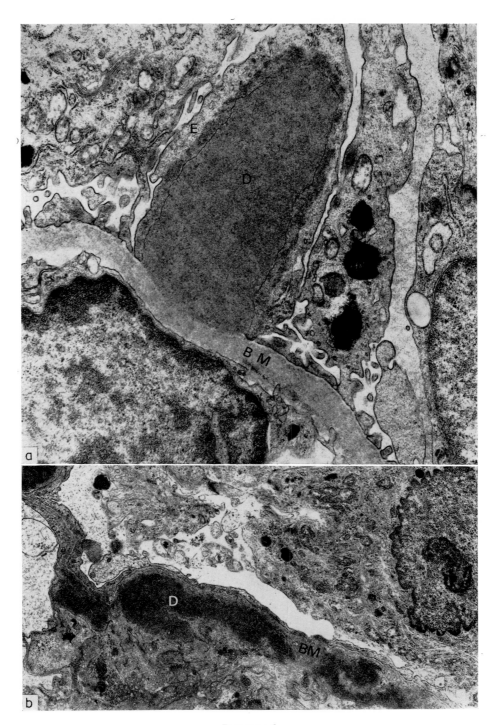

PLATE 23.6.

(a) This is an electron micrograph of part of a human renal glomerulus in a case of post-streptococcal proliferative glomerulonephritis. Situated on the capillary basement membrane (BM) and protruding from it into an epithelial cell (E) is a large conical deposit (D) of granular material which is an antigen–antibody complex ($\times$25,000).

(b) This electron micrograph shows part of a human renal glomerulus; the capillary basement membrane (BM) is thickened over much of its course by linear, dark deposits (D) along its sub-endothelial aspect. This may represent deposition of anti-GBM antibody ($\times$6000).

follow a perforating injury of the globe in which the uveal tract is involved. After some weeks, a diffuse lymphocytic infiltration may develop in the uveal tissues of the injured eye. At any time from about the third week to several years following the trauma, a similar lesion may appear in the other eye. Antiuveal antibodies have been identified in patients with such injuries and extracts of uveal tissue elicit a positive intradermal hypersensitivity test in these patients.

The commonest form of sequestration of antigen is in the tissue cells, although this cannot be as absolute as in the above example. Many cells of the body break down and are replaced, and it is difficult to be certain to what extent the reticuloendothelial system is familiar with the breakdown products. It is believed that if the first encounter of an antigen in an unsensitized subject is via the lymphoid cells then tolerance will result, but if it is via the macrophages then antibody formation will follow. Dosage of antigen is also likely to be of importance in relation to antibody formation and tolerance.

When autoantibodies are formed to the surface antigens of circulating cells, as is the case in some forms of haemolytic anaemia, it is clear that a pre-existing state of tolerance has broken down. Presumably these antibodies developed primarily because of changes in the antibody-forming system itself, but how this immunological homeostasis is upset is poorly understood. It is possible that new clones of lymphocytes may develop as a result of random somatic mutation. Under physiological circumstances, any newly formed clone of lymphocytes that reacts with one of the body's own tissues (and to which constituent the body has become immunologically tolerant) should be deleted. Therefore, it is necessary to postulate not only a mutation which produces the aberrant clone but also a failure of the deletion of the clone when it arises. Furthermore, any theory of autoimmune disease must account for the occurrence of the formation of autoantibodies not in a random manner but in groups. Thus in systemic lupus erythematosus, antibodies are formed not only to a considerable variety of different nuclear components but to multiple determinants in a single component such as DNA-nucleoprotein. In other diseases, notably in the organ-specific group of autoimmune disorders, i.e. chronic thyroiditis, pernicious anaemia, primary Addison's disease and hypoparathyroidism, there is both clinical and immunological overlap. Thus patients with idiopathic Addison's disease not only have a high incidence of antibodies specific for the cytoplasm of adrenocortical cells but also have antibodies specific for thyroid cytoplasm or gastric parietal cells. The multiplicity of antibodies involved makes it unlikely that the primary defect in this group of diseases is an abnormality of the many tissue constituents and there is no evidence that the antigens are shared between these different tissues. Further, when tissue is damaged, e.g. in myocardial infarction or in burns, there is only a transitory rise in antibodies to the myocardium or skin respectively, which does not lead to a progressive autoimmune disorder. Likewise, infection of the thyroid or testes by mumps virus and the destruction of the adrenal gland by tuberculosis are not associated with continual antibody formation against the respective tissues. One of the unexplained characteristics of the autoimmune disease is that the antibodies are continually formed over periods of many years. In autoimmune thyroid disease and in Addisonian pernicious anaemia, family studies show that the tendency to produce thyroid and gastric autoantibodies is controlled by an autosomal gene with incomplete penetrance showing a sex controlled bias. It is probable therefore that both the organ-specific group of autoimmune diseases, e.g., thyroid, adrenal, etc., and the organ-nonspecific group, e.g. SLE, are genetically determined disorders of immunological tolerance. This hypothesis is compatible with observations in experimental animals.

Genetic factors are of paramount importance in the occurrence of spontaneous autoimmune disease in experimental animals. Thus NZB mice, which develop autoimmune haemolytic anaemia and diseases which resemble systemic lupus erythematosus and glomerulonephritis, transmit the condition to their offspring. Mating these mice with other strains produces variants in the disease picture. In addition, in experimental animals Freund's adjuvants have a mutagenic effect on antibody-forming cells and act as a substitute for the genetic predisposition. The critics of the central-defect hypothesis argue that what is inherited in these animals is a susceptibility to virus infection and that chronicity of tissue damage is consistent with the nature of virus infection. Such a virus might show predilection for certain tissues or could be responsible for the abnormal behaviour of the antibody-forming system by invading the reticuloendothelial system.

Is the formation of autoantibodies always an abnormal process? A significant proportion of the population, especially females, develop thyroid and gastric circulating autoantibodies as they grow older. This is associated with subclinical chronic inflammation and a variable degree of atrophy of the corresponding tissues. This has given rise to the view that the development of autoimmunity is part of the ageing process (fig. 23.4).

As already mentioned, invading micro-organisms may sometimes carry antigens which are shared by certain tissues of the host, e.g. some group A β-haemolytic streptococci and cardiac antigens, group A type 12 β-haemolytic streptococci and renal antigens, and certain forms of *Esch. coli* 014 and colon antigen. If the appropriate forbidden clone has developed in the host, antibody formed in response to these antigens could give rise to

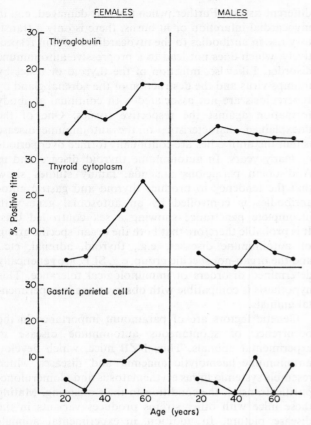

FIG. 23.4. The incidence of thyroid and gastric antibodies in 866 control subjects by age and sex.

rheumatic carditis, glomerulonephritis or ulcerative colitis.

The thymus has been implicated in the pathogenesis of autoimmune disease as it is essential for the development of the immunological system in early life and for its maintenance in the adult (vol. 1, p. 27.18). Suggestive evidence in support of this hypothesis is the abnormal histology of the thymus in certain disorders in man and experimental animals associated with autoimmunity. In particular, germinal centres are present in the thymic medulla in man and in animals with autoimmune disease. This used to be referred to as thymic hyperplasia, but is probably due to an autoimmune reaction against the thymus itself representing a deficiency of thymic function rather than the converse and is now called thymitis. Thus, neonatal thymectomy in NZB mice which are genetically destined to develop red cell autoimmunity with age, does not prevent or delay this process. Perhaps the thymus under normal circumstances is in some way responsible for the deletion of abnormal clones of lymphocytes that are self-reactive. How the thymus might achieve this is not understood and its role in autoimmunity is speculative.

Drug hypersensitivity

Adverse reactions to drugs are described throughout this volume where the individual drugs are described, and in chap. 32. While these reactions may be due to overdosage, drug interaction, unwanted but recognized pharmacological actions or secondary effects, in many instances the reaction is unpredictable and differs from the usual pharmacological effect. Such idiosyncrasies usually occur in only a small minority of individuals exposed to the agent. These reactions can occasionally be attributed to a genetically determined defect or abnormality in molecular structure of a body constituent or enzyme and are described under the topic of pharmacogenetics (p. 31.9). A larger number, however, are believed to be due to hypersensitivity in the immunological sense.

In some instances the immunological basis of the reaction has been established by the presence of an antibody demonstrated *in vitro* or by means of passive transfer. These have been referred to under the different types of immunological mechanisms believed to be involved. In many other cases the immunological mechanism is unknown. While these reactions are widely accepted as being allergic it is possible that a few may be shown subsequently to arise from genetic or other metabolic abnormalities which have not yet been revealed.

Hypersensitivity reactions to drugs are more prone to occur in children than in adults, and in females rather than males. Patients who exhibit reaginic reactions to other antigens appear to be particularly susceptible. The prolonged use of a multiplicity of drugs increases the severity and incidence of reactions. In those sensitized, severe reactions may be induced by very small doses. There is no clear relationship between reactions and chemical structure but cross sensitization between two or more drugs may occur. The possibility that hypersensitivity is due to a contaminant of a preparation of a drug, as has been suggested in the case of penicillin, rather than to the drug itself should also be kept in mind (p. 20.27).

In addition to anaphylactic and serum sickness-like reactions and to cytopenic blood reactions already described (pp. 23.1 & 3), the clinical manifestations of drug hypersensitivity are extremely varied but commonly affect the skin, liver, kidneys and connective tissues.

SKIN REACTIONS
These include pruritus, urticaria, the so-called exanthematous reactions such as generalized or local erythema and other circumscribed or bullous eruptions. They are caused by a large number of drugs which include phenazone and its related compounds, barbiturates, sulphonamides, phenylbutazone, thiazides, chloroquin, quinine, phenothiazines and sulphonylureas. Exfoliative dermatitis, in which the skin becomes inflamed with exfoliation

of the epidermal cells, is occasionally superimposed and may be serious. It is fortunately rare but occurs with heavy metals, barbiturates and sulphonamides. Some of these drugs may also induce photosensitivity.

THE KIDNEY

Sulphonamides, PAS, tetracyclines, erythromycin and phenindione have been incriminated in causing acute renal failure in which the walls of the arterioles are infiltrated with inflammatory cells, but the evidence is circumstantial. Proteinuria due to damage to the glomerular capillary wall may follow the use of troxidone, paramethadione, penicillamine, bismuth, mercury and gold.

THE LIVER

Intrahepatic cholestasis may be caused by a number of C-17 alkyl substituted testosterones including methyl testosterone and some oral contraceptives, e.g. norethisterone and norethynodrel. The mechanism of this reaction is uncertain, but it may represent an intoxication rather than a hypersensitivity reaction. On the other hand, the phenothiazines, nitrofurantoin and chlorpropamide induce an allergic intrahepatic cholestasis in which overgrowth of villi in the biliary canaliculi occurs and in which there is an infiltration of inflammatory cells.

Hepatic cell necrosis occurs in a small number of patients taking monoamine oxidase inhibitors, sulphonamides, phenindione, cincophen, PAS and erythromycin estolate. In some cases this reaction is associated with other features such as fever, joint pains, skin rashes, etc.

which suggest hypersensitivity, but again the evidence is circumstantial.

The possible role of drugs in inducing hypersensitivity reactions in polyarteritis nodosa and systemic lupus erythematosus is described on p. 30.12. Retroperitoneal fibrosis is a rare reaction to methysergide (p. 13.7).

TABLE 23.1. Classification and features of the genetically determined forms of immunological deficiency. After Hitzig W.H. (1968) *Proc. roy. Soc. Med.* **61**, 888.

Clinical findings	Type of immunological deficiency		
	Humoral	Humoral and cell-mediated	Cell-mediated
Onset	First years of life	First weeks of life	First weeks of life
Skin infections	+	+	+
Diarrhoea	− or +	+++	+
Monilia infection	−	+	+
Progress	Relatively benign	Fatal	Fatal
Lymphocyte count in blood	Normal	Reduced	Reduced
Immunoglobulins	Reduced	Reduced	Normal
Delayed hypersensitivity	Present	Absent	Absent
Plasma cells	Absent	Absent	Present
Lymphoid tissue	Normal	Abnormal	Abnormal
Thymus	Normal	Abnormal	Abnormal
Inheritance (p. 31.7)	Sex-linked	Autosomal-recessive and sex-linked	Autosomal-recessive

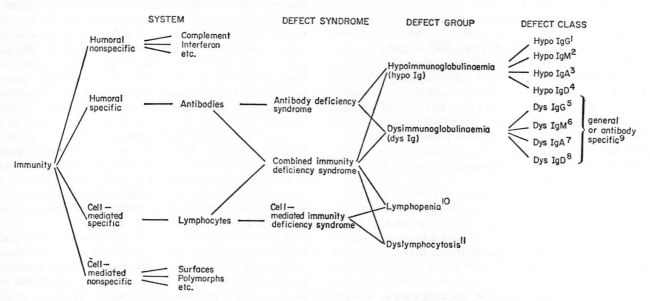

FIG. 23.5. A functional classification of the immunity deficiency states. Examples of nonspecific mechanisms are indicated but defects are not included. There is reason to believe that the eleven numbered parameters vary independently in these patients. After Soothill J.F. (1968) *Clinical Aspects of Immunology*, 2nd Edition, ed. Gell and Coombs. Oxford: Blackwell Scientific Publications.

Phenytoin and troxidone may also induce fever, enlargement of lymph nodes and skin rashes.

Immunological deficiency diseases in man

So important are the immunological mechanisms for survival that it is not surprising that patients are rarely seen suffering from defects of the mechanisms that lead to deficiencies. However, deficiencies of the humoral and cell-mediated components of the immunological system may arise and occur separately or together. Table 23.1 summarizes some of the features of the deficiencies and fig. 23.5 provides a more elaborate analysis of possible conditions.

DEFICIENCY OF HUMORAL IMMUNITY

A condition known as hypo- or agammaglobulinaemia arises as a sex-linked hereditary disorder. The lack of immunoglobulins is not absolute but the patients fail to respond to antigenic stimuli. However, delayed hypersensitivity and the capacity to react to a homograft are normal. It is not incompatible with survival for many years, though the patients are very susceptible to bacterial infections, particularly to pyogenic cocci. The analysis shown in fig. 23.5 is at present largely speculative but as the different immunoglobulins have different functions, deficiencies might be expected to produce different clinical pictures. Thus IgM deficiency is possibly associated with meningococcal meningitis and lack of IgA, which is secreted by mucous membranes, with gastrointestinal or respiratory tract infections. One possible explanation of such syndromes is abnormal functioning of the regulator genes determining Ig synthesis.

Maternal IgG passes across the placenta to the foetus during the third trimester of pregnancy. Premature babies may thus have some degree of hypogammaglobulinaemia and prophylactic IgG treatment may reduce the incidence of infections. Immunoglobulin deficiency may arise also in adults as a result of abnormal metabolism of serum proteins and this appears to occur in renal failure with uraemia where susceptibility to infection is increased. There is also evidence that in some patients the immunoglobulins are present in normal concentrations but are functionally defective (dysgammaglobulinaemia).

DEFICIENCY OF CELL-MEDIATED IMMUNITY

This condition is analogous to that which develops in thymectomized neonatal mice (vol. 1, p. 27.19). There may be severe lymphocytopenia and a predominance of reticulum cells in the lymphoid tissue, and the patient's lymphocytes are unable to respond by transformation, proliferation or differentiation following stimulation with antigens *in vitro*. On account of the deficiency in delayed hypersensitivity, affected children cannot reject skin homografts and do not respond in the normal way to antigens such as monilia. The child fails to thrive and there is wasting and diarrhoea. Moniliasis and viral infections arise and survival is usually brief. In a few individuals the lymphocyte count may be normal, but the cells are functionally incompetent (dyslymphocytosis).

In one hereditary type there is incomplete descent of the thymus gland embryologically; histologically the thymus shows general hypoplasia and disturbed structure, with a predominance of epithelial cells and reticulum cells, and absence of Hassall's corpuscles. Di George and his colleagues in 1968 described a distinct group of patients with isolated lymphopenia in whom multiple malformations resulted from a suppressed development of the third and fourth branchial pouches. In the first few days of life there is tetany attributable to hypoparathyroidism; if the infants survive this critical phase, lymphocytic incompetence is manifested later. The recognition of this type of immunological deficiency is of practical as well as theoretical importance as it should be correctable by replacement of the thymus. This in fact was demonstrated later the same year in two cases who were given transplants of fragments of human foetal thymus.

COMBINED DEFICIENCY STATES

Several types have been described in which there are combinations of agammaglobulinaemia and delayed hypersensitivity.

Abnormal immunoglobulin synthesis

In various proliferative and neoplastic disorders, mainly of the reticuloendothelial system, discrete components of immunoglobulins (M-proteins) may appear in the plasma. M-proteins are remarkably homogeneous. In an individual patient they belong to only one of the five immunoglobulin classes IgG, IgA, IgM, IgD or IgE, and contain light chains of either K or L type, never mixtures. Myeloma (p. 28.4) and Waldenstrom's macroglobulinaemia are the most important of these conditions and when associated with these diseases the proteins may be designated G-, A-, or D-myeloma proteins or M-macroglobulins (Waldenstrom). Abnormal proteins may occur also in the urine in these disorders. Bence Jones protein is found in the urine of about 50 per cent of patients with myeloma and 15 per cent of those with macroglobulinaemia. It consists of light chains only, usually dimerized, and in an individual patient these are either all K- or all L-chains (p. 22.11).

Heavy chain disease is a very rare disorder that occurs in association with rapidly progressive lymphomatous tumours. A dimer of the γ heavy chain which resembles the Fc fragment is present in the plasma and urine. No diseases with abnormal production of the heavy chains of immunoglobulins other than IgG have been found.

M-proteins are either abnormal proteins not present in the body in health or the result of excessive synthesis of a homogeneous protein which in health constitutes only a small proportion of normal protein molecules. The cellular basis for the homogeneity of M-proteins is probably increased synthesis by a single group or clone of lymphoid cells. Patients with abnormal immunoglobulin synthesis have an increased susceptibility to bacterial infections and particularly to bacterial pneumonia. This is partially the result of an impaired capacity to synthesize normal immunoglobulins and functional antibodies.

FURTHER READING

ANDERSON J.R., BUCHANAN W.W. & GOUDIE R.B. (1963) *Autoimmunity, Clinical and Experimental.* Springfield: Thomas.

ASHERSON G.L. (1968) Autoimmunity, in *Scientific Basis of Medicine.* London: Athlone Press.

DIXON F.J. (1968) The pathogenesis of glomerulonephritis. *Amer. J. Med.* **44,** 493.

GELL P.G.H. & COOMBS R.R.A. (1968) *Clinical Aspects of Immunology,* 2nd Edition. Oxford: Blackwell Scientific Publications.

GLYNN L.E. & HOLBOROW E.J. (1965) *Autoimmunity and Disease.* Oxford: Blackwell Scientific Publications.

IRVINE W.J. (1968) Immunobiology of the thymus and its relation to autoimmune disease, in *Modern Trends in Immunology,* vol. 2, p. 250, ed. Cruikshank & Weir. London: Butterworths.

—— (1968) Autoimmune and hypersensitivity phenomena in alimentary diseases, in *Recent Advances in Clinical Pathology,* ed. Dyke. London: Churchill.

—— (1967) Autoimmunity and endocrine disorders. *Practitioner,* **199,** 180.

SOOTHILL J.F., HOBBS J.R., HITZIG W.H. & KAY H.E.M. (1968) Symposium on immunological deficiency syndromes. *Proc. roy. Soc. Med.* **61,** 881.

TURK J.L. (1969) *Immunology in Clinical Medicine.* London: Heinemann.

Chapter 24
Drugs that suppress the immune response and inflammation

AGENTS WHICH SUPPRESS THE IMMUNE RESPONSE

Several stages are recognized in the development of the immune response on which drugs might act. These overlap but are sufficiently distinct to merit separate discussion. As described on p. 22.4, the initial stimulus is the exposure to an antigen, which may be a foreign macromolecule or a simpler compound (hapten) which produces an antigen after combination with endogenous protein. The animal or man responds by the synthesis of specific plasma antibodies which become bound to cells of lung, liver, skin and other tissues. These cells contain the inactive precursors or storage forms of several potent pharmacologically active compounds.

The binding of reaginic antibody by the tissues confers sensitization, for further exposure to antigen evokes a new and dramatic response. This is partly explained by the release of histamine and the slow reacting substance of anaphylaxis (SRS-A) and by the activation of the bradykinin precursor (p. 14.15 & 17.1). Without treatment

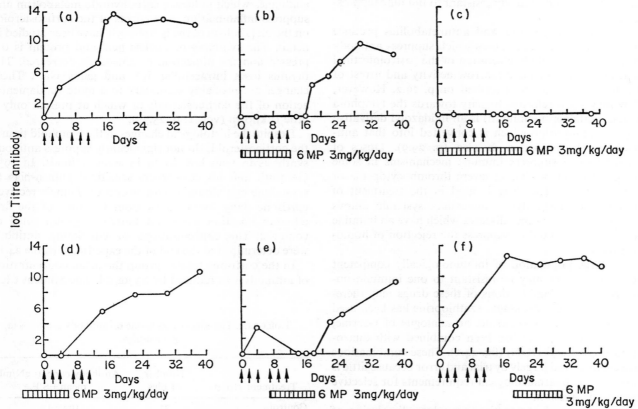

FIG. 24.1 Antibody response of rabbits to injection of antigen (bovine serum albumin) and 6-mercaptopurine (6-MP). Antigen injections shown as vertical arrows. (a) Control, antigen only, (b) 6-MP administration concurrent with antigen, (c) 6-MP administration extending over and beyond period of antigen administration, (d) 6-MP administration started before and stopped prior to completion of exposure to antigen, (e) 6-MP first given after three antigen injections (f) 6-MP given some days after antigen administration. (Schwartz R., Stack J. & Dameshek W. (1958) *Proc. Soc. exp. biol. & med.* **99**, 164.

24.1

they may lead to cell or tissue injury or death from inadequate tissue perfusion and hypoxia.

The response may be suppressed by drugs which act at any of the stages in this sequence. The majority of these drugs are fully described elsewhere and their pharmacological properties and metabolism are not repeated here.

Suppression of antibody synthesis

The plasma cells respond to antigen by synthesis of DNA, mitosis, morphological differentiation and the production of specific antibody. This sequence can be suppressed by **ionizing radiations** (p. 33.1), **alkylating agents** (p. 29.3), **antimetabolites** (p. 29.7) and **adrenocortical steroids** (p. 29.13) but the timing of the treatment is critical. **X-rays** and **busulphan** are most effective when given a few days before the antigen whereas the nitrogen mustards (p. 29.6) are most effective when given a few days afterwards. Fig. 24.1 shows the antibody response in rabbits given 6-mercaptopurine at varying times in relation to antigen exposure. Once established, antibody synthesis becomes relatively resistant to immunosuppressive agents.

Most alkylating agents and antimetabolites produce serious adverse effects at doses which suppress antibody synthesis; these include ulceration of the gastrointestinal tract, depression of bone marrow activity and arrest of gametogenesis and are described on p. 29.2. However, a few may show selective toxicity towards the lymphoid tissues. **Azathioprine** (imuran) is an imidazolyl derivative of 6-mercaptopurine which is converted into that antimetabolite by reduction *in vivo* (p. 29.9). Doses of 2–5 mg/kg/day suppress immune mechanisms in some patients without producing severe thrombocytopenia or agranulocytosis. The drug is used in the treatment of autoimmune haemolytic anaemia, systemic lupus erythematosus and other diseases which have an immune basis. It is also used to suppress the rejection of homograft tissue.

In a large population of immunologically competent cells a few clones may be resistant to one immunosuppressive agent. Combinations of these drugs may therefore be used with advantage; azathioprine has been used in conjunction with azaserine, an analogue of L-serine, and 6-mercaptopurine has been combined with duazomycin A (*N*-acetyl DON) (fig. 24.2). These combinations have been evolved largely by trial and error because little is known of the pharmacological requirements for selective immunosuppression.

Cortisone and hydrocortisone produce dissolution of lymphoid tissues within a few hours of the injection of pharmacological doses; the cell nuclei become pyknotic and the cytoplasm may be shed. The number of circulating lymphocytes falls and after one or two days treat-

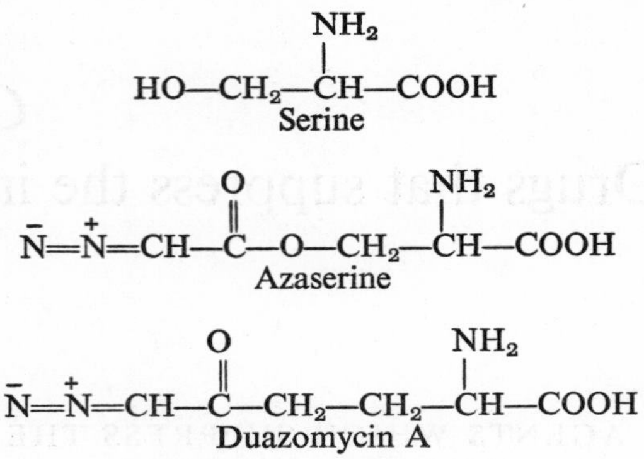

FIG. 24.2. Serine, azaserine and duazomycin A.

ment the weight of the thymus and lymphoid tissues is reduced. Rat lymph nodes in tissue culture show necrosis with low concentrations (3×10^{-7} M) of hydrocortisone. Time-lapse cinematography has shown that the small, mature lymphocyte is mainly affected. These effects are common to those natural corticosteroids and synthetic analogues which influence carbohydrate metabolism and suppress inflammation. The effects of the corticosteroids on the metabolism of the lymphocyte have been studied in detail. The synthesis of nucleic acid and protein is depressed and the utilization of glucose is decreased. The thymus loses intracellular K^+ and gains Na^+. These changes are probably secondary to a more fundamental action of the corticosteroids of which at present only a little is known (vol. 1, p. 25.35).

Despite the histological changes in the lymphoid tissues the corticosteroids do not significantly suppress antibody synthesis in man but do so in some animals. In 1952 Germuth and his co-workers sensitized guinea-pigs to crystalline egg albumin. One group of animals received cortisone daily for 30 days from the time of the first albumin injection whilst an untreated group acted as controls. The concentrations of circulating antibody were determined at the end of the experiment (table 24.1).

In the cortisone treated group the mean concentration of antibody was reduced by 83 µg/ml. The Student t test

TABLE 24.1. The effect of cortisone on antibody synthesis in guinea-pigs.

Treatment group	Number of pigs	Antibody conc. (µgN/ml) mean ± S.E.
Control	32	109 ± 17
Cortisone	17	26 ± 7
Number of observations (*n*)	49	

gives a probability (*P*) of less than o·oo1 for this difference; there is a 1 in 1000 chance that the difference between the two groups is due not to cortisone but to sampling error. However, immunization experiments in man and the monkey have failed to show inhibition of antibody synthesis and it is unlikely that these drugs benefit allergic subjects by this means.

Corticosteroids are especially useful in treating disorders of connective tissue associated with abnormal immune mechanisms (p. 30.9) and certain autoimmune disorders, e.g. thyroiditis, some haemolytic anaemias, ulcerative colitis, and primary biliary cirrhosis.

ANTILYMPHOCYTIC SERUM (ALS)

The selective suppression of lymphocytes has been achieved by immunological means. ALS can be prepared, e.g. by the injection of rat lymphocytes into rabbits. The rabbit serum produces a fall in the blood lymphocyte count when administered to a rat. Low counts are maintained for several weeks in animals receiving daily injections of antiserum. The count then returns to normal despite continued administration of antiserum.

The delayed hypersensitivity reaction is abolished and the survival of rat skin homografts is prolonged by the daily administration of ALS (fig. 24.3). The grafts remain healthy even after the lymphocyte count has returned to normal. A horse antiserum to dog lymphocytes has been shown to prolong the survival of kidney homografts. An antiserum to human lymphocytes, obtained by drainage of the thoracic duct, is being used to suppress the rejection of kidney homografts in man.

The immunosuppressive effect of ALS may depend on the coating of the host lymphocytes by antibody protein. It does not depend on the degree of lymphocytopenia. In order to avoid injecting large amounts of nonantibody protein, the active constituent of ALS which

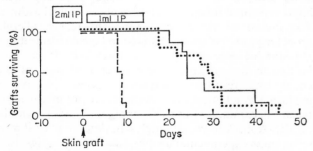

FIG. 24.3. Antilymphocyte sera and IgG prolong the survival of albino-strain rat skin grafts on hooded strain recipients. Two antisera each containing about 1 g of IgG/100 ml were given by intraperitoneal injection (continuous line and dots). Broken line represents control animals. After James (1967) *New Scientist*.

is an IgG has been purified by fractionation procedures consisting of salt precipitation and chromatography.

Reversal of tissue fixation of antibody

The binding of antibody by the tissues appears to be a physical phenomenon which is independent of metabolism. ^{131}I labelled globulin from antipneumococcal serum is bound by samples of guinea-pig lung *in vitro*. At 37° C the amount bound reaches a maximum in 2–3 hours. Although the extent of binding is reduced at 0°C, it is not affected by metabolic inhibitors or tissue damage. Binding is reversible and the rate of loss of antibody from the tissue is increased by the addition of nonantibody γ-globulin. Since the amount of antibody uptake required for sensitization is very small (less than 1 μg/g of wet tissue) it is unlikely that the clinical manifestations of tissue hypersensitivity would be influenced by treatment with γ-globulin from nonimmune subjects. No reports of relevant clinical investigations have been made.

None of the drugs which suppress the immune response are known to interfere with the binding of reaginic antibody by the tissues.

Depletion of stores of mediators

The quantitative importance of the different mediators of tissue hypersensitivity varies from species to species and from organ to organ in the same species. Histamine, the slow reacting substance (SRS-A) and bradykinin may be the most important agents involved in the pathogenesis of human bronchial asthma; histamine and bradykinin are probably also responsible for the features of urticaria in man.

The tissue stores of histamine may be depleted by pretreatment with compound 48/80 or other histamine liberators (p. 14.13). In some species this reduces the severity of a subsequent anaphylactic response but in the guinea-pig, for example, passive cutaneous hypersensitivity is not reduced; intravenous antigen still produces vasodilation and weal formation at the site of antibody injection. Even if subsequent allergic episodes were suppressed, the use of histamine liberators in human allergic subjects would be far too dangerous to contemplate. Morphine, for example, releases histamine tissue stores and may produce acute airway obstruction in asthmatic subjects (p. 5.49).

The corticosteroids deplete the histamine content of rat skin but it is doubtful whether this mechanism is responsible for their anti-allergic effects. In the guinea-pig for example, antigen challenge still evokes the release of histamine from the lung of a cortisone treated animal.

An analogy may be drawn between the decarboxylation of L-histidine to give histamine and the decarboxylation of L-dihydroxyphenylalanine (DOPA) to give dopamine. When the adrenergic tissues are provided with L-α methyl DOPA this is handled in the same way as DOPA and a false transmitter is produced (p. 15.32). Extending the analogy, it may become possible to produce a derivative of L-histidine which is utilized in the synthesis of a false mediator, a chemical analogue of histamine without its undesirable effects.

SRS-A cannot be extracted from the tissues of even a sensitized animal but is apparently formed from an inactive precursor after antigen challenge. On the basis of the response to antigen, it is inferred that the precursor is present in the lung, the heart and the great vessels. However no agents are known which deplete these tissues of SRS-A precursor.

The release of bradykinin from its parent protein occurs very rapidly in the presence of any of a wide variety of proteolytic and esterolytic enzymes; these include trypsin, and kallikreins from plasma, pancreas, salivary gland, intestinal mucosa and urine (p. 17.1). A similar enzyme is released from guinea-pig lung and skin on exposure to antigen. By the intravenous infusion of trypsin or kallikrein it is possible to deplete an animal of its circulating bradykinin precursor, but since this procedure also causes the release of the active peptide, it is unlikely to have any application in the treatment of hypersensitivity.

Removal of antigen challenge

Physicians treating allergy often try to identify the allergen and remove it from the patient's environment. Not uncommonly the responsible agent is a drug and occasionally this may have been injected in a depot form before the allergy was recognized. For example procaine penicillin may have provoked general anaphylaxis. The removal of the allergen in this situation is a special problem. The parenteral injection of a preparation of bacterial penicillinase has been used to convert the penicillin molecule into a nonantigenic derivative, but results are not satisfactory as the treatment itself carries an allergic risk.

Inhibition of the release of mediators

Little is yet known about the immediate events which follow the combination of antigen with tissue-bound antibody and cause the release of histamine, the activation of the SRS-A precursor and the production of the bradykinin-forming enzyme. It is possible that a series of enzymic reactions is involved and that future therapeutic agents will inhibit these enzymes. It has already been shown that chymotrypsin substrates and inhibitors reduce the release of histamine by antigen from sensitized guinea-pig lung.

Recently a new drug, **disodium chromoglycate**, has been developed. It is believed to inhibit the release of mediators at the time of antigen challenge. It is particularly effective in controlling bronchospasm induced by specific antigens. When the drug is given to an asthmatic subject before exposure to the antigen, protection may last for several hours while the drug has little effect if given after the antigen. In animal studies a similar capacity to inhibit passive cutaneous hypersensitivity to human reagins is shown when the drug is given simultaneously with the antigen, while it has no effect on the reaction of the skin to intradermal injection of histamine, 5-HT or bradykinin. It also fails to affect the skin lesions induced by SRS-A, and potent histamine liberators.

Disodium cromoglycate is inhaled as an aerosol in doses of 20 mg. So far, no adverse effects have been reported.

Disodium cromoglycate (intal)

Antagonists of the mediators

When anaphylaxis presents as an acute clinical problem the immediate aim is to give drugs which antagonize the effects of the mediators. These antagonists are the specific **antihistamines** (p. 14.16) and various drugs which have opposite actions to the mediators.

The specific antihistamines occupy the same tissue receptors as histamine without providing any stimulus to the effector cells. In organ bath experiments they reduce the size of a histamine response to an extent which depends on the relative molecular concentrations of histamine and antihistamine. The effects of histamine on tracheal and bronchial smooth muscle are antagonized *in vitro* and the intact guinea-pig may be partially protected from the effects of a histamine aerosol. In man the intravenous injection of the antihistamine **chlorpheniramine** (piriton 10 mg) quickly produces adequate tissue concentrations. The weal, the erythema and the itch of acute urticaria are reduced but there is no consistent improvement in lung function in acute bronchial asthma. The failure of the antihistamines to relieve allergic bronchospasm has been attributed to high concentrations of histamine close to the smooth muscle cells. It may also be due to the presence of the other mediators of the anaphylactic response. Bradykinin is rapidly inactivated in plasma by a kininase but its effects are not inhibited by the antihistamines. No specific antagonists of bradykinin or SRS-A are known, although salicylates may be shown to suppress experimental anaphylaxis in guinea-pigs. Fig. 24.4 represents an experimental model of bronchial muscle. A single dose of foreign protein, e.g. egg white or horse serum does little harm. A second dose, however, results in a severe anaphylactic response with bronchospasm which may be fatal. Whereas antihistamines pro-

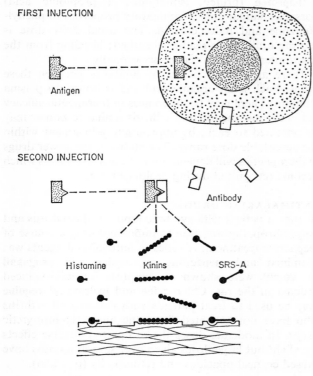

FIRST INJECTION

Antigen

SECOND INJECTION

Antibody

Histamine   Kinins   SRS-A

INJECTION OF ANTAGONISTS

Antihistamine   Aspirin

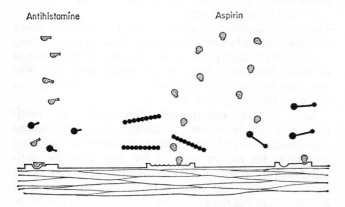

FIG. 24.4. Possible mode of action of antihistamines and aspirin in bronchospasm in guinea-pigs. Injection of antigen, e.g. egg white or horse serum, results in antibody production. After a second injection some weeks later the antigen-antibody complex results in the liberation of histamine, kinins and SRS-A all of which induce broncho-constriction. Antihistamines block the action of histamine and aspirin antagonizes the action of kinins and SRS-A. From Collier H. O. J. (1963) *Scientific American.* Offprint 169.

tect the animal to some extent, salicylates appear to augment the protection and they may do so by blocking the action of kinins and SRS-A on the bronchial muscle.

In clinical emergencies, drugs which act by producing effects which oppose the mediators are more effective than the specific antihistamines or aspirin. **Adrenaline** and **isoprenaline** (p. 15.15) and **aminophylline** (p. 5.39 and 15.13) are efficient bronchodilators in acute bronchial asthma. Adrenaline also produces constriction of the arterioles in the skin and the splanchnic area. Vascular permeability and oedema are reduced. Giant urticaria is relieved and where oedema threatens the airway, the risk of asphyxia is lessened. Despite their effectiveness these nonspecific antagonists have serious disadvantages. They are agonists in their own right, acting at receptors which differ from those occupied by the mediators, and their effects never precisely counteract those of the mediators. The dose of a sympathomimetic amine which relieves bronchospasm may produce systemic hypertension and potentiate rather than oppose the stimulation of the cardiac pacemaker which occurs in systemic anaphylaxis. Tachycardia and palpitations are frequently observed even when the amine is administered as an inhaled aerosol.

Hydrocortisone or the related steroids, **prednisone** and **prednisolone**, produce improvement in status asthmaticus within 12–24 hours but the mechanism is not known. Histamine aerosols still produce bronchospasm in asthmatic subjects receiving corticosteroids and the area of a wheal produced by intradermal histamine is not reduced. It has been suggested that the beneficial effects of these drugs in acute allergic states result from their anti-inflammatory actions (p. 24.6) and not from selective interference with any stage in the development of the anaphylactic response.

ANTI-INFLAMMATORY DRUGS

Inflammation and tissue anaphylaxis have many features in common. In each case the small vessels dilate, become more permeable and oedema develops. The affected tissue becomes infiltrated by leucocytes which are mainly neutrophil polymorphs in acute inflammation and eosinophil polymorphs in acute allergy. Pain is a characteristic feature of inflammation and itch of urticaria. In disease the two states often co-exist. In the study of drugs which influence the inflammatory response use is made of a variety of experimental models.

Experimental models of inflammation

Acute inflammation is commonly provoked by the injection of formaldehyde, egg white or dextran, or by local heating. The increase in blood flow may be estimated from the local temperature rise. Increase in permeability of the small vessels results in the extravasation of labelled protein which may be extracted and measured. The oedema is often estimated from changes in the volume of an inflamed paw, and the extent of the leucocyte infiltration is determined by tissue histology.

Chronic inflammation is measured by weighing the granuloma which develops around a cotton wool pellet or a subcutaneous bleb of croton oil. Local inflammation has been provoked by paper discs placed on the membranes of a chick embryo; the disc with its adherent inflammatory tissue is cut out and weighed. The pain of acute inflammation has been reproduced by the intra-arterial injection of possible chemical mediators and by their application to the base of a blister raised with cantharidin.

Each of these models has been used or suggested as the basis for a screening test to select agents which suppress the inflammatory response. They have also been used by biochemists interested in the chemical changes which accompany the inflammatory response.

Drugs which suppress the inflammatory response

Before discussing the possible modes of action of drugs which suppress inflammation it is necessary to summarize the agents concerned. These are grouped on the basis of their pharmacological properties rather than their chemical structures.

THE ANALGESIC-ANTIPYRETIC GROUP

Salicylic acid and **acetysalicylic acid** (aspirin, p. 5.53) are the most widely used remedies in minor inflammatory states and in the management of inflammatory joint diseases such as acute rheumatic fever or rheumatoid arthritis (p. 30.12).

Phenylbutazone (butazolidin) and **oxyphenbutazone** (p. 5.53) are acidic molecules also used to suppress the symptoms of inflammation in relation to joints. In absorption and distribution they resemble aspirin.

Mefenamic acid (ponstan) and **flufenamic acid** (fig. 24.5) both possess analgesic and anti-inflammatory activity in man. They are under trial in chronic rheumatoid arthritis and at the doses used (1 g/day) they appear to have similar therapeutic efficacy to aspirin and phenylbutazone.

Indomethacin (indocid), a substituted derivative of indolylacetic acid (fig. 24.5), was first prepared as a possible antagonist to 5-HT. Like aspirin it is rapidly absorbed from the upper gastrointestinal tract and reaches peak plasma concentrations in less than 2 hours. The drug is excreted in urine partly as a glucuronide. It is effective in acute gout and in about 30 per cent of cases of active rheumatoid arthritis in daily doses of 100 mg. In certain cases the joint swelling disappears as rapidly as with corticosteroids. Up to 50 per cent of patients experience adverse effects but these are usually mild and reversible. Occult gastrointestinal bleeding occurs but is said to be less than that due to aspirin. The usual daily dose is 25–75 mg.

Ibuprofen (brufen, isobutylphenyl propionic acid) possesses similar anti-inflammatory properties to phenylbutazone and indomethacin. The usual daily dose is 600 mg orally. It is readily absorbed; bleeding from the gastrointestinal tract occurs occasionally.

There are several points of similarity between these drugs. Each is an organic acid and is bound to plasma albumin. There may be differences in therapeutic efficacy but in chronic rheumatoid arthritis similar responses may be obtained to each, by appropriate adjustment within the acceptable dose range. The status of the newer drugs in therapeutics will depend upon the adverse effects which become recognized during prolonged use.

ANTIMALARIAL DRUGS

In 1951 a patient with systemic lupus erythematosus and polyarthropathy was seen to improve during a course of mepacrine treatment. A series of antimalarial agents was examined and **mepacrine**, **primaquine** and **proguanil** (p. 20.20) were shown to suppress formalin-induced oedema in the rat. **Chloroquine** and **hydroxychloroquine** may be used to treat patients with rheumatoid arthritis who have not benefited from the analgesic-antipyretic drugs. In moderate doses the recognized adverse effects are slight but large doses given over several months have caused corneal opacities and retinopathy (p. 20.20).

ADRENOCORTICAL STEROIDS AND THEIR SYNTHETIC ANALOGUES

The anti-inflammatory effects of pharmacological doses of **cortisone** and **hydrocortisone** were first studied clinically in 1948. With therapeutic doses the physiological effects of these hormones were exaggerated; fluid and salt retention produced weight gain, oedema, hypertension and even cardiac failure (p. 6.13).

The C-1, 2 unsaturated derivatives of cortisone and hydrocortisone, **prednisone** and **prednisolone** respectively, were shown to have the same salt retaining activity as the natural steroids but five times the anti-inflammatory potency. Five mg prednisolone and 25 mg hydrocortisone were equipotent in the suppression of inflammation but the former produced less salt retention. Many other derivatives have since been synthesized but prednisone and prednisolone still remain the most frequently prescribed systemic anti-inflammatory corticosteroids.

The introduction of a fluorine atom in the α-position at C-9 resulted in a group of highly active corticosteroid derivatives. The increase in potency was not however restricted to anti-inflammatory activity. In fact 9α fluorohydrocortisone or **fludrocortisone** proved to be the most active salt-retaining compound known. Further substitution at C-16 gave the potent anti-inflammatory agents **triamcinolone**, **dexamethasone** and **betamethasone** (p. 6.12).

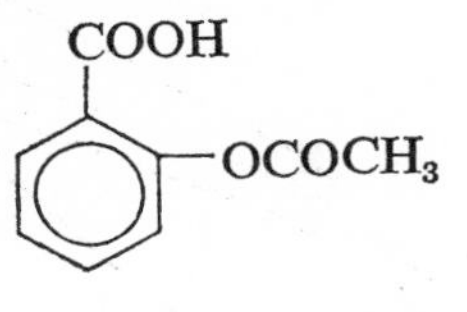

Acetylsalicylic acid

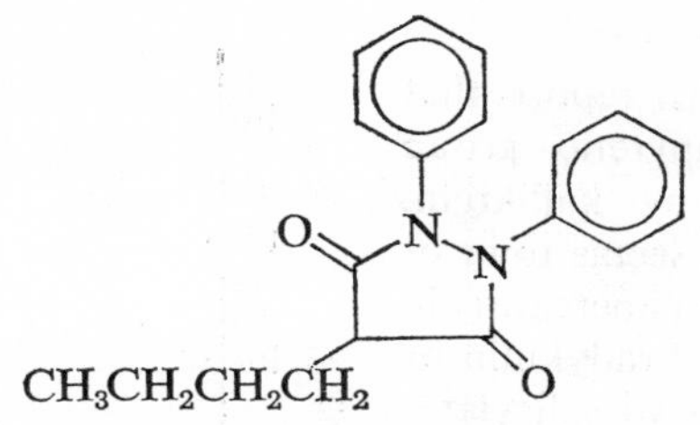

Phenylbutazone

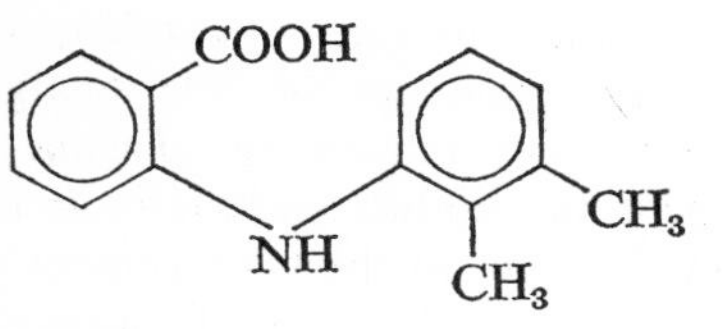

Mefenamic acid

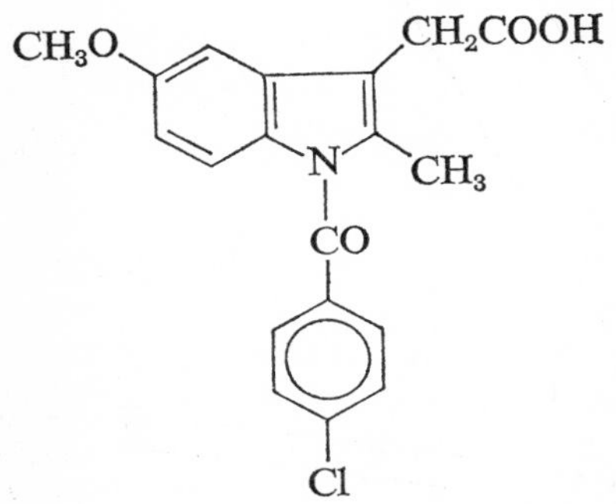

Indomethacin

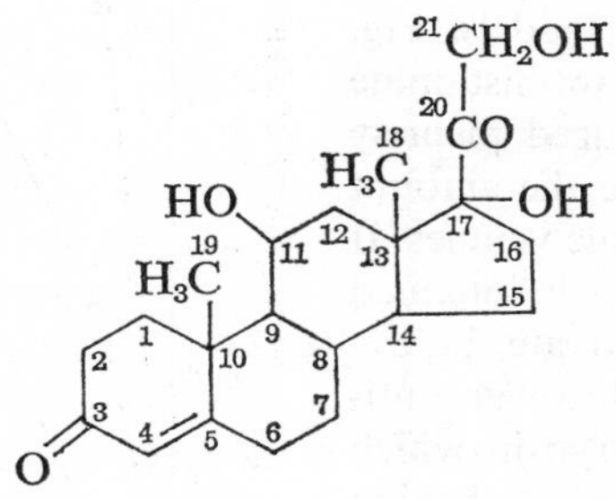

Hydrocortisone

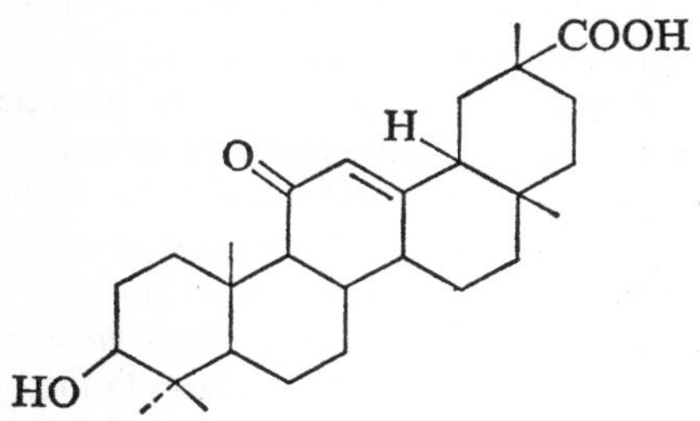

Glycyrrhetinic acid

FIG. 24.5. Chemical structure of some anti-inflammatory agents.

CARBENOXOLONE SODIUM

Carbenoxolone sodium (biogastrone) is a derivative of glycyrrhetinic acid (fig. 24.5) which shows a limited resemblance to hydrocortisone. It is an anti-inflammatory agent with salt retaining activity but no glucocorticoid effects. In controlled trials it has been shown to accelerate the healing of gastric ulcers (p. 10.5). Other anti-inflammatory agents have adverse effects on peptic ulceration, and it is likely that carbenoxolone promotes healing by a mechanism which is not directly linked to the suppression of inflammation. Weight gain and oedema may be prevented by diuretics. The potassium-depleting action of the drug should be offset by giving potassium salts.

ORGANIC GOLD COMPOUNDS

Several gold substituted sulphydryl compounds have been used to suppress inflammatory changes in active rheumatoid arthritis. **Sodium aurothiomalate** (myocrisin), for example, is given by weekly intramuscular injections. The plasma level of gold is steady during a course of injections but concentration occurs in the kidney and the excretion of protein in the urine is common. Exfoliative dermatitis and severe bone marrow depression occur but the incidence is low if the drug is stopped at the first signs of toxicity and withheld from elderly patients.

ENZYMES AND INHIBITORS

Systemic anti-inflammatory activity after oral ingestion has been claimed for preparations of trypsin, chymotrypsin and bromelains (proteolytic enzymes from the pineapple). The evidence is equivocal. The plasmin inhibitor **ε-aminocaproic acid** (p. 7.14) and the kallikrein antagonist **aprotinin** (p. 10.8) have both been tested in a few pathological states. Their role, if any, in the management of inflammatory conditions is not yet defined.

Possible mechanisms of anti-inflammatory action

During the first hour of an acute inflammatory response histamine can be detected in the exudate. At this stage the response can be delayed by the antihistamine drugs or by previous depletion of the tissue histamine stores with compound 48/80. Despite the delay, however, the intensity of the final response is not reduced. The intra-arterial injection of histamine evokes the release of kinin-forming enzyme from certain tissues. This also can be inhibited by the antihistamines.

The inflammatory response to experimental heat injury is suppressed by DOPA, dopamine and adrenaline. It is probable that the changes of acute inflammation are depressed by the release of catecholamines *in vivo*.

The proteolytic activity of inflamed tissue is probably an important factor in the initiation of kinin formation. ε-Aminocaproic acid probably owes its anti-inflammatory activity to the inhibition of the proteolytic activity of plasmin. Salicylates also have antiplasmin activity and sodium salicylate, phenylbutazone and indomethacin have each been shown to inhibit the proteolytic activity of inflamed rat paw. Chloroquine inhibits the proteolytic degradation of cartilage matrix.

Recent work has not confirmed the earlier reports that several members of the analgesic-antipyretic group inhibit the release of plasma kinins by kallikrein. Aprotinin inhibits kallikreins *in vitro* but seems to be of limited value in the management of acute pancreatitis in man. No effective, specific antagonists of bradykinin or kallidin are yet known. As already discussed salicylates suppress bronchospasm due to bradykinin and SRS-A in the guinea-pig and the combination of antihistamine and salicylates can be shown to reduce greatly the inflammatory exudate in some experimental models. Fig. 24.6 illustrates the influence of salicylates, antihistamine and histamine depletion in turpentine induced pleurisy in rats. Salicylates appear to help to reduce the amount of exudation of fluid through the walls of the venules. If chymotrypsin attains effective concentrations in inflamed tissues after ingestion then it may inactivate bradykinin and kallidin as it does *in vitro*. However anti-inflammatory effects are also claimed for trypsin which rapidly activates the bradykinin precursor whilst having no effect on the active peptide.

The salicylates also inhibit hyaluronidase and may thereby reduce the rate of depolymerization of the connective tissue ground substance. Gold salts stabilize the structure of connective tissue collagen by entering into combination with the protein chains and increasing the frequency of cross-linkage. However, salicylates, phenylbutazone and chloroquine all reduce the degree of cross-linkage at concentrations which occur *in vivo* during therapy.

The corticosteroids appear to protect the cellular components of inflamed tissues. Smaller numbers of disintegrating mast cells and fibroblasts are seen after their administration. It is possible that several of the non-steroidal anti-inflammatory agents may act partly by altering the distribution of the endogenous corticosteroids in favour of the tissues. In the rat for example, phenylbutazone displaces corticosterone from plasma protein and increases the size of the tissue corticosterone pool. This effect is restricted to those phenylbutazone analogues which have anti-rheumatic activity and is shared by sodium salicylate, flufenamic acid and indomethacin. The stimulation of ACTH secretion with increase in the plasma corticosteroid concentration and depletion of adrenocortical ascorbic acid has been demonstrated after large doses of salicylate in guinea-pigs. This does not occur after therapeutic doses in man however. The salicylates remain effective in the suppression of inflammation after adrenalectomy.

In the present state of knowledge, active drugs are found by screening hundreds of compounds in relatively crude tests of anti-inflammatory activity. After further laboratory tests a few are introduced into therapeutics and years later we begin to understand how they work.

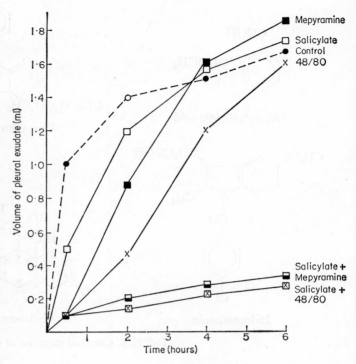

FIG. 24.6. Effects of various treatments on the development of turpentine induced pleurisy in rats. Systemic salicylates when given with antihistamine or after histamine depletion by 48/80 causes marked reduction in volume of the inflammatory exudate. Each remedy alone has little effect (see fig. 24.4). After Spector W.G. & Willoughby D.A.. *The Pharmacology of Inflammation* (1968) London: English Universities Press.

FURTHER READING

COLLIER H.O.J. (1963) Aspirin. *Scientific American Offprint No. 169.* San Francisco: Freeman.

GARATTINI S. & DUKES M.H.G. (1965) *Non-steroidal Anti-inflammatory Drugs.* London: Excepta Medica Foundation.

HITCHINGS G.H. & ELION G.B. (1963) Chemical suppression of the immune response. *Pharm. Rev.* **15**, 365.

KEELE C.A. & ARMSTRONG D. (1964) *Substances Producing Pain and Itch.* London: Arnold.

LIDDLE G.W. (1961) Clinical pharmacology of the anti-inflammatory steroids. *Clin. Pharm. & Thera.,* **2**, 615.

Chapter 25
Disorders of the cell

All disease is the result of damage, disablement and malfunction of the cells and tissues of the body. This chapter is concerned with the agents that damage cells and the mechanism of their noxious action, and the appearance, properties and behaviour of injured, dead and dying cells.

Disorders of the cell include:

(1) irreversible cessation of cellular activity and irreparable disorganization of cell structure both in cytoplasm and nucleus, which are together called cellular death or necrosis (Greek *nekros*, dead), and

(2) other less severe changes, which may herald necrosis but which alternatively may be signs of temporary or less serious derangement; these include,

   (a) swelling of the cell or its contained organelles,
   (b) disintegration and loss of cellular constituents,
   (c) aggregation, deposition or appearance of visible materials within the cell, and
   (d) abnormalities in metabolism, behaviour or function invisible by available techniques.

CAUSES OF CELLULAR DISORDER

Le corps de l'animal se compose de parties qui se détruisent et se renouvellent sans cesse. Augustus Waller, 1852.

The macromolecular fabric of the cell is in a state of dynamic equilibrium, with a continual balancing of anabolism and catabolism. By feeding or injecting animals with compounds labelled by ^{15}N, ^{14}C, ^{32}P and other isotopes, the incorporation and elimination of micromolecules in the cellular macromolecules can be traced. Such experiments show that proteins, nucleic acids and complex lipids are being continuously synthesized and degraded in living cells.

The cells of the body have to make good this persistent degradation; to do so they must be supplied with nutrients capable of replenishing, by their exergonic catabolism, the cellular stores of ATP and other high energy phosphate compounds. The energy available in high-energy phosphate bonds is essential for the replacement of individual components of the macromolecular fabric such as proteins, nucleic acids and phospholipids

and for the maintenance of cell membranes. Such micromolecules as amino acids also constitute the individual units from which the macromolecules are made. Moreover, the reactions in which the micromolecules engage are themselves usually dependent for their orderly sequence on the macromolecular fabric of the cell. For instance, the orientation of enzymes at mitochondrial surfaces is essential for the progress of oxidative phosphorylation, and the attachment of messenger RNA to ribosomes is a basic requirement for the synthesis of peptide chains from amino acids. Similarly, messenger RNA has only a limited span of life and must be constantly renewed by the replicating action of nuclear DNA (vol. 1, p. 12.4). Nuclear DNA exerts a crucial action on cellular survival and the loss of even one unique macromolecule of this archetypic substance may herald cellular death. The macromolecules of the cell thus provide a specific pattern essential for the interaction of micromolecules. As F. G. Hopkins observed in 1933: 'Life . . . in the downward course of energy-flow . . . imposes a barrier and dams up a reservoir which provides potential for its own remarkable activities'. To obtain this energy by catabolism the living cell requires an organization of great complexity.

To persist in the living state, the cell needs:

(1) a constant supply of nutrients, and
(2) an intact and permanent self-replicating structure.

All disorders of the cell are thus initiated by either:

(1) interference with behaviour or supply of micromolecules, or
(2) disorganization, disintegration or imperfection of the self-replicating fabric.

All lethal or irreparable cellular derangement begins in one of these ways. The main agents which cause these changes are:

(1) genetically determined defects,
(2) lack of essential nutrients,
(3) adverse physical environment,
(4) harmful substances, and
(5) living agents, which may be either the cells of the body itself or parasitic cells. These may act by creating conditions classifiable under 2, 3 and 4 or in some hitherto unsuspected manner.

20
25.1

GENETICALLY DETERMINED DEFECTS

Genetically determined diseases are discussed in chap 31. The manner in which cells are injured by genetic defects is therefore considered only briefly here. Inherited defects of the cell may consist in either invisible abnormality of genetic code or visible change of karyotype, i.e. a change in the appearance of the dividing chromosomes at metaphase.

Invisible abnormality of the genetic code

Genetic codes are determined by the linear order of purine and pyrimidine bases in the DNA molecules of the chromosomes (vol. 1, p. 12.10). A change of even one codon, composed of three such bases in adjoining nucleotides of a DNA chain, can alter the structure of one cellular protein by the substitution of one specific amino acid for another in a constituent peptide chain. Such an alteration can interfere with cellular activity, behaviour or structure, as the following examples show.

DEFECT IN ENZYMIC PROTEINS

Minute alteration in the structure of a protein can eliminate its activity as a specific enzyme and so delete part of the cell's metabolic equipment. Examples of metabolic defects due to such inherited lack of enzyme are **glycogen storage disease**, in which inherited absence of enzymes concerned with glycogen breakdown causes accumulation of glycogen (vol. 1, p. 9.10), and **phenylketonuria**, in which inherited absence of phenylalanine hydroxylase in hepatic cells causes accumulation of phenylalanine and phenylpyruvic acid. This accumulation is followed by mental impairment or idiocy (vol. 1, p. 11.24).

STRUCTURAL DEFECT PRODUCED BY ABNORMAL PROTEIN

Cellular structure can be severely injured by a change in the amino acid sequence of even one cellular protein. Thus the substitution of valine for glutamic acid as the sixth amino acid in each of the two β-peptide chains of haemoglobin results in the formation of **abnormal haemoglobin S** $\alpha_2\beta_2^{6\ val}$ instead of **normal haemoglobin A** $\alpha_2\beta_2^{6\ glu}$ (vol. 1, p. 11.9). This change is determined by the alteration of only one codon in the nuclear DNA of one chromosome. In an individual who is homozygous for the abnormal gene, haemoglobin S is formed. Unfortunately, in the reduced state haemoglobin S readily crystallizes out of concentrated solutions into long crystals, which grow mainly in one direction. When this happens within red blood cells, they become elongated or 'sickled' in shape and the patient suffers from **sickle-cell anaemia** (vol. 1, p. 38.10). Thus an inherited abnormality in even one codon, involving only one substituent amino acid in a protein molecule, can cause a major alteration in its behaviour with structural consequences to the cells.

Abnormal proteins produced by genetic abnormality can determine fundamental changes also in the structure of cell membranes; such abnormal membranes may aggregate to form lipoprotein deposits. This kind of genetic defect may account for the intra-cellular deposition of lipoproteins in cellular disorders like amaurotic family idiocy (p. 25.37).

Visible change of karyotype

A common type of visible abnormality of karyotype is the presence of one extra chromosome, no. 21 (trisomy 21), causing mongoloid idiocy or Down's disease (p. 31.17.) In this disorder the brain is small, the cerebral gyri are defective and the cortical neurones are irregularly crowded. How the extra chromosome causes imperfect neurogenesis and the other stigmata of the disease is obscure.

The karyotypes of the cells of malignant neoplasms are also often visibly abnormal. The number of chromosomes may be greater or smaller than the normal diploid number of forty-six. Thus chromosome counts from as low as 35 to as high as 250 have been observed in cells of human malignant tumours. Such cells may also have abnormally short or long 'marker' chromosomes. In chronic myeloid leukaemia, for instance, one of the small acrocentric chromosomes of pair 21 is replaced by the dwarf Philadelphia chromosome in which the long arm is largely missing (fig. 25.1). It is likely that malignant

(a)   (b)

FIG. 25.1. (a) Normal small acrocentric chromosomes pair 21. (b) Pair 21 in chronic myeloid leukaemia. The Philadelphia chromosome is on the right.

tumours result from somatic mutations which produce these new karyotypes. The mutant cells are thus inherently abnormal and this is possibly related to their invasive and metastatic powers, which are unfortunately transmitted to their descendants (p. 28.11).

LACK OF NUTRIENTS

The supply of nutrients to the cells of the body may be inadequate owing to,
 (1) poverty of diet,
 (2) defective absorption of nutrients,
 (3) deficiency of internal secretions,
 (4) interruption or retardation in supply of blood, or
 (5) defective penetration of nutrients into cells.

Poverty of diet

Of the three major foodstuffs, protein, carbohydrate and lipid, protein alone is commonly deficient to an extent capable of causing human disease. When the diet contains adequate amounts of protein, granules stainable by basic dyes are visible in the cytoplasm of the hepatic cells. These granules, discovered by Berg in 1912, contain protein, RNA and phospholipid; they are the part of the cytoplasm which synthesizes protein, and in the liver they are concerned specifically with making serum albumin. The EM shows them as the zones of rough-surfaced endoplasmic reticulum rich in ribosomes. After short periods of starvation, the granules disappear from the liver cells, but reappear when protein is supplied in the food. Loss of these granules is accompanied by loss of RNA from the cell. In addition, mitochondria disappear from the liver cells of rats fed diets low in protein (vol. 1, p. 11.29).

Chronic severe lack of protein in man may lead to **famine oedema**. Deficiency of amino acids impedes the formation of albumin by the cells of the liver, so that the concentration falls in the plasma and the lowered colloidal osmotic pressure contributes to the development of oedema (p. 26.11). When protein is fed, famine oedema slowly subsides at a rate probably determined by the rate of formation of the granules in the liver cells, without which synthesis of albumin cannot occur.

Prolonged partial deficiency of protein gives rise to the condition **kwashiorkor**, seen among malnourished children in Africa and America. The liver in this disease is enlarged and fatty and is depleted of protein and of RNA.

Acute massive hepatic necrosis occurs in rats fed for some months on a diet deficient in both selenium and vitamin E. Massive hepatic necrosis develops occasionally also in men working with nitroaromatic compounds such as trinitrotoluene. This may be due to the action of these substances in stimulating metabolism which increases the requirement of the liver cells for specific nutrients.

The role of dietary deficiencies in causing fatty deposition is considered on p. 25.33.

Defective absorption of nutrients

DEFICIENT ABSORPTION BY THE INTESTINE

In chronic malnutrition, defective absorption often arises as a sequel to lack of dietary protein. This is due to a failure to synthesize the proteolytic digestive enzymes, which are themselves proteins; incomplete digestion of protein and other nutrients follows. Atrophy of intestinal mucosa leads to failure to absorb even the small quantities of amino acids liberated by digestion of the scanty protein intake. Similarly, lack of lipase results in failure to absorb fat and this produces a fatty diarrhoea which further retards absorption of available protein. Thus a vicious cycle develops which accounts for severe

depletion of body protein and profound wasting of skeletal muscles. Failure to absorb folic acid and/or iron prevents the normal formation of red cells and leads to anaemia. Addison's pernicious anaemia is an example of failure in cell maturation due to faulty absorption from the gut of vitamin B_{12}. Primary failure to absorb nutrients, the **malabsorption syndrome**, leads to widespread abnormalities and deficiency in body minerals and vitamins.

DEFICIENT ABSORPTION OF OXYGEN

Although a patient may breathe normal air, he may fail to absorb sufficient oxygen into the pulmonary capillaries for the following reasons.

(1) Decreased pulmonary ventilation from drowning or occlusion of the larynx by foreign bodies prevents oxygen intake and is lethal. Paralytic poliomyelitis may destroy lower motor neurones in the brain stem and cervical cord and thus weaken or arrest respiratory movements. Reduction in pulmonary ventilation may result also from excessive doses of drugs which depress the respiratory centres (p. 9.1).

(2) Defective oxygen transfer may arise from the filling of alveoli with fluid or inflammatory exudate in acute or chronic lung disease. In these circumstances alveoli may be either underventilated or underperfused with blood. Such disturbances of ventilation/perfusion ratio (vol. 1, p. 29.21) are important causes of hypoxaemia.

(3) Lack of haemoglobin results in anaemia which limits severely the absorption of oxygen. Carbon monoxide also eliminates functional haemoglobin with particularly injurious consequences (p. 25.13). The mechanism by which hypoxia injures cells is considered along with cellular injury produced by ischaemia (p. 25.5).

(4) Oxygen lack arising from low Po_2 in high altitudes is discussed in vol. 1, p. 43.3.

Deficiency of internal secretion

Even though the blood receives nutrients from the bowel and oxygen through the lungs in sufficient amounts, it still may not contain all the substances required by many of the specialized cells of the body. An adequate complement of cell nutrients includes substances internally secreted by various groups of **fabricator cells**. These substances may be added in large amounts, such as glucose and fatty acids liberated by the liver and adipose-tissue, or they may be constituents formed in only small amounts by the specialized cells of particular endocrine organs, such as insulin and thyroxine. These substances added to the blood by specialized cells are necessary supplements for the nutrition of some or all of the tissues.

Interruption or retardation in supply of blood

Although the blood may contain adequate amounts of all the nutrients required by the cells, sufficient blood may fail to reach them. Insufficient blood supply is by far the most frequent cause of serious lack of nutrients and is the most important single determinant of the death and injury of cells. Reduction of the supply of blood to a tissue is called **ischaemia**.

Ischaemia may arise from a general failure of the circulation, a local occlusion of blood vessels or a combination of both these causes. It may be temporary or permanent. Permanent ischaemia, if severe enough, is followed by death of the affected cells.

GENERALIZED ISCHAEMIA

Arrest of the heart or ventricular fibrillation may occur suddenly due to occlusion of a coronary artery or may take place during general anaesthesia. In the former case, consciousness is lost rapidly owing to cessation of the supply of oxygen and glucose to the brain. A continuous supply of these nutrients is essential for the highly vulnerable grey matter and without them neurones rapidly suffer permanent injury. If the normal cardiac rhythm can be re-established within a few minutes there is a chance of full recovery, but complete cessation of circulation for more than 5 min is usually succeeded by irreparable damage to the cerebral cortex, so that consciousness never returns or personality is impaired, although the more resistant neurones in the brain stem may be unharmed.

Short episodes of loss of consciousness due to generalized ischaemia often follow complete heart block. William Stokes in his great book *Diseases of the Heart and Aorta*, published in 1854, described one of his patients suffering from these attacks with the words, 'On recovery, after all comatose symptoms have passed away, he remains for half an hour or an hour unable to recognize his most intimate friends and relations, even his wife he has mistaken for his mother.' Stokes rightly attributed these symptoms of disorientation and confusion, as well as the coma which preceded them, to defective supply of blood to the brain.

Fall in blood pressure with sudden failure of supply of blood to the brain may also follow acute haemorrhage, occlusion of the pulmonary artery and vasomotor failure as in fainting or syncope. Some serious accidents have occurred when patients have fainted in dental chairs; under these circumstances it is important to lower the patient's head so as to reduce the risk of cerebral ischaemia. If patients are kept upright for as short a time as 2 min after fainting, irreparable ischaemic injury to cerebral neurones may occur; these patients may never recover consciousness or may be restored to only a vegetative decerebrate existence.

LOCAL ISCHAEMIA

This may have three causes.
External compression of the nutrient vessels. For instance,

damage to muscle follows prolonged compression from plasters applied too tightly to fractures, or when collapsed masonry traps the victims of air raids.
Occlusive disease of the vascular wall. When the intima is thickened by atheroma or endarteritis the lumen may be so narrow as to obstruct an artery or arteriole. Spasm caused by hypertension or ergot poisoning may also occlude blood vessels.
Occlusion of the vascular lumen by thrombosis or embolus. This is often associated with occlusive disease of the vascular wall and is considered on p. 26.6.

COMBINATION OF GENERAL AND LOCAL ISCHAEMIA

Local retardation in supply of blood may not by itself be severe enough to cause necrosis of cells. Even when an artery is occluded, local collateral channels may provide sufficient nutrients to avert damage. But when there is coincident generalized ischaemia, extensive necrosis may occur in a tissue where the local supply is retarded.

Such a combination is illustrated in fig. 25.2. This shows massive necrosis of most of the cortex of one cerebral hemisphere caused by occlusion of the ipsilateral common carotid artery by a thrombus, in a patient suffering from coincident heart failure. In this case, when local partial ischaemia was superadded to general ischaemia, the collateral circulation to one side of the cortex through the Circle of Willis was insufficient to avert extensive cellular death in the zone where the supply of blood was most severely retarded; thus necrosis was confined to the grey matter on the same side as the obstruction.

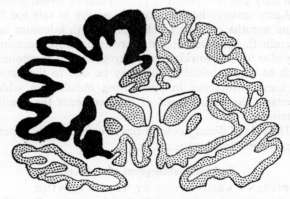

FIG. 25.2. Coronal section of cerebral hemispheres showing unilateral necrosis of cerebral cortex. Combination of general ischaemia from heart failure, and unilateral local ischaemia from occlusion of common carotid artery on one side has produced necrosis of most of the cerebral cortex on the same side. This necrosis is confined to the highly vulnerable grey matter and the less susceptible white matter appears uninjured.

Cellular injury produced by a similar combination of general and local ischaemia is illustrated in a patient who suffered from generalized ischaemia due to heart failure along with coincident local ischaemia caused by thrombosis of the right vertebral artery. Plate 25.1a, facing p. 25.6, shows neurones of the left cerebellar cortex which survived intact in spite of the general ischaemia. Plate 25.1b shows necrotic Purkinje cells and granule cells of the opposite right cerebellar cortex; these cells died because they were subjected to extreme lack of nutrients resulting from general ischaemia with superadded partial local ischaemia.

VISIBLE CONSEQUENCES OF ISCHAEMIA

Ischaemic atrophy and fatty change

When gradual in onset, ischaemia may cause contraction in the size of cells. This cellular atrophy commonly occurs in cardiac muscle when the coronary arteries are narrowed. The myocardial fibres shrink and eventually die; they are then replaced by connective tissue cells which can survive in the ischaemic zones, and these cells lay down collagen fibres. In this way ischaemic myocardium is replaced by fibrous tissue which impairs cardiac function (p. 27.4). Replacement of cardiac muscle by fibrous tissue owing to ischaemic atrophy is a common cause of chronic heart failure and may also lead to cardiac arrythmias. When partial ischaemia in the heart is not sufficiently severe to cause atrophy, droplets of globular fat may be deposited within the muscle fibres. This change also contributes to cardiac inefficiency.

Infarction

When ischaemia is sudden in onset, complete and permanent, it is followed rapidly by death of the cells throughout the affected tissue. When such an event occurs as a result of interruption in blood supply, it is referred to as infarction; the dead tissue is an **infarct**. Along with other cells damaged in the ischaemic tissue the endothelial cells of blood vessels are injured. Accordingly red blood cells entering the damaged tissue, through patent anastomotic arteries or by retrograde flow through veins, may escape through the injured capillary walls. For this reason the dead tissue may become stuffed with blood; this phenomenon gave rise to the word infarction (Latin *infarcire*, to stuff). Infarction is more fully described on p. 26.7.

DIFFERENTIAL VULNERABILITY TO ISCHAEMIA

Cells, tissues and organs differ markedly in their power to survive interruption or reduction of their supply of blood. While survival depends on local differences in blood supply which result in certain cells in a tissue or organ being more fortunately situated than their neighbours, there are real differences in metabolic requirements and demand for nutrients by different kinds of cell.

Local differences in supply of nutrients

The cells of the liver show **zonal vulnerability** to the generalized ischaemia of heart failure. The blood which supplies the hepatic cells percolates from branches of the hepatic artery and portal vein along the sinusoids which pass successively through zones 1, 2 and 3 to enter the central vein (vol. 1, p. 30.32). The cells in zone 3 thus receive blood which has just traversed zones 1 and 2, where it is milked of some of its nutrients. When the general circulation is adequate, blood reaching the central (zone 3) cells still contains sufficient oxygen and other nutrients, but when the percolation of blood through the hepatic spongework is retarded by heart failure, the central zone 3 cells do not receive an adequate supply. Thus a remarkable zonal distribution of progressively more severe injury develops; the best nourished peripheral zone 1 cells are unaffected, the partially maintained zone 2 cells show fatty change, while the most poorly supplied zone 3 cells are necrotic or atrophic (plates 25.1c and 1d, facing p. 25.6). Shrinkage of the dead and atrophic central cells and dilation of the central parts of the sinusoids account for the characteristic red mottling of the central zones in the 'nutmeg' liver of chronic heart failure.

The heart also shows zonal necrosis, atrophy and fatty change which result from local disparity in supply of nutrients to the cells of different regions. During systole the capillaries in the myocardium are narrowed or occluded when compressed by the contracting muscle. This effect is more severe and more prolonged in the inner parts of the ventricular muscle where intramural pressure becomes highest. Thus local coronary occlusion is likely to cause a more serious interruption in the supply of nutrients to the inner than to the outer myocardium. This accounts for the characteristic location of many cardiac infarcts in the inner subendocardial portions of the ventricular muscle (fig. 25.3). The more gradual processes of fatty deposition in the myocardial fibres, atrophy and replacement by pale fibrous tissue are, for similar

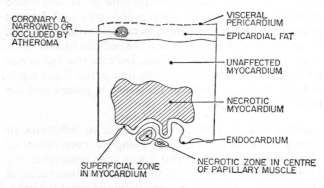

FIG. 25.3. Infarct of myocardium, showing typical location of necrotic heart muscle in the inner part of ventricular wall.

reasons, more pronounced in the inner than the outer myocardium.

Differences in cellular requirements
Differential vulnerability depends also on a real disparity in need for nutrients by different kinds of cell. Brown–Séquard in 1858 emphasized that of all organs the brain is most vulnerable to lack of oxygen. By perfusing limbs of decapitated animals with oxygenated blood he was able to reactivate muscles and nerves after several hours of circulatory arrest. But he found that the brain suffered irreversible loss of activity after a few minutes without flowing blood.

Epidermal cells survive for many hours at room temperature after the heart has stopped. Hair in fact continues to grow for some time after death. Excised skin and cornea remain alive for weeks if kept at 2–4°C. Cornea can then be used for homografting, while epidermis, although rejected by the homograft reaction if transferred to a patient of a different genotype (vol. 1, p. 27.13), can still be accepted as an autograft by its own original donor after storage for some weeks. At this low temperature, epidermal metabolism is so retarded that irreversible changes do not occur for a long time. Prolonged ischaemia in the living body, however, eventually causes necrosis of the skin. Thus external pressure is responsible for the dreaded bed sores which develop as a result of cutaneous ischaemia in bed-ridden patients who are badly nursed.

Striated muscle survives compression for up to 2 hr. Then the arrest of the circulation causes **ischaemic muscle necrosis**; a few hours later the dying muscle becomes oedematous with swollen regions of 'fish flesh' alternating with haemorrhagic zones. Whole limbs can survive arterial occlusion by tourniquet usually for periods up to 1 hr. This means that their nerve fibres as well as the muscles are relatively resistant to ischaemia.

Liver seldom shows infarction because of its dual blood supply by branches of both portal vein and hepatic artery. But if both are occluded, necrosis inevitably follows. Experiments with rats, in which the pedicles to liver lobes are clamped for varying periods, indicate that ischaemia up to 60 min produces reversible injury, but if ischaemia lasts for 2 hr the point of no return is passed and the injury is irreversible.

Renal tubular cells are also susceptible to ischaemia. In kidney transplant operations, complete deprivation of blood supply for one or two hours after removal of the organ from the donor results in reversible tubular cellular changes which cause temporary failure in renal function. More prolonged periods of ischaemia cause irreversible renal injury.

Macrophages and microglial phagocytes are exceptionally resistant to ischaemic injury. Thus, when ischaemia kills the centrilobular hepatic cells, macrophages filled with brown granules of haemosiderin survive among the dead hepatocytes in the central anoxic zones (plate 25.1d, opposite). Similarly, when neurones in cerebral cortex are killed by ischaemia, microglial phagocytes, which consume the remains of the more vulnerable neurones, survive for many months.

The secreting cells of the pituitary gland usually receive sufficient nutrients from the blood to cope with their various activities. Even generalized ischaemia does not usually single out the pituitary as a specially vulnerable organ. But in pregnancy the anterior pituitary cells are hypertrophied and excessively active; under these circumstances their demand for nutrients, including oxygen, is greatly increased. Thus severe postpartum haemorrhage may cause extensive pituitary necrosis because the enlarged active cells no longer receive sufficient nutrients. The necrosis of anterior pituitary cells is followed by pituitary hypofunction (Simmonds' disease, vol. 1, p. 25.15). This is characterized by atrophy of the ovaries, thyroid and adrenal cortex, with amenorrhoea, loss of pubic hair and low basal metabolic rate.

Nerve fibres in peripheral nerves are relatively resistant to ischaemia. Tourniquets applied for less than 1 hr give temporary paralysis followed by rapid recovery. Tourniquets applied for 2 hr cause axonal swelling and degeneration of myelin. The axon however, is, only reversibly injured and recovers in both structure and function in about 6 weeks. Tourniquets applied for longer periods produce complete degeneration of both axon and myelin. Recovery then occurs only by regrowth of new axonal material from the living nerve above the point of compression; this takes many months.

The cell bodies and dendrites of neurones, as opposed to axons, show unique vulnerability to ischaemia. Litten, in 1880, found that compression of the abdominal aorta in rabbits for 1 hr was followed by permanent paralysis of the lower limbs, although the kidneys survived this treatment; he suggested that the paralysis was due to ischaemic injury of the spinal cord. Paul Ehrlich and Brieger, in 1884, showed that after such aortic compression the spinal ventral horn cells were killed and that the grey matter became injured before the white matter was affected. Compression of the abdominal aorta for 20 min in cats or rabbits causes ischaemia which is followed by necrosis of the ventral horn cells. Neurones of the higher centres, as we shall see, are even more vulnerable to arrest in their supply of nutrients.

Cells thus vary greatly in their capacity to withstand a reduction of their blood supply. Probably those cells

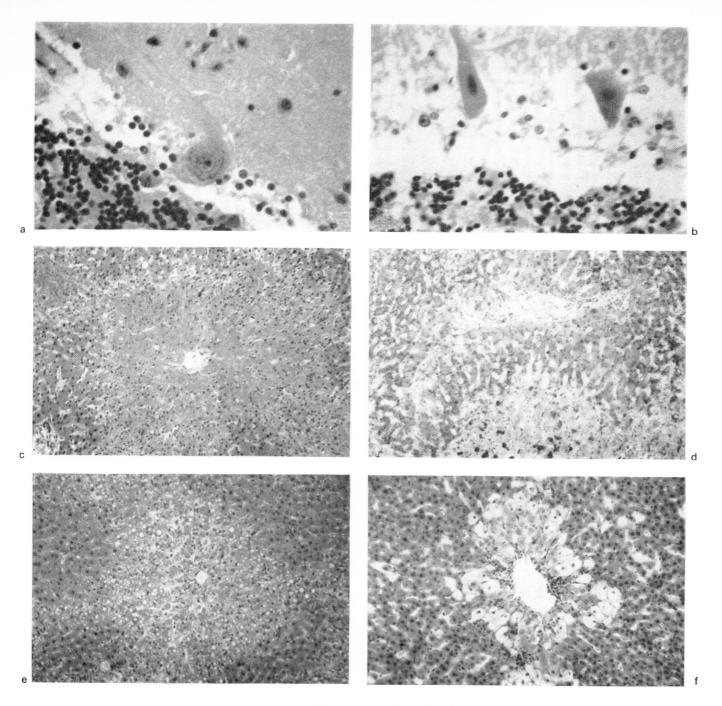

PLATE 25.1. Histology of cellular disorder.

(a) Normal cerebellar neurones from unaffected left cerebellar cortex for comparison with (b). Nissl granules visible in cytoplasm of Purkinje cell; also clearly defined nucleoli and chromatin in nuclei of Purkinje cell and granular cells. Haem. & eosin (×440).

(c) Liver cells injured by ischaemia due to heart failure; zonal distribution of cellular injury in lobule. The peripheral cells with pink cytoplasm are unaffected, while the most central cells around the central vein are more orange and necrotic. Haem. & eosin (×110).

(e) Rat liver lobule injured by CCl₄; peripheral cells unaffected, midzonal cells fatty, centrilobular cells necrotic and eosinophilic. Haem. & eosin (×110).

(b) Necrotic neurones from right side of cerebellar cortex injured by combination of general and local ischaemia; compare with (a). Purkinje cells are shrunken, the Nissl granules lost, and the nuclei shrivelled and homogeneous (pyknotic). Haem. & eosin (×440).

(d) Zonal distribution of liver cell damage as a result of ischaemia due to heart failure. The peripheral cells with pale pink cytoplasm are uninjured except for slight fatty change, the midzonal cells contain abundant droplets of fat (orange), while the centrilobular cells (at bottom of figure) are faintly coloured and necrotic; among these a few dark brown macrophages are seen. Sudan IV (×110).

(f) Rat liver lobule injured by CCl₄; peripheral cells unaffected, outer midzonal cells fatty (orange), inner midzonal cells swollen and hydropic, centrilobular cells necrotic. Sudan IV (×110).

which have the highest rate of metabolism, such as neurones, are the most readily injured. As the changes produced by ischaemia are likely to be most definite in the most vulnerable kinds of cell, the unique vulnerability of the neurone will be considered briefly before considering the general mechanism of ischaemic damage.

VULNERABILITY OF NERVOUS TISSUE TO ISCHAEMIA

Ischaemia interrupts the function of neurones and also destroys their life with great rapidity. These two effects must be carefully distinguished.

Arrest of function

Cessation of cerebral circulation in man for as short a time as 7 sec causes loss of consciousness, although usually no permanent damage results from even 100 sec of ischaemia. Similarly, dogs lose consciousness very rapidly after their cerebral circulation is arrested, even though they suffer no permanent injury from ischaemia lasting a few minutes. The electrical activity of the cerebral cortex of monkeys and cats disappears after ischaemia lasting for 10 sec, while the rate of consumption of oxygen by the cortex can be shown to have fallen after 30 sec. All these changes are at first reversible, and nervous activity and function recover completely provided the supply of blood is restored rapidly.

Onset of permanent neuronal damage

Controlled experiments on animals have provided more consistent results than the necessarily less systematic observations on man. Occlusion of the pulmonary artery by a clamp results in temporary arrest of the systemic circulation and enables complete cerebral ischaemia to be applied for accurately timed periods. When cerebral ischaemia is produced in cats by this technique, no permanent damage to neurones follows arrest of the circulation for up to 3 min. After arrest for 3·5–6 min, neurones in the frontal and occipital cortex are killed. The animals recover consciousness on re-establishment of the circulation, but they no longer recognize their keeper nor do they purr when stroked; they are able, however, to eat the food which they are offered. These experiments show that the frontal and occipital pyramidal cells are the most rapidly injured and that 'higher' functions such as power of recognition are the most vulnerable. Arrest of circulation for 8 min produces necrosis of the entire cerebral cortex, while successively longer periods of ischaemia injure the basal nuclei and finally the most resistant medullary centres.

In man more variable results have been reported. Cardiac arrest for 3 min in open heart operations causes permanent damage to the human brain at 37°C, but if the patient is cooled to 28°C, so as to depress cerebral metabolism, the brain can withstand periods of cardiac arrest up to 7 min with impunity. Following temporary cardiac arrest during operation and anaesthesia, cerebral ischaemia for up to nearly 2 min is usually compatible with full recovery, but even a small extension of this time may cause permanent damage. However, distressing examples of extensive necrosis of cortical and basal nuclear neurones have followed cardiac arrest under anaesthesia, when the period of complete ischaemia lasted only 1 min. Other factors such as previous nervous activity may account for these differences (see below).

Neurones thus differ among themselves in their extreme vulnerability to ischaemia, and varying rates of metabolism may determine these different degrees of susceptibility. It is clear, however, that cessation of function and of electrical activity caused by ischaemia need not produce any permanent damage. This shows that the survival of memory and other cerebral determinants of behaviour depend on macromolecular patterns rather than the more transient changes of electrical potential at neuronal surfaces. Function is irreparably injured only when the macromolecular fabric also suffers permanent damage.

MECHANISM OF ISCHAEMIC INJURY

In the brain there are scanty reserves of substrates for catabolism and ischaemia arrests the supply of two cardinal nutrients, glucose and oxygen. Which of these is paramount? Cerebral function is abolished by ischaemia in a few seconds, but cerebral tissue contains sufficient glucose to support even a high rate of anaerobic glycolysis for at least 3 min. On the other hand, the quantity of oxygen dissolved in the brain is sufficient to maintain cellular respiration for only about 10 sec. It is clear, therefore, that lack of oxygen and not lack of glucose is the immediate cause of loss of consciousness in cerebral ischaemia; this does not prove, however, that lack of oxygen rather than lack of glucose is the cause of permanent damage.

In less than 15 sec after vascular occlusion the oxygen within the cerebral cells is exhausted; there is then a sudden switch to anaerobic metabolism. In brain under these circumstances the glycolysis of glucose to lactic acid is greatly accelerated; in fact the rate of destruction of glucose by brain cortex in the absence of oxygen is three or four times as great as under aerobic conditions. In spite of this acceleration much less free energy is liberated (vol. 1, p. 9.18). The acceleration of the destruction of glucose in the absence of oxygen may be regarded as a vain effort on the part of the cells to gain energy from an uneconomic process. For a short time this acceleration may avert a fall in the level of ATP and it thus provides a temporary compensating mechanism, but without oxygen such a fall is inevitable. A factor which may make anaerobic compensation still less effective, in brain at any rate, is the local liberation of potassium ions by previous nervous activity or cell damage; potassium ions rapidly inhibit anaerobic glycolysis of cerebral cortex (p. 25.19).

A continuing supply of ATP and other compounds containing high energy phosphate bonds is necessary for cells of the brain:

(1) to enable the sodium pump to expel sodium from the neurones,

(2) to maintain the structure of cell membranes, and

(3) to initiate macromolecular synthesis.

When the cell is seriously depleted of ATP by ischaemia several changes are likely to follow.

(1) Na^+, Cl^- and water enter the cells, which swell. The entry of ions and swelling of the cells have been detected in the apical dendrites of cerebral pyramidal cells within 5 min of interruption of the blood supply. K^+ leave the cell.

(2) The membranes of the cell and its organelles become abnormally permeable and visible discontinuities appear. These changes become irreversible. Energy provided by ATP is probably necessary for the maintenance of lipoprotein membranes which actively decompose ATP. As neurones have the highest surface/volume ratio of all cells they suffer most rapidly irreversible injury by disintegration of their membranes through lack of ATP.

(3) Synthesis of macromolecules is retarded but catabolism goes on unimpeded.

(4) As a result of (2) catabolic enzymes previously inaccessible to their substrates may become accessible so that catabolism is actually accelerated.

(5) As a result of (3) and (4) loss of RNA and DNA occur. As soon as even one essential macromolecule of DNA disintegrates, cell injury is irreparable.

Changes in dead and dying cells are considered more fully on p. 25.22; this sequence of changes, resulting from ischaemic retardation in synthesis of ATP, may affect the cells of any tissue in the body and shows how ischaemia acts as the most common and most lethal cause in the pathogenesis of human disease as a whole.

Defective penetration of nutrients into cells

Even though the exacting assortment of substances which the cell requires reach its surface, one more hazard may still deprive it of effective nutrition; sufficient nutrients may fail to enter the cell or penetrate the organelles within it and the intracellular enzymes may not be supplied with sufficient substrates.

Such a defect in penetration of cells by glucose is partly responsible for disorders of metabolism caused by lack of insulin. This retards the entry of glucose into cells, and glucose accumulates in the extracellular fluid and blood (vol. 1, p. 25.40). The cells are thus deprived of glucose, although their outer surfaces are bathed with excessively saccharine fluid, a striking example of need in the midst of plenty. The catalytic effect of insulin in promoting entry of glucose applies especially to skeletal muscle and to lipocytes.

ADVERSE PHYSICAL ENVIRONMENT

Four physical agents which injure cells are considered; these are trauma, heat, cold and ionizing radiation.

Trauma

CONTUSION OR BRUISING

Trauma separates cells from each other more frequently than it tears individual cells asunder. Contusion or bruising tears blood vessels and leads to thrombosis by damaging vascular endothelium. Thus blood vessels, severed or occluded by trauma or compressed by haemorrhage, can no longer nourish the cells which they normally supply. Injury to the cells in bruised tissue is caused largely by lack of nutrients.

LACERATION AND RUPTURE OF CELLS

The cell envelope may be directly disrupted by violence. This happens readily in cells which are swollen by fat and which consist of globules of lipid covered by tenuous films of cytoplasm. The lipocytes of yellow bone-marrow are thus ruptured by fractures of bone; large drops of fat may then escape from the lacerated cells and be liberated into the blood. These fatty emboli can later occlude capillaries in lungs or brain. Fat embolism may be a

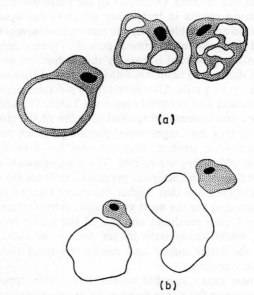

FIG. 25.4. Rupture of fatty liver cells. (a) Liver cells bloated by droplets of fat. (b) Coalescence of fat droplets from ruptured liver cells to form fatty cysts embedded in cellular remnants and connective tissue.

serious sequel of extensive fractures involving injury of yellow marrow (p. 26.6).

Liver cells in disease may also become bloated by droplets of liquid fat (fig. 25.4). Eventually the inflation by fat may be so gross as to burst the cells, when the fat from several cells coalesces into large extracellular cysts surrounded by cell remnants. The rupture of liver cells may possibly cause the intercellular connective tissue to condense, dividing up the surviving and regenerating liver parenchyma into variably sized masses of liver cells separated by bands of dense connective tissue containing fatty cysts. This series of changes, determined initially by rupture of fatty liver cells, may be a factor in the development of **portal cirrhosis** in which the portal circulation becomes obstructed and liver function is impaired.

DISSEVERED NEURONES

Owing to the great length and tenuity of its fibre the neurone is one of the few cells commonly severed by violence. Division of a nerve fibre is followed by damage both distal and proximal to the point of section.

Distal injury

The part of the fibre which is dissevered from its cell body undergoes **Wallerian degeneration**. Augustus Waller, in 1850, first established that the cell body is the 'nutritive centre' for the whole length of the fibre and he showed that the myelin sheath in the distal portion of divided fibres 'curdles into separate particles and that nervous conductility is lost along with this degeneration'. Irreversible degeneration of both axon and myelin occur distal to the point of section. Later work has shown that protein made in the cell body is continuously flowing down the axon in a viscous fluid, the axoplasm. Degeneration below the point of division is caused by cessation in the flow down the axoplasm of nutrients manufactured in the cell body and dendrites. In severe head injuries, even without visible external injury to the brain, numerous fibres may be severed by shearing forces and so produce coma and decerebrate rigidity. In peripheral nerves, prolonged compression as well as section may result in Wallerian degeneration below the point of trauma.

Proximal injury

Above the point of section (fig. 25.5) Wallerian degeneration progresses up the fibre only as far as the next node of Ranvier, i.e. to the uppermost part of the Schwann cell severed by the injury. Above this level the remainder of the axon, which is in continuity with the cell body, does not degenerate and its myelin sheath remains intact. Franz Nissl, in 1892, however, showed that after section of the axon the cell body swells and its perinuclear Nissl granules disintegrate; the nucleus takes up an eccentric position and is sometimes extruded from the

cell. These changes are called **Nissl degeneration** or **chromatolysis** (fig. 25.5). Most cells which retain their nuclei recover from this change in the course of a few weeks. After section it is likely that the proximal portion of the axon becomes sealed so that the continuously flowing axoplasm is dammed up. The swelling of the cell body is probably caused by rise of intracellular hydrostatic pressure owing to obstruction of axonal flow. Ramon y Cajal showed that section of cerebellar axons is followed by intense swelling of the Purkinje cells which become inflated into grotesque monstrosities distended with aqueous vacuoles.

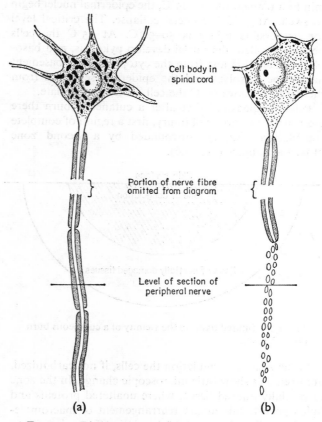

FIG. 25.5. Distal and proximal degeneration after section of a nerve fibre. (a) Cell body and myelinated fibre before division. (b) After section of fibre; Wallerian degeneration occurs distal to the plane of section and up the fibre as far as the next node of Ranvier, and Nissl degeneration is seen in the cell body proximal to the plane of section.

CEREBRAL CONCUSSION

Sudden cranial trauma may cause instantaneous coma which considerably outlasts the period of violence and is usually attended by amnesia of the accident itself. This kind of injury is called cerebral concussion. Concussion usually occurs without any macroscopic evidence of cerebral damage. However, careful microscopic observation of the neurones of concussed guinea-pigs shows that concussion is accompanied by agglutination and fragmentation of Nissl granules.

Effects of heat

Exposure of the body to high temperatures may cause grave and extensive cellular injury. Prolonged periods at high temperatures injure more severely than shorter exposures. Careful work by Peters and his colleagues on the application of a 'burning iron' at various temperatures for 1 min to the shaved skin of guinea-pigs established the range of temperature necessary to produce temporary or permanent epidermal damage. After exposure for 1 min to a temperature of 45°C, the epidermal nuclei begin to swell. At 50°C the nuclei collapse. The critical level for irreversible injury is 50–52°C. At 55°C the cells become swollen, the nuclei develop pyknosis, and basophilic material is lost from the cytoplasm; the basement membrane dissolves and the epidermis separates from the dermis. Above 60°C the cell proteins coagulate.

Peters emphasized that after a cutaneous burn there are usually two zones of injury, first a region of complete coagulation which is surrounded by a second zone of partial damage (fig. 25.6).

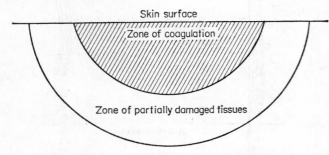

Skin surface
Zone of coagulation
Zone of partially damaged tissues

FIG. 25.6. Injured tissue in the vicinity of a cutaneous burn (after Peters).

In the zone of coagulation the cells, if not carbonized, are fixed and show little microscopic change. In the zone of partially injured tissue, where unaltered proteins and lipids persist, subsequent rearrangement of macromolecules as well as osmotic and autolytic effects give rise to more substantial signs of injury.

Moritz and Henriques studied the skin of pigs and men injured by tangential streams of hot water. The earliest sign of epidermal injury was swelling of the nuclei in the stratum spinosum. The chromatin in the swollen nuclei coalesced into crescentic masses; then the nuclei ruptured and the chromatin condensed into an irregularly shaped remnant separated from the remainder of the cytoplasm by a zone of clear fluid. The basal cells showed cytoplasmic swelling and vacuolation. These changes followed immediately on exposure to temperatures from 44–55°C. Above this temperature the cells did not swell but shrivelled slightly and showed little microscopic

alteration. The rate at which irreversible injury was sustained increased rapidly with rise in temperature. Thus, exposure for 6 hr to a temperature of 44°C was required to produce transepidermal necrosis; this was the lowest temperature to cause irreversible injury. For each degree rise of temperature between 44° and 51°C, the time required to produce irreversible injury diminished by about one-half. At 51°C transepidermal necrosis occurred in 3 min.

DENATURATION AND COAGULATION OF PROTEINS INCLUDING ENZYMES

Inactivation of enzymes is an important result of rise in temperature. Enzymes differ in their susceptibility to heat and those concerned with anabolism are more susceptible than those concerned with hydrolytic fission. Indeed phosphatases are so resistant to heat that they may remain active after embedding of tissues in molten wax at 56°C. By selective interference with anabolic processes, heat may result in a rise of intracellular concentration of small molecules which after heating continue to be formed by the still active hydrolytic enzymes. This may account for the rise of internal osmotic pressure and swelling of cells heated to between 44°C and 55°C. Above 60°C the cell proteins coagulate and no enzymes remain active.

Denaturation of protein attached to DNA may be responsible for the spectacular effects of heat on the nuclei of epidermal cells, in which the dispersed chromatin of the interphase nucleus is clumped into a crescentic mass marginated against the nuclear membrane. Removal of structured water bound to protein or DNA may take part in this denaturation so that the tenuous helices of partially uncoiled DNA are clumped or coiled into condensed pyknotic remnants.

Denaturation of proteins by heat is in part responsible for thermal disintegration of cell membranes. Heat may expel structured water which is normally bound as a hexagonal lattice by hydrogen bonding to the proteins of cell membranes. When this aqueous lattice is eliminated, active groups in the proteins become exposed and molecular rearrangement and disintegration of the membranes follow.

DISINTEGRATION OF LIPOPROTEIN MEMBRANES

Heilbrunn suggested that heat injures by altering the physical state of intracellular lipids. He measured the viscosity of crustacean ova by observing the rate at which these cells can be separated into clear and turbid zones by centrifugation; heating to temperatures below the point of coagulation of proteins caused a sudden rise in viscosity associated with melting or solution of the intracellular lipids. Such a change in cell lipids is likely to dislodge oriented phospholipids from lipoprotein membranes and so cause disintegration of cell membranes and organelles. At higher temperatures heat may also dissociate the lattices of structured water which stabilize the proteins on the outer surfaces of lipoprotein membranes; thus thermal disintegration of the membranes may involve denaturation of protein as well as disorientation of lipids.

Exposure of the body to intense heat causes profound changes in red blood cells. Moritz and his colleagues showed that haemoglobin escapes from red cells of pigs exposed to hot air at 180°C, while the red cells disintegrate into minute spherical masses (microspherocytes). Sevitt found similar changes in severely burned human patients (fig. 25.7). Thermal disintegration of red cells to form small spherical globules probably results from partial disruption of their lipoprotein membranes along with disarray of oriented phospholipids which form an integral part of the red blood cell surface.

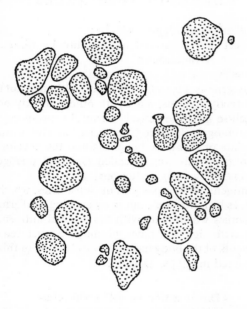

FIG. 25.7. Blood film from a patient with recent severe burns, showing microspherocytes (after Sevitt).

DISLOCATION OF INTRACELLULAR EQUILIBRIUM BETWEEN ANABOLISM AND CATABOLISM

Heat increases the velocity of chemical reactions so that the action of hydrolytic enzymes, which are relatively resistant to thermal inactivation, may be accelerated. Heat may also increase the accessibility of hydrolytic and glycolytic enzymes to their substrates by causing partial disintegration of lipoprotein membranes. But it is likely that anabolism of protein, which requires precise orientation of ribosomes on rough-surfaced endoplasmic reticulum, is inhibited by disorientation of their membrane lipids. Uncompensated acceleration of catabolism may thus contribute to loss of basophilic material (RNA) from cytoplasm of epidermal cells.

Effects of cold

Cold causes irreversible cell injury and much of the damage arises indirectly from ischaemia of the chilled tissues. However, extreme cold also exerts a direct injurious action.

INDIRECT DAMAGE CAUSED BY ISCHAEMIA

Immersion of a limb in cold water gives rise to local vasoconstriction and ischaemia. Cell damage follows as a direct result of a defective supply of nutrients. In limbs, the first cells to be injured are those of the vascular endothelium. When the temperature again rises, the circulation of blood is re-established and plasma leaks out into the tissue through the damaged endothelium and basement membrane of small vessels. Oedema and vesiculation of the skin follow, together with skin necrosis if the ischaemia has been prolonged. Immersion of limbs for long periods in cold water thus produces swelling and blistering with a variable extent of necrosis; in World War I this condition frequently occurred in soldiers living in water-logged trenches and was called **trench foot.**

More intense cold freezes the exposed parts; this injury is called **frostbite.** The direct effect of freezing is superimposed on the indirect effect of ischaemia, but the ischaemia itself is even more severe after freezing than after mere cooling, since thrombosis occurs in the damaged blood vessels. The necrotic tissue in frostbite becomes blackened owing to decomposition of haemoglobin liberated from extravasated red blood cells.

DIRECT DAMAGE TO CELLS BY FREEZING

When slices of liver tissue are frozen very rapidly by immersion in liquid propane at −175°C, minute crystals of ice are formed both within the cells throughout cytoplasm and nucleus, and also in the extracellular fluid. Trump and his colleagues who conducted these experiments showed that after this treatment, discontinuities appeared in the external cell membranes and also in the mitochondrial membranes, while the endoplasmic reticulum was vesiculated and degranulated; the nuclei became shrunken and uniform in staining.

When liver tissue is frozen more slowly by dry ice at −79°C, no crystals of ice form within the innermost cells which cool at the slowest rate, but large extracellular crystals of ice are produced in the spaces outside the cells. After this slower freezing, the mitochondrial membranes appear undamaged and no ribosomal degranulation occurs, although the plasma membrane shows discontinuities and the cisternae of the endoplasmic reticulum are vesiculated. Slow freezing, although not causing so much disorganization of the cells, temporarily shrivels them by extracting water.

These observations account for the intensely necrotizing action of rapid freezing.

One method by which the formation of ice crystals injures cells is probably by extraction of water into the growing icicles. If this water comes from the free water of the cell no lasting damage may result. But if the water converted into ice crystals is taken from bound cell water, then the cell membranes may disintegrate. The essential water of the cell is probably bound and structured in the form of lattices held together by hydrogen bonds and firmly attached by bonding through the oxygen and nitrogen atoms of the membrane proteins. If this peripheral lattice of stabilizing water is removed, the proteins of the membranes become disarranged and denatured. The membranes may also be damaged by concentrated saline formed temporarily within and outside the cells following partial freezing of tissue and cell fluid. Lovelock showed that the membranes of red blood cells are damaged by exposure to high concentration of saline so that the cells haemolyse when reintroduced to isotonic saline after this treatment. High concentrations of saline formed during freezing may thus contribute to the disintegration of lipoprotein membranes.

Ionizing radiation

The mechanisms by which ionizing radiation injures cells are considered here only briefly as the biological effects of radiation are discussed fully in chap. 33.

Cellular damage is initiated by displacement of electrons and protons from atoms within the cells so that a pair of oppositely charged ions is produced by each displacement. These ionized atoms tend to decompose. There are two views as to why this decomposition is harmful to the cell, the target theory and the toxigenic theory.

TARGET THEORY

If the ionized substance or target is a molecule of DNA, irreparable damage may be inflicted by its decomposition or alteration. The result may be death of the cell, inhibition of mitosis or an invisible molecular change in the karyotype. Such a latent change may be followed by a succession of mutations at mitosis. Most of these mutants are probably not viable or are suppressed, but eventually a viable mutant may result which produces a clone of successful cells with invasive properties. The target theory thus explains the development of malignant neoplasms in the thyroid gland and other organs, which may occur many years after the therapeutic use of ^{131}I (p. 6.8).

The view that radiation injures by its action on DNA is supported by the fact that radiation inhibits mitosis and exerts a selectively lethal action on all cells with a high rate of mitosis, i.e. intestinal epithelium, haemopoietic and lymphoblastic cells. Ionizing radiation also causes injury to the chromosomes when applied to cells in mitosis (p. 33.4).

TOXIGENIC THEORY

The ionization of cell water by radiation leads to the formation of free peroxy radicals such as $HO_2^\cdot$ (p. 31.3). If formed in the cell, these radicals would be highly toxic by the oxidation of the SH groups of proteins and coenzymes to the SS forms. That such a toxigenic action is in fact exerted by large doses of X-rays is indicated by the observation that reduced glutathione and hypoxia can diminish the harmful effects of radiation. Thus newborn mice, which normally can withstand anoxia for 20 min, are protected from otherwise lethal doses of X-rays by deprivation of oxygen during irradiation, while after such irradiation in the presence of air the mice die with gross cutaneous necrosis.

HARMFUL SUBSTANCES

Harmful substances injure cells by:

(1) direct action on cell architecture by disarray of orientated macromolecules,

(2) interference with enzymic action,

(3) toxigenesis, i.e. some substances, although not themselves directly noxious, react with others already present in the cell to generate actively harmful substances,

(4) carcinogenesis (oncogenesis), i.e. harmful substances may initiate or stimulate neoplasia and the development of tumours in this way is called chemical oncogenesis (Greek *onkos*, swelling or tumour), and

(5) antigenic action, i.e. certain substances, which may themselves be innocuous, injure by exciting the formation of antibodies which react with the original antigen. This may be a foreign substance or may be liberated from constituents of the body itself. Harmful action of this kind is considered in chaps. 22 & 23.

Direct action on cell architecture

Substances which react with specific groups in cell membranes (fig. 25.8) can disintegrate or even dissolve

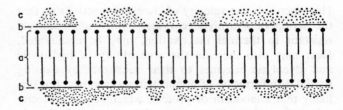

FIG. 25.8. Cell membrane composed of: (a) bimolecular film of orientated phospholipid molecules with their polar ends external, (b) adherent films of protein (covering phospholipid), and (c) structured water attached to films of protein.

parts of this complex structure; compounds which probably act in this way are considered first. Harmful substances react also with nuclear DNA and a few examples of this action are discussed.

SAPONIN

Saponin and other surface-active agents, like sodium taurocholate, lyse red blood cells and liberate their haemoglobin; saponin also injures the surface membranes of leucocytes and liberates enzymes such as alkaline phosphatase and esterase from the damaged cells. Saponin is a glycoside which combines specifically with sterols and precipitates them. It causes lysis probably by reacting with cholesterol in the cell membranes and thus disturbs the orientation of the lipids in the laminar micelles. Dramatic changes in the EM appearance of cell membranes occur when red blood cell ghosts, chick liver cells, Rous sarcoma virus or lecithin/cholesterol films on water are treated with saponin; a hexagonal lattice-like structure becomes visible in each case. This lattice is probably produced by saponin combining with sterols in the cell membranes to form a hexagonal lipid reticulum surrounding less dense aqueous spaces; these latter zones are permeable and hence haemoglobin can escape from the saponin-treated red cells. These findings imply a close similarity between the membranes of different kinds of cell.

LEAD SALTS

Lead ions precipitate proteins by forming bridges between sulphydryl and carboxyl groups in adjacent peptide chains of protein. Lead ions are rapidly taken up by red blood cells *in vitro* and *in vivo*. The cells become more fragile and lysis occurs as they impinge on each other and against the capillary walls in the flowing blood; severe anaemia may follow. These changes probably depend on disarray of orientated protein molecules in the red cell envelope. Potassium ions as well as haemoglobin escape from the injured red cells. The anaemia of chronic lead poisoning may depend partly on interference with synthesis of haemoglobin, as well as on excessive fragility of red blood cells.

Lead poisoning also causes paralysis due to demyelination of peripheral nerves. In guinea-pigs poisoned by lead acetate, internodal segments of the peripheral nerves show loss of myelin as well as some axonal degeneration; the velocity of nerve impulses is simultaneously diminished.

CORROSIVES

Sulphuric acid chars organic molecules by removing the elements of water. Many other corrosive substances such as hydrochloric acid and ammonia also harm by dehydration; even without charring these less violent corrosives rapidly remove the structured water which stabilizes the surfaces of lipoprotein membranes. When the aqueous lattice is removed, the proteins become denatured.

CARBON TETRACHLORIDE

This poison, when inhaled, ingested, or injected in toxic amounts, causes acute necrosis as well as conspicuous fatty change in the liver. It is a powerful solvent for phospholipids, but its toxicity probably depends also on activation inside liver cells, promoting autocatalytic peroxidation of the ethylenic double bonds in phospholipids. This view is supported by the fact that antioxidants like α-tocopherol can protect against its harmful action. In any case it is likely that CCl_4 causes disarray of phospholipids and lipoproteins in the membranes of cell organelles such as the endoplasmic reticulum and other laminar micelles which are responsible for the dispersion of fat. The cells may thus be irreversibly injured or show fatty change.

The livers of rats poisoned by CCl_4 show extensive centrilobular necrosis, zone 2 hydropic change, and also fatty deposition (plates 25.1 e and f, facing p. 25.6). The cells in zone 3 near the centres of the liver lobules, which are the least well supplied with nutrients, are the most severely injured and peripheral cells in zone 1 may show no signs of injury.

The earliest alteration detected by the EM consists of swelling of the cisternae of endoplasmic reticulum into vesicles followed by dispersal of the ribosomes. With the light microscope, this latter change is seen as a dispersal of cytoplasmic basophilia. Synthesis of protein is inhibited by dislocation of ribosomes from the endoplasmic reticulum. Damage to mitochondria and lysosomes occurs late in liver cell injury by CCl_4. Death of the cell may be due to extensive irreversible damage to membranes or an indirect result of inhibition of protein synthesis. The greater vulnerability of the centrilobular zone 3 cells may be determined by a lower normal level of phospholipid in these relatively hypoxic central cells or to a poorer supply of α-tocopherol. The mechanism of fatty change caused by CCl_4 is considered on p. 25.31.

ALLOXAN

Alloxan injected into animals causes necrosis and disappearance of β-cells from the pancreatic islets followed by hyperglycaemia due to lack of insulin, along with ketosis and sometimes coma. It is not known why alloxan singles out the β-cells of pancreatic islets for this highly necrotizing action. Alloxan reacts rapidly with the α-amino groups of proteins and thus forms aldehydes from the decomposed portions of protein molecules. An action of this kind might be expected to cause widespread disintegration of cell membranes, but in fact damage is confined to pancreatic and renal cells.

$$\text{Alloxan} \quad + \quad \text{Amino acid} \quad \longrightarrow \quad \text{Aldehyde} \quad + R-\overset{O}{\underset{H}{C}} + CO_2 + NH_3$$

Alloxan   Amino acid   Aldehyde

In the β-cells of rat pancreas, insulin is contained within small cytoplasmic vesicles covered by lipoprotein membranes which are coloured dark crimson by paraldehyde-fuchsin after treatment with $KMnO_4$; the cytoplasm of the β-cells thus appears to be stuffed with crimson granules (β-granules). In the normal pancreatic islet, the β-cells cohere to each other as contiguous polyhedral epithelial cells grouped in columns or cords to form a sponge work perforated by numerous capillaries (plate 25.2a, opposite), but 5 hr after injection of alloxan the β-cells have shrunk into spheroidal cells and their epithelial contiguity is lost (plate 25.2b, opposite). Many of these contracted and separated cells are still filled with crimson granules and in some of them nuclear pyknosis is visible. By 25 hr after injection of alloxan most of the nuclei of the injured β-cells have disappeared although the cytoplasmic granules are preserved. By 48 hr after injection all the β-cells have vanished from the islets and the injected rats have become diabetic.

Although the mechanism by which alloxan kills the β-cells is unknown, it is likely that injury is determined by a rapid reaction between alloxan and protein on the cell surfaces; this possibly involves change in permeability and surface tension of the external membrane so that water is extruded and the cells shrink into spherical necrotic remnants. Another theory is that alloxan destroys SH groups which are present in high concentration in β-cells.

THE ACRIDINE DYES AND THE NITROGEN MUSTARDS

These are toxic substances which combine with DNA and RNA and which exert a specifically injurious action on dividing cells, such as intestinal epithelium and bone marrow. The chromosomes of the dying cells are clumped at metaphase. The injury so much resembles that produced by ionizing radiation that they are called **radiomimetic poisons**. Because of the vulnerability of actively dividing myeloblasts to the nitrogen mustards, these substances are used in treating leukaemia (p. 29.4).

DIMETHYL NITROSAMINE

$$\begin{array}{c} CH_3 \\ CH_3 \end{array}\!\!\!\searrow\!\!N-N=O$$ causes centrilobular necrosis of liver cells in rats and mice. This substance methylates DNA and RNA in the liver cells; indeed after injection of dimethyl nitrosamine labelled with ^{14}C, radioactive 7-methyl guanine was isolated by Magee and Farber from the nucleic acids of the liver cells. It is thus likely that dimethyl nitrosamine exerts its harmful action by converting guanine in nucleic acids into 7-methyl guanine.

Guanine nucleotide   7-Methyl guanine nucleotide

Interference with enzymic processes

Poisons may interfere directly with intracellular enzymic action. This interference depends on:

(1) denaturation of enzymes,

(2) specific disablement of their catalytic groups, and

(3) competitive inhibition by mimicry of substrate.

Most of these enzymic disorders deprive the cell of metabolic reactions essential for its maintenance and so may be succeeded by disintegration of structure.

DENATURATION OF ENZYMES

Corrosive poisons and heavy metals, which disorganize the fabric of the cell and its membranes, also denature enzyme molecules and may immediately arrest all enzymic processes. Hence these agents act as fixatives and preserve or stabilize because they preclude autolytic enzymic action.

SPECIFIC DISABLEMENT OF CATALYTIC GROUPS

Carbon monoxide injures primarily by competing with oxygen for haemoglobin and thus causes cellular hypoxia. This substance, however, also combines with the iron in cytochrome oxidase and so prevents the donation of electrons to molecular oxygen; thus the absorption of oxygen by cells as well as by haemoglobin is inhibited. Oxidations in cerebral neurones are specially susceptible to this inhibition and these cells rapidly suffer irreparable damage.

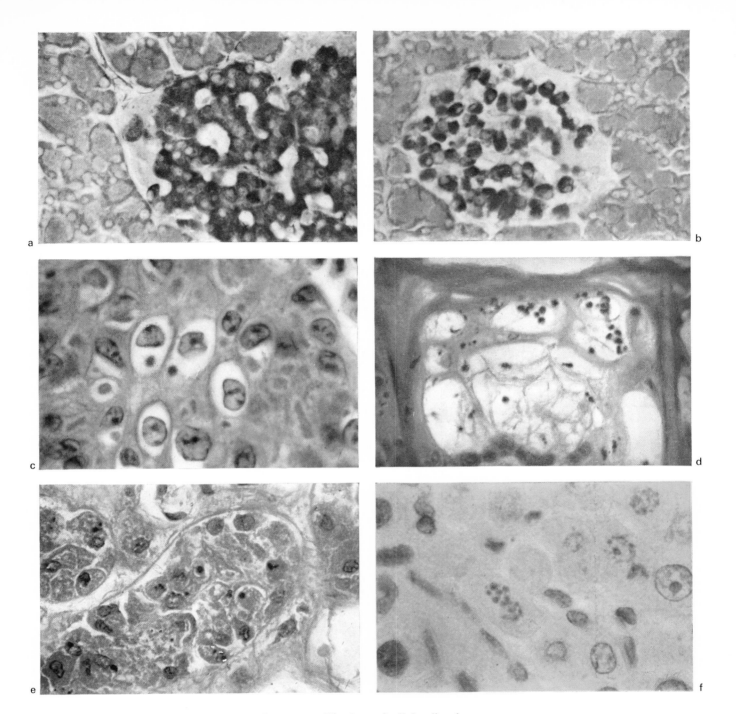

PLATE 25.2. Histology of cellular disorder.

(a) Normal rat pancreatic islet; β-cells form cords of contiguous epithelial cells stuffed with crimson granules. PPF–MeB (×440).

(b) Rat pancreatic islet 5 hours after injection of alloxan; β-cells have shrunk and separated from each other. PPF–MeB (×440).

(c) Rabbit epidermal cells infected by vaccinia virus; epithelial cells are swollen and contain eosinophilic cytoplasmic inclusion bodies. Haem. & eosin (×1100).

(d) Rabbit epidermal cells infected by vaccinia virus; a later stage than shown in (c). The upper epidermal cells are grossly inflated by aqueous vacuoles. Haem. & eosin (×430).

(e) Renal tubular cells from human kidney in a case of poisoning. The cells are desquamated from their basement membrane; their cytoplasm is eosinophilic and disintegrating, and some nuclei are karyorrhectic, i.e. broken up into small granules. Haem. & eosin (×690).

(f) Rat liver cells injured by CCl_4; nuclear karyorrhexis is prominent, and the granules of disintegrating chromatin are rich in DNA. Feulgen (for DNA) counterstained picric acid (×1100).

Cyanide also combines with the catalytic iron group of cytochrome oxidase and, like carbon monoxide, eliminates the active unit concerned with transfer of electrons to molecular oxygen; cellular oxidation thus cannot proceed and the main supply of energy to cells ceases. Without oxidation of glucose, neurones convert glucose to lactic acid at a greatly increased rate. In animals poisoned by cyanide the concentration of lactic acid in the brain rises, and slices of cerebral cortex exposed to cyanide form large amounts of lactic acid even in the presence of oxygen. But the supply of energy from this accelerated glycolysis is not sufficient to maintain neuronal integrity. Thus small doses of cyanide cause coma and convulsions with irreversible cerebral damage, although the rest of the body is unharmed. Larger doses are followed by arrest of the heart and of respiration within a few seconds.

Arsenious oxide and arsenites act by eliminating the catalytic SH groups of coenzyme A and of lipoic acid amide, which are both essential coenzymes for the oxidative decarboxylation of pyruvic acid (vol. 1, p. 9.12). The arsenite ion (derived from arsenious oxide) forms a stable complex with lipoic acid amide by removal of its active SH groups.

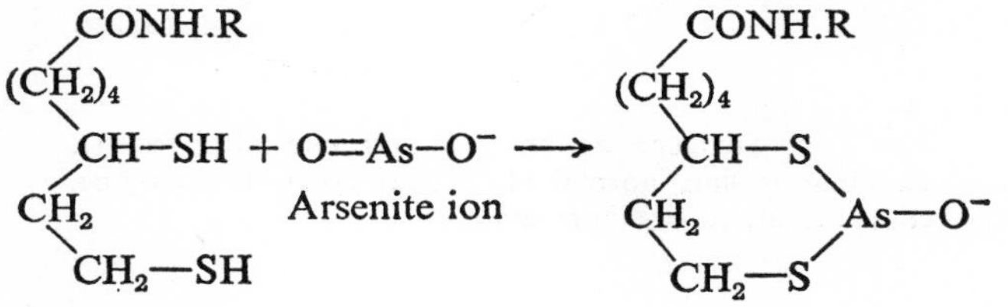

In the absence of active lipoic acid amide, pyruvic acid accumulates and is therefore detectable in the tissues and in the blood in arsenic poisoning. Since the oxidative decarboxylation of pyruvic acid is an essential stage in the oxidation of glucose, many cells are deprived of their main source of energy. Injury to the epithelial cells of stomach and small intestine accounts for the vomiting and diarrhoea in the initial stage of acute arsenic poisoning. This is succeeded by coma and convulsions owing to neuronal damage after the poison is absorbed. In chronic arsenic poisoning widely disseminated neuronal injury occurs. Damage to peripheral nerves results in paraesthesia and paresis, while injury to the cerebral neurones accounts for terminal 'idiotic apathy'.

COMPETITIVE INHIBITION BY MIMICRY OF SUBSTRATE

Substances with a constitution similar to the substrate of an enzyme can inhibit it competitively (vol. 1, p. 7.10). *Fluorocitrate* thus inhibits the utilization of citrate by competitive inhibition of the enzyme aconitase; in this way it interrupts the citric acid cycle in brain and so eliminates the main source of energy. Peters has shown that intracerebral injection of minute doses of fluorocitrate (less than 1 μg) kills rats in convulsions. It is thus one of the most poisonous substances known. When injected into rats fluorocitrate causes citric acid to accumulate in enormous quantities in heart, brain and kidneys.

Fluorocitrate may injure cells not only by interrupting their supply of energy, but also because the accumulated citrate decreases ionized calcium, so causing an increase in nervous excitability followed by convulsions.

Aminopterin is a 'mitotic' poison and so is specially lethal to dividing cells. It is similar in constitution to folinic acid N^5 formylTHF, an essential catalyst for the synthesis of DNA.

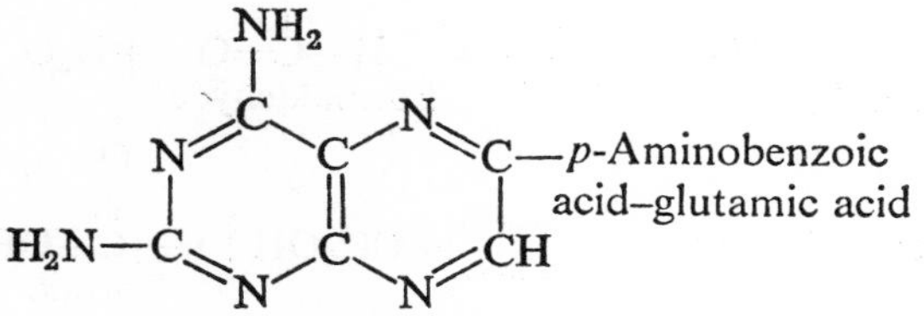

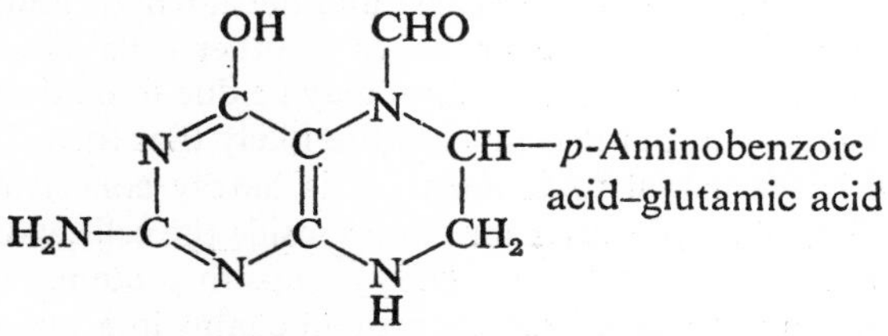

When injected into mice, it inhibits mitosis of the rapidly dividing epithelial cells of the intestinal mucosa and so kills them. Aminopterin also suppresses cell division in the bone marrow of leukaemic patients (p. 29.7). Aminopterin probably interferes with the mechanism by which N^5 formylTHF normally acts as a donator of single carbon units in the synthesis of DNA. Thus replication of DNA is inhibited and mitosis is prevented. Aminopterin also interferes with the actual process of mitosis; when it is added to cultures of chick embryo cells, the chromosomes rapidly clump and this interferes with the transition from metaphase to anaphase. This action also probably depends on competitive interference with the activity of N^5 formylTHF and can be prevented by the addition of large amounts of this substance.

Toxigenesis

Substances which are themselves not directly noxious may react with materials in the body to form other substances which are actively harmful. Thudichum, in 1884, suggested that insanity might be caused by 'effects on the brain substance of poisons fermented in the body'. In some instances enzymes convert foreign substances which are themselves innocuous, into highly toxic derivatives; in other cases the foreign substance may be an enzyme itself which liberates a toxic product on reacting with substances in the body. The ultimate toxic product may disorganize cell architecture directly or interfere with enzymic processes or act in some unknown manner.

METHANOL

Methanol would be no more toxic than its higher homologue ethanol but for its intracellular oxidation by alcohol dehydrogenase to the highly toxic formaldehyde and the further conversion of formaldehyde to formic acid.

$$CH_3OH - 2H \xrightarrow[\text{dehydrogenase}]{\text{Alcohol}} \underset{\text{Formaldehyde}}{H-\overset{\overset{H}{|}}{C}=O} + H_2O$$

$$2H-\overset{\overset{H}{|}}{C}=O + H_2O \xrightarrow[\text{mutase}]{\text{Aldehyde}} CH_3OH + H-\overset{\overset{O}{\parallel}}{C}-OH$$
$$\underset{\text{acid}}{\text{Formic}}$$

Both the alcohol dehydrogenase and the aldehyde mutase occur in liver cells and probably in other cells as well. The harmful action of methanol may be due to oxidation to formic acid, but it is much more likely that formaldehyde is the actual toxic agent. It is hardly conceivable that formaldehyde, after formation inside the cells, would not react immediately with NH_2 groups in proteins; this would cause linkage between protein chains in a manner similar to fixation. Formaldehyde itself is a highly necrotizing poison.

In poisoning by methanol there is initial inebriation, presumably due to the direct action of the alcohol, followed by coma. Patients who recover from coma may be blind owing to injury to the ganglion cells in the retina and degeneration of the optic nerves. The retinal injury and widespread cerebral damage which follow methanol poisoning are probably caused by the products of its oxidation; formaldehyde may thus act as an intracellular fixative with devastating effect.

FLUORACETATE

Rats injected with 5 mg of this substance become rigid and develop convulsions. The animals may die from asphyxia during a convulsion; otherwise they usually collapse and die from heart failure within 24 hours. Fluoracetate is not directly toxic; it inhibits no enzymic action itself, but by entering the citric acid cycle of metabolism, in the same way as acetate or acetyl coenzyme A, it is converted into the highly toxic fluorocitrate, already discussed on p. 25.15. This synthetic action, in which the active fluoro-2C compound mimics acetyl

coenzyme A (normal active 2C compound in fig. 25.9) and thus combines with oxalacetate to form fluorocitrate, heralds disaster for the cell. Peters aptly called the formation of fluorocitrate a lethal synthesis.

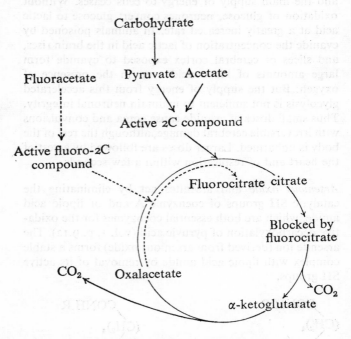

FIG. 25.9. Toxigenic action of fluoracetate (after Peters). Continuous line, normal citric acid cycle; broken line, course followed by fluoracetate.

LECITHINASE OF VENOMS

Snake venoms contain an enzyme which splits lecithin by hydrolysing the linkage of fatty acid to the β-C atom of glycerol, so that a β-hydroxy compound **lysolecithin** is formed (vol. 1, p. 10.4)

Lysolecithin lyses red blood cells and causes intravascular haemolysis. Thus the lecithinase of venoms, which is not itself directly injurious, reacts with the lecithin in blood to produce the harmful lytic agent lysolecithin.

Carcinogenesis (oncogenesis)

The correct term for the production of tumours in general is **oncogenesis**. Carcinogenesis means simply the production of carcinomata, but this term is frequently used as a substitute for oncogenesis, since most of the tumours first produced experimentally were malignant epithelial tumours.

Harmful substances may induce neoplasms. Sir Percival Pott, in 1775, described carcinoma of the scrotum in chimney sweeps and he suggested that this tumour is caused by the action of soot. Since that time some human and animal neoplasms have been shown to arise from contact with various substances.

HYDROCARBONS

Neoplasms of the skin are found among men who come in contact with oils and tars formed by thermal decomposition of coal, shale and mineral oil. Usually the neoplasms begin as benign papillomata; later malignant change may occur if exposure to the irritant continues. If the exposure ceases before malignant change has occurred, the benign tumours may regress or may remain dormant for years and later become frankly malignant as squamous carcinomata.

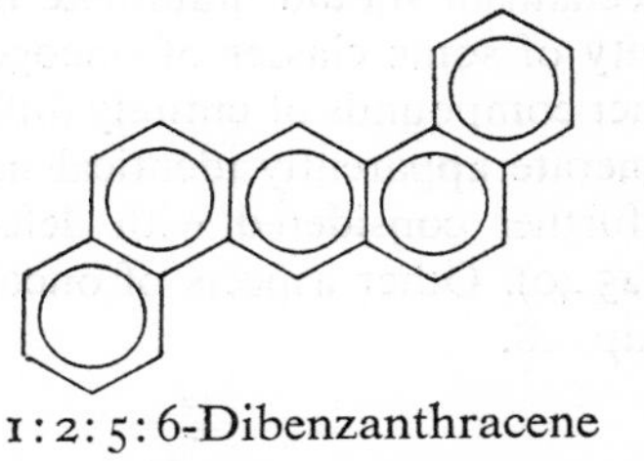

1:2:5:6-Dibenzanthracene

By painting various hydrocarbons on the skin of mice, Cook and Kennaway showed that many are oncogenic. They found first that 1:2:5:6-dibenzanthracene produces tumours and later showed that small changes in chemical structure can greatly affect the oncogenic activity (table 25.1.)

Table 25.1. Influence of chemical structure on oncogenic activity of derivatives of 1:2-benzanthracene.

Name of compound	Structure	Oncogenic activity
1:2-Benzanthracene	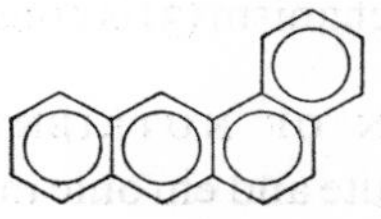	Nil
5-Methyl-1:2-benzan-thracene	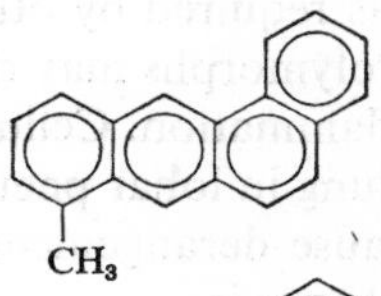	Active
10-Methyl-1:2-benzan-thracene	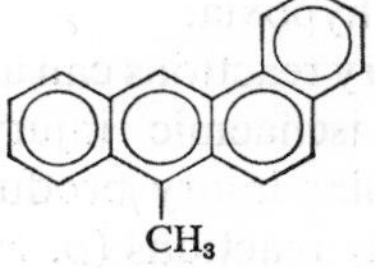	More active
9-10-Dimethyl-1:2-benzanthracene	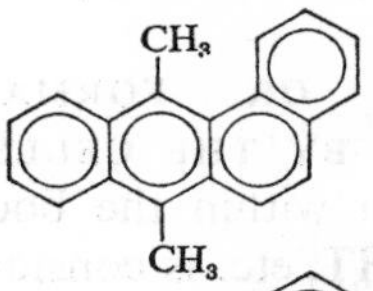	Extremely active
9-10-Dihydro-10-methyl-1:2-benzanthracene	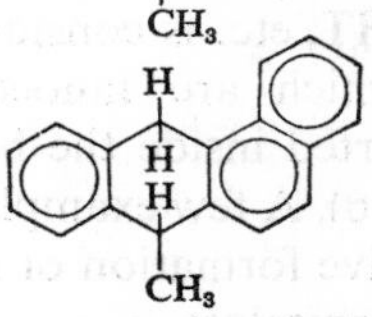	Nil

Later they isolated two isomeric pure hydrocarbons from the products of distillation of gasworks pitch; these hydrocarbons were found to be 3:4-benzpyrene and 1:2-benzpyrene. The former is intensely oncogenic when

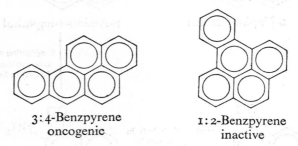

3:4-Benzpyrene   1:2-Benzpyrene
oncogenic   inactive

painted on the skin of mice, while the latter is inactive. 3:4-Benzpyrene is probably responsible for much of the oncogenic potency of industrial hydrocarbon mixtures. It is also possible that hydrocarbons play a part in causing human neoplasms even among those not specially exposed to industrial hazards. 3:4-Benzpyrene is present in tobacco smoke and in diesel-oil fumes and it may be formed also by heating cooking fats. 3:4-Benzpyrene is thus an inveterate enemy of man.

ORGANIC AMINO COMPOUNDS

The incidence of neoplasm of the bladder among those working in the manufacture of aromatic dyes is at least twenty-five times as great as in the general population. 2-Naphthylamine and benzidine have been specially

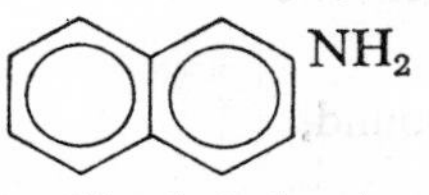

2-Naphthylamine 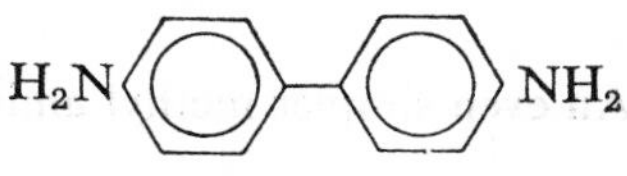   Benzidine

incriminated as causes of this kind of industrial cancer, which includes both papilloma and carcinoma of the bladder.

Experiments on mice indicate that 2-naphthylamine is not directly carcinogenic when implanted into the bladder wall, but that 2-amino-1-naphthol is active under these conditions. It seems likely that 2-naphthylamine, when absorbed by man, is converted into 2-amino-1-naphthol in the liver. This substance is then conjugated with glucuronic acid and excreted by the kidney. Unfortunately, the resulting glucuronide is hydrolysed in the renal tubules by renal glucuronidase, so that the highly carcinogenic 2-amino-1-naphthol is reformed and discharged into the bladder after concentration by tubular reabsorption of water. In this way enzymic action within the body converts 2-naphthylamine into an actively harmful substance (fig. 25.10), to which the bladder epithelium is exposed in concentrated solution.

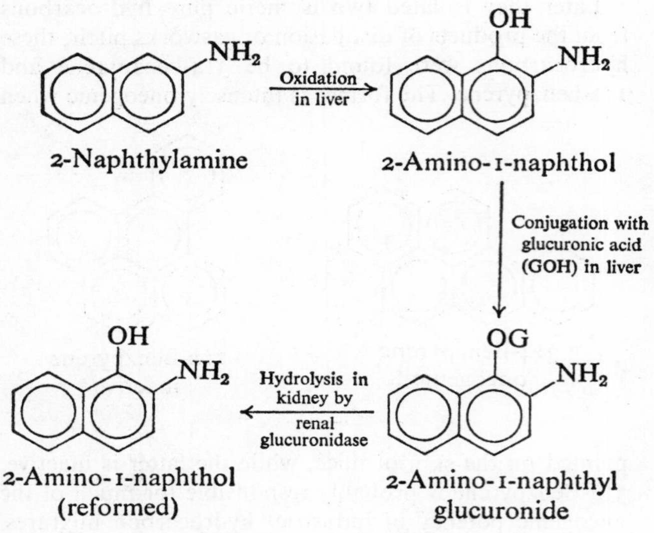

FIG. 25.10. The conversion of 2-naphthylamine to 2-amino-1-naphthol which is finally released to act on bladder epithelium.

Both rats and mice develop malignant tumours of hepatic cells and bile ducts when fed the azo dye, butter yellow, i.e.

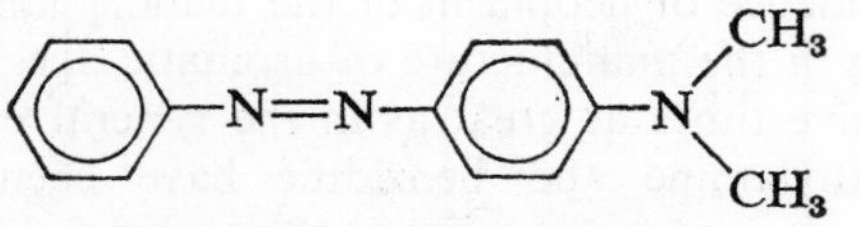

p-Dimethyl aminoazobenzene

An even simpler methyl amino compound,

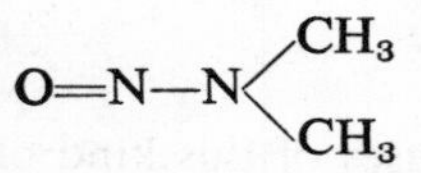

Dimethyl nitrosamine

causes hepatic and renal tumours in rats, mice and hamsters. Renal tumours occur in some animals after even a single dose of dimethyl nitrosamine. It is possible that its oncogenic properties depend on its capacity to methylate nucleic acids; this action might initiate somatic mutation with the production ultimately of potentially malignant cells.

ARSENIOUS OXIDE AND ARSENITES

Arsenious oxide, formerly used in the treatment of human skin diseases and chronic leukaemia over long periods, may cause hyperkeratosis followed eventually by squamous carcinoma of the skin. Potassium arsenite painted on the skin of mice is also oncogenic.

MECHANISMS INVOLVED IN CHEMICAL ONCOGENESIS

The mode of action of chemical oncogens has not so far been fully explained. The paramount difficulty is to account for the exceedingly wide variety of substances which possess activity. Although small changes in structure may exert large effects on activity, as in substituted benzanthracenes and azo dyes, substances so dissimilar in constitution as As_2O_3 and 3:4-benzpyrene both lead to squamous carcinoma when applied to the skin. Any valid theory of mechanism should illuminate this paradox of high specificity of some classes of oncogenic substance, while yet other compounds of entirely different composition may generate apparently identical neoplasms. This question is further considered with defects of cell behaviour (p. 25.40). Other aspects of oncogenesis are discussed in chap. 28.

LIVING AGENTS

Living agents which injure cells are either cells of the body itself or parasitic cells.

Injury by the cells of the body itself
These can injure by the following mechanisms:
(1) depriving other cells of essential nutrients,
(2) liberating or forming harmful substances, and
(3) forming antibodies which react specifically with their antigens to cause subsequent cellular damage.
Of these three mechanisms only (1) and (2) are discussed here, since mechanism (3) is considered in chaps. 22 and 23.

DEPRIVATION OF NUTRIENTS BY BODY CELLS
The cells of acute and chronic inflammatory exudates may utilize nutrients required by other cells which are therefore injured. Polymorphs may thus cause cellular damage in purulent inflammation. Cellular exudates which fill the alveoli of the lung in lobar pneumonia and in pulmonary tuberculosis cause derangements in pulmonary function which lead to hypoxia.

Inflammatory reactions can also produce vascular stasis and lead to ischaemic injury. Vascular stasis plays a part in cellular injury produced by cold and by local hypersensitivity reactions (p. 22.20).

LIBERATION OR FORMATION OF HARMFUL SUBSTANCES BY THE CELLS OF THE BODY ITSELF
The liberation within the body of substances such as histamine, 5-HT, etc. is considered on pp. 14.12 & 16.3. Substances which are innocuous in themselves may also be converted inside the body into actively harmful agents (p. 25.16). A few examples are now given of liberation or excessive formation of harmful substances by the tissue cells themselves.

Potassium

The normal concentration of potassium inside cells is about thirty times as great as that in blood plasma and intercellular fluid. Extensive cellular injury, including lysis of red blood cells, releases K^+ which are toxic to both heart and brain. K^+ liberated from lysed red cells following severe burns may cause death from cardiac arrest due to hyperkalaemia. Such intravascular lysis occurs also in drowning by fresh water. When fresh water is aspirated into the lungs, it is rapidly absorbed by osmosis into the blood, where it causes haemodilution with lysis. This dilution lowers $[Na^+]$, while $[K^+]$ is raised owing to release from the lysed red cells. The Na^+/K^+ ratio in the plasma falls to a level which is toxic to cardiac muscle and which produces ventricular fibrillation. This is the usual cause of death in drowning by fresh water, which is thus much more rapidly lethal when inhaled, than salt water. K^+ are liberated from damaged red blood cells in severe lead poisoning and thus add to the toxic action of lead itself.

In the brain after a cerebral haemorrhage or haemorrhagic infarction, K^+ are probably liberated from hypoxic neurones as well as from extravasated red cells. This liberated potassium may thus further injure the neurones by inhibiting anaerobic glycolysis (fig. 25.11) so

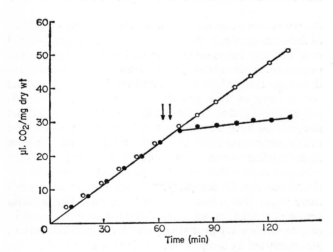

FIG. 25.11. Effect of addition of K^+ on rate of anaerobic glycolysis of slices of rabbit cerebral cortex. Both series of points record normal anaerobic glycolysis in two parallel experiments up to the period between the arrows, when KCl (●) was added to give a final concentration of 50 mEq/litre; ○, no KCl was added.

depriving them of their last remaining source of energy. Locally liberated K^+ may thus aggravate neuronal injury initiated by ischaemia.

Potassium ions are also released from dying fibres of striated muscle. After ischaemic muscle necrosis, due to

prolonged compression of limbs, $[K^+]$ in the plasma rises, sometimes to lethal levels of 8–10 mEq/litre.

Myoglobin

Following prolonged compression of limbs, myoglobin also leaks out of dead muscles. It is in part excreted in the urine, but is also transformed into acid haematin which is precipitated in the renal tubules as a brown granular deposit. This precipitate may occlude renal tubules and contribute to acute renal failure which occasionally follows injuries of this nature.

Bilirubin

In haemolytic disease of the newborn there is excessive destruction of red blood cells which are injured by adsorbed maternal antibodies (vol. 1, p. 26.20). As well as being grossly anaemic, the child may be severely jaundiced. The concentration of plasma bilirubin may rise to 50 mg/100 ml. This bilirubin, which is held in the plasma in loose association with albumin, passes freely through the poorly developed blood–brain barrier of newborn infants. The bilirubin which enters the brain stains various zones in the grey matter a deep yellow (**kernicterus**, nuclear jaundice). The zones most usually coloured are the subthalamic and medullary nuclei, the globus pallidus and patchy areas in the cerebral cortex. In these yellow zones many of the neurones are necrotic and shrivelled and are intensely coloured by adsorbed bilirubin. Neuronal damage in haemolytic disease of the newborn is in part caused by the toxic action of bilirubin, since similar shrunken yellow neurones are produced in kittens by injection of bilirubin. In baby rabbits, however, the cerebral neurones can be coloured by injected bilirubin only if the brain is first injured by hypoxia. It is possible, therefore, that in human neonatal jaundice the neurones are first damaged by hypoxia and are then selectively coloured by bilirubin.

Similar damage may occur when sulphonamides or other drugs which displace bilirubin from protein binding are given to pregnant women or newborn infants (p. 12.18).

Haemoglobin S

The production of this abnormal haemoglobin has already been described (p. 25.2). The sickled red cells which contain it are more viscous than normal cells and so occlude the smaller blood vessels; this stasis is followed by thrombosis and ischaemic necrosis. Infarction is thus common in sickle-cell anaemia and occurs typically in the lungs, spleen and bones, while ischaemic ulcers form on the legs. The retardation of circulation caused by the viscous sickled red blood cells further increases the amount of reduced haemoglobin; this promotes further crystallization and sickling which results in further stasis. Thus a vicious cycle of sickling and stasis is initiated.

Injury by parasitic cells

These can injure by the following mechanisms:

(1) depriving other cells of nutrients,
(2) liberating harmful substances,
(3) harmful antigenic actions, and
(4) intracellular growth.

DEPRIVATION OF NUTRIENTS CAUSED BY PARASITIC CELLS

Many parasites interfere with the nutrition of cells by altering their blood supply. Notable examples are malignant tertian malaria and hookworm infestation. Red blood cells parasitized by *Pl. falciparum* adhere to one another and so may occlude capillaries in the internal organs and especially in the brain, causing the coma which is the dreaded complication of malignant malaria. Hookworms, by sucking blood from their attachment to the intestinal mucosa, can cause a severe anaemia which impairs the functions of cells in many organs, especially the heart. Many bacterial infections can lead to severe ischaemia by producing stasis, septic thrombi and localized necrosis.

LIBERATION OF TOXIC SUBSTANCES BY PARASITES: BACTERIAL EXOTOXINS

The production of bacterial exotoxins and their nature are described on p. 18.30.

Clostridium welchii, which grows in the anaerobic medium of traumatized infected muscle, produces an α-toxin with a necrotizing action. The toxin hydrolyses lecithin and other phospholipids in lipoprotein membranes. The α-toxin is in fact a phospholipase which splits lecithin into diglyceride and phosphoryl choline (vol. 1, p. 10.3). This action disintegrates the lipoprotein membranes on the surface of cells and of their internal organelles, and it results in cellular death and the lysis of red blood corpuscles. In muscle, fatty deposition occurs in the dying fibres. This is probably initiated by destruction of phospholipid which normally emulsifies the intracellular fat. Without the emulsifying phospholipid, the dispersed and invisible fat creams into visible globules. The organism produces other enzymes which ferment the muscle glycogen to produce bubbles of gas within the infected fibres. In this way the muscle becomes crepitant; this condition is called gas gangrene (p. 18.65).

Clostridium botulinum produces an exotoxin which is one of the most powerful of all known poisons. One mg of the toxin of *Cl. botulinum* type A can kill 300×10^6 mice. It acts on the unmyelinated terminals of cholinergic fibres in muscle and in spinal cord and prevents the release of acetylcholine (p. 4.5). In the disease **botulism**, death is caused by the action of the toxin in paralysing the muscles of respiration and deglutition.

Clostridium tetani also releases an intensely poisonous protein and 1 mg can kill 70×10^6 mice. The toxin, when it reaches the central nervous system, increases reflex activity to cause the convulsive spasms of skeletal muscles characteristic of **tetanus**. Death is generally due to spasm of the respiratory muscles. The toxin is specifically adsorbed by nervous tissue and may act by diminishing synaptic resistance or by interfering with inhibitory impulses.

Corynebacterium diphtheriae produces a powerful exotoxin and 1 mg of this toxic protein can kill 10^4 guinea-pigs. It exerts a highly necrotizing effect on cells and when *C. diphtheriae* grows in the fauces, its toxin is liberated and kills the local mucosal cells (p. 18.62). Absorption of the toxin is followed by fatty deposition in and necrosis of heart muscle with cardiac failure and arrest. The toxin also acts on myelinated nerve fibres to cause degeneration and paralysis; demyelination is initiated by disruption of lipoprotein membranes in the mesaxonal portion of the Schwann cells. The intensely necrotizing action of the toxin on cells has not been fully explained, but experiments with human cancer (HeLa) cells in culture show that the toxin interferes with the synthesis of cell protein.

Streptococcus pyogenes produces several exotoxins. Two of these, streptolysin O and streptolysin S, haemolyse red cells and also cause severe cellular injury. Streptolysin O produces cardiac arrest when perfused in low concentrations into isolated rat hearts, and the loss of myocardial contractility is irreversible. Streptolysin O also kills polymorphs, and motion pictures taken by phase–contrast microscopy have shown rapid and extensive lysis of their cytoplasmic granules; the cells then round up and their nuclear lobes swell and fuse together. These changes occur within 5 min of exposure of the polymorphs to streptolysin O. Streptolysin S has similar effects but these begin after a latent period of 30 min. The harmful action of these exotoxins (especially the cardiotoxic effect of streptolysin O) probably plays an important part in illness caused by streptococcal infection (p. 25.26).

LIBERATION OF TOXIC SUBSTANCES BY PARASITES: BACTERIAL ENDOTOXINS

The production of endotoxins is described on p. 18.30. Although their pathogenic effect is often important it depends on relatively large amounts of toxin being released by disintegrating organisms which are essentially invasive and thus grow and divide in abundance within the body. It is possible that some of the harmful effects of endotoxins depend on the development of hypersensitivity.

Salmonella typhi produces an endotoxin which is a

complex of lipopolysaccharide and protein. It is a disintegrated portion of the antigenic mozaic of the bacterial surface and is much less toxic than bacterial exotoxins; however, as little as 1 μg can cause fever in man after intravenous injection. This effect is indirect and probably depends on the injurious effect of the endotoxin on polymorphs. Saline extracts of normal polymorphs contain a rapidly acting pyrogen which causes fever by direct effect on the heat regulating centre in the brain. By damaging polymorphs the endotoxin of *S. typhi* probably releases this direct pyrogen. The characteristic leucopenia of typhoid fever is caused in part by the injurious action of the endotoxin on polymorphs, but probably depends also on the temporary suppression of myeloblastic tissue in bone marrow by mononuclear hyperplasia. The endotoxin is doubtless responsible for the necrosis of mononuclear cells in typhoid lesions, although these tightly aggregated cells may also die through lack of nutrients. Necrosis of these masses of mononuclear cells in the lymphoid follicles of the small intestine is succeeded by extensive ulceration of the mucosa.

The endotoxin of *P. pestis* probably acts on blood vessels and so causes intense shock and vasodilation.

Gram-negative bacilli such as the *Shigellae* of dysentery, *Esch. coli* and *Ps. pyocyanea* also liberate endotoxins when they disintegrate. *Esch. coli* can produce bacteriaemia which may be followed by a fall in blood pressure and collapse due to liberation of endotoxins. Similar endotoxins may be formed by contamination of distilled water by Gram-negative bacilli; even though the distilled water is subsequently sterilized before it is used to make up solutions for intravenous injection, intense rigors and bouts of fever follow their use (p. 18.30).

Mycobacteria possesses a cell wall rich in lipids, some of which contain the branched chain fatty acid phthioic acid, $C_{26}H_{52}O_2$ (3-13-19-trimethyl tricosanoic acid). When phthioic acid is injected into guinea-pigs it causes accumulation of mononuclear cells and giant cells, followed by necrosis. It is likely that this toxic lipid contributes to the necrotizing action of tubercle bacilli (p. 21.16).

HARMFUL ANTIGENIC ACTION BY PARASITES
The classical example is tuberculin, a protein which is liberated from disintegrated tubercle bacilli; it exerts highly damaging effects on the tissues of animals sensitized by previous infection with tubercle bacilli, but is innocuous to the tissues of unsensitized animals (p. 21.16). The cells of sensitized animals react by acute inflammation which may produce stasis and ischaemic necrosis, but tuberculin also directly harms sensitized cells. Thus tuberculin reduces the motility of macrophages and polymorphs from sensitized animals; this interference with motility can impair the survival of cells in culture. It is thus reasonable to suppose that tuberculin,

liberated from tubercle bacilli growing in the tissues, can kill epithelioid cells of tuberculous exudates owing to reaction with specific antibody in the cells.

The necrotic process probably depends on three factors:

(1) the avascularity of tuberculous exudates,
(2) the directly harmful action of phthioic acid and other lipids, and
(3) injury of sensitized cells by tuberculin.

As described on p. 21.17, epithelial cells in sensitized and immune animals kill tubercle bacilli within them more readily than cells in non-sensitized animals.

Another example of antigenic action is provided by lobar pneumonia, due to the pneumoccus. In this disease there is a synchronous outpouring of exudate into the infected pulmonary alveoli; the fact that this action is rapid and that it occurs mainly in adults, who presumably have suffered from previous infection by pneumococci, suggests that the tissues are sensitized by previous pneumococcal infection and thus contain antibodies which react with antigens liberated from the pneumococci. The resultant exudate interferes with oxygen transfer and can cause cellular hypoxia (p. 23.1).

INTRACELLULAR GROWTH OF PARASITES
Profound cellular injury can follow intracellular growth of parasites.

Intracellular protozoa
As described in chap. 19, the malaria parasites all grow inside human red blood cells which they rupture after schizogony; the merozoites are then liberated into the plasma and infect further red cells. As each batch of infected red cells is ruptured the patient suffers bouts of rigors followed by fever. Severe anaemia follows repeated attacks. Whether toxins from the plasmodia or those from the products of the ruptured red cells are responsible for the fever is unknown. The schizonts of *Plasmodium falciparum* exert a further and far more detrimental effect by causing vascular occlusion.

INTRACELLULAR PATHOGENIC BACTERIA
Neisseria meningitidis (p. 18.71) and *Neisseria gonorrheae* (p. 18.72) multiply inside polymorphs and their cytoplasm becomes stuffed with numerous diplococci. Only when the bacteria die are their endotoxins liberated; the polymorphs then become necrotic.

Tubercle bacilli grow inside mononuclear phagocytes. Although these at first appear to be uninjured, their surface properties are altered and many of them fuse to form multinucleate giant cells containing the bacilli (p. 21.17). Later the mononuclear cells are killed and disintegrate into caseous debris. *Myco. leprae* is less harmful to the mononuclear phagocytes which ingest it; the 'lepra cells', which densely infiltrate the dermis in nodular leprosy, are mononuclear cells which are packed with vast numbers of these intracellular mycobacteria. The pathogenicity of *Myco. leprae* is so low that the mononuclear cells survive intense parasitism for a long time.

INTRACELLULAR GROWTH OF RICKETTSIAE

Rickettsia prowazekii, the causative organism of epidemic typhus, grows and multiplies in the endothelial cells of capillaries, especially those of the brain and the skin. The infected endothelial cells swell and proliferate and thrombi form on their surfaces. The capillaries therefore become occluded and the surrounding tissues are injured by ischaemia. In the brain characteristic aggregates of microglial mononuclear cells coalesce around the occluded capillaries to produce 'typhus nodules'. Cerebral ischaemia resulting from capillary occlusion probably accounts for the profound stupor and confusion which are so typical of typhus fever (p. 18.85).

INTRACELLULAR GROWTH OF VIRUSES (p. 18.102).

This is a potent cause of cellular injury, although viruses can infect cells without obvious damage. Why viral replication is so necrotizing to some cells in which viruses multiply is obscure. Perhaps the replication of viral DNA or RNA exhausts the supply of available nucleotide units needed for replenishment of the cell's own nucleic acid, or else the formation of viral protein may compete with the synthetic anabolism of cell proteins. Cytopathic effects produced by viruses on cells in culture include:

(1) contraction into spherical necrotic remnants with pyknotic nuclei (poliovirus),

(2) coalescence to form multinucleated syncytia (herpes and measles viruses),

(3) formation of cytoplasmic inclusions followed by cell disintegration (vaccinia),

(4) formation of intranuclear inclusions (adenoviruses, herpes and measles viruses), and

(5) transformation into neoplastic cells (polyoma virus).

Similarly, when viruses replicate in cells within the body the visible changes induced are varied. These include cellular proliferation (poxviruses), cellular swelling and vacuolation, loss of Nissl granules in motor neurones (poliovirus), and the formation of inclusion bodies in cytoplasm or in nucleus (poxviruses, plate 25.2c and d, facing p. 25.14). These changes may be succeeded by extensive cellular death, as can happen in the epidermis in smallpox.

UNKNOWN PATHOGENIC MECHANISMS

Some pathogenic micro-organisms which produce cellular injury form no known toxin, and do not appear to interfere with cellular nutrition, nor do they penetrate into cells. Thus *Leptospira icterohaemorrhagiae*, the cause of Weil's disease, produces liver and skeletal muscle cell injury by some entirely obscure mechanism. There is occasional hepatic cell necrosis and Zenker's degeneration of muscle is also seen (p. 25.25).

NATURE OF CELLULAR DISORDER

Until cellular physiology and biochemistry are better understood and the fusion of these sciences with cytology and cytochemistry becomes more perfect, a satisfactory classification of cellular disorder will not be possible.

Structural and architectural damage on the one hand and interference with chemical and physical processes on the other can be considered separately. That such a demarcation is invalid, however, is obvious when it is remembered that metabolism and behaviour are inextricably dependent on cell structure. For the sake of simplicity three principal types of cellular defect are discussed, realizing that many derangements involve events in more than one of these descriptive compartments and that each type of disorder may be attended by the others in its wake.

The three kinds of defect are:

(1) disintegration of the fabric of the cell,

(2) intracellular aggregation or deposition, and

(3) invisible derangements of metabolism, function or growth.

DISINTEGRATION OF THE MACROMOLECULAR FABRIC OF THE CELL

Mechanism of disintegration

Disintegration of the cell fabric depends on two kinds of process, macromolecular disarray and chemical fission.

MACROMOLECULAR DISARRAY

This consists of disorientation of macromolecules with disruption of cell membranes and organelles followed later by denaturation of proteins. This is a physicochemical phenomenon, which arises by the direct action of adverse physical conditions, e.g. heat, or noxious substances, e.g. saponin, or indirectly through cessation of the exergonic reactions necessary for stabilizing orientated macromolecules. The initial phases of macromolecular disarray may, of course, involve chemical changes, like the removal of phosphoryl choline from lecithin by the α-toxin of *Cl. welchii* (p. 25.20), as well as physicochemical changes, such as the loss from membranes of structured water by the action of heat or freezing (p. 25.10). But even when initiated by a chemical change, the fundamental mechanism is physical disorganization of macromolecules.

CHEMICAL FISSION

Lesions of this kind consist of chemical decomposition of macromolecules into smaller units of low molecular weight and commonly arise from derangement in the normal intracellular equilibrium between anabolism and catabolism.

Retardation of anabolism

Anabolism of macromolecules is a process which is readily deranged by structural damage, because spacial alignment in nucleus and in ribosomes is essential for the replenishment of RNA and protein. Synthesis of these substances is normally continuous so as to keep pace with their normal catabolism. Anabolism may be interrupted also by interference with the supply of nutrients which provide synthetic units and also the fuel for the exergonic reactions producing ATP.

Acceleration of catabolism

Excessive catabolism may occur when the structural barriers which curb the full accessibility of catabolic enzymes to their substrates are removed. In the living cell many of the disruptive enzymes are locked away inside organelles such as lysosomes. Moreover, the free water necessary for hydrolysis may not be available. Structural injury to the fabric may thus accelerate catabolism by making hydrolytic enzymes more accessible and by allowing ingress of water necessary for hydrolytic fission; indeed, osmotic entry of water may promote a vicious cycle of catabolism.

Although changes in the cytoplasm and nucleus occur simultaneously as a result of cell injury, we shall for convenience first consider cytoplasmic disintegration, then nuclear disintegration and finally the fate of the remnants.

Cytoplasmic disintegration

This involves many kinds of change, which may occur simultaneously, in succession or as isolated events; these changes include:

(1) injury and lysis of cell membranes,
(2) aqueous swelling and vacuolation,
(3) chromatolysis and loss of cytoplasmic basophilia,
(4) mitochondrial disintegration, and
(5) changes in other cytoplasmic constituents.

INJURY AND LYSIS OF CELL MEMBRANES

Focal expansions and interruptions in the plasma membrane of liver cells and formation of fine vacuoles within the cells are the earliest signs of injury visible by EM in liver cells after occlusion of their blood supply; the microvilli which project from the cells at their sinusoidal border also disappear. Later, the endoplasmic reticulum frag-

ments, its cisternae dilate, and the mitochondria swell (p. 25.25). All these changes are reversible, provided the circulation is restored within 1 hr of occlusion, but if ischaemia lasts for 2 hr no recovery occurs.

Permeability of injured cells

Necrosis makes cell membranes completely permeable. Dying cells, however, may for a time remain semipermeable and during this phase osmotic swelling can occur. But as soon as the membranes of the cell and of its internal organelles become fully permeable, further osmotic swelling is precluded. Thus cells which are rapidly killed show little swelling *post mortem* or may shrink in size (plate 25.2b, facing p. 25.14).

Lysis

When the plasma membrane of injured cells disintegrates sufficiently for large molecules to escape, then cellular lysis is said to have occurred. When red blood cells are lysed, their haemoglobin escapes and serves as a visible indicator of lysis. Uncoloured large molecules, such as enzymes, also diffuse out of lysed cells.

Ischaemic injury

As described on p. 25.8, ischaemia causes fragmentation of the external membrane of cells and is a potent cause of lysis with escape of large molecules. After infarction of the heart, lysis of the external membranes permits aspartate aminotransferases and lactic dehydrogenase to escape from the dying cardiac fibres into the blood. A rise in the levels of these enzymes in serum thus gives diagnostic confirmation of myocardial infarction.

Injury of cells by heat

Heat causes lysis of cell membranes. We have seen how red blood cells in burned patients break up into microspherocytes with the escape of haemoglobin. Freezing also lyses red cells and damages cell membranes (p. 25.11).

Harmful substances and toxins

When saponin lyses red blood cells and polymorphs, haemoglobin escapes from the former and hydrolytic enzymes from the latter. Lead salts also lyse red blood cells by combining with the membrane proteins, so that their membranes become brittle to the trauma of the normal circulation. Staphylococcal leucocidin makes the surface membranes of polymorphs more permeable, so that both K^+ and cellular granules are extruded through the disintegrated membrane. Streptolysin O fragments the lysosomes within the polymorphs (pp. 18.68 & 70).

AQUEOUS SWELLING AND VACUOLATION

Swelling of the cytoplasm with watery fluid may be a prominent feature of injured cells. Part of this change is caused by vesiculation of the cisternae of endoplasmic reticulum and by swelling of mitochondria, but the earliest change detectable, for example in liver cells damaged by ischaemia, is the formation of small aqueous vacuoles close to the cell membrane and injury to the cell membrane itself. Lysosomes may swell later.

Lack of nutrients
Lack of nutrients, especially oxygen, is a potent cause of aqueous swelling. After arrest of the circulation in rabbits, the pyramidal cells of cerebral cortex and the Purkinje cells of cerebellum swell within 3–6 min and sodium chloride and water enter the cells. When rats are killed by asphyxia, vacuoles of water are found in their liver cells 20 min after death, provided the animals are not bled between death and dissection; this change may be more prominent in previously starved rats. If the pedicles of lobes of the liver in rats are ligated, fine intracellular vacuoles, visible by EM, are formed near the sinusoidal borders and swollen blebs appear at the cell surfaces within 15 min of the onset of ischaemia. Large vacuoles of water are found in human liver cells after death from asphyxia and starvation.

Poisons
In the livers of rats poisoned by carbon tetrachloride, conspicuous aqueous swelling with vacuolation occurs in the midzonal (zone 2) cells. This vacuolation starts by dilation of the cisternae of the endoplasmic reticulum and of the mitochondria. Eventually the cells become intensely vacuolated (plate 25.1f, facing p. 25.6); the centrilobular (zone 3) cells, however, usually die without vacuolation.

Toxaemia and infection
Sublethal doses of diphtheria toxin cause aqueous swelling in the hepatic cells of guinea-pigs. Infection by poliovirus may give rise to aqueous swelling in the anterior horn cells of spinal cord. Vaccinia and variola viruses produce characteristic 'ballooning' degeneration of epidermal cells (plate 25.2d, facing p. 25.14).

Mechanism of aqueous swelling
Entry of water into injured cells probably depends on osmotic absorption. The internal osmotic pressure of healthy cells is equal to that of the external fluid, but after cell injury the internal osmotic pressure may exceed the external for two reasons.

(1) In cell injury the net catabolism of macromolecules and of smaller substances such as ATP produces a rise of internal osmolality; this causes water to enter the cells by osmosis.

(2) Healthy cell membranes largely exclude Na^+ and Cl^- from the internal milieu; these extracellular ions are excluded actively by a sodium pump which depends for its energy on ATP. Thus when exergonic reactions stop

through lack of nutrients or when the membrane is directly damaged, Na^+ and Cl^- enter the injured cells; water is then drawn into the injured cells with these ions by osmosis.

This dependence of aqueous swelling on osmosis means that it occurs only when the cell membranes retain their semipermeable nature. When they are so severely injured as to become completely permeable, osmosis and aqueous swelling are precluded. Usually after death human and animal cells are not grossly swollen or vacuolated, because *post mortem* ischaemic damage disintegrates cell membranes before substantial osmotic absorption can take place.

CHROMATOLYSIS AND LOSS OF CYTOPLASMIC BASOPHILIA
Chromatolysis means disintegration or loss of the cytoplasmic aggregates of basophilic material which are so prominent in cells capable of intensely active synthesis of protein. Such basophilic zones, typified by the Nissl granules of neurones and the granules of Berg in hepatic cells, are now known to be composed of numerous cisternae of rough-surfaced endoplasmic reticulum lying in parallel and covered on their outer surface by ribosomes. The anionic phosphate groups of RNA make these zones strongly basophilic and thus account for their intense colouration by cationic dyes like pyronin, methylene blue and the metallic dye lake of haematoxylin. Disintegration or loss of these basophilic zones has long been regarded as a hallmark of cellular injury.

Neurones show temporary disintegration of Nissl granules and dispersal of ribosomes after excessive activity. On recovery the dispersed ribosomes become reattached to the endoplasmic reticulum and the Nissl granules reform. Reversible loss of Nissl granules from ventral horn cells of the spinal cord occurs in animals after long periods of muscular activity. Einarson and Krogh demonstrated loss of basophilia in the cerebral neurones of human patients who had died in acute delirium. Section of axons similarly causes temporary disintegration of Nissl granules (Nissl degeneration) in the cell bodies from which the severed axons arise. Permanent disintegration of Nissl granules occurs in dying cells. Thus the basophilic zones disappear completely in neurones killed by ischaemia; plates 25.1a and 1b, facing p. 25.6 illustrate chromatolysis of this kind caused by ischaemic necrosis in Purkinje cells of the cerebellum. Similar disappearance of Nissl granules occurs in neurones injured by poliovirus. Fig. 25.12a shows normal motor neurones of the human hypoglossal nucleus stained by pyronin; intensely coloured Nissl zones are prominent. Fig. 25.12b shows motor neurones, stained by pyronin, from the hypoglossal nucleus of a child who died of bulbar poliomyelitis; practically all the Nissl granules have disappeared.

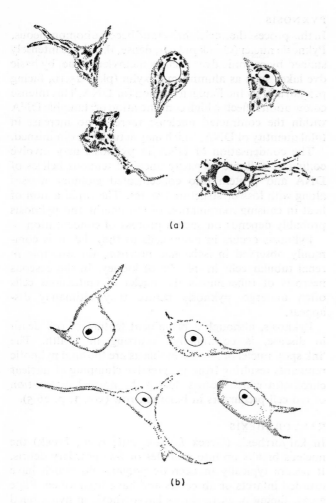

(a)

(b)

FIG. 25.12. Neurones of human hypoglossal nucleus stained by pyronin (× 1000). (a) Normal; prominent Nissl granules rich in RNA. (b) Bulbar poliomyelitis; chromatolysis with disintegration and loss of Nissl granules.

Hepatic cells lose their basophilic cytoplasmic zones also when injured. Thus after poisoning by carbon tetrachloride the centrilobular zone 3 cells of the livers of rats show loss of basophilia (plate 25.1e, facing p. 25.6). Observations by EM show that this change begins with detachment of ribosomes from the endoplasmic reticulum and these at first lie free in the cytoplasmic matrix.

Chromatolysis thus consists of initial dispersal of ribosomes, probably without any immediate hydrolysis of RNA. The first change indeed may be in the membranes of the endoplasmic reticulum, causing detachment of ribosomes. Later the dispersed RNA disappears. This may be due to excessive hydrolysis by ribonuclease, which becomes fully accessible to its substrate as a result of destruction of membranous compartments or which is liberated from ruptured lysosomes. But it is also possible that RNA, when dissociated from conjugation with protein, is lost by diffusing out of the dying cells.

MITOCHONDRIAL DISINTEGRATION

Mitochondria are highly sensitive to adverse conditions. In normal cells they are usually filamentous or sausage shaped. After cellular injury they swell into spherical vesicles and may agglutinate into clumps or be transformed into droplets of lipid before they finally break up into granules and disappear, i.e. **chondriolysis**.

Ischaemia is a potent cause of mitochondrial damage. When myocardial ischaemia is produced in rabbits by ligating small branches of the coronary arteries, the mitochondria in the ischaemic fibres become swollen before the myofibrils show signs of injury. Similarly, after tourniquets are applied to the limbs of mice both the mitochondria and the tubules of endoplasmic reticulum in the muscle fibres swell and disintegrate before the contractile material is destroyed. Mitochondria contain the enzymes concerned with cell respiration. Succinic dehydrogenase can readily be located in cardiac fibres by histochemical methods in the mitochondria between the contractile fibrils. In human cardiac infarcts succinic dehydrogenase disappears from the dying fibres and is lost within 8 hr of the onset of ischaemia.

CHANGES IN OTHER CYTOPLASMIC CONSTITUENTS

Eventually, dying cells become homogeneous and eosinophilic and lose all indications of internal structure. If aqueous swelling does not occur early in the course of injury such amorphous cellular remnants may persist for a long time.

Striations of cardiac and skeletal muscle disappear from dying fibres. When tourniquets are applied to the limbs of mice for 2 hr the ischaemic leg muscles die and show the following sequence of changes after removal of the tourniquets:

(1) saccules of endoplasmic reticulum and mitochondria swell and disintegrate,

(2) Z discs between the sarcomeres disappear, and

(3) contractile material of fibrils disappears.

In typhoid fever, patches of necrosis develop in striated muscles. Here, the fibres lose all structure and become glassy and eosinophilic (**Zenker's hyaline degeneration.**)

Lysosomes in dying cells may be injured. Thus in cerebral neurones damaged by ischaemia, the lysosomes, identified by their high content of acid phosphatase, swell and later disappear. In liver previously injured by ischaemia the lysosomal enzymes, cathepsin, ribonuclease and desoxyribonuclease, are found to be located in the supernatant fluid when the liver tissue is subsequently homogenized and centrifuged; when normal liver is similarly treated, these same enzymes are found in the centrifugate of lysosomal particles. These observations suggest that release of lysosomal enzymes occurs in ischaemic injury to the liver cells. But this release may have occurred after homogenization because the lysosomes of ischaemic tissue are more readily ruptured. Indeed careful observation by cytochemical methods indicate that release of lysosomal enzymes in ischaemic liver cells is a relatively late phenomenon in the course of cell death and cannot contribute to the early changes in cell membranes and organelles.

The **granules of polymorphs** are membranous saccules rich in enzymes. **Degranulation** occurs rapidly during phagocytosis of bacteria; under these circumstances the cell remains actively motile. Weissmann showed that streptolysin O causes complete degranulation of polymorphs within a few minutes. The granules rupture into the cell cytoplasm and then filamentous processes grow out from the cell membrane; the cytoplasm rounds up and motility disappears. If the granules of polymorphs are regarded as lysosomes, it is possible that the liberation of the enzymes of these lysosomes into the cytoplasm of the injured cells may contribute to damage produced by streptolysin.

Nuclear disintegration and injury

Many of the adverse conditions which destroy cytoplasmic structure simultaneously cause injury to the nucleus. These changes in the nucleus include swelling, homogenization and clumping of chromatin, pyknosis, karyorrhexis, karyolysis and karyokinetic injury.

SWELLING, HOMOGENIZATION AND CLUMPING OF CHROMATIN

Swelling of nuclei is the first sign of injury in epidermal cells exposed to excessive heat; later the chromatin clumps into crescentic masses attached to the margins of nuclear membranes. Streptolysin O damages polymorphs rapidly and the lobes of the nuclei swell and fuse together within a few minutes of contact.

The serum of patients suffering from systemic lupus erythematosus (p. 30.12) contains an abnormal globulin (LE factor) which can exert a uniquely harmful action on nuclei. This LE factor is probably an antibody to a constituent of nuclei, which, after being specifically absorbed by nuclei, rapidly damages them. When normal polymorphs and lymphocytes in the buffy coat of human blood are exposed *in vitro* to LE factor, some of their nuclei swell and become homogeneous. Later they are extruded from the damaged cells and these swollen, homogenized nuclei are taken up by uninjured polymorphs, which are then seen to contain spherical homogeneous inclusions rich in DNA. These polymorphs, containing products of phagocytosis of nuclei, are called **LE cells**. Lymphocytes and polymorphs, when observed under phase-contrast microscopy, are seen to suffer nuclear swelling and homogenization within 5 sec of exposure to LE factor.

PYKNOSIS

In this process the nuclei shrivel and become homogeneous. Pyknotic nuclei (Greek *pyknos*, dense, thick) are intensely stained by cationic dyes such as methylene blue, by basic dye lakes such as alumhaematoxylin (plate 25.1b, facing p. 25.6) and by the Feulgen method for DNA. This intense colouration reflects a high concentration of stainable DNA within the contracted nucleus; there is no increase in total quantity of DNA, which may actually be diminished.

The condensation of DNA in pyknosis may involve coiling or collapse of partly uncoiled tenuous helices of DNA and protein into concentrated globular masses along with loss of structured water. The rapid action of heat in causing margination of chromatin and pyknosis probably depends on such a process of condensation.

Pyknosis occurs in many cells as they die. It is commonly observed in ischaemic necrosis, for example in renal tubular cells in infarcts of kidney. In the caseous necrosis of tuberculosis the nuclei of epithelioid cells often undergo pyknosis before they ultimately disappear.

Pyknosis, although a prominent feature of cell death in disease, is continually occurring in health. The 'ink spot' nuclei of late normoblasts are the final pyknotic remnants resulting from progressive clumping of nuclear chromatin which occurs during the normal maturation of red cell precursors in bone marrow (vol. 1, p. 26.5).

KARYORRHEXIS

In karyorrhexis (Greek *karyon*, nut; *rexis*, break) the nucleus breaks up into granules or fine powdery debris. It occurs typically in necrotic polymorphs which have invaded infarcts or abscesses and have been killed. Plate 25.2e, facing p. 25.14 shows karyorrhexis in dying renal tubular cells; the granules of the necrotic nuclei are coloured intensely by alumhaematoxylin owing to their high content of DNA. Plate 25.2f shows karyorrhexis in dying cells from the liver of a rat poisoned by CCl_4; the granules of aggregated chromatin are strongly Feulgen-positive.

The nature of karyorrhexis is obscure. One possibility is that the unravelled DNA of each chromosome of the normal interphase nucleus becomes coiled up by injury to form a separate granular mass. This could account for the kind of karyorrhexis shown in plate 25.2f where the granular remnants are no smaller than the Barr bodies of normal female cells. But in tuberculous caseation, where karyorrhexis produces minute granules of Feulgen-positive material, each individual chromosome must be subdivided into innumerable fragments.

KARYOLYSIS

In this process the nucleus dissolves away (Greek *karyon*, nut; *lysis*, solution); its capacity to be stained both by basic dyes and by the Feulgen method for DNA diminishes progressively and later the nucleus disappears altogether. Karyolysis may be primary or secondary; thus it may be the initial change in nuclear disintegration or, alternatively, it may be a sequel to pyknosis and karyorrhexis.

The mechanism of disappearance of DNA probably involves hydrolysis by deoxyribonuclease; thus during incubation of rat liver *in vitro* there is a loss of DNA which occurs in parallel with a fall in the number of stainable nuclei.

Karyolysis takes place continuously even in the healthy body. In the normal process of keratinization in human skin the cells of the stratum granulosum lose their nuclei by karyolysis at the same time as they are transformed into the cornified scales of the horny layer. Plate 25.3a, facing p. 25.28, shows this process of karyolysis in normal skin stained by haematoxylin and eosin. This synchronous loss of nuclei from the cells is accompanied by disappearance of all DNA stainable by the Feulgen method. In certain disorders of the skin such as psoriasis, keratinization is disturbed and scaly lesions develop in which nuclear karyolysis is incomplete and laminar nuclear remnants, stainable by the Feulgen method, persist even in the outermost horny layer (parakeratosis).

Karyolysis is also the final fate of nuclei in cellular death caused by disease. It is conspicuous in ischaemic necrosis of cardiac muscle fibres. In these cells there is usually no intermediate karyorrhexis or pyknosis, but the nuclei of polymorphs which invade infarcts usually suffer karyorrhexis before they disappear. In tuberculous exudates the nuclei of dying epithelioid cells often show pyknosis or karyorrhexis initially before all nuclear remnants vanish in the terminal karyolysis of caseation.

KARYOKINETIC INJURY

The nuclei of dividing cells are specially susceptible to injury by ionizing radiation as well as by certain specific harmful substances. When severe, this kind of damage involves clumping of the chromosomes at metaphase with necrosis of the cell; this injury is specially evident in the columnar epithelium of the small intestine of animals after large doses of ionizing radiation or following treatment with mitotic poisons like aminopterin. This type of nuclear damage is sometimes termed pyknonecrosis.

Ionizing radiation

Nuclear DNA appears to be the principal target for the injurious action of radiation and it is likely that during mitosis DNA passes through a specially vulnerable phase. Irradiation of dividing cells in culture with microbeams of α-particles from polonium-coated needles, or of protons from electrostatic generators, under phase-contrast microscopy, enables the effects of irradiating different parts of the cell to be studied. The chromosomes are the most vulnerable parts of the dividing cells; indeed

doses of radiation much larger than those which cause chromosomal injury produce no ill effect if directed on to the cytoplasm alone or on to the mitotic spindle. The susceptibility of the chromosomes increases from prophase to metaphase. After irradiation of the condensed chromosomes at metaphase, 'sticky' bridges appear between them so that their separation is delayed at anaphase. With larger doses the nuclear membranes fail to reform at telophase or the chromosomes clump, with pyknonecrosis, at metaphase.

Small doses of radiation temporarily inhibit mitosis without killing the dividing cells; frequency of mitosis is diminished for a time. When squamous carcinoma in human patients is irradiated with intermediate doses of X-rays insufficient to cause immediate necrosis, mitosis in the tumour is temporarily suppressed and damage to the chromosomes becomes visible in most of the neoplastic cells when they begin to divide again. This damage consists of breaks in the chromosomes or lagging of separation in anaphase. Later, however, apparently normal mitosis resumes, but nevertheless the tumours often subsequently disappear. It is thus likely, as suggested by Mitchell, that irradiated nuclei of tumours suffer a latent macromolecular lesion. Latent injury to the nucleus may be responsible also for the late development of neoplasms from apparently normal cells; thus carcinoma of the thyroid may appear in adults many years after irradiation given in childhood to cause regression of an enlarged thymus gland. Latent or molecular change in DNA may thus ultimately result in development of malignant mutant cells.

Karyokinetic poisons

The **radiomimetic poisons** such as the nitrogen mustards and aminopterins (p. 29.4) ape the effects of radiation; they cause clumping of chromosomes in metaphase and also impede the onset of anaphase. **Colchicine** is sometimes called a **spindle poison**; it impedes the development of the fibrillar material of the achromatic spindle and arrests mitosis in metaphase. Colchicine is a valuable tool in the study of human chromosomes; if it is added to cell cultures one to two hours before fixation of the cells many cells are trapped in metaphase and numerous mitotic nuclei become available for chromosomal analysis.

Reversible injury and death

Reparable disintegration may follow adverse conditions insufficient in duration or severity to cause lethal injury. Thus, although initial disintegration of the cell membranes begins in liver cells within half an hour of ligation of the pedicle of a liver lobe, full recovery of the cells occurs if the blood supply is restored within one hour of vascular occlusion (p. 25.6). Similar reversible change occurs in the cell bodies of neurones when their axons are cut; the cell bodies swell initially and their Nissl granules temporarily disintegrate, but later the cell bodies recover completely.

Irreparable disintegration accompanied by permanent cessation of activity is synonymous with cell death or necrosis. A cell may be regarded as dying when disintegration has progressed beyond the point of possible return to the normal structure and equilibria of life. Unfortunately this point cannot be detected by inspecting a cell after fixation. Thus Krogh produced irreparable ischaemic injury in the ventral horn cells of the spinal cord in rabbits by clamping the aorta for 1 hr. Yet the first microscopic changes became visible in the neurones 1 hr later; by then the Nissl granules were no longer sharp in outline and minute vacuoles had appeared. Later the Nissl granules disintegrated completely and the nuclei disappeared; within 24 hr many of the cells decomposed into faintly stainable shadows. It is clear, therefore, that immediately after ischaemia the cells had suffered an invisible injury which left an irreparable imprint on them. The nature of such latent though lethal injuries is obscure. It is possible that either lipoprotein membranes have so far disintegrated as to be incapable of reformation subsequently, when the supply of energy is restored, or some unique molecule of nucleic acid has been lost.

Fate of remnants in dead and dying cells

The fate of necrotic remnants is of three kinds, persistence, autolysis, and heterolysis.

PERSISTENCE

Persistence of the remnants in a physically altered state but with little chemical decomposition of protein or lipid is the commonest immediate sequel to necrosis. Autolysis is impeded by two factors, the lack of free unstructured water for hydrolysis and the inaccessibility of catabolic enzymes to their substrates.

Coagulative necrosis (see also p. 25.42)

As disintegration of lipoprotein membranes proceeds, semipermeability is abolished; water is not absorbed into the dying cell by osmosis, and hydrolytic catabolism is arrested. Later the enzymes become denatured and inactivated, and the cell is transformed into a mummified mass of denatured protein. This sequence of events is the essence of the so-called **coagulative necrosis**. It is well seen in the centrilobular cells of rat liver after injection of CCl_4; as these cells die, their nuclei disappear or show karyorrhexis (plate 25.1e, facing p. 25.6), but their cytoplasm remains rich in protein and is even more intensely coloured than that of normal cells by anionic dyes like eosin and erythrosin.

Denaturation of protein involves unravelling of folded

chains along with exposure of active groups and their mutual aggregation. This change occurs in pieces of rat liver when transplanted into the peritoneum of other rats of the same strain. The transplanted liver cells die because of ischaemia and then become more opaque owing to denaturation with aggregation. Opacification is a basic feature of coagulative necrosis and is thus common in infarcts; the opaque dead cells do not transmit light and so reflect it to give a whitish appearance. The dead cells of infarcts are characterized by their abundance of cytoplasmic protein which persists although DNA and RNA disappear. Conspicuous persistence of protein is responsible for the intense colouration of necrotic kidney cells in infarcts stained by Danielli's tetrazo method which colours the phenolic tyrosine groups of proteins (plate 25.3b, opposite).

Caseous necrosis (see also p. 25.42).

Infection by tubercle bacilli may cause extensive lethal effects. Epithelioid cells of exudates die and disintegrate into a granular material of cheese-like consistency in which both cellular structure and outline have vanished (p. 21.17). Even though all nuclear remnants ultimately disappear, abundant protein remains in an amorphous denatured state. Caseous material is intensely coloured by Danielli's tetrazo method for protein. Owing to exposure of basic $-\overset{+}{N}H_3$ groups of the denatured protein of caseous material, the anionic dye erythrosin is selectively absorbed so that caseous foci are intensely coloured by it (plate 25.3c).

Persistence of denatured protein and lipoprotein in necrotic tissue emphasizes the importance of macromolecular disarray as opposed to chemical fission as the principal kind of initial disintegration in dying cells.

AUTOLYSIS

Disappearance of RNA and DNA commonly occurs in necrotic cells despite persistence of protein. Disintegration of basophilic zones in necrotic cytoplasm is accompanied by loss of RNA; how far this loss of RNA is by diffusion or due to enzymic destruction by ribonuclease liberated from lysosomes is uncertain. Deoxyribonuclease, also liberated from lysosomes, may contribute to the loss of DNA which occurs in karyolysis.

Autolysis of protein probably depends on the availability of free water in the dying cell before the hydrolytic enzymes become denatured. This process is minimal in rapidly killed cells where semipermeability of the surface membrane is destroyed. When injury is not sufficiently severe to destroy this semipermeability, aqueous swelling may occur with entry of water into the injured cell. Simultaneously the hydrolytic enzymes may become accessible to their substrates as intracellular compartments are broken down in the injured cells. Hydrolysis

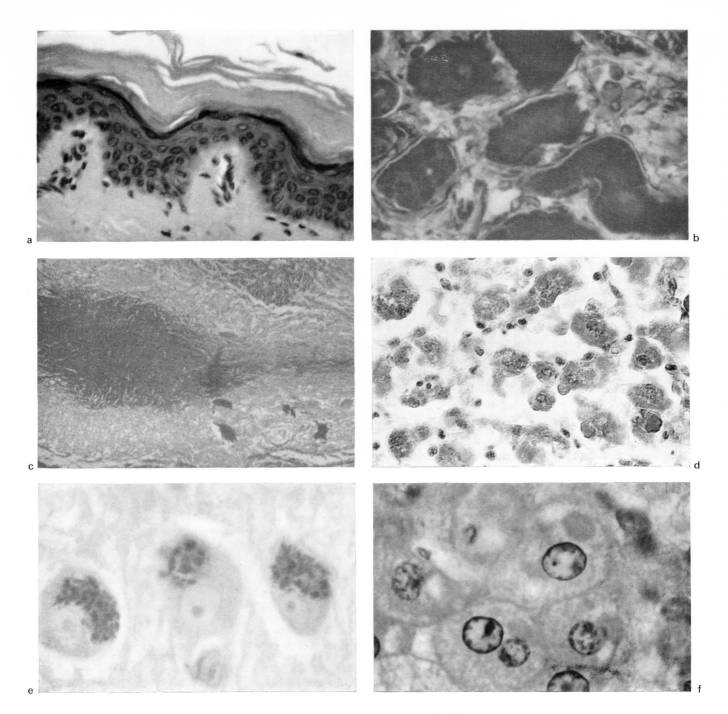

PLATE 25.3. Histology of cellular disorder.

(a) Normal human epidermis; karyolysis of nuclei occurs as the cells keratinize. Haem. & eosin (×430).

(c) Tubercle in a lymph node. Stained by anionic dye erythrosin which is bound intensely by protein (probably denatured) in caseous material and in giant cells (×110).

(e) Normal neurones from inferior olivary nucleus of a man aged 62. Abundant cytoplasmic granules of lipofuscin intensely coloured by periodic acid-Schiff technique (×1100).

(b) Renal tubules from infarct of kidney stained by Danielli's tetrazo method for protein. Conspicuous persistence of intensely coloured denatured protein in necrotic tubular cells (×440).

(d) Infective hepatitis; human liver cells filled with droplets of fat. Sudan IV (×400).

(f) Rat liver cells injured by CCl_4. Deposition of eosinophilic denatured protein as rounded bodies in cytoplasm of centrilobular hepatocytes. Haem. & eosin (×1100).

of protein ensues, along with the formation of numerous micromolecules of peptides and amino acids. Liberation of enzymes from lysosomes has been suggested as a cause of autolytic damage in dying liver cells.

HETEROLYSIS

In this process the dead cells are consumed by others. It is well seen in old infarcts and traumatic lesions of the cerebral cortex. Here cerebral histiocytes surround the dead neurones and consume them (neuronophagia). The necrotic grey matter is then liquefied into cystic spaces. This process is called softening or **malacia** (Greek *malakia*, softness); it is a typical example of liquefactive necrosis.

In infarcts of the cerebral cortex the remnants of the dead neurones, which may persist for months, are eventually entirely consumed; the necrotic grey matter is then replaced by cystic cavities containing cerebral histiocytes which are stuffed with granules, the remnants of the vanished neurones. The granules in the histiocytes contain a lipoprotein stainable by the PAS method (vol. 1, p. 13.3) and Sudan black. The granules may be derived by aggregation of the lipoprotein membranes of the disintegrated cells. This memorial to the vanished cells persists when all else is gone.

INTRACELLULAR AGGREGATION OR DEPOSITION

In derangement of this kind normal dispersed liquid or colloidal compounds of the cell become visibly aggregated, or abnormal liquids or colloids enter from outside or are formed *de novo* and then coalesce to give visible deposits. This aggregation or deposition may be due to interference with normal dispersion or to accumulation of the deposited material to such excess that it cannot be held in the dispersed state. Indeed interference with dispersion may so retard normal utilization and excretion that accumulation in excess becomes a consequence as well as a cause of deposition.

Accumulation of colloidal or liquid deposits may thus arise equally from disorganization of dispersion or from initial excess. The excess may depend on acceleration of entry, on formation and synthesis or on retardation of excretion and metabolism. The surplus of deposited material may be so gross as to inflate the cell with massive aggregations of apparently inert material. Deposition may be associated also with the growth or replication of intracellular parasites as exemplified by the inclusion bodies so frequently formed in cells infected by viruses.

Deposition of fat (triglyceride) and its determinants

The appearance of visible droplets of liquid fat in the cytoplasm is one of the most prominent features of disordered cells. In health, such droplets are seldom visible

and cannot be demonstrated in the normal cells of liver kidney or heart muscle. The fat in these tissues is not normally in a form capable of dissolving dyestuffs of the Sudan group. This invisible or concealed fat can, however, be extracted from the tissues by mixtures of lipid solvents and estimated by chemical methods.

The lipocytes of areolar tissue, on the other hand, contain droplets of liquid fat which have the capacity to dissolve the Sudan dyes; this visible fat displays the properties of a liquid, which forms a separate phase from the rest of the cytoplasm.

Cells which in health are devoid of visible fat may in disease contain spherical droplets of liquid fat in abundance; this fat, like that of the lipocytes, is in liquid form capable of being coloured by the Sudan dyes. This appearance is referred to as **fatty change**.

STATE OF INTRACELLULAR FAT

Fats and oils are not soluble in water but in the cell they may be so finely dispersed as to be invisible by microscopic methods. This capacity of cells to hold triglycerides in dispersion probably depends on the presence of phospholipids and proteins. Triglycerides, being hydrophobic, are prevented from dispersion in water by enormous interfacial forces. In living cells, therefore, unless dispersing agents are available, fats tend to aggregate into large spherical droplets, thus diminishing interfacial surfaces to a minimum.

Phospholipids, unlike fats, possess a hydrophilic portion in their ionizable phosphate and choline groups. In the cell, they form **laminar micelles** in which the polar ends are in contact with water or protein but the hydrocarbon chains are occluded internally and shielded from contact with the aqueous phase of the cytoplasm (fig. 25.13). Micelles of this type incorporate fats and oils

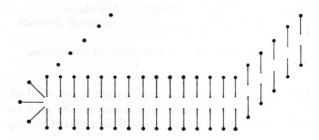

FIG. 25.13. Laminar micelle of phospholipid. Polar groups external in contact with aqueous phase, non-polar hydrocarbon chains occluded internally.

which by themselves are insoluble and indispersible in water. Thus, a mixture of phospholipid and neutral fat becomes readily dispersible (fig. 25.14). Intracellular invisible fat may thus be dispersed in the micelles of phospholipid and protein (fig. 25.15). Another possibility is

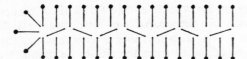

FIG. 25.14. Fat molecules in laminar micelle of phospholipid.

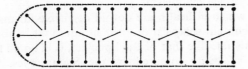

FIG. 25.15. Fat held in laminar micelle of phospholipid stabilized by adherent film of protein.

that a complex of fat with protein alone enables the fat to be dispersed simply as a lipoprotein. In either case the hydrophobic nonpolar fat is dispersed by being held out of contact with the aqueous phase of the cytoplasm.

The ratio of fat to phospholipid and protein thus plays a critical part in determining whether visible globules of fat occur in the cell or not. Excess of fat beyond the amount which can be accommodated in laminar micelles or lipoprotein complexes causes globular fat to be deposited. Similarly, lack of phospholipid and of protein promotes the same transition from dispersed to globular fat. As soon as globular fat makes its appearance there exists an equilibrium between it and dispersed fat (fig. 25.16).

Dispersed fat		*Globular fat*
Invisible or masked held in micelles or lipoprotein complexes	$\xrightarrow[\text{Phospholipid; protein}]{\text{Cholesterol}}$	Visible as spherical droplets

FIG. 25.16. Equilibrium between dispersed and globular fat.

In many normal cells this equilibrium is not reached, since all the triglycerides are dispersed as invisible micellar and lipoprotein fat. This is the situation in cells of healthy liver, kidney and heart muscle.

Once the threshold for deposition is passed, either excess of fat or lack of phospholipid and protein pushes the equilibrium from left to right so as to cause further deposition of visible droplets. Doubtless these visible droplets of fat are surrounded by unimolecular films of phospholipid which are held at the interphase so as to diminish interfacial tension to a minimum; in this way the visible fat of the cell is also held out of direct contact with water (fig. 25.17). Such an equilibrium between dis-

persed and globular fat probably exists in the lipocytes; in these cells it is known that fat exists in two compartments, a small compartment (dispersed fat) associated with the other cytoplasmic constituents and a large compartment of visible globular fat. As the ratio of fat to phospholipid and protein increases, the phospholipid and protein available for stabilizing the fat droplets in the manner shown in fig. 25.15 becomes less, so the size of the droplets increases. Finally, the lipocyte appears as a large single globule of fat surrounded by a tenuous film of cytoplasm.

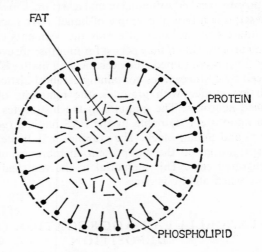

FIG. 25.17. Spherical globule of fat covered by a unimolecular film of orientated phospholipid with external adherent protein.

Another cellular constituent which may affect the equilibrium between dispersed fat and globular fat is cholesterol. This substance is known to antagonize the power of phospholipid to emulsify fat. It is thus likely that increase of intracellular cholesterol tends to push the equilibrium shown in fig. 25.16 from left to right and to promote the deposition of globular fat.

Visible globular fat is temporarily at least outside the zone of active transport and metabolism. Dispersed fat, on the other hand, is readily available for mobilization out of the cell and also for participating in enzymic reactions within the cell. Experiments on lipocytes have supported this concept of the dynamic cellular reactivity of dispersed fat. Thus centrifugal fractionation of lipocytes exposed to [14C-I] palmitic acid demonstrates that the dispersed cytoplasmic fat, not present in the visible droplets, rapidly incorporates the radioactive fatty acid, while the globular fat of the visible droplets only slowly assimilates it. Moreover, the dispersed fat of lipocytes has a much more rapid turnover than the fat present in the liquid globules.

The dominant position of dispersed fat in cell economy is emphasized in fig. 25.18. It is clear that dispersed fat

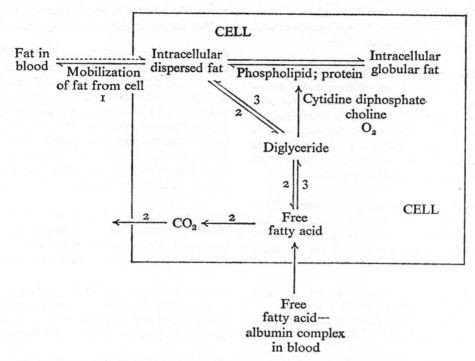

FIG. 25.18. Intracellular relation between dispersed fat and globular fat. Dispersed fat is the form in which fat is, (1) transported from the cell, (2) hydrolysed and oxidized, and (3) formed *de novo* from free fatty acid.

has a unique importance, since it is the form in which fat is:

(1) transported out of the cell (route 1),
(2) hydrolysed to FFA and then oxidized (route 2), and
(3) formed *de novo* in the cell from FFA (route 3).

The concept of an equilibrium between dispersed and globular fat, as well as the realization that dispersed fat is the form used for mobilization and metabolism, helps to envisage the mechanisms of fatty deposition in disease. Visible droplets of fat are formed when a certain ratio of fat to phospholipid and protein is surpassed or if the action of these substances in dispersing fat is impeded. It is thus clear that fatty deposition can arise in two principal ways:

(1) by interference with dispersion of fat, either from diminution in the quantity of phospholipid and protein or by annulment of their emulsifying action, and

(2) by quantitative increase of intracellular fat to an extent which cannot be accommodated in micelles or lipoprotein complexes; this usually depends on substantial accumulation of fat without compensating increase in phospholipid and protein.

Moreover, only invisible micellar or lipoprotein fat is likely to participate in metabolism and transport. Transition of dispersed to globular fat, which involves diminution in the quantity of the reactive form, thus impedes the removal of fat from the cell. This interference with removal promotes accumulation of fat; this happens even when fat is not entering the cell as such, since fat is formed *de novo* in the cell from FFA and from carbohydrate. Thus defective mobilization of fat itself results in accumulation of excess fat, and this promotes further deposition of visible globular fat.

INTERFERENCE WITH DISPERSION OF FAT

Lack of phospholipid inside the cell interferes with dispersion through a deficiency of the principal emulsifying agent. Thus in striated muscle affected by gas gangrene, fat is deposited because of destruction of stabilizing phospholipid by the exotoxin of *Cl. welchii* (p. 25.20). Also, as a result of poisoning by CCl_4, phospholipid in liver cells is probably altered by lipoperoxidation so that its dispersing power is diminished (p. 25.13).

Lack of choline and lack of inositol in the diet deprive the cell of essential constituents for the fabrication of phospholipids; thus deficiency of either of these substances in the diet of rats causes fatty deposition in the liver. Lack of choline may be conditioned by lack of methionine which provides labile methyl groups for synthesizing choline. These substances are referred to as lipotropic compounds.

Lack of oxygen interferes with synthesis of cytidine diphosphate choline which is an essential requisite for the synthesis of phospholipid (vol. 1, p. 10.18). This may be studied in liver slices by measuring the rate of incorporation of ^{32}P added to the medium into the phospholipids; lack of oxygen interrupts this incorporation. In this way it may impede dispersion of fat.

Lack of protein can also interfere with dispersion of fat, since protein as well as phospholipid is probably necessary for stabilizing dispersed fat. When rats are fed on a diet deficient in protein, visible fat rapidly appears in the hepatic cells even when methionine is supplied so as to provide for synthesis of choline; Best and his colleagues found that this deposition is accompanied by little or no increase in the total content of fat in the liver.

Excess of cholesterol fed to rats causes their liver cells to become bloated with fat. Cholesterol antagonizes the power of phospholipids to emulsify fats and in this way probably impedes their dispersion and so promotes deposition.

INITIAL QUANTITATIVE INCREASE IN INTRA-CELLULAR FAT AND ITS ACCUMULATION
This arises in two ways, firstly by excessive formation and entry of fat, and secondly by retardation of removal or excretion of fat.

Excessive formation and entry of fat
Hypoxia may cause excessive formation of fat within the cell from FFA, especially in cells of liver and heart muscle. FFA enters these cells from the blood and then has three major fates (fig. 25.19): (1) oxidation to CO_2, (2) conversion to phospholipid, and (3) conversion to fat.

It is clear that hypoxia eliminates route 1. Also, since oxygen is necessary for the synthesis of cytidine diphosphate choline, it eliminates also route 2. Thus hypoxia

effectively diverts the metabolism of FFA along route 3, so that fat accumulates in the hypoxic cells.

Lack of choline, by interfering with synthesis of cytidine diphosphate choline, may similarly divert FFA away from route 2 and along route 3. Indeed the addition of cytidine diphosphate choline to homogenates of rat liver impedes synthesis of fat as measured by the incorporation of ^{14}C-labelled glycerol into the liver triglycerides. Thus lack of choline may contribute to fatty deposition both by accelerating the formation of fat and by interfering with dispersion; choline deficiency probably does not play a role in human disease.

Discharge of depot fat, as in starvation, in diabetes, and in other wasting diseases, causes a rise in FFA in the blood and so may result in excessive entry of FFA into the liver with acceleration of fat formation along route 3.

Excessive entry of preformed fat may also contribute to accumulation in cells. This may occur in the liver in diabetes and also in histiocytes, when they ingest extracellular droplets of fat liberated from dead tissues.

Retardation of removal and excretion
All factors which interfere with dispersion retard the removal of fat from the cell and thus cause further deposition of visible intracellular fat. Cell injury may also interfere with the structural channels of excretion of fat from the cell by destroying the tubules of endoplasmic reticulum. Retardation of removal, however, can promote deposition only when fat is actually being formed in the cell or is entering from outside. Thus, when cell damage is so severe as to interrupt the synthesis of triglyceride

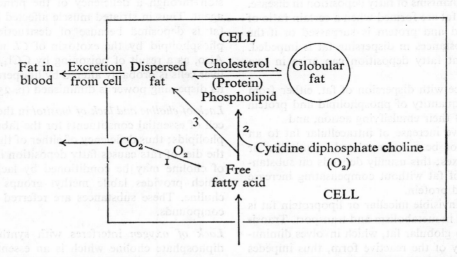

FIG. 25.19. Major intracellular fates of FFA in liver cells and cardiac muscle fibres. (1) Oxidation to CO_2; (2) conversion to phospholipid; (3) conversion to fat.

from FFA, retardation of removal cannot give rise to deposition.

Fatty deposition in disease

Cells are frequently exposed to circumstances which cause intracellular deposition of fat. Indeed, disease may both interfere with dispersion and excretion of fat and at the same time accelerate the formation of fat within the cell. Diseases and disorders associated with fatty deposition include cellular hypoxia, malnutrition, diabetes, poisoning and infection.

CELLULAR HYPOXIA

Intracellular deposition of fat results from generalized ischaemia in heart failure, from local ischaemia due to arterial occlusion or from severe anaemia. The cells of the liver and of the heart are specially susceptible.

Liver

In congestive heart failure the flow of blood along the sinusoids is retarded and when it reaches the central (zone 3) cells it is depleted of oxygen; the central cells may receive so little oxygen that they die, while the partially hypoxic zone 2 cells show conspicuous deposition of globular fat (plate 25.1d, facing p. 25.6). Two factors contribute to this fatty change. Firstly, the hypoxia causes intracellular lack of phospholipid and of protein, owing to interference with synthesis, and thus impedes dispersion of fat. Secondly, hypoxia inhibits the oxidation of FFA and also retards its conversion to phospholipid; the metabolism of FFA is therefore diverted along route 3 of fig. 25.19 to form excess of neutral fat. In the zone 2 cells, which show intense fatty change, hypoxia is sufficient to cause diversion of FFA to fat but is not sufficiently severe to kill the cells and so interrupt this metabolic conversion altogether, as happens in the most profoundly hypoxic central cells which thus contain less fat (plate 25.1d, facing p. 25.6). The typical 'nutmeg liver' of heart failure accordingly shows a tripartite zonal pattern; the most hypoxic central regions contain dilated congested sinusoids bordered by atrophic or necrotic cells, the partially hypoxic zone 2 cells are fatty, while the peripheral cells (zone 1) are unaffected.

Cardiac muscle

Hypoxia is a common cause of fatty deposition in cardiac muscle fibres. As in the liver sinusoids there is progressive depletion of oxygen from the blood as it passes along the capillaries which supply the cardiac fibres. The fibres situated near the arteriolar ends of capillaries are best supplied with oxygen, while the fibres placed near the terminations of capillaries in venules are nourished by more hypoxic blood. Thus anaemia and chronic progressive coronary occlusion may cause a zonal or patchy deposition of fat in cardiac muscle; in this condition the fatty change occurs in the regions where the cardiac fibres

21

are most hypoxic. Moreover, contraction of the heart contributes to the hypoxia, since during each systole the capillaries are temporarily closed. This occlusive effect is greatest in capillaries nearest to the ventricular cavities where intracardiac pressure is highest during systole. For this reason fatty change is usually more pronounced in the inner than the outer portions of ventricular muscle; in these visibly fatty parts there is a quantitative increase in the amount of extractable fat. Fatty deposition in ischaemic heart muscle is sometimes very prominent at the margins of regions where more severe hypoxia has caused necrosis. Between the necrotic and the unaffected fibres there is thus a zone of partial hypoxia where the fibres show intense fatty change.

FATTY DEPOSITION CAUSED BY MALNUTRITION

Acute starvation causes increased hydrolysis of fat in adipose tissue followed by a rise in the level of FFA in the blood. Excessive entry of FFA into the liver cells accelerates the formation of fat and is followed by accumulation with deposition. By feeding mice with linseed oil labelled with deuterium, Best and his colleagues succeeded in fattening mice with labelled tissue fat. These animals were then starved or injected with anterior pituitary extract and accumulation of hepatic fat labelled with deuterium followed. These experiments showed in a novel manner that fat deposited in the liver in starvation contains fatty acids derived from depot fat.

Chronic malnutrition is usually associated with deficiency of protein in the diet. This in itself interferes with dispersion of fat and causes its deposition in the liver (p. 25.32). Enlarged fatty livers are common in malnourished children in the tropics suffering from kwashiorkor. Usually these livers are also severely depleted of protein.

FATTY DEPOSITION IN HUMAN DIABETES

Lack of insulin in the juvenile type of diabetes is associated with severe wasting. As in starvation, FFA rises in the blood and more enters the liver. There, however, glycerokinase, absent from adipose tissue, ensures synthesis of triglyceride from FFA and glycerol. Quantitative accumulation of fat thus follows together with deposition of visible fat in the liver. In uncontrolled diabetes there is severe lipaemia due to the failure of adipose tissue to store fat. Lipaemia may then cause excessive entry of fat itself into the liver and thus result in further fatty deposition.

In the milder type of diabetes encountered in middle aged corpulent patients, the pancreas usually secretes insulin in significant amounts. In these patients there is probably excessive discharge of FFA from overloaded adipose tissue; this FFA is similarly converted to fat in the liver cells by esterification.

Hypercholesterolaemia is usual in all forms of diabetes;

this is probably another factor in hepatic fatty change, since cholesterol impedes the action of phospholipid in dispersing fat.

POISONING AND INFECTION
Carbon tetrachloride

After large doses of CCl_4 a characteristic pattern of cell injury develops in the liver lobules; a sequential transition is displayed from the centre to the periphery of each lobule through successive zones of cells. Plate 25.1e & f, facing p. 25.6, shows a typical sequence with fatty change most marked in zone 2.

Sometimes fatty change is more widespread and affects the central cells as well, but the peripheral cells are usually

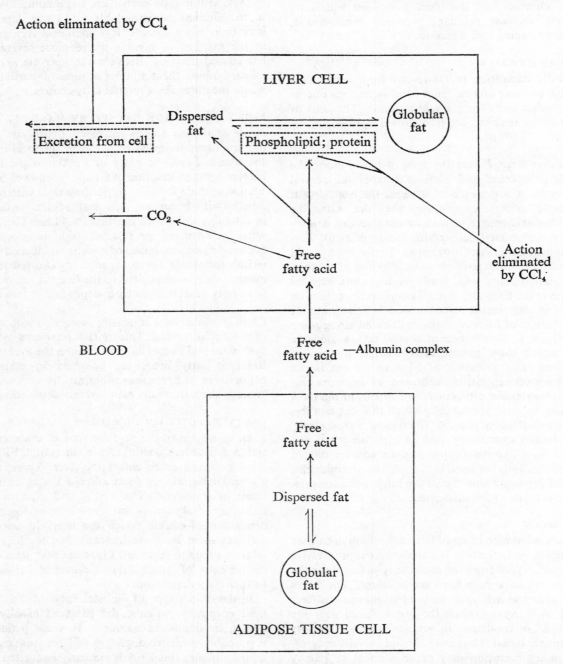

FIG. 25.20. Deposition of globular fat in liver damaged by CCl_4. By altering or decomposing phospholipid and so disintegrating lipoprotein micelles, CCl_4 converts dispersed fat into globular fat and prevents excretion of fat from the cell. Fat, however, continues to be formed from FFA and then becomes trapped as globular fat.

unaffected. This lobular distribution of cell injury suggests that lack of oxygen or of some other nutrient, such as α-tocopherol, contributes to damage (p. 25.5). If CCl_4 injures by initiating the decomposition or removal of phospholipid and thus disintegrating membranes and micelles, injury would be most severe in those cells which are in any case relatively deficient in phospholipid such as the central zone 3 cells of the lobule. The sharp zonal transition from unaffected to extremely fatty zone 2 cells may correspond to a ratio of fat to phospholipid which must be exceeded before visible droplets begin to form. Once visible deposition occurs, the excretion (mobilization) of fat from the cells is retarded and accumulation follows along with further deposition. There is evidence that CCl_4 also impedes the synthesis of protein in the liver cells by dislocation of ribosomes from the endoplasmic reticulum (p. 25.13); this action may also interfere with dispersion and so contribute to deposition. The most intense deposition is produced when interference with dispersion and continuous conversion of FFA to fat in the liver cells proceed simultaneously; then fat continues to pile up and pass into visible globules. This FFA itself is derived from the fat of adipose tissue, as demonstrated elegantly by Best. Mice fattened with linseed oil labelled with deuterium were exposed to CCl_4 vapour; the fat accumulated in their livers was rich in labelled fatty acid which must have come from the stores in their adipose tissue (fig. 25.20).

In the necrotic central zone 3 cells less fat is deposited because death arrests the conversion of FFA to fat.

Ethanol
Chronic alcoholism sometimes causes severe hepatic fatty change followed by cirrhosis. This effect is probably indirect and due to defective dietary intake of proteins and lipotropic factors. Thus when a man drinks a bottle of gin daily, he may eat little else. Careful experiments by Best and his colleagues indicate that ethanol ingested over long periods by rats conditions a deficiency of lipotropic factors and suggest that, provided adequate amounts of choline or methionine are included in the diet eaten, ethanol *per se* does not cause chronic fatty change. Acute intoxication by ethanol may, however, directly cause deposition of fat in the liver. Ashworth showed that when rats are fed large quantities of ethanol dissolved in oil, intense hepatic fatty change develops without any interference with synthesis of liver protein. It is possible that ethanol in large amounts may dissolve phospholipid and thus interfere with dispersion of fat or else promote excessive production of acetic acid followed by accelerated synthesis of fat.

Bacterial and viral infection
Intracellular fatty deposition is frequently visible in the organs of patients who die as a result of acute bacterial infection. Prolonged fever with anorexia and malnutrition may contribute to fatty deposition in these cases. In gas gangrene, droplets of fat occur in the fibres of the infected skeletal muscles and their content of fat is quantitatively increased. This deposition with accumulation doubtless depends on the α-toxin of *Cl. welchii*, which decomposes lecithin (p. 25.20) and thus interferes with the dispersion of fat. Viral hepatitis may cause intense fatty change in liver cells (plate 25.3d, facing p. 25.28).

Disintegration of myelin
The lipids sphingomyelin, cerebroside, lecithin and free cholesterol in the myelin sheath are orientated as bimolecular laminar micelles and are hydrophilic; when the myelin degenerates hydrophobic globular lipid is produced. A valuable means of distinguishing these products of degeneration is the Marchi reaction.

MARCHI REACTION
All cellular lipids have the capacity to dissolve osmium tetroxide (OsO_4). Dissolved OsO_4 reacts with the ethylenic bonds to produce black OsO_2 (or H_2OsO_4) which colours the lipids black. When potassium chlorate is mixed with OsO_4 it also dissolves in the lipids, provided they are hydrophilic, and effectively prevents reduction of OsO_4 to OsO_2. Hydrophobic lipids, on the other hand, cannot dissolve $KClO_3$, so they are blackened by a mixture of $KClO_3$ and OsO_4 just as effectively as by OsO_4 alone. This reaction differentiates hydrophilic lipids which remain uncoloured from hydrophobic lipids, including globular fat, which are coloured black (Adams). Thus normal myelin, which does not blacken (Marchi negative), is conveniently distinguished from degenerated myelin, which blackens (Marchi positive).

Sudan IV also distinguishes between normal and degenerating myelin, since it fails to stain the hydrophilic micellar lipids of normal myelin, but colours intensely the hydrophobic droplets formed by disintegration of the myelin sheath.

During the first phase of Wallerian degeneration, 3–7 days after section of a nerve, the myelin sheath below the point of section swells and fragments into 'ellipsoids' bounded by a double contoured envelope of myelin which surrounds a central aqueous space. During this phase no histochemical changes occur in the lipids of the myelin, which are still hydrophilic and Marchi negative. The axon of the severed nerve below the point of section simultaneously disintegrates into short filiform fragments each enclosed by an ellipsoid of degenerating myelin (fig. 25.21).

During the second phase of Wallerian degeneration, 7–15 days after section, the ellipsoids decompose into droplets of liquid lipid. These droplets are hydrophobic, Marchi positive, and are coloured by Sudan IV. Chemical and histochemical methods show that these

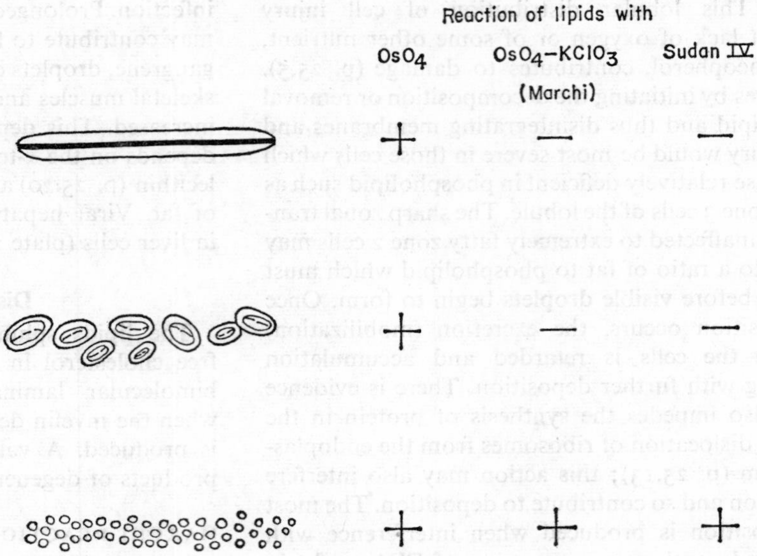

	Reaction of lipids with		
	OsO_4	OsO_4-KClO_3 (Marchi)	Sudan IV
Intact segment of a myelinated fibre with central axon	−	+	−
Degeneration, first phase, ellipsoids of myelin, fragments of axon	−	+	−
Degeneration, second phase, droplets of hydrophobic lipid	+	−	+
Degeneration, third phase, phagocytosis of hydrophobic lipid	+	−	+

FIG. 25.21. Wallerian degeneration in distal portion of a severed myelinated nerve fibre, showing change from hydrophilic myelin to hydrophobic globular lipid.

droplets are composed mainly of **cholesterol esters**. This change from hydrophilic to hydrophobic lipid entails the decomposition of the orientated laminar micelles of the compressed Schwann cell membranes into droplets of cholesterol ester. Although the precise chemical changes involved in this decomposition are unknown, the transformation is of great interest as it indicates the fate of the lipids of cell membranes when they disintegrate en masse. Recent work by Petrescu indicates that much of this conversion occurs within the invading phagocytes.

In the final or third phase of Wallerian degeneration these droplets of cholesterol ester are removed by phagocytes which invade the degenerating nerve.

Demyelination in the CNS, as observed in the plaques of disseminated sclerosis, probably consists of a similar change from hydrophilic micellar lipids into liquid droplets of hydrophobic cholesterol ester.

Deposition of cholesterol ester and fat in arteries

Atherosclerosis is a condition in which irregular fibrous thickening of the intima of arteries develops, coupled with deposition of lipids in this thickened layer. This process of thickening and deposition occurs usually in sharply defined plaques which appear as characteristic creamy patches visible on the inner surfaces of the arteries

(atheroma). In human atherosclerosis the most marked deposition of lipids takes place in the deepest part of the intima immediately adjacent to the internal elastic lamina (fig. 25.22), although deposition may be much more widespread and may even extend into the media.

The lipids in atheroma are deposited both within and

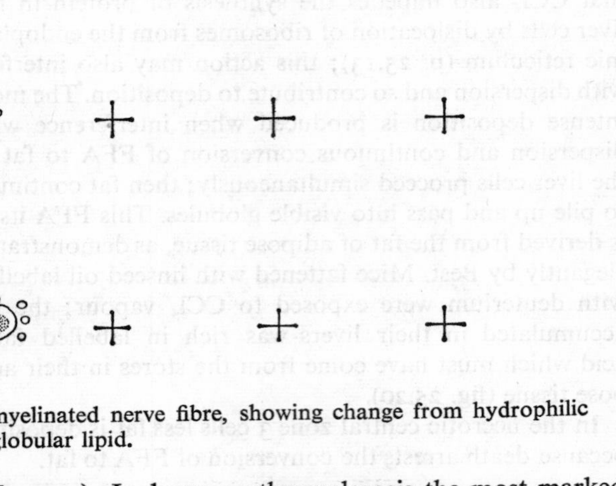

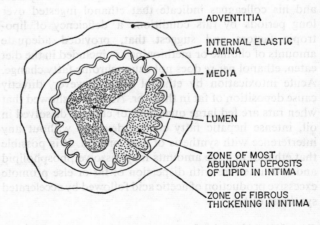

ADVENTITIA

INTERNAL ELASTIC LAMINA

MEDIA

LUMEN

ZONE OF MOST ABUNDANT DEPOSITS OF LIPID IN INTIMA

ZONE OF FIBROUS THICKENING IN INTIMA

FIG. 25.22. Atheroma in an artery. The most abundant deposition of lipid is in the deep part of the intima; the deposited lipids are both intracellular and extracellular.

between the cells in the intima of the affected arteries. The intracellular deposits consist of droplets of cholesterol ester and triglycerides. The extracellular deposits also contain cholesterol ester and triglycerides, but in addition include solid crystals of cholesterol.

The liquid droplets of cholesterol ester and of fat are readily stained by Sudan dyes, but these do not stain the solid crystals. Droplets of cholesterol ester and also solid crystals of free cholesterol are birefringent and appear brilliantly illuminated when examined between polaroid glasses. The intracellular deposits are located inside round and stellate histiocytes and also within fusiform fibrocytes.

The cause of atheroma is unknown but some of the factors which affect it indicate that the mechanisms involved include excess cholesterol and intimal hypoxia.

EXCESS OF CHOLESTEROL

Atheromatous deposits appear in the arteries of rabbits fed with cholesterol. In man, hypercholesterolaemia, which is occasionally an inherited disorder, occurs in such diseases as diabetes and hypothyroidism, and is often followed by severe and precocious atheroma. Cholesterol is itself a constituent of the deposited lipids and thus probably exerts a direct effect on deposition, but it may also interfere with dispersion of lipids by antagonizing the emulsifying action of phospholipid.

INTIMAL HYPOXIA

The deepest zone of the intima, immediately inside the internal elastic lamina, is the most hypoxic part of the arterial wall and is also usually the site of the most abundant deposition of lipids. The hypoxia in the outer intima probably becomes even more severe when the effective distance through which arterial oxygen must diffuse is increased by localized mural thrombosis. The deposition of lipid is probably determined by

(1) excessive entry or formation of lipids, due to increased entry of lipids from the blood in hyperlipaemia and hypercholesterolaemia, or to diversion of metabolism by hypoxia;

(2) inhibition of removal of lipids, due to interference with dispersion of lipids by lack of protein or phospholipid (in hypoxia) or by excess of cholesterol.

Two of the commonest sites for human atheroma are the coronary and cerebral arteries, and ischaemic injury to the heart and to the brain as a result of atherosclerosis is the commonest cause of death in men over 40.

Deposition of complex lipids

NEURONAL LIPOFUSCIN

Neurones which die are not replaced and the metabolic activity of those which survive is lifelong. Even without functional impairment, however, time alone exerts an effect on neurones by causing the progressive deposition of clusters of yellowish granules of **lipofuscin** or 'wear and tear' pigment. This deposition is universal in mankind and appears to be occurring continuously in nerve cells, heart and liver as well as other organs (p. 36.5).

Prominent masses of lipofuscin are present in the pyramidal cells of the cerebral cortex, in spinal ventral horn cells and in the cell bodies of the hypoglossal nuclei in the elderly and aged. In the neurones of the olivary nucleus, however, this deposition occurs much earlier in life and by middle age these cells contain abundant and uniform clusters of coarsely granular lipofuscin (plate 25.3e, facing p. 25.28).

Neuronal lipofuscin contains both protein and lipid. Lipofuscin is coloured intensely by Sudan black and also by the PAS method which stains the granules a vivid rose red. The presence of complex lipid, which is possibly glycolipid, in lipofuscin accounts for its intense colouration by these stains. Prolonged extraction with alcoholic-ether partially removes the lipids of lipofuscin; unfortunately this does not imply that old age can be averted by copious draughts of alcoholic fluids.

A material very similar to lipofuscin is deposited in the neurones of rats and monkeys fed on diets deficient in vitamin E; this is probably due to autoxidation of lipid normally inhibited by Vitamin E (vol. 1, p. 10.10). Einarson suggested that similar autoxidation over long periods of time accounts for the deposition of lipofuscin in old age. Autoxidation of the membrane lipids of the cell surface and organelles may thus interfere with dispersion and so cause aggregation of the disorganized lipoprotein laminae into globular lipofuscin, which then accumulates as an indestructible remnant throughout the perennial course of neuronal life. This process would thus be specially prominent in the neurone, with its relatively immense area of cell surface.

AMAUROTIC FAMILY IDIOCY (TAY–SACHS DISEASE)

This disease, caused by a rare abnormal recessive gene, leads to idiocy and blindness associated with deposition of excessive amounts of complex lipoprotein containing both ganglioside (vol. 1, p. 10.5) and cholesterol in the neurones of the brain and retina. The cerebral neurones swell into grotesque forms bloated by copious deposits. This change occurs in the cell bodies and also in the apical dendrites of pyramidal cells which develop bizarre swellings filled with lipid. The ganglion cells of the retina are also filled by these deposits, which give a creamy appearance to the retina, but as the optic fibres degenerate, the central fovea becomes more transparent than usual so that the red reflex of the choroid causes the foveal area to appear as a 'cherry red' spot on the creamy retinal background. Under EM the cytoplasm of the cerebral neurones appears filled with laminated spheroids; these bodies are about 1 μm in diameter and have a laminar periodicity of 5–6 nm. It is likely, therefore, that there is a basic abnormality in the array of lipoprotein membranes which produces these laminar aggregates in the neurones; this deposition is later followed by degeneration of axons and disintegration of their myelin sheaths.

HUNTER SYNDROME (GARGOYLISM)
This inherited abnormality is described on p. 30.6.

The mental defect is possibly due to the deposition of a complex lipid in the cerebral neurones which become stuffed with granules composed of ganglioside and protein (fig. 25.23a). A striking neuronal abnormality is the presence of fusiform swellings on the axons of the cerebellar Purkinje cells; these enlargements are filled by granules of lipid, stainable by Sudan black (fig. 25.23b).

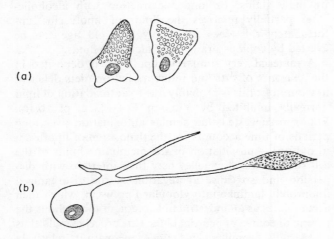

(a)

(b)

FIG. 25.23. Hunter syndrome in a child aged 4 years. (a) Spinal ventral horn cells; frozen section. Stained PAS (× 300). (b) Cerebellar Purkinje cells with fusiform swelling on a dendrite; wax embedded section. Stained Sudan black (× 300).

Deposition of protein
Disorders of cells may produce deposits in which protein is the dominant constituent. Such deposition may be due to aggregation of the original cellular protein or may result from excessive formation or entry of abnormal protein.

ACTION OF METALS
Metals can aggregate protein so as to deposit within the cell a metallic-protein complex. These metals include iron and copper.

Iron is stored within cells as **ferritin**, a macromolecule with an electron-dense centre rich in iron surrounded by a shell of protein. Normally ferritin is dispersed in the cytoplasm, but when iron is present in excess the mole-cules aggregate into brown granules of haemosiderin which are coloured dark blue by potassium ferrocyanide. Phagocytes which destroy red blood cells contain both dispersed ferritin and also granules of haemosiderin, which appear by EM as aggregates of ferritin and are often situated inside saccular organelles called siderosomes. In haemolytic anaemia granules of haemosiderin and also dispersed ferritin accumulate in the hepatic parenchyma as well as in phagocytic cells. In the hereditary disease **haemochromatosis**, iron is absorbed into the body in excess and haemosiderin slowly accumulates in the cells of many organs. In the liver cells numerous electron-dense particles of ferritin are visible by EM both dispersed through the cytoplasm and aggregated as granules of haemosiderin. This deposition is eventually associated with hepatic cirrhosis. Deposition of haemosiderin also damages the myocardial fibres with resultant heart failure, while involvement of the pancreatic islets leads to the development of diabetes.

Copper occurring in excess in the cells causes **hepato-lenticular degeneration (Wilson's disease)**, in which a copper-protein complex is deposited in liver cells and probably also in the neurones of the corpus striatum. In the liver this eventually produces cirrhosis, while degeneration of striatal neurones causes tremor and rigidity. Copper also accumulates in brown granules deposited near the corneal limbus to give a characteristic brown ring sometimes visible in the outer cornea, the Kayser–Fleischer ring. The basic determinant of this disease is congenital absence or deficiency of **caeruloplasmin**, the α_2-globulin-copper complex of normal plasma. Without caeruloplasmin there is a rise of free copper in the blood along with excessive entry into the tissues. This disease is caused by a recessive gene (pp. 31.5 & 10.13).

ACTION OF ORGANIC POISONS
When rats are injected with CCl_4 hyaline eosinophilic inclusions rich in protein appear in the cytoplasm of centrilobular liver cells. This change is probably a prelude to necrosis and involves aggregation of protein along with denaturation to an intensely acidophilic material. Later these eosinophilic masses occupy most of the cytoplasm of the necrotic cells. Fat is deposited simultaneously with protein and alteration of phospholipid in lipoprotein membranes probably initiates these changes (plate 25.3f, facing p. 25.28).

A very similar material, **Mallory's alcoholic hyaline,** is deposited as irregular eosinophilic spherules in the liver cells of chronic alcoholics. This material is rich in protein and is probably derived from disorganized mitochondria and endoplasmic reticulum. Chronic alcoholism may act by causing lack of lipotropic factors (p. 25.35). Hartroft observed deposition of a similar substance in livers of rats fed on a diet deficient in choline. It seems likely that lack of phospholipid in the hepatic cells of chronic alcoholics may thus result in deposition both of protein as 'alcoholic hyaline' and of liquid globules of fat.

EFFECTS OF VIRAL INFECTION

Inclusion bodies rich in protein are formed in many cells by viral infection and are situated in the cytoplasm or in the nucleus.

Cytoplasmic inclusion bodies

Infection by the poxviruses often produces spheroidal eosinophilic masses in the cytoplasm of epidermal cells. These sometimes enlarge to occupy most of the cytoplasm. Plate 25.2c, facing p. 25.14, shows eosinophilic inclusions which are rich in protein in rabbit epidermis infected by vaccinia. The elementary bodies of the virus, which contain DNA, are elaborated within the inclusion bodies, which consist mostly of protein, whether derived from the host cytoplasm or from the virus; the elementary bodies are fabricated in these specialized zones of cytoplasm where the local protein is aggregated by viral action. Cytoplasmic inclusions produced by the reoviruses are actual arrays of viral elementary bodies (nucleoprotein). But in some viral infections cytoplasmic inclusions are mere aggregates of host-cell protein produced by cellular injury. Thus the **Negri bodies**, produced in hippocampal neurones and Purkinje cells infected by the 'street virus' of rabies, are spherical deposits of host cell protein. Also in yellow fever the entire cytoplasm of dying liver cells may aggregate into hyaline masses rich in protein, called **Councilman bodies**.

Nuclear inclusion bodies

Infection by viruses of the herpes group and by measles produces type A intranuclear inclusions. These are large hyaline eosinophilic masses of protein which occupy most of the nucleus except for a peripheral clear zone separating them from the nuclear membrane. Although these inclusions may indicate the zone where viral replication originally occurred, the final eosinophilic remnant is probably an aggregate of degenerate cell protein. Type B intranuclear inclusions are small spheroidal aggregates of protein which are visible within the nuclei of neurones infected by poliovirus, which itself replicates in the cytoplasm. These type B inclusions must therefore be regarded as deposits of protein produced indirectly by viral infection. Adenoviruses, which replicate within the nucleus, produce large intranuclear arrays of viral nucleoprotein arranged in twenty-sided microcrystalline icosahedra. Inside the nuclei of cells infected by adenoviruses crystals of protein distinct from the elementary bodies of the virus may also be deposited.

EXCESSIVE ENTRY OF PROTEIN

After experimental intraperitoneal injections of egg white,

the egg ovomucoid, a glycoprotein, is excreted through the renal glomeruli and is later reabsorbed by the renal tubules. During this process of reabsorption of ovomucoid the tubular cells contain conspicuous granules of glycoprotein which stain intensely with the PAS method. The reabsorbed ovomucoid is thus partly deposited as granules in the renal cells. Similarly in disease in man associated with proteinuria, hyaline eosinophilic droplets of protein may be seen in the cells of the convoluted tubules.

Phagocytic cells can ingest the entire nuclei of lysed or vanished cells. Ingested homogeneous masses containing protein and DNA are visible in polymorphs of blood treated with serum containing the anti-nuclear LE factor of lupus erythematosus (p. 25.26).

EXCESSIVE FORMATION OF PROTEIN

Large amounts of globulin are formed in plasma cells during the synthesis of antibodies. When these globulins contain antibody to a specific antigen like diphtheria toxoid, the antibody can be detected by preliminary adsorption of added antigen followed by subsequent pin-pointing of the adsorbed antigen with specific fluorescent antibody (sandwich technique). Sometimes the fabrication of antibody within plasma cells is so excessive that hyaline masses of protein (Russell bodies) are deposited in their cytoplasm (p. 21.11).

Deposition of glycogen

Excessive deposition of glycogen occurs in certain cells in diabetes. Although lack of insulin impedes the entry of glucose into skeletal muscle, it does not interfere with penetration of glucose into liver, heart muscle and pancreatic islets. Thus in diabetic hyperglycaemia the cells of these organs contain excessive glucose, which is deposited as glycogen in the cytoplasm of cardiac muscle fibres and pancreatic insular cells, and also as characteristic intranuclear 'vacuoles' in liver cells. Deposition of glycogen within cells is seen also in glycogen storage disease (pp. 25.2 & 31.9).

INVISIBLE DERANGEMENTS OF METABOLISM, BEHAVIOUR AND GROWTH

Metabolic defects of the cell

Up till now we have considered visible disintegration of the cell or visible aggregation and deposition of materials within it. Invisible defects in metabolic activity are now discussed briefly.

Many defects of metabolism cause the accumulation of soluble substances in the tissue fluids. Indeed excesses in the blood and urine of soluble substances, insufficiently absorbed or liberated by cells in excess, have been extensively investigated in metabolic disease. But it is well to remember that such accumulation merely reflects more fundamental derangements of the cells themselves. Thus hyperglycaemia of diabetes partly reflects failure of the cells to absorb glucose; the hyperbilirubinaemia in hepatic jaundice indicates that damage to hepatic cells has interfered with the uptake of bilirubin, synthesis or transport of bilirubin glucuronide and thus interrupted the normal process of disposal and excretion (vol. 1, p. 31.10).

Metabolic defects of cells include:

(1) retardation of absorption of substances by the cell,

(2) acceleration, retardation or diversion of chemical processes within the cell, and

(3) retardation of excretion of substances by the cell.

RETARDATION OF ABSORPTION BY THE CELL

This may be due to defective ingestion by the cell as in Addisonian pernicious anaemia; in this disease vitamin B_{12} is imperfectly absorbed by the cells of the intestinal mucosa. Defective cellular penetration of glucose is caused by lack of insulin. Defective renal tubular re-absorption of the amino acids cystine, lysine, arginine and ornithine results in cystinuria; in this inherited defect the relatively insoluble cystine crystallizes out of the urine and leads to the formation of urinary calculi.

ACCELERATION, RETARDATION OR DIVERSION OF CHEMICAL PROCESSES WITHIN THE CELL

When the rate of formation of any metabolite is accelerated so as to outpace its rate of disposal, then this metabolite accumulates in excess. For instance, in gout the rate of formation of uric acid in the cells is increased so that excretion from the body cannot keep pace with it; uric acid, therefore, accumulates and is later deposited in tissues as crystals of sodium urate. Recently this excessive formation of uric acid has been successfully curbed by treatment with allopurinol (p. 29.9), which inhibits the oxidation of hypoxanthine and xanthine to uric acid. In alkaptonuria the normal disposal of homogentisic acid, formed from tyrosine, is abolished or retarded; homogentisic acid therefore accumulates and is excreted in the urine (vol. 1, p. 11.24). In **phenylketonuria** the hereditary deficiency of the enzyme phenylalanine hydroxylase in the liver cells retards or deletes the normal oxidation of phenylalanine to tyrosine; phenylalanine therefore accumulates and some of it is diverted along an alternative path to phenylpyruvic acid, which is then excreted in the urine (vol. 1, p. 11.24). Ketosis in diabetes and starvation arises by a disproportionate metabolism of triglycerides, so that acetoacetic acid is formed in excess by hepatic cells.

RETARDATION OF EXCRETION OF SUBSTANCES BY THE CELL

Defective disposal of fat in fatty deposition shows how retardation of excretion can cause accumulation; here the basic fault is probably a defect in dispersion of fat.

Defects of function

ELECTRICAL ACTIVITY

Both electrical activity of the cerebral cortex and consciousness are rapidly abolished by hypoxia. These effects follow within a few seconds of curtailment in the supply of energy to the neurones; irreversible injury to the cells occurs more slowly. In cerebral concussion the electrical activity of the cerebral cortex diminishes or ceases and consciousness is lost simultaneously. Often there is no macroscopic evidence of cerebral damage, although the Nissl granules in some of the neurones are rapidly agglutinated and fragmented. Death of neurones immediately abolishes their electrical activity; thus thermocoagulation at 80°C of the cerebral cortex of monkeys immediately and permanently deletes the characteristic potential changes in the injured cortical region. Similarly the electrical activity of myocardial fibres is abolished by infarction of heart muscle.

MEMORY

Repetitive patterns of electrical activity at the neuronal surface, which are themselves determined by mutually aligned and complementary mosaics of lipid and protein molecules, may provide the physical basis for memory and thought. In concussion, disalignment of these lipid and peptide patterns at cell surface membranes would account for coma and arrest of electrical activity. Also this traumatic disalignment may interrupt the process of synthesis of the complementary, and inherited, peptide patterns which are responsible for the continued re-creation of their counterpart lipid patterns; thus the transient lipid patterns derived from recently received impressions would never become catalogued into the archives of permanent memory. This type of mechanism would explain why concussion is so frequently followed by **retrograde amnesia** for events immediately preceding the accident, while memory for long past episodes is unimpaired. Just as in old age, when memory of recent happenings may fade rapidly, concussion erases the traces of recent memory more readily than those of remote memory.

Neoplasia

Neoplasia is a derangement of growth and is discussed in chap. 28. The basic disorder in neoplastic cells involves a somatic mutation with either visible or invisible (molecular) change of karyotype. The change to fully malignant cells which are both invasive and metastatic probably occurs in several stages. Rous and his colleagues showed that the application of chemical carcinogens to the skin of rabbits is followed by a sequence of changes:

(1) hyperkeratosis,

(2) the appearance of several papillomata in the keratotic area, and

(3) the change of one of the papillomata to a carcinoma.

If the carcinogen ceases to be applied at any stage before (3), the lesions regress. However, reapplication either of the carcinogen or of less specific irritants such as turpentine rapidly revives the papillomata in the same sites as before. These observations led Rous to suggest that a latent change occurs in the cells and to call the specific substances which cause the latent change initiating agents, and the less specific irritants which determine the final change to malignancy promoting agents. The change towards malignant neoplasia may be determined by a highly specific chemical or physical initiating agent which causes a somatic mutation. The mutant cells may be unstable and so tend to mutate further. Further mutants are usually not viable or are suppressed by more robust normal contemporaries, but if the latter are put at a disadvantage by adverse and possibly non-specific promoting agents, a potentially malignant mutant may be put at an advantage and so survive. The initial mutation may be an invisible macromolecular change in DNA, although pre-malignant changes in, for example, human uterine cervical epithelium usually involve visible change of karyotype.

VISIBLE EFFECTS OF CELL INJURY

Changes in diseased tissues which are visible to the naked eye at autopsy or to microscopic examination only, include:

(1) alterations in size, colour, opacity and consistency which are directly determined by intracellular events, and

(2) indirect intercellular reactions to cell injury such as congestion, haemorrhage and oedema.

These changes provide a useful indication of cell damage, but they are notoriously deceptive in assessing the actual state of the damaged cell.

Post mortem change

Visible changes caused by cellular disintegration in the body after death must be carefully distinguished from those which occur *ante mortem* in diseased tissues of the living body. Most of the cells of internal organs examined at autopsy are already dead. Although the lipoprotein membranes of these dead cells are disarranged, changes detectable by the naked eye or by routine microscopy do not occur for many hours. Usually autopsies are performed on refrigerated bodies or within 24 hours of death; under these circumstances *post mortem* disintegration is not readily detectable, although some tissues are perceptibly softened.

Post mortem disintegration or **autolysis** proceeds at different rates in different tissues; it is relatively slow in brain and relatively rapid in kidney and intestine. When a dead body remains at room temperature for 4 days the kidneys are softened into a semifluid consistency; microscopic examination of the fixed tissue shows that the cells of the convoluted tubules are disintegrated, although relatively little change is seen in the glomeruli and collecting tubules. In the convoluted tubules the cells are separated from one another, and their nuclei disappear. The liver is flabby and shows intercellular fissures; however the dissociated hepatic cells are remarkably intact, and the majority of their nuclei, although small, are still stainable by haematoxylin.

Ante mortem change

If degeneration or death of cells occurs during the patient's life, *ante mortem* changes alter the appearance of the tissues and cells so that they may be differentiated from those in which changes have occurred only after the patient's death. Visible changes determined by *ante mortem* cellular disorder include the following.

AQUEOUS SWELLING

Injured or dying cells can absorb water and swell as long as their osmotic properties remain intact. *Post mortem* swelling is usually not discernible because semipermeability is rapidly lost. However, sometimes *ante mortem* cellular swelling and vacuolation may result in enlargement of the injured tissue visible at autopsy. Thus infarcts of the cerebral cortex often appear swollen; such swelling is best detected by comparison of the necrotic cortex with unaffected grey matter from the opposite hemisphere. This change is probably caused by vacuolation of neurones and their dendrites and also by swelling of oligodendroglia as a result of cerebral ischaemia. On microscopic examination such swollen cortex is seen to have disintegrated into loose spongy tissue perforated by numerous lacunae.

The term **cloudy swelling** was originally applied by Virchow to a change which he observed in renal tubular cells in glomerulonephritis; these cells, when examined in sections of unfixed and unstained tissue, appeared swollen and granular. Unfortunately, this term has since been applied indiscriminately as an imaginary condition wished on the cells of any organ which appeared soft or swollen at autopsy; it was supposed to indicate that the cells had suffered injury during the patient's life. When dying cells swell they become more transparent and not more opaque, probably because their intracellular organelles become enlarged. When cells suffer coagulative necrosis they do indeed become opaque, or cloudy, owing to denaturation of intracellular protein. This 'cloudy' change, however, is quite independent of swelling and may indeed be accompanied by shrinkage. In any case cloudiness and swelling of cells before fixation cannot be deduced from microscopic examination of stained sections of fixed tissue, nor can the size of cells be judged by naked eye inspection of tissues at autopsy. The term cloudy swelling should therefore be discarded.

FATTY CHANGE
Deposition of liquid droplets of globular fat in the cells of liver and myocardium makes these tissues yellowish in appearance and greasy to touch. The fatty cells are turbid and opaque and their distribution may produce a conspicuous pattern of pale zones alternating with apparently normal tissue.

Liver
In diabetes, in alcoholism and in malnutrition the liver may appear uniformly fatty, but if cirrhosis supervenes the yellowish regions are subdivided by grey or pinkish strands of compressed connective tissue. In infective hepatitis zonal centrilobular fatty change produces a prominent lobular pattern. Heart failure also causes patterned fatty change in the liver; the pale fatty regions of the lobules are peripheral or midzonal and they present a striking contrast to the dark red centrilobular zones of ischaemic atrophy, necrosis and congestion.

Heart
Deposition of fat in the myocardial cells was vividly described by William Stokes in 1854: 'the substance of the ventricle was softened, most easily broken by the finger, and of a pale yellowish colour . . . the scalpel was greased in cutting the muscular substance'. This fatty change is usually most conspicuous in the inner parts of the myocardium which are relatively the most ischaemic. Fatty change may uniformly affect continuous zones of myocardium or the fatty myocardial fibres may occur in clusters so as to give a speckled pattern.

FATTY INFILTRATION
This condition is described here because the term is often confused with fatty change. It is, however, not a disorder of cells; it indicates simply an increase of adipose tissue in an organ by infiltration of groups of lipocytes among the parenchymal cells. This is seen usually in association with general obesity, and in these circumstances is found commonly in the heart.

HYALINE
This term is often used to describe an eosinophilic homogeneous, rather structureless material which can be seen microscopically in tissue in certain conditions. It is a descriptive term and has no constant biochemical connotation. The appearance is usually found in connective tissues, especially in the walls of small blood vessels in high blood pressure, diabetes and old age, or in old

fibrous scars. It is also commonly employed in the description of **alcoholic hyaline**, described on p. 25.38, and of hyaline droplets of reabsorbed protein in renal tubules.

COAGULATIVE NECROSIS
In this condition the cells become hardened and opaque like ground glass, and their nuclei are lost by karyolysis. Tissues composed of these necrotic cells become indurated and opacified. Wagner, in 1864, described coagulative necrosis of the respiratory passages in diphtheria, while Weigert noted a similar state in epidermis over smallpox pustules. Coagulative necrosis occurs in the tracheal epithelium after exposure to NH_3 and other corrosive gases. It was at one time thought that fibrinogen entered the dead tissue and clotted within it to form fibrin which hardened the tissue. This indeed probably happens in diphtheria to produce the yellowish grey 'false membrane' which is composed of fibrin, necrotic epithelial cells and polymorphs. But in most tissues coagulative necrosis is due to denaturation of the cells' own protein, which congeals to make them homogeneous and opaque. The outline of the dead cells is usually preserved and they are intensely coloured by acidic dyes such as eosin and erythrosin owing to exposure of $-NH_3^+$ groups in the side chains of the unravelled denatured proteins.

In pale infarcts of the kidney and spleen, ischaemia causes coagulative necrosis of continuous masses of cells. The necrotic zones are whitish owing to expression of blood and are also opaque and hard. Such pale infarcts are usually surrounded by a red zone of inflammation. Coagulative necrosis of the cells occurs also in red infarcts of cerebral cortex, lung and intestine; the striking feature of these lesions, however, is their brown-red colour produced by extravasation of red blood cells. Indeed the colour of red cerebral infarcts was graphically likened to the dregs of wine ('la lie de vin') by Léon Rostan in 1823.

In congestive cardiac failure ischaemia produces coagulative necrosis of the centrilobular cells of the liver. The dead cells shrivel, become eosinophilic and lose their nuclei, while the intercellular sinusoids become dilated and filled with red cells. This produces dark red colouration of the centrilobular zones to give the typical 'nutmeg' pattern in the livers of patients dying with chronic heart failure. This spectacular lobular pattern is primarily determined by congestion and not by cellular death, although the intralobular contrast is heightened by fatty change which gives a pale appearance to the midzonal or peripheral regions.

CASEATION OR CASEOUS NECROSIS
In this process tuberculous exudates and neighbouring tissue are transformed into creamy-white cheesy débris (Latin *caseus*, cheese) (p. 21.16). All cell outlines vanish

and the nuclei also disappear (karyolysis) or disintegrate into basophilic granules (karyorrhexis). The cytoplasmic remnants are granular and eosinophilic. Later calcium salts may be absorbed by caseous foci, which then become hard and chalky white (calcification).

GUMMATOUS NECROSIS

This sequel to cell death occurs in tertiary syphilis (p. 21.19). The dead cells coalesce into a rubbery mass called a gumma (Latin *cummi*, gum), which is pale brown or creamy-white in colour. Some of the cell outlines remain and the cells do not disintegrate into the amorphous granular débris seen in caseation. Zones of gummatous necrosis occur within the typical diffuse lesions of tertiary syphilis and therefore become surrounded by dense greyish white fibrous tissue.

GANGRENE

Dead tissues, when exposed to bacteria, have a low resistance to infection; they subsequently become blackened. This change is called gangrene. The black colour is caused by conversion of haemoglobin and myoglobin into dark pyrrol pigments. Dry and wet types of gangrene are recognized, and are described on p. 26.10.

Gas gangrene

This specific disintegration of striated muscle follows infection by pathogenic clostridia. The exotoxins secreted by *Cl. welchii* and *Cl. oedematiens* kill the muscle fibres as well as causing fatty deposition within them. Enzymes from the clostridia then ferment muscle glycogen to produce bubbles of gas beneath the sarcolemma; the dead muscle becomes crepitant. Subsequent decomposition of muscle proteins, including myoglobin, by saprophytic *Cl. histolyticum* and *Cl. sporogenes* finally converts the muscle into a greenish-black deliquescent mass.

LIQUEFACTIVE NECROSIS

This process occurs typically when dead cerebral neurones are consumed by microglial phagocytes and cerebral grey matter is replaced by softened spongy tissue containing cystic cavities filled with fluid. Infarcts of the cerebral cortex begin to show this liquefaction after a few weeks and are later transformed into brown or greyish zones of softening, where phagocytic cells called 'compound granular corpuscles' erode the dead neurones. Ultimately all remnants of the neurones are consumed by these phagocytes, which become stuffed with lipoprotein granules probably derived from the lipoprotein membranes of the vanished neurones.

Conclusion

The fate of lipoprotein membranes of necrotic cells in liquefactive necrosis of nervous tissue is an appropriate theme on which to conclude this chapter, as it emphasizes how macromolecular disorientation and disarray will increasingly be studied in the cytopathology of the future.

The lipoprotein mosaic which forms the cell membrane requires for its maintenance a continuous supply of energy in the form of ATP derived from cell respiration. Neurones, which have the greatest surface/volume ratio and the greatest relative membrane area of all cells, thus require the highest rate of supply of energy. This exceptional demand accounts for the unique vulnerability of the neurone to ischaemia. Irreversible injury to this extensive array of orientated lipoprotein at neuronal surfaces therefore rapidly follows ischaemia. But the vast lipoprotein mosaic in the dead neurones, although disarrayed, is resistant to catabolism and becomes aggregated into granules of lipoprotein which persist inside cerebral phagocytes in zones of liquefactive necrosis. The most vulnerable of cells thus leave the most lasting memorial.

> The thorns he spares when the rose is taken;
> The rocks he leaves when he wastes the plain.
> The wind that wanders, the weeds wind-shaken,
> These remain.
>
> Algernon Charles Swinburne

FURTHER READING

ADAMS C.W.M. (1965) Demyelination: morphology, histochemistry and biochemistry, in *Neurohistochemistry*, ed. C.W.M. Adams. Amsterdam: Elsevier.

BANGHAM A.D. *et al.* (1962) Action of saponin on biological membranes. *Nature* **196**, 952.

BASSI M. & BERNELLI-ZAZZERA A. (1964) Ultrastructural changes of liver cells after reversible and irreversible ischaemia. *Exp. molec. Path.* **3**, 332.

DIXON K.C. (1965) Ischaemia and the neurone, in *Neurohistochemistry*, ed. C.W.M. Adams. Amsterdam: Elsevier.

—— (1967) Events in dying cells. *Proc. roy. Soc. Med.* **60**, 271.

EINARSON L. & KROGH E. (1955) Variations in the basophilia of nerve cells associated with increased cell activity and functional stress. *J. Neurol. Neurosurg. Psychiat.* **18**, 1.

VAN HARREVELD A. (1961) Asphyxial changes in cerebellar cortex. *J. cell. comp. Physiol.* **57**, 101.

HIRSCH J.G., BERNHEIMER A.W. & WEISSMANN G. (1963) Motion picture study of the toxic action of streptolysin on leucocytes. *J. exp. Med.* **118**, 223.

KAROW A.M. & WEBB W.R. (1965) Tissue freezing: a theory of injury and survival. *Cryobiology* **2**, 99.

KEMP N.H., STAFFORD J.L. & TANNER R. (1964) Chromosome studies during early and terminal myeloid leukaemia. *Brit. med. J.* **i**, 1010.

KERR J.F.R. (1965) A histochemical study of hypertrophy and ischaemic injury of rat liver with special reference to changes in lysosomes. *J. Path. Bact.* **90**, 419.

MORITZ A.R. *et al.* (1947) Studies on thermal injury. *Amer. J. Path.* **23**, 695 & 915; *Arch. Path.* **43**, 466.

SPRIGGS A.I., BODDINGTON M.M. & CLARKE C.M. (1962) Chromosomes of human cancer cells. *Brit. med. J.* **ii**, 1431.

TROWELL O.A. (1946) The experimental production of watery vacuolation in the liver. *J. Physiol.* (*Lond.*) **105**, 268.

Chapter 26

Some disorders of the circulation

Disorders of the circulation include a number of conditions in which the blood distributed by the heart to the tissues is inadequate in amount. They arise as a consequence of diseases of the heart and blood vessels, and as a result of disorders which alter the volume and distribution of the blood and body fluids. They include congestive heart failure, shock and disturbances in water and electrolyte balance. Because these constitute an important part of clinical medicine and arise in a number of systemic diseases, their discussion is postponed to vol. 3. In this chapter selected circulatory abnormalities which may affect individual tissues are described. They are haemorrhage, thrombosis and embolism, ischaemia and infarction, and congestion.

Haemorrhage

Haemorrhage is brought about by rupture of blood vessels, veins, capillaries or arteries. It may result from injury, from the erosion of a vessel wall by an inflammatory or neoplastic process, from peptic ulceration or from rupture of an aneurysm, which is a localized dilation of a blood vessel. Arterial degenerative disease, often occurring together with high blood pressure, is sometimes associated with haemorrhage, especially intracerebral haemorrhage. Other arterial diseases such as polyarteritis (p. 30.12) or syphilis (p. 21.19) may have similar consequences. Raised venous pressure, associated with varicose ulceration, may cause venous haemorrhage.

Capillary haemorrhages occur in septicaemia and certain forms of poisoning, and also in blood diseases, e.g. leukaemia and thrombocytopenia, and in some deficiency diseases, e.g. scurvy and lack of vitamin K.

The compensatory changes which occur in the cardiovascular system as a result of haemorrhage vary with the volume of blood lost. They have the effect of maintaining the arterial and venous blood pressures (vol. 1, p. 28.40).

As every ambulance worker knows, arterial blood spurts from a torn vessel, whereas venous blood flows more steadily. The site of a haemorrhage is obviously important. If bleeding takes place from a skin surface or mucous membrane, the blood is discharged from the body, which thereby loses not only blood cells and plasma but also the iron of haemoglobin ordinarily retained in the reticuloendothelial cells and used again in blood formation. Conversely, haemorrhage into the body tissues or cavities usually induces organization of the damaged tissue with eventual fibrosis; the haemoglobin is broken down into its constituent parts and the iron is retained in the body. In some instances where a large amount of blood is extravasated into the tissues, there is a measurable increase in serum bilirubin. Potassium is also liberated from the red blood cells and may accumulate in the blood, especially if the renal circulation is reduced and urine output falls or ceases (p. 25.19). Obviously blood shed into the tissues occupies space and this may be of serious consequence, e.g. within the skull. A large mass of blood extravasated into the tissues is called a **haematoma**.

The spontaneous arrest of haemorrhage is the result of several factors which include the contraction of the vessel wall and alterations in the rate of the blood flow and in the behaviour of the platelets (vol. 1, p. 26.14). Vascular contraction is seen when arteries are divided and is an effective means of reducing the arterial calibre, aiding local coagulation. On the other hand, where a vessel is incompletely severed, retraction may widen the breach in the arterial wall and delay coagulation. Arteries with thickened, fibrosed walls, due to disease or age, may fail to contract and haemorrhage may be severe. Capillary vessels may close down independently of their arterioles; venous contraction, if it occurs at all, is ineffectual in controlling haemorrhage.

Thrombosis

Thrombosis is the process of coagulation of circulating blood within the vascular system. It results in the formation of a solid or semi-solid substance called a **thrombus** from the constituents of the blood. Thus thrombosis is always a vital process and it is pathological in its occurrence and in its effects. Clotting, on the other hand, is the term for coagulation of blood after it is shed from the vessels, but it occurs also within the heart and vessels in certain circumstances after death.

STRUCTURE OF A THROMBUS

The structure and appearance of a thrombus differ

from those of a clot in several ways. Essentially a thrombus consists of platelets, fibrin and red corpuscles in varying proportions and differing patterns. For instance, some thrombi are formed mainly of platelets and fibrin and are called **pale** or **white thrombi**, whereas others have large numbers of red corpuscles enmeshed in the fibrin and are described as **red thrombi**. Most thrombi are mixed in type. Thrombi which form rapidly are red, while those which form more slowly are white or pale. Frequently those colour distinctions are noticeable in gross specimens, especially in aneurysmal sacs where laminated thrombi tend to form (plate 26.1a, opposite. There are no corresponding patterns in clotted blood. Thrombi often contain accumulations of polymorphs in large numbers, whereas in a clot the leucocytes are present in proportion to their numbers in the circulating blood. Thrombi are firm, dry and friable compared with clots which are soft and jelly-like.

Thrombi often have a rounded head which is pale, being composed mainly of platelets, and is adherent to the intima, and a long thin tail which is red, consisting of erythrocytes and fibrin, and is only loosely attached to the vessel wall.

The recognition of thrombosis as a vital phenomenon obviously precludes the name 'postmortem thrombosis' to describe the clots which occur often after death in the cardiac chambers and in wide vessels, where the bulk of the blood is relatively large.

CAUSES OF THROMBOSIS
Over 100 years ago, Virchow stated that three factors were essential for thrombus formation:
(1) abnormality of the vascular endothelium,
(2) alterations in the rate, force and direction of the blood flow locally, and
(3) changes in the constitution of the blood.
All three factors may contribute to a thrombosis in different degrees.

Gross abnormalities of the vascular endothelium occur in degenerative diseases such as atherosclerosis and consequently in arteries the endothelial factor is frequently dominant. Surrounding inflammation, as from an abscess, may involve vessel walls and produce endothelial damage, as may intrinsic inflammatory disease of the vascular wall, e.g. due to polyarteritis and thrombo-angiitis obliterans. Infiltration of the vessel wall by malignant tumours is another source of endothelial damage.

The influence of variations in the rate of blood flow and of turbulence is illustrated by the frequency with which thrombi are found in dilations and culs-de-sac, e.g. in aneurysms, where laminated thrombi form, and on cardiac valves which are deformed, e.g. by rheumatic fever, and on abnormal vascular communications, e.g. patent ductus arteriosus, where thrombi consisting largely

of platelets are often deposited. Stasis and changes in rate and direction of blood flow are particularly important in the initiation of thrombosis in the heart, especially in the atria. In venous thrombosis, the relatively slow rate of the circulation is the most important factor, and this is obvious in the condition of varicose veins of the legs, where dilation of the vessels reduces the flow markedly.

Important changes in the constitution of the blood follow trauma and bleeding as after surgery and childbirth, after removal of the spleen and in some blood diseases. Injury and bleeding cause consumption of clotting factors and of platelets. The clotting factors are sometimes replaced transiently in excessive amounts; the platelet replacement is achieved by increased marrow activity and the young platelets pouring into the circulation maximally about the seventh to the tenth day are more adhesive than older platelets. The spleen appears to control maturation and release of blood cells from the bone marrow; hence in the first week or two after surgical removal of the spleen there may be an exceedingly high platelet count in the blood, leading to a thrombotic tendency. The rare blood diseases accompanied by a tendency to thrombus formation possess this characteristic for various reasons, e.g. abnormally high platelet numbers, agglutinins tending to clump the red cells (cold agglutinins) and increased viscosity (erythraemia).

FORMATION OF A THROMBUS
The formation of a thrombus begins by the deposition of platelets on the vascular intima, a phenomenon largely attributable to the release of adenosine diphosphate by the platelets themselves; the demonstration of this apparently specific action of ADP has formed a most important modern contribution to the study of clotting *in vitro* and of thrombosis *in vivo*. Aggregation at the earliest stage is reversible but the rapid appearance of minute amounts of fibrin binds the platelet mass together and is associated with alteration in the platelets known as viscous metamorphosis (vol. 1, p. 26.14). Nevertheless, electron microscopy has shown that these changes in platelets vary according to their situation in the aggregate. Fibrin formation is accompanied by degranulation of platelets, but even in the later stages when platelet disintegration may occur in some parts of a thrombus, vesicles formed by the intact platelet plasma membranes can be identified by EM (non-granular bodies).

The small mass of platelets projects into the lumen, and fibrin and red blood cells are laid down in varying amounts. The rough surface of this mass then leads to a further deposition of platelets and the process is self-perpetuating. The alternating layers of platelet deposition and red blood cells may appear on section as waves of pale and red lines, the **lines of Zahn**.

Whether or not a fibrin and red cell thrombus is formed depends much on local circulatory conditions.

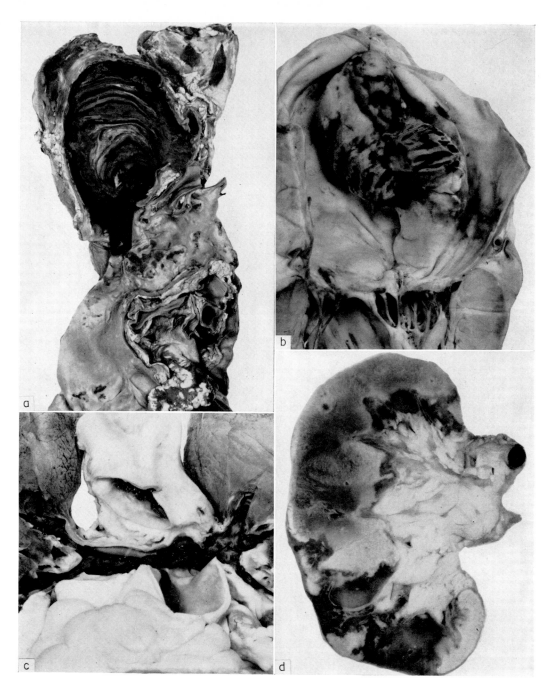

PLATE 26.1.

(a) A syphilitic aneurysm of the arch of the aorta, showing laminated thrombus filling the sac.

(b) The left atrium in this case of rheumatic valvular disease of the heart contains a large, ovoid, adherent thrombus, projecting from its attachment into the atrial lumen. Note the thickened, fibrosed and distorted mitral cusps.

(c) A large venous embolus is seen in the right and left branches of the pulmonary artery, blocking the large intrapulmonary branches of both these vessels.

(d) This section of a kidney shows several pale infarcts, affecting mainly the cortex but to a lesser extent the medulla, and being in general wedge-shaped. A cross-section of the renal artery in the hilar fat shows a thrombus in its lumen.

For instance, if an arterial wall is punctured by a needle, as occurs during an aortogram, the site of the puncture fills with a platelet plug but a mural thrombus is rare, probably because of the rapid blood flow in the vessel. On the other hand, a large thrombus may form on an atherosclerotic abdominal aorta where ulcerated plaques provide sites for platelets to adhere. In large vessels, the thrombus usually remains plastered as a plaque against the wall of the vessel, whereas in small arteries continuation of the process may lead to an occlusive thrombus which blocks completely the direct blood flow to the part or tissue supplied by the affected vessel.

Experimental and clinical observations emphasize the significance of local circulatory dynamics in determining whether or not thrombus formation takes place, but it is an oversimplification to accept these as the only factors. The contributions of fibrinolysins and the natural anticoagulants are probably also of considerable influence. Fibrinolysins can be demonstrated in blood vessel walls but not much is known of their concentration or how far they can limit thrombus formation; fibrinolysin derived from plasminogen is active in the circulating blood in the removal of formed thrombus. Mast cells with their basophilic cytoplasmic granules which contain heparin are present along the adventitial sheaths of blood vessels but their contribution to the prevention of thrombosis is not known.

CARDIAC THROMBOSIS

Thrombosis may occur within the chambers of the heart and in the coronary arteries. The cardiac valves are frequent sites of thrombi; here they are known as **vegetations**, and are essentially of two types. In one variety they form small warty nodules of pinhead size along the lines of contact of the cusps. Vegetations of this nature are found in acute rheumatic endocarditis; they are composed mainly of platelets. In bacterial endocarditis the vegetations are bulky, friable structures comprised mainly of fibrin, platelets and polymorphs, but also containing the causative organisms; they are attached to the valves by inflammatory granulation tissue, and at these sites the endocardium has been destroyed. The location of the lesions depends on valvular deformities, either acquired through previous rheumatic inflammation or congenital in origin, and thus they are most often seen on the mitral and aortic cusps.

In addition, thrombosis may take place within the cardiac chambers as a reaction to endocardial damage. Myocardial infarction is much the commonest cause and thrombus forms on ventricular endocardium in contact with necrotic myocardium unless and sometimes even if anticoagulants are used to prevent it. As a rule this thrombus is firmly adherent to the endocardium but it is friable in its superficial parts. By the process of organization, endocardial thrombus may be transformed into firm scar tissue which may strengthen the infarcted wall; unorganized thrombus is a source of emboli (p. 26.5). The assessment of the advantages and risks of endocardial thrombus has led to controversy as to the use of anticoagulants in the treatment of myocardial infarction.

Thrombus forms also on the atrial endocardium when it is damaged. Rheumatic endocarditis is the most important cause, and the left atrium is the more frequent site (plate 26.1b, facing p. 26.2); the combination of atrial dilation and endocardial roughening, together with irregular blood flow, in the functional disorder of atrial fibrillation which often occurs in rheumatic mitral disease, provides ideal conditions for thrombosis. The thrombus often forms on the septal endocardium from which it protrudes into the atrial cavity; sometimes it forms a stalked mushroom-shaped structure, the top of which may become detached to constitute a **ball thrombus**, free in the atrial blood. The tip of the left atrial appendage is another important site of thrombus formation in atrial fibrillation. Experience has shown that when this arrhythmia has been present for some time there is a risk of embolism from the thrombus, especially when the cardiac rhythm is restored to normal.

The relatively large capacity of the cardiac chambers makes them particularly prone to blood clotting after death; clots of this nature are usually dark in colour, shiny and soft. If the red cells have separated from the plasma, the clots are pale yellow (chicken fat). They are not adherent to the endocardium, being thus distinguishable from true thrombi, and from **agonal thrombi** which form in the right ventricle just before death when patients have been seriously ill for some time. Agonal thrombi are adherent to the endocardium at their point of origin which is usually toward the apex of the ventricle, and they extend into the main stem and sometimes along the major divisions of the pulmonary artery. They are usually firm in consistency.

ARTERIAL THROMBOSIS

Lesions of the vascular intima are the major factors involved in arterial thrombosis, and of these conditions atherosclerosis (p. 25.36) is of prime importance.

This condition is a degenerative condition of arteries which is present to some extent in practically everyone of middle age, and increases with time. In many individuals, however, it begins much earlier than this. It affects the aorta (plate 26.2a, facing p. 26.6) and its branches, and in addition the larger branches of systemic arteries including the coronary, cerebral and renal arteries. It is the most important disease of arteries, and is responsible for much of the pathology of old age (p. 36.2). It takes the form of the deposition of large fat-containing cells and free lipid in the intima (p. 25.36), with associated intimal fibrosis and thickening, vascularization and haemorrhage. These lesions develop originally as smooth yellow plaques; later the endothelial surface may break down and the lipid material is extruded. The roughened surface now present may lead to the formation of thrombus.

According to one concept, the **thrombogenic hypothesis**, the formation of atheroma is due to repeated mural thrombosis, but whether or not this is always true, there is no doubt that the majority of atherosclerotic plaques grow by the continuing incorporation of thrombus which forms on their surfaces. Obviously, those plaques whose surfaces have eroded, are specially prone to thrombus formation and in many plaques minute cracks and fissures can be seen with fragments of thrombus in them, potential sites for the growth of an occlusive thrombus (plate 26.2b, facing p. 26.6).

Thrombus formation is an accompaniment also of inflammatory arterial lesions, such as polyarteritis nodosa (p. 30.12) and the other various forms of arteritis which tend to affect smaller vessels and may be due to autoimmune reactions. As a rule these lesions incorporate fibrinoid necrosis of the arterial wall as a localizing thrombotic factor. Direct involvement of an artery in an inflammatory process, as in an abscess or a tuberculous lesion, is not common, but may lead to the development of thrombosis.

Thrombosis may occur also in a segment of an artery after arterial spasm. An example is seen in the thrombotic occlusion of interlobular branches of renal arteries after shock following retroplacental haemorrhage in pregnancy. Spasm of those vessels may persist for periods of hours, and when subsequently the blood enters the ischaemic vessel after the spasm has passed off, thrombosis may develop at that site. This may be a mechanism of production of renal cortical necrosis.

Trauma to arteries rarely induces thrombosis unless the vessels are already diseased, e.g. in atherosclerotic arteries. The consequences of injuries to arteries naturally depend on the extent of the damage and on the condition of the vessel at the site of injury. In the case of muscular arteries which are otherwise normal, the partial severance of the vessel by a wound from an external instrument or its penetration by a sharp edge of bone may be followed by a traumatic aneurysm in which thrombosis occurs. In the development of such a lesion, the leak from the artery is contained by investing structures to form a haematoma which by its organization produces a saccular dilation. Aneurysms of this nature are generally of the category named 'false aneurysms', i.e. the sac is formed not by the arterial wall proper but by reactive fibrous tissue.

VENOUS THROMBOSIS

Possibly on account of their thin walls with relative lack of muscle, endothelial damage sufficient to initiate thrombosis is of fairly frequent occurrence in veins.

Intimal thickening leading to stenosis and thrombosis sometimes develops in veins after prolonged infusion of saline or other fluids. Indeed, the progressive occlusion of veins is occasionally a source of difficulty when life is sustained by intravenous therapy or by repeated haemodialysis. Inflammation, however, is probably the principal cause of endothelial damage in veins; although theoretically inflammation and subsequent thrombosis, i.e. thrombophlebitis, may develop in any vein, there are several veins especially susceptible to this. The venous sinuses of the skull, notably the sigmoid sinus and the cavernous sinus, are occasionally affected. The former may thrombose as a direct result of the spread of inflammation through the roof of the middle ear in suppurative otitis media, or by the extension of thrombosis along its mastoid tributaries in acute mastoiditis. Cavernous sinus thrombosis is a recognized possible extension of orbital inflammation and of inflammation of the territory drained by the veins of the nasal mucosa. But these hazards have been greatly reduced by modern treatment. Phlebitis of the veins of the leg, however, is still relatively common and occurs as an accompaniment of varicosities in these structures; infection usually enters subsequent to repeated injury and, once established, is difficult to treat.

Although endothelial damage is important aetiologically, slowing in the rate of blood flow is the dominant factor in venous thrombosis. Venous flow lacks the force and vigour of arterial flow, and its relative slowness is easily exaggerated by every dilation and tortuosity. Thrombosis is thus a complication of varicose veins and of rectal haemorrhoids in the systemic circulation, and occurs also in the pulmonary vessels in the altered haemodynamics of pulmonary hypertension.

Venous thrombosis of deep leg veins not associated with inflammation, i.e. phlebothrombosis, is a hazard of immobilization and is seen typically after major surgery, following prolonged bed rest and in patients suffering from paralysis, e.g. hemiplegia. Dissection of a fatal case often shows that the thrombus has begun in the deep veins of the gastrocnemius muscles, and a common finding is a long thrombus extending from the posterior tibial veins through the length of the femoral vein proximally. The influence of a tributary stream of blood is shown by the fact that the thrombus may not extend beyond the entrance of the great saphenous vein.

After accidental or surgical injury, there is an increase in the number and the adhesiveness of blood platelets. By daily platelet studies, Helen Payling-Wright showed that in the three first postoperative weeks, the increased platelet count, the adhesiveness of the platelets and the incidence of venous thrombosis follow the same pattern, reaching a maximum about the tenth day. The most important danger of thrombosis in the leg is that of pulmonary embolism (p. 26.5).

Venous thrombosis may, of course, occur as a complication of blood conditions involving a clotting abnormality; there is a small but significantly increased risk of venous thrombosis in women who use oral contraceptives (p. 12.9). **Thrombophlebitis migrans** is a condition in which there is recurrent thrombosis in veins in different parts of the body. It is found most commonly in patients with malignant disease, particularly carcinoma of the pancreas. An increase in tissue thromboplastin produced by the tumour is probably responsible. **White leg (phlegmasia alba dolens)** is the name given to a thrombophlebitis of the femoral and external iliac veins which sometimes occurs after childbirth. It is a painful condition and slow to resolve. The exact nature of the lesion is not clear, but there may be associated lymphangitis.

ARTERIOLAR AND CAPILLARY THROMBOSIS
Thrombosis in the microcirculation occurs locally in inflammatory lesions, heat, cold and electrical injuries and possibly as part of the homograft reaction. Widespread thrombosis throughout the microcirculation, called **disseminated intravascular coagulation**, may also occur in shock, septicaemia, severe hypertension, hypersensitivity reactions and occasionally *de novo*. This complication makes an important contribution to disturbances in function in these conditions.

FATE OF THROMBI
The fate of a thrombus depends to some extent on whether or not it is infected. A thrombus which is bacteriologically sterile is referred to as bland. A bland thrombus in a superficial vein which has formed as a result of a trivial injury, e.g. a needle puncture or a prolonged saline infusion, is usually removed by lysis within a short time and the lumen restored, but in general an occlusive thrombus becomes canalized in the following manner. Endothelial cells derived from pre-existing endothelium first grow over both ends of the thrombus; capillary buds from these cells and also from the endothelium of the vessel beneath the thrombus penetrate the thrombus, unite with each other and produce new capillaries which ramify in the thrombus. Monocytes also elongate to become endothelial cells and fibroblasts. However the reaction is basically of endothelial origin (plate 26.2c facing p. 26.6).

In the case of arteries occluded by thrombus, recanalization takes place from components internal to the internal elastic lamina. Ultimately the vessel may become completely recanalized and the lumen restored to normal function; sometimes there is differentiation within the organizing thrombus and even smooth muscle may develop inside the elastic lamina. The thrombus may become a mass of fibroblastic and collagenous tissue penetrated only by small capillary channels; this is notably the case in mural thrombi which do not occlude the vessel. In

this way the thrombus finally becomes a structureless thickening of the intima, covered by endothelium which has grown over it from the pre-existing endothelium of the vessel; it often contains remnants of blood such as haemosiderin and lipid substances.

An endocardial thrombus following a myocardial infarct tends to organize to a dense white collagenous substance, but there is little or no organization of a laminated thrombus in an aneurysm.

If a thrombus is infected there is a superimposed inflammatory reaction which not only deters organization but may lead to fragmentation of the thrombus and encourage embolism.

Embolism
An embolus is a portion of some abnormal material which is transported in the blood or lymph and is impacted in a blood or lymph vessel at another site. Several substances may form emboli, e.g. a thrombus, atheromatous material, micro-organisms, tumour cells, fat cells, rarely amniotic fluid and trophoblast fragments, or air. The most common emboli come from a thrombus and these illustrate many aspects of the process.

Arterial thrombotic emboli may take origin on the left side of the heart, e.g. from a thrombus in the left atrium and auricle or on the endocardium of the left ventricle, or from valvular vegetations. They may arise also from a thrombus on the surface of an aortic atheromatous lesion.

Venous thrombotic emboli usually come from a large vein, such as the femoral vein, or less commonly from the right side of the heart, generally the atrium; they may be derived from the right ventricle as when an endocardial thrombus follows a cardiac infarct. Venous thrombi are carried to the lungs, where they form a pulmonary embolus. This may be large enough to occlude the main pulmonary artery, a condition which is usually fatal, or one or both of the two main branches of this artery (plate 26.1c, facing p. 26.2). In this case, the lesion is again likely to be fatal, but prompt surgical removal of the embolus may be life-saving. Often smaller emboli block intrapulmonary branches of the arteries, and these sometimes lead to infarction of the lung.

Passage of a venous embolus to the right atrium, through a patent foramen ovale to the left atrium, and thence to the systemic circulation with impaction in an artery is known as **paradoxical embolism**.

Emboli derived from a thrombus are usually enlarged by secondary thrombosis at the site of impaction.

Occasionally, fragments of **atheromatous material** from a plaque in the aorta may break off and form emboli. Branches of the renal artery, in particular, may be seen to be blocked by material containing cholesterol (cholesterol embolism).

Emboli of micro-organisms may arise in the course of

many infective conditions. The organisms may cause multiple small pyaemic abscesses at their points of arrest. This occurs in infective endocarditis or as a complication from abscesses or foci of acute infection, e.g. acute osteomyelitis.

Emboli of neoplastic cells are of great importance in the blood spread of malignant tumours (p. 28.7).

Fat embolism occurs most commonly as a result of the entry of marrow fat into the circulation after trauma to bone; occasionally trauma to or even inflammation and necrosis of adipose tissue has the same result. After a fracture, pieces of haemopoietic marrow may be found in pulmonary vessels. Fat embolism is said to occur occasionally in cases of fatty liver; here rupture of the distended cells presumably releases the fat into the circulation. Fat embolism occurs in the form of large numbers of separate globules capable of occluding capillaries. The capillaries in the lungs and central nervous system are the main sites of their arrest. Emboli, when present in large numbers, may produce respiratory distress and may lead to disturbance of consciousness and sometimes coma. Minute capillary haemorrhages may be seen in the pleura or found on microscopic examination of the brain. Emboli may be found also in the renal glomeruli but seldom disturb function (plate 26.2d, opposite). Detection of fat emboli involves the use of sections cut on the freezing microtome and extensive use of this technique shows that they are common after bone trauma; in most cases they produce no signs or symptoms.

Amniotic fluid embolism is rare. It is caused by the entry of amniotic fluid into the blood stream at the placental site as a result of pressure from uterine contractions. Acute respiratory distress and sudden death usually follow. It is possible that these features arise from the high thromboplastin content of the amniotic fluid, which may lead to thrombosis of small systemic and pulmonary vessels and to fibrinogenopenia. Trophoblastic fragments also may be found in the pulmonary capillaries of pregnant women; they are believed to disappear by lysis and are not known to be harmful.

Gaseous emboli occur occasionally when a large amount of air enters the circulation as a result of therapeutic procedures. For instance, the accidental opening of a large vein during a surgical operation in the neck may allow air to enter the vessel as a result of the negative pressure of the thoracic cavity. Rarely, air may enter the circulation in the course of intravenous transfusion and this has been known to occur also during a single intravenous injection, although again very rarely. Air embolism has followed attempted criminal abortion.

In fatal cases of air embolism death is due to the obstruction of the right ventricle and pulmonary artery by a frothy mixture of air and blood, or to a similar obstruction of intrapulmonary arteries. To demonstrate this lesion at post mortem examination, the heart must be opened, attached to the thoracic organs and under water, so that the escaping air bubbles may be seen. Obviously, for frothing to take place the amount of air injected must be large, and it has been estimated that about 200 ml of air are needed to produce a fatal outcome.

Caisson disease is a form of gas embolism and is an occupational risk of men required to work in air under pressure, when the gases of the air go into solution in the fluids of the body (vol. 1, p. 43.6). On rapid decompression, nitrogen is released as small gaseous emboli, which may lodge in any capillary system of the body with corresponding ischaemic effects; in the nervous system bubbles of gas can produce permanent lesions. Involvement of the internal ear leads to vertigo and damage to the muscles and joints gives rise to the painful condition known as **bends**.

EFFECTS OF EMBOLISM

Embolism cuts off partially or completely the blood to the tissue supplied by the affected vessel. The result obviously depends upon the degree of anastomosis between this vessel and those adjacent to it, but either ischaemic atrophy or complete infarction of the tissue usually occurs.

Ischaemia

Ischaemia is defined as a reduction in the blood flow to an organ or tissue and is often due to narrowing or closure of its arteries; this reduces or cuts off the supply of oxygen and nutrients to the cells with consequences which are discussed on p. 25.4. The development of ischaemic lesions is influenced by anatomical and physiological factors as well as by the nature of the pathological factor responsible.

Some arteries lack adequate collateral channels and are known as end arteries, a name given by Cohnheim in the last century. The retinal, splenic and renal arteries have no effective collateral circulation and they are called **absolute end arteries**. Other arteries are known as **functional end arteries** (vol. 1, p. 28.15); there is some degree of anastomosis or potential for forming anastomoses, but this is usually insufficient to maintain the vitality of the part if the artery is occluded. The coronary arteries are examples of this type. In a third group of arteries, an obstruction usually leads to ischaemic lesions of some degree, despite anastomotic and collateral channels; they are the cerebral, carotid and mesenteric arteries. The liver and lungs are in a special class, as they each have a double blood supply, thus providing some blood even when a major vessel is blocked.

Collateral channels exist at the capillary level, and in the presence of obstruction to a main arterial blood supply such anastomotic vessels dilate, carrying blood from an uninvolved capillary bed to that supplied by the obstructed vessel.

Ischaemia may result from vasoconstriction, or from

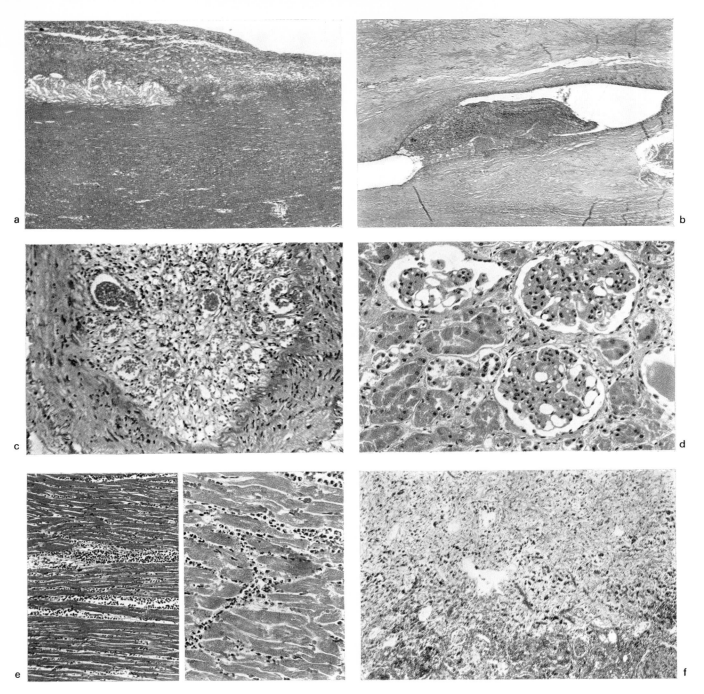

PLATE 26.2. Histology of circulatory disorders.

(a) Part of an atheromatous plaque in the aorta. Most of the aortic wall seen consists of media, but at the top left, intimal thickening is present and in this plaque, particularly in its deepest layers, are clear vacuoles, previously filled by lipids, and sharp clefts, the site of deposition of cholesterol crystals. Haem. & eosin ($\times 40$).

(c) An organized and canalized thrombus in an artery. Haem. & eosin ($\times 100$).

(e) Myocardial infarction. The left half ($\times 100$) shows a low power view of the necrotic myocardium; hypereosinophilia of fibres, lack of nuclei, and polymorph infiltration are seen. The right half ($\times 250$) shows loss of striations and nuclei of the dead muscle fibres, together with the infiltrating polymorphs. Haem. & eosin.

(b) This section of part of a coronary artery shows an atherosclerotic intima and a central lumen partially occluded by a thrombus superimposed upon the atherosclerosis. Organization of the thrombus is proceeding. Haem. & eosin ($\times 25$).

(d) Fat embolism in the kidney. Three glomeruli exhibiting great distension of several capillaries by round, clear vacuoles are present. These have contained neutral fat, dissolved out in the processing of the tissue. Haem. & eosin ($\times 200$).

(f) Pulmonary infarction; part of a true pulmonary infarct which is being organized. The lower part of the field shows haemorrhagic infarcted tissue from the region as yet unorganized; the remainder shows fibroblastic granulation tissue, with deposition of brown haemosiderin granules. Haem. & eosin ($\times 60$).

partial or complete obstruction of an artery by a thrombus or embolus. The relative importance of vasoconstriction is often difficult to estimate. Experimentally it was demonstrated visually by Byrom that vascular spasm occurs in the cerebral circulation in the encephalopathy of hypertensive rats; it is believed that this may occur also in hypertensive human beings. Vasoconstriction of the digital arteries on exposure to cold is a physiological response and may be so severe in some people as to cause Raynaud's disease. Vasoconstriction can sometimes be demonstrated in the coronary circulation by the use of angiograms, although it is difficult to conceive of spasm in vessels which are severely damaged by atherosclerosis or by calcification. Reflex constriction of renal arteries probably contributes to the production of acute renal failure following severe blood loss. In the main, however, the most common basis of ischaemia lies in:

(1) primary arterial disease, predominantly atherosclerosis or arteriosclerosis and less commonly calcification of the media (Mönckeberg's sclerosis),

(2) thrombosis, almost invariably associated with arterial disease, and

(3) embolism.

The different causes modify the result in several respects, and especially determine whether the onset of ischaemia is sudden or gradual, and whether the occlusion is partial or complete.

GRADUAL ISCHAEMIA

This is usually a consequence of stenosis due to progressive primary arterial degenerative diseases, most frequently of atherosclerotic origin. If the vessel involved is an end artery, as for instance a major branch of a coronary artery, the cells furthest removed from the blood supply atrophy and die; they undergo dissolution and disappearance and are replaced by excess fibrous tissue. It is a general principle that specialized cells undergo this change more rapidly than cells with less exacting metabolic requirements (p. 25.6). If the artery is not an end artery, the effect of gradual narrowing depends on the capacity of the collateral vessels. For example, progressive stenosis of a femoral artery is potentially less serious if the site of the lesion is distal to the origin of the profunda branch; similarly the relative freedom of the peroneal artery from disease adds to its important role in preventing ischaemic lesions of the toes. Further, the capacity of any group of anastomotic channels to dilate is dependent on their freedom from disease; generalized calcification of the media, for instance, prevents the vascular flexibility characteristic of a healthy circulation.

Secondary arterial disease associated with narrowing of the lumen is also of importance in the production of ischaemia. In the condition of endarteritis obliterans, which occurs in association with chronic inflammatory lesions such as peptic ulceration or chronic tuberculosis,

there is progressive narrowing of arterial branches by concentric multiplication of the endothelial cells. This lesion is also an important local consequence of irradiation (p. 33.7).

The functional consequences of gradual ischaemia are for the most part those of acclerated loss of specialized cells, but in one situation at least the effect may be of another nature. This is in the kidney, where partial renal ischaemia leads to the structural changes of atrophy of nephrons with fibrosis, but the functional effect is not limited to loss of renal tissue and is complicated by the development of high blood pressure.

RAPID ISCHAEMIA

Sudden occlusion of an artery may be due to the impaction of an embolus or to the formation of thrombus on an existing lesion. In either event, rapid ischaemia of the tissues supplied by the vessel results and the severity and extent of the lesion is governed by the anatomy of the part. Occlusion of an end artery is followed by the structural change known as infarction; the types of infarct are discussed below. Sudden occlusion of an artery which is not an end artery has very variable results, dependent on the collateral channels. For example, surgical ligation of an internal carotid artery to reduce the risk of rupture of an aneurysm of the Circle of Willis may be well compensated in a young person because of the capacity of the other carotid artery and of the collateral vertebral and orbital circulations. In an older person, however, occlusion of a common or internal carotid artery may produce serious ischaemic damage to the brain because these collateral arteries have become narrowed.

The effects of ischaemia are directly related also to the oxygen requirements of the tissue concerned. Tissues of high metabolic activity are least able to withstand oxygen lack. Consequently the effect of ischaemia is relatively severe in the cerebral cortex, since the neurones are unable to survive deprivation of oxygen for more than about three minutes (p. 25.7).

Clinicians are familiar with the remarkable way in which tissues may recover from ischaemia. To some extent this is due to the gradual expansion of collateral channels which can restore vitality to cells on the periphery of an ischaemic lesion. Occlusive thrombi and emboli may be canalized and the lumen of a vessel reopened. In cerebral ischaemia, neurones which have escaped the ischaemic process may be capable of taking over the function of those which have suffered damage.

Infarcts

Infarcts are formed when deprivation of blood to a part or the whole of an organ by obstruction of an artery, usually an end artery, leads to necrosis of the dependent tissue. They are described as either pale or red (haemorrhagic) in appearance, and as bland or septic in nature. **Pale infarcts** occur in organs where the affected artery is an end artery with little anastomosis, e.g. spleen, kidney and heart, and **red infarcts** usually in organs with some anastomosis between vessels, or a double circulation, e.g. lung. However, as the description of the infarct as pale or red depends simply upon the amount of blood in the lesion, all infarcts are red at their inception, although this phase may be very transient.

Septic infarcts derive their infection either from the tissue in which the infarct has occurred, or from an infected embolus which is the actual cause of the infarction.

Microscopic structure
Infarcted tissue shows diffuse haemorrhage in the first few hours and later, after approximately 24 hours, cytoplasmic eosinophilia and nuclear pyknosis occur; nuclei may also undergo karyolysis. The cells then begin to fragment; although cellular outline may be retained for a time an amorphous granular mass eventually results. A polymorph infiltration develops some hours after the initial infarction, and is generally confined to the periphery of the lesion.

Fate of infarcts
Organization to scar tissue begins at the periphery of the infarct, usually several days after the initial lesion, when capillaries begin to grow in from the adjacent living tissue. Given time, the infarct may become completely converted to dense fibrous tissue; however, in some large infarcts a central portion of unorganized necrotic tissue may remain for a very long time, possibly permanently. There is a tendency for calcium to be laid down in necrotic tissues (dystrophic calcification), and this process may occur in infarcts too large to be completely organized. Before and during the process of organization, the red blood cells in the infarct become broken down, and granular pigments, including haemosiderin, are formed; these impart a yellow or orange colour to the necrotic tissue. The haemosiderin can be seen lying free or within macrophages in the lesion.

PALE INFARCTS
Splenic infarcts generally affect only part of the organ and follow the occlusion of a major branch of the splenic artery within the spleen; where several branches have been occluded, as for instance by emboli, several infarcts of different ages are often present. The infarcts are pyramidal in shape, with the apex towards the splenic pedicle; when cut across they are wedge-shaped and often appear almost white against the dark splenic pulp. As a rule they involve the capsule, and there may be a few flakes of fibrin on the surface of the infarct. Septic splenic infarcts are soft and there is a superficial fibrinous exudate (localized perisplenitis). In time, they usually

organize and contract, capillaries and fibroblasts invading the infarct from the adjacent tissue. Functionally these infarcts have little effect on the health of the patient but to the clinician and to the pathologist they suggest the presence of a source of emboli, probably on the left side of the heart, e.g. bacterial endocarditis or thrombus on the site of a cardiac infarct. Thrombotic occlusion of branches of the splenic artery is uncommon, but may occur in erythraemia and in leukaemias.

Renal infarcts have the same general pattern as those of the spleen and are pale and wedge shaped on section (plate 26.1d, facing p. 26.2). When a relatively large branch of the renal artery is occluded, the apex is close to the renal pelvis. Microscopically, the infarct shows typical coagulation necrosis in which the anatomical structure of the kidney is retained for a time, although the cell nuclei have disappeared. Usually a narrow rim of renal tissue remains immediately under the capsule, from which it draws its blood supply. The infarcts organize as in the spleen, with resultant deep scars and pits in the cortex. Infarcts of the kidney are often caused by emboli arising from a thrombus in the left ventricle or atrium, or on atheromatous lesions of the aorta or renal artery.

Infarcts of the myocardium (plate 26.2e, facing p. 26.2) are among the most important and common diseases of men and to a lesser extent of women in prosperous communities. With few exceptions, the lesion is due to atherosclerosis of the coronary arteries with or without superimposed occlusive thrombus. The affected portion of the myocardium is suffused with blood about 12 hours after the occlusion, and thereafter becomes pale; by the third or fourth day the yellow colour of the dead tissue demarcates it from the healthy muscle. Immediately adjacent to the necrotic tissue there is a zone of hyperaemia from which organization subsequently develops, transforming the infarct into a scar. Local factors greatly influence the extent of the vascular reaction and consequently the density of the scar tissue. If the infarct involves the epicardium, there is a fibrinous pericarditis, usually localized. Involvement of the endocardium provides a site for the formation of a thrombus which then becomes a potential source of emboli. Organization of mural thrombus, however, produces a dense, white, firm endocardial scar which may strengthen the cardiac wall. A complete infarct of the whole thickness of the ventricular wall may be followed by rupture of the heart. Cardiac infarcts are almost always ventricular, the left ventricle, the cardiac apex and the interventricular septum being often involved.

RED OR HAEMORRHAGIC INFARCTS
Pulmonary infarcts follow occlusion of a branch of a pulmonary artery, but this does not always produce infarction, because of the presence of the bronchial circulation.

Often they are wedge shaped on section but sometimes they are sufficiently extensive to occupy most of a lobe, simulating the red consolidation of pneumococcal pneumonia. In pulmonary hypertension, thrombosis may occur in a branch of a pulmonary artery which is atherosclerotic, but most pulmonary infarcts arise from emboli and are due to the release of thrombus from the veins of the leg or pelvis, or from the right side of the heart. In the latter case the lungs are probably already congested and this favours infarction; it is difficult experimentally to induce pulmonary infarcts in the absence of pulmonary congestion. Indeed, obstruction of an artery in an otherwise normal lung may involve intra-alveolar haemorrhage and ischaemia of affected alveolar walls, but not true infarction. The haemorrhagic nature of pulmonary infarcts, when they occur, is due to the bronchial arteries which continue to supply blood to the alveoli; haemorrhage into the alveoli takes place through the devitalized capillary walls and the air spaces are literally stuffed with blood. Fibrinous pleurisy develops locally over the infarcted part, and may cause pain.

True pulmonary infarcts develop usually in patients who are gravely ill, and then autopsy seldom shows much evidence of organization. If the patient survives, organization occurs, accompanied by absorption of some of the alveolar haemorrhage and by the expansion of closed but still viable alveoli, so that most of the affected lung tissue may be restored to normal. However, a small pulmonary scar may often be seen (plate 26.2f, facing p. 26.6).

Infarcts of the intestine are haemorrhagic and commonly follow interruption of the blood supply by mechanical means such as volvulus, strangulation of a hernia or intussusception, or by thrombosis of the superior mesenteric artery. These conditions are all surgical emergencies. Infarction is much commoner in the small intestine than in the colon.

The superior mesenteric artery supplies the small intestine and the proximal half of the colon; the remainder of the colon is supplied by the inferior mesenteric artery. Anastomosis between these arteries is by way of the superior left colic branch of the inferior mesenteric artery with the middle colic artery, and is insufficient to sustain the intestinal circulation if the superior mesenteric artery is suddenly closed (vol. 1, p. 30.45). The intimate supply to the intestine is by a series of intercommunicating arterial loops which increase in number as the bowel is approached. They provide a good collateral circulation except in their most distal parts, where the short straight vessels connect the distal loops with the bowel itself.

In elderly patients, a thrombus in the aorta may block the orifice of the superior mesenteric artery, or alternatively thrombus may form in the main stem of the artery when it is affected by atherosclerosis. Embolic occlusion of the artery or one of its large branches by a thrombus from the left atrium or from the aorta may occur.

Mechanical obstruction generally acts first on the veins which collapse and may thrombose, while the arteries continue to pump blood into the bowel wall. Ultimately the circulation stops and the arteries are also obstructed. The vessels in the wall of the bowel are dilated and congested; fluid and blood exude into the wall and into the lumen of the gut. The bowel wall becomes necrotic and is invaded by micro-organisms from the lumen.

Infarcts of the nervous system most frequently affect the brain and result from atherosclerosis. As the sites of occlusion are important, a reminder of the main features of the arterial supply to the brain is given. Four main arteries supply the brain, the two internal carotid and the two vertebral arteries (vol. 1, p. 24.70). These anastomose in the Circle of Willis. This is formed in front by the two anterior cerebral arteries joined together by the anterior communicating artery, arising from the internal carotids. It is formed behind by the posterior communicating arteries arising from the basilar artery, itself formed by the junction of the two vertebral arteries. Except in the Circle of Willis, the only anastomoses in the arterial supply are by the small vessels of the investments of the brain and by the capillaries throughout the brain. The communication between the two internal carotid arteries is barely adequate for one alone to maintain the cerebral circulation. However, in young healthy subjects, ligation of one internal carotid artery is not necessarily followed by ischaemic lesions of the brain.

When an infarct occurs in the brain, the degree of atherosclerosis of the Circle of Willis and its branches is often very gross. On the other hand, it is recognized that almost one-half of cerebral ischaemic lesions can be accounted for by atherosclerosis situated outside the skull. Common extracranial sites are the origins of the internal carotid arteries, and the vertebral arteries, usually between their origin and their entry into the transverse processes of the sixth cervical vertebra. Inside the skull, the commonest site is in the middle cerebral arteries.

Ischaemic lesions of the brain in most instances represent the effects of disease involving several arteries rather than a single local vascular occlusion (p. 25.4). For example, although one internal carotid artery may be occluded without producing an infarct, the blood supply to the frontoparietal lobe on that side is necessarily seriously reduced and any superimposed lesion may lead to ischaemic change. Stenosis of a right internal carotid artery may be followed by an ischaemic lesion on the left side, if that hemisphere is already inadequately supplied with blood through stenosis or occlusion of a left internal carotid artery. Disease involving both carotid and vertebral arteries is common in old people, and in some patients a sudden movement of the neck may be sufficient to produce transient ischaemia of the brain. Cervical spondylosis with torsion of the vertebral arteries may be an important contributory factor. Occlusion due to embolism occurs occasionally, the commonest cause being detachment of portions of atheromatous material or of thrombus on atheromatous lesions of the larger carotid arteries. Emboli from the endocardium in myocardial infarction and from thrombus in the left atrium in mitral disease can also be responsible. Bacterial endocarditis may be a source of infected thrombus.

Inflammatory change involving the small intracranial arteries may be followed by thrombosis. Endarteritis as a result of cerebrovascular syphilis, tuberculosis and even of pyogenic infection is recognized. Similarly, trauma and irradiation can produce narrowing of these vessels.

Infarcts of the brain may involve grey matter or white matter or both; they may be mainly in the cortex or they may be situated deeply in the region of the basal nuclei. They may be pale and difficult to detect if recent, but some are haemorrhagic. The commonest sites for an infarct are in the portion of the brain supplied by the middle cerebral artery. The lesion consists of necrotic, oedematous tissue which looks and feels distinctly soft compared with the solid normal brain tissue in relation to it. Some petechial haemorrhages may be seen. In both the grey and white matter the lesion usually ultimately liquefies and may in time form a small cyst containing clear fluid.

Infarcts of the liver are uncommon. Although by virtue of its double circulation through the portal vein and hepatic artery the liver would appear to be an obvious site for red infarcts, both red and pale types occur. Interruption of the hepatic artery by accidental ligation, embolus or thrombus usually gives rise to pale infarcts. They may occur in any lobe as sharply defined zones of coagulative necrosis. Red infarcts are caused by arrest of the portal circulation by thrombosis of a branch of the portal vein, usually from its involvement in a metastatic tumour.

Gangrene

This is a term used to describe a form of necrosis or infarction in which bacterial infection is also present (p. 25.43).

The bacteria involved are mainly those which grow easily in dead tissues; usually several organisms are present, and many may be saprophytes. The affected tissues become black and an unpleasant odour is produced.

Infection is most likely to be superimposed on ischaemic necrosis when the ischaemia involves skin or a mucous membrane such as that of the intestine, so that micro-organisms can easily reach the tissue.

Gangrene is conventionally divided into wet and dry types. However, only the wet type should strictly be designated as gangrene; the term **dry gangrene** is used to describe a type of ischaemic necrosis which occurs in the distal parts of limbs, usually the leg, as a result of ob-

struction to the circulation, in the absence of any complicating bacterial infection. This condition is found mainly in cases of primary arterial disease in elderly subjects. The tissues gradually become purple and ultimately black. The part is dry, shrunken and virtually mummified. If infection does occur, the condition is one of **wet gangrene,** as seen in other tissues such as intestine.

Gas gangrene results from infection by anaerobic organisms and is described on p. 25.43.

Congestion and oedema

Congestion is a term commonly used to describe the condition in which the tissues contain an increased amount of blood within their vessels. It may occur either as a reactive vasodilation or hyperaemia from physiological or pathological stimuli, or the blood may accumulate passively in the venous capacitance vessels due to inadequate drainage with reduced venous return to the heart. This is invariably pathological in origin.

Reactive vasodilation is associated with dilation of arterioles and capillaries and with the opening of vessels which in the uncongested state are collapsed and empty. This occurs physiologically in the skeletal muscles during exercise, in the skin and mucous membranes on exposure to warmth and to ultraviolet radiation, though in the latter case the capillary dilation is delayed for some hours, and in the gastric mucosa in response to the ingestion of food. Pathologically, commonplace examples are seen in acute inflammation and repair (p. 21.2). The active hyperaemia of the early stages of acute inflammation leads to redness and warmth of the part, but when the small vessels are fully dilated the rate of blood flow is reduced and stasis develops (p. 21.4). In addition, reactive hyperaemia occurs following the relief of an arterial obstruction, such as surgical ligature. **Passive congestion** connotes an increased quantity of blood in dilated venous channels and is invariably associated with reduction in the rate of blood flow, leading sometimes to cyanosis from the high proportion of reduced haemoglobin. Passive congestion is of two kinds, local and general. The local type is due to obstruction to the venous return from a part, e.g. by venous thrombosis, by pressure from a tumour, or by surrounding fibrosis; it is associated with distension of collateral venous channels and often with oedema. The general type involves all of the pulmonary or systemic circulation and is always due to a diminished output of blood by the heart; pulmonary congestion tends to occur when the output of the left ventricle is reduced, and systemic or peripheral congestion when that of the right ventricle falls. Very often congestion affects pulmonary and systemic vascular beds together and such changes are cardinal features of heart failure.

Oedema is the term used to describe the presence of excess fluid in the interstitial or intercellular spaces.

Local oedema arises from a local increase in permeability of the small capillaries and venules, e.g. in response to local inflammation or following an injection of histamine (p. 14.5), or because there is obstruction to the flow of lymph or venous blood draining a part of the body. The accumulation of fluid is due to disturbance in the balance of factors in Starling's hypothesis (vol. 1, p. 28.24). The normal difference in the colloid osmotic pressure (COP) between the interstitial fluid and that of the plasma is narrowed when inflammation occurs or histamine is given; the capillary hydrostatic pressure, now unopposed by difference in the COP, causes fluid to migrate from the vascular compartment to the interstitial spaces. In local venous and lymphatic obstruction the oedema develops because of an absolute rise in pressure within the small vessels.

Local oedema due to venous obstruction is associated with passive congestion of venous channels, and the aetiological factors are mentioned on p. 26.10. Oedema resulting from lymphatic obstruction, i.e. **lymphoedema**, may be due to fibrosis of the tissues in which the lymphatics run; this occurs after irradiation and after infection, especially if associated with venous thrombosis. Malignant obstruction of lymphatic channels is a common cause, and surgical removal of groups of lymph nodes, e.g. axillary lymph nodes in cases of breast carcinoma, may lead to blockage of the draining lymphatics and consequent oedema. In some countries, *Wurchereria* infection is a common cause of lymphatic blockage. Lymphoedema, if of long duration, tends to lead to fibrosis of the affected tissues, which become indurated (p. 19.33).

Pulmonary, systemic and generalized oedema are due to a similar sequence of events in the general circulation. Thus a rise in intracapillary pressure (left or right heart failure) or a fall in the intravascular COP from a reduced concentration of plasma proteins causes generalized oedema. The latter may occur in famine oedema, in severe protein-losing kidney and gastrointestinal disease and in liver disease. When the primary event is transudation of fluid from the vascular compartment with a low capillary COP, the ensuing oligaemia stimulates retention of sodium and water by the kidney, by mechanisms mediated by the volume control system (vol. 1, p. 33.17). Water and salt then accumulate in the body. When the primary event is a reduced cardiac output, venous pressure in the left or right atria or both rises; generalized pulmonary or peripheral oedema or both occur, and this is again maintained by renal retention of water and salt; this is mediated by a number of factors which include changes in renal perfusion pressure and vasoconstriction, and aldosterone and vasopressin release. The pathogenesis of congestive heart failure will be described more fully in vol. 3.

Oedema and visible swelling of the tissues does not occur until the interstitial fluid pressure rises from its normal average value of slightly less than atmospheric pressure to atmospheric pressure and above. Generalized oedema is not clinically recognizable until the interstitial fluid volume increases by about 10 per cent of normal when the affected parts, e.g. the limbs, swell. The skin is distended and pressure of a finger on the affected area leaves a depression on the surface (pitting oedema). Accumulations of fluid within the body cavities are often referred to in special terms. **Ascites** means accumulation of fluid within the peritoneal cavity and **hydrothorax** and **hydropericardium** refer to accumulation of fluid between the layers of the pleura or pericardium.

On histological examination oedema can be most easily seen in the interstitial connective tissues, where separation of the fibres is demonstrable.

FURTHER READING

DIBLE J.H. (1966) *The Pathology of Limb Ischaemia*, chap. 2. Edinburgh: Oliver & Boyd.

FRENCH J.E. (1967) Electron microscopy of thrombus formation, in *Modern Trends in Pathology*. London: Butterworths.

MITCHELL J.R.A. (1968) Platelets and thrombosis. *Sci. Basis Med.* 266.

POOLE J.C.F. (1964) Structural aspects of thrombosis. *Sci. Basis Med.* 55.

Chapter 27
Tissue and organ growth and its disturbances

The factors which initiate, control and limit the normal growth of cells, and therefore of tissues and organs, are little understood. In animals, growth of the entire body continues from conception until maturity and then in general ceases. However, individual organs and tissues may undergo a period of rapid growth after this time, as in the process of repair following damage, or as a response to hormonal or other biochemical stimulation or to an increased work-load. Not all body cells are capable of dividing after birth or childhood; as indicated in vol. 1, p. 13.1, cells may be classified into three categories in relation to this capacity.

(1) Some cells divide rapidly and regularly throughout life; the epithelium of the gastrointestinal tract, pulmonary alveoli, and of the epidermis are examples.

(2) Some cells divide continuously from birth until adult life, but after this do so only slowly to replace the cells being worn out by normal wear and tear; these cells may, however, divide rapidly to produce adequate regenerated tissue following trauma or disease. The liver is a good example.

(3) Other cells, which may divide for a little time after birth, rapidly lose this ability. Cardiac muscle and nervous tissue are examples.

In the adult, the rate of cell division is balanced with the rate of ageing and decay; only in this way can the size of the organ or tissue be kept approximately constant.

Regeneration of tissues

The repair and regeneration of unspecialized **connective tissue** is discussed on p. 21.12, with special relation to inflammation. This process illustrates also the intermutability of different cell types in connective tissue during regeneration and cellular proliferation. For example, in the organization of a thrombus through the medium of granulation tissue, the cells arise mainly from angioblastic elements, the endothelial cells lining the intima of the vessel; in spite of this, the resulting tissue is identical with that formed in the organization of an inflammatory exudate, where the cells involved arise from both fibroblastic and vascular sources. Again, in the repair of a fracture, if immobilization is poor, a false joint or pseudoarthrosis may result, complete with synovium.

Regeneration of **epithelial tissue** is a simpler process than that of connective tissue. No intermediate reparative or granulation tissue is formed and there is direct replacement by proliferation of cells which have survived the injury or the pathological process which destroyed the tissue. Regeneration is evoked by destruction of cells, and the presence of blood clot or other organic debris which is so important in connective tissue repair, does not stimulate epithelial proliferation. Examples of epithelial regeneration are seen in the epidermis after a skin wound, in the increase in amount of residual liver tissue after experimental hepatectomy or following liver necrosis in human disease (plate 27.1a, facing p. 27.2), or after removal of part of a kidney in a growing animal.

After partial hepatectomy in rats, there is a marked increase in the number of dividing cells which rapidly reaches a peak within 30–40 hours. The increased mitotic activity throughout the remaining tissue continues at a high rate until the organ once more approaches its normal size. The regeneration of hepatic tissue is accompanied by increased numbers of polyploid cells (vol. 1, p. 12.16) and in addition individual cells tend to be larger than normal. The rate of regenerative hyperplasia is directly related to the amount of tissue removed and is unaffected by the administration of growth hormone or of cortisone. Reproduction of the highly organized architecture of the liver is deficient to a varying extent, but bile ducts, blood vessels and connective tissue as well as hepatocytes are regenerated. However, deficiencies are common in epithelial regeneration in many organs and a reconstituted epidermis, for instance, may be permanently thinner than normal and usually fails to regenerate its specialized appendages, the sweat and sebaceous glands and hair follicles.

Lining epithelia of the gastrointestinal, respiratory and urinary tracts usually regenerate completely after acute ulceration. Regeneration over a chronic gastric or duodenal ulcer may be only partial.

In the condition of acute tubular necrosis of the kidneys, one of the causes of acute renal failure, foci of damage to the basement membrane of the renal tubules are seen, often associated with necrosis of a few tubular epithelial lining cells. As the patient recovers and these foci heal, regeneration of the cells takes place from surrounding cells, and mitotic figures can be seen in the tubules of such kidneys.

REGENERATION OF SOME SPECIALIZED TISSUES
Muscle fibres have limited powers of regeneration, and in fact myocardial fibres cannot regenerate at all. Skeletal muscles regenerate to some extent by proliferation of satellite cells (vol. 1, p. 15.6), and smooth muscle can undergo hyperplasia, as is seen in the uterus during pregnancy. In skeletal muscle, large syncytial masses with marginal sarcolemmal nuclear proliferation may be seen at the ends of severed fibres, and it is believed that these may join to re-establish continuity of the fibres.

In the repair of a **fractured bone**, the first stage is organization of the haematoma with the necrotic tissue and inflammatory exudate which are in varying degree present between the ends of the broken bone. This is accompanied by mononuclear cell phagocytosis of necrotic material. Organization is effected by granulation tissue derived from periosteum, endosteum and marrow. The proliferating connective tissue cells act as fibroblasts in the early stages, but later revert to osteoblastic function. Associated with the fibrillar collagenous material there now appears a hyaline, amorphous ground substance, which becomes osteoid tissue as a result of the activity of osteoblasts. This is laid down on both aspects of the periosteum and in the fractured medullary canal, gradually extending to replace most of the nonspecific granulation tissue. Some cartilage may develop in the tissue at this stage. Calcium is now deposited in the osteoid; this may be associated with phosphatase activity, resulting in supersaturation of tissue fluids by calcium and phosphate (vol. 1, p. 16.10). The tissue is quite soft at this stage, and is known as **callus**. The new bone formed has no regular structure, and is essentially woven bone. This bone is now partly resorbed by osteoclasts with concomitant laying down of calcium salts in an orderly fashion in the osteoid to form lamellar bone, which is then remodelled. The end result depends entirely on the stresses to be borne by the bone.

If immobilization of the broken bone is poor, excessive cartilage tends to be formed at the site of fracture. Repair of a fracture depends on provision of an adequate blood supply, and where this is poor by reason of traumatic damage, or because the patient is elderly and has arterial disease, the callus formed may remain fibrous or cartilaginous or too little bone may be laid down.

Regeneration of **nervous tissue** differs in the central nervous system from that of peripheral nerves. In the former no functional regeneration occurs, although it is possible that this is due more to the lack of proliferative capacity of the myelin-producing cells, the oligodendroglia, than to inability of the nerve cells themselves to regenerate. The other neuroglia proliferate to repair lesions in the central nervous system.

The degenerative processes occurring in peripheral nerves after injury have been alluded to on p. 25.9; regenerative changes begin while such degenerative lesions are progressing. The Schwann cells proliferate and move from the torn ends of the nerve into the intervening space; into this mass of cells neurofibrils grow from the proximal end of the nerve. At the same time, the endoneurial connective tissue proliferates and fibrosis develops outside the Schwann cells. Some of the growing neurofibrils within the Schwann cell mass now acquire a myelin sheath and gradually enlarge out of proportion to the others, extending until they join up with the fibrils of the peripheral end of the torn nerve. Thus the functional capacity of the nerve is at least partially restored, though not all the fibres are reconstituted.

POSSIBLE MECHANISMS OF REGENERATION
It has been demonstrated that if the circulation of a rat which has undergone partial hepatectomy is anastomosed to that of a normal rat for a sufficiently long period, DNA synthesis is stimulated in the liver cells of the normal rat. This suggests some hormonal control of regeneration which acts specifically on the cells of the affected organ. These substances have been called **chalones** and are either mitotic stimulants released by the removal of tissue or inhibitors of mitosis which, if the organ or tissue is of normal size, restrict mitotic activity to the appropriate rate. Evidence that chalones act as inhibitors of mitosis has been obtained by Bullough who damaged the epidermis on one side of a mouse ear. In such a case the mitotic rate in the epidermis rises abruptly at the site of damage. However, the mitotic rate of the undamaged epidermis on the other surface of the ear, 1 mm distant, rises also. In addition, the mitotic rate of the undamaged epidermis is highest after the epidermis on the damaged side has been removed entirely. Since the mitotic activity is most marked when the source of the chemical messenger is removed, it is argued that the substance is an inhibitor and is normally present in cells and tissues. Attempts to isolate chalones have been only partially successful but the epidermal substance is believed to be a protein with a mol. wt. of about 25,000.

It has been shown also in plants and experimental animals that ultrasonic irradiation can stimulate the regenerative process; ultrasound appears to increase enzyme activity and thus the metabolic rate of cells, and it is suggested that this may be due to the mechanical compression effect of the sound waves in breaking molecular bonds.

Hyperplasia and hypertrophy
Hyperplasia is an increase in the size of a tissue or organ above normal due to an increase in the number of constituent cells; one type of hyperplasia is the process discussed above, which can be described as regenerative

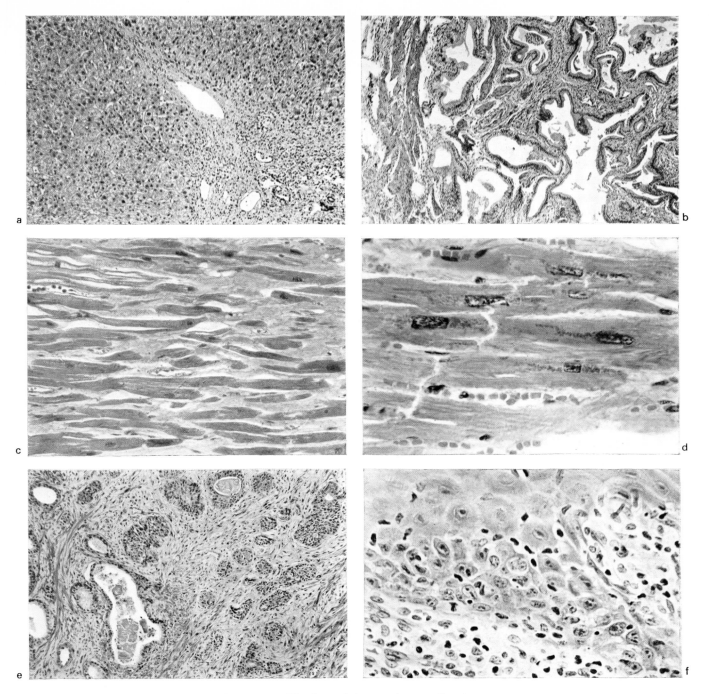

PLATE 27.1. Histology of tissue and organ disorders.

(a) Nodules of regenerating liver tissue from a patient who had developed a form of focal hepatic necrosis; the normal lobular structure is lost. Haem. & eosin (×85).

(c) The individual myocardial fibres are undergoing atrophy and are being replaced by connective tissue. Haem. & eosin (×190).

(e) This field from a prostate gland shows normal prostatic acini to the left and small solid foci of metaplastic squamous epithelium to the right. Haem. & eosin (×75).

(b) The field shows hyperplastic gall-bladder mucosa in a case of chronic cholecystitis. Epithelial proliferation has led to the protrusion of glands into the substance of the muscle coat, to the left of the picture. Haem. & eosin (×65).

(d) Brown atrophy of the heart; the myocardial fibres are slightly shrunken, and show large amounts of the pigment lipofuscin at the poles of the nuclei. Haem. & eosin (×450).

(f) A focus of aberrant hyperplasia of the epidermis; the deeper layers of the squamous epithelium show pleomorphism and variation in size of cells, and their orientation and relation to adjacent cells is disturbed. Haem. & eosin (×475).

hyperplasia. **Hypertrophy** means an increase in the size of individual cells and may cause enlargement of an organ itself, although it is often associated with hyperplasia. It is important to distinguish clearly between these two processes, since some types of mesodermal cell, such as cardiac muscle fibres, do not possess the capacity to proliferate and therefore respond to increased work load only by hypertrophy. There are many causes of these two processes, but most commonly they are induced by an increase in functional requirements.

Endocrine stimulation may be an aetiological factor; anterior pituitary growth hormone produces a mixture of hypertrophy and hyperplasia in the liver similar to that which occurs after excision or destruction of hepatic parenchyma. Physiological hyperplasia occurs in the gonads at puberty and in the breast during lactation. Oestrogens lead to hypertrophy of the myometrium but cause hyperplasia of the endometrium and vaginal epithelium. A single injection of oestrogen leads to an almost immediate synthesis of both messenger and transfer RNA, ribosomes and protein, resulting in a burst of mitotic activity within 24 hours. Treatment of certain diseases in the male by female sex hormones may cause the patient's breasts to enlarge.

Hormones are evidently concerned also to some extent in regenerative hyperplasia. If one kidney is removed, the remaining kidney undergoes compensatory hyperplasia, but it has been shown experimentally that hypophysectomy prevents this response, which is thus hormone dependent. The operation of normal feed back mechanisms may also lead to hyperplasia. Thus in chronic renal disease, which is associated with reduced concentration in serum calcium, hyperplasia occurs in the parathyroid glands.

Another example of a response to increased functional demands is the hyperplasia of the bone marrow seen in many forms of anaemia and physiologically in those who live at high altitudes.

The condition of glandular prostatic hyperplasia and fibroadenosis of the breast are epithelial hyperplasias of no known cause.

Hyperplasia commonly occurs as a result of chronic irritation; long standing inflammatory processes of the skin are associated with epidermal hyperplasia, e.g. at the edge of a varicose ulcer; hyperplasia of gall bladder mucosa is often seen in chronic cholecystitis (plate 27.1b, facing p. 27.2). Rarely, anomalies of vascular supply such as arteriovenous fistulae are responsible for hyperplasia. This is sometimes seen strikingly in children; a limb in which such a fistula is present grows disproportionately large. The mechanism is presumably that of increased blood supply and improved tissue nutrition.

The commonest and most important form of pure hypertrophy is that seen in the myocardium when it performs extra work; this is seen in the left ventricle in hypertension or under the haemodynamic handicap of valvular disease, and in the right ventricle in cases of chronic lung disease and of mitral valve stenosis. The heart may become more than twice normal size and individual myocardial fibres several times normal size may be formed. The process is not unlimited, however, and the controlling mechanisms are unexplained. Inability of the coronary vascular supply to increase beyond a certain point and to sustain further cytoplasmic increase seems likely to be a key factor.

Indeed, a common accompaniment of myocardial hypertrophy which has been present for some time is replacement fibrosis; numbers of the enlarged muscle fibres atrophy and disappear because of lack of sufficient blood supply, and their place is taken by collagen fibres.

A similar type of pure hypertrophy is seen in skeletal muscles where it is produced by frequent use, as in athletes, or by occupations involving heavy manual work. Of course, this type of response can properly be regarded as a physiological adaptation and the same is true of the combined hypertrophy and hyperplasia which occurs in the uterus in pregnancy.

Where smooth muscle is involved, the causative factor is nearly always a mechanical obstruction distal to the site of hypertrophy. Important examples occur in the hollow viscera, particularly the alimentary canal, where obstructive or stenosing lesions increase the work of the muscularis proximally, leading to varying degrees of hypertrophy and hyperplasia (plate 27.2, facing p. 27.4). A similar mechanism holds good in the urinary bladder if there is obstruction to the outflow of urine, most commonly caused by prostatic enlargement.

The importance of hyperplasia lies not merely in its aetiology, but in that it may undergo a transmutation to become **neoplasia** or new growth; then hyperplastic growth becomes transformed to tumour growth. It appears, in simple metaphor, that if a tissue 'gets enough practice at growing' it becomes unable to revert to a more stable condition and keeps on growing. This growth is now unco-ordinated with and unrelated to the needs of the body as a whole and is thus an abnormal form of cellular proliferation which is recognized as neoplasia or tumour formation.

It is to the possibility of transmutation to tumour formation that hyperplasia owes much of its importance as a topic in pathology; it may be a **premalignant lesion** (p. 28.11); some of the most important tumours in the human subject, such as carcinoma of the breast and prostate, commonly supervene upon a pre-existing hyperplasia.

Atrophy, hypoplasia and aplasia

Decrease in size of an organ or tissue is called **atrophy** and is distinguished from the conditions of **hypoplasia** and **aplasia** which are of developmental origin.

Atrophy may result theoretically from a reduction in

the size or in the number of the constituent cells of an organ or tissue, or from both; a combination of the two factors is probably most common.

Several features are commonly seen on microscopic examination of atrophic tissues. In the earlier stages, the tissue may appear to be hypercellular because more cells than normal are seen in one microscopic field. In many cases cellular atrophy is accompanied by a replacement of the parenchymal tissue by fibrous tissue, by fat or both. There is often a sparse infiltration of the connective tissue by lymphocytes. In addition, the atrophic cells frequently accumulate in their cytoplasm lipofuscin or lipochrome, which is present normally in cells to a much less extent (vol. 1, p. 13.16).

LOCALIZED ATROPHY

As might be expected, conditions opposite to those which produce hypertrophy and hyperplasia give rise to **atrophy**, so that important causes are reduced work-load and diminished vascular supply. The commonest example of atrophy induced by reduced work-load, **disuse atrophy**, is seen in the skeletal muscles following inactivity due to immobilization for treatment of a fracture. Changes in the related bones occur also and protein loss from the osteoid matrix is followed by loss of minerals. Another important though less common form of disuse atrophy is seen in exocrine glands such as the salivary glands or pancreas where obstruction of the duct stops functional activity. The result is atrophy and ultimate disappearance of a substantial amount of the secretory tissue. At the same time, the connective tissue component or stroma shows a gradual increase, a relationship which is very common in tissues undergoing atrophy.

What may be considered as disuse atrophy is observed where part of the function of a tissue is taken over by a drug being administered therapeutically. Thus, in patients receiving long term treatment with cortisone, adrenocortical atrophy gradually develops, while patients given thyroxine show atrophy of the thyroid gland. These substances act by inhibiting the release of ACTH and TSH respectively (vol. 1, pp. 25.22 & 37).

Interference with the nerve supply of tissues is associated with another form of atrophy, well seen in skeletal muscle following lower motor neurone lesions affecting the related peripheral nerve or the ventral horn cells, as in poliomyelitis. It is possible, however, that **neuropathic atrophy** is really only a form of disuse atrophy.

Atrophy due to reduced vascular supply, **ischaemic atrophy**, is most commonly seen in the parenchymatous organs, particularly the heart, brain and kidneys and may occur when atheroma and arteriosclerosis reduce the lumina of the vessels. In the brain cortical atrophy results, with loss of nerve cells, and in the kidney the comparable lesion is glomerular shrinkage or loss, tubular atrophy

and associated increase in connective tissue. The condition commonly occurs in the myocardium (plate 27.1c, facing p. 27.2) where atheroma of the coronary arteries gradually cuts down the input of nutrients to the myocardial fibres so that they dwindle in size and finally disappear in piecemeal fashion, leaving only groups of cells separated by fibrous tissue which is correspondingly increased.

The myocardium suffers from a completely different form of atrophy known as **brown atrophy** (plate 27.1d, facing p. 27.2). The term is descriptive, the heart becoming small and unusually dark brown in colour, while the epicardial fat acquires a curious gelatinous character. The coronary vessels do not share in the atrophy, and so as the heart shrinks they gradually become tortuous, because a given length of artery has to fit between two points which are approaching each other. Histologically, individual myocardial fibres become thinned, but most characteristic is the accumulation within the fibres, around the poles of the nuclei, of granules of lipofuscin. Brown atrophy occurs commonly in wasting diseases such as cancer, chronic sepsis or tuberculosis and in old age (p. 36.5). In the event of successful treatment, however, it is reversible, like disuse atrophy, whereas ischaemic atrophy of the heart cannot be reversed since myocardial fibres which have disappeared cannot be regenerated even if the vascular supply could be restored. Brown atrophy of the heart may be associated with a similar lesion in other organs.

Pressure atrophy is common and has been recognized from an early stage in the history of pathology; it affects the tissues around growing tumours, expanding cysts and aneurysms. But a widely held view is that atrophy in these conditions is caused by compression of blood vessels, so that the lesion is really a form of ischaemic atrophy. This may be valid in many instances, but it may not always be so. For example, secondary tumour growing vigorously in the liver is quite often intimately admixed with the liver cells rather than forming an expanding globular mass. Hence, liver cells and tumour cells share a common environment so far as availability of blood supply is concerned. Yet while the tumour cells grow actively the liver cells show a marked degree of atrophy and this must surely be a true example of pressure atrophy. Erosion of the vertebral column by an expanding aneurysm of the arch of the aorta is another, less common, example of pressure atrophy.

Atrophy may sometimes be found in organs when no cause is immediately obvious (idiopathic atrophy). The decrease of parenchymal tissue in such an organ may be associated with an increase in mononuclear cells, and under these circumstances an autoimmune aetiology has been suggested (p. 23.7). Examples of this are atrophic gastritis, and atrophy of the adrenal cortex and thyroid gland.

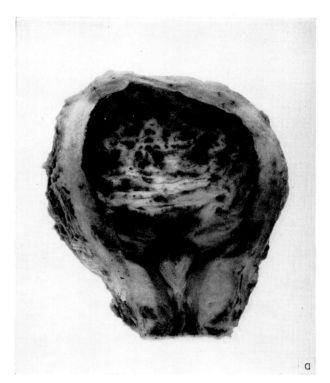

PLATE 27.2. Hypertrophy and hypoplasia.

(a) Bladder and prostate. The wall of the bladder is thicker than normal due to hypertrophy of the muscle coat; prominent trabeculae of hypertrophied muscle can be seen on the mucosal surface, which shows also much congestion. The hypertrophy is due to enlargement of the prostate gland, which has obstructed the urethra and therefore the outflow of urine.

(b) Kidneys removed at necropsy from a middle-aged man. The right is much smaller than the left but shows no other significant lesion apart from a scar near the upper pole, probably the result of old infarction. This illustrates the process of hypoplasia, since no acquired cause for the small size of the kidney was found.

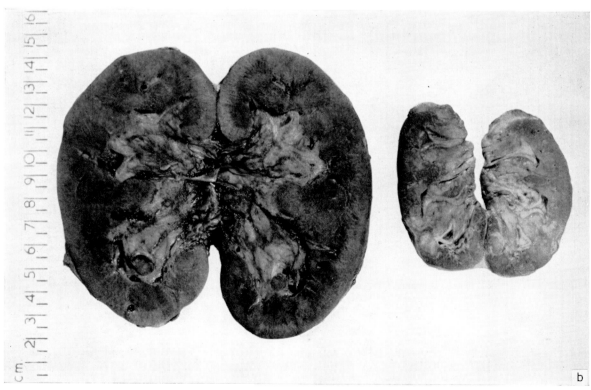

Atrophy has a physiological aspect in that some tissues atrophy with age but too early to be regarded as a change of senescence. Atrophy of the thymus is progressive in childhood and adolescence, while the lymphoid tissue of the body diminishes throughout adult life, and the ovaries, uterus and breasts atrophy from the menopause into senescence. These changes in the genital organs are related to alteration in endocrine influence on the tissues, but the cause of the lymphoid atrophy is uncertain. There are many examples of physiological atrophy in foetal life and in early infancy, such as the disappearance of the thyroglossal duct and of the ductus arteriosus.

GENERALIZED ATROPHY

So far all the varieties of atrophy discussed have been local, i.e. restricted to a particular organ or tissue affected by abnormal conditions such as ischaemia or disuse. But atrophy may occur also in a general form. Most obvious is that seen in simple starvation. The fat depots are the first to undergo atrophy, and later a gradual reduction in the size of organs, **microsplanchnia**, occurs. This second phase of starvation atrophy is remarkably selective, the gastrointestinal tract, liver and heart showing most loss of tissue, while the CNS is virtually unaffected.

Starvation of this order is little seen in Western countries, however, where generalized atrophy is much more commonly due to malignant diseases. In cases of advanced cancer, a combination of wasting, weakness and anaemia is common and is known as **cachexia**. The cause is uncertain but may be partly low food intake. Another view is that malignant tissue elaborates a specific toxin or toxins; no such factors have so far been identified, and it is more probable that any toxins produced are the result of ulceration with infection, a common complication of tumours in any hollow viscus. Although tumours have great powers of growth, they have virtually no power of repair. Once their surface is ulcerated, it remains so, and infection follows almost inevitably.

Generalized atrophy occurs also in extreme old age. In this condition and in the wasting of chronic disease, the cells of the affected organs and tissues tend to accumulate an excess of lipofuscin pigment.

The term **hypoplasia** is used to describe the condition in which an organ develops incompletely, and never reaches the full size or maturity of the normal adult organ. Two aspects are involved and usually co-exist, failure to achieve full maturity embryologically and failure to grow to adult size as the rest of the body tissues and organs are growing. Any organ may be involved in this condition, but it is more commonly seen in some than in others. One kidney may be hypoplastic, and represented by a small organ which reveals histologically a normal structure, or in addition foci of embryologically immature tissue (plate 27.2b, facing p. 27.4). It may be pointed out here that when at autopsy one kidney is found to be

smaller than the other, and smaller than normal, it may be difficult to be certain whether this is due to hypoplasia, or to acquired unilateral disease such as pyelonephritis or ischaemic vascular disease. Further, it is interesting that a small, hypoplastic (or aplastic) kidney may possess an artery of normal size, and also a normal pelvis and ureter, since these arise from different embryological structures.

Aplasia is the extreme form of hypoplasia; it implies that the organ involved has not developed at all, or is represented by a structure which may be a small, rudimentary, almost unidentifiable organ or simply a nodule of fatty and fibrous tissue. The term **agenesis** may be used when no trace of an organ is present. While this condition may affect any organ, it is probably seen most commonly in paired organs, a well known example again being the kidney. This is an important point to remember in clinical practice, for it is incumbent upon the surgeon, before performing nephrectomy for disease or trauma, to ensure that the patient has a fully developed organ present on the other side. Other paired organs which may be affected with relative frequency are the testes and ovaries. Obviously if a single organ important to development, such as the pituitary or thyroid, is aplastic or even severely hypoplastic, the individual may show widespread abnormalities, often incompatible with extrauterine life.

It should be noted that the term 'aplasia' is sometimes used in another sense; it is applied to the cessation of haemopoietic activity in the bone marrow, leading to aplastic anaemia.

Metaplasia

This process owes much of its practical importance to its tendency to undergo malignant transformation. The term metaplasia means altered form, and the process may be defined as the transformation of one type of fully differentiated tissue into another. Important examples, from a practical standpoint, occur in epithelial tissues, and usually involve conversion to a less highly specialized or organized type of epithelium, generally following a period of chronic inflammation. Thus in the bronchial tree, the respiratory epithelium of the large bronchi may become converted to stratified squamous epithelium and in the urinary bladder the same change may affect the transitional epithelium. In the stomach, loss of the highly specialized cells of the glands and their replacement by mucus-secreting cells is known as intestinal metaplasia and is a common feature of the condition of chronic gastritis.

In all these examples of metaplasia there is an increased tendency for neoplasia to supervene. The transformed tissue evidently acquires some form of biological instability so that metaplastic foci may often be described as precancerous. As in all biological matters, however, the rule is not absolute; for example, while squamous metaplasia in the prostate is not uncommon in relation to infarcts and abscesses in that organ, squamous carcinoma (the malignant tumour of squamous epithelium) is rare (plate 27.1e, facing p. 27.2). Again in the pancreas, where squamous metaplasia of the ducts is sometimes found associated with chronic inflammation or obstruction, squamous carcinoma is rare.

While epithelial metaplasia usually involves a change to a less specialized or complex type of epithelium, the rule is not universal and an important exception occurs in the urinary bladder in the condition of cystitis cystica, which is a metaplasia associated with a chronic inflammatory lesion. In this condition the transitional epithelium grows downwards in solid clumps into the submucosa. Some of the clumps may eventually become detached; a central space appears and the cells acquire mucus-secreting properties so that the end result is a glandular mucous membrane. The process occurs also occasionally in the ureters and is called **glandular metaplasia** (or ureteritis cystica). If cancer supervenes in this condition the tumour is of glandular type, and the cells continue to produce mucus.

Malignant transmutations from hyperplasia and metaplasia occur not abruptly, but gradually. The epithelial cells show first minor nuclear abnormalities, with increase in size and chromatin content. Later, these features become more marked, cells show variation in size and shape, mitotic figures are seen in increasing numbers, and loss of polarity appears, i.e. the normally regular orientation of cells at right angles to their basement membrane becomes blurred or obliterated. These aberrant cellular changes are sometimes referred to as **dysplasia** (plate 27.1f, facing p. 27.2).

The surface cells of the serous sacs, the mesothelium, also possess remarkable potential for metaplasia similar to that just described. In peritonitis it is common to find the surface cells of the peritoneum cuboidal or columnar, in contrast to their normal very flat form. If the peritonitis has been protracted it is not unusual to observe downward budding of the mesothelium with formation of glandular spaces rather similar to the appearances of cystitis cystica. This vigorous growth in the peritoneum may be accompanied by a great deal of aberration in the cells, of the kind that would generally be regarded as precancerous, but so far as is known this metaplasia does not lead to tumour growth, possibly because it is usually short-lived. Nevertheless it can lead to great diagnostic difficulty for it may in a biopsy so mimic tumour growth in a patient suspected of having an abdominal neoplasm as to make a definite decision impossible.

In general the pleura and pericardium are less versatile in metaplasia than the peritoneum, and glandular formations are rare, but cuboidal or columnar transformation of the surface cells is quite common.

Much interesting and fundamental work with the serosa has been done in animal experiments. It has been shown, for instance, that if both ovaries are excised, regeneration may occur from the pedicles, or even from the adjacent peritoneum. The flattened cells of the serous membrane may look inert, but this observation, as well as the metaplastic changes described above, indicate that this is not so. Pregnancy has been reported in women who have undergone bilateral oophorectomy (surgical removal of both ovaries) and the regenerative process seen in animals affords the only likely explanation of the phenomenon.

Metaplasia occurs very commonly in connective tissues, with the important distinction, however, that it rarely leads to tumour formation. Deposition of calcium salts is common in old scars, in the walls of old abscesses and in the walls of degenerate arteries. In all such situations this may be followed by the development of bone, often with a fully formed marrow element which may contain haemopoietic cells.

In the repair of fractures, something similar to metaplasia may occur; this is the formation of a **false joint** at the site of a non-united fracture (p. 27.1). Constant movement leads to excessive formation of cartilage, and if movement is prolonged a synovial membrane develops and indeed quite a faithful reproduction of the structure of a normal joint. It is obvious that this is an adaptive process in which tissues are formed which are appropriate to the local environment, i.e. one of movement, although movement is not normally found at that site in the body. Appreciation of this sort of adaptation is the key to understanding metaplasia, and to an awareness of the plasticity and intermutability of many cell types in the body. It is convenient for descriptive purposes to distinguish the different types of cell which go to make up the adult body and, of course, some cells can never change; nerve cells are a good example. However, it is doubtful whether the full range of possibilities of transmutation is yet known; a hindrance to the expansion of our knowledge is a tendency to cling too grimly to the idea that only a very limited intermutability is possible. It is well to remember that the entire body is derived from a single cell and that every cell in the adult body must contain the genetic information necessary to form a complete body. It is hardly surprising if some of this enormous potential occasionally appears, under suitable conditions of environment, in a process which may fairly be likened to that produced in the embryo by the action of organizers or inducers (vol. 1, p. 18.47).

Metaplasia is surely nothing more than the response of living tissues to alterations in their environment and so is one of the most basic biological processes in human pathology.

FURTHER READING

CAMERON G.R. (1962) Healing in organs, in *General Pathology*, 3rd Edition, ed. H.W. Florey. London: Lloyd-Luke.

BULLOUGH W.S. (1968) The control of tissue growth in *The Biological Basis of Medicine*, vol. 1, ed. E.E. Bittar & N. Bittar. New York: Academic Press.

FLOREY H.W. & JENNINGS M.A. (1962) Healing, in *General Pathology*, 3rd Edition, ed. H.W. Florey. London: Lloyd-Luke.

HARRIS H. (1962) Cell Growth and Multiplication, in *General Pathology*, 3rd Edition, ed. H.W. Florey. London: Lloyd-Luke.

WALTER J.B. & ISRAEL M.S. (1967) Disorders of growth, in *General Pathology*, 2nd Edition. London: Churchill.

WILLIS R.A. (1962) Regeneration and repair, and metaplasia in, *The Borderland of Embryology and Pathology*, 2nd Edition. London: Butterworths.

Chapter 28
General pathology of tumours

Under normal conditions, many tissues of the body are continuously replaced by proliferation of their constituent cells to make good normal wear and tear. When tissue has been destroyed by injury or disease, repair and regeneration come into play as described in the previous chapter, and involve proliferation of cells at a much increased rate. Sometimes however, and usually without obvious cause, a proliferation of cells occurs which exceeds that of repair or hyperplasia. It begins and continues indefinitely with no apparent relation to the growth and maintenance of the body tissues, leading to the development of a tumour mass; this often extends without regard to normal microanatomical boundaries, breaking through basement membranes and breaching the walls of small blood and lymphatic vessels. This is the state of **neoplasia** (new growth) or tumour growth. Frequently, the process becomes established in a single focus, but sometimes there are adjacent satellite foci. Occasionally, the abnormal growth process is systematized, a form seen particularly in the reticuloendothelial system where, for instance, bone marrow throughout the body may be involved in the leukaemias which involve neoplastic overproduction of leucocytes.

The cellular proliferation ranges in degree from one so slight as to be just abnormal to that of wild growth, in which a mass of tumour cells extends destructively into adjacent tissues; in the latter case complete removal of the tumour is difficult, since the surgeon cannot judge accurately how far to dissect in order to ensure removal of all neoplastic cells. Should any such cells remain, the tumour will very probably grow again (**recurrence**). In addition, in such cases, breaching of blood and lymphatic vessels leads to the transport of cells far beyond the limits of the original or primary tumour. Between these two extremes tumours exhibit varying rates of growth, varying tendencies to destroy surrounding tissues and varying rapidity of invasion of lymphatic and blood vessels. Some grow to a large size, while others never progress beyond the stage of being just visible macroscopically; some produce early clinical symptoms, and others are not known to have been present until autopsy. Nevertheless, it is possible to divide tumours into two main groups, described as benign and malignant. At one end of the spectrum the **benign** or **simple** tumour is clinically significant mainly by virtue of its increasing size and the pressure it exerts on other tissues, and at the other end is the **malignant** tumour, or **cancer**. It should be appreciated that tumours occur which are not easily placed in either category, and that some tumours may change their character from benign to malignant over a period of time. A common problem for the pathologist is that of assigning a tumour to one or other of the groups, thus enabling the clinician to treat it as effectively as possible.

When a malignant tumour invades lymphatic or blood vessels, the cells carried to other parts of the body may grow to form a secondary tumour, and this process is known as **metastasis**. Surgical removal of the primary tumour is then, in general, of no avail.

Malignant tumours may kill by destroying tissues, by interfering with physiological functions, by causing haemorrhage or ulceration and infection, or by secondary starvation. These are more likely when metastatic spread has occurred. Malignant tumours usually grow relatively rapidly, but in some cases there may be long periods during which growth is slow; on very rare occasions malignant tumours regress spontaneously. The common picture of cancer is that of a painful disease; however, pain is uncommon in the early stages, although it often becomes severe later. Malignant tumours are responsible for about one-fifth of all deaths in Britain.

The first part of this chapter gives a classification and general description of human neoplasms. Apart from the broad division into benign and malignant tumours, the classification is **histogenetic**, i.e. it is based on the tissue of origin of the lesion as far as this can be ascertained by gross and microscopical investigation. Reference is then made to biological, epidemiological and behavioural aspects of tumours.

Benign and malignant tumours

Table 28.1 lists the main differences between benign and malignant neoplasms, but these are not always clear-cut. General rules provide guidance in the diagnosis of malignancy in many cases, but they are not entirely adequate, singly or collectively, as a means of assessing the future behaviour of a tumour, and it is this aspect which is most important. Classifying a tumour is not an academic exercise but provides information which influences the treatment of the patient and assists in making a prognosis, i.e. a forecast of how the lesion may be expected to behave.

The structure of a tumour, as seen in histological preparations, is often a good guide to its biological behaviour. Tumours which reproduce the structure of their

TABLE 28.1. Comparison of characteristics of benign and malignant tumours.

	Benign	Malignant
Structure	Well differentiated, resembling tissue of origin	Tendency to loss of structural and cellular differentiation; may be anaplastic
Manner of growth	May possess a fibrous capsule produced by pressure on surrounding tissue	Unencapsulated; invades surrounding tissue
Rate of growth	Slow and may cease	Usually rapid
Mitotic figures	Absent or scanty	Usually more numerous
Metastatic growth	Absent	Often present
Clinical effects	Limited to mechanical or hormonal effects	Usually lethal, due to widespread destruction of tissues and metastasis

tissue of origin are likely to be benign, while those in which the parent architecture is poorly preserved are likely to be malignant. This loss of architectural organization in neoplastic growth, known as **dedifferentiation**, may reach such a degree that the parent structure is no longer recognizable. In such cases there is usually not only structural dedifferentiation but also a lack of differentiation of the cells themselves, i.e. the cells cease to resemble the normal cells of the parent tissue. For example, the cells of a carcinoma of the stomach may exhibit little evidence of gland formation and lose their columnar appearance; they vary in size and shape, i.e. exhibit **pleomorphism**. Mitotic figures are numerous and may be of abnormal form. Tumours which totally lack architectural and cellular differentiation are described as **anaplastic**.

However, dedifferentiation does not always accompany malignancy. For instance, malignant tumours of the thyroid may be so well differentiated as to be almost indistinguishable from normal thyroid tissue.

The formation of a capsule round a tumour, due to compression of adjacent tissue by the expanding mass of cells, and increase of fibrous tissue at the periphery, is usually associated with a benign growth. It is certainly a reassuring feature when present, for malignant tumours are not encapsulated; encapsulation, however, is often absent from tumours which are unquestionably benign, particularly those arising in the connective tissue. In contrast, malignant tumours, which lack a capsule, do not only compress but also invade the surrounding tissues, insinuating themselves between tissue cells, eventually destroying and replacing them.

The rate of growth of a tumour is usually a moderately reliable guide to its biological status. Rapid growth generally indicates malignancy, but the means of assessing it are open to error. Sometimes a sudden increase in size may take place over a few days, which may be due to haemorrhage into the tumour and not to tumour growth.

The growth rate of a neoplasm may be assessed from a study of the histological appearances and in particular from the numbers of mitotic figures observed. One difficulty is that if the mitotic cycle is short, few mitotic figures may be seen in the histological section; equally, if the mitotic cycle is retarded, as may happen if the tumour is growing where there is little space to expand, large numbers of mitotic figures may be seen in the telophase as daughter cells form, and give a false impression of the true growth rate.

The occurrence of metastatic growths invariably indicates malignancy, for it demonstrates that the tumour cells have the growth potential to enter vessels, to be conveyed to distant sites and to establish themselves there. Benign tumours do not metastasize. Generally, the expectation of life is short once a secondary focus becomes demonstrable by clinical or radiographic examination, but a focus which is not clinically obvious may lie dormant for years. This, of course, can be recognized only retrospectively. Unfortunately it is never possible to tell in advance whether a tumour will give rise to this type of silent metastatic lesion. The ability to metastasize is mainly responsible for the great difficulty in curing malignant tumours. Eventually, vital structures are damaged by tumour growth in or near them.

Tumours which appear identical on gross and histological examination may, in fact, be very different biological entities in regard to growth rate and occurrence of metastasis. Thus the histological appearance of a tumour is a fallible means of assessment, but as yet no better method is available.

Benign neoplasms kill the patient only occasionally, usually by accident of position. Obviously a tumour growing within the cranial cavity, however slowly, will eventually cause death and the designation 'benign' for such a tumour is clearly a misnomer. Occasionally a functionally active benign tumour of glandular tissue may cause serious disease or even death; e.g. an adenoma of the parathyroid gland associated with increased rate of secretion of parathyroid hormone produces hypercalcaemia which may reach a fatal level, and a tumour of chromaffin tissue (phaeochromocytoma), nearly always benign, can secrete catecholamines (p. 15.3). In general, however, benign neoplasms may be present for many years and cause little more than inconvenience; some varieties, especially those arising in connective tissue, may actually become static after years of slow growth.

The site of a tumour may contribute to an accurate forecast of its behaviour; a malignant epithelial tumour of the large intestine carries a much better prognosis than one in the stomach or in the bronchus, but the reason for this difference is by no means clear. It is important, also, to have clinical information about the patient before attempting to make an accurate diagnosis in an individual tumour; a lesion which might in an adult be diagnosed as a malignant melanoma of the skin on its histological appearance can be regarded as benign when it occurs in a child.

CLASSIFICATION OF TUMOURS

The **histogenesis** of a neoplasm denotes the particular tissue from which it has arisen, and is the basis on which the major classification of tumours is made. As a general rule tumours are named so as to indicate their probable histogenesis, their anatomical site and also whether they are benign or malignant. In anaplastic tumours, however, the histogenesis may be impossible to determine, occasionally to the extent that it cannot even be decided whether a tumour is of epithelial or connective tissue

origin; then the diagnosis can be no more precise than 'anaplastic malignant tumour'.

Table 28.2 is a simple and workable classification. It is, of course, by no means a comprehensive list of neoplasms but merely indicates how the more common and representative of them may be grouped; many tumours are omitted which will be discussed in detail in the clinical parts of this book. Furthermore, some tumours are difficult to classify accurately, since none of the three germ layers gives rise to any single well-defined group of neoplasms. It is not proposed to consider all the categories of tumours in an encyclopaedic fashion, but merely to discuss the general scheme, giving a few relevant examples.

Most tumours may be placed in one of two main groups, those arising from epithelial tissues, and those from connective tissues. This grouping does not imply any specific embryological origin. Ectoderm gives rise to epithelial elements, e.g. epidermis, and probably also to arrector pili muscles and the smooth muscle of the iris; endoderm is the layer of origin of some epithelia, e.g. the intestinal mucosa, but probably also of the thymus. Some other epithelia, e.g. renal and testicular, and all the connective tissues of the body, are mesodermal. The classification of endothelia and mesothelia is discussed in vol. 1, p. 17.3. Although as lining tissues they may be called epithelia, they arise from mesoderm, and tumours developing in them resemble connective tissue rather than epithelial neoplasms. In addition, the cells possess

TABLE 28.2. A classification of the commoner tumours.

	Benign	Malignant
TUMOURS OF EPITHELIAL TISSUE		
Glandular epithelium	Adenoma	Carcinoma
Surface epithelium	Papilloma	
TUMOURS OF CONNECTIVE TISSUES		
Fibrous tissue	Fibroma	Fibrosarcoma
Adipose tissue	Lipoma	Liposarcoma
Cartilage	Chondroma	Chondrosarcoma
Bone	Osteoma (existence doubtful)	Osteosarcoma
Muscle	Rhabdomyoma (existence doubtful) (striated muscle)	Rhabdomyosarcoma
	Leiomyoma (smooth muscle)	Leiomyosarcoma
Vessels	*Haemangioma	Haemangiosarcoma
	*Lymphangioma	Lymphangiosarcoma
Reticuloendothelial and		Leukaemias
haemopoietic tissue		Lymphosarcoma
		Reticulum cell sarcoma
		Plasma cell myeloma
		Hodgkin's disease
TUMOURS OF NERVOUS TISSUE	Glioma (p. 28.4)	Glioma; glioblastoma
	Some nerve sheath tumours	Some nerve sheath tumours
TUMOURS OF EMBRYONIC ORIGIN		
Totipotent cells	Benign teratoma	Malignant teratoma
Abnormal organogenesis		Nephroblastoma (kidney)
		Medulloblastoma (brain)
		Neuroblastoma (sympathetic nervous system)
Trophoblast	Hydatidiform mole	Chorion carcinoma

* More commonly regarded as hamartomata, rather than neoplasms (see text).

phagocytic properties, like cells of the reticuloendothelial system, which is mesodermal. These lining tissues therefore tend to be regarded as a connective tissue rather than an epithelium by pathologists, and their tumours are classified as such.

Benign epithelial tumours are called **papillomata** if growing on a free surface and **adenomata** if growing in a solid glandular epithelium. According to the type of epithelium, three kinds of papilloma exist, **adeno-papilloma**, e.g. from colon (plate 28.1a), **transitional cell papilloma**, e.g. from bladder, and **squamous cell papilloma**, e.g. from skin.

All malignant epithelial tumours are known by the term **carcinoma**, which may be accompanied by a descriptive adjective or prefix according to the type of epithelium from which the tumour has originated, or with reference to the structure of the growth. Thus, a **squamous carcinoma** (plate 28.1b) originates in squamous epithelium and has a recognizable squamous structure; an **adenocarcinoma** (plate 28.1c), originating in glandular epithelium, shows differentiation into glands, and a **transitional cell carcinoma** arises in and resembles transitional epithelium. A **papillary adenocarcinoma** may arise by malignant transformation of a papilloma, and exhibits some degree of papillary structure, as well as glandular epithelium.

Benign tumours of connective tissue are named according to their tissue of origin, **fibroma, lipoma, chondroma**, etc. and their malignant equivalents are designated by the term **sarcoma** with appropriate prefix where the tissue of origin can be identified. Thus malignant tumours of fibrous tissue, cartilage and bone are called **fibro-chondro-** and **osteosarcoma** respectively.

Tumours of connective tissue are all of mesodermal origin; muscle is also mesodermal, and although it is not strictly speaking a connective tissue, its tumours are classified in this group. In fact, muscle tumours behave in general in the same way as connective tissue tumours.

As mentioned previously, the identity of the parent tissue may be in doubt in anaplastic malignant tumours of epithelial or connective tissue origin, and a purely descriptive nomenclature may have to be adopted. For example, a carcinoma may be called a spheroidal cell carcinoma with reference to its constituent cells, and this type was formerly referred to as carcinoma simplex. An undifferentiated sarcoma may also be described as a spindle cell or round cell sarcoma.

MALIGNANT TUMOURS OF THE
RETICULOENDOTHELIAL SYSTEM
The clinical and pathological characteristics of this group are very different from those of other sarcomata. Those arising from tissues which form white blood cells, the **leukaemias**, may be myeloid (granulocytic) or lymphoid (lymphocytic). In these conditions the blood contains large numbers of white cells, sometimes of primitive nature. An important tumour affecting the bone marrow is the **plasma cell myeloma** (myelomatosis or multiple myeloma). In this disease the bone marrow becomes packed with plasma cells, often focally, and the deposits may cause discrete osteolytic lesions of the bone, 'punched out' defects being visible on radiological examination, particularly in the skull. Soft tissue masses of plasma cells may also be present.

Other tumours involve the component parts of the RE system throughout the body. The two most important are **reticulum cell sarcoma** (reticulosarcoma) and **lymphosarcoma**. These arise from the two main cell types in lymphoreticular organs, the reticulum cell and the lymphocyte or lymphoblast. They usually involve many or all lymph nodes, the spleen, sometimes the liver and the bone marrow, and masses of the neoplastic cells may be found in other tissues. Cases of lymphosarcoma may be associated with a leukaemia of lymphoid type.

A relatively common disease of the reticuloendothelial system is **Hodgkin's disease** (lymphadenoma). There has been controversy as to whether this is really a neoplasm, for unlike most tumours the abnormal tissue consists of cells of very varying types; the main cell is the reticulum cell, but lymphocytes, eosinophils, characteristic giant cells and fibroblasts are also involved. However, its general course, behaviour and fatal termination are those of a neoplasm, and it is now generally considered as such. It involves lymph nodes, spleen, liver, bone marrow and sometimes skin and other soft tissues.

Abnormal immunoglobulins appear in the plasma in many patients with plasma cell myeloma and other malignant tumours of the reticuloendothelial system. These are called M-proteins and include the Bence–Jones protein which sometimes occurs in the serum and urine of patients with plasma cell myeloma (p. 23.12).

GLIOMATA AND SOME NERVE SHEATH TUMOURS
Gliomata are tumours of the neuroglia and of the ependyma, and most arise from astrocytes, oligodendrocytes and ependymal cells, which are neuroectodermal in origin. Microglia are thought to be of mesodermal origin (vol. 1, p. 14.6) but are very rarely the parent cell of tumours. Gliomata are usually regarded as malignant, irrespective of their other characteristics, because those in the brain if untreated lead to death from increased intracranial pressure, and those in the spinal cord are usually fatal because of damage to its tissues. However, the more rapidly growing and pleomorphic of these tumours are often called **glioblastomata**. The tumours vary greatly in their speed of growth and in the degree of invasion of surrounding brain tissue, and they never metastasize outside the central nervous system. In this respect they differ from other malignant tumours. Some nerve sheath tumours, e.g. neurilemmomata, which arise from

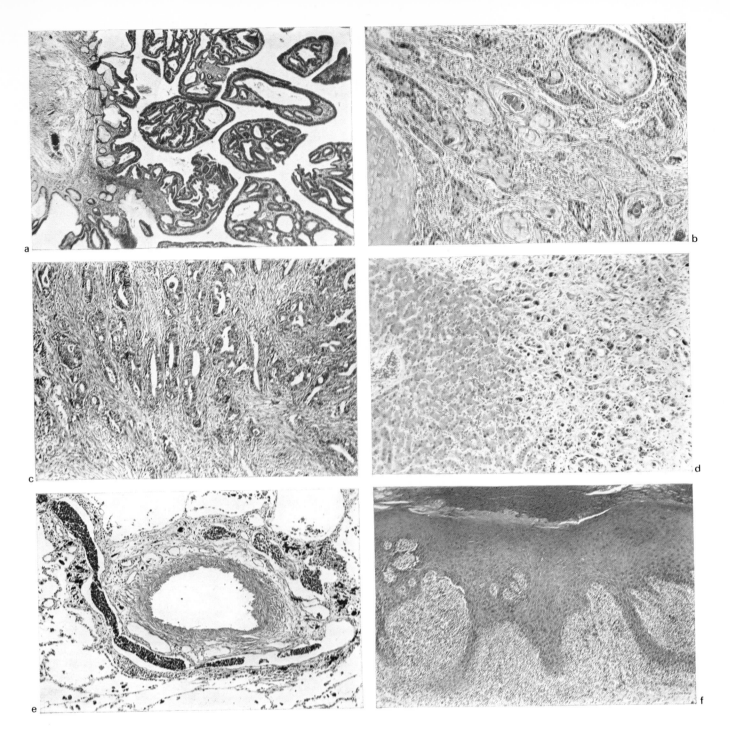

PLATE 28.1. Histology of tumours.

(a) Part of a benign adenopapilloma of colon, showing the pedicle or stalk cut in cross-section on the left of the picture. The glandular acini are less regular than normal but do not invade the pedicle. Haem. & eosin (×50).

(c) Field from an invading adenocarcinoma. The acini are poorly formed compared with those in (a). Haem. & eosin (×50).

(e) Invasion of perivascular lymphatics by an anaplastic carcinoma of bronchus. The masses of darkly staining tumour cells almost completely fill the dilated lymphatics. Haem. & eosin (×55).

(b) Squamous carcinoma invading the wall of a bronchus. The deeply staining red material is keratin, forming centrally in the cell masses and indicating moderate differentiation. A plate of cartilage which remains uninvaded is seen at lower left. Haem. & eosin (×50).

(d) A metastatic focus in liver from a gastric carcinoma; the tumour is generally anaplastic but shows occasional glandular acini. Haem. & eosin (×75).

(f) Leukoplakia. This premalignant lesion of squamous epithelium involves excessive keratin formation (hyperkeratosis), epithelial hyperplasia, and irregularity of the cells of the basal layers. The dense subjacent chronic inflammatory cell infiltration is an important feature. Haem. & eosin (×40).

Schwann cells, are also of neuroectodermal origin; they are usually benign.

TUMOURS OF EMBRYONIC ORIGIN

In addition to the two main groups of epithelial and connective tissue tumours, a third group consists of tumours of developmental type, often arising from embryonic cells which are capable of differentiating into tissues from more than one germ layer. They may be subdivided into three groups:

(1) teratomata,
(2) tumours associated with aberrant development of one organ, and
(3) chorion carcinoma.

Teratomata arise from embryonic cells which can develop into tissues of any of the three germ layers and usually occur in the younger age groups. They are sometimes present at birth, but may not become obvious until middle age; the primitive cells must then have remained inactive since intrauterine life. Some of these tumours are benign, but many are malignant; the presence and degree of malignancy is reflected in the degree of differentiation and structural organization of the tissues in the tumour. If all the tissues present are well differentiated, the tumour is probably benign, and its removal effects a complete cure. However, some of these tumours are composed of less well differentiated tissues. In some cases carcinomatous or sarcomatous tissue can be recognized but the tumour may contain bizarre anaplastic cells, whose origin cannot be identified. A well defined group of teratomata differentiate essentially along ectodermal lines, producing well formed epidermis, with sebaceous and sweat glands, hair and even teeth. Bone and cartilage may be found in the connective tissue. These lesions are often cystic and are called **dermoid cysts**; they grow particularly in the ovaries. The testes may also be the site of teratomata, and here the tumours are usually malignant.

Tumours due to a defect in the embryonic development of a single organ occur in infancy or early life, or may develop in intrauterine life. They are all malignant. A tumour of the kidney, the **nephroblastoma** or Wilm's tumour, is one of these. It includes connective tissue and epithelium and primitive tubules can be seen differentiating from the malignant connective tissue cells. Mesodermal tissues such as muscle may also be present. Other tumours of this kind are the **neuroblastoma**, found mainly in the adrenal medulla, and the **retinoblastoma**, which occurs in the eye.

Chorion carcinoma arises from trophoblast. A benign lesion from the same source is named **hydatidiform mole.** Chorion carcinoma usually occurs after a pregnancy, which may have been normal or abnormal, but it may sometimes develop in a teratoma, e.g. in the testis.

A **hamartoma** is a congenital malformation, usually causing a swelling, which may present clinically as a neo-plasm. It may resemble a tumour in the sense that it exists as a slowly growing mass of abnormal tissue. The tissues involved are mature, and are appropriate to the organ where the lesion occurs, but they are not organized in the normal way, presumably due to some defect in development, but are arranged irregularly; unlike a teratoma a hamartoma never contains tissues foreign to the site in which it is growing. Lesions which fall into this category are the haemangioma and the lymphangioma; the hamartoma of the lung consists of cartilage, connective tissue and epithelium, and the hamartoma of the kidney is a mixture of mature connective tissue, fat, and occasionally other tissues. These lesions do not become malignant and give rise to symptoms only because of their space-occupying characteristics. There is, however, a malignant tumour of blood vessels, the **haemangiosarcoma**, but it is doubtful if it ever arises in a hamartomatous haemangioma.

General appearances of tumours

MACROSCOPIC APPEARANCE

Benign epithelial tumours of papillary type are usually rounded, cauliflower-like growths possessing a stalk of varying length and made up of discrete papillary processes which are usually thin and delicate; decrease in length with increasing solidity of the processes and stalk may indicate malignant change. Adenomata are well defined, rounded lesions in the substance of the parent tissue, often more solid than the normal tissue.

Benign connective tissue tumours are usually pale, solid, well defined structures, and may resemble the parent tissue, e.g. chondroma.

Malignant tumours vary a great deal in their macroscopic appearance; in cases of early malignancy in a hitherto benign tumour, no naked eye change may be seen. Usually, however, a malignant tumour can be seen to be invading surrounding tissues, and breaching fascial, tissue or organ surfaces. Many carcinomata appear pale yellow and rather friable, whereas sarcomata may be greyish pink. Adenocarcinomata from mucus-producing tissues such as the colon may themselves contain much mucus, and are referred to as mucoid.

Malignant tumours, especially sarcomata, often show foci of necrosis and haemorrhage. If a tumour is situated in the wall of a hollow viscus, it often ulcerates and becomes infected; haemorrhage may occur. It is strange that although tumours possess great powers of growth they have little power of repair and once their surface has become ulcerated, healing rarely occurs.

HISTOLOGICAL STRUCTURE

Papillomata (plate 28.1a, facing p. 28.4) consist of simple or complex elongated processes which possess fibrovascular cores, and are covered by the epithelium from which the lesion is arising. The processes unite in a stalk, which attaches the papilloma to the parent surface. Some papillomata, particularly in the colon and bladder, tend to undergo malignant change, and the cores of the processes and the stalk must be examined for evidence of infiltration by malignant epithelial cells, since such invasion is important evidence of this change. The epithelial lining of the processes may also show aberration and increasing hyperplasia of cells, both of which suggest malignant change.

Adenomata occur in solid organs such as adrenal cortex, pituitary, kidney and parotid gland. They are sometimes functional, and lead to hypersecretion of hormone or other substance produced by the organ, and their structure is usually similar to that of the parent organ, but they may show some irregularity of glandular architecture, increased mitotic activity, and the presence of solid masses of undifferentiated cells; these features suggest malignant change.

Benign connective tissue tumours appear histologically similar to the tissue from which they arise; fibromata consist of interlacing bundles of elongated cells and fibres, and vary to a considerable extent in their relative content of cells and collagen fibres. A tumour of smooth muscle, or **leiomyoma**, exhibits interlacing or whorled bundles of smooth muscle cells, and contains also fibrous tissue which may be so abundant as to justify the name **fibroleiomyoma**. These tumours are extremely common in the uterus, where they are often called **fibroids**. It should be noted that special staining may be necessary to distinguish collagen fibres from muscle in tissue sections. Leiomyomata occur in several organs and tissues, and probably arise in some cases from the tunica media of small arteries.

In benign connective tissue tumours, as in those of epithelial type, malignant change may supervene and must be looked for in aberration of cell type, lack of differentiation of architecture, increased mitotic activity and early invasion of surrounding tissues.

Malignant tumours, as previously described, may show any degree of dedifferentiation both in cellular appearance and general tissue architecture. Some adenocarcinomata may retain the ability to secrete whatever substance or substances were produced by the normal organ, and exert functional effects by virtue of a hormonal secretion. Other adenocarcinomata have the ability to produce mucus; cells of such tumours may resemble a signet-ring, the cytoplasm being virtually replaced by a globule of mucus which pushes the nucleus to one side; such cells are called **signet-ring** cells.

Well differentiated sarcomata reproduce to some extent the tissue of origin, for example, a chondrosarcoma may show large foci of aberrant but recognizable cartilage. As differentiation decreases, the cells become characterless, spindle-shaped or ovoid.

Pleomorphism of cells and high mitotic activity are usually apparent in malignant tumours. Foci of necrosis are common, and indeed in some cases almost the whole tumour may be necrotic; this feature is usually considered to be due to rapid growth of the lesion outstripping the growth of its blood supply. However, some local failure of haemodynamic adaptation in the tumour is a more probable cause. Examination of tissue sections of malignant tumours may show tumour cells in lymphatics or in blood vessels, and this may constitute a guide to prognosis.

Occasionally, a diagnosis of malignancy may have to be made on the appearance of the cells alone. For example, under the microscope a focal lesion of the skin may show epidermal cells which are abnormal in shape and size, and have enlarged nuclei, with increased mitotic activity. These cytological features may be so marked as to justify a diagnosis of malignancy and the condition is called a **carcinoma-in-situ**. Such a lesion may occur in other organs but is probably commonest in squamous epithelium.

Carcinomata possess a supporting fibrovascular stroma for their epithelial cells, said to be derived from the normal stroma of the parent tissue. In some carcinomata, particularly those of the breast and stomach, the proportion of connective tissue present may often greatly exceed that of the tumour cells and the term scirrhous is used to describe such disproportionate growth of fibrous stroma. Traditional names for such tumours are scirrhous carcinoma of the breast and leather bottle stomach. The latter term was derived from the fancied resemblance of the thickened and indistensible stomach to a leather bottle.

In sarcomata, on the other hand, since the neoplasm originates in connective tissue, the stroma is not a separable component.

Invasion by malignant tumour

The greatest single obstacle to the effective treatment of malignant tumours is their ability to grow invasively and to metastasize. It is, therefore, appropriate to consider further what is known of the mechanisms underlying these two aggressive biological characteristics. Invasive growth is the more important of the two, for without it there can be no metastasis. An early concept of invasive growth was that the malignant cells simply followed the lines of least resistance. In a malignant tumour the cells grow between fascial planes; they also grow into lymphatics and veins but only rarely into arteries or other tissues which offer greater physical resistance. Cartilage in particular is rarely invaded. This concept was replaced by a hypothesis in which the tumour cells play a more active role.

MOTILITY OF CELLS
This theory held that the cells possessed the faculty of

amoeboid movement whereby they made their way through the tissues, but most of the evidence was derived from tissue culture, an environment in which many cells exhibit greater capacity for movement than *in vivo*. Further, doubts soon arose as to the identity of the motile cells in culture, many of which were believed to be histiocytic or macrophagic in nature and derived from the stromal or connective tissue component of the tumour rather than from the tumour cells themselves. It was further noted that cells which possess motility under normal conditions, such as leucocytes and macrophages, tended to move in the tissues as individuals, whereas tumour cells by contrast tended to extend through the tissues as solid columns or trabeculae and not as single units.

CELL ADHESIVENESS

Associated with the idea of motility in tumour cells is that of 'diminished mutual adhesiveness' which implies that malignant tumour cells adhere less to one another than do normal cells. Abnormalities at the cell surface have been demonstrated in tumour cells; for example, surface electrical charges have been found to be greater than normal in cells of tumours which metastasize readily, while a decreased intracellular concentration of calcium ions has been noted. It has not, however, been shown that these alterations are in fact part of a mechanism leading to a loss of mutual adhesiveness and in any case such a loss, while it might facilitate the start of movement by tumour cells through tissues, seems unlikely to contribute anything to the movement itself.

OTHER THEORIES

Another popular hypothesis of recent years has been the concept of elaboration of lytic products by the tumour cells. According to this idea, the cells produce extracellular lytic agents capable of dissolving or partially destroying the ground substance mucopolysaccharide of the tissue being invaded. As early as 1946, hyaluronidase had been invoked as such a possible factor and more recently other enzymes, notably aminopeptidase, have come under scrutiny, but no convincing evidence has been produced that such a mechanism plays a major role in invasive growth.

Of considerable interest is the behaviour of malignant tumours in relation to blood vessels. Malignant tumours of the bronchus frequently invade capillaries and veins and not uncommonly the pulmonary arteries, but only rarely do they invade systemic arteries. The fact that the frequency of invasion bears a constant and inverse ratio to the intravascular pressure has prompted investigations of the extent to which this might influence the invasive growth. It was found, experimentally, that when the intraluminal blood flow is abolished in an artery, its

resistance to invasion by tumour is lost; since the experiment does not interfere with viability of the arterial wall it seems that the resistance of arteries to tumour invasion is largely if not entirely due to the pressure within them. Furthermore, whatever role may be played by the active mechanisms suggested above, one key factor in invasive growth is clearly the hydrostatic pressure in tissues and the tensions created.

ROUTES OF SPREAD

Certain broad differences are observed in the routes of spread followed by carcinomata and sarcomata. Carcinomata tend to invade primarily lymphatics, frequently setting up metastatic tumours in regional lymph nodes at a comparatively early stage, while invasion of blood vessels leading to haematogenous spread with more distant secondary growths tends to occur much later. It is, of course, possible that some at least of the blood spread in carcinomata occurs because all lymph eventually drains into the blood and may carry tumour cells with it. Sarcomata, in contrast, tend to spread primarily by invasion of the blood stream with early production of distant secondary growths, very frequently in the lungs. This difference probably depends upon the close relation between tumour cells and blood vessels in sarcomata and the greater opportunity for blood vascular invasion. In a sarcoma the cells grow from one cell type only, which gives origin to the tumour and also to its vasculature. In many sarcomata the vascular channels appear merely as sinusoids lined by tumour cells, and there is maximal chance for the cells to invade the vascular spaces. Carcinomata consist only partly of neoplastic cells, the vasculature being carried in a distinct connective tissue stroma. Stroma and vessels are probably not part of the neoplasm itself but the result of a non-neoplastic reaction of the surrounding normal connective tissues. The validity of this concept is uncertain, but it helps to explain the less frequent invasion of the blood stream by carcinomata.

Haematogenous spread

The thinner walls of veins and capillaries and their lower intravascular pressure render them more vulnerable to invasion than arteries. For this reason the lungs are probably exposed to circulating neoplastic cells in most cases of malignant tumour. This does not mean that secondary deposits develop in the lungs in every case, since tumour cells can apparently pass through the pulmonary capillary network without establishing metastatic foci. What factors determine the impaction and subsequent development of cells in the lungs are not understood. Occasionally a small group of tumour cells is seen in the lungs surrounded by a fibroblastic and chronic inflammatory cell reaction.

Presumably in most cases tumour cells carried in

venous blood pass through the lungs and are distributed to peripheral organs in the arterial supply. In some cases blockage of veins by a tumour may lead to the reversal of blood flow in adjoining venous channels and this may enable neoplastic cells to reach other nearby tissues without passing through the lungs. Occasionally a tumour, e.g. carcinoma of the kidney, invades a large vein, in this case the renal vein, leading to the development of a mass of thrombus and tumour, which may block the vein and give rise to pulmonary embolism.

Venous spread from malignant tumours of the gastrointestinal tract is by means of the portal venous system to the liver; this organ is, therefore, often the site of secondary growths in such cases (plate 28.1d, facing p. 28.4). Tumours in other systems, such as the genito-urinary tract, also frequently metastasize to the liver, which is probably metabolically suitable as a tissue for the growth of neoplastic cells.

The type of blood vessel in which a tumour embolus impacts may determine the fate of the tumour cells. If impaction occurs in a small artery or arteriole with a relatively thick wall, the embolus may become organized and the tumour cells destroyed before there is time for them to penetrate the vessel wall. If impaction occurs in a thin walled capillary or venule, invasion and subsequent secondary growth is facilitated.

Lymphatic spread
The extent of lymphatic spread to regional lymph nodes is of great significance in the prognosis after surgical removal of a neoplasm. Tumour cells may be seen in lymphatics in histological sections (plate 28.1e, facing p. 28.4), although it does not necessarily follow that secondary deposits will be found in regional lymph nodes examined at the same time. Once tumour has reached the first line of the regional lymph nodes, it may be carried from them to more distant nodes, and in some cases may reach most of the groups of lymph nodes in the body. Certain types of carcinoma, such as carcinoma of the lung, may spread to involve many groups of nodes, including the superficial groups, before the primary tumour has produced significant clinical features; thus the patient may present with clinical features suggesting a primary lesion of lymph nodes.

Sometimes lymphatic spread occurs in a retrograde fashion, i.e. obstruction of lymphatics by tumour may cause the lymph flow to be reversed, and the tumour is carried to groups of nodes which would under ordinary circumstances not be involved.

Transcoelomic spread
While spread by lymphatics or by blood vascular channels constitutes the major part of remote spread of tumour, there are several other routes. Chief among these is transcoelomic spread, in which tumour cells are shed into a serous cavity and become implanted on the serosa itself, often with extension into subjacent parenchyma. This may happen when a carcinoma of the stomach or colon, for example, spreads after growing through the wall of the organ to the peritoneal surface. Secondary growths may occur on any part of the serous membrane, often in large numbers. Carcinomata of stomach or colon may lead in this way to large secondary growths in the ovaries, often bilateral, though there is, of course, no actual peritoneal covering on the ovaries. This secondary tumour is often distinguished by a mucus secretion and much stromal proliferation, giving a characteristic picture to which the term **Krukenberg tumour** is given. It must be added, however, that some authorities believe the Krukenberg tumour arises by lymphatic or blood spread to the ovary from the primary site. Transcoelomic spread may be observed also in the pleural cavity and, more rarely, in the pericardial sac.

Implantation
Implantation on epithelial surfaces is noted particularly in the renal tract but occurs occasionally in the bronchial tree. Viable tumour cells are carried by the flow of urine in the one instance and the passage of air in the other, to sites often at a relatively great distance from the primary tumour, and succeed in forming a satellite focus of tumour growth at the point of implantation. Cerebral tumours sometimes behave in a similar way and may produce seedling metastatic foci or implants in the walls of the ventricles or on distant meningeal surfaces.

Cerebral tumours form a special category in regard to metastatic growth. For all practical purposes secondary deposits never occur outside the CNS, despite the fact that some glial tumours are highly malignant and grow rapidly.

Cytological investigation
As might be expected, where a malignant tumour is growing in the wall of a hollow viscus or serous cavity, or in the wall of a natural passage such as a bronchus, some of the growth occupies the lumen and great numbers of cells are shed from the surface. Techniques exist for the identification of tumour cells in sputum, effusions into the serous sacs, in gastric washings and smears obtained directly from accessible surfaces, notably the cervix uteri. This method is known as **exfoliative cytology**. It is possible in these specimens to recognize the more aberrant tumour cells, showing marked nuclear hyperchromatism and an increased nuclear–cytoplasmic ratio; difficulty arises with those which are less aberrant, for cells which are merely hyperplastic may show quite as much aberration as well differentiated tumour cells. In conditions not themselves malignant, but which tend to develop into a malignant state, e.g. metaplasia, cells of very aberrant appearance may be shed. Infection is one of

the commonest causes of epithelial hyperplasia, and chronic infection and inflammation may be associated with metaplasia, so that accurate identification of malignant cells is frequently difficult. While exfoliative cytology is a useful screening technique, a definitive diagnosis should be confirmed by more reliable means, such as biopsy, whenever possible.

Biology of cancer

As already indicated, malignant neoplasms differ markedly in their origin and clinical course. Because it is difficult to generalize about their behaviour the conception of 'cancer' as an entity is perhaps more likely to mislead than to clarify thought. The one feature which all malignant neoplasms exhibit, and which to a lesser extent benign neoplasms also show, is a failure of tissue homeostasis which controls the cell mass of any tissue and the magnitude of its functional contribution. The essential feature of the neoplastic condition is loss of this control mechanism. Theoretically a tumour might arise as a result of an increase in the mitotic rate or a diminution in the rate of maturation, ageing or disposal. There are arguments which suggest that both factors are responsible and, as in the case of normal tissues, a balance is ultimately struck between cellular proliferation and cell death. In some tumours this point is reached relatively early and the growth remains small; in others it is not reached until the extent of the whole tumour is so massive that it cannot be supported by the organism. The role of chalones (p. 27.2) in the growth of cancer is speculative. It has been suggested that in the case of epidermal tumours in rabbits there is reduction in the concentration of tissue chalone inhibiting mitosis, rather than an inability to respond to it, and a similar claim has been made in the case of experimental leukaemia in mice. This is an important area for further research.

There are many agents or factors which can cause or predispose to neoplasia, some of which can be studied directly in experimental animals. In man this is not possible, but the incidence of a number of natural neoplasms is closely associated with particular environmental factors and in some instances it is reasonable to assume that the neoplasm arises directly as a result of their influence.

An important concept in the aetiology of cancer is the existence of 'field change'. This implies that a change takes place over a wide extent of tissue or organ concerned which makes it prone to develop foci of malignant growth at a later date, in response to some stimulus, as yet undefined. This process may be of the nature of the initiator–promotor mechanism suggested as operative in chemical carcinogenesis. In several cases where such 'field change' is suspected, the tumour is seen to arise not in a single focus but in many foci in the tissue at risk, such as the skin or the mucosa of the bronchial tree. Incidentally, the existence of field change often makes complete local removal of a tumour a matter of great difficulty since it may be impossible to say how much tissue needs to be removed in order to prevent recurrence. Indeed, recurrence, which is essentially a clinical entity, meaning the re-appearance of a tumour at or near its previous site, is often not due to incomplete removal but to the fact that neoplastic change has supervened or been promoted in the area of field change beyond the original excision. It is also possible to interpret this and other evidence on the view that removal of part of a tumour or a metastatic growth stimulates growth of tumour which remains, in the same way as removal of part of a liver stimulates the rest of the organ to increase its growth rate (p. 27.1). This effect has been shown experimentally and may also occur in man.

Five aspects of aetiology are now to be discussed: (1) chemical carcinogens, (2) physical agents, (3) viruses, (4) premalignant states, and (5) genetic factors.

CHEMICAL CARCINOGENS

As described on p. 25.16, Sir Percival Pott, already well known for his classic description of the common fracture of the ankle, reported in 1775, cases of carcinoma of the skin of the scrotum in chimney sweeps, which he attributed to their occupation; at work their clothes became soaked in the tarry deposits left in chimneys by the low grade coal then used in domestic fires, and this readily accumulated in the corrugated scrotal skin. Some hundred years later the first paraffin cancers of the skin were recognized and these early clinical observations were the springboard for modern cancer research. They led to efforts in the latter part of last century to produce cancer in experimental animals by painting the skin with tar. It was not, however, until 1914 that two Japanese workers, Yamagiwa and Ichikawa, reported the development of papillomata and carcinomata in the skin of rabbits' ears after long continued application of tar.

This work focused attention upon the importance of **chemical carcinogens** or cancer-producing agents. It was also noted that carcinomata sometimes developed in areas of hyperkeratosis of the skin seen in patients who had been treated for a long time with arsenic, then the main remedy for syphilis, and in workers using arsenic commercially. Carcinoma of the urinary bladder was observed in aniline dye workers. Characteristic features of these occupational cancers were the occurrence of the disease in only a small proportion of the exposed population, sometimes after long exposure amounting to ten years or more, and the fact that in some instances the tumours appeared years after the worker had given up his hazardous employment. These observations fostered the idea that some essential preliminary change was a prerequisite for the development of malignant disease and that after a long latent period this might give rise to neoplasia. Kennaway and his co-workers identified the first chemically pure polycyclic hydrocarbon carcinogen, 1,2,5,6-dibenzanthracene, by examining the fluorescence spectra of many tars and oils known to be carcinogenic. It was shown experimentally that after exposure of a tissue to such a carcinogenic agent for a short period of time, transient changes occurred which did not in themselves lead to tumour formation and regressed, leaving no trace. However, there remained a state of proneness or predisposition to tumour formation, which could be stimulated subsequently by a wide range of nonspecific irritant substances such as phenols, turpentine, chloroform, non-ionic detergents and croton oil, to produce tumour growth. A two-stage mechanism was thus envisaged, the first being that of **initiation** by the carcinogen, and the second a phase of **promotion** by the nonspecific irritant agent. These promoting agents were sometimes referred to as co-carcinogens. In the years that have followed, large numbers of carcinogenic polycyclic hydrocarbons have been identified, and the process continues.

Other important groups of substances possessing carcinogenic properties are given on p. 25.17. There has been little progress in the attempt to relate chemical structure with carcinogenic ability, and as yet the various groups of chemicals used in experimental carcinogenesis are not known to have anything else specific in common.

Some human tumours have been related to intake of specific substances, but in only a few cases is convincing evidence adduced. Some of those environmental chemical factors are discussed in the section on epidemiology of tumours (p. 28.15). Tobacco, asbestos and nickel are among the substances involved.

The mechanism of chemical carcinogenesis is unknown. Some believe that the main action is between the surface of the cell and the chemical, and others that DNA is involved in the reaction. The cell surface theory would seem to be important in explaining the immunological association of tumour growth, whereas involvement of DNA would explain genetic changes in the cells. The basis of the reaction between alkylating agents and DNA is given on p. 29.3.

PHYSICAL AGENTS

Ionizing radiations are well known to be carcinogenic (p. 33.6). The early pioneers of radiology were unhappily their own experimental animals and cases of squamous carcinoma of the skin were by no means rare in these workers. In more recent times a higher incidence of leukaemias among radiologists than among the general public has been noted. Radiological examination of the abdomen in pregnant women contributes to the incidence of leukaemias in early childhood. A classical example of the carcinogenic action of radioactive material occurred in a group of workers in the USA who developed sarcoma of bone following ingestion of radium and meso-

thorium; this was the result of using their lips to put a fine point upon their brushes while painting the dials of luminous watches. Ultraviolet radiation is evidently also of importance as a carcinogenic agent, though less marked in its effect than X-radiation, and a high incidence of carcinoma of the skin in exposed areas among outdoor workers in countries where there is much sunshine has long been familiar to dermatologists (p. 28.16).

Heat may be carcinogenic. Inhabitants of Kashmir, who in the very cold winters were in the habit of binding small charcoal braziers to their abdomens, were liable to develop squamous carcinoma of the abdominal wall.

VIRUSES

An important milestone in research on the cause of cancer occurred in 1911 when Peyton Rous transmitted a spindle-cell sarcoma in birds by means of a cell-free filtrate, and thereby first demonstrated the production of tumour growth by a virus. Subsequently a number of similar tumours were discovered by Rous and others, and in 1935 Shope described the virus-induced papilloma of the rabbit. Since then a large number of malignant diseases, carcinomata, sarcomata and leukaemias, which can be transmitted in animals by viruses have been described.

Negroni and Harris isolated a micro-organism which they thought was of viral nature from cases of human leukaemia but it has been shown that this is in fact a mycoplasma, and its aetiological connection with leukaemia is very doubtful. The occurrence of patients with leukaemias in clusters would support the hypothesis that an infective agent, possibly a virus, is responsible. So far, statistical analysis has shown that most clusters which have been reported could occur by chance.

The **milk factor** of Bittner is thought to be viral in nature. Bittner found that if the litters of a strain of mice which had a high incidence of mammary carcinoma were given to foster-mothers of a strain with low incidence, the number of such tumours developing in these litters was less than would have been expected; the converse was found also to be true. The **polyoma virus** was discovered during investigations on the viral aetiology of mouse leukaemia. This virus differs from other oncogenic viruses in that it can produce several different types of tumour and is active in many species.

Several types of adenovirus are oncogenic.

In man a **papova** virus (p. 18.95) is certainly the agent responsible for infectious warts. A rapidly growing tumour, apparently of lymphoreticular type, occurs in African children, known as the **Burkitt lymphoma**, named after the surgeon whose field observations first defined this entity. The geographical distribution of this tumour suggests that it may be due to an arthropod-borne virus (p. 18.95). Particles having the structure of herpesvirus have been found in some of the nuclei of the lymphoma cells and antibodies to the virus have been found in the sera of patients suffering from the tumours. However, it has not been possible to prove conclusively that this virus is the cause of the tumour. A recurring difficulty in work of this type is that viruses are frequently to be found in tissues where they occur apparently as 'passengers', so that the identification of a virus in regular association with a tumour does not necessarily mean that the tumour is caused by the virus.

How a virus acts as a carcinogen is not understood, but it probably involves an action on the genetic apparatus of the cell. Most of the tumour viruses known at present appear as diseases of laboratory animals. However, the fowl leukaemias are important economically in the poultry industry.

The viral aetiology of malignant disease in man has not been fully established, but as the avian and murine leukaemias have been shown to be due to viruses, it is not unlikely that at least some of the types of human leukaemia also stem from viral infection. The proof of such speculation is difficult since it has been shown in animals that the only indication of viral activity in a tumour may be the presence of either a new antigen or a viral specific messenger RNA. This is relatively simple to detect when the infecting agent is known. Erroneous conclusions may arise due to the presence in human tumours of viruses unrelated to the clinical condition. This may result from a diminished humoral and cellular response in patients with established malignant conditions; for example they may be poor interferon producers (p. 18.108).

PREMALIGNANT STATES

It has already been pointed out that chemical and physical carcinogens may act slowly and that neoplasia may follow long after the last exposure to them. There exist several pathological conditions, particularly long continued irritation or trauma, which tend to develop into a malignant tumour. Several examples of malignant neoplasm in man appear to be causally related to previous disease or chronic irritation in the same region associated with a variety of pathological processes.

In the days when many men smoked clay pipes over periods of years, carcinoma of the lower lip was common, perhaps due to repeated heating of the mucosa. Some carcinomata of the buccal cavity have been said to be associated with the presence of broken teeth, causing repeated trauma to the mucous membrane of the mouth and tongue.

In chronic varicose ulcers, there may be epidermal hyperplasia at the margins, as a result of attempts to re-epithelialize the ulcer floor; this may be the site of a squamous carcinoma of the skin. Likewise in ulcerative colitis, a chronic relapsing disease in which multiple ulceration of the colon occurs over long periods of time

with regenerative hyperplasia of the intervening mucosa, carcinoma occurs much more frequently than in the general population. Presumably the induced hyperplasia in these examples is transformed over a period of time into neoplasia.

Another change sometimes associated with chronic irritation which frequently develops into malignancy is metaplasia (p. 27.15). In most examples of this process, a specialized epithelium is transformed into one more resistant to trauma, usually squamous epithelium. The best known example of this is the squamous change seen in the bronchi of many heavy smokers; this is probably the mode of origin of carcinomata of the lung in many cases.

The development of a carcinoma of the breast is often preceded by a condition known as fibroadenosis. This disease sometimes involves proliferation of the cells lining the ducts of the breast (epitheliosis) which can progress into neoplasia.

Certain diseases of squamous epithelium, of known or unknown aetiology, involve changes in the cells which in many cases herald the development of malignant change. Such a condition occurring in the skin is known as **senile keratosis**, a misleading name, since it does not develop only in old people. In mucous membranes, such as that of the mouth, it is referred to as **leukoplakia** (plate 28.1f, facing p. 28.4). This latter condition used to be thought to be due to syphilis.

Finally, benign tumours may on occasion become malignant, and there are some which are particularly prone to do so. Papillomata of the large intestine and of the bladder are among the most important.

All of these conditions which are known to be complicated in a significant proportion of cases by the development of a malignant tumour are referred to as **premalignant** or **precancerous**; their diagnosis on biopsy material is a warning to the clinician that precautions should be taken against the development of malignancy, e.g. by a wide excision of the lesion.

GENETIC FACTORS

There is no doubt that an hereditary predisposition to the development of some neoplasms exists. For example there are strains of mice in which the great majority of the females develop mammary carcinoma. Since deaths from cancer in man are common, it is not surprising that the belief that heredity is an important cause of human cancer is widespread. Good evidence to support this view is not available in most cases, however. Some uncommon conditions are undoubtedly inherited, e.g. multiple polyposis of the colon, in which the mucosal papillomata often become malignant (p. 31.3). The evidence that heredity plays an important part in the aetiology of any of the common malignant diseases of man is slight, but not entirely negligible, e.g. carcinoma of the stomach occurs most frequently in persons of blood group A (p. 31.12).

Malignant disease certainly involves transformation of the genetic material of the affected cells. For over fifty years the **mutational theory** of the causation of cancer has implied that the essential change in neoplastic cells is an alteration in their genetic material in a way which increases their mitotic rate. For long the mutational theory and the other theories of the aetiology of neoplasia were regarded as being more or less mutually exclusive, but it is now appreciated that all tumour-producing agents, whether chemical, physical or viral, probably operate by producing an alteration in the genetic material of the cell; each may alter the DNA in such a way as to give rise to a new type of cell with different biological properties, constituting a neoplastic cell. The abnormalities of mitosis and sometimes of chromosome number observed in most rapidly growing tumours have suggested that the essential abnormality in tumour growth is located in the genetic material of cells but there are still difficulties in regarding neoplastic transformation as of the same character as spontaneously occurring mutations. The greatest of these is that spontaneously occurring mutation is generally a sudden and complete event, whereas the evidence from tumour growth indicates that neoplastic transformation is frequently gradual, often, for example, supervening upon pre-existing hyperplastic or metaplastic states, as discussed on p. 28.11.

Chromosomes and neoplastic disease

For many years microscopic examination of tissue sections has shown abnormal mitosis in malignant neoplasms in man and animals. Later, abnormalities of chromosome number and form were shown to occur in many animal tumours. Similar observations in man were impracticable, because of the lack of methods for the study of human chromosomes. Nevertheless, the demonstration by various methods of abnormal variation in the DNA content of human tumours implied the existence of **aneuploidy** or variation in chromosome numbers in these cells.

Since human chromosome studies became possible in 1956 (vol. I, p. 12.15), variations in the chromosome number and form have been observed in many malignant neoplasms, notably acute leukaemia, a malignant disease of the RE system, and carcinoma of the cervix. It seems likely that similar changes occur in most or all malignant tumours, and their demonstration depends on the adaptation of existing techniques to particular tumours. With the exception of myeloid leukaemia in the chronic phase, and possibly some other malignant RE system tumours, the chromosome changes which have been found are varied and nonspecific and few cases of any one neoplasm have shown identical changes. The significance of these nonspecific changes remains un-

certain. Some believe them to be a consequence of neoplastic change and unrelated to its occurrence. Others regard them as the visible and variable concomitants of a more subtle change, possibly a true mutation, which has already brought about malignant transformation.

In some malignant neoplasms with gross and varied chromosomal changes, long and careful studies have demonstrated the existence of several distinct cell lines. Each line may be represented by several cells even in quite small samples, and may be distinguished from each other by characteristic chromosomal abnormalities. In some of these cases it is possible to show how one line has been derived from another by an aberration of cell division. These results provide an explanation for the natural history of malignant neoplasms, which usually lead to death, even if temporarily alleviated by surgery, radiotherapy or chemotherapy. Such therapeutic failure may depend on the appearance of a cell line with a genotype unaffected by the therapeutic agent. This continuing evolution of new cell lines provides an explanation for the eventual appearance of a resistant cell line as long as cells of the original tumour persist, however sensitive the tumour may be initially to chemotherapy.

Chronic myeloid leukaemia is the only neoplasm in which a specific chromosomal abnormality regularly occurs. This is the **Philadelphia chromosome**, which is apparently due to a loss of chromosomal material from the long arm of one chromosome of the pair 21. This is not a constitutional abnormality and is found only in cells of bone marrow origin and in cells presumably originating in the bone marrow but present in the spleen. In the chronic phase of the disease it is usual to find the Philadelphia chromosome without other abnormality. This aberration, however, appears to predispose the cells which carry it to further chromosomal change, since others generally appear later in the course of the disease. This is the usual finding at the stage of metamorphosis, when what has previously behaved with low grade malignancy takes on more obviously malignant features.

It is of interest in relation to the causation of leukaemia that in chronic myeloid leukaemia part of one chromosome of the pair 21 is apparently lost, while mongols who have a greatly increased liability to develop acute leukaemia have an extra chromosome of the same pair. These findings suggest that chromosome 21 carries gene loci concerned with the production of leucocytes.

The cytogenetic evidence associating abnormality of a chromosome of pair 21 with chronic myeloid leukaemia is present in almost all cases of the disease, and the change itself is very similar from case to case. Less constant change, involving a chromosome of the pairs 17–18, has recently been described in a minority of cases of RE system tumours.

The metabolism of tumours

In 1926 Warburg wrote a book, *The Metabolism of Tumours*, in which the thesis is presented that malignant cells have greater glycolytic activity than normal cells, but that the respiratory or oxidative activity is not increased but may be diminished. This has been conceived of as an adaptation to partially anaerobic conditions, which may be present in a tumour when the multiplication of the tumour cells precedes the growth of the supporting connective tissue which carries the blood supply. There can be little doubt that the actively growing cells in a neoplasm may move into areas where the Po_2 is diminished. Damage to the electron transport system may occur and lead to increased use of glycolytic mechanisms to provide the energy needed for the growing cells.

Forty years after its publication, Warburg's thesis is still in dispute. While many tumour cells have an increased capacity to break down glucose with formation of lactic acid, difficulties of measuring respiratory activity of tumour and normal cells under comparable conditions make it less certain whether there is an impairment of oxidation. Thus, there remains a doubt as to whether a change in the manner in which the cells derive their energy is an essential feature of the neoplastic process.

Neoplasia is certainly associated with changes in the synthetic capacity of the cells. These may be attributable to changes in DNA content which occur with chromosome abnormalities. As already described, neoplasia is often associated with dedifferentiation of the characteristic cellular and tissue structure and in these tumours losses of enzymic activity have been detected. A deletion theory postulates that malignant cells escape from the general homeostatic controls of the body because they have lost certain specific functions. These functions have not been identified and the theory remains vague.

One aspect of tumour metabolism which has clinical significance concerns the nonessential amino acid asparagine which is readily synthesized by normal mammalian cells. Certain tumour cells lack this ability and are susceptible to the enzyme asparaginase which breaks down asparagine to aspartic acid. Since asparaginase does not interfere with the metabolism of normal cells, its therapeutic use has been suggested. Asparaginase given intravenously causes regression of some experimental tumours and remissions have been reported to occur in acute lymphoblastic leukaemia in man. This may represent the first therapeutically useful demonstration of a qualitative biochemical difference between normal and malignant cells (p. 29.13).

However, while malignant cells may lose certain synthetic capacities, they may also acquire others. A striking example of the development of new properties in neoplastic cells is the clinical observation that occasionally tumours of a variety of different types, but not arising from endocrine tissues, have proved to be hormonally active. Hypoglycaemia has occurred with connective tissue tumours and with carcinoma of the liver; Cushing's syndrome has been noted occasionally in cases of oat-cell carcinoma of the lung which may secrete an ACTH-like substance and cause adrenocortical hyperplasia. Increased thyroid function may be associated with chorion carcinoma; carcinoma of the kidney and lung may secrete substances with parathyroid hormone activity which produce hypercalcaemia. Carcinoma of the lung may also secrete a vasopressin-like polypeptide which leads to water retention. The explanation of the anomalous production of hormones is conjectural, but it seems likely that in malignant neoplasms a wider spectrum of competence is conferred upon the cells. The entire body is derived from a single cell in which must be vested all the genetic coding necessary for the wide variety of metabolic activities which the fully differentiated organism represents. Growth with failure of differentiation may enable cells to perform metabolic functions not possessed by their normal progenitors.

Some other systemic effects of tumours are not hormonal in nature. They include a curious variety of effects such as pigmented lesions of the skin, generalized pigmentation and dermatitis, recurrent venous thrombosis due to the production of thromboplastins by the tumour, anaemia associated with reduced concentration of serum iron and red blood cell haemolysis, fibrinogenopenia with bleeding, eosinophilia, pruritus, pyrexia, cerebral and cerebellar degeneration, peripheral neuritis, inflammatory cell infiltration, atrophy and necrosis of skeletal muscle, periosteal thickening and increased osteoid formation affecting long bones, a myasthenia gravis-like syndrome and amyloidosis. Some of these are associated with several different kinds of tumours, while others are particularly or specifically related to a single type or limited number of neoplasms.

The possibility that malignant cells synthesize some specific toxic agent or agents arises from these observations and from the fact that cancer patients, particularly in the later stages of the disease, often show the clinical picture of cachexia, a combination of wasting, weakness and anaemia. As has been noted earlier, however, tumours develop frequently in situations where they may undergo ulceration with consequent haemorrhage and infection and they may occlude hollow viscera leading to stagnation of their contents, often followed by infection. No specific toxic metabolite has been identified in tumours and the systemic effects are clearly not due to a single cause. They appear to arise from a number of metabolic, haematological and immunological abnormalities which probably occur as secondary phenomena.

Immune responses to neoplastic cells

The antigenic make-up of tumour cells can be shown

experimentally to undergo simplification and they may lose some of the antigens of the cells from which they were derived, during dedifferentiation. This phenomenon may explain the fact that certain tumours can be successfully transplanted into more than one genetically distinct host.

However, there is also evidence that neoplastic cells provoke an immune reaction in the animal in which they arise; the most convincing comes from experiments in which a chemically induced tumour is transplanted into mice belonging to a pure line, with the same genotype.

A tumour is induced in mouse A by a chemical carcinogen and is then transplanted into mice B–D. If these animals are all syngenic with mouse A, the transplant takes and a new tumour grows. If these tumours are then surgically removed and B–D mice are later given a second transplant of the tumour from mouse A, this transplant may not take and the mice may be said to be specifically immune to this particular tumour.

Whether or not immunity is demonstrated depends on the size of the challenging dose. If this is large, e.g. a visible piece of tumour inserted with a trochar, the immunity is inadequate and the transplant usually takes. If the dose is small, e.g. some 50–100 thousand tumour cells injected subcutaneously, most immune animals reject it, although such a dose would give rise to a tumour in the majority of unimmunized animals.

Oncogenic viruses (p. 18.108) have been shown regularly to induce the formation of new antigens in tumour cells although it is not clear whether these antigens represent viral antigens associated with the cell or new antigens brought into being by the viral infection.

Nearly all the animal tumours that have been tested, whether provoked by a chemical carcinogen or by a virus, or arising spontaneously, have been shown to contain antigens which produce specific immune responses. Chemical carcinogens produce tumours which possess antigens specific to each individual tumour, not to the chemical, whereas in virus-produced tumours the antigen is specific for the virus. As in transplantation immunity, the host resistance appears to be brought about mainly by the cytotoxic effect of lymphocytes on the tumour cells, i.e. cellular immunity.

It is reasonable to postulate that human tumours may provoke similar immune reactions, although only a minority have been shown to be caused by chemical agents. Indeed clinical and pathological findings in man are consistent with the presence of immune responses to neoplastic cells; many tumours induce a cellular reaction of plasma-cells and lymphocytes which infiltrate the tissue at the edge of the advancing mass of malignant cells. There is no doubt, as has been mentioned, that an infiltration of lymphocytes and plasma cells is often seen around an invading tumour. These may be said to be troops in retreat. Had they been victorious, it is unlikely that the tumour would have come to the pathologist's attention.

Another attractive hypothesis, albeit with little factual support, is the concept that neoplasia occurs in the tissues and organs of the body much more frequently than is generally supposed. The cells so formed are recognized as 'foreign' by the body's immunological mechanisms and are destroyed before they become sufficiently numerous to form a tumour. Only an occasional lesion 'gets away' and develops to form a clinical tumour.

Suppression of the immune response by drugs used to modify the response to organ transplantation are associated with an increased incidence of tumours of the reticuloendothelial system and the higher incidence of malignant neoplasms in the elderly may be related to impaired immunity mechanisms. The possibility exists of utilizing the immune reaction as a means of bringing about rejection of tumours in humans although the problem is fraught with ethical and practical difficulties.

IMMUNOLOGICAL THEORY OF INVASION

This seeks to explain the characteristics of malignant disease on the basis of loss of hypothetical agents known as identity proteins or self-marker molecules by the tumour cells, enabling them to mingle with a special kind of freedom in foreign tissue, such as when metastatic foci are set up. The idea is attractive although it depends also upon the hypothesis that tissue boundaries in embryogenesis are defined by an immunological incompatibility. Since the existence of this mechanism is conjectural, the immunological concept of malignant metastasis must be regarded as hypothetical.

METASTATIC SPREAD IN HUMAN PATHOLOGY

The student will not have attended many post mortems on persons dying of malignant disease before he is struck by the fact that secondary growths occur predominantly in certain situations and that some other organs and tissues in the body are only rarely involved. Frequent sites of secondary tumour growth are lymph nodes, lungs, liver, brain and skeleton, while the spleen and the skeletal muscles enjoy relative immunity. Some of this distribution may be attributable to the arrangement of the circulation. From a primary tumour in any part of the body, liberated cells which enter the venous system are carried to the lungs; cells from primary tumours of the gastrointestinal tract entering the portal vein must reach the liver. However, it is difficult to explain why certain tumours show a tissue predilection for the establishment of their secondary growth; thus carcinoma of the lung metastasizes frequently to the adrenal glands and the brain, and carcinoma of the prostate shows a marked tendency to metastasize to bone. Lacking any real understanding of the factors involved which cannot be explained on such simple grounds as distribution of circulation, we take refuge in a 'seed and soil' theory. This suggests that the differences are in part explicable on the basis of the varying metabolic requirements of tumour cells of different types and the availability of those requirements in the various organs and tissues of the body to which tumour cells may be conveyed. However, it seems likely that some other mechanisms are involved. The period immediately following the impaction of a tumour embolus must surely be a crucial one in determining its ultimate fate. It is possible that if the embolus consists of no more than a few thousand cells, the local cellular immune response is sufficiently vigorous to destroy them.

The immune hypothesis might help to explain why secondary tumours are found infrequently in the spleen, which is well equipped to mount an effective cellular immune response. A tumour embolus might be expected to be peculiarly vulnerable there, since it might stick in the long penicillar arterioles, whose thick walls could provide an effective barrier to the penetration of the tissues by the neoplastic cells.

It is not so easy to provide a plausible explanation of the rarity of secondaries in skeletal muscle. Perhaps the tumour cells are not able to settle in any one site, but tend to be moved on through the blood stream by the contraction of the muscle fibres.

Finally it is evident that in malignant disease, large numbers of circulating tumour cells fail to become established as metastatic foci, for the frequency with which circulating tumour cells can be seen microscopically in blood vessels greatly exceeds the frequency of secondary remote growths.

Hormone dependence

It has long been known that certain tumours are to some extent hormone dependent. For example, in many cases of carcinoma of the breast, regression of the tumour follows bilateral adrenalectomy and oophorectomy, which withdraws adrenocorticosteroids, oestrogen and progesterone from the body. Prostatic carcinoma, similarly, often regresses for a long period during administration of oestrogen, and the same effect can be obtained by castration, now rarely performed therapeutically. Thus breast carcinoma is said to be dependent on oestrogen and progesterone, and prostatic carcinoma on androgens. Unfortunately, this dependence is never complete and growth usually reasserts itself after a variable interval. Prostatic carcinoma often responds well, however, and may regress completely. These facts surely provide some clue as to how tumour cells, already in metastatic sites, may remain dormant, sometimes for 10 years or even more. Spontaneous remission or even regression of a primary tumour is similarly possible, but much more rarely recorded, perhaps since treatment of some kind is almost invariably given for primary tumours, and any improvement ascribed to it.

Epidemiology of malignant disease

Although the biology of malignant disease is obscure, the epidemiological approach (chap. 35) has shed much light on factors associated with causes, and has suggested methods of prevention. Indeed, this approach may be the most hopeful towards control of a group of diseases which collectively cause more than one in five deaths in Britain and other countries with similar living standards.

Mortality rates from most forms of malignant disease increase with age, but there are some exceptions; for example, nephroblastoma is peculiar to early childhood. The age-specific incidence is bimodal in leukaemias, Hodgkin's disease and malignant neoplasms of brain and bone; all are commoner in childhood and after middle age than in early adult life. This and histological differences of the lesion in children and adults suggests the possibility of a different aetiology or pathogenesis. Recent epidemiological surveys in the USA have revealed the existence of two types of Hodgkin's disease; the 'juvenile' form is relatively less common in the south, suggesting an environmental cause. In forms of malignancy known to follow exposure to a carcinogen, the interval between exposure and onset may be brief or prolonged, and the 'dose' may be small or great. In general the dose-response relationship is uniform; for example, among survivors of the nuclear bombs used at Hiroshima and Nagasaki in 1945 the incidence rates for leukaemias fell directly in proportion to their distance from the point of the explosion and emission of ionizing radiation.

Descriptive epidemiology has implicated both 'constitutional' (i.e. genetic or inborn) factors such as ethnic origin, blood group and secretor status, and environmental factors such as geography and occupational exposure to carcinogens. When analytical epidemiology is applied, some of the associated factors are seen to be forms of human behaviour. If this could be changed the incidence could be reduced. The subject is diffuse; to comprehend it one must almost consider each condition separately. However, some patterns are emerging, and some risks can be defined. These include exposure to irradiation, the use of tobacco in any form and prolonged occupational contact with certain types of chemicals. Environmental or behavioural factors often act most powerfully upon individuals with certain inborn characteristics. Thus basal cell carcinoma of the skin (rodent ulcer) occurs most frequently in the equatorial zones (where ultraviolet irradiation in sunlight is maximal) among people whose skin is lightly pigmented; outdoor occupations and the cult of sunbathing predispose to its development. In tropical Queensland the incidence of rodent ulcer is over forty times greater than among people of comparable genetic stock in England and Wales. In Florida, the incidence is at least ten times greater among fair-skinned people than among negroes. Malignant melanoma of the skin is similarly distributed; its incidence is highest among people of Celtic origin, and exposure to sunlight appears to be a predisposing factor even though the primary melanotic lesion may originate on an unexposed skin surface.

OCCUPATIONAL FACTORS

Chimney sweeps' carcinoma of the scrotum has already been mentioned (p. 28.9); carcinoma of scrotal skin also follows occupational exposure to shale oil and lubricating (mineral) oil used in cotton spinning. Numerous industries have since been shown to carry an occupational risk of exposure to carcinogens in processes which make use of coal tar derivatives. These include the manufacture of aniline dyes and synthetic rubber. The responsible agents are the naphthylamines and benzidine; they are excreted in the urine and the bladder is a common site for the occurrence of papillomata which often become malignant.

Malignant neoplasms occur at various sites in those occupationally exposed to irradiation. For generations the miners of Saxony and Bohemia had a high incidence of carcinoma of the lung because of their exposure to radioactive pitchblende.

The first generation of medical men to work with Rontgen rays and radium included many who died of leukaemia and other malignancies. Exposure to quite small doses of diagnostic X-rays has since been shown to enhance the risk of malignant disease (p. 35.13). Other substances implicated in occupational carcinomata include arsenic and asbestos, both of which are associated with an increased incidence of carcinoma of the respiratory tract. This occurs also among smelters, perhaps from inhaled fumes. Exposure to organic solvents such as benzol is associated with an increased incidence of leukaemias. Woodworkers and furniture makers have a high incidence of carcinoma of the nasal mucosa and antrum, presumably due to inhaled wood dust or fumes from polishing fluids. Occupational exposure to nickel and the habit of sniffing snuff, a form of dried cured tobacco, are also associated with a high incidence of carcinoma of the nasal mucosa and antrum.

TOBACCO AND MALIGNANT NEOPLASMS

Almost all the evidence incriminating tobacco as a health hazard has come from epidemiological studies. Those which associate cigarette smoking and carcinoma of the lung are described on p. 35.11; pipe smokers and tobacco chewers are prone to carcinoma of the buccal cavity and tongue. Clemmesen demonstrated a significant excess of carcinoma of the bladder among cigar smokers in Denmark. This indicates that tobacco contains a carcinogen excreted in the urine. *Health consequences of smoking*, a review published annually by the US department of Health Education and Welfare, contains statistical evidence for an association between consumption of tobacco and carcinoma at most common sites in the respiratory, gastrointestinal and genitourinary tracts. Carcinogens have been isolated from tobacco and cause skin cancer when painted on rats, while malignant change has been experimentally induced in the respiratory epithelium of animals exposed to inhalation of tobacco smoke. The cause and effect relationship can be regarded as proven unequivocally. Many doctors, including most epidemiologists, have given up smoking. It remains only to convince an unwilling public that the seductive weed is dangerous.

CLIMATE AND SEASON

Following the demonstration by Cridland that the incidence of Hodgkin's disease was highest in winter, it was shown that the onset of symptoms of leukaemia and many other childhood malignant diseases occurred significantly more often in summer months than at other times of the year. Workers in the southern hemisphere have been less successful in demonstrating seasonal variations in incidence of, or death from, malignant disease, but have had to use smaller numbers. Lea demonstrated that death rates from carcinoma of the breast are inversely correlated with mean annual temperature. The significance of these observations is uncertain.

CARCINOMA OF THE GASTROINTESTINAL TRACT

Local irritation, as from carious teeth or ill-fitting dentures, may contribute to carcinoma of the buccal cavity. Apart from tobacco smoke, hot food and drink may be implicated and so may strong and unrefined alcohol. Carcinoma of the buccal cavity is common in India among those who chew betel, but it has been shown that if the quid contains no tobacco, neoplasms do not occur. Also found in the Indian subcontinent is carcinoma of the hard palate, a very rare condition in other parts of the world. It occurs among smokers of chutta, a cigar with the lighted end in the mouth. Carcinoma of the pharynx and oesophagus occur predominantly among smokers and heavy drinkers.

There is profuse and confusing data on the epidemiology of carcinoma of the stomach. Incidence is highest in USSR, Chile, Japan, Austria and Finland in that order, and lowest among the white population of the United States, Australia, New Zealand and Canada. In Britain the incidence is high in N. Wales and N.E. Scotland. When international rates are compared, there is a high correlation between the incidence of carcinoma of the stomach and carcinoma of the colon. Carcinoma of the stomach is commonest in the lower socio-economic classes, but in all countries the incidence is falling. Reviewing this evidence, Wynder pointed out that it fits the hypothesis that a dietary factor is implicated. High intake of carbohydrate, and relatively low intake of fats and of

TABLE 28.3. Epidemiology of malignant disease. M.R., mortality rate; I.R., incidence rate.

Site and type of malignancy	Per cent of cancer deaths in Britain	I.R. in Britain per 100,000 population		Inborn, inherited, and genetic factors	Environmental factors	Behavioural factors
		M	F			
Buccal cavity, pharynx	1·5	0·5	0·2			Tobacco (M.R. × 6–10 with pipe, chewing tobacco) Alcohol (unrefined spirits)
Nasopharynx, antrum	rare				Industrial: woodworkers, French polishers, nickel smelters	Tobacco, snuff, M.R. × 2–4 among smokers
Oesophagus	2·5	5·9	2·6			Tobacco (M.R. × 4 if used in any form). Alcohol
Stomach	12·2	29·6	18·1	20% higher incidence in blood group A	Geographical: USSR, Chile, Japan, Austria, Finland, N. Wales, N.E. Scotland. Trace elements (Zn, Cu, Cr, Co)	Social Class: V > I Diet: high intake unrefined CHO, low intake fats, fresh fruit and vegetables. Tobacco: all forms M.R. × 2
Colon	8·5	17·9	23·7	Familial polyposis, autosomal dominant (p. 31.3)		10% of cases of ulcerative colitis→Ca colon
Rectum	5·1	17·1	13·7			
Liver (primary)	0·7	3·0	3·7	?Ethnic: Negro. Haemachromatosis liver disease	?Geographical: ?sequel of infective or nutritional liver disease	Absorption of excess iron from cooking pots
Pancreas	4·3	8·8	6·8	20% higher incidence in blood group A		Tobacco: M.R. × 2 if 20+ cigarettes/day
Larynx	0·7	4·8	0·7			Tobacco: M.R. × 12–18 if 20–40 cigarettes/day
Trachea, bronchus, lung, pleura	25·0	92·1	15·5	?Inherited factors (p. 34.12)	Industrial: radioactive ore; chromates, nickel, iron smelters, asbestos. Geographical: urban, atmospheric pollution, M.R. × 6. Asbestos (mesothelioma of pleura) Radiation: antenatal X-ray M.R. +40% ?Ultraviolet irradiation (sunlight)	Tobacco: M.R. × 20–30 if 20+ cigarettes/day. Social class: V > I
Bone	0·5	1·1	0·8			
Malignant melanoma	0·5	1·3	2·5	Ethnic: Celtic		
Skin	0·4	33·8	26·7	Ethnic: fair complexion	Ultraviolet irradiation (sunlight) therefore geographical. Industrial: exposure to soot (esp. scrotum)	Sunbathing. Outdoor occupation I.R. × 20–40
Breast	9·2	0·6	65·8	?Ethnic: European : Japanese M.R. = 4 : 1. Length of reproductive life (early menarche, late menopause, short or absent pregnancy/lactation intervals)	Latitude: high incidence in high latitudes. ?Mean annual temperature	Social class: I > V. Artificial feeding of infants
Cervix uteri	2·3	—	21·8	?Ethnic: European, Negro. Peak incidence at menopause for Europeans, 15 years postmenopausal for Jews		Social class: V > I. High parity. Poor hygiene. Uncircumcized sex partner. Early age of 1st intercourse, frequent intercourse, multiple sex partners
Corpus uteri	1·1	—	14·1			
Ovary	3·0	—	14·6			
Prostate	3·6	22·3	—	Ethnic: European : Jew : Japanese = 4 : 2 : 1		Social class: I > V. Uncircumcized M.R. × 2. ?Sexual customs
Bladder	3·3	17·7	5·9		Industrial: aniline dyes, processed rubber (electric cable industry), naphthylamine, benzidine. Geographical (parasitic): Bilharziasis	Tobacco: M.R. × 2–3 among cigar and cigarette smokers
Kidney	1·4	4·9	2·6			
Brain, nervous tissue	1·8	6·2	4·3	Retinoblastoma, autosomal dominant	Radiation: antenatal X-ray. Season: summer+	
Thyroid	0·3	0·6	1·9		Radiation: use of radioisotopes	
Lymphosarcoma	1·2	4·3	3·0		Burkitt's lymphoma: ?virus with insect vector	
Hodgkin's disease	0·8	2·7	1·9		Season: maximum incidence in winter	Social class: I > V
Leukaemias	2·7	6·8	5·3	Possibly some associated genetic defects	Season: maximum incidence in summer. Radiation: nuclear fallout; antenatal X-ray M.R. +40% (p. 35.00). ?Clusters: ?virus.	Social class: I > V

fresh fruit and vegetables is a common factor in countries where the incidence of carcinoma of the stomach is highest. Increasing use of canned and processed foods may be related to declining incidence. However, inborn characteristics, notably blood group A (p. 31.9), and other environmental factors, including the concentration in soil of trace amounts of copper, cobalt, zinc and chromium, also appear to be implicated.

CARCINOMA OF REPRODUCTIVE ORGANS

Carcinoma of the breast occurs most commonly in Northern Europe, North America and Australasia, and least commonly in Japan. This distribution correlates closely with international differences in breast feeding practices. Prolonged periods of lactation (17 months or more during reproductive life) are statistically associated with a reduced incidence, and women who had an early menarche and a late menopause have a higher than average incidence.

Population studies of normal women on the island of Guernsey have shown that those who subsequently developed breast cancer had abnormalities of urinary 17-hydroxycorticosteroids and androgens before the clinical appearance of their tumours. This suggests that an endocrine abnormality, albeit slight, may predispose to the development of the tumour. By the extension of such studies it may be possible in the future to isolate 'high-risk' groups from the general population.

Differences in the incidence of carcinoma of the cervix were first thought to be related to ethnic origin. The condition was observed to be much commoner among Gentiles than among Jews. Further study revealed the important aetiological role of poor hygiene, low socio-economic status, multiparity and the uncircumcized state of sexual partners. The uncircumcized state has also been shown to be associated with an incidence of carcinoma of the prostate about double that in circumcized men. Smegma, the secretion which collects under the prepuce, contains a carcinogen. International comparisons complicate this story; carcinoma of the prostate is especially uncommon among Japanese men, who are uncircumcized. It has been suggested that culture and custom may play a part. The Japanese man's approach to his sex life is forthright and direct; he does not indulge in preliminary love-play with the accompanying prolonged sexual congestion characteristic of courtship in the western world. If this suggestion is true, and if there are social class differences in sexual behaviour in Britain, they might account for the fact that carcinoma of the prostate is commonest in social class I, and least common in social class V. Epidemiologists will not add to their popularity if they suggest yet another addition to the list of potentially harmful activities which already includes smoking and drinking.

The above account and other epidemiological evidence are summarized in table 28.3.

FURTHER READING

AMBROSE E.J. & ROE F.J.C., eds. (1966) *The Biology of Cancer*. New York : van Nostrand.

AZZOPARDI J.G. (1966) Systemic effects of neoplasia, in *Recent Advances in Pathology*, 8th Edition, ed. C.V. Harrison. London : Churchill.

DOLL R., PAYNE P. & WATERHOUSE J. (1966) *Cancer Incidence in Five Continents*. Berlin: Springer.

FAIRLEY G.H. (1969) Immunity to malignant disease in man. *Brit. med. J.*, i, 467.

MACPHERSON I. (1967) Recent advances in the study of viral oncogenesis. *Brit. med. Bull.* 23, 144.

US Public Health Service (1967) *The Health Consequences of Smoking*. Washington : US Department of Health Education and Welfare.

WALTER J.B. & ISRAEL M.S. (1965) *General Pathology*, 2nd Edition, chapters 26–31. London : Churchill.

WYNDER E.L. (1967) On the epidemiology of gastric cancer, in *Racial and Geographical Factors in Tumour Incidence*, ed. A. A. Shivas. Edinburgh : University Press.

Chapter 29
Chemotherapy of malignant disease

The first successful attempt at cancer chemotherapy was based on the observation that potassium arsenite or Fowler's solution had a beneficial effect on the coat and appetite of sick horses. By an obscure process of deduction, this led Lissauer to use it to treat leukaemia in 1865. Although Ehrlich placed such empirical treatment on a scientific basis, no further advance of any importance was made until World War II. Then, the similarity which was observed between the effects of mustard gas used in the war and those of X-rays in destroying rapidly growing tissues induced Auerbach and Robson to test similar compounds for their mutagenic effects. The results showed that these drugs act on the chromosomal material and this discovery led to the synthesis of many new compounds which affected cell division. These compounds, variously called **nucleotoxic** or **radiomimetic**, are mostly alkylating agents (p. 29.3). Their introduction was closely followed by the discovery of **antimetabolites**, substances which interfere with the normal metabolic processes of the cell. Of greatest therapeutic importance were the folic acid antagonists, which also provided a key to the study of chromosome metabolism, but antipurines, antipyrimidines and glutamine antagonists have all been tried with varying degrees of success in the treatment of cancer. In addition, corticosteroids, sex steroids, some radioactive substances and a miscellany of other drugs which do not fit into precise groups are used in the treatment of cancer.

THEORETICAL APPROACH

The differences between malignant and normal cells might provide a specific point of attack for drugs. However, as discussed on p. 28.13, cancer cells appear biochemically to be remarkably similar to normal cells, and few fundamental differences have so far been found. Nevertheless tumour cells may show abnormally high rates of protein synthesis, anaerobic glycolysis, nucleic acid metabolism and cell division. Furthermore, some malignant cells are dependent on asparagine and this may prove a useful point of attack. These features and the high rate of cell division provide the main target for cytotoxic drugs.

EXPERIMENTAL SCREENING OF DRUGS

Animal testing of drugs is on the whole empirical and the results frequently show little correlation with the efficacy of the same drugs in man. Mice and rats are normally used because they have a short life span, and are easy to rear and keep. However, hamsters, chicks, frog embryos and *in vitro* biochemical and tissue culture tests are also employed.

Theoretically, drugs may be tested in animals on three types of cancers, i.e. spontaneous, induced and transplanted growths. Transplants are generally used, since it is difficult to obtain at any one time sufficient animals with suitable spontaneous tumours showing the same degree of tumour growth. Transplantable tumours are usually naturally occurring tumours which can be transplanted from one animal to another. A tumour is removed from a donor, cut into small pieces and inserted under the skin, into the peritoneal cavity or elsewhere in the recipient. It is then allowed to grow and is subsequently transferred to other animals, and thus maintained for further use. Such a progression may change the characteristics of the tumour, so that ultimately it bears little resemblance to the original. For example, the average number of chromosomes in the Walker tumour has varied between 52 and 64, over 10 years. Despite this, transplants are reliable test objects for drug screening.

In the hope that an active substance will be discovered by empirical investigation, the Cancer Chemotherapy National Service Centre (CCNSC) in the United States, tests annually tens of thousands of compounds. In Britain, because money is not available on the same scale, far fewer compounds are screened. The results have been disappointing. Since the introduction of large screening programmes, only drugs with moderate advantages over those previously available have been discovered. Drugs effective in one test are frequently not effective in a second and compounds producing prolonged remissions, if not complete regressions of tumours in animals, may have little or no action in man. The ultimate solution may come from a better understanding of the cause and progress of the disease, though an empirical approach may still prove useful.

CLINICAL TRIALS

The decision to use an unproven, but potentially useful drug in the treatment of a disease where an established drug is available is never easy. The problem is more difficult when the untreated disease is fatal and a drug which prolongs the life of the patient for a brief period, is already available. With notable exceptions, however, most known anticancer drugs produce only short remissions. In these circumstances, little can be lost by trying a new substance. While clinical trials may thus be justified, assessment of their value gives rise to further problems.

(1) There is an enormous scatter in the length of time of survival of the patients; thus it is difficult to assess whether or not their lives have been prolonged.

(2) Most patients receive a combination of treatments. Surgery and, if the disease is widely disseminated, radiotherapy are used, frequently in combination, chemotherapy merely providing an adjunct to such a regimen. Only if it is known beyond doubt that other methods are ineffective is chemotherapy used alone. Sometimes, combinations of drugs are tried and this complicates assessment still further.

(3) Although malignant tumours account for 17 per cent of all deaths in Britain, any particular cancer is uncommon in any one hospital. This makes controlled trials difficult, unless organized on a national basis.

CLINICAL TOXICITY

Inherent in the use of nonspecific cytotoxic drugs is the danger that all cells which are proliferating rapidly are liable to attack. Thus, a number of toxic effects occur with all such drugs, the most common of which are as follows.

Bone marrow

Blood-forming elements are destroyed, and a fall in the platelet, red or white blood cell count may occur soon after the start of treatment. Regular blood examinations are, therefore, an essential part of management if serious complications are to be avoided. A depression in the number of circulating reticulocytes, which require only 48 hours for their formation, gives the earliest indication of toxicity and may warrant stopping treatment. A fall in the number of circulating white blood cells may render the patient vulnerable to infection and thrombocytopenia may be followed by severe or fatal haemorrhage.

Gastrointestinal tract

The mucosal cells of the alimentary tract are continually replaced by active division. Inhibition of their replication results in nausea, vomiting, diarrhoea and, in severe cases, intestinal perforation and haemorrhage. Dryness, soreness or ulceration of the lips and oral mucosa are early signs of toxicity.

Sex glands

A direct action on the germinal epithelium of the testis may cause sterility, but the effect is temporary if the drug is stopped. It is thought that a block occurs in the early stage of spermatogenesis. In women temporary amenorrhoea occurs.

Foetus

There is evidence that some drugs have a teratogenic action in man, but remarkably few cases of abnormality have been observed. Cytotoxic drugs should not be given during the first 3 months of pregnancy and, if possible, should be avoided throughout the remainder of pregnancy.

Skin and appendages

Cell division in the dermal skin layer may be impaired causing dermatitis and pruritus. Alopecia is caused by many drugs and women should be warned of this possibility. Fortunately the hair usually returns when treatment is stopped. Atrophy of finger nails is a common effect.

Tumour

Ironically, immense destruction of large areas of tumour may itself cause fatal shock by releasing unidentified toxic substances into the circulation. There is also accumulating experimental and clinical evidence that cytotoxic drugs, used for prolonged periods, may cause increased incidence of primary neoplasia especially lymphoma. It is not known, however, whether the malignant conditions are due to somatic mutations induced by the drug, or whether they are caused by a virus which has invaded the host during the suppressed immune response.

Methods used to reduce toxicity

A number of techniques are employed to prevent or reduce systemic toxicity, particularly of the bone marrow. On the whole, these have been disappointing, and some degree of toxicity is usually unavoidable.

Intra-arterial injection provides a means of giving small doses of the drug with high local concentrations at the tumour site, but is only suitable for circumscribed tumours of the extremities, e.g. head, neck and limbs.

Regional perfusion is a technique, in which the blood leaving the tumour is recirculated into the supplying artery instead of returning straight into the general circulation. This is done by a small pump worn by the patients. Larger amounts of drug can be given and, in the case of perfused extremities, only small quantities of drug reach the rest of the body. One major advantage of this method is that local conditions can be modified to enhance the antitumour activity of the drug. For example, raised Po_2 and temperature both increase the efficacy of mustine; triiodothyronine may also be used to increase the metabolic rate of the tumour.

The use of tourniquets is another but less effective method of preventing escape of the drug into the circulation.

The injection of autologous bone marrow provides some degree of protection of the bone marrow. Between 400 and 500 ml of bone marrow are removed prior to treatment and diluted with Ringer's solution and dextrose. The bone marrow cells are then returned to the body several hours after treatment when the drug has been inactivated or excreted. Thus, even if damage has occurred to the bone marrow which remained, the autotransplanted tissue is unharmed. The main danger with such treatment is infection, as the white cell count may be low for several days.

Antidotes, where they exist, can provide further protection and, if used in conjunction with perfusion and infusion techniques, help to reduce systemic toxicity. Examples include N^5 formylTHF (folinic acid) when using methotrexate (p. 29.8), thymidine with 5-fluorodeoxyuridine and thiosulphate or cysteine with alkylating agents. Antidotes are of little value in treating toxicity following systemic administration of the drug, since efficacy against the tumour is correspondingly reduced.

Alkylating agents

These substances are called radiomimetic because of the similarity of their effects to those produced by high energy radiations. Drugs from this class currently used in the treatment of malignant disease fall into four groups, depending on the active chemical configuration (table 29.1); of these the mustards are by far the most important.

TABLE 29.1. Alkylating agents and their active groups used in the treatment of malignant disease.

Mustards	β-chloroethylamino	$-NHCH_2CH_2Cl$
Methanesulphonates	methanesulphonoxy	$-OSO_2CH_3$
Ethyleneimines	ethyleneimino	$-N\begin{smallmatrix}CH_2\\\\CH_2\end{smallmatrix}$
Epoxides	epoxide	$-CH\overset{O}{\diagup\diagdown}CH_2$

In the highly active alkylating agents these functional groups appear at least twice (bifunctional) and sometimes more than this (polyfunctional). Duplication is an essential feature of high activity.

Sulphur mustard, synthesized in 1854, is the substance from which the whole range of synthetic nitrogen mustards, and more recently the **methanesulphonates, epoxides** and **ethyleneimines,** have been derived. Sulphur mustard

was used in chemical warfare during World War I. This prompted investigation into the nitrogen derivatives, which was intensified in World War II. Nitrogen mustard was first used in the treatment of human cancer in 1942, and its beneficial effect on Hodgkin's disease was shown by Jacobson in 1943. Synthesis of less toxic alternatives did not follow until later.

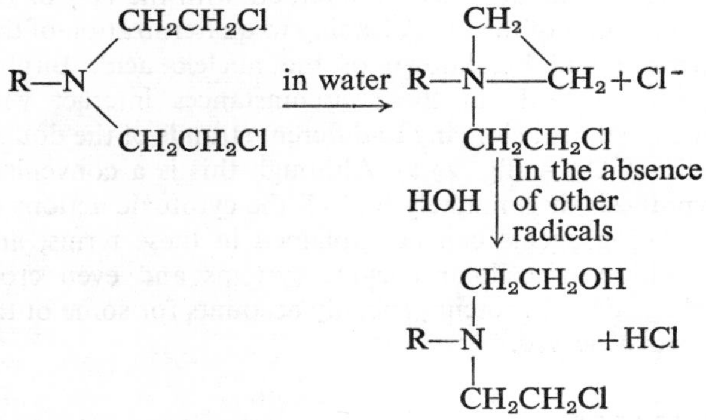

$$R-N\begin{smallmatrix}CH_2CH_2Cl\\\\CH_2CH_2Cl\end{smallmatrix} \xrightarrow{\text{in water}} R-N\begin{smallmatrix}CH_2\\|\ \ CH_2+Cl^-\\CH_2CH_2Cl\end{smallmatrix}$$

$$\xrightarrow[\text{radicals}]{\text{In the absence of other}} R-N\begin{smallmatrix}CH_2CH_2OH\\\\CH_2CH_2Cl\end{smallmatrix} +HCl$$

FIG. 29.1. Cyclization of mustine hydrochloride.

All alkylating agents attack biologically important radicals, e.g. hydroxyl, phosphate and carboxyl. This is a direct reaction in all but the tertiary amines, which are by themselves relatively inert. Mustards, as crystalline hydrochlorides, rapidly undergo cyclization to the ethyleneimonium derivative, which in turn alkylates both organic and inorganic radicals (fig. 29.1).

The exact mechanism of the cytotoxic action of these substances, apart from that of alkylation, is still a matter of dispute. They cause structural damage to chromosomes

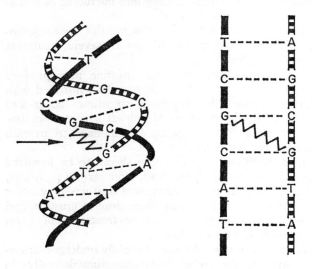

FIG. 29.2. Bifunctional mustards and double helix of DNA. The bases of DNA are represented by their initial letters and the alkyl chain by the zig-zag line. The affected base sequence on either strand is guanine–cytosine. From Brooks P. and Lawley P.D. (1964) *Brit. med. Bull.* **20**, 91.

at the time of their replication during interphase, which becomes visible only when the cells reach a later stage of mitosis. Nuclear abnormalities appear, cell growth is inhibited, and degeneration occurs. Since during inter-interphase, the nuclear DNA becomes exposed and is particularly vulnerable to attack, the mustard has the opportunity of interacting with it. The currently held theory is that the mustard interacts with the N-7 of the guanine unit of the DNA leading to quaternization of this nitrogen and breakdown of the nucleic acid. Bifunctional mustards in these circumstances interact with guanine units belonging to different strands of the double helix of DNA (fig. 29.2). Although this is a convenient hypothesis, it is unlikely that all the cytotoxic actions of alkylating agents can be explained in these terms, and inhibition of cellular enzyme systems and even cross linkage of cell protein probably accounts for some of the effects observed.

MUSTARDS

Mustine (nitrogen mustard, HN2, mechlorethamine, mustargen) is an extremely irritant substance which can

$$CH_3-N \begin{cases} CH_2CH_2Cl \\ CH_2CH_2Cl \end{cases}$$

Mustine

be given only intravenously. Extravasation into the soft tissues produces severe and painful necrosis, and it is usually better to inject the drug into the tubing of a fast-running intravenous infusion.

The main hazards in the use of mustine are thrombocytopenia and leukopenia. If they are severe, treatment must be stopped.

For 8 hours after injection, mustine may produce nausea and vomiting, but this may be controlled with chlorpromazine. Skin eruptions sometimes occur and herpes zoster is common. Menstrual irregularities frequently arise, but no permanent damage to ovarian function has been reported.

In dogs ^{14}C-mustine has been shown to be localized around the auditory nerve, and, after carotid perfusion, around the optic nerve. Permanent deafness may occur after treatment with a large single dose of mustine, and optic nerve damage may follow treatment of brain tumours by cerebral perfusion.

Mustine is water soluble and rapidly undergoes transformation to the cyclic ethyleneimonium derivative in either acid or alkaline solution. This occurs in a few minutes, and then the molecule can react with a number of inorganic and organic radicals. Hence the solution must always be prepared immediately before injection.

This rapid breakdown also explains why techniques to localize the drug are of value, and why the use of tourniquets affords some protection to the bone marrow.

Mustine is the treatment of choice when Hodgkin's disease is disseminated and unsuitable for X-ray therapy.

It is often used in combination with other alkylating agents, and more recently it has been used in conjunction with methylhydrazine (p. 29.13) and vinblastine (p. 29.11) in an attempt to prolong the period of remission.

With less predictable results mustine is used in the treatment of other malignant reticuloses and in chronic leukaemia, either alone or with corticosteroid therapy. Symptomatic relief has also been reported in the treatment of carcinoma of the bronchus, ovary and breast, and in the suppression of intrapleural and intraperitoneal malignant disease causing effusion.

Mustine is given in doses of 0·4 mg/kg of body weight as a single intravenous injection, or in divided doses over 2–4 days. This can be repeated only after the bone marrow has recovered completely, which may take at least 6 weeks. In the treatment of malignant effusions mustine can be given directly into the body cavity involved. Overdosage and gross toxicity can be counteracted by giving sodium thiosulphate.

Cyclophosphamide (endoxana, cytoxan) is a nitrogen mustard molecule linked via the nitrogen atom to a

$$\begin{array}{c} H_2C-NH \\ H_2C \quad O=P-N \begin{cases} CH_2CH_2Cl \\ CH_2CH_2Cl \end{cases} \\ H_2C-O \end{array}$$

Cyclophosphamide

cyclic phosphoric acid esteramide, which masks the action of the mustard; hence its description as a 'latent mustard'. The rationale behind the synthesis of this compound is interesting if disappointing. Neoplastic tissues are known to possess high phosphatase and phosphoramidase activity, capable of splitting the cyclophosphamide molecule to release the active mustard moiety. It was thought that activation of the compound would thus occur preferentially within the tumour. Unfortunately both liver and plasma also activate the drug so that adverse effects are greater than expected. There is also evidence that it is not after all a mustard which is released.

One advantage of cyclophosphamide is that the level of phosphoramidase activity in megakaryocytes is low, so that thrombocytopenia is not common. Also, since at the time of injection the mustard is masked, it is not an irritant to the veins.

The main adverse effect is alopecia which, although worse than with the other mustards, is usually reversible. In addition it produces nausea and vomiting, but no more so than do other mustards.

Cyclophosphamide is readily absorbed when given orally and maximum plasma levels are obtained within 1 hour. After an intravenous dose, about 14 per cent of unchanged drug can be recovered from the urine but little from the faeces. Distribution studies show high concentrations in tumour tissues, although in animals large amounts have also been found in kidney, liver and spleen.

It has been used to advantage in Hodgkin's disease but is more effective in lymphoproliferative diseases such as lymphosarcoma and chronic lymphocytic leukaemia. In multiple myeloma it is also one of the most successful treatments, probably because it can be tolerated over a long period.

It is often effective on tumours of epithelial origin, a fact which can be correlated with its tendency to produce alopecia and ridging and atrophy of finger nails. It sometimes appears to cause improvement in bronchial and breast carcinoma and in disseminated neuroblastoma in children, where no other treatment is of value.

The recommended dose is 100–150 mg/day either by the intravenous or oral routes. Some, however, prefer a high initial dose of 300–400 mg/day for 3–7 days followed by 100–150 mg/day indefinitely.

Chlorambucil (leukeran, phenylbutyric mustard, C.B. 1348) can be given by mouth and is the slowest acting and least toxic of all the nitrogen mustards in clinical use. Nausea and vomiting are the commonest adverse effects, but occur only after high doses. Cytotoxic effects on the bone marrow and lymphoid organs are similar to other mustards and may necessitate reduction in dosage and, in severe cases, cessation of treatment. Little is known of its distribution, metabolism and excretion in man.

Chlorambucil

Chlorambucil is regarded as the treatment of choice in chronic lymphatic leukaemia. Its slow onset of action does not immediately endanger the bone marrow, and it has been used in Hodgkin's disease and other reticuloses where there is no pressing need for rapid onset of clinical effect. Some success has been obtained in the treatment of macroglobulinaemia and ovarian carcinoma.

The recommended dose is 5–10 mg in a single daily dose for 3–6 weeks, followed by a maintenance dose of 2–4 mg/day unless toxic effects develop.

Uramustine (uracil mustard, U. 8344) is more potent than chlorambucil. It is a derivative of the 5-halogenated uracils, which are pyrimidine antimetabolites. It was synthesized in the hope that the mustard moiety would not be released until it reached an area of high nucleic acid production, i.e. high cell reproduction, where the pyrimidine base would be taken up. While this does occur, the reaction lacks specificity.

Uramustine

It can be given by mouth, but it is not regarded as an important drug, although it has been used in Hodgkin's disease, chronic myeloid leukaemia and some reticuloses.

Melphalan (phenylalanine mustard, alkeran) the L-isomer, and the racemic mixture used by Russian

Melphalan

workers (known as merphalan or sarcolysin) both have advantages over other mustards, particularly in the treatment of melanomata. The L-isomer is much more active than the D-isomer, which may indicate that it is incorporated into the normal amino acid pathways. Although basically similar in action to other alkylating agents, it rarely causes nausea and vomiting and alopecia has not been reported. The therapeutic ratio is relatively high.

Melphalan is well absorbed when given orally, but it may be given intravenously. In the blood it has a half-life of 105–120 min, compared with 14 min for mustine. Radioactive studies have shown that it is distributed in the protein of the cytoplasm in a number of organs, notably the kidney.

It is used in disseminated radio-resistant Hodgkin's disease, as an alternative to chlorambucil or cyclophosphamide. In the treatment of multiple myeloma, small doses given for long periods produce remissions and prolong life.

The greatest successes with melphalan so far have been in the treatment of malignant melanomata. Regional perfusion of the foot, accompanied by surgery, has produced some striking results (plate 29.1, facing p. 29.6). In the treatment of melanoma of the pelvis and more complex sites relief of intractable pain may be achieved, but leakage into the general circulation may lead to bone marrow depression.

The initial daily dose is 0·05–0·1 mg/kg orally for

2–3 weeks. A maintenance dose ranging from 2 mg/day to 2 mg twice a week is then recommended so that the leucocyte count remains around 3000–3500/mm³.

METHANESULPHONATES

Busulphan (myleran) is unique in that it attacks specifically cells of the myeloid series. Compared with the mustards, the reaction with DNA is more sluggish, and *in vivo* its main action is the removal of thiol groups from proteins or peptides. Evidence in rats suggests that it prolongs the intermitotic interval, so that cells divide normally but less often. This explains why qualitatively there appears to be little interference with cell division or maturation. Toxic reactions mostly affect cells of the myeloid series, and thrombocytopenia may occur with doses over 10 mg. However, unlike mustards, few if any adverse effects are seen in the gastrointestinal tract and lymphoid tissue. Other adverse effects include nausea, amenorrhoea, impotence, sterility and skin pigmentation.

$$CH_3—\overset{\displaystyle O}{\underset{\displaystyle O}{\overset{\|}{\underset{\|}{S}}}}—OCH_2CH_2CH_2CH_2O—\overset{\displaystyle O}{\underset{\displaystyle O}{\overset{\|}{\underset{\|}{S}}}}—CH_3$$

Busulphan

Busulphan is well absorbed when given orally and disappears rapidly from the circulation. After interaction with thiol groups of proteins, hydroxytetrahydro-thiophene sulphone is produced, which is then excreted mainly in the urine. No unchanged drug is found in the urine.

Remissions have been reported with chronic myeloid leukaemia in 85–90 per cent of patients and are comparable with those obtained with ³²P therapy or X-irradiation. However, the drug is frequently used as a second choice when patients no longer respond to radiation. It has also been used with some success in polycythaemia vera, where the platelet depression which it produces may be beneficial.

Busulphan is given as a single daily dose of 0·06 mg/kg. This is continued for as long as is necessary to bring about remission as assessed by white cell counts. A second course of treatment 6–18 months later may be required.

Mannitol myleran is an example of the group of drugs

$$CH_3—\overset{O}{\underset{O}{\overset{\|}{\underset{\|}{S}}}}—OCH_2\underset{HO}{CH}\underset{OH}{CH}CH\underset{HO}{}\underset{OH}{CH}CH_2O\overset{O}{\underset{O}{\overset{\|}{\underset{\|}{S}}}}—CH_3$$

Mannitol myleran

described as polyols which are large molecular derivatives of drugs known to be effective in malignant disease.

These drugs were synthesized and tested after the observation that tumour cells had a greater capacity than normal cells to take up large molecules by pinocytosis. There are some exceptions, which include cells of the reticuloendothelial system, the intestinal epithelium and kidney tubules. Both in England and Russia this has stimulated research in the hope that a compound with a greater specificity of action will be found. The clinical use of mannitol myleran is similar to that of busulphan.

ETHYLENIMINES

Tretamine (triethylene melamine, TEM) was first synthesized in Germany in the fabric industry to produce strengthening of long fibre chains by cross linkage. This, and the fact that the ethylene–imine stage is known to be an intermediate in HN2 reactions made it a logical choice for cancer chemotherapy to cross-link chromosome fibres.

Tretamine

It is much less reactive than mustine and its use is hampered by the fact that it is readily polymerized in acid solution. This occurs in the stomach and as a result it is about half as effective by this route as when given intravenously. If sodium bicarbonate is given at the same time, effective doses with predictable absorption can be achieved. However, severe damage to bone marrow and other adverse effects may follow its use and many believe that it should no longer be used in clinical practice.

Thiotepa (triethylene thiophosphoramide) acts by liberating ethyleneimonium ions intracellularly, but its use is hampered by erratic absorption when given by mouth.

Thiotepa

In man, following administration of ³⁵P-thiotepa, 80–93 per cent of the activity found in the urine was due to inorganic phosphorus, indicating almost complete breakdown to the active ethyleneimonium ions. The drug is well tolerated and less toxic than the nitrogen mustards, although anorexia, nausea and vomiting may occur.

Used in a variety of diseases, it is most valuable as an adjuvant to surgery in carcinoma of the breast and ovary.

The drug is available as a sterile powder in a vial containing 15 mg of thiotepa, with sodium chloride and sodium bicarbonate, enough to ensure alkaline pH and is dissolved in 1·5 ml of sterile water for injection. The usual intravenous or intramuscular dose for adults is 10 mg/day for 5 days followed by a maintenance dose of 5–20 mg/week. Single weekly injections into body cavities of between 5–60 mg are used to control malignant effusions. When the white blood cell count falls below 3000/mm³, therapy should be stopped.

Triaziquone (trenimon), in *in vitro* experiments using cultures of malignant tissues, has a potent cytostatic

Triaziquone

action, one part in 10^9 stopping mitosis within 24 hours. It inhibits both glycolysis due to a reduction in the content of NAD, and also respiration due to inhibition of acyl activation. These are unlikely to be the primary causes of its cytotoxic action, and evidence suggests an effect on the nucleic acids of the nucleolus. Its toxicity is similar to the other ethyleneimonium derivatives, but the risk of a local irritant action is greater.

It is of little use in malignant blood disorders. It is of most value in the local treatment of malignant effusions associated with carcinomata and in the regional perfusion of tumours.

Doses range from 0·2–0·5 mg given intravenously or into the tumour or body cavity.

EPOXIDES

Ethoglucid (triethylene glycol diglycidyl ether, epodyl) is a bisepoxide. These compounds inhibit growth of the Walker carcinoma in rats, but are generally too toxic for

Ethoglucid

clinical use. Renewed interest has been shown recently in bisepoxides in an attempt to find a safe derivative which could be used in the manufacture of synthetic resins. As a result some of the compounds which had been previously ineffective when given intraperitoneally were shown to be effective when given intravenously. Ethoglucid is a colourless, slightly viscous liquid. It is rapidly removed

from the blood after intravenous injection, having a half life of only 10–15 min. The drug is then found in all tissues except the liver. Intravenous injection may be followed by a transient hypotension, nausea and vomiting for 24 hours, but this is less severe than with other alkylating agents; haematological depression follows 2–3 weeks later.

Local perfusion of carcinoma results in swift relief of pain and the patient experiences a feeling of well-being This symptomatic relief outweighs objective improvement which is often difficult to assess. Local nerve destruction probably accounts for the relief of pain which is rarely permanent. It has recently been employed to treat tumours in the head and neck and it reduces the need for surgical drainage in malignant effusions.

An intra-arterial dose related to the size of the tumour is recommended. This may vary from as little as 2–5 ml into the head and neck to three or four times this amount in other sites.

Antimetabolites

Antimetabolites which interfere with the metabolism of four different groups of substances, i.e., folic acid, purines, pyrimidines and glutamines are used in cancer chemotherapy. In the normal process of mitosis a cell must double its DNA content before division into two daughter cells can occur. Thus any interference with the necessary metabolic processes prevents the cell from reaching this state of mitotic preparation.

FOLIC ACID ANTAGONISTS

Folic acid, an essential dietary factor, is converted in the body to the coenzyme tetrahydrofolic acid (THF), a conversion brought about by folate reductase. Inhibition of this enzyme restricts the availability of THF for cellular functions involving the transfer of one carbon unit. This affects primarily the production of thymidylic acid, inosinic acid and some of the precursors of RNA and DNA (vol. 1, chaps. 12 & 26).

Methotrexate (amethopterin) holds an honoured position in tumour chemotherapy since a closely related com-

Methotrexate

pound, aminopterin, produced in 1948 the first striking remissions in acute leukaemia (p. 25.15). It has also produced cures in chorion carcinoma.

Methotrexate exerts a strong inhibitory action on folate reductase. Since this is a competitive inhibition one would expect to be able to antagonize it with folic acid. However, in the concentration which it is possible to obtain physiologically this does not occur, but N^5 formylTHF (folinic acid) can be used instead, and clinically this substance has limited efficacy in the treatment of methotrexate overdosage, provided it is given within 4 hours.

As with the alkylating agents, use of the drug is accompanied by toxic effects on other rapidly dividing cells. The most severe are the reduction in the platelet and leucocyte counts, which follows the marrow depression which must be produced to treat the leukaemia. Diarrhoea is also common and if treatment is not stopped haemorrhagic enteritis, intestinal perforation and death may ensue. Milder effects include dermatitis, alopecia and hepatic dysfunction, all of which appear to be reversible. Methotrexate and other folic acid antagonists interfere with development of the foetus by an action on the embryonic mesenchyme and should be avoided during pregnancy whenever possible.

When given by mouth, methotrexate is rapidly absorbed and between 60–90 per cent of the drug is excreted unchanged in the urine within 12 hours. In the blood about 50 per cent of the drug is bound to plasma proteins. Since the kidney is obviously important in excretion of the drug, care is needed in treating patients with renal insufficiency. Any drug not excreted in this way is excreted in a metabolized form, although it can still be detected in the human kidney after several weeks and in the human liver after several months. ^{3}H-methotrexate is slowly transported into cells where it probably becomes bound to folate reductase.

Methotrexate does not cross the blood–brain barrier. It is of no value in treating neoplasms of the CNS. It is second to steroid therapy and mercaptopurine in the management of acute leukaemias in children and induces substantial remissions when administered over a period of 3 weeks, but ultimate regression is certain.

In chorion carcinoma and related trophoblastic tumours in women it is of established value, and remissions of 5 years or more are common. The success is explained partly by the nature of the tumour; since chorion carcinoma, a rare gonadotrophin-producing tumour, is derived from foetal membranes, it may be regarded as a transplanted neoplasm. This may make it particularly susceptible to drug treatment, a possibility given weight by the fact that other drugs have proved successful in the treatment of resistant cases, e.g. chlorambucil, actinomycin D and vinblastine.

Methotrexate may be used in regional perfusion of the head and neck and in the treatment of carcinoma of the breast but it has little part to play by itself. Recommended oral doses in acute leukaemias are 2·5–5·0 mg/day in children and 2.5–10.0 mg/day in adults. In chorion carcin-

oma oral doses of up to 30 mg/day are given for 5 days, or if continuous intra-arterial infusion is used, as much as 50 mg/day may be given for 10 days. Toxicity may be prevented by injection of N^5 formylTHF every 4–6 hours.

ANTIPURINES

These drugs were discovered as the result of planned investigation of substances which might impede nucleic acid synthesis. The only important member of the group, 6-mercaptopurine, was synthesized in 1952 and used clinically in 1954. So far no derivative has superseded this drug, but there are still many untried possibilities which may be of value either in malignant disease or as immunosuppressive agents.

Mercaptopurine (6-mercaptopurine, puri-nethol) is an

Mercaptopurine   Adenine

antagonist of adenine and hypoxanthine to which it is chemically related. It appears to interfere with purine metabolism in several ways:

(1) by transformation to the thio analogue of inosinic acid it inhibits the formation of succinoadenylic acid from inosinic acid, and its conversion to adenylic acid,

(2) by competition with hypoxanthine for the inosinic acid pyrophosphorylase enzyme system, and

(3) by inhibiting the incorporation of formate and glycine during purine biosynthesis.

These biochemical interactions make a simple explanation of the mode of action of mercaptopurine impossible, but they can be related more closely to subsequent cellular effects. The most important interaction is the formation of the ribonucleotide, thioinosinic acid, as cell resistance to drug action is related to the inability of cells to perform this conversion. The outcome of this and the other metabolic disturbances is an interference with nucleic acid synthesis and ultimately cell division. Inhibition of cell division in bone marrow and gut leads to leucopenia, thrombocytopenia and anaemia, and anorexia, nausea, vomiting and diarrhoea. Gross toxicity produces hepatic cell necrosis and jaundice occurs in a third of all patients treated.

Oral mercaptopurine is readily absorbed into the blood stream where its half-life is about 90 min. The loss from the blood is due partly to cellular uptake and partly to metabolic degradation. Both the unchanged form and the metabolites are rapidly excreted by the kidneys. The most important metabolite is 6-thiouric acid, formed by xanthine oxidase. This has led to an investigation of

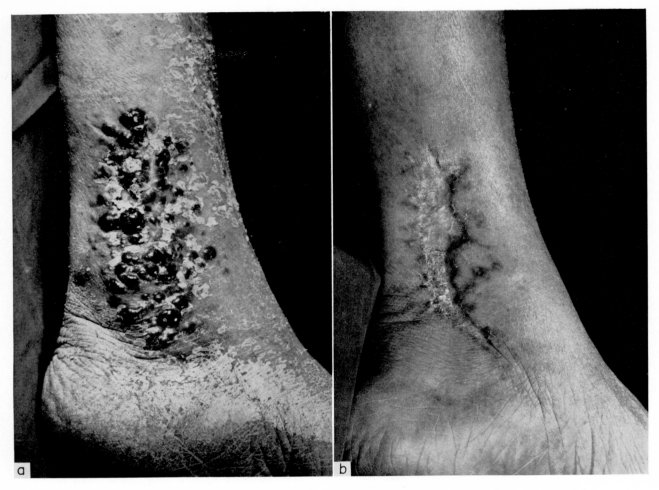

PLATE 29.1. Malignant melanomata (a) before perfusion with melphalan and (b) more than 1 year later. This is an exceptionally good regression which unfortunately is uncommon. By permission of Mr C.I. Cooling of the Royal Marsden Hospital.

substances which inhibit xanthine oxidase and thus prolong the action of the mercaptopurine. One such compound which competes with hypoxanthine and mercaptopurine for the enzyme is **allopurinol** (4-hydroxypyrazolopyrimidine; zyloprim). This has been tested clinically as a possible potentiator and is also useful in the treatment of gout where it reduces the formation of uric acid.

The main use of mercaptopurine is in the treatment of acute leukaemias in children. Without treatment the average time of survival after diagnosis is 3–4 months. With the drug this has been increased to 15 months and some children survive for 2 years or more. In adults remissions are not as good. Although the drug is of some value in myeloid leukaemia it produces less consistent results and is not as easy to use as busulphan. The drug is also valuable in the treatment of the homograft reaction in tissue transplantation.

Corticosteroid induced remissions of leukaemias may be prolonged by its use. Given orally or by intramuscular injection a typical dose is 2–5 mg/kg/day.

Azathioprine (imuran, BW 57–322) is a derivative of 6-mercaptopurine and was developed in the hope that substitution of the sulphydryl group would limit the

Azathioprine

physiological degradation caused by oxidation of this group. This proved to be the case, but the resulting drug offers no advantage in the treatment of leukaemias over the parent compound. Its value as an immunosuppressive agent is discussed on p. 24.2.

ANTIPYRIMIDINES
The basic unit of the DNA molecule is thymine (5-methyluracil) linked as the deoxyribonucleotide (thymidylic acid) to other units of the DNA helix. Since the methyl group of the thymine provides the connection with the nucleotide, it was thought that substitution of this group might interfere readily with the subsequent synthesis of DNA. This occurs with the fluorine derivative 5-fluorouracil, and with the fluorine or iodine derivatives of the ribonucleotide, 5-methyldeoxyuridine. Both substances are incorporated into the normal metabolic pathways and subsequently inhibit the synthesis of DNA.

Fluorouracil (5-fluorouracil) is converted in the body to the corresponding ribonucleoside and ribonucleotide, the former being converted to 5-fluoro-2'-deoxyuridine-5'-phosphate. This substance then inhibits the synthesis of DNA, but it has no selective action on tumour cells

and hence produces severe adverse effects. Furthermore, the nucleotide which is formed is a very toxic substance and it is readily incorporated into the DNA molecule. To overcome this the 5-fluorodeoxyuridine was introduced and its actions are described below.

Fluorouracil

Mild overdosage causes anorexia and nausea, which is followed by stomatitis and diarrhoea, and may lead to intestinal necrosis and perforation. The most frequent blood disturbance is leukopenia. It produces its maximum effect between the 10th and 15th days, but disturbance of liver and renal function may complicate the picture by interfering with normal drug metabolism. Occasionally alopecia, nail changes, dermatitis, atrophy of the skin and more rarely neurological manifestations occur.

Given intravenously it is catabolized in a similar manner to uracil to give 5-fluoro-5,6,-dihydrouracil. The ring is then opened to give N-carbamyl-α-fluoro-β-alanine which is subsequently converted to CO_2 and urea. Studies in man using a single intravenous dose of 2-^{14}C fluorouracil indicate that in 24 hours only 11 per cent of the radioactivity is excreted in the urine but 63 per cent is expired as CO_2. Following intravenous infusion the amount excreted increases to 90 per cent.

The drug is of value as a palliative treatment in certain types of advanced carcinoma particularly of the breast, gastrointestinal tract, female genital tract and in the head and neck. Beneficial effects are rarely seen in other tumours, or in leukaemias, except sometimes in children.

The pronounced toxic effects of the drug make treatment of the debilitated patient impossible, and in treating tumours in the head and neck, continuous infusion techniques are used to help overcome the toxicity.

It is given intravenously in single injections at a dose of 15 mg/kg over 5 days. This dosage is safe provided renal and hepatic function are normal but may cause serious toxicity if they are not. It is possible to assess liver function by measuring the capacity of a subject to produce $^{14}CO_2$ following a dose of 2-^{14}C uracil.

After a 4 week interval a second course of treatment may be given but, in patients who do not show gross toxicity with the first course, four additional injections of 7·5 mg/kg may be given on alternate days immediately following the 5-day course.

5-Fluorodeoxyuridine has a direct action on the thymidylate synthetase system, but *in vivo* it is readily converted to 5-fluorouracil, and therefore has a similar toxicity.

Weight for weight it is half as active as the parent compound. Clinically it has little if any advantage over

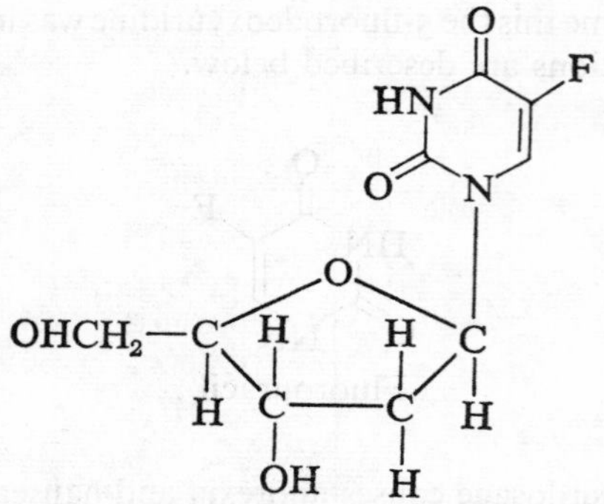

5-Fluorodeoxyuridine

fluorouracil and similarly an iodine derivative recently introduced has no particular advantages.

6-Azauridine is given intravenously and is converted intracellularly to 6-azauridylic acid which in turn inhibits the enzymatic formation of uridylic acid. Clinically,

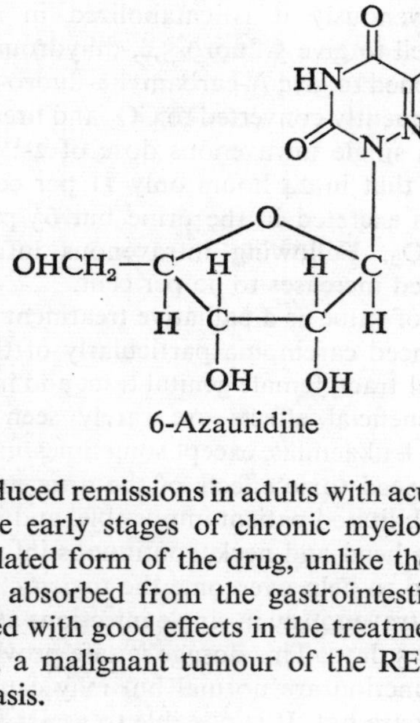

6-Azauridine

it has produced remissions in adults with acute leukaemia, and in the early stages of chronic myeloid leukaemia. The acetylated form of the drug, unlike the parent compound, is absorbed from the gastrointestinal tract and can be used with good effects in the treatment of mycosis fungoides, a malignant tumour of the RES in the skin, and psoriasis.

GLUTAMINE ANTAGONISTS

These substances inhibit several amino transfer reactions in which glutamine is the amine donor, and is of importance in inhibiting the enzyme responsible for the formation of the ribonucleotide of formylglycinamide. There are two main compounds, **azaserine** and *N*-**acetyl DON** (*N*-acetyl-6-diazo-5-oxo-L-norleucine, duomycin). Both have been disappointing in the treatment of cancer but *N*-acetyl DON is of value as an immunosuppressive agent (p. 24.2).

Spindle poisons

COLCHICINE DERIVATIVES

Colchicine is an alkaloid found in the corm and seeds of *Colchicum autumnale* (autumn crocus, meadow saffron) coming originally from Colchis in Asia Minor. It was first used in the sixteenth century for the treatment of gout and is still a useful drug for this condition. Around 1900

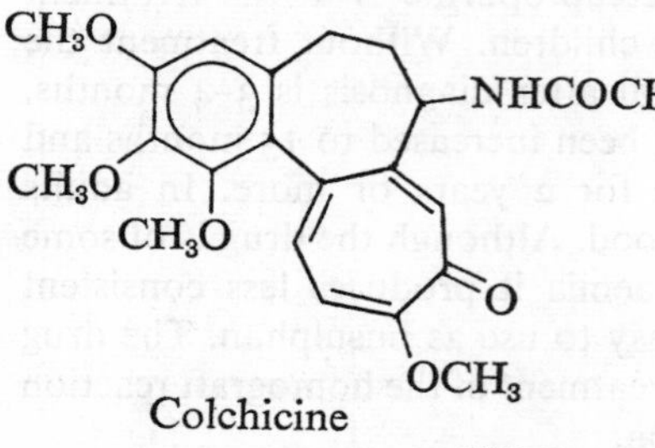

Colchicine

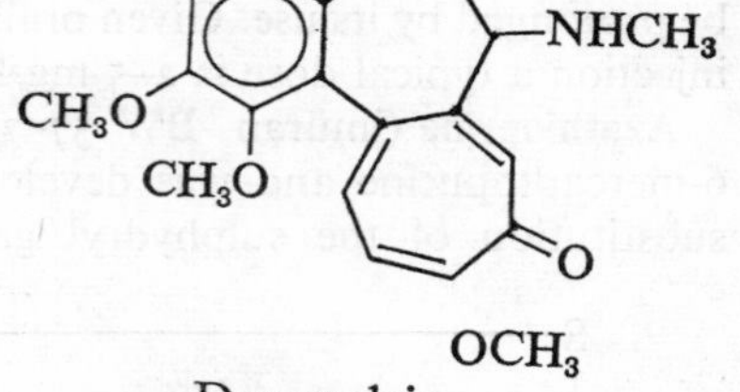

Demecolcine

(*N*-deacetyl-*N*-methylcolchicine)

it was shown to affect mitosis, and in 1937 Dustin found that metaphase was arrested due to incomplete spindle formation. This results in abnormal nuclear configurations and cell death. Clinically colchicine has a low therapeutic ratio and is of no value in the treatment of neoplastic disease. However, it is a useful research tool.

Attempts to improve the therapeutic ratio resulted in the introduction of **demecolcine** (*N*-deacetyl-*N*-methylcolchicine) a derivative also found in *Colchicum autumnale*. It has been used only in clinical trials so far without startling results but it may provide a stepping stone to a more successful drug in the future.

Demecolcine appears to cause more damage to polymorphonuclear leucocytes than does colchicine, although it appears to act in a similar manner. Given orally in a dose of 3–10 mg/day it has proved useful in myeloid leukaemia, but it is less effective than folic acid antagonists, alkylating agents and busulphan. Adverse effects include alopecia, liver damage, bone marrow depression and gastrointestinal disturbance.

VINCA ALKALOIDS

The periwinkle plant (*Vinca rosea*) from which these alkaloids are derived possessed a folklore reputation in the West Indies as an oral hypoglycaemic agent. This prompted an investigation in 1949 to confirm this belief and to isolate the active principle. No hypoglycaemic action was discovered, but crude plant extracts induced a rise and then a fall in the number of circulating leuco-

Velbamine part
Vindoline part

Vincristine and Vinblastine *CH₃ instead of CHO

cytes. By 1958 workers in Canada had shown this to be due to the alkaloid vinca leucoblastine, now called vinblastine, and after purification this substance was subsequently introduced as a cytotoxic agent. However, tests on leukaemia in mice revealed that the crude extract of *Vinca rosea* had a greater action than vinblastine. This led in 1961 to the discovery of another alkaloid, vincristine. In all, four alkaloids of this type are present in the plant extract.

The two active drugs differ structurally only in that vincristine has a formyl group in the dihydroindole portion of the molecule as opposed to a methyl group in vinblastine. This minor difference in structure accounts for wide differences in their clinical properties.

Their exact mechanism of action is not known, but both compounds, like colchicine, produce a powerful anti-mitotic action and arrest cell division in metaphase by inhibiting spindle formation. However, both compounds also interfere with glutamic acid metabolism in the citric acid cycle and the effect on mitosis can be modified by the concomitant administration of glutamic acid.

Vinblastine has been used for some years in the treatment of neoplastic conditions. Weekly intravenous doses starting at 0·1 mg/kg and increasing by 0·05 mg steps at weekly intervals to 0·30 mg/kg have produced good remissions in a number of diseases. It is very irritant locally and precautions must be taken to avoid extravasation. Although expensive compared with the mustards, it is useful when resistance to these has occurred. The drug is cleared rapidly from the blood following intravenous injection and is probably taken up selectively by neoplastic tissue. Metabolism is by the liver and excretion by way of the bile.

Significant improvements have been obtained in Hodgkin's disease, even in advanced cases unsuitable for X-ray therapy and resistant to nitrogen mustards. It is, however, much less effective in reticuloses and leukaemias. In chorion carcinoma it is of particular value since beneficial effects can be obtained when the disease no longer responds to methotrexate.

Toxicity includes loss of hair, gastrointestinal disturbances, stomatitis, bone marrow depression and to a varying degree other adverse effects characteristic of cytotoxic drugs. In addition it may induce effects peculiar to the vinca alkaloids; these include paraesthesia (especially around the mouth), temporary mental depression, loss of deep tendon reflexes and more rarely headaches, psychoses and convulsions.

Vincristine (oncovin) has been used with success in a number of diseases, some of which do not respond to vinblastine. It is marketed as a powder, which is made up as a sterile solution and given intravenously. The usual weekly dose is 0·01 mg/kg which is one-tenth the starting dose of vinblastine. It can be increased at weekly intervals by 0·01 mg/kg to a maximum of 0·05 mg/kg. Clinically it is less effective than vinblastine in the treatment of Hodgkin's disease, but whereas vinblastine has no worthwhile effect in acute leukaemias, vincristine produces good remissions. In combination with prednisone in children it has been described as about 80 per cent effective. It also has some application in the treatment of reticulum cell sarcoma, and tumours of the breast, lung and testis.

Toxic effects include the usual cytotoxic disturbances but the main effects are neurological. Paraesthesia is profound; the deep tendon reflexes are lost, and neuritic pain may be severe. In addition muscle weakness may occur, with foot drop, ptosis and double vision. These toxic effects are fortunately not seen in children, but adult patients are often unwilling to return for further treatment.

Antibiotics

Since the production in 1940 of actinomycin A, the first crystalline antibiotic to be extracted from a species of *Streptomyces*, many related substances have been evolved, some with potent antitumour activity. On a molecular basis they are the most potent antitumour agents which have yet been used. The most important of the group, actinomycin D, is described in detail but some others are worthy of a mention. Its structure is given on p. 20.14.

Actinomycin C (sanamycin), is a mixture of actinomycins C₂, C₃, and D and was the forerunner to actinomycin D. It was used initially with beneficial results in the treatment of reticuloses because of its very low bone marrow toxicity but was subsequently replaced by actinomycin D. However, it has been used with steroids in the management of kidney graft operations.

A more recent introduction, of Japanese origin, is

mitomycin C (p. 20.15). However, it produces severe toxic effects including gastrointestinal disturbance, bone marrow depression and alopecia. In Hodgkin's disease and recticulum cell sarcoma it has produced beneficial effects, but it is regarded as a suitable treatment only where all else fails.

A more recently introduced antibiotic is **mithramycin** which is effective in treating metastatic embryonal sarcomata and chorion carcinoma of the testis, where it is said to produce excellent remissions. It is not yet an established drug and because of its toxicity is used with extreme caution. Even more recently another antibiotic **rubidomycin** was introduced for the treatment of acute leukaemias in man. Extensive trials have shown it to produce satisfactory remissions even when used alone. So far, cardiotoxicity causing death in 10 per cent of the patients, and bone marrow aplasia represent the major forms of toxicity.

The above antibiotics are all potentially useful substances but the most important compound at the present is **actinomycin D** (dactinomycin) which apart from its antibiotic effects is of main interest as a radiosensitizing agent.

Its use after X-irradiation may produce erythema and dermatitis at the sites of X-ray exposure, and potentiate the effect of the radiation for up to one year after exposure. It is thought to produce its biological effect by reacting with guanine in the helical configuration of DNA and, although no similar action occurs with RNA, the binding with DNA in effect inhibits the synthesis of RNA by preventing the transcription of DNA dependent m-RNA. The change in physical characteristics of the DNA molecule can be used to advantage in the study of cellular biochemistry.

Clinically, like other cytotoxic drugs, it inhibits all rapidly proliferating cells. It induces atrophy of the thymus, spleen and other lymphoid tissues, and produces toxic manifestations on the gastrointestinal tract, bone marrow, skin and hair follicles.

Actinomycin D has been most useful in conjunction with X-ray therapy in the treatment of tumours of mesodermal origin, particularly nephroblastomata in children. Some success has also been reported in the treatment of sarcomata in children.

Actinomycin D is available as freeze dried powder. Orally it is much less potent than when given by parenteral injection, but given in this way the dose is 3–10 mg/kg/ day. Intravenously a dose of 15 mg/kg over 5 days is suggested, and this can be repeated after a suitable interval. As with the mustards it is safer to administer the drug by injecting it into the tubing of an intravenous infusion.

It is also of some value in the suppression of the immune response in tissue transplantation.

In adults 'triple therapy' with actinomycin D, methotrexate and chlorambucil has produced objective remissions in resistant testicular and ovarian tumours, and in chorion carcinoma, but in other neoplastic diseases only temporary remissions have been obtained.

Miscellaneous drugs

This group includes a number of drugs both old and new which do not fit into a classification based on structure or mode of action.

Urethane (ethyl carbamate), commonly used as an

$$
\begin{array}{c}
NH_2 \\
| \\
C{=}O \\
| \\
O{-}C_2H_5
\end{array}
$$

Urethane

anaesthetic for experimental animals, has a profound action against certain cancers in rats and mice. It appears to produce its effects by interfering with the biosynthesis of pyrimidine. It was used in the treatment of chronic myeloid leukaemia and plasma cell myeloma, but it is now only infrequently used, having been replaced by cyclophosphamide and chlorambucil.

METHYLHYDRAZINES

These are very recently introduced drugs having been shown experimentally to prolong interphase, to produce chromosome aberrations and to cause breakage of the chromatids. It is likely that they produce their effect by the intermediate formation of peroxide in much the same manner as ionizing radiations are thought to act (p. 33.3). Such peroxide can in turn act on the DNA by the intermediary of —OH radicals, but exactly how the DNA is modified is unknown.

Procarbazine (*N*-4-isopropylcarbamyoyl benzyl-*N*-methylhydrazine; natulan) has produced good results in the treatment of Hodgkin's disease which is resistant to alkylating agents and vinblastine. It can be given orally (50 mg three times a day, increased to 200–400 mg/day in the adult) or intravenously. Adverse effects include nausea and vomiting; drowsiness and disorientation frequently follow the use of methylhydrazine, and some patients experience flushing when drinking alcohol.

OTHER DRUGS

A large number of compounds are tried annually in the clinical treatment of cancer. Of these only a few can be regarded as useful, and not until clinical experience extends over many years is it possible to include them in a list of standard drugs. However, it is worth mentioning four groups of compounds which have recently given impressive results in clinical trials. They are **hydroxyurea, methylglyoxal guanylhydrazone, torephthalanilides** and **sodium vanadate**. It is impossible to predict the ultimate value of these compounds in medicine.

ASPARAGINASE

The amino acid asparagine can be synthesized by normal mammalian cells from other more basic constituents but certain malignant tissues lack this ability and are dependent on a supply from the host (p. 28.13). Sufficient quantities of asparaginase for use in man have been obtained following the discovery that asparaginase is produced in large quantities by certain strains of *Esch. coli*. Encouraging remissions in some patients have occurred following its use in the treatment of acute lymphoblastic leukaemia, although its use in other leukaemias and Hodgkin's disease has proved less satisfactory. Adverse reactions include anorexia, nausea and weight loss, and symptoms related to the action on protein synthesis such as hypoproteinaemia and oedema; following a second course of treatment, acute hypersensitivity reactions may occur.

One interesting feature is that, by means of an *in vitro* test, it is possible to predict with some degree of reliability whether or not the patient will respond.

Hormones

A number of naturally occurring and synthetic hormones have been used in the treatment of malignant conditions. Their action is probably more specific than other forms of treatment, but as a result they are of value only in a limited number of conditions. Hormone dependent organs are especially affected, although in no case has a cure been obtained. Five types of hormones are used: corticosteroids, androgens, oestrogens, progestagens and thyroid hormones, of which the first three are of greatest importance.

CORTICOSTEROIDS

These reduce the ability of lymphocytes to undergo mitosis; they are consequently of value in the treatment of acute leukaemias in children and of lymphosarcoma. They may be used alone or in conjunction with cytotoxic compounds but, with notable exceptions, they are usually less effective in reducing the lymphocyte count and the volume of the tumour mass than the alkylating agents. In children with acute leukaemias remissions ranging from 2 weeks to 9 months have been obtained in 30–50 per cent of cases although some authorities put this figure as high as 70–80 per cent. The remission rate may be even higher in combination with vincristine. Only 10–20 per cent of adults respond to such treatment.

In some individuals resistance develops, but cross resistance does not occur, and this fact constitutes a good reason for then using vincristine, cyclophosphamide and methotrexate in turn. Another reason is the long-term toxicity which follows steroid therapy (p. 6.13).

Corticosteroids also play a useful role in the treatment of the anaemia, haemolysis and thrombocytopenia of cancer which generally increases as the disease progresses (p. 7.8). Corticosteroids are also useful in the palliative treatment of cancer of the breast. **Prednisone** and **prednisolone** are the most frequently used and are given in a daily dose of 20–60 mg.

ANDROGENS AND OESTROGENS

These drugs are of value in the treatment of cancer of the prostate and of the breast. Both organs are dependent on hormones for their normal growth, function and morphological integrity and carcinomata arising from them are to some extent hormone dependent.

The effects of the two hormones are best described by considering the two diseases individually.

Cancer of the prostate

Apart from surgical removal of the gland, which is possible in only 5 per cent of cases, treatment can be effected by reducing the output of natural androgens by castration or by giving oestrogens.

In the 1930's it was noticed that at puberty the prostate became rich in acid phosphatases. It was then shown that in cases of metastatic carcinomata the plasma phosphatase activity became elevated, but fell after castration which also caused shrinkage of the prostate. Androgens were shown to stimulate prostatic growth and the production of acid phosphatases by prostatic acinar epithelium. Thus a high level of acid phosphatase in the blood is evidence that prostatic carcinoma is present and a fall in the level of this enzyme provides a good index of the success of treatment.

Castration, either alone or with subsequent oestrogen therapy, constitutes a severe psychological trauma, the severity of which depends on the age of the patient. Sexual impotence is a common result.

Some of these disadvantages are avoided by oestrogen therapy. Oestrogens act partly by inhibiting the normal control of the pituitary over the androgenic secretion of the testes and partly by a direct antagonism of the action of androgens on the prostatic tissue. The result is a prompt relief of pain, regression of tumour masses, increase in appetite, weight gain and a feeling of well-being. Unfortunately some patients do not respond, whilst others relapse after initial improvement. This is due to the presence or subsequent development of cells which do not depend on androgens for their development.

The oestrogen of choice in prostate cancer therapy is **stilboestrol** given in a dose of 5 mg orally three times a day, although **ethinyloestradiol** (1–2 mg/day) has also been used.

Adverse effects include gynaecomastia, atrophy of the testes, gastrointestinal disturbances, and occasionally oedema of the inguinal region and lower limbs. Oestrogen therapy has led to breast carcinoma in the male.

Cancer of the breast

Surgery and irradiation remain the best methods of treatment but, where dissemination is wide androgen or oestrogen therapy is useful. In cancer developing before the menopause the best results are obtained with methods that reduce the natural oestrogen level. These include ovariectomy and adrenalectomy, and the administration of androgens or corticosteroids. However, when the natural oestrogen activity is low, as in cancer occurring ten or more years after the menopause, oestrogen treatment is preferred. Administration of oestrogens before this may make the cancer worse.

The androgen of choice is **testosterone proprionate** given intramuscularly three times a week at doses of 50–100 mg, but oral **fluoxymesterone** (5 mg four times a day) is an alternative (p. 12.11). The adverse effects of androgens particularly disliked by women are those causing masculinization. Initially it is limited to the growth of facial hair and deepening of the voice, both of which effects are reversible provided treatment is stopped. However, if continued, the patient may develop the male pattern of baldness, acne, prominent muscles, veins and body hair, and hypertrophy of the clitoris; all these are largely irreversible. Hypercalcaemia is an important complication of oestrogen therapy. To control this, a large fluid intake is advised, but it may in addition be necessary to give intravenously a chelating agent such as sodium edetate (disodium EDTA p. 10.12).

Oestrogen therapy is best effected with stilboestrol at doses of 10–15 mg/day orally. The most prominent adverse effect is nausea which may appear at breakfast time like the 'morning sickness' of pregnancy. The symptom can, however, be avoided if dosage is increased slowly from the outset of treatment.

PROGESTATIONAL HORMONES

These are used predominantly in the treatment of endometrial carcinoma previously treated by surgery and radiotherapy. Progesterone derivatives have also been reported to be of benefit in the treatment of carcinoma of the kidney.

THYROID HORMONES

Thyroid hormones, by suppressing the pituitary feedback mechanism, reduce the activity of the thyroid gland. This fact has been known for many years and, in the small percentage of patients suffering from well defined tumours of the thyroid gland, it gives excellent results.

The limiting factors in their use are the general metabolic effects they produce. Nevertheless this has been overcome to some extent by the use of the proprionic and acetic acid derivatives of thyroxine and tri-iodothyronine.

Radioactive drugs

The use of the term radioactive drug is perhaps misleading since they are drugs only in the broadest sense. The two most frequently used substances are radioactive isotopes of normal body constituents, i.e. iodine and phosphorus. Compounds which can be more correctly termed drugs include radiogold and, more recently, labelled substances which are taken up specifically by tumour tissues, e.g. menaphthone sodium diphosphate (synkavit).

The magnitude of the effect produced is related to the ionizing power of the radiations. Thus γ-radiation, although it penetrates some distance, produces little change along its path, but α-particles produce considerable ionization and damage. Ionization means that electrons are ejected from the molecules through which the radiation passes. Radiations interfere with cellular division, and the intracellular formation of peroxide may be partly responsible for their action (p. 33.3).

The greatest limitation in the use of radioactive isotopes is the lack of specificity with which they are taken up by malignant tissue, except in certain cases. Only recently have these difficulties been systematically tackled, and the use of menaphthone sodium diphosphate to some extent overcomes them.

Sodium phosphate (^{32}P) is a β-emitter with a half-life of 14·3 days, producing an average tissue penetration of about 2 mm. It is supplied in sterile form for injection and is distributed throughout the body fluid. Given orally, 25 per cent is excreted in the faeces.

Uptake by the body cells depends primarily on their rate of turnover, and in rapidly dividing cells this is high. High activity is thus found in bone marrow, spleen and lymph nodes and in sites where metabolic turnover is high, e.g. liver. Eventually the ^{32}P, by continued turnover leaves the soft tissue cells and some finds its way into the bone. This provides additional radiation of the bone marrow which may in turn cause haematological depression.

^{32}P is probably of greatest value in the treatment of polycythaemia vera where the overproduction of erythrocytes, platelets and leucocytes are all inhibited. Dosage ranges from 2·5–5 millicuries given in one injection.

A number of **isotopes of iodine** are currently available for clinical use. ^{131}I emits predominantly β-particles and some γ-rays; its half-life is 8 days. ^{125}I has a half-life of 60 days, whilst ^{132}I has a half-life of only 2–3 hours. ^{131}I, with its β-emission penetrating tissue to about 2 mm and its convenient half-life, is the most useful isotope.

TABLE 29.2 Drugs used in the treatment of cancer.

Disease	Drug(s) of choice	Second line drug	Other drugs shown to be partially effective
Cure			
Chorion carcinoma	Methotrexate	Chlorambucil Actinomycin D Vinblastine	Mithramycin N-acetyl-DON
Useful Remissions			
Hodgkin's disease	Alkylating agents	Vinblastine Vincristine Methylhydrazine	Uracil mustard Tretamine
Acute leukaemia in children	Corticosteroids Mercaptopurine	Vincristine Methotrexate Cyclophosphamide	Other alkylating agents
Chronic lymphocytic leukaemia	Chlorambucil	Corticosteroids	Vinblastine
Chronic myeloid leukaemia	Busulphan	Mercaptopurine	Alkylating agents Demecolcine Vinblastine
Lymphosarcoma	Alkylating agents	Corticosteroids	Melphalan
Reticulum cell sarcoma	Alkylating agents Vincristine Methylhydrazine	Methotrexate	Actinomycin D
Plasma cell myeloma	Melphalan	Cyclophosphamide Corticosteroids	—
Nephroblastoma	Actinomycin D + X-irradiation	Cyclophosphamide Vincristine	—
Carcinoma			
Breast (premenopause)	Testosterone Fluoxymesterone	Corticosteroids	Alkylating agents Fluorouracil Thio-tepa } Triple Vinblastine } therapy
Breast (postmenopause)	Oestrogens	Corticosteroids	Alkylating agents Thiotepa
Prostate	Oestrogens		
Polycythaemia vera	^{32}P	Busulphan	Alkylating agents
Poor Remissions			
Acute leukaemias in adults	Steroids Mercaptopurine	Methotrexate Vincristine	Asparaginase
Neoplastic effusions	Alkylating agents locally	^{198}Au	—
Carcinoma			
Bronchus	Alkylating agents	Corticosteroids Vincristine	
Ovary	Alkylating agents especially chlorambucil	Oestrogens	Thiotepa Triaziquone
Uterus	Progestogens	Alkylating agents	Thiotepa
Thyroid	^{131}I		
Gastrointestinal tract	Fluorouracil	Thiotepa	
Head and neck	Ethoglucid, fluoroucil, mustine by local perfusion.	—	—

Radioiodine is taken up selectively by the thyroid gland, and it is used mainly to test thyroid function; in higher doses thyroid tissue is destroyed. A thyroid function test requires in the region of 5–50 microcuries of ^{131}I, treatment of thyrotoxicosis about 5–15 millicuries, destruction of the normal gland between 25–50 millicuries, and destruction of malignant thyroid tissue is achieved with 60–100 millicuries. Such treatment is particularly convenient since all that is required is a small drink of water containing radioactive sodium iodide. The radioiodine accumulates in the thyroid gland and in any secondary thyroid tissue.

Unfortunately use of radioiodine in metastatic conditions of the thyroid has so far proved disappointing because the metastases take up very little of the ^{131}I, despite attempts to stimulate it by TSH.

Radiogold (^{198}Au) is supplied as a colloidal suspension of particles ranging in size from 3–7 nm in diameter. It emits mainly β-particles and some γ-rays, and has a half-life of 2·7 days. It is given by injection directly in the body cavities for palliative treatment of neoplastic effusions. Therapy is expensive and, since the average dose is quite high (between 35–150 millicuries), the patients become a severe radiation hazard to the hospital staff. On the whole its use provides no advantage over that of alkylating agents.

Since 1948 when it was realized that **tritiated menaphthone sodium diphosphate** (tetra-sodium 2-methyl-1:4

Tritiated (T) menaphthone
sodium diphosphate

naphthaquinol (T) diphosphate, TRA 72, synkavit) became concentrated selectively in tumour tissue, a number of radioactively labelled derivatives have been investigated. Of these, tritium labelling has proved the most successful since it has the optimum specific activity to deliver a therapeutic dose of radiation. Specific activity, measured as the ability to destroy tumour tissue, is dependent on the nature of the isotope (in terms of half-life and energy of its emissions) and the selectivity with which it is taken up by tumour cells.

The radioactive half-life of tritium is around 12 years, but the biological half-life is very much less, about 13

days in tumour cells, and 3–6 days in normal tissue. The β-emissions of tritium have an average tissue penetration of 0·9 μm with a maximum of 6 μm (less than the diameter of most human cells) which gives it excellent properties for a specific localized action. It appears that three atoms of tritium attached to the molecule provide the optimum curative dose of irradiation, but only that with one atom of tritium/molecule has been tried clinically.

Clinical studies have been confined so far to patients in whom conventional methods of treatment do not offer a chance of cure or useful palliation. The drug is usually given by intra-arterial injection. In an investigation of forty-eight patients, nearly all of whom were seriously ill with advanced, recurrent, radio-resistant or refractory malignant disease, thirteen useful palliations were produced. It is probable that use of the compound containing three atoms of tritium/molecule will be more effective.

Other radioactively labelled compounds which have aroused considerable experimental interest are tritiated thymidine and tritiated stilboestrol but no information on their clinical effect is yet available.

Treatment of choice

Table 29.2 indicates the foremost drug available for the treatment of individual tumours. Other drugs, which are used when either the first is ineffective or when the patient develops resistance, are also given, and additional drugs which may produce some effect are mentioned in the fourth column. The choice of drug is made difficult by the practice of using sequential and multiple methods of treatment involving up to five different drugs. In addition, it is important to remember that drug therapy is often of secondary importance to surgery and/or radiation therapy and often used only in disseminated conditions, or where other treatment fails.

FURTHER READING

BROOKS P. & LAWLEY P.D. (1964) Alkylating agents. *Brit. med. Bull.* **20**, 91.

HALL T.C. (1962) Chemotherapy of cancer. *New Engl. J. Med.* **266**, 178–85, 238–45 and 289–96.

KENNEDY B.J. (1966) Chemotherapy for Cancer, in *Modern Treatment*, vol. 3. New York: Harper.

MITCHELL J.S. ed. (1965) *The Treatment of Cancer.* London: Cambridge University Press.

ROSS W.C.J. (1962) *Biological Alkylating Agents.* London: Butterworth.

TIMMIS G.M. & WILLIAMS D.C. (1967) *Chemotherapy of Cancer, the antimetabolite approach.* London: Butterworth.

Chapter 30
General pathology of connective tissue and intercellular matrix

The organs of the body are held in continuity and contiguity by connective tissue which, like the steel framework of a reinforced concrete building, is inconspicuous, ubiquitous but indispensable (vol. 1, chap. 16). Unlike the steel skeleton of a skyscraper with its passive relationship to piping, telephone cables and drains, mammalian connective tissue is active in the metabolism of the organs which it supports. Indeed, in some homeostatic activities, such as the maintenance of the concentrations of plasma calcium and phosphate, the connective tissues play a critical role.

The connective tissues form a system which, like the reticuloendothelial system, is widely dispersed. This scattered arrangement means that there are few disease processes in which connective tissue components are not secondarily involved. Connective tissue is also a site of primary localized or generalized disturbances, the majority of which are acquired, and due to trauma, infection and neoplasia. More rarely, there occur hereditary abnormalities of connective tissue, some of which can be classified as inborn errors of metabolism.

Rheumatism is an ill-defined word derived, through ancient French, from a term meaning a 'watery discharge'; it is by common consent the clinical description for a miscellany of diseases, all of which cause pain in bones, joints or ligaments. With few exceptions the rheumatic diseases are disorders of the connective tissue system. Because the term **connective tissue disease** is more soundly based anatomically and physiologically, it is suggested as a substitute for the word rheumatism.

Table 30.1 is given as an *aide-mémoire* to the composition of the connective tissue.

BASIC PATTERNS OF CONNECTIVE TISSUE RESPONSE IN DISEASE

Disturbances of growth
Aplasia of connective tissue is exemplified by the failure of a limb bud to develop; the skeleton fails to form, perhaps under the influence of some exogenous chemical such as thalidomide (p. 12.17). Incomplete formation of bones and limbs is a form of connective tissue **hypoplasia**.

Metaplasia, the transformation of one tissue into another during adult life, is encountered in several circumstances, e.g. when haemopoietic bone marrow becomes replaced by fibrous tissue.

Connective tissue cells retain a capacity for dedifferentiation and for proliferation. In muscle also, regeneration is known to occur to a greater degree than was previously imagined. Connective tissue **hyperplasia** occurs when excess callus forms at a site of fracture repair owing to defective immobilization and in a severe form in keloid formation (p. 30.4). Benign and malignant neoplasms of connective tissue also occur (p. 30.15).

Atrophy of connective tissue is a common part of the ageing process and is a feature of many diseases which are treated by rest, e.g. in limb immobilization. The administration of adrenocorticosteroids may induce atrophy of connective tissue, e.g. in the dermis. By contrast, **hypertrophy** of connective tissue cells is infrequent. Increase in size of individual cells may be encountered in hereditary disorders such as the mucopolysaccharidoses (p. 30.5).

Mucoid change, fibrinoid, basophilic body formation and collagen sclerosis
These changes occur in the course of systemic connective tissue diseases and particularly in those in which the immunological mechanism is disordered. Over the years they have been identified and named on the basis of their appearance in tissues prepared by classical histological methods. These disturbances are, however, poorly understood, but are thought to represent fundamental alterations in connective tissue structure related to causes of the individual systemic disorders. Their recognition provides a means for the pathological diagnosis of these diseases.

MUCOID CHANGE
Connective tissue may change to resemble primitive mesenchyme, the tissue in localized myxoedema or in Wharton's jelly of the umbilical cord. Tissue which is the site of mucoid change stains more deeply than normal with haematoxylin; ground substance accumulates, presumably synthesized by the altered cells. Such mucoid

TABLE 30.1. Composition of connective tissue. Cells, fibres and ground substance are united to form a connective tissue system; like the reticuloendothelial system, it is widely dispersed and components are found in all organs.

CELLS	Young form	Mature form	Main structural characteristics	Main properties of young cells
Primitive mesenchymal cell, derived from embryonic mesoderm	Fibroblast	Fibrocyte	Much endoplasmic reticulum; vesiculate nucleus: prominent nucleolus	Synthesis of collagen, reticulin, elastin and ground substance
		Mast cell	Much endoplasmic reticulum: metachromatic granules	Metabolism of mucopolysaccharide and heparin synthesis
	Chondroblast	Chondrocyte	Much cytoplasmic glycogen and fat	Synthesis of collagen, chondroitin sulphates, non-collagenous protein
	Osteoblast	Osteocyte	Much endoplasmic reticulum; alkaline phosphatase activity	Similar to those of chondroblast + alkaline phosphatase activity and modulation of process of calcification
		Osteoclast	Often multinucleate	Bone resorption
	Lipoblast	Fat cell or lipocyte	Eccentric nucleus and lipid-laden cytoplasm	Storage of lipids
	Synovioblast	Synovial cell: Type A	Surface villi and vacuolated cytoplasm	Phagocytosis; lysosomal activity
		Type B	Abundant endoplasmic reticulum	Synthesis of hyaluronic acid

FIBRES	Chemical composition	Physical form	Site of synthesis	Main properties	Staining characteristics
Collagen	Three helical chains of amino acids of which about 13% are hydroxyproline and 13% proline	Macromolecules form tropocollagen fibrils: arranged extracellularly in bundles	Within vacuoles of connective tissue cells, in relation to endoplasmic reticulum	Confers strength, rigidity, stability on connective tissues	Red with van Gieson, blue with Mallory, purple-brown with silver
Reticulin	Collagen fibrils coated with glycoprotein. Amino acids of fibrils as in collagen	Delicate bundles of fibres lying among ground substance	As for collagen	Structural support for blood vessels; forms basis of reticulo-endothelial system	Black with silver, blue with Mallory
Elastin	Little hydroxyproline; associated lipid + polysaccharide	Broad laminae of fibres	In vacuoles of fibroblasts and smooth muscle cells. Cu-containing enzyme needed	Resistance to tension and support of connective and smooth muscle cells	Brown with orcein and dark blue with resorcinol methods

GROUND SUBSTANCE	Structure	Properties	Origin
*Mucopolysaccharides**	Polyanionic polymers. Chains of repeating disaccharide units. Hyaluronic acid and chondroitin sulphate	Basis of ground substance, viscosity and lubricating qualities of synovial fluid	Synthesized by cells such as fibroblast, chondroblast
Non-collagenous protein	Protein molecules to which are attached the mucopoly-saccharides	With mucopolysaccharides, provide basis of connective tissue ground substance	Synthesized by cells of parent tissue
Glycoproteins	Mucopolysaccharide–protein complexes. Usually <4% carbohydrate	Associated with connective tissue fibres	Associated with collagen and reticulin fibrils
Interstitial fluid	Does not differ significantly from that of other tissues; water and electrolytes are bound to mucopolysaccharides		

* For the revised and now recommended chemical nomenclature, see postscript on p. XVII.

change is seen in a typical form in the small visceral arteries in **systemic sclerosis**, a progressive disease which may involve the connective tissues in all organs. The skin is most obviously affected (scleroderma) and becomes hard and leathery. The vascular change affects the intima; cells, which may be fibroblasts or smooth muscle cells, proliferate and the lumen of the vessel narrows as the ground substance increases. The appearances closely resemble those seen in renal interlobular arteries in the accelerated phase of systemic hypertension. An accumulation of mucoid material is present in the aortic media in the Marfan syndrome (plate 30.1a, facing p. 30.4).

The special staining reactions which identify mucoid change are those which are used to define connective tissue mucopolysaccharides. In sites such as normal cartilage, aorta, skin and umbilical cord, these give characteristic reactions which distinguish them from other tissue polysaccharides like glycogen. They are essentially negative with the periodic acid–Schiff (PAS) reaction. With dyes such as toluidine blue and methylene blue they display metachromasia, and a violet appearance is produced. The connective tissue mucopolysaccharides resist diastase, unlike glycogen, and give a positive reaction with Hale's colloidal iron method and with alcian blue.

THE FIBRINOIDS

In many diseases, tissues show zones of amorphous, granular material which stain deeply with eosin and resemble fibrin. In 1880 Neumann named this amorphous material fibrinoid and described its presence in the walls of ruptured aneurysms, in endocarditis and in inflammatory reactions on serous surfaces, such as pericarditis. Subsequently, aggregates of a similar material were encountered at the base of active peptic ulcers (plate 30.1b, facing p. 30.4), in the injured walls of arterioles in accelerated hypertension (plate 30.1c), and in the lesions in a variety of systemic connective tissue diseases (table 30.2).

Besides the eosinophilia, the principal staining characteristics of fibrinoid are as follows: (1) a positive PAS reaction which suggests the presence of a polysaccharide component; (2) a bright red colour beautifully seen in Lendrum's modifications of the picro–Mallory methods, which imply a fibrin content, and (3) with silver impregnation, a yellow brown colour. It is refractile but not birefringent and does not fluoresce in ultraviolet light. It also exhibits metachromasia.

During the past 20 years, chemical, immunological and EM investigations have shown that fibrinoid in different diseases is composed of a variety of substances which look similar after the crude processes of fixation and staining. Fibrinoid resists digestion by glycolytic enzymes and is hydrolysed by pectinase but not wholly by hyaluronidase. Polyamino sugars are present and sometimes DNA. The

TABLE 30.2. The sites of occurrence and probable chemical nature of the materials which have been called fibrinoid.

Sites	Chemical nature
Inflammatory reactions	
Bacterial endocarditis	Fibrin
Active peptic ulcers	Fibrin
Miscellaneous processes	
Generalized Schwartzmann reaction (18.31)	Fibrin and other proteins
Around mature placental villi	Fibrin
Tissue death	
Arteriolar injury in accelerated (malignant) hypertension	Fibrin; globulins
Aneurysmal sacs	Fibrin
Immunological reactions	
Rheumatoid arthritis	Fibrin
nodule	Low hydroxyproline content
Rheumatic fever	
Aschoff body	γ-Globulin
pericarditis	Fibrin, albumin γ-Globulin
nodule	? Degraded collagen; Mucopolysaccharide
Systemic lupus erythematosus (SLE)	γ-Globulin; DNA
Polyarteritis nodosa	Fibrin; other plasma proteins

metachromatic component is destroyed by testicular hyaluronidase.

Table 30.2 sets out some of the present knowledge of the probable chemical nature of fibrinoid in different conditions. Plate 30.1d illustrates fibrinoid in rheumatoid synovitis.

As a result of these studies much of the significance of the fibrinoids as a basis for defining disease has been lost. In the systemic acquired connective tissue diseases (p. 30.9), the presence of fibrinoid can no longer be accepted as supportive evidence that the disease is of immunological origin, a concept which appeared to follow from the demonstration that fibrinoid is a characteristic feature of experimental type III Arthus hypersensitivity arthritis in rabbits.

The term fibrinoid belongs to an age of pathology before the cryostat, the integrating microdensitometer and the technique of immunofluorescence. These can be used to establish the chemical identity of eosinophilic aggregates in damaged tissues, and the tissue reactions seen with the diagnostic microscope can be translated with increasing confidence into exact biochemical and biophysical language. A more complex, more cumbersome terminology results, but this is the price of progress. In spite of this, the term fibrinoid will probably continue to be used to describe a characteristic appearance under light microscopy in a variety of diseases, as a matter of diagnostic convenience.

BASOPHILIC BODY FORMATION

In systemic lupus erythematosus (SLE, p. 30.12), aggregates of basophilic material, which can be shown by the Feulgen reaction to be of nuclear origin, accumulate in the tissues; they have a high content of DNA. These haematoxylin bodies range in size from masses which pack the lymph node sinusoids near sites of nodal necrosis (plate 30.1e, opposite) to small, compact structures 4–12 μm in diameter, located e.g. in foci of necrosis in glomerular tufts. The basophilic body is a hallmark of this strange disease. It is of particular interest because of its resemblance to the nuclear material phagocytosed by the polymorphs in the lupus cell phenomenon, an artefact exploited in the diagnostic LE cell test (p. 25.26). It seems probable that basophilic bodies form as a result of nuclear injury caused by immunoglobulins such as the LE cell factor which have a specificity for the basic histone of nuclear DNA-protein.

The finding of basophilic bodies in tissues therefore indicates that injury at this site may have resulted from the action of antinuclear antibody. The demonstration of the LE cell phenomenon and of autologous antinuclear antibodies in SLE strongly suggests that tissue injury has been caused by antibodies formed by the patient against components of his/her own cells, an autoimmune reaction. The presence of these antibodies in the serum is of diagnostic importance in this disease and they may occasionally be found in the related diseases, rheumatoid arthritis, systemic sclerosis, dermatomyositis and polyarteritis nodosa. However, basophilic bodies are not recognizable in tissue lesions except in SLE. Nucleophagocytosis (but not true LE cell formation) has been recognized in patients given drugs such as penicillin, hydrallazine and phenolphthalein. The ingested nuclear material does not resemble the LE cell precisely; for example, the inclusion does not have a homogeneous, ground-glass appearance. The cells found in these circumstances are named 'tart' cells. Occasionally a drug sensitivity reaction accompanied by a true positive LE cell test may be the first sign of the disseminated disease.

COLLAGEN SCLEROSIS

In many disturbances of connective tissues, there is a tendency for hyperplastic fibroblasts to form excess collagen. This collagen sclerosis, or fibrosis, found typically in old scar tissue, is prominent also in the lesions of systemic sclerosis where it affects both the skin and the viscera; fibrosis occurs around splenic penicillar arteries in SLE. In rheumatic fever, fibrosis is responsible for cardiac valvular deformity and in rheumatoid arthritis it accompanies the formation of the 'pannus' which marginally replaces articular cartilage. One result of fibrosis in rheumatoid arthritis is ankylosis of the affected joint.

Collagen sclerosis is part of the reaction called **keloid formation**. A keloid is a localized hyperplasia of fibroblasts and tends to occur in relation to incompletely healed wounds or injuries such as burns and abrasions. Keloid formation is more common in Negroes than in the fair skinned and in some communities the process has been encouraged for cosmetic reasons, by deliberately interfering with healing. Although keloids may arise from radiation injuries, paradoxically the tissue of a keloid is quite sensitive to therapeutic irradiation. Histologically, the exuberant fibrous tissue formation of a keloid is confined to the middle and deeper layers of the dermis. There are broad, interlacing bundles of collagen and fibroblasts, but as time passes fewer cells remain than in normal scar formation and elastic fibres are not present. Dermal appendages are lost and there is progressive secondary thinning of the overlying epidermis. Although the reaction is primarily one of dermal fibrous tissue of mesenchymal origin, squamous carcinomata of epithelial origin are unexpectedly frequent at sites of keloid formation. Why malignant tumours of connective tissue do not occur under these circumstances is not known.

Ageing

Old age is the inevitable sequel to all forms of life, at least in the environmental conditions which prevail today. The ageing of connective tissue becomes a disease process only if it is abnormally rapid.

All components of connective tissue change with time. With advancing age the ratio of mucopolysaccharide to collagen falls steadily. The fibre content of connective tissue therefore increases with age, a characteristic not only of normal tissues, but also of scars; the abundant sulphated mucopolysaccharide of the young scar, easily defined by its metachromasia, is replaced by increasingly dense collagenous material of decreasing vascularity. The pallor, progressive shrinking and deformity of ageing scars are familiar to all. In cartilage, a continuous reduction in the proportion of chondroitin 4-sulphate accompanies a steady increase in the proportion of polymerized keratosulphate. An intimate relationship exists between the protein-polysaccharides of connective tissue ground substance and the proteins of mature collagen and reticulin which also change with time. Individual fibres enlarge and increased numbers of cross-linkages form between adjacent fibrils. Aged connective tissue is more compact than young; it is also less cellular.

Effects of age on these changes are seen most readily in organs with the highest content of connective tissue. Thus, hyaline articular cartilage, which is blue-white and almost translucent in youth, becomes opaque and yellow with age. At the same time aged cartilage loses its compressibility; it is less effective as a cushion against

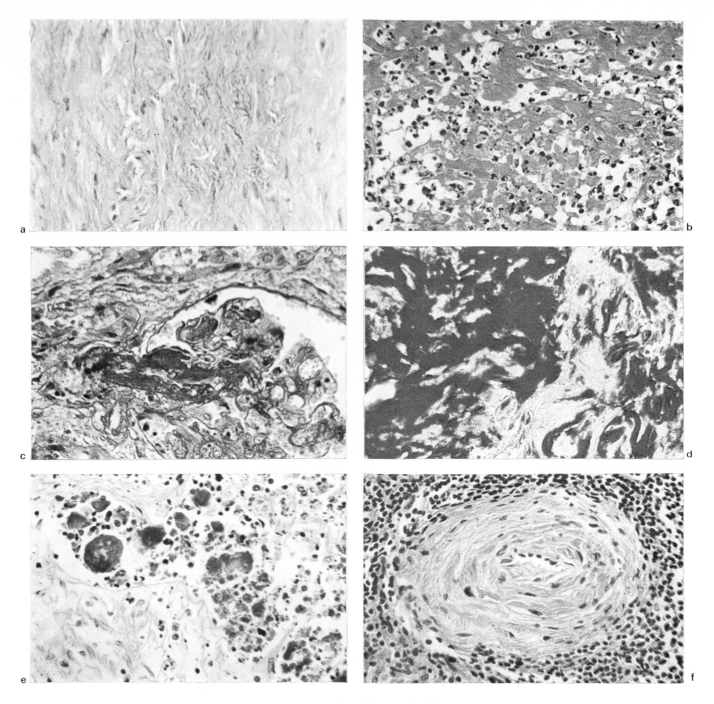

PLATE 30.1. Lesions of connective tissue.

(a) Mucoid change in aorta in the Marfan syndrome. There is an excess of pink (metachromatic) material between blue-staining collagen and elastic fibres, and smooth muscle cells. The staining reactions are characteristic of those seen in mucoid material and primitive mesenchymal ground substance. Toluidine blue (×415).

(c) Glomerular arteriole showing fibrinoid in accelerated hypertension. Fibrinoid, staining bright red, extends from the wall of the arteriole into the vascular pole of the glomerulus. The material is an extracellular accumulation of plasma proteins including fibrin; it mingles with the residue of injured vascular smooth muscle cells. Picro–Mallory (×310).

(e) Basophilic bodies in a lymph node in systemic lupus erythematosus. Irregularly shaped, blue-staining masses of nuclear material are seen lying in the cortical sinuses of a partly necrotic lymph node. Haem. & eosin (×345).

(b) Fibrinoid at the base of an active peptic ulcer. This field shows an accumulation of pink-staining material on the floor of an active ulcer. The fibrinoid seen in this situation is mainly fibrin. Haem. & eosin (×310).

(d) Fibrinoid in synovial tissue in rheumatoid arthritis. Bright red-staining fibrinoid material in this case includes fibrin and γ-globulin; it lies among the swollen, inflamed synovial connective tissue. Picro–Mallory (×310).

(f) Collagen sclerosis in penicillar arteriole in systemic sclerosis. Surrounding the media is an increased number of layers of advential collagen fibres and fibrocytes. The appearance of the inner part of the vessel suggests that there is also an excess of subendothelial collagen. Haem. & eosin (×310).

mechanical stress and strain and becomes increasingly susceptible to injury. These changes are associated with a gradual decrease in the rate of division of chondrocytes with resulting hypoplasia and atrophy. The reduction in hyaluronic acid synthesis by synovial tissue, which is a feature of senility, contributes to the inferior lubricating properties of ageing synovial fluid. Physical changes in cartilage structure combined with decreased ease of movement culminate in the degenerative process called osteoarthrosis.

Elastic tissue synthesis is also changed in old age. In the dermis, elastic fibres are smaller but apparently more numerous than in youth. The skin loses its elasticity and remains wrinkled when compressed; the dermal collagen assumes basophilic staining characteristics. The sum of these changes is described as **senile elastosis**, a condition closely reproduced by the effects of ionizing radiation. This resemblance is of interest since it is possible that cosmic and other background radiation may be factors in the molecular changes associated with old age.

Measurement of tissue mucopolysaccharide and of collagen at any given age shows that the relative amounts of connective tissue ground substance, of collagen fibres and of tissue parenchyma remain remarkably constant in the face of a wide variety of changes. In pregnancy, a steady increase and subsequent abrupt decrease in uterine smooth muscle is paralleled by corresponding changes in collagen. Again, an experimental incision of the liver may lead to the rapid formation of new collagen; as liver cells regenerate, the collagen content diminishes until a normal ratio of parenchyma to stroma is restored. This balance can be upset by agents such as carbon tetrachloride which injure hepatocytes; there is a failure to reabsorb collagen just as there is a failure in hepatocytes to regenerate.

The constancy of the proportion of connective tissue components to parenchyma at a single age, and the changes in the ratio of ground substance to fibres as age advances, are subject to endocrine control and altered in diseases of the endocrine glands. In myxoedema, acromegaly and Cushing's syndrome, for example, the connective tissue components change in amount and in character. In myxoedema, there is an accumulation of mucopolysaccharide; the skin becomes coarse and thickened. In acromegaly, there is excess connective tissue formation, a change seen particularly clearly in bone where the disturbance results in the heavy jaw and broad hands (vol. 1, p. 25.13). In Cushing's syndrome, poor wound healing, a feature also observed when corticosteroids are given in large doses for therapeutic reasons, is accompanied by a curious form of obesity and by the development of striae in tense skin.

Developmental changes in connective tissue and the process of ageing are influenced by the vagaries of nutrition; these matters are referred to again on p. 30.8.

INHERITED DISORDERS OF CONNECTIVE TISSUE

A number of rare, inherited diseases which affect the muscles, skeleton and organs, including those of the cardiovascular and nervous systems, have been known for many years. These diseases are now classified together as the main structure affected is the connective tissue system (table 30.3).

The Marfan syndrome
Some of the more obvious characteristics of the Marfan syndrome can be appreciated by watching the ball play of the Harlem 'Globetrotters'. Essential factors for success at basketball are suppleness and great height, especially if the height is exceeded by the span of the outstretched arms. The ability to grasp the ball in one hand is dependent on enormously long 'spider' fingers (arachnodactyly). The 'disease' is familial and the inherited characteristics include prolapsed lenses, patellar dislocation and congenital cardiac disease, but all are seldom present together. Young adult males with Marfan's syndrome occasionally die suddenly and unexpectedly from dissecting aortic aneurysm; patent interatrial septum is common. Much more frequently, the genetic characteristics of the disease are expressed incompletely, and a chance observation of a skeletal deformity such as funnel sternum draws attention to the condition.

The pathological features of Marfan's syndrome are mysterious; there is presumably a fault in morphogenesis so that although individual connective tissue components such as ground substance protein-polysaccharides and collagen are not demonstrably abnormal, their arrangement as ligaments, tendons and bones is altered, and the shape and physical strength of these structures changed. To the skeletal defects and the presence of cardiac anomalies is added an accumulation in the media of elastic arteries of a metachromatic material which partially replaces smooth muscle and connective tissue, weakening the vessel wall and occasionally culminating in spontaneous rupture. This condition is known as medial mucoid degeneration. It may also be encountered in the absence of the Marfan syndrome.

The mucopolysaccharidoses
Hunter in 1917 and Hurler in 1919 independently described two forms of a group of inherited disorders of connective tissue metabolism. Table 30.3 lists the six categories of disease now included under the title of mucopolysaccharidoses. They are characterized by an excessive urinary excretion and possible excessive synthesis of one or other of the polyamino sugars which

TABLE 30.3. Inherited disorders of connective tissue. This extraordinary group of inherited disorders includes the mucopolysaccharidoses which are now the object of active chemical and cytological study. Except in the Morquio syndrome, dermal fibroblasts contain metachromatic mucopolysaccharide and chemical analysis of connective tissue and urine reveals the precise abnormality. Presumably the defect(s) in the genetic code responsible for these changes will eventually be known.

McKusick includes, in addition to the disorders shown in this table, inborn errors of metabolism such as alkaptonuria (p. 31.9) and homocystinuria (p. 31.9) which are more generally classified as hereditary metabolic diseases. Several inborn errors of metabolism involve connective tissue secondarily because of the predilection for connective tissue of an abnormally retained metabolite; they are not primary diseases of connective tissue. For the revised and now recommended chemical nomenclature, see postscript on p. XVII.

Disease		Nature of inherited disorder	Principal pathological changes
Eponymous designation	Fundamental name		
Marfan syndrome	Arachnodactyly	Abnormal morphogenesis of organs with high connective tissue content	Long arm span relative to height; spider fingers; ectopia lentis; funnel sternum; cardiac defects; dissecting aortic aneurysm
Hurler syndrome	Mucopolysaccharidosis I	Excess excretion and possibly synthesis of chondroitin sulphate B and heparitin sulphate with faulty fibroblast differentiation	Dwarfing; deformity; mental retardation; early death
Hunter syndrome	„ II	Excess excretion and possibly synthesis of chondroitin sulphate B and heparitin sulphate	Gargoylism; hepatosplenomegaly; mental deterioration; deafness
Sanfilippo syndrome	„ III	Excess excretion heparitin sulphate	Mental deficiency; premature death
Morquio syndrome	„ IV	Excess excretion keratosulphate	Dwarfing; flat vertebrae; herniae
Scheie syndrome	„ V	Excess excretion chondroitin sulphate B	Claw hands; aortic valve disease
Maroteaux–Lamy syndrome	„ VI	Excess excretion chondroitin sulphate B	Retarded growth; hepatosplenomegaly; bone deformities
Ehlers–Danlos syndrome	Hyperelastosis cutis	Hyperelastic skin, which is brittle and heals poorly; easy bruising; pseudotumours (calcified lipomata)	Excess dermal elastic tissue, but individual collagen and elastic fibres normal; increased dermal and vascular mucopolysaccharide; lipomata
Ekman–Lobstein syndrome	Osteogenesis imperfecta Infantile	Blue sclerae; large thin skull; multiple congenital fractures	Defective formation of bone in membrane; osteoporosis; small but fully calcified bone trabeculae
	Adult	'Brittle bones'; nerve deafness (otosclerosis); visceral anomalies; ready fracturing of bone	Insufficient bone matrix which forms abnormally; osteoporosis; osteoarthrosis
Groenblad–Strandberg syndrome	Pseudoxanthoma elasticum	Yellow papules on skin; impaired vision; hypertension; peripheral vascular disease; gastrointestinal bleeding	Widespread disturbance of connective tissue fibre formation; collagen fibres are fragmented and calcified; elastin is widened and twisted

normally form the polymerized polysaccharide component of the connective tissue protein-polysaccharides.

The syndrome is recognized in childhood, when, after a few months of normal development, there is failure to grow, deformity and mental retardation, and enlargement of the liver and spleen. The ugly facial appearance of these children led to the unhappy term 'gargoylism'.

The underlying metabolic abnormality is an accumulation in the viscera, brain, heart and arteries of a water-soluble mucopolysaccharide. In the cornea, for example, which often becomes opaque, there are abnormal metachromatic granules; the renal glomerular epithelial cells become large and vacuolated. There is some evidence that tissue lipids increase in the nervous system. The presence of vacuolated, mucopolysaccharide-laden 'gargoyle' cells in the tissues causes faults in local metabolism. This gives rise to the cardiac, cerebral and bone lesions, and so is responsible for the mental defect and physical deformity.

Chemical analyses of tissues show that chondroitin sulphate B and heparitin sulphate are present in excess; they are found in large quantities in the urine and defective excretion does not apparently account for the tissue accumulations.

The mucopolysaccharidoses are fascinating and fortunately rare examples of the manner in which inherited defects in the synthetic use of the basic components of ground substance by connective tissue cells lead to widespread changes in the structure of the skeletal and supporting tissues; involvement of the connective tissue components of many organs results in death from visceral disease.

The Ehlers–Danlos syndrome (hyperelastosis cutis)

Through the ages, circuses and exhibitions have profited from the fascination of monstrosities and malformations for the man in the street. There has always been a particular attraction in watching the double-jointed India rubber man who can hyperextend his fingers and wrists, draw out the skin of his neck into bat-like webs and touch the tip of his nose with his tongue. Fortunately, perhaps, the casual observer is not aware that these changes are accompanied by defective wound healing, a bleeding tendency, lipomatous tumours of the soft tissues and often death from rupture of an artery.

Underlying this ancient disease, which was described in the seventeenth century, is an inherited disorder of dermal connective tissue. Excess of elastin and a diminution in collagen is suggested. Although the EM appearances of the collagen and elastic fibres are normal, a defect in the formation of collagen bundles is possible. The subcutaneous lipomata tend to become calcified. The bleeding tendency and a failure of simple incised wounds to heal properly has been attributed to inadequate support from surrounding connective tissue and to the presence of weak-walled vessels. However, the fact that a Factor XII (Hageman) deficiency has been noted in one case suggests that an inherited defect in blood coagulation may be present. The scars which form when hyperelastotic skin heals are as thin as cigarette paper.

The Ekman–Lobstein syndrome (osteogenesis imperfecta)

The names 'osteogenesis imperfecta' or 'fragilitas ossium' have the sanction of custom, and it is occasionally overlooked that the infantile and adult forms of this genetic bone disease are clinically and historically distinct (table 30.3).

McKusick recounts that Ivar the Boneless, the ninth-century Scandinavian invader of England, was an early sufferer from the disease. He was carried into battle on shields and had cartilage where bone should have been. The congenital form of the disease, with numerous intra-uterine fractures, short limbs, blue sclerae and thin skull, is often incompatible with postnatal life. The adult form of the disease may pass unrecognized or may be diagnosed only when nerve deafness due to accompanying otosclerosis, eye changes or fracture are investigated later in life.

The underlying disorder is a defect in the formation and growth of bone trabeculae, probably the result of failure in the maturation of collagen. It is suggested that the basic change in the collagen which is formed may be due to an abnormal amino acid sequence, genetically determined. The bone trabeculae found at the epiphysis of a long bone in a case of congenital osteogenesis imperfecta are small, misshapen and often fractured or distorted. When the whole bone is broken, healing begins actively, but the healed bone is again liable to fracture. Calcification of bone matrix proceeds normally and there is therefore no evidence of osteomalacia. Osteoporosis may, however, be recognized.

The defective formation of the collagen of the bone matrix in the bony labyrinth leads to a localized form of osteogenesis imperfecta; the dense but abnormal bone synthesis culminates in otosclerosis and nerve deafness. The blue sclerae result from an abnormal orientation of collagen fibres which absorb light of longer wavelength more completely than blue light.

The Groenblad–Strandberg syndrome

Confluent, symmetrical intradermal plaques found at the flexures of the body, gastrointestinal bleeding, angioid streaks in the retina, hypertension and peripheral vascular insufficiency together comprise a rare syndrome in which, at first, it might seem difficult to pin-point a fundamental inherited disorder of connective tissue.

The most obvious pathological disturbance is an aggregation of fibres in the deeper dermis with the staining characteristics of elastin. The fibres become fragmented, basophilic and calcified. Their presence accounts for the confluent plaques at the skin flexures. Little is known of the vascular changes in this disease; arterial elastic tissue is said to be granular and fragmented. In the eye there may be sclerosis of the choroidal vessels. It is still disputed whether elastin or collagen fibres are fundamentally abnormal. That the disease is a disturbance of collagen is suggested by investigation of skin by frozen section and EM techniques; that elastin is at fault is suggested by a resemblance to the degeneration found in senile elastosis, after irradiation and trauma (p. 30.8) and by histochemical studies of the abnormal fibres. The elucidation of this obscure problem will come when more is known of the relationship between normal collagen and elastin formation.

ACQUIRED DISORDERS OF CONNECTIVE TISSUE

In this section, the manner in which connective tissues may be disorganized in the course of incidental acquired diseases is considered; next, primary acquired disturbances of connective tissue are discussed.

The connective tissues are immediately influenced by any significant disturbance of the major metabolic pathways. Starvation, avitaminosis, intestinal malabsorption, uraemia and hypopituitarism are examples of diseases which change protein and carbohydrate metabolism, and electrolyte and fluid balance. The resultant disturbances of connective tissue may escape notice because attention is concentrated on the presenting features of the parent disease.

Injury

The majority of injuries involve connective and other tissues simultaneously. However, in certain instances, as in the fracture of bones (p. 27.2) and in the rupture or cutting of a tendon, most of the injured tissue is of mesodermal origin.

When an epithelial surface such as the skin undergoes any trauma other than the slightest abrasion, the subepithelial connective tissue is disrupted. As healing occurs, the behaviour both of epithelial and of mesodermal cells determines the pattern by which the injured organ is restored to normal. Where restoration is incomplete, scar formation occurs and this process is, of course, a function of cells of mesodermal origin.

In the healing of a clean, incised skin wound such as a surgical incision, the dermal and subcutaneous connective tissue reactions to injury are not seen immediately; they follow the epithelial cell proliferation which begins during the first 24 hours. A particularly vigorous response is elicited in the normally inert subcutaneous fat; slightly less activity is recognized in the loose connective tissue which surrounds the skin appendages. Three to five days may elapse before new collagen synthesis is evident in clean incised wounds, but the intracellular synthesis of collagen precursors begins before this time.

An immediate result of direct injury to loose connective tissue is a 'softening' of the ground substance; it swells, changes in staining characteristics and becomes susceptible to penetration by micro-organisms. Where mast cells are present, their granules swell and are discharged, presumably with local release of 5-HT, heparin and histamine. When the inflammatory stimulus persists, macrophages accumulate in response to chemotaxis (p. 21.9). Cells capable of multiplication in response to injury may persist into adult life in small numbers in all connective tissues. They are transformed and assume those cellular characteristics by which we recognize fibroblasts; that is, they begin to synthesize the protein

precursors of collagen in relation to an abundant endoplasmic reticulum and are found to be only slowly motile, moving, in experimental conditions, a few micrometers in one hour compared to the much larger distances crossed by a macrophage. Young motile bipolar fibroblasts seen under these conditions throw out cytoplasmic processes which fuse with those of neighbouring cells and, in the favourable nutritional environment provided by an abundance of young capillary buds, begin to lay down the protein-polysaccharides of ground substance. Into this matrix are secreted the molecules of collagen precursor, which mature in the interstices of the ground substance. In this way young scar tissue is formed. Scar tissue formation can progress adequately only in the presence of a number of essential metabolites such as ascorbic acid and adrenohormones such as corticosteroids. Corticosteroids given therapeutically may delay healing.

Infection

The very nature of the connective tissue system, its ubiquitous character and subtle organization, means that, with the exception of bones and joints, connective tissue is rarely the primary site of infective processes. Osteomyelitis and arthritis of bacterial and fungal origin are well recognized, but they are no longer common in Britain. Nevertheless, the whole character of several common diseases is determined by the responses of the connective tissue cells, fibres or ground substance to the infecting agents.

The influence of microbial products upon connective tissue may be exemplified by reference to the hyaluronidase of β-haemolytic streptococci, the collagenase of the *Clostridia* and the fats and proteins of the *Mycobacteria*.

Nutritional and metabolic diseases

An adequate intake of vitamin C is essential for the normal role of connective tissue in the healing of wounds. In scurvy, collagen formation is impaired and scar tissue cannot be formed normally; indeed, old scars may break down and wounds re-open.

CONNECTIVE TISSUE IN SCURVY

Ascorbic acid (vitamin C) is essential for normal human collagen metabolism and is probably necessary both for the synthesis of normal connective tissue matrix and for the integrity of old, healed wounds. Man, monkey and guinea-pig lack the enzyme necessary to convert L-gulonolactone to L-ascorbic acid; the majority of other mammals can synthesize the vitamin.

In vitamin C deficiency there is a defect in the synthesis of collagen due to inadequate hydroxylation on fibroblast ribosomes of peptides containing proline. Fibroblasts are few, and contain lipid droplets and many round, dilated cisternae in the ribosome-deficient endoplasmic reticulum. Tissue hydroxyproline is an accurate reflection of collagen content; in scorbutic guinea-pigs there is a pronounced reduction of hydroxyproline in skin and bone. Collagen synthesis in experimental granulomata in scorbutic animals is deficient and the local injection of vitamin C into implanted polyvinyl sponges in such animals stimulates the rapid formation of abundant collagen. Tropocollagen, the salt-soluble intracellular precursor of insoluble mature extracellular collagen, is deficient in scorbutic guinea-pig skin. There is diminished formation of hydroxyproline from proline in the connective tissue of these animals.

The explanation for the unexpectedly rapid new formation of collagen when vitamin C is given to scorbutic animals is now evident; studies with labelled amino acids show that hydroxyproline is deficient and that proline-containing protein accumulates on the fibroblast ribosomes and may even be secreted extracellularly, as 'protocollagen'. This is not a collagen precursor, but when vitamin C is given there is rapid hydroxylation of the protein bound to ribosomes which is then secreted as collagen. Within 12 hours of giving vitamin C to a deficient animal, the ribosomes begin to show normal orientation on the endoplasmic reticulum; smooth cisternae appear and collagen is synthesized and directly secreted through the plasma membrane, probably not via the Golgi apparatus.

In addition to deficient collagen synthesis, it is likely that there is an abnormality in connective tissue matrix in scurvy. Guinea-pig studies show that there is diminished galactosamine synthesis, and perhaps increased degradation of polymerized mucopolysaccharides. Impaired galactosamine synthesis is probably due to a block in the UDP-*N*-acetylglucosamine 4-epimerase reaction.

Other nutrients assist in the formation and maintenance of connective tissue in foetal life. A variety of disorders of connective tissue, including cranial and vertebral deformities, can be produced in young rabbits born of mothers who have been fed on unbalanced diets grossly lacking in vitamin A.

However, it is doubtful if dietary deficiencies contribute significantly to the aetiology of any important connective tissue disorder of man apart from scurvy.

Immunological diseases

Klemperer in 1942, in a classic paper, postulated that the anatomical and physiological evidence for the existence of a connective tissue system carried with it the corollary that, as with other systems, there exist system diseases. He showed that changes in the structure of collagen and the occurrence of 'fibrinoid' (p. 30.3) were characteristic features in the disseminated conditions, systemic sclerosis and systemic lupus erythematosus; he considered that these were primarily disorders of the fibrous proteins of connective tissue, and named them the 'diffuse

diseases of collagen'. It was a short and acceptable step to the phrase 'collagen disease' or 'collagenosis'; although these terms are widely used in clinical practice, biochemical and biophysical studies have provided no evidence that fibrous proteins are primarily disturbed in these disorders, and the term 'immunological connective tissue disease' represents the modern view.

The development of fibrinoid is a characteristic histological feature of type III Arthus hypersensitivity (p. 22.20). Since fibrinoid is found also in cases of rheumatic fever, rheumatoid arthritis and the related diseases systemic lupus erythematosus, systemic sclerosis, polyarteritis nodosa and dermatomyositis, it seems possible that these also may be of immunological origin. Much evidence now supports this hypothesis, and it is believed that the pathological features of these diseases and their variants may indeed be caused, directly or indirectly, by the injurious action of antibodies or of antibody-forming cells, or by some perversion of the immunological system. At the present time the consensus of opinion is against the idea that a primary change in the immunological system leads to all of these disorders. The theory was proposed by Burnet that a clone of lymphoid cells might emerge, through random mutation, capable, by virtue of their immunological competence, of reacting with and consequently injuring connective tissue cells in many parts of the body.

This mode of origin was suggested for rheumatoid arthritis; in this disease numerous features such as enlarged lymph nodes, a hyperactive reticuloendothelial system, and the presence of circulating antibody (the rheumatoid factor) against native immunoglobulin and of plasma cells and fibrinoid in the synovial tissues combine to support the idea that this is a 'disorder of the immunological mechanism' or even an autoimmune disease (p. 23.7). The clonal selection theory is, however, not unanimously accepted.

Today there is more support for the alternative hypothesis that rheumatoid arthritis, like polyarteritis nodosa and rheumatic fever, may be caused by an exogenous agent like a virus or bacterium. However, the way in which extrinsic antigens cause tissue damage in these three diseases is quite distinct. In polyarteritis nodosa a chemical, acting as a hapten, induces specific hypersensitivity to foreign protein. When the sensitized patient is next exposed to this antigen, an immediate or a delayed hypersensitivity response causes tissue injury. In rheumatic fever, vascular, cardiac and perhaps joint cells share an antigenic determinant with the Group A β-haemolytic streptococci; antibodies formed against the streptococci injure the tissue cells (fig. 30.1). In rheumatoid arthritis, it is suspected that an infective agent of low virulence, lodged in the joint cells, alters cell antigenic structure so that these altered antigens come to be regarded as foreign; an immunological reaction of auto-

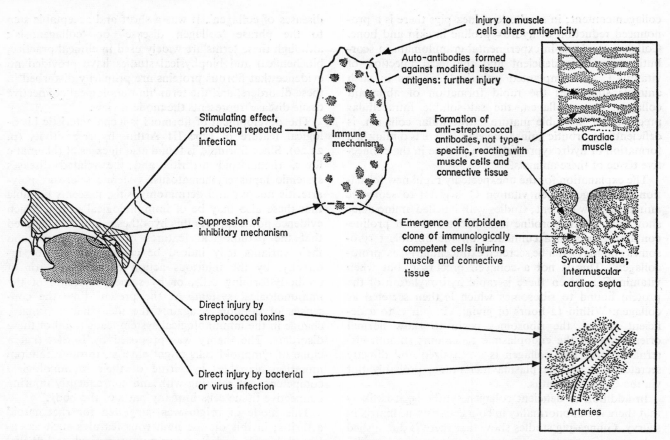

Stimulating effect, producing repeated infection

Immune mechanism

Suppression of inhibitory mechanism

Direct injury by streptococcal toxins

Direct injury by bacterial or virus infection

Injury to muscle cells alters antigenicity

Auto-antibodies formed against modified tissue antigens: further injury

Formation of anti-streptococcal antibodies, not type-specific, reacting with muscle cells and connective tissue

Emergence of forbidden clone of immunologically competent cells injuring muscle and connective tissue

Cardiac muscle

Synovial tissue; Intermuscular cardiac septa

Arteries

FIG. 30.1. Some possible ways in which the pathogenesis of rheumatic fever may be explained. The most probable of these involves a cytotoxic immunological reaction at the surface of cardiovascular cells due to a sharing by these cells of an antigenic determinant also present in Group A β-haemolytic streptococci, infection with which is the initial step in the disease.

immune type is set up against them and recognizable tissue injury results.

In systemic lupus erythematosus, there is evidence of an inherited abnormality of the immunological mechanism; the patient may display several varied immunological disturbances which commonly include antinuclear factor activity (p. 23.5), greatly increased γ-globulin synthesis, drug hypersensitivity, haemolytic anaemia and tissue lesions of delayed hypersensitivity type.

It is, therefore, reasonable to group together rheumatoid arthritis, rheumatic fever, polyarteritis nodosa, systemic lupus erythematosus, dermatomyositis and systemic sclerosis, but to abandon the idea that they are collagen diseases. It is, however, still justifiable to regard them as systemic disorders of mesenchymal tissue, and the varied pathological changes encountered are probably the results of disturbances producing immunological disorders which lead to tissue injury. The basic changes encountered in the more common of this group of diseases are now discussed.

RHEUMATIC FEVER

The fundamental disorder in rheumatic fever is not understood. The disease often follows infection with a Group A β-haemolytic streptococcus. An interval of two or more weeks between the infection and the onset of arthritis suggests that the characteristic lesions (table 30.4) are the result of an immunological reaction to the products of the infecting organism; there is no evidence that the lesions are due directly to bacterial infection. The streptococcal component is shared by many Griffith types of organism; unlike acute glomerulonephritis, no single type is particularly associated with rheumatic fever. The cytotoxic effect is mediated in part by antibody and in part by a cellular response. The disease, which is much less common than formerly, causes lesions of the articular, cardiovascular and nervous systems. The lesions result from a series of microscopic changes, which are probably due to an interaction between an antigenic component of the patient's tissues and cellular or circulating antibodies formed against components of the cell wall of the infecting streptococci. The manner in which streptococcal and tissue antigens cross-react is important in pathogenesis.

The immunological evidence, much of which is based on immunofluorescence microscopy, shows that γ-globu-

TABLE 30.4. The immunological diseases of connective tissue.

Disease	Principal target organ	Nature of immune reaction	Postulated cause	Main pathological changes	Main chemical changes
Rheumatic fever	Heart (all parts), synovial joints	Hypersensitivity to component of streptococcus, the antigenic structure of which is in part shared by heart tissue	Group A β-haemolytic streptococcal infections	Fibrinoid, vasculitis, carditis, synovitis, chromatophilic substance, nodules, Aschoff bodies	C-antigens and antistreptolysin-O titre elevated (p. 18.67)
Rheumatoid arthritis	Synovial joints, subcutaneous tissue	Delayed hypersensitivity reaction to altered synovial tissue antigen	Corynebacteria, mycoplasmas, inherited predisposition	Fibrinoid, granulomatous nodules, vasculitis, plasma cell exudation, polyserositis, synovitis	Hypergamma-globulinaemia with rheumatoid factors and antinuclear factors
Systemic lupus erythematosus	Small blood vessels, renal basement membranes	Inherited or acquired change in sensitivity or selectivity of immunological system	Drug sensitivity, ultraviolet light, prolonged skin disease	Fibrinoid, focal lymphoid necrosis, basophilic body formation, vascular endothelial change, collagen sclerosis	Hypergamma-globulinaemia with antinuclear factors, LE cells (p. 25.26)
Polyarteritis nodosa	Muscular arteries	Delayed hypersensitivity	Drugs such as sulphonamides	Fibrinoid, vasculitis	Hypergamma-globulinaemia
Systemic sclerosis	Skin, smooth muscle, renal connective tissue	Unknown	Premature ageing of connective tissue fibres	Fibrinoid, collagen sclerosis	Hypergamma-globulinaemia
Dermatomyositis	Skin, skeletal muscle	Unknown	Unknown	Myositis, collagen sclerosis	Not known

lin, probably of antibody nature, is bound to the sarcolemma of cardiac muscle cells. A cross-reaction between antiserum prepared against streptococcal cell wall and cardiac myofibrillar sarcoplasm and arterial smooth muscle is demonstrable. The fibrinoid found on the pericardial surface is a fibrinous inflammatory exudate although the fibrinoid present in damaged blood vessel walls and in cardiac muscle is at least partly γ-globulin.

Four histological changes are commonly found.

(1) There is a sterile exudative inflammatory reaction, especially of cardiac valves and small arteries.

(2) **Chromatophilic substance** is seen in the intermuscular connective tissue matrix, due to focal changes in the staining characteristics of the ground substance.

(3) **Subcutaneous rheumatic nodules** with swollen, oedematous centres, and margins in which histiocytes are arranged radially, are seen in zones of connective tissue exposed to minor trauma. These nodules are large and usually visible macroscopically.

(4) **Aschoff bodies** appear within myocardial, subendocardial and subepicardial connective tissue. These are focal histiocytic cellular aggregates which form near small blood vessels; fibrin-like material and giant-cells are seen.

One of the most important results of cardiac inflammation in rheumatic fever is healing, with scar tissue formation, of the valves and subvalvular tissue. The scar tissue contracts with time, the valve orifices become abnormally narrow (stenotic) and the valve cusps distorted and incompetent. The surgical operation of mitral valvulotomy is widely practised to relieve mitral valvular stenosis, the most common and most serious of the cardiac complications, and during the operation portions of the left atrial appendage may be taken for histological study. The results of investigations of this kind have shown that Aschoff bodies are often present in the perivascular connective tissues within heart muscle or beneath the endocardium in the hearts of patients in whom clinical examination, erythrocyte sedimentation rates and other laboratory tests suggest that the rheumatic process is inactive. These findings have thrown doubt on the older view that Aschoff bodies are a sensitive index of active cardiovascular disease in rheumatic fever.

This evidence may be taken in conjunction with demonstrable interactions between antistreptococcal antibodies and the cardiovascular tissues. The sites at which these reactions can be shown to occur is not confined to those at which Aschoff bodies are found. The widespread distribution of antistreptococcal antibody on or within cardiac muscle cells may also help to explain cases in which death results from cardiac failure during acute rheumatic fever. When the focal Aschoff body was considered to be of prime significance, it was difficult to understand how such an inconspicuous, localized injury could lead to heart failure. The evidence that damage to cardiac muscle cells mediated by circulating antibodies may be much more subtle and widespread helps to explain the mechanism of unexpected deaths as well as to illuminate the specificity of the antistreptococcal response.

RHEUMATOID ARTHRITIS

In this common disease there is good evidence of antibody formation against an altered native immunoglobulin; the IgM antibody formed in this way, the **rheumatoid factor**, is found both on and in the cells resembling plasma cells which lie within the synovial tissues, and also in the plasma, where it exists as a loose complex with the IgA antigen. It is supposed that this macroglobulin is synthesized by plasma cells. The antibody may be detected by adding the patient's serum to sheep red blood cells which have been sensitized with anti-sheep red blood cell antibodies obtained from a rabbit (Rose-Waaler test). Agglutination occurs in 50–60 per cent of patients with rheumatoid arthritis, but it is also increasingly positive with advancing age.

How and why focal immune or autoimmune reactions occur in rheumatoid arthritis, and their exact relationship to the pathogenesis of the disease, remains obscure. As rheumatoid arthritis evolves there develop:

(1) a plasma cell and lymphocytic synovial reaction,
(2) subcutaneous rheumatoid nodules or granuloma,
(3) arteritis and amyloidosis, and
(4) nonspecific pericarditis and pleurisy.

It is likely that the syndrome of rheumatoid arthritis with anaemia, hyperglobulinaemia, diminished resistance to infection and a propensity to form amyloid, is the result of a hitherto unsuspected infection which leads to hyperplasia of the reticuloendothelial system, and to striking changes in immunological responsiveness. It is also possible that the clinical disease is not a pathological entity but a number of disorders linked together on the basis of common clinical features.

SYSTEMIC LUPUS ERYTHEMATOSUS

The pathological findings in this strange disease are also due to a series of fundamental disturbances in cell biology. There seems to be an unusual responsiveness to native and to foreign antigens. It has been suggested that the reaction to native antigens towards which the patient's immune system is normally tolerant and to other exogenous or altered endogenous antigens reflects a change in the entire pattern of immunological responsiveness, caused perhaps by random somatic mutation, by an inherited abnormality of antibody protein synthesis, or by hypersensitivity to chemical agents such as penicillin or hydrallazine.

The main histological disturbances are as follows.

(1) **Fibrinoid** appears in affected tissues such as small blood vessels, skin and kidney; these eosinophilic zones contain γ-globulin and depolymerized DNA.

(2) **Focal necrosis** of lymphoid tissue, often accompanied by aggregates of haematoxyphilic material derived from broken down cell nuclei, can be shown by the Feulgen reaction for DNA (plate 30.1e, facing p. 30.4).

(3) **Vascular changes** in the small blood vessels often result in a thickened intima, endothelial plaques and fibrinoid; in fact the disease was at one time thought to be a primary disorder of the vascular system.

(4) **Collagen sclerosis** may result either as a primary response around the splenic arteries or secondarily, following the organization of zones of fibrinoid change and tissue necrosis (plate 30.1f, facing p. 30.4).

The LE factor responsible for the formation of LE cells (p. 25.26) and other antibodies specific against nuclei (p. 23.5) are detectable in the blood of over 90 per cent of patients with SLE.

POLYARTERITIS NODOSA

Arteritis is a feature of several of the immunological disorders of connective tissue. In addition, inflammatory diseases of muscular arteries caused by immunological sensitivity exist independently; the prototype disease is polyarteritis nodosa. This first attracted attention because of the bead-like nodules on systemic arteries, visible to the naked eye, and due to aneurysmal expansion of the vessels. However, in many cases it is now recognized that the lesions are too small to be seen by the naked eye.

It is now held that polyarteritis nodosa is an immunological disorder, analogous with rheumatic fever; classification with the systemic immunological connective tissue diseases is accepted chiefly because of the arteritic changes which occur in occasional cases of rheumatoid arthritis and systemic lupus erythematosus. Evidence that a hypersensitivity reaction is involved in polyarteritis is of three kinds.

(1) *Clinical:* asthma, often an allergic disorder, is a common associated feature.

(2) *Immunological:* bacterial infection may occur two to three weeks before the onset, which suggests a hypersensitivity reaction. Drugs such as arsenic, sulphonamides and penicillin, and horseradish have been shown to be antigenic determinants causing autoimmune

responses in some cases. Plasma cells, presumed to be immunologically competent, are seen in the lesions, and in the walls of injured vessels γ-globulin, fibrin and complement have been demonstrated.

(3) *Experimental:* many procedures, such as the injection of foreign proteins into rabbits and rats, the long continued administration of sulphonamides or the immunization of rats against homologous arterial extracts, have demonstrated that antigenic sensitization can cause polyarteritis.

The fundamental lesion is focal necrosis of segments of the walls of small arteries and of arterioles. Swelling and oedema first mark the affected sites, and eosinophilic material containing plasma proteins accumulates beneath the endothelium. Necrosis of smooth muscle cells in the medial coat progresses to disintegration of elastic laminae and of the reticular framework of the vessel. Healing and fibrosis of the wall may be complicated by aneurysmal swelling. A cellular infiltrate accompanies the medial changes; the presence of many eosinophils is unusual, but these cells are common in cases in which the pulmonary vessels are affected.

Amyloidosis

In a wide variety of human and animal diseases, hereditary and acquired, infectious and neoplastic, a glycoprotein called **amyloid** is laid down among connective tissue ground substance. EM shows that the material is in the form of very fine fibrils; these are deposited within basement membranes and reticulin framework and especially between vascular endothelial cells and their basement membranes, and in relation to the capillary basement membrane of renal glomeruli. Amyloid is found in connective tissue in many parts of the body and is often deposited in association with the collagen fibres in the hepatic space of Disse (vol. 1, p. 30.32).

The name amyloid, like many others in pathology, is a misnomer; it was applied by Virchow because the material gave the same blue colour reaction to iodine after treatment with sulphuric acid as did starch (Latin, *amylum*). In this way, Virchow excluded the protein component which he knew to be present. The word 'amyloid' is now used merely as a convenience; a more precise title such as 'idiopathic fibrillar glycoproteinosis' would be cumbersome.

In all forms of amyloid a microfibrillar structure has been shown, and the fibrils have a high protein content. Thus, when material from an amyloid-rich organ is fractionated by density gradient centrifugation, the amyloid fraction has a nitrogen content of about 15 per cent, similar to that of most proteins. Contrary to early belief, IgG and IgM immunoglobulins are not part of the protein fraction of amyloid although they may be associated with amyloid deposits in a nonspecific manner. The polysaccharide component is composed of neutral

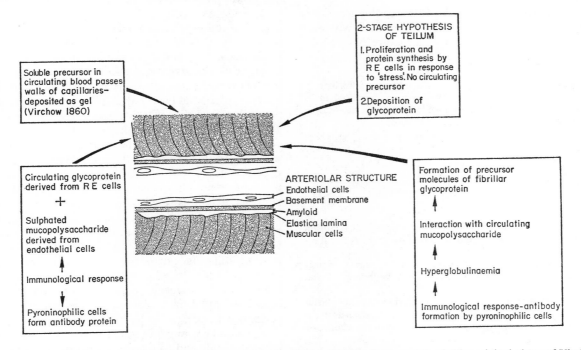

FIG. 30.2. Four possible mechanisms by which the formation of amyloid has been explained. The original views of Virchow can now be discounted, but it is not yet certain whether amyloid as recognized pathologically is an exaggeration of fibrillar glycoprotein formation which normally accompanies ageing or a perverted, abnormal form of protein synthesis.

sugars and sialic acid but not the amino sugars, characteristic of the mucopolysaccharides.

Amyloid can readily be recognized by light microscopy, when it is abundant in tissues such as liver or spleen. In haematoxylin and eosin-stained paraffin sections, amyloid appears as a pale eosinophilic, rather hyaline substance. Recognition is aided by a nonspecific affinity which amyloid displays for Congo red, and by metachromasia with methyl violet. A green birefringence which amyloid deposits exhibit after interaction with Congo red is apparently specific, and is an intrinsic property of the microfibrils. Another dye, thioflavine-T, which has an affinity for amyloid, fluoresces yellow in ultraviolet light; primary fluorescence, recognized by ultraviolet microscopy of the tissue to be studied, without added fluorochrome dyes, is not demonstrable. The EM shows that the fibrillar structure is due to the presence of laterally aggregated filaments which are about $7 \cdot 5$ nm in diameter, with a periodic beading at $10 \cdot 0$ nm intervals in the long axis.

It has for some years been customary to classify amyloid on the basis of its supposed causes. Thus amyloid may be secondary to some chronic infectious or suppurative disease such as pulmonary tuberculosis, or to rheumatoid arthritis, or may have no apparent predisposing condition, when the description primary is used. There are both hereditary and acquired varieties, and the deposits may be localized to one organ, or are generalized (table 30.5).

This classification loses much of its meaning when it is realized that wherever amyloid is found, and whatever the cause, the same microfibrillar structure is recognizable, and that stated differences in sites and in staining

TABLE 30.5. Causes of amyloidosis. In all forms a fibrillar protein, distinct from antibody globulin, is deposited in connective tissues. Why such a wide variety of diseases leads to this disorder is not known.

Hereditary:
  (1) familial Mediterranean fever,
  (2) febrile urticaria,
  (3) accompanying cardiomyopathy or neuropathy.

Acquired:
  (1) secondary; amyloidosis of general visceral distribution occurring in diseases such as rheumatoid arthritis or tuberculosis;
  (2) localized; a single nodule constitutes the whole clinical syndrome in a site such as the larynx, subcutaneous tissue or heart;
  (3) para-amyloid; amyloid deposited during the neoplastic growth of vigorously protein-synthesizing cells such as those of plasma cell myeloma; also encountered in the stroma of tumours such as medullary carcinoma of thyroid;
  (4) primary; amyloid of general distribution but not associated with any recognizable underlying disease.

reactions between primary and secondary amyloidosis are inconsistent. Whether there are significant differences in chemical structure between different samples of amyloid is not known but is unlikely.

The immediate cause or causes of amyloid deposition are not understood (fig. 30.2). Secondary amyloidosis is the most common variety in Britain, and is most often associated with rheumatoid arthritis. The features of this disease which may be related to amyloid formation are reticuloendothelial hyperplasia and hyperactivity, excessive γ-globulin synthesis, lymphoid hyperplasia, plasma cell proliferation and autoantibody formation.

Therapeutic antisera are commonly made by the prolonged, repetitive injection of horses with appropriate antigens; animals used in this way develop amyloid. In experimental animals, bacterial and protozoal antigens can also induce amyloidosis. This, together with the frequency of amyloid in patients with long-standing suppurative disease, suggests that an immunological mechanism is concerned with amyloid formation. However, amyloid itself does not include antibody protein and it seems likely that it is an incidental by-product of the reticuloendothelial cells which are hyperactive in antibody synthesis. The view that plasma cells are involved in this process receives support from the high incidence of a variety of amyloid, para-amyloid, in plasma cell myeloma, a neoplastic disease of the plasma cell series. The role of a soluble, circulating precursor of amyloid was considered by Virchow and is still invoked, but evidence now suggests that circulating material found in the γ-globulin fraction is derived from amyloid previously synthesized by reticuloendothelial cells.

In essence, amyloid is a fibrillar protein laid down in connective tissue ground substance and a product of reticuloendothelial cells. It is most abundant in organs such as spleen and liver in which these cells are numerous. Reticuloendothelial cells synthesize amyloid fibrils when they are immunologically hyperactive. The cells which form antibody globulin, the plasma cells, do not form amyloid, but antibody globulin may be found incidentally attached to amyloid deposits. Amyloid is not a mucoprotein, but the nature of its carbohydrate moiety suggests that it is a glycoprotein. This glycoprotein is synthesized intracellularly, presumably by endoplasmic reticulum, and is extruded into nearby ground substance in much the same way as collagen is formed. The numerous precipitating causes for amyloidosis are so varied that it has been suggested that amyloid protein synthesis is a normal reticuloendothelial cell function which only occasionally becomes excessive and which increases, perhaps with age.

In secondary amyloidosis, the liver, kidney, spleen, adrenal glands and to a lesser extent the gastrointestinal tract are mainly affected. In primary amyloidosis, when no obvious cause is present, it is usually reported that the distribution is mainly in heart, gastrointestinal tract, tongue and muscles, but in some cases the secondary type of distribution occurs without any obvious known cause.

EFFECTS

In general, the affected organs increase in size, and become pale in colour, appearing waxy or translucent. As the amyloid accumulates between cells, these atrophy and may disappear; this is probably related to interference with their nutrition. However, in some organs little functional change may be obvious; amyloidosis of the liver does not often lead to significant hepatic failure. In the kidneys, however, amyloid material so obliterates glomerular capillary structure that renal failure often ensues; in the earlier stages of renal amyloidosis the affected glomerular capillary basement membranes allow excessive amounts of protein to pass through and proteinuria is common. Amyloidosis of the adrenal glands is a rare cause of Addison's disease (vol. I, p. 25.31).

NEOPLASTIC DISEASES

As in other tissues it is difficult to draw the line between the processes of hyperplasia and benign neoplasia.

Benign tumours are named in accordance with the cell type from which they arise, for example, fibromata, chondromata, lipomata and osteomata. The features of these neoplastic diseases may sometimes be difficult to distinguish from inflammatory granulomata, from the components of scars and from hyperplastic processes, and may be indistinguishable from certain malformations and congenital anomalies. One example of this confusion is the angioleiomyoma or congenital fibrovascular anomaly of the kidney, in which a circumscribed zone of primitive hyperplastic blood vessels, often arterial, lies among connective tissue containing smooth muscle bundles and lipoid cells. This rare abnormality is a hamartoma, but behaves like a slowly growing neoplasm, and contains young connective tissue cells which individually are indistinguishable from those of normal fibrofatty tissue.

Malignant tumours are called **sarcomata**. Untreated, they may grow to a large size, and the name describes their fleshy appearance when cut across. A suffix designates their supposed cellular origin, e.g. fibrosarcomata, myxosarcomata, osteosarcomata and liposarcomata.

All the connective tissues are derived from embryonic mesoderm. At first this germ layer consists of undifferentiated cells dispersed in ground substance and this is called mesenchyme. Later these mesenchymal cells aggregate and differentiate to form bone, cartilage, blood, lymph, fibrous tissue and fat. Some mesenchymal cells are believed to remain throughout life in the interstices of all connective tissues, where they retain a capacity for differentiation to fibroblasts, synovioblasts and other young connective tissue cells. Primary malignant tumours of connective tissue may arise from this stem cell itself, when they are called mesenchymomata, or they may come from any of the more specialized derivative cells, giving rise to fibrosarcomata, chondrosarcomata, etc.

All primary malignant tumours of connective tissue are uncommon, and many are very rare. Only the most common are described here. For accounts of the rarer malignant connective tissue tumours the student is referred to the list of works for further reading at the end of this chapter.

The primary tumours of synovial tissues are described on p. 30.16.

BENIGN TUMOURS

Fibromata are among the most frequent of human neoplasms; they are found beneath skin surfaces and serous membranes and also within the viscera. When the tumours lie among normal connective tissues, they are not always sharply circumscribed and in the skin, for example, may merge with dermal collagen. However, surgical removal is not followed by recurrence.

Fibromata are small, pale nodules of firm consistency, grey-white on section. Their nondescript appearance makes it difficult to distinguish them from scar tissue and keloid. Microscopically, they are formed of bundles of fibroblasts lying in a collagenous matrix and may be distinguished from fibrosarcomata by their size, cellularity and the cytological features of the component cells.

Desmoid tumours are localized masses which occur in the rectus muscles of parous women. They arise in scar tissue, but in spite of local evidence of infiltration do not recur after excision. Desmoid tumours are composed of fibroblasts or fibrocytes and collagen fibres; they have many of the characteristics of keloids (p. 30.4) and, like keloids, include numerous collagen fibres which appear larger than normal and have a hyaline appearance.

Xanthomatous tumours of connective tissue are common; they are aggregates of fat-containing histiocytes in a fibroblastic stroma. Associated with the local accumulation of fat, many multinucleated (Touton) giant cells form; their nuclei are arranged in a ring, and they give these small circumscribed yellow-orange nodules a characteristic microscopic appearance. The tumours are often very vascular and the pigmentation is in part due to haemosiderin.

Xanthomata may be associated with high plasma cholesterol levels as in essential hypercholesterolaemia; other types, like the **xanthelasma** of senile skin, seem to form as part of the ageing process.

It is difficult to draw a dividing line between fibrous xanthomata, giant cell tumours of tendon sheaths, which are small yellow-orange nodules found in relation to synovial tissue, and the **sclerosing haemangiomata**, found in the skin mainly of the lower limbs. The component cells of the sclerosing haemangioma which, as its name suggests, contains many small vascular channels, resemble fibroblasts but often contain much lipid. This tumour has poorly defined margins, merges with the surrounding dermal connective tissue but shows no tendency to recur after excision. As with so many of the benign tumours of connective tissue, it is difficult to be certain that the lesion is neoplastic.

Lipomata are common in the middle-aged and elderly. They are composed of fat cells, indistinguishable from those of normal adult adipose tissue, which form lobulated masses in the subcutaneous tissues and elsewhere. They grow steadily to a large size, but show little or no tendency to become malignant. Occasionally an eccentric patient will cling to his large disfiguring lobulated mass, as though it were an eye or a limb and refuse excision.

Lipomata resemble large masses of shining yellow adipose tissue so closely that their neoplastic nature is often disputed.

MALIGNANT TUMOURS

Many of these come to include cells which have differentiated in a particular direction; for example, the presence of osteoid, of cartilaginous matrix or of much intracellular fat allows a neoplasm to be placed in the categories of osteogenic sarcoma, of chondrosarcoma or of liposarcoma respectively, in spite of the fact that most cells in the tumour cannot be distinguished from fibroblasts or even from primitive mesenchymal cells.

In some instances tumour cell differentiation is poor, or has advanced in several directions simultaneously. In these circumstances the dominant cell of the tumour resembles the young mesenchymal cell or exhibits features of, for example, bone-forming, cartilage-forming and also fat-forming cells. Under these conditions, when it is not possible to classify the tumour precisely, the term **mesenchymoma** is used.

Fibrosarcomata are comparatively slowly growing tumours composed of fibroblasts of relatively uniform character arranged in broadly interlacing bands or in angulated groups. They are most common between the ages of 20 and 50 years and occur with equal frequency in males and females. Collagen is formed, the amount varying inversely with the rate of growth of the tumour. Large, lobulated fibrosarcomata appear in regions such as the thigh or shoulder. There is direct infiltration of nearby tissues and the tumours tend to recur after local excision. Fibrosarcomata resist ionizing radiations and after a period of years an exacerbation of growth usually leads to metastasis in lung.

The cytological features of fibrosarcoma may charac-

terize the end stages of differentiated malignant tumours such as liposarcomata in which each local recurrence may lead to a reduction in differentiation.

Liposarcomata are most common in old men but may occasionally be found in young persons of either sex; they arise in situations such as the leg where there is relatively little normal fat. They do not seem to develop from previous lipomata or in sites where lipomata are common. By the time the tumour is diagnosed a large lobulated mass may have formed. Microscopically, stellate (mesenchymal) and spindle (fibroblastic) cells are frequent; mitotic figures are uncommon. Lipid droplets are found in abundance in many tumour cells and multinucleated giant cells may form. Local recurrence after excision is usual and the degree of differentiation diminishes with time so that eventually the tumour may be indistinguishable microscopically from a fibrosarcoma.

Myxosarcomata are rare. The component cells resemble those of the primitive mesenchyme; there is much metachromatic ground substance. Local recurrence and a fatal outcome are the rule.

TUMOURS OF SYNOVIAL ORIGIN

The word ganglion describes a common multiloculated swelling containing mucoid material, found on the dorsum of the wrist or hand, often causing local discomfort. The tumour, strictly not neoplastic, may be removed surgically for cosmetic reasons or for diagnostic purposes (bronchogenic carcinomata occasionally metastasize to the bones of the hand). Ganglion may recur and complete surgical excision is difficult. However, spontaneous disappearance is not uncommon. Microscopically, the lining of the cystic spaces resembles flattened synovial tissue, but it is rare indeed for any evidence of continuity with a joint or tendinous synovial space to remain by the time excision is performed.

Benign synoviomata or **giant cell tumours of tendon sheaths** occur on the small joints of the fingers and toes, and less commonly on other joints, as small, slowly growing, firm, painless nodules. The extensor and flexor surfaces of the index, middle and ring fingers are most commonly affected. The circumscribed nodules have a pale appearance but are flecked orange-yellow on section because of their content of lipid and of haemosiderin. The structure bears some resemblance to a xanthoma, but the main body of the giant cell tumour is composed of spindle-shaped fibroblasts and much collagen. Synovial clefts are seen, narrow spaces lined by synovial cells and free from blood. Numerous histiocytes containing fat and haemosiderin are present, together with many multinucleated giant cells, from which the name of the tumour is derived; their origin is not entirely clear but some may be formed by fusion of histiocytes. These giant cell tumours tend to recur locally following excision, but malignant change is never seen when the site is a small joint. When microscopically benign synoviomata occur in joints such as the knee, where synovial sarcomata are known to develop, there is some reason for regarding the benign and malignant conditions as different phases of the same process.

In larger synovial joints giant cell synovial tumours are rare. In sites such as the elbow and knee, however, there occurs a more diffuse lesion affecting all parts of the joint and having rather the characteristics of a fibrovascular inflammatory reaction. This diffuse, brown-pigmented lesion, in which localized zones may resemble the giant cell tumour of the finger joints, is called **pigmented villonodular synovitis**. The condition is slowly progressive but is not premalignant.

Synovial sarcomata are very uncommon. They arise most often in the knee joint and in its associated tendon sheaths and bursae, but other parts of the leg may be affected. The usual age of the young adults who develop this disease is 30 years; males suffer more commonly than females. No predisposing or causative factors are known. Microscopically, the tumours range from extremely poorly differentiated cellular structures to better differentiated fibroblastic masses within which are well-defined clefts lined by fleshy synovial cells. The two main cell types of the tumour, the stromal and the cleft cells, may perhaps correspond to the type A and type B cells of the normal synovia (table 30.1). Although very cellular, these tumours do not respond to ionizing radiation. They grow slowly but inexorably, and both local recurrence and distant metastasis are the eventual outcome. Premature exploratory operations predispose to spread.

FURTHER READING

COHEN A.S. (1965) The constitution and genesis of amyloid, in *International Review of Experimental Pathology*, vol. 4, p. 159. New York: Academic Press.

DUBOIS E.L. (ed.) (1966) *Lupus Erythematosus*. New York: McGraw-Hill.

FITTON JACKSON S. (1964) Connective tissue cells, in *The Cell*, vol. 4, p. 387, ed. Brachet J. & Mirsky A.E. New York: Academic Press.

FITTON JACKSON S., HARKNESS R.D., PARTRIDGE S.M. & TRISTRAM G.R. (1965) *Structure and Function of Connective and Skeletal Tissue*. London: Butterworths.

GARDNER D.L. (1965) *Pathology of the Connective Tissue Diseases*. London: Edward Arnold.

— (1969) *Textbook of the Rheumatic Diseases*, ed. Copeman, W.S.C. 4th Edition. Edinburgh: Livingstone.

GLYNN L.E. & HOLBOROW E.J. (1965) *Autoimmunity and Disease*. Oxford: Blackwell Scientific Publications.

KLEMPERER P., POLLACK A.D. & BAEHR G. (1942) Diffuse collagen disease; acute disseminated lupus erythematosus and diffuse scleroderma. *J. Amer. med. Ass.*, **119**, 331.

McKUSICK V.A. (1966) *Heritable Disorders of Connective Tissue*, 2nd Edition. Saint Louis: C.V. Mosby.

SCHUBERT M. & HAMERMAN D. (1968) *A Primer on Connective Tissue Biochemistry*. Philadelphia: Lea & Febiger.

STOUT A.P. & LATTES R. (1967) Tumours of the soft tissues, section 11, fasicle 5 of *Atlas of Tumour Pathology*, 2nd Series. Washington: Armed Forces Institute of Pathology.

Chapter 31
Genetic factors and disease

An account of the principles of human genetics and of normal human chromosomes is given in vol. 1, pp. 12.15 & 38.1. This chapter is concerned with the manner in which genetic factors and visible chromosomal aberrations may determine the presence of disease. Clinical descriptions of the important diseases, in which genetic factors are mainly responsible, will be given in vol. 3.

GENETIC AND ENVIRONMENTAL FACTORS IN DISEASE

Although genetics is one of the fundamental biological sciences, its wide relevance to medicine has been acknowledged only recently. In the past, medical genetics appeared to be concerned largely with forecasting the familial occurrence of rare diseases, all more or less beyond the scope of preventive medicine or effective treatment. The number of diseases known to be determined genetically has now increased greatly, and there is a growing acceptance of the idea that a disease of genetic aetiology is not necessarily unaffected by treatment, whether prophylactic, palliative or curative. Furthermore, no human disease is without genetic aspects, although these vary greatly in the contribution they make to the occurrence and natural history of particular diseases. The relevance of genetic factors to all diseases, and their variation in importance from one disease to another, may be seen by considering the following spectrum of conditions:

Genetic factors
Haemophilia
Phenylketonuria
Diabetes mellitus
Schizophrenia
Rheumatoid arthritis
Essential hypertension
Coronary artery disease
Carcinoma of breast
Peptic ulceration
Tuberculosis
Trauma
Environmental factors

That no disease is purely genetic or environmental in origin may be seen from consideration of the ends of this spectrum. Environmental factors play no known part in determining the occurrence of haemophilia, but the course of the disease depends, amongst other factors, on the frequency of injury and the availability of blood transfusion. Similarly, phenylketonuria is simply determined as an autosomal recessive, but its most damaging effect may be prevented by modification of the diet of the affected child. At the other end of the spectrum, the occurrence of trauma may be influenced by intelligence which appears to be partly inherited. Tuberculosis provides an example of the varying assessments in recent medical history of the relative roles of genetic and environmental factors. Before the discovery of the tubercle bacillus, the concept of an hereditary consumptive diathesis was commonly used to explain the high incidence of pulmonary tuberculosis in certain families. When the disease was better understood this was thought to be due solely to environmental factors such as close proximity to an infective case in a family, or to poverty and malnutrition which may diminish resistance. While the pre-eminence of environmental factors is unquestioned, twin studies have shown that in fact genetic predisposition to tuberculosis does exist. In the middle of the spectrum are a number of common diseases of unknown aetiology. The sickness and death occasioned by any one of them, e.g. diabetes mellitus, schizophrenia or hypertension, probably outweighs the combined effects of all the diseases, in which a genetic factor is the prime cause. None of these common diseases is simply inherited, yet genetic factors operate in each.

DIFFICULTIES IN THE STUDY OF HUMAN GENETICS

Human inheritance is of obvious interest to man, yet the study of human genetics has progressed much more slowly than that of many other species. The small size of human sibships and the long generation time are good reasons for this. In addition, the mobility of human populations and the long reproductive life of the human female may make impossible the study of a complete sibship, let alone several generations. In industrialized countries with rapidly growing and mobile populations, such as Australia or Canada, there are particular difficulties, especially in the study of genetic diseases manifest only in later life, e.g. Huntington's chorea.

Further difficulties arise when the dividing line between normality and disease is uncertain, as in essential hypertension and schizophrenia. In these and other conditions, lack of precise diagnostic criteria may result in several different pathological entities with different genetic mechanisms being mistaken for a single disease. The Hunter–Hurler syndrome is a rare disease in which there are corneal opacities and deafness as well as cardiac abnormalities and mental and physical retardation (p. 30.6). Two distinct modes of inheritance have now been detected, a sex-linked recessive form (Hunter's syndrome) in which corneal opacities do not occur, and an autosomal recessive form (Hurler's syndrome) in which deafness is relatively uncommon. Similar heterogeneity of the syndrome may well be responsible for the difficulty in studying the genetic factors in diabetes mellitus, hypertension and many other diseases.

FAMILY HISTORIES AND HUMAN PEDIGREES

A detailed family history is the basis of all enquiry into the genetic factors in disease. As this takes time and trouble, it should be considered as a special investigation. Cryptic notes such as 'No family history of hypertension or diabetes' which are often seen in hospital records are almost without value. If a family history is being compiled as a basis for genetic counselling, it is best to have both parents or prospective parents present. At least one hour should be set aside for the interview but much longer may be needed if sibships are large or if the memory or intelligence of those interviewed is defective. Each parent and each sibling should be considered separately noting the name, year of birth, year of death and the number and sex of children. The married and the maiden names of women should both be noted. The questions to be asked about the health of each person and the cause or circumstances of death vary with the disease suspected or recognized in the family. If it is planned to pursue the enquiry by seeking doctors' records, hospital notes or death certificates then the home address at the time of death or illness will be required. Abortions and neonatal deaths should be specifically sought in each sibship.

How far an enquiry of this kind is pursued depends on the information required and other individual circumstances. Few people know much about their forebears apart from their grandparents and their parents' sibships. Where information is less complete than is required the patient may be given a list of questions in writing and a second interview arranged after an opportunity has been given for consultation with older relatives. Neither interview should be hurried. Systematic questioning without undue haste often elicits information which the patient has forgotten and which would otherwise have

been lost. Tact is needed when the question of illegitimacy, adulterous cohabitation or incest arises.

Autosomal dominant inheritance

In simple autosomal dominant inheritance, a phenotypic effect is attributed to the presence of a single dominant allele (D) which is responsible for the inherited trait, in contrast to the recessive allele (d) which is not. If the allele responsible for the dominant trait is rare then an individual with the appropriate phenotype is usually heterozygous (Dd) at the genic locus in question. The homozygous condition (DD) for any rare allele occurs much less often, usually in the progeny of two heterozygotes. If the allele D determines the presence of a disease or other abnormality, we may talk of persons with the appropriate phenotype as being affected. Strict interpretation of the definition of dominance requires that, in general, the individual of genotype Dd should be of the same phenotype as regards the effects of the alleles Dd, as is the individual of genotype DD. If the allele D is rare, or if it has an adverse effect on the reproductive capacity of those who carry it, then the phenotypic effect of the genotype DD may never have been observed and the true dominance of the allele D may never have been proved. We return to this aspect of assumed dominant inheritance when discussing inheritance of intermediate type (p. 31.6).

Table 31.1 gives some diseases inherited as autosomal dominants. Some of the features of this type of inheritance are illustrated by a pedigree of a family with **spherocytic haemolytic anaemia** (fig. 31.1), also known as hereditary spherocytosis and in the past as acholuric jaundice. The erythrocytes are thicker than normal and so become

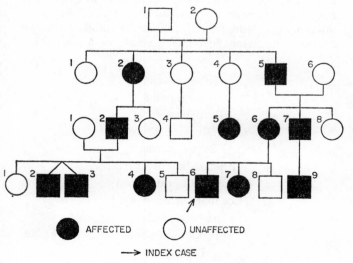

FIG. 31.1. Possible pedigree of hereditary spherocytosis, illustrating autosomal dominant inheritance.

TABLE 31.1. Some diseases usually inherited as autosomal dominant traits.

Disease	Chief features
Elliptocytosis	Erythrocytes appear oval; usually harmless but may lead to anaemia
Spherocytic haemolytic anaemia	Increased fragility of erythrocytes; may lead to haemolytic anaemia with splenomegaly and jaundice
Von Willebrand's disease	Haemorrhagic disease with a capillary defect and a low level of antihaemophilic globulin
Neurofibromatosis	Multiple tumours of peripheral nerves and patchy brown pigmentation of skin
Huntington's chorea	Progressive mental deterioration starting at age 30–40 years. Choreiform movements
Marfan's syndrome	Connective tissue disorder (p. 30.5)
Ehlers–Danlos syndrome	Connective tissue disorder (p. 30.7)
Osteogenesis imperfecta	Connective tissue disorder (p. 30.7)
Polycystic disease of the kidney	Cystic replacement of kidneys with slowly developing renal failure
Peutz–Jeghers syndrome	Gastrointestinal polyposis with mucocutaneous pigmentation
Polyposis of the colon	Polyposis of colon; a precancerous condition
Tylosis	Hyperkeratosis of the palms and soles, associated with liability to cancer of the oesophagus
Polydactyly	Extra digits on hands and feet
Hepatic intermittent porphyria	Swedish form; overproduction of porphyrins in the liver which may be precipitated by barbiturates
Haemorrhagic telangiectasia	Multiple telangiectases which rupture and may cause haemorrhage
Familial periodic paralysis	Attacks of flaccid paralysis associated with a low serum potassium

more nearly spherical. Their life span is reduced and an increased rate of destruction may lead to anaemia with jaundice and splenomegaly. Although the disease is sometimes obvious in childhood, it is commonly latent until adolescence or adult life. Family histories suggest a genetic cause for the disease and no environmental cause has been found although environmental factors, e.g. pregnancy or infection may aggravate the condition.

The pedigree shows that the disease is neither sex-linked nor sex-limited since males and females are often equally affected. In general, affected individuals have one affected parent who may be either the father or the mother. Consanguinity is no more common in such families than in the community from which they are drawn. If the family studied is large, it may be possible to show that in affected sibships the proportion of affected to unaffected individuals does not deviate significantly from the ratio of 1 : 1. These features serve to identify the unifactorial auto-

somal dominant inheritance and to distinguish it from both autosomal recessive inheritance or some kind of multifactorial inheritance. Obviously, the detection of the positive features of autosomal dominant inheritance requires that a sufficiently large family should be available for study, usually including more than one generation. It must depend too on the disease either being obvious or readily diagnosed.

The medical history is not a satisfactory criterion for the diagnosis of spherocytic haemolytic anaemia. Many affected individuals are not anaemic, and in others the evidence of haemolysis may be detected only with difficulty. In some circumstances it may be adequate to identify spherical erythrocytes in a peripheral blood film or to accept a history of splenectomy if more stringent criteria are satisfied in the case of other members of the same family. The specific abnormality underlying spherocytic haemolytic anaemia is unknown, but latent cases in affected families may be detected by demonstrating a reduction in erythrocyte life span even in the absence of anaemia, together with increased fragility of the erythrocytes when incubated *in vitro*.

It happens not infrequently that an individual, or even several siblings, known to be affected by a condition usually inherited as an autosomal dominant, has two apparently unaffected parents (fig. 31.1). There are several possible explanations for this observation. Firstly, one of the parents may indeed be affected, but this can be established only after detailed laboratory or clinical investigations. These might include measurements of erythrocyte fragility in spherocytosis, special assays of porphyrin or aminolaevulinic acid in urine or faeces in the hepatic porphyrias of both Swedish and South African types, and clinical and biochemical observations of the patient after exercise or the administration of insulin and glucose in familial periodic paralysis. If such tests are positive the patient has the disease in a partially expressed form. If the results of this type of investigation are negative, it must be concluded that the parents are of normal phenotype and unaffected by the disease. A second explanation is that the offspring may be illegitimate. This cannot be excluded but may be confirmed by the demonstration of a genetic factor not possessed by either the mother or the reputed father. The knowledge of the use of blood grouping for this purpose is so widespread that a woman with an uneasy conscience may refuse to allow the taking of a blood sample.

Two remaining explanations are that the disease may have arisen as a consequence of a fresh mutation, either gonadal in one of the parents, or somatic in the affected individual. It is usually impossible to confirm or refute the validity of either of these possibilities.

Full knowledge of the occurrence of diseases inherited as autosomal dominant traits may be impossible because the condition only becomes manifest after childhood, e.g. the skin and mucosal lesions in haemorrhagic telangiectasia and the benign tumours in neurofibromatosis. In Huntington's chorea the mean age of onset of the clinical features is 35·5 years with a standard deviation of 12·4 years, and there is no known way of detecting this condition before these appear. As a consequence, in an affected family, it is usually impossible to state which of the individual members will be affected. In the past, when the average expectation of life was not much more than the average age at onset of the disease, pedigrees must have been even more incomplete since many potential patients died of other causes before the disease developed.

PENETRANCE AND EXPRESSIVITY IN HUMAN DISEASE

These two terms, which describe different aspects of the phenomenon of variability of gene effect have already been described (vol. 1, p. 38.5). Penetrance denotes the frequency with which a gene or gene complex produces a discernible effect in the phenotype of those who carry it. If half those of the appropriate genotype show any effect, then the gene or gene complex is said to show 50 per cent penetrance. In human genetics many statements about penetrance must be regarded as provisional since more sensitive methods of examination may show a particular gene to be penetrant in an individual in whom it was once regarded as nonpenetrant. In hepatic porphyria of Swedish type, new methods of measuring aminolaevulinic acid and porphobilinogen enable subclinical cases to be detected. Such cases are said to show a low degree of expressivity by comparison with their relatives who have obvious clinical manifestations and readily detectable porphobilinogenuria. Expressivity then relates to the degree of effect of the gene in producing clinical disease in a particular individual. A nonpenetrant gene has no expressivity, but a penetrant gene may show great variation in expressivity. For example, in families with a gene for polydactyly, some members may have well developed additional digits on all four extremities, some may have both normal and abnormal extremities and in others an extra digit may be so small as to be barely recognizable.

Variations in gene effect probably depend on interaction between the gene or gene-complex in question and either other genes or the environment. In some instances it may depend simply on the presence or absence of interacting genes; in others it may depend on a complex balance of many factors, genetic and environmental. Consequently, although it is often convenient to talk of the penetrance and expressivity of a particular gene, both are best regarded, not as attributes of a particular gene, but of the whole genotype and the environment. In human disease differences in gene effects should suggest a need to identify the factors in the genotype and the environment which determine the differences.

Autosomal dominant and intermediate traits show great differences in penetrance and expressivity, as do sex-linked genes in heterozygous females such as those for colour blindness and haemophilia. In contrast, sex-linked genes in males and autosomal recessive traits are usually much more constant in their effects.

CODOMINANCE

The genetics of the human ABO blood group system illustrate an important variant of simple dominant and recessive inheritance. The position is set out in table 31.2.

TABLE 31.2. The ABO blood groups.

Genes	Genotypes	Phenotypes	Antigens in erythrocytes	Antibodies in serum
A	AA AO	A	A	anti-B
B	BB BO	B	B	anti-A
O	AB OO	AB O	A+B none	neither anti-A and anti-B

Both A and B are dominant with reference to O and the heterozygotes AO and BO can be distinguished from the homozygotes AA and BB only by family studies. The heterozygote AB shows neither dominance nor recessivity and both antigens are present. The two alleles are then said to be codominant.

In fact, this is an oversimplified account of the genetics of the ABO blood groups. Most human erythrocytes also contain the antigen H and the amount present in any individual is related to the ABO group. Cells of group O contain most and cells of group AB the least. H substance is believed to be the basic material from which A and B antigens are made under the influence of the appropriate gene. Since H substance is present in the cells of persons of genotype AB, it cannot be regarded as the product of the O gene. An anti-H antibody may occur in some people of genotypes A, B and AB but it is of little importance in human disease or blood transfusion. Another complication which does have practical importance is the occurrence of subgroups of A (vol. 1, p. 26.18). Although for most purposes A_2 can be regarded as a weaker form of A_1, it shows the same codominance with B as does A_1, so that individuals of genotype A_2B have both A_2 and B antigens in their erythrocytes.

Obvious codominant inheritance is uncommon and has not been detected in the case of alleles determining structural features. Its rarity is probably more apparent than real. When gene action is better understood it may be that many instances of intermediate inheritance (p. 31.6) will be seen as examples of codominance. Thus the inheritance of the sickle cell trait has often been cited as an example of intermediate inheritance. The heterozygote (Hb^S/Hb^A) shows an abnormality in the shape of erythrocytes which is harmless. The homozygote (Hb^S/Hb^S) has a similar abnormality of the erythrocytes associated with a severe haemolytic anaemia, coming on in early childhood. Viewed in this way the gene for haemoglobin S can be regarded as an intermediate gene. When the gene products in the various genotypes are considered it is seen to be an example of codominance. The homozygotes, Hb^A/Hb^A and Hb^S/Hb^S, have haemoglobin A and S respectively in their erythrocytes. The heterozygotes have both.

Other instances of intermediate inheritance, as well as situations sometimes described as examples of incomplete dominance or incomplete recessivity, may be recognized as examples of codominance when the gene products are as easily and specifically determined as are the ABO blood groups and haemoglobins A and S.

Autosomal recessive inheritance

TABLE 31.3. Some diseases usually inherited as autosomal recessives.

Disease	Chief morphological features
Albinism	⎫ See table 31.7; most of the inborn
Phenylketonuria	⎬ errors of metabolism are inherited
Galactosaemia	⎭ as autosomal recessive traits
Hurler's syndrome	Connective tissue disorder (p. 30.5)
Ellis–van Creveld syndrome	Connective tissue disorder. Dwarfism, polydactyly, atrial septal defect
Wilson's disease	A disturbance of copper metabolism affecting the liver, brain, kidneys and cornea (p. 25.38)
Laurence–Moon syndrome	Biochemical defect unknown. Mental retardation, hypogonadism, adiposity, retinitis pigmentosa
Mucoviscidosis	Fibrocystic disease of the pancreas. Viscid secretions of mucous glands throughout body
Amaurotic familial idiocy (Tay–Sachs disease)	Accumulation of ganglioside in brain leading to progressive mental deterioration, with blindness and deafness (p. 25.37)
Spinocerebellar ataxia	Degeneration of the cerebellum

Table 31.3 gives some diseases usually inherited as autosomal recessives. Traits inherited in this way are not obvious in the heterozygote but manifest in the homozygote who generally is the child of heterozygous parents. Except in the rare event of a mating of two homozygotes, affected individuals have unaffected parents and may have affected sibs but themselves have normal children. These and other features of autosomal recessive inheritance are shown in fig. 31.2, a pedigree of a family

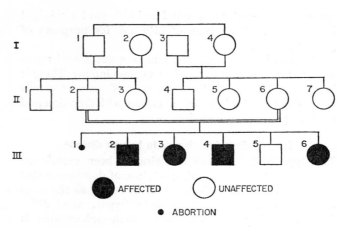

FIG. 31.2. Possible pedigree of phenylketonuria, illustrating autosomal recessive inheritance.

with phenylketonuria. The enzymic defect has already been described (vol. 1, p. 11.24). Although rare, it is now well known because surveys are carried out in many countries to detect affected individuals at or soon after birth. The development of the mental defect may be prevented or made less serious if a diet low in phenylalanine is begun within the first few weeks of life. At later ages this treatment becomes progressively less effective and is worthless after the age of 6 years.

The pedigree (fig. 31.2) shows affected males and females. As with all rare conditions inherited as recessives, there is a strong possibility of consanguinity in affected families, e.g. the first-cousin marriage (II 2 and II 6). Such a marriage may bring together two recessive alleles carried in a single dose by a grandparent. The rarer the gene in question the more likely is consanguinity. Not all instances of an abnormal child having normal parents are to be explained by recessive inheritance. It may be due to a new dominant gonadal mutation in one parent, to a fresh combination of alleles at two or more loci or to the operation of environmental factors other than by the production of a fresh mutation.

The gene for phenylketonuria is certainly recessive as far as the causation of obvious disease is concerned. It is incompletely recessive in its effects on the metabolism of phenylalanine. A phenylalanine tolerance test can detect heterozygotes since on average twice the plasma phenylalanine level of normal controls is reached when they are given the same dose of phenylalanine by mouth. Heterozygotes do not excrete phenylpyruvic acid in the urine and so cannot be detected by the method commonly used for homozygotes. Their plasma phenylalanine levels are usually only a little higher than normal whereas homozygotes have values up to 20 times above normal. In many other inherited diseases now regarded as of recessive nature, future studies may show recessivity to be more apparent than real. The opportunity to detect the heterozygous carrier is unusual and hitherto for this and other reasons it has been of little use for purposes of genetic counselling.

Mucoviscidosis is the most common autosomal recessive trait in man and occurs in 1 in 2000 infants. There is increased viscosity of the secretions of mucous glands throughout the body which interferes with digestion and leads to pulmonary infection.

Intermediate inheritance in human disease

This type of inheritance has already been mentioned with regard to the strict interpretation of dominance and in consideration of codominance. In so far as the term intermediate implies that the heterozygote must differ from both homozygotes, intermediate inheritance is probably common in man. Since the term does not imply that the effect in the heterozygote is halfway between the effects in the homozygotes, it may be applied to any condition, usually regarded as inherited as a recessive, in which the heterozygote is detectable. In this sense the genes for phenylketonuria, galactosaemia and haemophilia may be regarded as showing intermediate rather than recessive effects in at least some heterozygotes. As methods of study become more sensitive the number of such recessive conditions and the proportion of heterozygotes showing intermediate effects may be expected to increase. The same trend in refinement of study and detection of gene effects may be expected to show that codominance rather than intermediate inheritance is a more apt description of many of these gene effects. Thus the heterozygote HB^S/Hb^A shows a recessive effect of the gene HB^S as regards the production of haemolytic anaemia, an intermediate effect as regards erythrocyte morphology and codominance when the actual gene products are the criteria of gene action.

There are at present no such complexities in considering β-thalassaemia as an example of intermediate inherit-

ance. While the basic defect is not fully understood it seems to be an inability to synthesize sufficient haemoglobin A. This results in the production of hypochromic erythrocytes showing poikilocytosis and the target cell abnormality. Since these abnormal cells have a reduced life span and the ability of the bone marrow to produce them is restricted, haemolytic anaemia results. A defect may arise in the synthesis of either the α or β chains of haemoglobin A ($\alpha_2\beta_2$), giving rise to α- or β-thalassaemia. By way of physiological compensation other haemoglobins, the synthesis of which is unaffected by the genetic defect, may be present. In both conditions a major form is recognized in homozygotes and a minor form in heterozygotes.

The relationship of the genotype to the resulting disease in both α- and β-thalassaemia is shown in table 31.4.

The transmission of an intermediate gene, as exemplified by that for β-thalassaemia, is relatively simple. Persons of all three possible types, the heterozygote and both the homozygotes can be distinguished without complex investigation. Mating of a heterozygote with a normal person results on average in equal numbers of heterozygous and normal offspring. The mating of heterozygotes results, on average, in homozygotes with β-thalassaemia major, heterozygotes with β-thalassaemia minor and normal homozygotes in the proportions 1 : 2 : 1.

Both the inheritance and the haematological findings are greatly complicated where a gene for thalassaemia, α or β, coexists with a gene for one of the β chain variants of haemoglobin A, such as haemoglobins S, C, D or E. Such situations are common in the world population and are major causes of morbidity, mortality and foetal death.

INTERMEDIATE INHERITANCE REVEALED BY A RARE HOMOZYGOTE

Other examples of intermediate inheritance, of great significance if rare occurrence, are provided by some un-

TABLE 31.4. Genotypes, resulting disease and effects on haemoglobin synthesis in the thalassaemias.

Genotype	Disease	Impaired synthesis	Other haemo-globins present
β-Thalassaemia			
Homozygote	β-thalassaemia major Severe disease Most die in childhood	Hb A ($\alpha_2\beta_2$)	Hb F ($\alpha_2\gamma_2$) Hb A$_2$ ($\alpha_2\delta_2$)
Heterozygote	β-thalassaemia minor Mild or compensated haemolytic anaemia Variable in severity Heterozygous advantage is postulated (see vol. 1, p. 38.10)	Hb A ($\alpha_2\beta_2$)	Hb F ($\alpha_2\gamma_2$) —some cases Hb A$_2$ ($\alpha_2\delta_2$) —most cases
α-Thalassaemia			
Homozygote	α-thalassaemia major Incompatible with extra-uterine life Stillbirth	Hb A ($\alpha_2\beta_2$) Hb F ($\alpha_2\gamma_2$)	Hb Bart's (γ_4) Hb H (β_4)
Heterozygote	α-thalassaemia minor No significant disease	No obvious impairment	Hb Bart's (γ_4) —in newborn only

common diseases ordinarily regarded as due to genes of dominant effect. Because of their rarity they are usually seen only in the heterozygote. When the exceedingly rare homozygote does occur, as a result of the mating of two heterozygotes, the homozygote may be found to be much more severely affected, at variance with the accepted definition of dominance. Haemorrhagic telangiectasia is regarded as being inherited as an autosomal dominant. Small vascular lesions appear on the skin and mucous membranes and give rise to haemorrhage. It is rarely manifest in childhood and even in old age the lesions are still small. The only known child of two heterozygotes was presumably homozygous (fig. 31.3). The child had

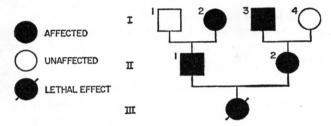

FIG. 31.3. Pedigree of haemorrhagic telangiectasia with **a** rare homozygote, the child of affected parents, who was especially severely affected. After Snyder L.H. & Doan C.A. (1944) *J. Lab. clin. Med.* **22**, 1211.

one large telangiectatic lesion at birth and others appeared within a few days. Haemorrhages began in the first month and the child died before the end of the third month of life. At autopsy there were large telangiectases of skin and mucous membranes as well as multiple haemangioendotheliomata in internal organs. This single case provides good grounds for regarding the gene for haemorrhagic telangiectasia as being, in fact, intermediate in effect rather than dominant. Analogous situations have been recorded in other apparently dominant conditions.

Intermediate inheritance is probably more common than is realized because true frequency is at present obscured by the rarity of the homozygous state for some genes of dominant effect and by the imperfections of methods for the detection of heterozygotes for some genes of recessive effect. Conversely, complete dominance and recessivity may be less common in relation to human disease than has been accepted in the past.

Sex-linked inheritance

The X chromosome carries other genes, besides those concerned in sex differentiation and function. Most mutant forms of these genes giving rise to disease are recessive. Consequently, the diseases are not manifest in heterozygous females with the normal allele on a second X chromosome, but only in males who may be

described as hemizygous for the allele on their single X chromosome. Some diseases inherited as X-linked recessives are listed in table 31.5.

TABLE 31.5. Some diseases usually inherited as X-linked recessives.

Disease	Chief features
Childhood progressive muscular dystrophy (Duchenne type)	Progressive degeneration of skeletal muscles with weakness
Haemophilia (Haemophilia A)	Deficiency of antihaemophilic globulin leading to bleeding disorder
Christmas disease (Haemophilia B)	Deficiency of Christmas factor leading to bleeding disorder
Familial agammaglobulinaemia	See p. 23.12
Aldrich's syndrome	Sometimes low IgM, thrombocytopenia, diarrhoea and proneness to infection (p. 31.11)
Glucose-6-phosphate dehydrogenase deficiency	Increased liability to induced haemolysis (p. 31.10)
Nephrogenic diabetes insipidus	Lack of responsiveness of renal tubules to ADH
Colour blindness	Inability to distinguish between shades of red and green. (vol. 1, p. 24.60)
Hunter's syndrome	Connective tissue disorder (p. 30.5)

The characteristics of sex-linked recessive inheritance are seen in the pedigree of a family in which childhood progressive muscular dystrophy (Duchenne type) occurred (fig. 31.4). Only males are affected. Affected individuals may have affected male siblings but have normal parents. The mothers of affected individuals commonly have affected brothers and maternal uncles. In affected sibships half the males manifest the disease and half the females are heterozygous carriers. A heterozygous female married to a normal male transmits the mutant gene to half her sons who manifest the disease and to half her daughters who, like herself, are heterozygous carriers but appear normal. In the pedigree none of the affected males had offspring, as is usual because of the severity of this disease and the early age of onset. In sex-linked recessive conditions in which affected males reproduce, all their daughters are heterozygous carriers and all their sons normal. This follows because all sons receive their father's Y chromosome and all daughters receive their father's only X chromosome.

As the biochemical defect in progressive muscular dystrophy is not known, attempts to detect heterozygous carriers have met with little success. Abnormal aldolase and creatine kinase levels in serum are poor guides, but electromyography may be more reliable.

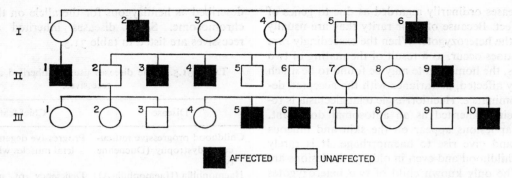

FIG. 31.4. Possible pedigree of childhood progressive muscular dystrophy, illustrating sex-linked recessive inheritance.

There is a group of diseases (table 31.6) each of which shows more than one form of Mendelian inheritance although the patients may be clinically indistinguishable. In a minority of families with progressive muscular dystrophy the mode of inheritance is as an autosomal recessive. It is in such families that most of the reported female cases of the disease have occurred. Understandably, they gave rise to much confusion before it became clear that autosomal inheritance might operate in some families. Such confusion was heightened when female cases occurred sporadically and the pattern of inheritance in the particular family could not be established.

Not all female cases of progressive muscular dystrophy can be accounted for in this way. At least one female child with this disease had the abnormal sex chromosome constitution XO, and so, like an affected male, could be described as hemizygous for the abnormal gene. An analogous finding has been described in an apparent female with haemophilia found to have the sex chromosome constitution XY and other findings justifying a diagnosis of testicular feminization. Obviously, when a female manifests a condition which is usually sex-linked, the possibility of an abnormal sex chromosome constitution must be considered. Apart from this possibility, females with X-linked recessive conditions may in fact be homozygous for the mutant gene, usually being the offspring of

TABLE 31.6. Clinically indistinguishable conditions showing two forms of Mendelian inheritance.

Gaucher's disease	Autosomal dominant and recessive
Achondroplasia	Autosomal dominant and recessive
Childhood progressive muscular dystrophy (Duchenne type)	Sex-linked and autosomal recessive
Limb-girdle muscular dystrophy	Autosomal recessive and autosomal dominant
Retinitis pigmentosa	Sex-linked and autosomal recessive

an affected male and a heterozygous female. This is known to have occurred in haemophilia, colour blindness, glucose-6-phosphate dehydrogenase deficiency and sex-linked ichthyosis, but not in progressive muscular dystrophy.

Sex-limited inheritance

Autosomal inheritance is said to be sex-limited if the same genotype is differently expressed in the two sexes. Sex limitation is said to be complete if the gene in question is expressed in one sex only. Where the gene effect is greater in one sex, the gene is said to show partial sex limitation or sex influence; and the same term may be applied to describe more frequent expression in one sex than in the other.

Complete sex-limitation is rare in man, but would explain pedigrees of testicular feminization. This rare condition is transmitted by females but expressed only in genotypic males, giving rise to one form of pseudo-hermaphroditism. Affected individuals are phenotypic females in whom most female secondary sex characteristics develop despite their having testes instead of ovaries and the male sex chromosome constitution XY. Baldness is a second example of complete sex limitation although the mechanism of inheritance is not clear, probably because of the variability of expression in affected males. The gene in question is apparently dominant in males and recessive in females. Since the gene is extremely common, the occurrence of bald females may be explained by their being homozygous for the postulated gene.

Partial sex limitation is much more common, being found usually in diseases the inheritance of which cannot be simply explained. Thus gout, cleft lip (both with and without cleft palate), and megacolon (Hirschsprung's disease) are all more frequent in males. Some congenital abnormalities having a complex genetic component such as anencephaly, spina bifida and congenital dislocation of the hip are more frequently expressed in females.

Sex-limitation with expression only in males may, in a single sibship, be confused with sex-linked inheritance.

The distinction is easily made if two generations are studied since in sex-limited inheritance the affected male transmits the gene to his sons.

Inborn errors of metabolism

This term was first used in 1908 by Garrod, a London physician who later succeeded Osler as Regius Professor of Medicine at Oxford. Garrod had studied four rare disorders, and his relatively simple clinical, family and chemical observations led him to propose a new concept in human pathology. He suggested that in alkaptonuria, albinism, cystinuria and pentosuria there was a block in a metabolic process due to an inherited deficiency of a specific enzyme. Table 31.7 shows that since Garrod's day the number of known inborn errors has multiplied; the basic principles he enunciated may operate in many diseases in which the error of metabolism is incompletely

TABLE 31.7. Some inborn errors of metabolism.

Clinical condition	Enzyme abnormality
Alkaptonuria	Homogentisic acid oxidase (vol. I, p. 11.25)
Cystinuria	Unknown (vol. I, p. 33.10, 11.22)
Pentosuria	Unknown
Galactosaemia	Galactose-1-phosphate uridyl transferase (vol. I, p. 9.11)
Phenylketonuria	Phenylalanine hydroxylase (vol. I, p. 11.25)
Argininosuccinaciduria	Argininosuccinase
Acatalasaemia	Catalase (p. 31.11)
Adrenogenital syndrome	Several types, each involving different adrenocortical hydroxylases (vol. I, p. 25.32)
Hypophosphatasia	Alkaline phosphatase
Goitrous cretinism (one type)	Dehalogenase (vol. I, p. 25.21)
Congenital hyperbilirubin-aemia	Glucuronyl transferase (vol. I, p. 31.10)
Glycogen storage disease	Several types, each involving a different enzyme (vol. I, p. 9.10)
Methaemoglobinaemia (one type)	Methaemoglobin reductase (vol. I, p. 26.6)
Favism and congenital nonspherocytic haemolytic anaemia (one type)	Glucose-6-phosphate dehydrogenase (vol. I, p. 26.8 also vol. 2, p. 31.10)
Congenital nonspherocytic haemolytic anaemia (one type)	Pyruvate kinase
Porphyria: congenital erythropoietic form	?Porphobilinogen deaminase and uroporphyrin isomerases
Swedish variety of hepatic type	Enhanced activity of δ-aminolaevulinic acid synthetase (vol. I, p. 26.6)
Hartnup disease	Unknown
Albinism	Tyrosinase
Homocystinuria	Cystathionine synthetase (vol. I, p. 11.22)

understood or the affected enzyme unknown. Some congenital structural abnormalities may be due to inborn errors of metabolism, the significant disorder occurring only at a particular stage in intrauterine development. More recently, the principle of the inborn errors of metabolism has been seen to operate in some untoward reactions to drugs, giving rise to the term pharmacogenetics (see below).

Most of the inborn errors of metabolism are inherited as autosomal recessive traits, but there is a growing list of those in which heterozygotes may be detected. In them the pathological effects of the gene are absent but the metabolic abnormality can still be demonstrated, though to a lesser degree than in homozygotes. Thus in galactosaemia heterozygotes can be detected by showing diminished galactose-1-phosphate uridyl transferase activity in erythrocytes (table 31.8). This partial deficiency is not associated with any pathological consequence, but its detection is of great value in the study of the disorder.

TABLE 31.8. Galactose-1-phosphate uridyl transferase activity in the erythrocytes of normal homozygotes and individuals heterozygous for the gene determining galactosaemia. From Donnell G.N. *et al.* (1960) *Pediatrics*, **25**, 572.

Enzyme activity in erythrocytes (μM uridyl diphosphate glucose utilized/ml erythrocytes/hour)					
Normal Homozygotes			Heterozygotes		
No.	Mean	S.D.	No.	Mean	S.D.
106	5·9	1·01	25	2·9	0·83

No inborn error of metabolism can yet be treated by substitution for the defective enzyme. When successful therapy is practicable it may depend on sparing the defective metabolic process by manipulation of the diet, as in galactosaemia and phenylketonuria. In favism and acute porphyria the consequences of the defect are minimized by avoiding environmental factors which may precipitate pathological effects (p. 31.10). Cortisone therapy in the adrenogenital syndrome substitutes for the failure to produce cortisol, and by a physiological feedback reduces the endogenous activity leading to the production of abnormal quantities of adrenocortical androgens. Worthwhile therapy is possible in only a few of the disorders but the successes foster the hope that in other inherited disorders the pathological consequences may no longer be inevitable.

Pharmacogenetics

Pharmacogenetics is the study of genetically determined variations in the response to drugs. Prior to 1957 it was commonly believed that the wide variation in the response to drugs was in all instances a continuous variation represented by a unimodal curve approaching a normal

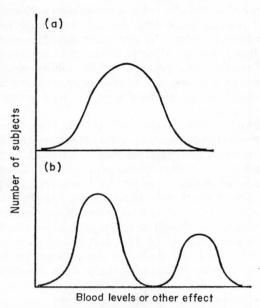

FIG. 31.5. Patterns of response to drugs, (a) continuous and (b) discontinuous variation.

distribution. More recently it has become clear that in some instances the distribution of responses is bimodal (fig. 31.5) or even trimodal and the possibility has been raised that each type of response might represent a genetically determined phenotype, the population being polymorphic (p. 31.13). In terms of clinical response such a discontinuous variation is often revealed as an unusual, adverse or toxic reaction to a drug.

SUXAMETHONIUM (SUCCINYLCHOLINE) SENSITIVITY

Most pharmacogenetic discoveries have resulted from the unexpected occurrence of adverse effects. Suxamethonium sensitivity is an example. The drug is used in anaesthesia as a short-acting muscle relaxant (p. 5.69), but in some patients it gives rise to a prolonged period of paralysis and arrest of ventilation. Normally the drug is hydrolysed rapidly by the serum pseudocholinesterase. Sensitive individuals have abnormally low levels of activity of this enzyme and a similar deficiency is also present in many of their close relatives. Later it was discovered that the enzyme in affected individuals had certain unusual characteristics and the delayed inactivation of the drug was not due simply to low levels of normal enzyme. The local anaesthetic dibucaine inhibits the activity of the normal enzyme but not of the abnormal one and this difference provides the basis of a method of investigation of suxamethonium sensitivity. In normal subjects dibucaine produces about 79 per cent inhibition but only 16 per cent inhibition in suxamethonium-sensitive individuals who account for 1 in 1000 to 1 in 5000 of the general

population. A third group of individuals in whom dibucaine produces inhibition of the order of 62 per cent is found among the relatives of those showing suxamethonium sensitivity. The simplest explanation of these findings is that sensitive individuals are abnormally homozygous, the majority of the population normally homozygous, and the intermediate group heterozygous. In fact the situation appears to be more complex and more than two alleles may occur.

Thus suxamethonium sensitivity has so much in common with the inborn errors of metabolism that it may be considered to be one. The inherited abnormality appears to have had no deleterious effect until suxamethonium had been synthesized and used in clinical anaesthetic practice. The same cannot be said of all inborn errors of metabolism with pharmacogenetic aspects.

UNWANTED EFFECTS OF OTHER DRUGS

The Swedish type of hepatic porphyria, acute intermittent porphyria, possibly due to increased activity of δ-aminolaevulinic synthetase (table 31.7), may appear clinically only after administration of certain drugs, particularly barbiturates. The features include abdominal and muscle pains, paralysis, mental disorders, vomiting and electrolyte disturbances. The means by which drugs aggravate this genetically determined disorder are unknown. Deficiency of glucose-6-phosphate dehydrogenase (G6PD), which is a key enzyme in the hexose monophosphate pathway (vol. 1, p. 9.8), results in severe haemolytic anaemia after ingestion of the bean *Vicia fava* (vol. 1, p. 26.8). In the same individuals the antimalarial drug primaquine, phenacetin, aspirin, sulphonamides, nitrofurantoin, probenecid and other drugs may all provoke haemolytic anaemia. A number of different forms of G6PD deficiency exist and some are unassociated with any clinical abnormality. In Mediterranean people the enzyme may possess several functional peculiarities, e.g. low Michaelis constant, and be present in greatly reduced amounts. Detection of G6PD activity is carried out in field studies by measuring the decolorization time of a solution of brilliant cresyl blue or by estimation of the ability to reduce methaemoglobin in the presence of methylene blue. Results have shown that deficient individuals constitute a small group of the population. Activity of G6PD is reduced by primaquine in those carrying the defect. Thus if sensitive and non-sensitive red blood cells are incubated with primaquine in glucose, the concentration of reduced glutathione (GSH) falls only in the abnormal cells. The fall in GSH content of sensitive cells is believed to reflect inability to metabolize glucose and is related to the increased fragility and ensuing haemolysis. Reduced G6PD is not the only cause of drug induced haemolysis. An abnormal haemoglobin has been found in a European family who developed haemolysis after treatment with sulphonamides, and its presence may represent a possible explanation for unusual haemolytic responses in patients of North European origin.

Not all pharmacogenetic studies are prompted by the occurrence of adverse effects. Nevertheless this is the usual reason and the occurrence of a few individuals possessing abnormalities in their metabolic handling of a drug is liable to lead to untoward effects, as doses of drugs are usually decided on the basis of the therapeutic response and the occurrence of minimal toxic effects in the majority. The possibility of genetic factors determining plasma salicylate levels after administration of aspirin has not been confirmed. In contrast, genetic factors have been shown to determine important differences in the metabolism of the antituberculosis agent isoniazid. Studies of plasma levels of the drug after intravenous administration of a standard dose revealed that some people achieve high, and others low, plasma levels and that the distribution of plasma levels is bimodal. The drug is excreted in the urine only after acetylation and those who have unduly high plasma levels are believed to have defective powers of acetylation. Studies of purified acetyl transferase from livers of rapid and slow acetylators have not shown significant differences in their Michaelis constant and other characteristics and the difference between the phenotypes therefore appears to be due to differences in the amount of enzyme present rather than due to qualitative differences in the enzyme. It is not known if these findings are relevant to the efficiency of treatment of tuberculosis since isoniazid is rarely used alone for this purpose. On the other hand, slow acetylators are known to be four times more likely to develop isoniazid neuropathy. Family studies indicate that slow inactivation of isoniazid is inherited as an autosomal recessive character.

Polymorphism is also believed to exist in the acetylation of hydrallazine, occasionally used in the treatment of hypertension, sulphadimidine and possibly other sulphonamides, and phenelzine used in the treatment of depression. Adverse effects of hydrallazine (p. 8.10) and phenelzine occur mainly in slow acetylators.

Genetically determined enzyme deficiencies or abnormalities have also been discovered affecting catalase, alcohol dehydrogenase and the mechanism of hydroxylating phenytoin (p. 5.59) used in the treatment of epilepsy. Acatalasia was discovered in Japan when hydrogen peroxide was used in the treatment of oral infection. If hydrogen peroxide was applied to the affected tissues a brownish colour appeared instead of bubbles of oxygen as would be expected. This was subsequently traced to absence of catalase in the tissues, particularly but not exclusively affecting Asians. Adverse effects of phenytoin therapy following a small dose, i.e. nystagmus and ataxia, have been shown to occur in a single family in whom there is a relative inability to hydroxylate the drug.

Purified enzyme studies from human livers have shown two forms of alcohol dehydrogenase which possess different pH optima, activities and other characteristics. Difficulty in obtaining alcohol dehydrogenase from living subjects makes family studies virtually impossible and so far there is no evidence to suggest that individuals with the higher enzyme activity are able to oxidize alcohol more quickly.

The potential value of genetically determined drug reactions in understanding the origin of disease is illustrated by the discovery that a marked rise of intraocular pressure occasionally follows the use of corticosteroid eye drops. In a population of healthy volunteers the rise in intraocular pressure following instillation of corticosteroid into the conjunctival sac was found to have a bimodal distribution. The offspring of patients suffering from glaucoma which is a major cause of blindness in temperate countries were then studied and almost all of them showed an abnormal rise in intraocular pressure. Pedigree studies suggest that intraocular pressure is controlled by a pair of allelic genes which determine low and high intraocular pressures and that different combinations of these genotypes can determine the pressure response (p. 35.8).

Individual families have also been discovered who are resistant to anticoagulant drugs and, although there is no information on the incidence of this response, it is believed to be inherited either as an autosomal dominant or as an X-linked dominant.

The discovery of discontinuous patterns of response to drugs indicates the existence of polymorphic genetic systems and permits the use of drugs to uncover unsuspected genetic differences. It seems likely that more such differences will be demonstrated as new drugs are discovered and used clinically.

Immunogenetics

Genetic and other methods have established the occurrence of a number of syndromes in which there is an inherited deficiency in the immunological response. These are comparatively rare but it is likely that others are so far unrecognized. As described on p. 23.11 they are due to deficiencies in humoral and cellular responses and their inheritance is given in table 23.1.

In other immunogenetic disorders in which liability to infection is the prominent clinical feature the mechanism is more difficult to define. These include Aldrich's syndrome in which recurrent infections, diarrhoea and thrombocytopenia are prominent and in which low IgM is only sometimes present. Inherited abnormalities of leucocytes which have reduced bactericidal activity has also been discovered but these individuals show no evidence of depression of antibody production.

The possibility that hypersensitivity reactions to drugs are also determined genetically must also be kept in mind

(p. 23.10). Experimental work in rats shows differences in their immunological response to large molecular weight dextrans and egg white given intraperitoneally. Hyperreactivity has been shown to be an autosomal dominant characteristic. The reactive rats have a tenfold rise in blood histamine concentration while nonreactive rats showed no rise. It is possible that human subjects who develop a hypersensitive reaction to dextran or other drugs without previous exposure may represent a rare human phenotype. The role of genetics in the development of autoimmune disease is discussed on p. 23.9.

Genetic linkage and association

Gene loci situated on the same chromosome are said to be linked loci. In the fruit fly *Drosophila* the linkage groups have been mapped out in detail on the chromosomes. In the mouse there are a number of clearly defined linkage groups not yet related to specific chromosomes (vol. 1, p. 38.5). In man only one major linkage group, the genes located on the X chromosome, has so far been demonstrated (p. 31.20). However, it has been possible to establish five pairs of autosomal linkages in man:

(1) Lutheran blood groups and ABO secretor status, i.e. the antigens of the ABO blood groups found in saliva,

(2) the Rh blood groups and elliptocytosis,

(3) ABO blood groups and the nail–patella syndrome, a rare disorder with deformed nails and absent patellae,

(4) Duffy blood group and congenital zonular cataract, and

(5) transferrin and serum cholinesterase.

Linkage studies are concerned with the topographical situation of gene loci on the chromosomes; they have no direct relevance to the causation of disease although the characters studied include some diseases. The most useful characters used in linkage studies are the **genetic markers**. Marker genes are chosen for the high frequency of their alleles in the population under study, simple inheritance and the ease with which the effects of the alleles can be detected.

Genetic association is said to occur when two different phenotypic features are found in the same individual, more often than can be accounted for by chance. Some associations are of course largely independent of genetic influences, e.g. the association of malnutrition and liability to tuberculosis or between smoking and bronchial carcinoma. Genetic association arises when there are two or more distinct effects of an allele, e.g. the arachnodactyly, aortic regurgitation and dislocation of the optic lens, all occurring in Marfan's syndrome (p. 30.5). Association may be seen in a population which is stratified with much nonrandom mating. Thus in both Australia and the United States there is an evident association between glucose-6-phosphate dehydrogenase deficiency and thalassaemia, diseases which are determined by genes at loci on different chromosomes. Both the alleles determining

these diseases are more common in people of Mediterranean origin than in people of Northern European stock. The frequent association of the two characters in the same individual is attributable to incomplete social assimilation of people of Mediterranean origin.

At first glance it may seem that significant association of two characters in the same individuals in a population is evidence of true linkage. In fact, it is quite the reverse. In particular families, closely linked characters may occur in the same individuals for several generations, but the process of crossing over ensures that even the characters determined at closely linked loci show no such association in the general population, if random mating is the rule. Several associations have now been clearly established between genetic markers and diseases, but the way in which the genetically determined character makes for increased liability to the disease is still not clear. Most of the significant associations have been demonstrated by several studies in various populations. Some which are still inconclusive may yet be confirmed with greater or lesser degrees of certainty by further studies, especially if the data collected in different populations are homogeneous and so may be pooled.

BLOOD GROUPS AND DISEASE
Most of the investigations of these associations have been negative. Table 31.9 gives the positive results which are established firmly, others which seem likely, and some which available data suggest may be positive but which require further study.

TABLE 31.9. ABO blood groups, secretor status and associations with disease.

Established associations

Group O	Duodenal ulcer
Non-secretor	Duodenal ulcer
Group A	Carcinoma of stomach

Probable associations

Group O	Gastric ulcer
Group O	Stomal ulcer (i.e. after gastro-enterostomy)
Nonsecretor status	Gastric ulcer
Nonsecretor status	Stomal ulcer
Group A	Pernicious anaemia
Group A	Tumours of salivary gland
Group O	Infection with Asian influenza virus, A_2
Nonsecretor status	Rheumatic fever
Group O	Rheumatic fever

Possible associations

Group A	Gall stones
Group A	Carcinoma of uterine cervix
Group A	Smallpox
Group B	Plague

The associations of blood group A with both carcinoma of stomach and pernicious anaemia are of interest because, even before these had been demonstrated, the two diseases themselves had been shown to have a significant connection.

The most striking of the established associations are those of duodenal ulcer with blood group O and nonsecretor status. The effects of the various combinations of alleles at these two loci show a graded association with duodenal ulcer. People of group O who are nonsecretors are most susceptible, and secretors of blood groups A, B or AB are least affected. Those of groups A, B or AB who are nonsecretors and those of group O who are secretors are intermediate in liability, and in that order. The relative strengths of these associations make it unlikely that the liabilities to duodenal ulcer are due solely to absence in nonsecretors of a direct effect on the mucosa by the group-specific substances, providing protection against acid digestion. If it were so, nonsecretors of group O and nonsecretors of groups A and B would not be expected to differ in their liability to duodenal ulcer, as in fact they do. The hypothesis of a direct protective effect was an obvious possibility to consider. In fact, the association may depend on some concealed or intermediate effects of the alleles determining blood group and secretor status. How these effects are exerted in the causation of duodenal ulcer is further obscured by the many other factors that may be in part responsible for this disease.

Genetic polymorphism and disease

Individual men and women with clear and distinct qualities, such as the presence or absence of a blood group and the ability or inability to distinguish red from green, exist together and interbreed freely to form a single population. This commonplace observation is the basis of genetic polymorphism. This has been defined by Ford as 'the occurrence together in the same habitat of two or more discontinuous forms of a species in such proportions that the rarest of them cannot be maintained merely by recurrent mutation'. The definition excludes differences in height or intelligence which show continuous variation and the differences between human groups not originating in the same habitat. It also excludes both the effects of rare harmful genes manifest in the heterozygous state and the effects of harmful recessives, both of which tend to be eliminated by selection and maintained only by fresh mutation.

The occurrence of polymorphisms implies the operation of factors of natural selection albeit less powerful ones than operate against the obvious genetic anomalies. One such form of selection which may operate where a polymorphism depends on a single pair of alleles, implies an advantage for the heterozygote over both homozygotes. This seems to be the form of selection which has operated in those human polymorphisms which are even partially

understood. Selection and advantage in human populations suggest differential fertility, the consequences of disease and advantages or disadvantages, not recognizable as diseases, in particular environmental conditions. The identification of these selective factors is made difficult by the long human generation-time and the radical changes that have occurred in the human environment, mainly as a result of man's own manipulations. Possible advantages include increased resistance to malaria and other infectious diseases, increased fertility and increased chance of survival in famine, due to increased stores of fat.

Heterozygous advantage in the form of increased resistance to *Plasmodium falciparum* malaria is likely in both the sickle cell trait and glucose-6-phosphate dehydrogenase deficiency. No heterozygous advantage has been identified in ABO and Rh blood group polymorphisms and some heterozygotes are at a special disadvantage in their liability to haemolytic disease of the newborn. The different antigen frequencies which occur in different parts of the world or even in different districts of the British Isles (vol. 1, p. 26.17) indicate that the factors determining selectivities must have been powerful at one time but may now be obscured by changes in the environment. For example, they might have been conveyed by means of resistance to an infectious disease which improved nutrition, or better sanitation has rendered less important. The known associations between the ABO blood groups and duodenal ulcer and gastric carcinoma are not likely to have had much selective influence since most of the mortality they cause occurs after the reproductive age. On the other hand, in the past they may have produced significant mortality at earlier ages.

MULTIFACTORIAL INHERITANCE AND DISEASE

The terms **multifactorial** and **polygenic** are commonly used as synonyms in describing inheritance. The number of gene pairs involved may be only two but it is required that the effect of any pair must be small in relation to the total variation. Hence in polygenic inheritance the frequency distribution curve must be continuous. Classical examples of this form of inheritance in man are provided by height, intelligence and the number of skin ridges in fingerprints.

Multifactorial inheritance probably operates in a great many common diseases which run in families. One difficulty in its investigation is that in most diseases only the presence or absence of disease can be scored, so that a discontinuous distribution is found. Since a continuous distribution of susceptibility to the disease is believed to underlie this finding it has been described as a quasi-continuous variation. One of the few human diseases which may be characterized by measurement of a single feature is essential hypertension in which high blood pressure develops in patients who are free from renal or endocrine disease. Despite this advantage its study is not free of difficulties inherent in measurement of blood pressure and in the definition of the populations to be studied. There is still controversy as to whether there is a continuous distribution of human blood pressures which would suggest that essential hypertension is determined multifactorially, or whether blood pressure shows a bimodal distribution consistent with essential hypertension being inherited as a Mendelian character. That genetic factors are important in causing essential hypertension is shown by the high incidence of the disorder in identical twins. That diabetes is also partly genetically determined is indicated by studies of the frequency of the disease in monozygotic twins and among relatives of affected individuals. One survey has shown that in 65 per cent of identical twins either both or neither were affected, while only 20 per cent of nonidentical twins were concordant. Similarly the incidence of diabetes among first degree relatives of young diabetics (sibling, offspring and parents) was found to be over ten times greater than that in relatives of nondiabetic individuals. In contrast the difference in incidence of diabetes in the relatives of diabetics over 70 years was only 1·5 times that of the controls. These results indicate the increasing effect of environmental factors on the older age groups. The pattern of inheritance of diabetes is believed by some to be autosomal recessive but many others believe it to be an example of multifactorial inheritance. More accurate methods of detecting occult cases of diabetes or those who will develop diabetes in the future (prediabetes) are likely to assist in resolving the problem.

Chromosomal abnormalities

It was only in 1956 that the normal human chromosome number was clearly shown to be 46 and the first human chromosomal abnormalities were reported in 1959. There followed a very rapid accession of knowledge, so that many came to regard human cytogenetics as constituting the major part of the study of human genetics in relation to disease. The rate of discovery of new chromosomal abnormalities has now become slower and it seems unlikely that any common aberration, dependent on variation in chromosome number or gross variation in chromosome form, remains to be described. Other abnormalities, especially in neoplastic cells, may be discovered when more sensitive methods of study are developed. Chromosome mapping based on the study of chromosomal abnormalities already known may be expected to progress slowly. Progress has also been made in establishing the frequency in various populations of the commoner abnormalities associated with abnormalities of phenotype, as well as of apparently harmless variation in chromosome form. These studies will be greatly aided by the improvement of methods, at present being developed, for the automatic scanning and analysis of karyotypes.

ABNORMALITIES OF CHROMOSOME NUMBER

The commoner constitutional chromosome aberrations associated with aberrations of phenotype are all abnormalities of chromosome number. Most arise as a consequence of an error at meiosis, known as nondisjunction (vol. 1, p. 38.11), which results in an ovum or sperm with one chromosome more or less than the normal number of 23. When such a gamete fuses with a normal one, a zygote with 45 or 47 chromosomes is produced, instead of one with 46 chromosomes. The results of these errors are exemplified for the commoner sex chromosome abnormalities in table 31.10. Only the consequences of

TABLE 31.10. The origins of some of the commoner sex chromosome abnormalities from fusion of normal and abnormal gametes to produce abnormal zygotes. The known autosomal trisomies are due to analogous errors.

Normal Male 46 chromosomes, XY	Normal Female 46 chromosomes, XX	
	Gametes	
Normal Sperm 23 chromosomes, X	Normal Ova 23 chromosomes, X	Normal Zygotes 46 chromosomes, XX
23 chromosomes, Y	23 chromosomes, X	46 chromosomes, XY
Abnormal Sperm 24 chromosomes, XY	Normal Ova 23 chromosomes, X	Abnormal Zygotes 47 chromosomes, XXY
22 chromosomes, O	23 chromosomes, X	45 chromosomes, XO
Normal Sperm 23 chromosomes, X	Abnormal Ova 24 chromosomes, XX	Abnormal Zygotes 47 chromosomes, XXX
23 chromosomes, Y	22 chromosomes, O	45 chromosomes, YO (nonviable)

nondisjunction at the first meiotic division in one parent are shown. Nondisjunction may also occur at the second meiotic division or at both. The range of abnormal zygotes is further increased by the possible occurrence of meiotic nondisjunction in both parents to yield two abnormal gametes.

Individuals with the sex chromosome constitution XXX are said to be triple-X. The term **trisomic** (having three chromosomes of a pair instead of the normal two) is usually reserved for the corresponding autosomal abnormalities. Individuals of sex chromosome constitution XO are monosomic for X. Monosomy for autosomes is theoretically possible but only one living case is known. Most are presumably incompatible with life, like the YO state.

MOSAICISM

Not all individuals with constitutional chromosomal abnormalities are homogeneous as regards the chromosome complement of their body cells. Those that have two or more cell lines of recognizably different chromosome constitution are known as mosaics. This state may arise as a consequence of either nondisjunction or anaphase lagging leading to chromosome loss at mitotic division, some normal cells already being present (vol. 1, 38.11). Alternatively, secondary nondisjunction may occur in an abnormally constituted zygote or foetus giving rise to normal cells.

THE CAUSES OF CONSTITUTIONAL CHROMOSOMAL ABNORMALITIES

The causes of nondisjunction and anaphase lagging are unknown. Exposure to ionizing radiations may increase their frequency but there is no evidence that radiation exposure is responsible for constitutional chromosomal abnormalities in human subjects.

Whatever the basic causes of nondisjunction, mongolism (p. 31.17) is related to the age of the mother. For women having children before the age of 20, the risk is 1 in 2300, which increases after the age of 45 to 1 in 46. There is a similar association with the much rarer trisomy 17–18 and possibly with the still rarer trisomy 13–15. The relationship of X chromosome abnormalities to maternal age is less clear cut. The birth of XXY males and XXX females is probably related to maternal age. In the case of XO females, no such relationship has been demonstrated. The frequency of mosaicism in XO individuals suggests that these arise, not so much because of a meiotic error in the maternal ovary, as following a mitotic error in the zygote.

CHROMOSOMAL ABNORMALITIES OTHER THAN ABNORMALITIES OF NUMBER

Almost all these abnormalities are secondary to chromosomal breakage. If a chromosomal fragment is without a centromere (acentric), it may persist but is liable to be lost at succeeding divisions. A chromosome which has lost a fragment is said to have undergone partial deletion.

Exposure to ionizing radiation is the best known cause of chromosomal breakage and the consequent losses and rearrangements. Both viruses and some chemical agents can produce identical effects, but the importance of these agents and spontaneous breakage, as causes of chromosomal abnormalities in man, is unknown.

The common sex chromosome abnormalities

The recognition of persons with numerical abnormalities of the X chromosome is greatly simplified by the occurrence of sex chromatin and the ease with which it is examined. This is equally true when the individual is a patient in whom clinical features suggest X chromosome abnormality, or when large populations are surveyed in attempts to establish the frequency of these abnormalities. Recognition of sex chromatin preceded the demonstration of sex chromosome abnormalities in man by about 10 years. In 1949 Barr and Bertram showed that females of various mammalian species had, in many cells, a characteristic condensation of nuclear chromatin (the Barr body) lying on the inner aspect of the nuclear membrane (plate 31.1a–d). No similar body was seen in normal males. Several groups of patients, in whom an abnormality of sexual differentiation or function was recognized clinically, were then examined. The most important findings were that abnormal females with Turner's syndrome were sex chromatin negative like normal males, and that abnormal males with Klinefelter's syndrome were sex chromatin positive like normal females.

The numerical relationship between the number of sex chromatin bodies which may be demonstrable in a cell and the number of X chromosomes it carries is shown in table 31.11. The number of sex chromatin bodies is ob-

TABLE 31.11. The numerical relationship between the X chromosome and the sex chromatin body.

Phenotype	Sex chromosomes	Number of sex chromatin bodies
Normal male	XY	0
Normal female	XX	1
Turner's syndrome	XO	0
Testicular feminization	XY	0
Klinefelter's syndrome	XXY	1
,,	XXXY	2
,,	XXXXY	3
Triple-X female	XXX	2
—	XXXX	3
—	XXXXX	4

viously one less than the number of X chromosomes. It must be emphasized that the possible number of sex chromatin bodies is not invariably demonstrable. A buccal smear (vol. 1, p. 12.16) from a triple-X female may contain 10 per cent of cells with two chromatin bodies and 30 per cent with one, no sex chromatin being identifiable in the remaining 60 per cent. In an XXXXX female, only 1 per cent of cells could be seen to have four sex chromatin bodies (plate 31.1d, facing p. 31.16).

Quite apart from this striking numerical relationship, the size of the sex chromatin body may parallel the size of the X chromosome where one of these is morphologically abnormal. Many aspects of this remarkable relationship between the X chromosome and sex chromatin are explained by the **Lyon hypothesis.** According to this theory, in any somatic cell, only one X chromosome is genetically active. Any other X chromosomes assume the form of a ball of chromatin, the sex chromatin body, in which form they produce little or no messenger RNA and so remain metabolically largely inactive. The hypothesis accounts for the relationship between numerical abnormalities of the X chromosome and the number of sex chromatin bodies. It also explains several otherwise unaccountable phenomena in human and animal cytogenetics and genetics. The essentials of the theory are generally accepted. Reservations concern mainly whether or not the whole of the X chromosome is inactivated and whether inactivation is effective during a part or all of the life of the cell. Obviously, if inactivation affected the whole chromosome throughout the life of all cells, XO and XXX or XXXXX females would not differ in phenotype.

KLINEFELTER'S SYNDROME

The discovery that some males have 47 chromosomes and the sex chromosome constitution XXY was the first demonstration of a constitutional chromosome abnormality in man. The presence of the sex chromatin body is in keeping with their having two X chromosomes like normal females. The male phenotype is in accord with their having a Y chromosome like normal males.

XXY males account for 2/1000 live male births. Before puberty they may show no specific clinical abnormality. After puberty the diagnosis may be suggested by their very small testes. It may be established by examination of a buccal mucosal smear for sex chromatin. Probably most males with XXY Klinefelter's syndrome are not diagnosed as such. They are psychologically male and are sterile but not impotent. Consequently, many first seek medical advice because of infertility. Most patients are mentally healthy, although the incidence of mental defects and possibly of behavioural abnormalities is greater than normal.

Some males with Klinefelter's syndrome are mosaics of sex chromosome constitution XY/XXY. They may have a lower incidence of sex chromatin in buccal mucosal smears and may be fertile.

A relatively small proportion of patients have the sex chromosome constitution XXXY, XXXXY, XXYY, or are mosaics with cell lines of these sex chromosome constitutions. These males are generally more severely affected than XXY individuals. Their sex chromosome constitution may be suggested by the occurrence of a few buccal mucosal cells with two or even three sex chromatin bodies (plate 31.1b & c), although most of the cells have only a single body.

TURNER'S SYNDROME

Females with this condition account for 0.4/1000 live female births. They are probably much less common in the population at all ages, since they have a high neonatal mortality. The most conspicuous clinical feature is short stature. Adults are almost invariably less than 5 feet in height. Webbing of the neck and other congenital defects are often present. Patients may seek advice because of primary amenorrhoea and failure of development of secondary sex characteristics. These are related to a constant abnormality of the ovaries, which consists of ridges of recognizable ovarian stroma without ova or follicles.

Diagnosis of Turner's syndrome is suggested by the clinical features and may be confirmed by examination of a buccal mucosal smear for sex chromatin, most patients being chromatin negative. The most common finding on chromosome study is 45 chromosomes and the sex chromosome constitution XO. Mosaicism is more common than in the other X chromosome abnormalities. The cell lines most commonly coexisting with the XO cell line have the sex chromosome constitution XX, XXX or one normal X and one morphologically abnormal X chromosome (X plus abnormal X). Mosaics may be chromatin positive and it is likely that examples of Turner's syndrome without menstrual abnormality or infertility are in fact mosaics.

THE TRIPLE-X SYNDROME

The unremarkable phenotype of the triple-X female accounts for the fact that the condition was the last of the common X chromosome aberrations to be discovered. Like so many findings in human cytogenetics, this was foreshadowed by the finding of triple-X females (called 'super-females') in *Drosophila*, 30 years before. The known association of X-chromosome aberrations with sexual abnormality led to the study of a young woman with unexplained secondary amenorrhoea. She was found to have two sex chromatin bodies in some cells of a buccal mucosal smear (plate 31.1b, opposite). Studies revealed 47 chromosomes, the additional chromosome being almost certainly a third X chromosome. These results are typical of those obtained in triple-X females. Mosaicism is much less common than in XO Turner's syndrome. Most triple-X females show no obvious deviation from the normal female phenotype. There is an association with mental retardation but it is much less strong than in Klinefelter's syndrome. Some have unexplained secondary amenorrhoea, but most give a normal menstrual history and seem of normal fertility. It is of interest that all the children of triple-X mothers so far studied have a normal chromosome constitution. On average, half the female offspring might be expected to be XXX and half the males XXY. Since this is not so, their XX ova must either be nonviable or at a great disadvantage.

Triple-X females account for about 1·2/1000 live female births. Since no special mortality is known, this may approximate to their frequency in the female population at all ages. Most are undiagnosed and unsuspected.

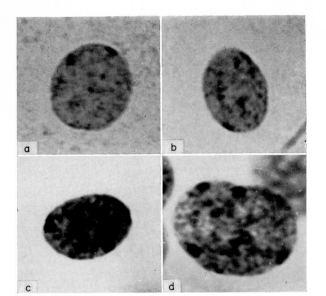

PLATE 31.1.

Sex chromatin bodies in the nuclei of human buccal mucosal cells. They may be distinguished from nonspecific chromocentres by their size, shape and position on the nuclear membrane. a, b, c and d contain respectively one, two, three and four sex chromatin bodies.

(e) Karyotype from a female mongol with 46 chromosome and a 13–15:21 chromosomal translocation. (See karyotype of a normal human cell, vol. 1, plate 12.1, p. 11.14.)

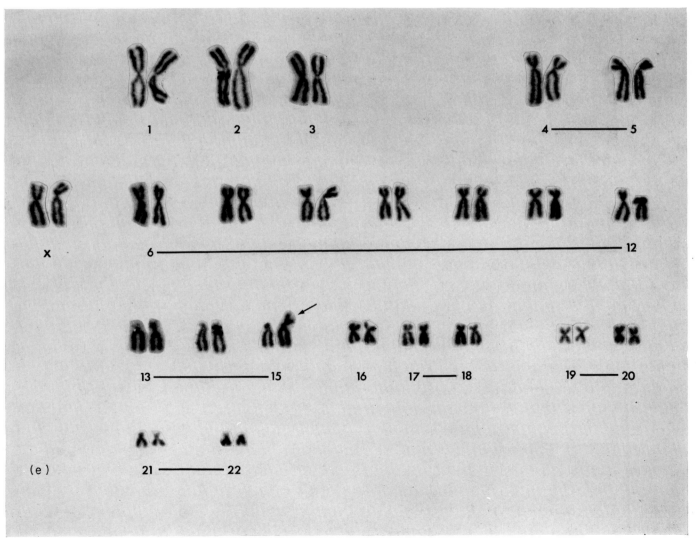

THE XYY SYNDROME

Until recently only a few males with two Y chromosomes had been described. XXYY males, who on buccal smear examination are chromatin positive, do not seem to differ in phenotype from cases of XXY Klinefelter's syndrome. XYY males are chromatin negative and consequently much less easily detected. A surprising number of XYY men were found in an institution for the mentally ill and retarded, all of whom had criminal convictions. Of 315 individuals studied, 16 had chromosomal abnormalities, and in 9 the abnormality was the XYY sex chromosome constitution. This number was more than the previously reported total in the world literature. As a group, they were taller and had been convicted at an earlier age than the other inmates of the institution. Much more work is needed on the XYY state, including assessment of the phenotypes of those in the general population, before any generalization can be offered about the XYY syndrome.

Common autosomal abnormalities

MONGOLISM (TRISOMY 21 OR DOWN'S SYNDROME)
Mongols are mentally defective and have a variety of physical defects, cardiac abnormalities being common. The name is derived from a supposed resemblance of their features to those of Mongolian people. In addition to the characteristic flat face, mongols usually have a large, often protruding, fissured tongue and a short stature. The grade of mental defect varies, but mongols are generally friendly, cheerful and easy to manage. Mongolism is the only common disorder associated with an autosomal aberration. The incidence at birth is about 1·5/1000 live births, and it is equally common in males and females. The prevalence in the population is much less because of the mongols' increased mortality, mainly due to congenital cardiac abnormalities and a special liability to infection. In addition, they have a 20-fold increase in their liability to acute leukaemia.

About 90 per cent of mongols show a definite trisomy for chromosome 21. Most are probably trisomic in all cells, but a small proportion are mosaics with the proportion of trisomic and normal cells varying from one individual to another and from one tissue to another in the same individual. Trisomic-normal mosaics account for 3–10 per cent of trisomic mongols. Mosaicism can never be excluded since only three tissues are usually available for chromosome studies. Most mosaics do not differ obviously in phenotype from the homogeneously trisomic.

A variety of cytogenetic aberrations have been found amongst the 2–5 per cent of mongols who are neither simple trisomics nor trisomic/normal mosaics. Some have aberrations involving other chromosomes, as well as trisomy for chromosome 21, and some are complex mosaics. The common feature in all is the presence of at least a part of an additional small acrocentric chromosome. It is not always certain, as far as microscopic appearances go, that the extra chromosomal material is derived from one of the larger pair of small acrocentric chromosomes (pair 21). In some instances it could equally well be derived from the smaller pair (pair 22) but it seems unlikely that there are two classes of mongols dependent on trisomy 21 and trisomy 22, respectively. Even if the mongol chromosome is eventually shown to be one of the smaller pair, it will probably continue to be called pair 21.

Translocations and familial mongolism
The most common cytogenetic finding in mongolism, other than simple trisomy 21 or trisomy 21/normal mosaicism, involves a translocation between a chromosome of the group 13–15 and a chromosome of the pair 21. This probably occurs in 2–4 per cent of all mongols. It has attracted attention because of its association with a special liability of some women to have mongol children and with even more obvious familial mongolism.

Long before the chromosomal abnormality in mongolism was demonstrated in 1959, it was appreciated that the occurrence of mongolism was, in general, related to maternal age. It had even been shown to be independent of the age of the father. Where more than one mongol occurred in a family, the association with maternal age was found to be weak. The pedigree of such a family is shown in fig. 31.6. The index case (III 2) was a mongol and a younger brother, also a mongol, was already dead. A maternal aunt (II 3) had also had a mongol child (III 1). There was an unusual history of neonatal death in the mother's sibship but no other recognized instances of mongolism.

The index case was shown to have only 46 chromosomes; not all of these were normal, one chromosome of the group 13–15 being replaced by a medium submetacentric chromosome; a similar finding in a female mongol is shown in plate 31.1e, facing p. 31.16. The appearance of the abnormal chromosome is consistent with its being the product of a fusion between a chromosome of the group 13–15 and a chromosome of the pairs 21–22. This fusion necessarily involves some loss of material from the short arm of both chromosomes and the centromere of one of them. Individuals with this chromosome constitution have in fact the equivalent of an additional chromosome of the pair 21, in keeping with their mongol phenotype. This interpretation seems the more likely when the mothers of such individuals are examined. In the family shown in fig. 31.6 the mothers of mongols (I 1, II 3, and II 6) each had 45 chromosomes. They then have the same submetacentric chromosome replacing one of the group 13–15 as is found in their mongol offspring, but only three discrete chromosomes of the pairs 21–22. In keeping with their essentially normal phenotype, these women have an essentially normal complement of genetic

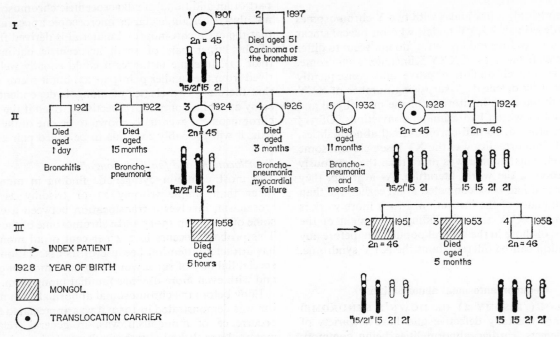

FIG. 31.6. Pedigree of familial mongolism due to a familial chromosomal translocation. After Carter C.O. *et al. Lancet* (1960) ii, 678.

material, apart from the minimal deletions which must have occurred from the short arms of both the translocated chromosomes.

The heterozygous carriers of a chromosomal translocation may produce several kinds of gametes at meiosis. Some are normal, some give rise to a translocation carrier like the affected parent on fertilization by a normal gamete, some are obviously not viable and some give rise to a translocation mongol. One study based on reports of 40 women with this type of translocation revealed 82 children of normal phenotype, 35 of them translocation carriers, 29 translocation mongols, two trisomic mongols and 25 stillbirths or abortions. In addition there were 14 other mongol children whose chromosome constitution was not established. This experience indicates that on average a woman with such a translocation may be expected to have mongol children, normal children of normal chromosome constitution and normal children who are translocation carriers like herself in equal proportions. She is also more likely to abort spontaneously or have stillborn children. The greatly increased risk of having mongol offspring is the reason why every effort should be made to discover translocation carriers so that appropriate genetic advice may be given. Translocation should be suspected when a mongol is born to a young mother, or if a woman gives a history of familial mongolism. However, not all young women who have mongol children are translocation carriers. In fact, only about 7 per cent of those who have mongol children

before the age of 30 have a chromosomal abnormality themselves, a 13–15: 21 translocation being the commonest of these.

Males too may of course be carriers of this translocation. They may transmit the balanced translocation to their children but these children are much less likely to include mongols than are the children of matings in which the female is the translocation carrier. Similarly, marriages in which the male is the translocation carrier show no obvious excess of stillbirths or miscarriages. The aberrant sperm of such males must be much less often viable than ova carrying the same chromosomal abnormality.

Other constitutional chromosomal abnormalities lead to an increased liability to have mongol children. One of these is maternal trisomy 21/normal mosaicism, the mother herself usually being of normal phenotype. Another is a translocation between two chromosomes of the pairs 21–22. In this case, in contrast to the 13–15:21 translocation, the abnormality is generally transmitted through the father. The birth of mongol children with 46 chromosomes and this type of translocation shows a marked association with advancing paternal age.

TRISOMY 13–15

The clinical features of this condition were described as long ago as 1882 but did not gain general recognition until the discovery of the associated chromosomal abnormality in 1960. The frequency of trisomy 13–15 in liveborn children is unknown, but a combined frequency for trisomy 13–15 and trisomy 17–18 of 0·7 per 1000 births has been suggested. The relative frequency of trisomy 13–15 in abortuses indicates that it is less compatible with normal intra-uterine development than either trisomy 17–18 or mongolism. All the children are apparently deaf and mentally retarded and have numerous other abnormalities. Most of them die in the first month of life and few survive as long as one year.

It is not known which chromosome of the group 13–15 is involved in this syndrome. Whichever it may prove to be, consideration of the clinical features suggests that the syndrome is homogeneous, i.e. if the trisomy is of, say, chromosome 13, then trisomy 14 and 15 are not commonly live-born. Children with double autosomal trisomies including trisomy 13–15 may not have the characteristic clinical features.

TRISOMY 17–18

Unlike trisomy 13–15 this condition was not recognized as a syndrome before the chromosome abnormality was first detected in 1960. The clinical findings may seem to be fairly characteristic, but they are often detected in new born children in whom no chromosomal abnormality is found, so they are certainly non-specific. The child is usually of low birthweight and mental retardation is invariable. The ears are commonly malformed. Cardiac abnormalities are a common cause of death.

The frequency of trisomy 17–18 at birth is unknown, but it is probably more common than trisomy 13–15. It is a much less common finding amongst abortuses with chromosomal abnormalities, so presumably trisomy 17–18 is more apt to undergo continued intra-uterine development. There is a marked preponderance of females at birth but they do not appear to live longer than males. Death usually occurs after a few weeks of life although mean survival is probably longer than in trisomy 13–15.

The chromosome involved in the trisomy has not been identified conclusively as 17 or 18 but most of those who feel that it can be identified, regard it as 18. Mosaicism for trisomic and normal cells has been described in children who are phenotypically indistinguishable from those in whom there is no evidence of mosaicism.

No causal factor has been identified in trisomy 17–18, other than an association with advancing maternal age. Exposure of the mother to radiation and other environmental factors have been suggested as causes, but have not been confirmed.

CRI-DU-CHAT SYNDROME

Apart from the autosomal trisomies, this is at present the only clinically recognizable autosomal abnormality. Its frequency is unknown. Most examples have been found amongst mentally retarded children in institutions or in the newborn. From birth these children have a peculiar mewing cry which has given the syndrome its name. Other congenital abnormalities are common. Mental defect is more severe than in mongolism, and the other congenital abnormalities are commonly less conspicuous than in trisomy 13–15 and trisomy 17–18.

This syndrome is associated with a partial deletion of the short arms of a chromosome of the pairs 4–5, almost certainly one of the smaller pair 5. There is no evidence that the lost portion of the chromosome may be translocated to another chromosome. In one case the deletion presumably occurred in the course of formation of a ring chromosome. Studies of genetic markers in this syndrome have failed to establish any detectable gene locus on the deleted part of chromosome 5. The cause of the deletion is unknown and no association has yet been demonstrated between parental ages and the occurrence of the *cri-du-chat* syndrome.

CHROMOSOMAL ABNORMALITIES AND SPONTANEOUS ABORTION

Table 31.12 shows that in one study about 20 per cent of spontaneous abortions were found to have major chro-

TABLE 31.12. Chromosome anomalies among 227 spontaneous abortions. After Carr D.H. (1967), *Amer. J. Obstet. Gynec.* **97**, 283.

Chromosome abnormality	No.
Trisomy 3	1
Trisomy 4–5	1
Trisomy 6–12	2
Trisomy 13–15	6
Trisomy 16	8
Trisomy 17–18	1
Trisomy 19–20	1
Trisomy 21–22	6
Trisomy E and trisomy G	1
Triploid—69 chromosomes	9
Tetraploid—92 chromosomes	2
XO	12

mosomal abnormalities. There can be little doubt that they were the cause of the abortions. It is interesting to compare these results with the abnormalities found in liveborn children. The XXY and XXX states are amongst the most common chromosomal abnormalities in liveborn children, yet they are not represented among the abortions. In contrast, the most common single finding in the abortions is the XO state, which ranks only fourth in the liveborn. Trisomy 16 and triploidy are excessively rare in life but common in aborted foetuses. Amongst the findings in spontaneous abortions, tetraploidy, trisomy 3, and trisomy 4–5 have not been described in the living.

Chromosome mapping in man

The process of localizing particular genetic factors to particular chromosomes has progressed only slowly in man. The only certain knowledge is of loci on the X chromosome. The Xg blood group, which is X-linked (vol. 1, p. 38.7) provided a genetic marker which can be used in linkage studies to determine the relative positions on the X chromosome of the gene loci. Previously, the only X-linked character with the properties of a marker was colour blindness, which is too rare to be of much use. Unfortunately the Xg blood group has proved less helpful than was originally expected, mainly because its locus is at one end of a long chromosome and distant from the loci for other useful characters. Direct cytological observations have as yet made no useful contribution to these studies, generally because of the lack of a demonstrable gene-dose effect for the characters studied. Thus a triple-X female has no higher plasma levels of antihaemophilic globulin or Christmas factor, or of erythrocyte glucose-6-phosphate dehydrogenase activity than has a normal female. Also it has not been possible to demonstrate any abnormality of a genetic marker in a female with a partially deleted X chromosome. If this should prove possible, consideration of the two findings, cytogenetic and clinical or immunological, might make it possible to establish the position of the locus or loci in question on the normal X chromosome.

GENE LOCI ON THE Y CHROMOSOME IN MAN

Formerly the Y chromosome in man was believed to be largely inert genetically. This view was based on an analogy with *Drosophila*, in which species an XXY individual is a functionally and phenotypically normal female and one of sex chromosome constitution XO a phenotypic male although infertile. With the finding that in man XXY, XXXY and XXXXY individuals are phenotypic males, albeit infertile, this view was no longer tenable. Although some masculinizing genes are probably carried on autosomes, the most active are likely to be carried on the Y chromosome. Nevertheless, the complexity of sex determination in man is indicated by the condition, **testicular feminization**, in which sex reversed males of sex chromosome constitution XY have testes, but otherwise a female phenotype including breast development and female external genitalia. This condition is probably determined either by a mutant gene on the X chromosome behaving as a recessive, or as an autosomal dominant character with sex limitation.

These observations, important as they are, provide no basis for accurate mapping of the Y chromosome. The phenotypic features concerned are all probably determined by genes at several loci and so are unsuitable as genetic markers. So too are the phenotypic features of increased height and a tendency to criminal behaviour which might have been associated with the possession of more than one Y chromosome. As has already been pointed out, studies of XYY and XXYY men have been biased, especially as regards their behaviour, by the selection of mentally retarded or criminal populations.

More valuable general conclusions about gene loci on the Y chromosome, which are nevertheless lacking in the specificity needed for linkage studies, have been provided by observations on individuals with structural abnormalities of the Y chromosome. Two phenotypic females with sexual infantilism and primary amenorrhoea were found to have a chromosome constitution which included only one X chromosome and an abnormal Y chromosome with no short arms, but with two long ones. These observations suggest that the male determining genes on the normal Y chromosome are carried on its short arms and that those on its long arms are not primarily concerned with sexual development or function.

It has been suggested that the genes determining various congenital abnormalities are likely to be Y-linked. The only gene accepted as Y-linked in man is that for hairy pinna of the ear (vol. 1, p. 38.8).

MAPPING THE AUTOSOMES IN MAN

While correlation of visible chromosomal aberrations and phenotypic features has been fruitful in mapping the chromosomes of other species, in man this approach has so far been unrewarding. Human mitotic chromosomes are smaller than the giant salivary gland chromosomes which are so useful in *Drosophila*; the human phenotype is also more complex than the relatively simple phenotype of maize. Furthermore, in other species, breeding experiments, not practicable in man, may elucidate the phenotypic changes associated with chromosomal abnormalities.

Most but not all of the attempts to locate specific loci on human chromosomes have been made by seeking a gene-dose effect for particular enzymes in trisomic individuals. These depend for success on the presence of three 'doses' of a particular structural gene being revealed by a 50 per cent increase in the activity of its enzyme. This may only be expected if the synthesis of the enzyme is determined solely at loci on the one chromosome and takes no account of the position and activity of the postulated regulator gene. Even if these objections are invalid, detection of an increase in enzyme activity in trisomy would depend on dosage-compensation being absent or ineffective. Furthermore, it would merely indicate that the structural gene in question may be present somewhere on the triplicated chromosome without giving any more specific indication of its position. Results so far suggest that in man genetic control of even so specific a phenotypic feature as the activity of a particular enzyme is more complex than the control of even gross features in *Drosophila* and maize.

Increased activity of several enzymes has been found in

both the leucocytes and erythrocytes of individuals trisomic for chromosome 21. The first enzyme activity to be studied in mongols was that of alkaline phosphatase in polymorphs. This was prompted by the knowledge that activity of the enzyme is usually decreased in those cells in patients with chronic myeloid leukaemia. If this was due to the loss of the appropriate gene locus from the Philadelphia chromosome, then mongols, being trisomic for the chromosome, might show an excess activity. They do indeed show some increase and the genetic control of alkaline phosphatase activity in polymorphs, although complex, may well involve a locus on chromosome 21.

It is of interest that for many of the enzymes assayed in the erythrocytes and leucocytes, trisomic mongols show an increase while translocation mongols do not. This might be explained by the loss of the gene loci in question in the process of chromosomal translocation, but seems unlikely when the same results are obtained for several different enzymes. A second possibility is that the difference is due to a positional effect whereby the triplicated gene fails to exercise its normal effect in translocation because of its altered position with reference to other genes. Such a positional effect has been recognized and studied in other species. These findings are of considerable interest, not only because of their relevance to mapping human chromosomes, but also because of their possible implications for both mongolism and chronic myeloid leukaemia, and in the mongols' increased liability to develop acute leukaemia. Despite their importance they defy interpretation at present.

Another approach to mapping the autosomes in man is to study individuals with chromosome deficiencies, who may be expected to show deficiency or absence of a specific feature such as activity of an enzyme, or even some more gross phenotypic abnormality. This approach has been used in individuals with deletion of the short arms of a chromosome of the group 17–18 as a constitutional abnormality. It has thus been established that the loci for the Rh and MNSs blood groups are not normally present on the deleted fragments. Unfortunately, but understandably, chromosomal deficiencies are much less common than trisomic states both as regards the number of individuals affected and their range of chromosomal aberrations. Nevertheless, families with balanced translocations offer an especially worthwhile opportunity for detailed study. Each translocation implies two chromosomal deletions, and the occurrence of these in families may provide several individuals for study, all with identical deletions.

FURTHER READING

BAIKIE A.G. (1965) Chromosomal abnormalities, in *Recent Advances in Paediatrics*, 3rd Edition ed. Gairdner D. London: Churchill.

CLARKE C.A. (1964) *Genetics for the Clinician*, 2nd Edition. Oxford: Blackwell Scientific Publications.

— (1969) *Selected Topics in Medical Genetics*. London: Oxford University Press.

EVANS D.A.P. (1969) Genetic factors in drug therapy, in *Scientific Basis of Medicine Lectures*. London: Athlone Press.

FORD E.B. (1965) *Genetic Polymorphism*. London: Faber.

HARRIS H. (1962) *Human Biochemical Genetics*. Cambridge: The University Press.

KALOW W. (1962) *Pharmacogenetics: Heredity and the Response to Drugs*. Philadelphia: Saunders.

MCKUSICK V.A. (1967) *Mendelian Inheritance in Man: Catalogs of Autosomal Dominant, Autosomal Recessive and X-linked Phenotypes*. London: Heinemann.

ROBERTS J.A.F. (1970) *An Introduction to Medical Genetics*, 5th Edition. London: Oxford University Press.

SORSBY A. (1953) *Clinical Genetics*. London: Butterworth.

STANBURY J.G., WYNGAARDEN J.B. & FREDRICKSON D.S. (1965) *The Metabolic Basis of Inherited Disease*, 2nd Edition. New York: McGraw-Hill.

STERN C. (1960) *Principles of Human Genetics*, 2nd Edition. San Francisco: Freeman.

Chapter 32
Hazards from poisonous substances in a modern society

The title may suggest that such hazards did not exist in older societies, but this is incorrect. Animals have evolved in an environment abounding in the poisonous products of some of their botanical contemporaries. Only by bitter experience did people discover that while one type of toadstool was a tasty addition to the diet, another like *Amanita phalloides* might form part of the last meal taken by their friends or relatives. Even now the hungry inhabitants of certain parts of the world, when reduced to eating cycad nuts, soak them first in water for a few days. They offer the water to the hens to drink and, if the hens die, the nuts are soaked for longer to remove the poisonous cycasin. This is a glycoside which is acutely hepatoxic and highly carcinogenic for mammals when ingested. Whether or not the mutagenic action of this type of carcinogen has played any part in evolution cannot be assessed, but at least evolution took place in an environment containing it and other natural carcinogens.

The pyrrolizidine alkaloids are widespread in plants of many different types that grow all over the world and are well known as liver poisons and carcinogens. Such plants are the source of many 'bush teas', and medicines made in homes which cannot afford the products of the pharmaceutical industry. Even in countries where synthetic drugs are consumed in vast quantities, herbalists still make a living and ragwort (*Senecio jacobea*), a rich source of one of the carcinogenic alkaloids, can be bought as a remedy for numerous ailments.

While an advanced society may relish the tasty products of the fungal decomposition of various wholesome foods like cheese, other fungi abound on the staple foods of those in less developed communities. The products of one of these, aflatoxin, from certain strains of *Aspergillus flavus*, is a most active chemical carcinogen and is present in all kinds of crops harvested and stored under conditions of high humidity.

What role natural poisons of this type play in the genesis of disease in communities that are not exposed to modern synthetic chemicals is uncertain. However, the irregular distribution of primary carcinoma of the liver in different parts of the world suggests that a natural carcinogen might be at work in some places.

Although efforts are now being made to obtain records of the incidence of diseases and causes of death in simple rural communities before these become changed by urban and industrial development, it is difficult to collect the background data needed to assess the aetiology of particular diseases in these populations, and it is not possible to say whether, from a toxicological point of view, it is safer to live in a sylvan or an urban jungle.

In an industrialized country, man is exposed to a wide range of synthetic chemicals used in manufacture and transport, in farms and gardens, in food preparation and preservation and in medicine. The sick and all too often the healthy are exposed to the dangers of adverse effects of drugs which may be caused by overdosage, drug interaction, unwanted secondary effects or be due to idiosyncrasy arising from genetically determined enzymic deviations (p. 31.9) or hypersensitivity (p. 23.10).

Irrespective of its origin, a poison is defined as any substance which, when introduced into or absorbed by the living organism, injures health or destroys life. The toxicity of a substance consists of its capacity to do this and the toxic hazard represents the probability that it will lead to injury or death.

FACTORS DETERMINING THE HAZARD TO HEALTH
In a modern community, a number of different factors must be taken into consideration in trying to assess toxicological risks.

(1) The **toxicity of the compound** depends on the nature of the adverse biological effects which it produces when absorbed into the body by any route.

(2) The **numbers and age of the population** exposed to the compound and liable to absorb it are important. A lung irritant in an urban atmosphere is a greater danger to the elderly, whose lungs have lost their elasticity and capacity for repair, than it is to the young. On the other hand, if the toxic substance is a carcinogen, there is likely to be a latent interval of 10–20 years or more between exposure and the appearance of the disease, so the younger age groups are at greater risk than the elderly.

(3) The **size of the dose** acquired at each exposure to a toxic compound obviously affects the nature of the response. The orchard worker who sprays peach trees with an insecticide may handle large drums full of concentrate once or twice a year, and each time be at risk of acute intoxication if the pesticide is misused. On the other hand, those who enjoy the fruit and ingest minute quantities

many times each year, are never in any danger of acute poisoning from residues of the spray that may be present. A person may absorb several times a day many grams of a potentially toxic drug taken as a medicine, but only occasionally a microgram of some potentially toxic constituent of a plastic wrapping of food.

(4) The **frequency and duration of exposure** to a toxic chemical are important in determining its effects. Few, if any, poisons are totally cumulative and the body possesses biochemical mechanisms for destroying many of them (p. 2.11). The exposure to noxious substances is usually intermittent. Thus metabolic and excretory mechanisms may be able to prevent a poison accumulating to dangerous levels in the tissues of any person who spends, say, only 8 hours a day for 5 days each week at a place of work where exposure occurs.

Students reading the 10th edition of this book may be facing other problems, such as those arising from the hazards of a continual exposure to toxic material in spacecraft bound for distant planets where no intermission of exposure may be possible for long periods. The dangers then are more likely to arise from minor degrees of cerebral failure rather than from liver necrosis.

(5) **Ease of recognition** of the signs of exposure helps to prevent over exposure and ensure treatment of the earliest and reversible manifestations of poisoning. Ease of recognition usually depends on the nature of the premonitory or early symptoms of poisoning in a group known to be exposed, e.g. in an occupation or as patients receiving drugs. However, among the general population exposure may not be recognized or, in the case of household remedies, the taking of drugs may not be known. The symptoms and signs of poisoning may then be thought to be diseases of more conventional or unknown origin. In the case of Pink disease, once quite common in infants, it took 40 years from the time of the first description of the disorder for the recognition that it resulted from an exposure to mercury which was present in 'teething powders' then on general sale.

ACUTE POISONING

Some biochemical disturbances

Some accounts have been given already of the mechanisms of acute cell injury due to poisoning with **carbon monoxide, cyanide** and **fluoracetate** (p. 25.14, 15 & 16). In the case of cyanide and carbon monoxide, the brain, the tissue most dependent for survival on a continuous supply of oxygen, is primarily affected. In both cases, if poisoning is not fatal, recovery may be complete, but residual disability depends on the amount of cerebral structural damage that follows the hypoxia. Further examples of poisons which disturb specific mechanisms are now given.

A variety of substances can produce cyanosis which may be severe enough to be fatal. A well known example of this type of compound is **aniline**. This is present in some waterproof marking inks and has been known to poison infants clad in recently marked napkins which had not been washed before use. The cyanosis produced by aniline and other aromatic compounds is due to the oxidation of haemoglobin to methaemoglobin. Methaemoglobinaemia is sometimes seen following the use of phenacetin and nitrites.

The high energy phosphate bonds in ATP are formed by oxidative phosphorylation which can be uncoupled by a number of poisons, the best known being the **dinitrophenols** and **dinitrocresols**. Cells so poisoned use increasing amounts of energy to produce the required amount of ATP and the excess is dissipated as heat. Dinitrocresols (DNOC) have no useful therapeutic purpose and attempts to use them for obesity led to a number of fatalities. More recently these drugs have been used as herbicides, e.g. **dinoseb**. Workers exposed to DNOC develop symptoms with alarming suddenness which reflect the increased metabolism, e.g. restlessness, tachycardia, perspiration and fever. Coma and death may ensue but recovery when it occurs is rapid and complete.

The role of acetylcholine in nervous activity is dependent not only on the ability of the nerve cells to produce it rapidly, but also on the capacity of acetylcholinesterase to destroy it almost instantaneously. This enzyme is sensitive to a number of inhibitors, including the **carbamates**, of which **eserine** (p. 4.6) and **propoxur** an insecticide are the best known examples, and the **organophosphorus compounds**, e.g. DFP (p. 4.6). The organophosphorus compounds have been extensively studied because some are very poisonous and have a potential role as war gases, and some are used as insecticides, e.g. **parathion**. These compounds are poisons because acetylcholinesterase cannot distinguish them or their metabolites from acetylcholine. The enzyme is carbamylated or phosphorylated and then is unable to remove the accumulating acetylcholine. This disturbs nerve function and the animal is poisoned. When inhaled or ingested, the effects are those of severe cholinergic stimulation combined with disturbance of the central nervous system. Sweating, salivation, weakness, intestinal colic, bradycardia and bronchospasm may be followed by constriction of the pupil, muscular fasciculation, convulsions, respiratory failure and death. If death does not occur, recovery is complete. Carbamate insecticides inhibit cholinesterase for much less time than do organophosphorus compounds and so are potentially less dangerous.

Treatment of intoxication with carbamate or organophosphorus insecticides includes the use of atropine which antagonizes the muscarinic effects of acetylcholine and of **pralidoxime**, a cholinesterase reactivator. Pralidoxime is a quaternary ammonium compound (hydroxy-iminomethyl-1-methylpyridinium) which is given slowly intravenously in a dose of 1–2 g.

Certain of the organophosphorus compounds like **triorthocresyl phosphate** can produce delayed structural damage in cells of the central nervous system. This capacity to produce permanent damage is not related to their ability to inhibit cholinesterase but possibly to their action on other esterases which play a role in maintaining the integrity of the neurone. There have been hundreds of cases of permanent disability resulting from the ingestion of triorthocresyl phosphate, usually as an accidental contaminant in food. In Morocco in 1959, the sale of stolen aircraft lubricants as a cheap cooking oil might have gone undetected but for the fact that the oil contained triorthocresyl phosphate as an anticorrosion agent. Consumption of the oil led to an outbreak of poisoning at first resembling an epidemic of an acute virus infection like poliomyelitis. Then unusual epidemiological features pointed to an outbreak of food poisoning. From this and other outbreaks of poisoning from triorthocresyl, many victims remain disabled for life as a result of loss of neurones.

Poisons like **tetraethyl lead**, a lipid-soluble antiknock additive to petrol, can produce striking changes in brain function and behaviour that resemble a psychosis. Severe cases develop convulsions, but if death does not occur recovery is complete and the disturbance of brain metabolism is only temporary. Poisons which produce violent convulsions may be fatal by reason of the ensuing asphyxia. A complex chlorinated naphthalene derivative, **dieldrin**, a powerful insecticide, caused many cases of poisoning among men spraying it in houses. No one died and the victims and their colleagues developed an unusual indifference to its effects. While their wives might complain when they had convulsions in bed during the night, many of the men who dropped their equipment at the start of a seizure at work picked it up and carried on when consciousness returned, scarcely aware of what had happened to them. Nothing is known about the biochemical basis of this curious effect.

Thus poisons can produce rapidly fatal effects by disturbing the biochemical mechanisms linked to the minute-to-minute survival of cells particularly in the nervous system. However, the effects are usually reversed rapidly, structural damage is slight or absent, and recovery is often complete.

Poisons producing structural damage to tissues

A large group of poisons and drugs have a selective action on certain organs, commonly the brain, liver, kidney or bone marrow. The liver is the organ most heavily exposed to a poison absorbed by the portal system from the gut. The kidneys are susceptible to poisons concentrated and excreted in the urine. The lungs and upper respiratory tract suffer first from exposure to irritant gases and highly reactive substances like **nitrous fumes, sulphur dioxide** and **phosgene**, which may never reach the blood and the rest of the tissues. Paradoxically **paraquat** (dimethyl dipyridilium), widely used as a weedkiller which is not volatile, exerts its most serious toxic effect on the lungs when ingested. Some days after a small dose, proliferation of the bronchiolar epithelium occurs which progressively reduces pulmonary function and is usually fatal. On the other hand **chloroform** may be absorbed through the lungs without injuring them but may lead to liver damage as a sequel to anaesthesia. The importance of the site of action in determining the significance of a toxic effect is obvious when comparing the results of cell death in brain and liver. Whereas neurones have no capacity to regenerate, the liver may be restored after widespread cell destruction by many agents. Although the glomeruli of the kidneys cannot be replaced much tubular damage can be repaired effectively.

DAMAGE TO BRAIN

Poisons that selectively damage the brain are rightly feared. **Carbon disulphide** is widely used in the rayon industry. Where ventilation in the factories has been inadequate workers have been poisoned, causing a variety of irreversible conditions in the CNS which have led to dementia and premature senility. Part of such damage may be due to accompanying vascular injury, but the action of carbon disulphide is not understood.

Whereas mercury vapour may give rise to reversible damage in the CNS, **methyl** and **ethyl mercury salts**, used extensively as fungicides, can damage limited parts of the cerebral and cerebellar cortex in a highly selective way; while the victim may retain normal mental acuity he develops gross ataxia, blindness, dysarthria and other irreversible lesions. **Methanol** is well known as a cause of permanent blindness by destruction of the retina. As described on p. 25.16 this may be brought about by formaldehyde liberated by the alcohol dehydrogenase in the retina. This enzyme preferentially oxidizes ethanol and so ethyl alcohol is the recommended treatment for people known to have drunk methanol. Such treatment may prevent but will not, of course, reverse retinal damage. It is the ethanol that preserves the eyesight, if not the insight, of the red biddy drinker.

Another poison with a striking action on the nervous system is **manganese**. Miners exposed heavily to manganese oxide in poorly ventilated mines develop a syndrome like Parkinson's disease. The basal nuclei are affected. The inability to reproduce the condition in experimental animals has prevented study of the mechanism of these specific toxic effects. Neither time nor drugs seem able to effect a cure for the condition. Liver damage is also often present.

DAMAGE TO THE LIVER

Damage to the liver from toxic agents is particularly liable to occur because of its position in relation to alimentary absorption and because it is the main site of metabolism of many compounds.

Carbon tetrachloride has been the subject of detailed studies and as a prototype of cellular injury is described on p. 25.14. Although not a powerful liver poison it usually kills people by causing tubular necrosis with acute renal failure rather than by hepatic cell damage. Sometimes it kills in apparently innocent circumstances. People have been fatally intoxicated by cleaning the stains from their clothes with a household cleaner containing carbon tetrachloride immediately on their return from a cocktail party. It is safer to allow the stains to dry and to oxidize the alcohol in the blood before using the chemical for this purpose. Another agent which causes hepatic cell necrosis is **tetrachlorethane** used as a solvent. The consumption of the fungus *Amanita phalloides* under the impression that it is an edible mushroom causes death from complete liver necrosis within a few days. The causal agent is a cyclic polypeptide called **phalloidin**, but the mechanism of its toxicity is unknown. **Yellow phosphorus** may be present in some rat poisons and causes liver cell necrosis. A similar effect may arise in children accidentally eating large quantities of **ferrous sulphate** (p. 7.2). Other well recognized drugs which may lead to liver necrosis include **cinchopen, tetracyclines** when given in large doses intravenously, **paracetamol, chloroform**, and some **monoamine oxidase inhibitors.**

Abnormalities of the villi of the intrahepatic biliary ducts associated with intrahepatic cholestasis and jaundice occasionally occur with **phenothiazine derivatives** and certain **steroids**, e.g. C-17 alkyl substituted compounds of testosterone including methyl testosterone and norethandrolone (p. 12.13); the reaction to the phenothiazines represents a hypersensitivity, that due to the steroids, is probably an intoxication. The possible role of contraceptive steroids in inducing liver damage is discussed on p. 12.10.

Poisons which lead to cell death are of less significance if the target is the liver as this organ possesses an amazing capacity to regenerate. However, in some cases scar tissue may play an important part in preventing restoration of function, and cirrhosis develops especially if the liver is repeatedly damaged by exposures to toxic materials. The action of poisons on the liver usually causes jaundice when the cell destruction is widespread or in the event of intrahepatic biliary obstruction. In less severe cases liver function studies may demonstrate unsuspected abnormalities. If life is spared, complete recovery from the effects of a poison that damages the liver is usual.

DAMAGE TO THE KIDNEY

The kidney is susceptible to toxic damage for a variety of reasons. Renal blood flow and oxygen consumption are high and damage is easily produced by agents which induce cellular hypoxia. The kidneys are the channel of excretion of many drugs and the selective reabsorption of water and salt exposes the renal tubular cells to a level which may be many times that in the systemic blood.

Mercury poisoning is the oldest and best understood type of nephrotoxicity. Mercuric chloride was once widely used as a disinfectant and had some popularity with would-be suicides. Mercury vapour may be inhaled in a laboratory and some pesticides contain mercury. Although widely distributed throughout the tissues, it is concentrated in the kidneys where it induces proximal tubular cell degeneration and necrosis. Exactly how mercury causes cellular destruction is not known and binding to thiol groups is not the whole explanation. A similar reaction may follow intoxication with **organic mercurial diuretics** and may result in acute renal failure (p. 11.6). Poisoning with **gold** and **arsenic**, which were once used widely in therapeutics, may induce similar lesions. Reference has already been made to the effect of **carbon tetrachloride** and renal tubular necrosis may follow exposure to **chlorates**, used as weedkillers, **tetrachlorethylene** used in dry cleaning, and **ethylene glycol** (antifreeze). Ethylene glycol may owe its toxic properties to being converted to oxalic acid in the body. Nephrotoxicity to therapeutic agents includes a wide range of drugs used clinically. The role of **sulphonamides** in inducing renal damage is discussed on p. 20.15. Other potentially nephrotoxic antibacterial agents include **streptomycin, kanamycin, polymyxins** and **amphoterecin**. Chronic exposure to **lead, phenacetin**, and possibly to **aspirin** can lead to chronic renal failure. Renal hypersensitivity reactions to drugs are described on p. 23.4.

DAMAGE TO BONE MARROW AND BLOOD DYSCRASIAS

Little information exists on the ways in which some poisons damage the bone marrow. Depression of function with aplasia of the marrow may follow exposure to drugs which are known to be safe for the great majority of people. Thus each time this toxic reaction arises it comes as an unpleasant surprise; only after the occurrence of a number of such incidents perhaps over some months or years is it recognized that exposure to a certain drug carries this particular risk. Unfortunately the drugs known to cause marrow aplasia and aplastic anaemia in this way cannot be made to produce the same effects in laboratory animals. It seems certain that a few people are more sensitive to the marrow damaging effects of some drugs, perhaps due to an unrecognized genetic defect, either of drug detoxication or marrow metabolism. **Chloramphenicol** is the most important offender but **hydantoin anticonvulsants, troxidone, sul-**

phonamides, **phenylbutazone**, **gold** and **perchlorates**, may also be responsible.

Apart from radiation, there is one compound that damages marrow in both animals and people whenever the dose is great enough. This is the common solvent **benzene** which has poisoned many people in industries when it has been used without the appropriate safety measures. No one has yet identified the metabolite which is likely to be responsible.

The **alkylating agents** can also produce marrow aplasia in people and animals when given in the appropriate doses. These compounds (p. 29.3) attack all dividing cells. Where the dose is not immediately lethal from an effect on the lining of the intestine, damage to the marrow may ultimately cause death of the animal. The mode of action has been studied intensively because these compounds have potential value as chemotherapeutic agents for cancer, including leukaemias. Unfortunately, contrary to popular belief, cancer cells do not divide unduly rapidly when compared to some normal tissue cells and many of these agents have a more selective action on other dividing cells, such as developing sperm. In appropriate doses they can induce sterility in male insects and male rats or mice without in any way reducing competitive vigour, a term used by the entomologists. They seem to act by inducing lethal mutations in the developing sperm and this can be quite transient. Doubtless when female professors of pharmacology outnumber the male, there will be an increased interest in the possible use of such compounds as contraceptives so that the toxic hazards of pill taking may be more evenly distributed among the sexes.

In excessive doses the germinal layers of the testis may be destroyed by alkylating agents. There may well be other compounds which exert unrecognized toxic effects on the testis. Studies on compounds damaging fertility indicate the limited value of microscopic studies in detecting any but gross changes in spermatogenesis.

While depression of all the cellular constituents of marrow (aplastic anaemia) is one of the most lethal consequences of drug intoxication, a fall in the total white count (granulocytopenia) is the most common. The mechanism again is unknown but serum antibodies which agglutinate leucocytes have been detected in granulocytopenia after administration of a number of drugs (p. 23.3). Similarly thrombocytopenia with bleeding into the skin and elsewhere is a further example of marrow failure due to drug hypersensitivity (p. 23.10).

The occurrence of acute haemolytic reactions due to a genetically determined decrease in the G-6-P dehydrogenase activity in red blood cells and brought about by oxidative agents and drugs is discussed on p. 31.10. Over forty drugs are known to act in this way in sensitive individuals. Haemolysis due to hypersensitivity reactions to drugs is discussed on p. 23.3. A number of drugs also induce haemolysis by mechanisms that are unknown. These include phenacetin, organic arsenical compounds, amphetamine, antihistamines and mephensin; methyl chloride and naphthalene (present in some air conditioners) may also do so.

CUMULATIVE AND CHRONIC POISONING

There is a widespread fear, by no means confined to non-medical and unscientific circles, that chemical substances not classified as poisons on the basis of acute toxicity tests may act as chronic or long term poisons. The demonstration that a substance is not acutely poisonous, even in large doses, does not exclude the possibility that it might have deleterious effects if taken in small doses over long periods.

Even in the case of substances known to be acutely poisonous, it may be necessary to try to establish a safe dose that may be absorbed repeatedly over long periods. The safe use of many chemicals in industry is based first on estimations of the concentrations to which persons may be exposed during their work, and secondly on making sure that their working conditions do not allow this to be exceeded.

When a toxic material gains access to the tissues in doses that are not immediately and obviously injurious, several things may happen to it. It may be excreted unchanged in the urine, if it is freely soluble in water. If a man takes a dose of fluoracetate (p. 25.16) that does not poison him, his urine may kill guinea-pigs which are much more sensitive to this poison. If the toxic material is not freely soluble in water but tends to partition into lipid, it is not readily excreted by the kidney. If there was no mechanism to dispose of such substances, mammals would probably never have evolved, for their progenitors would have died from an accumulation of unwanted lipid-soluble materials that had been ingested in their diet from other living things. The mechanisms which prevent the body being thus overwhelmed by a surfeit of lipid-soluble chemical debris reside principally in the liver and probably to a significant extent in the cells of the gut and kidney. These reactions are mainly oxidative and conjugating mechanisms and convert lipid-soluble into water-soluble materials (p. 2.17). From the liver the substance is then passed directly into the blood and hence into the urine, or is excreted into the bile and reaches the gut. It may be excreted in the faeces in some cases after further degradation, or be partly reabsorbed and re-excreted. Provided the compound is never present in concentrations that damage the tissues, i.e. in poisonous doses, there is no reason why such a mechanism of degradation, water solubilization and excretion should not operate indefinitely. It is continually in operation for dealing with tissue metabolites and unwanted ingredients of food.

THE DISPOSAL OF DDT

Not all drugs or foreign compounds are attacked with equal speed and vigour by solubilizing enzymes. If the compound is very insoluble in water but highly lipid-soluble and is only slowly converted by the liver enzymes, it may accumulate in the fat. The best known example of this type of compound is the insecticide dicophane or DDT. This compound has been used on an enormous scale to control insects of importance in agriculture and public health. For such purposes it is quite safe and there is no need for any special protective measures. However, its chemical persistence has led to its presence in human food. Its chemical stability seems to have posed problems for the liver as well as nature lovers, because when ingested in small quantities not all is metabolized rapidly or excreted, but some is laid down in neutral fat. As the amount in the fat rises, so does the level in the blood including that reaching the liver. At the higher concentrations the liver enzymes work more effectively and more DDT is metabolized and excreted. The concentration in the body fat at any one time reflects the level of intake over a preceding period of time and not the accumulation throughout life. Doubtless other substances can be stored in fat in a similar way if their solubility in water and fat and rate of metabolism by the liver are appropriate. However, the preoccupation of some authorities with the hypothetical long term effects of pesticides ensures that until other scares replace them, much attention will be paid to DDT and kindred substances. This will lead to a fuller understanding of the possibilities of chemicals producing cumulative and chronic poisoning, as well as revealing some of the extraordinary adaptive capacity of the mammalian liver for eliminating foreign chemicals (p. 2.11 and 10.9).

THE DISPOSAL OF LEAD, RADIUM AND MERCURY

Some poisons may accumulate in the tissue because they can neither be excreted rapidly enough nor rendered readily water soluble. Lead can cause poisoning if the rate of intake by mouth exceeds a certain level. At or below 2 mg/day it is mostly excreted in the faeces and the small proportion that is absorbed appears in the urine. If the rate of ingestion rises, then the level in the urine rises because more is absorbed; if this exceeds around 0·15 mg Pb/l, absorption is assumed to be excessive and potentially dangerous. The lead is laid down in bone and it exerts its first detectable effects on the maturation of red blood cells and the formation of haemoglobin. Some lead can be laid down and retained indefinitely in the bones without exerting a toxic effect. However, rapid mobilization, as occurs in acute intercurrent disease, can raise the blood levels and produce systemic poisoning. **Radium** is also laid down with calcium in bone and if the radiation is not great enough to produce bone marrow damage, it may at a later date produce bone sarcomata. There are other bone-seeking radioactive isotopes of special concern to those who have to assess the hazards from long term exposure to small quantities of radioactive materials and environmental contaminants, e.g. nuclear explosions and accidents (p. 33.3).

Mercury has a predilection for the kidney and accumulates in the tubules if the level of absorption is too great to keep pace with excretion. It is probable that mercury is excreted as a water-soluble cystine complex and as long as the concentration of mercury is not high enough to damage the tubules, excretion can probably continue indefinitely without harm. It is usual to assess the exposure of man in industries using mercury by determining urinary mercury. Other things being equal, it will be those men in a group who are not excreting mercury who may be more severely poisoned than those with a high urinary level.

DISPOSAL OF DUSTS

There is another group of potentially toxic materials that depend upon a completely different excretory mechanism for protecting the body from cumulative poisoning. These materials are the dusts and other particulates. When particles above 7–10 μm in diameter are inhaled, they are trapped in the nose or upper respiratory tract and pass into the nasopharynx to be swallowed in due course. The majority of particles below 7 μm penetrate to the lungs. Some may be removed by bronchial cilia and pass up the trachea to be swallowed. Others are ingested by phagocytes and these may also be excreted via the trachea or pass through the lungs into the lymphatics. Although the lungs and draining lymph glands of city dwellers are stained black by the carbon which they inhale during a life-time in such an environment, this does not produce significant injury to the lungs. In other words, the excretory mechanism of the respiratory tract is adequate to prevent damage from the particulates inhaled from a normal environment. If the mechanism is overloaded, for example, by a working life spent in a dusty mine, lung function may be damaged by the mass of coal that collects in it, but coal itself is a relatively inert material inside tissues. Other dusts such as **silica** in certain forms, and **asbestos** in particular, are not inert and the cells that ingest such particles are damaged or killed and a chronic progressive inflammatory lesion develops which may destroy the functional lung tissue. In the case of asbestos the lesion may become malignant (p. 28.17). Exposure is not always occupational and mesothelioma have developed in women whose only exposure to asbestos arose from brushing their husbands' clothes. **Beryllium oxide** dust may also provoke a serious tissue reaction, mainly in the lungs, even when inhaled in small doses compared with the amounts necessary to produce damage from silica

(p. 21.20). Beryllium as a dust in the form of beryl can apparently be inhaled with impunity which is just as well since the air of cities where much coal is burnt may contain beryllium in this form in quantities which would be unacceptable in a factory making or handling beryllium as its oxides. The biochemical basis for the toxic effects of silica, asbestos, beryllium oxide and other dusts is not understood. The first step appears to be damage by the ingested particles to the macrophages that remove them from the lungs. The damaged cell products may be partly responsible for the lesion but the particles themselves are reingested after they have been liberated by the dissolution of the macrophages which they have killed. Some particles, for example **cotton fibre dust**, do not cause structural damage to lung tissues as a result of ingestion by macrophages but lead primarily to functional changes associated with bronchospasm, presumably from liberation of biologically active amines or similar compounds. A type IV hypersensitivity reaction may also play a part in the case of silica and beryllium (p. 23.7).

BASIS OF CHRONIC POISONING

Chronic effects from poisoning may therefore follow the production of structural damage from either single or repeated doses or from the accumulation of the toxic material itself until dangerous concentrations are reached in the tissues.

As mechanisms of poisoning become better understood, it may be possible to recognize more cases where the cumulative effect is due to the persistence of a biochemical lesion so that restoration to normal is slower than the rate at which the poison reaches the biochemical target. The coumarin anticoagulants are not powerful acute poisons but repeated doses produce cumulative effects. Organophosphorus compounds poison by inhibiting cholinesterases. A proportion of the enzyme inhibited by a single dose is restored to activity within a few hours but some remains permanently inactivated and can only be replaced by the synthesis of new protein. The organophosphorus compound itself may be so unstable that it persists only for a few minutes but repeated daily doses may poison the animal if the rate of replacement of cholinesterase does not keep pace with the amount destroyed by each dose of inhibitor. In suspected poisoning the determination of cholinesterase in the serum and red blood cells is of value in diagnosis.

The possibility of being able to foretell whether a poison will be likely to produce chronic or cumulative effects even though the poison itself does not persist in the tissues will depend upon more knowledge of its mechanism of action. Thus alkylating agents can produce striking cumulative effects on the developing sperm when the repeated doses are at levels quite without effect on the bone marrow or gut. From their chemical properties it is extremely unlikely that these agents themselves can persist

for more than a very short time after entering the circulation. Presumably in the testis there must be some constituent that reacts readily with very low concentrations of the alkylating agent and which can only be restored or replaced slowly.

LETHAL SYNTHESIS

The metabolic systems which help to detoxify and hasten the excretion of potentially toxic materials are discussed on p. 2.11. However, the chemical changes which these enzymes induce may not always render a compound less toxic even if they do make it relatively more soluble in water. **Tetraethyl lead**, a useful fuel additive for the petrol engine, is itself biologically inert. The mammalian liver contains enzyme systems which readily remove ethyl radicals to form the triethyl lead ion, which can be excreted. Unfortunately it is one of the most active inhibitors of oxidative phosphorylation that is known and so interferes with brain metabolism. In the attempt to get rid of the inert tetraethyl lead, the liver produces an active poison for the brain. The well-known organophosphorus insecticide **parathion** has practically no action against cholinesterase but both insects and mammals have enzyme systems which convert the P=S bond to P=O and the resulting **paraoxon** is one of the most active inhibitors of cholinesterase and appreciably more water soluble than parathion. **Malathion** is a more interesting insecticide which is much more poisonous to insects than it is to mammals. Like parathion it must be transformed to **maloxon** by conversion of P=S to P=O before it becomes a poison to either. However, malathion has an ester group and when this is hydrolysed it ceases to be an inhibitor of cholinesterase even when it is oxidized. The livers of mammals are rich in this esterase so that when malathion is absorbed it is rendered inert before it can be oxidized. Insects lack this esterase and so are killed.

The mammalian liver has enzyme systems that carry out readily the reaction known as *N*-demethylation which, under some circumstances, may fulfil an important role in the body's economy. If, however, the inert material dimethylnitrosamine is introduced, *N*-demethylation results in the formation of a very unstable monomethylnitrosamine which in turn decomposes to liberate diazomethane. This is extremely reactive and if liberated inside liver cells can either kill them or in small doses produce damage that eventually leads to the development of cancer (p. 25.18). Metabolic processes which convert an inactive molecule into a poison can sometimes produce an active drug, which is excreted in the urine where it may be identified. Perspicacious manufacturers may then make the metabolite and sell it as a drug; thus paracetamol is obtained from phenacetin (p. 2.13) and oxyphenylbutazone from phenylbutazone (p. 5.58). The conversion of an inert molecule to a toxic one need not only take place in the liver and the conversion of fluoracetate to fluorocitrate by the citric acid cycle in the kidney and other tissues has been described (p. 25.16).

It will be obvious that any understanding of the mechanism of action of poisons depends on a detailed knowledge of the body's biochemical processes and the sites at which physiological disturbances or cellular damage may occur. That a poison may only be generated by the metabolic processes inside cells or even special organs makes it impossible to rely on the less differentiated animals, tissue cultures, etc., to provide a basis for distinguishing poisonous from nonpoisonous compounds.

Production of cancer by poisons

Probably one of the most dreaded sequelae of exposure to a poison is the possibility that cancer may be produced. This may be an occupational hazard of those who survive acute effects of such an exposure and it is a preoccupation of those who worry about others exposed to 'foreign chemicals'. Some aspects of chemical carcinogenesis are discussed on p. 25.16 and 28.9. 2-Naphthylamine is known to produce bladder tumours in men exposed to it in various industries where it is made or used. As a result this compound is no longer made in Britain. Complex polycyclic hydrocarbons which produce skin cancer in some species (p. 25.17) are believed to be the active agents in tar or soot cancer in man. Asbestos and radiation are other known causative agents of cancer in man and animals (p. 28.17 and p. 33.6).

Apart from those animal tumours known to be caused by viruses, it is possible that all tumours are the result of exposure to one or more chemical carcinogens. Since the cause of much cancer remains a mystery, it is natural that much work has been done on the reactions between chemical carcinogens and the tissues in which tumours will eventually appear as a result of the administration of such compounds. It is generally believed that cancer, if it has a chemical aetiology, follows only after a prolonged exposure to the aetiological agent. This is undoubtedly true for man in the case of cigarette smoking, for abstention reduces the probability of an individual developing a bronchial cancer within a few years. What in fact this late repentance may do is to increase the latent period between exposure to the carcinogen and the development of the tumour. However, the study of chemical carcinogens in the laboratory has provided many examples of tumours following only a single dose of the carcinogen which may itself be a highly reactive compound that does not persist in the tissues for more than an hour or so. Yet the animal will not develop cancer until a year or more later. Of particular interest in this connection is the sensitivity of the newborn animal to some carcinogens of this type. The problems involved in identifying the biochemical changes that occur immediately the carcinogen is given and establishing the connection between events in a few cells months or years later presents

obvious difficulties, so that a speedy solution to the question of the biochemical basis of the carcinogenic action of chemicals is improbable. The important lesson from such studies is that if a significant proportion of human cancer is due to exposure to some chemical carcinogen this may be a result of prolonged and repeated exposure as in the case of cigarette tobacco or it may be the result of single or occasional exposure which may be completely forgotten by the time the tumour appears many years later. Moreover, chemical carcinogens may be of natural origin and some of these are certainly as active against animals as any produced by the chemist. As already discussed, people in primitive communities away from industrial hazards may be just as severely exposed to chemical carcinogens as city dwellers and industrial workers. The high incidence of liver cancer in young people in some parts of Africa and Asia bears witness to this.

As in physiology, so in cancer research, a study of natural poisons may prove profitable.

Atmospheric pollution

The air we breathe is not only contaminated by dusts but also by liquids (vapours) and gases. A polluted atmosphere commonly contains all three, but it is probably the gases which do the most damage. Concentration of noxious substances is likely to be high when atmospheric conditions produce fog in an industrial area in which toxic products of combustion can accumulate. This commonly occurs when warm moist air is trapped beneath an inversion layer of colder air, and under these circumstances there is little or no wind to disperse the resulting smog (smoke plus fog). Epidemics attributed to atmospheric pollution occurred in the Meuse Valley in Belgium in 1930, in Donora, Pennsylvania, in 1948 and in London in 1952. In the last, the smog lasted a full week, during which there were very large numbers of cases of acute exacerbations of chronic bronchitis, and of acute respiratory complications of other chronic disease such as congestive heart failure. About 4000 more than the expected number of deaths occurred that week in London and most of them were attributable to the effects of the smog. As in the other epidemics, sulphur dioxide was incriminated and its concentration reached a level of 3·7 mg/cubic metre; in the previous twenty years it had never exceeded 2.2 mg/cubic metre. SO_2 is the most widespread toxic gas in urban polluted atmosphere, but other gases may also reach toxic levels. Incompletely combusted petroleum products are chiefly responsible for the ill-effects which accompany the notorious Los Angeles smog, of which the main clinical manifestations are conjunctival irritation and mucosal congestion affecting mainly the upper respiratory tract. Quite possibly there are delayed effects of chronic exposure to atmospheric pollution. The evidence for an association with malignant disease of the respiratory tract, carcinoma of the lung in particular, is not convincing, but further study is needed before this can be excluded.

TESTING FOR TOXICITY

Before people are wittingly exposed to new chemical substances whether as remedial drugs, placebos, food additives, cosmetics, domestic preparations or during the course of their occupations, toxicity should be investigated so that risks attending exposure can be assessed.

To reveal the precise mode of action of a toxic material is a worthy ambition but it is rarely achieved. However, with the slowly growing knowledge about how some poisons act, it should become easier in the future to compare the toxic effects of new compounds in a useful and informative way with the effects of the few well studied ones. While it is to be hoped that the long term study of toxic substances will continue in some laboratories, the main effort must be directed to acute toxicity tests on mammals; in this way within a short time information may be obtained that enables a decision to be made whether to expose people to a new compound.

Some people hanker after a recipe for tests which will enable the toxicity of a new compound to be established. It is possible to prescribe precise means by which a particular aspect of toxicity may be recorded and compared over a whole range of compounds. Conditions such as those appropriate for a bioassay may be established. However, this is not an appropriate method for studying the toxicity of a new compound. This thinking may, however, explain some of the idolatry attached to the LD50. It may be important to determine this to two places of decimals in a bioassay but such precision is superfluous in a general study of toxicity. What is far more important than the numerical data is some account indicating the nature of the reactions in the poisoned animals and particularly the speed and degree of recovery in the 50 per cent that survived.

Only the outline of a procedure for determining the toxicity of a new compound can be described. In general, the aim is to determine the lethal dose to laboratory animals given the compound by various routes and to try to decide the cause of death. If death is rapid and recovery in the survivors speedy and complete, it is unlikely that pathological examinations will reveal much. They are essential where death is delayed or recovery slow and incomplete. Cumulative effects must be determined by repeated doses of fractions of the LD50 at different intervals from hours to days depending upon the proposed uses of the material being tested. If a toxic effect can be identified and in some way measured, the slope of the dose/response relationship should be established and the size of the maximum no-effect dose determined. If this maximum noneffective dose over a short period is established, it may

be necessary to confirm that it is also a nontoxic dose when given over a longer period. There is a tendency to believe that the longer such a test is carried out the more valuable is the information derived from it. Unfortunately, but not unexpectedly, laboratory animals like people grow old and suffer from a variety of degenerative disorders and infections. If, therefore, a test is continued in laboratory rats for their average life span of five score weeks and ten, the subjects will be old and diseased so that it will be difficult to recognize any but the most striking manifestations of a toxic effect of a drug. One such easily recognized pathological lesion is a tumour, so that old animals may be used in tests for carcinogenicity when the number of tumours in the dosed animals can be compared with the number in the controls.

SPECIES DIFFERENCES

The purpose of toxicity tests on laboratory animals is not to make the world safer for rats and mice but to reduce risks to people. What interpretation can be put upon the findings in animal studies? Are there one or more species whose reactions closely resemble those of man? A sensible guide in testing a new compound is to see what, if any, are the species differences in the acute toxic dose. If mice, guinea-pigs, dogs, cats and monkeys all respond in a similar way to a dose comparable on a body weight basis to the LD50 for a rat, then it is reasonable to assume that man will respond in the same way. Species differences are unlikely when the toxic compound acts directly upon a biochemical process common to living matter. Species differences may vary strikingly when the compound under examination is not itself toxic but becomes metabolized to release the toxic moiety. The routes and rates of metabolism of a compound may vary from species to species. Again species differences may be more striking if the drug has a selective action on one organ or a specialized biochemical system. Wherever possible extensive toxicity studies should be carried out on a species that metabolizes the compound in the same way as man. This advice presupposes that man has been exposed to the compound and that this has happened before a full picture of its toxic potential has been obtained. For a potentially useful drug this is done usually because it is also necessary to establish that the drug is effective before expending a great effort in time and cost to find out what its toxic effects may be. For other materials such as potential food additives or substances to which exposure may occur in industry, careful observations must be made on people exposed to them in early stages to assess their full effects and the degree of protection needed.

In general there are no rules for a choice of species for tests to improve the predictability of toxic effects on man. Problems of extrapolation would not be solved if monkeys were used. For example, man is extremely susceptible to triorthocresyl phosphate which can be given in large doses to monkeys without apparently damaging the nervous system. On the other hand, the cow and barn-yard fowl respond to it like people do. Admittedly experience with primates in toxicity studies is still limited and is likely to remain so until a suitable type can be bred and reared satisfactorily in laboratories. The expense involved might have the beneficial effect of reducing the worship of large numbers in toxicity studies and greater attention might be given to more careful study of fewer animals.

GENETIC DIFFERENCES

The study of large groups of the conventional laboratory species can be wasteful because their response on the whole is remarkable uniform. However, wild rats differ from laboratory rats in their sensitivity to some rodenticides and black rats may differ in this respect from brown rats thus making rat eradication by poisoning difficult. Among different strains of mice, including pure lines, striking differences in response to pharmacological agents have been recorded but the biochemical basis for these differences is not known. One reason for using large groups of animals is to provide an opportunity of detecting the occasional unusual reactor. There is so little evidence of the profitability of this exercise that its value must be seriously questioned. It may be necessary to use large numbers in a group so that sufficient survive for a reasonable life-span in tests for carcinogenicity but this reflects the poor life expectation of the animals often used in such tests.

In man on the other hand it is the abnormally reacting individual who again and again appears when large numbers are exposed to different drugs. While there is a well-established genetic basis for individuals who are unduly sensitive to suxamethonium (p. 31.10) or liable to develop polyneuritis when given isoniazid (p. 31.11) and haemolysis when given primaquine and other oxidant drugs (p. 20.20), a similar basis has not yet been shown to account for the development of the great majority of cases of aplastic anaemia, blood dyscrasias, skin reactions and other unexpected and sometimes severe ill effects in a minority of people given certain drugs. The possibility, however, that these are genetically determined or represent hypersensitivity reactions which are genetically determined cannot be excluded.

VALUE OF TOXICITY TESTS ON ANIMALS

In underlining the limitations of toxicity tests on animals as indices of what may happen in man, the need to carry out such tests is not questioned. Tests on animals show up common and widespread toxic effects. The capacity of a compound to produce obvious damage to vital organs is revealed and in many cases nothing more is heard of such compounds because they are of no value as drugs or food additives. However, no matter how satisfactory the findings on animals may be, they do not prove the compound will be free from adverse effects on man. They can only indicate that it is justifiable to expose people to the compound in order to discover whether a safe dose for the animals is also nontoxic for man. Anything learnt about the mechanism of toxic effect in the animals leads to search for a similar effect in people.

An analysis of the results of toxicity tests on rats and dogs of a series of drugs was recently compared with the reports from doctors giving the same drugs to patients. It was concluded that animal tests gave a reasonable degree of predictability of likely side effects. Of course, tests on animals, at least the conventional ones, usually give little indication of subjective effects such as headache or nausea. Whereas rodents cannot vomit, dogs and cats may do so on slight provocation. While nausea and vomiting may be a disappointing response to the administration of a new drug it represents the first step to reducing the chances of a more serious or permanent injury from a more complete absorption of the compound.

A difficult problem may arise when a compound is being tested for toxicity and is found to be a chemical carcinogen when given by one or more different routes of administration. If a proposed food additive produces tumours in animals when added to the diet, it is easy to decide that the compound is unsuitable for adding to food for human consumption. If the compound is one to be used in industry, steps must be and normally are taken to protect those who use the compound from any significant exposure to it. The ideal solution is to find a noncarcinogenic substitute. When the compound under test is a possible drug the decision is difficult. Were the new drug merely to be an addition to the host of tranquillizers competing with each other inside and outside the patient, there is no problem. If the drug was proposed for the treatment of cancer or some other rapidly fatal disease for which no remedy yet existed, a trial on patients in spite of the effects on the animals would be carried out. Greater difficulties arise when the drug is clearly a useful one and the relevance of the tests on the animals not immediately obvious. Iron dextran (p. 7.3) has been in use for several years and found to be a valuable and safe method of giving parenteral iron. It was then discovered by chance that repeated injections into rats or mice could lead to the development of sarcomata at the site of injection. However, to produce the tumours the injections had to be multiple and the dose much larger in relation to body weight than when used in treating patients. Furthermore, the animals were not anaemic and did not need the iron. The drug persisted in their tissues and the tumours developed from the cellular reaction. On the other hand, iron dextran is rapidly withdrawn from the tissues of anaemic patients and no local tissue reaction is aroused. This underlines the need to look closely into the conditions under which tests for toxicity on animals have been carried out and compare them with the conditions under which people will be exposed to the agent under test. Controversy still rages as to whether a chemical considered for use in human food should be rejected because it gives rise to tumours in the tissues of animals at the site of subcutaneous injection. The subcutaneous route has not yet been proposed as a normal means of giving nourishment to man. It can therefore be argued that testing food additives by subcutaneous administration has no relevance to the assessment of any potential toxic hazards they may possess. When the food additive under consideration happens to be a colouring agent, it might be argued that it is of no biological value so that an adverse response in any test, however irrational, should be grounds for rejecting its use. However, the interpretation of the results of animal tests should be separated from considerations of the expediency of using the substance under test. The risks should be balanced against the benefits as in the case of drugs. The benefits of having food brightly coloured clearly cannot be assessed highly.

Future trends

As more and more new chemicals are examined for toxic properties, compounds with possibly unique effects are being discovered; some may be turned to man's advantage. A toxic compound may be useful in the control of pests or disease organisms; there is also the possibility of using such poisons as tools in studying biochemical and physiological processes. It is to be hoped that these poisons will be made available to research workers in physiology and biochemistry.

Another recent development is the greater interest in studying the reaction of animals to toxic substances. When death and the study of tissues from dead animals cease to be the main criteria for assessing toxicity and are replaced by biochemical studies in the poisoned animal, the methods of detection of toxic effects become more precise. What starts as a test for detecting a change in a sick animal in which a large part of a vital organ is destroyed may gradually become a means of detecting the first biochemical departure from normal. This is excellent progress until the stage of interpretation of these findings in terms of potential hazard is reached. If a poison kills an animal when it inhibits 95 per cent of the activity of a certain enzyme, it is reasonable to conclude that an inhibition of 5 per cent, assuming measurements can be made to this degree of accuracy, represents the earliest detectable effect. It indicates that exposure to and absorption of the toxic agent have taken place. However, if the inhibition does not progress, can such an exposure be considered to be a threat to health if there are no symptoms? If a 5 per cent inhibition is considered a permissible degree of exposure, at what level of inhibition, before symptoms and signs appear, is it necessary to reduce or eliminate further exposure? Without the biochemical test, symptoms would have been the only yardstick.

In other instances the first biochemical response of the organism to exposure to a compound might be a defence mechanism rather than a toxic or deleterious effect. If the liver enlarges at the same time as its complement of metabolizing enzymes increase their activity, is this a dangerous or desirable reaction? Is this a true work hypertrophy or a protest by the liver at receiving an unnecessary chemical insult? There are no answers to these questions at present but they illustrate the difficulties of drawing satisfactory conclusions about dangers to health from sensitive responses to foreign compounds. These difficulties have been illustrated more fully by work on the effect of noxious material on higher nervous activity.

The effects of ethanol, anaesthetics and sedatives on higher nervous activity are obvious and are the outstanding pharmacological effect of such drugs in appropriate doses. This effect may be studied in animals. Such behaviour studies will almost certainly provide a sensitive index for detecting the toxic effects of substances that primarily affect the brain. However, in some parts of the world where the teaching of Pavlov has been predominant, the conditioned reflex is considered to represent the functioning of higher nervous activity. Studies on a variety of toxic substances have been carried out using the effect on the conditioned reflex as an indication of a toxic effect, and it is claimed that exposure to a variety of compounds whose main toxic effect may be on the lungs, on the liver, on the kidneys or other organs and tissues show that doses ineffective on the target organ may still have an effect on the conditioned reflex. For this reason many recommendations for the safe level of toxic substances to which people may be exposed in industry are set much lower in the USSR than in the USA. Such tests may also be devised on man. For example, exposure to an irritant gas may affect the finer EEG pattern. If such responses are made into conditioned reflexes, it may be possible to elicit them by exposing the subject to a concentration of SO_2 one tenth or less of the least concentration that can be detected by smell. These responses in the EEG may be a sensitive means of detecting the reaction of an irritant substance with receptors in the respiratory tract but it can hardly be sustained that such a level of exposure is a potentially toxic hazard. Thus it becomes necessary to distinguish an effect or a reaction arising from the contact of a toxic substance with the tissues from a toxic or potentially deleterious effect.

Until recently the fact that people were being exposed to dangerous materials was only recognized when they died in significant numbers and at post mortem unusual pathological findings were seen. Now the estimation of the safe level of the commonly used solvent trichlorethylene is based on psychological assessment; are workers unduly quarrelsome, bad tempered and irritable at home? While the pathologist's slab may be replaced by the marriage bed as the object of study of toxic effects, the findings from the latter present more serious problems of interpretation.

Adverse effects will, of course, never even be considered in a differential diagnosis if enquiries are not made about the patients' occupations or the nature of any drug treatment they may be receiving for other conditions. For female patients it is said that a lead on medication may be obtained by asking them to empty their bags on the consulting room table, but of course men also receive and take drugs. Both sexes may meet toxic solvents at their work.

If an actual or potential exposure to drugs or industrial poisons is established, it is important to be able to differentiate the signs and symptoms that might be the result of poisoning from those that could be the evidence of a disease not known or suspected to be the result of any poisoning. Finally, it is important to bear in mind that the evidence of an exposure to drugs or industrial poisons may not necessarily only take the form of a complete shut down of function in important organs like the liver, kidneys or bone marrow but may result in less drastic departures from the normal. For poisons whose main or sole point of action is the central nervous system, it is possible to envisage all kinds of subtle effects from doses that do not lead to functional damage that is obvious to the nearest bystander.

While the mechanisms of toxicity offer a challenge to pharmacologists, physiologists and biochemists, it is clear that intelligent study of things that threaten life go hand in hand with greater knowledge of the factors that maintain and support it.

FURTHER READING

ALDRIDGE W.N. ed. (1969) Mechanisms of toxicity. *Brit. med. Bull.* Volume 25, No. 3.

ALLISON A.C. (1968) Lysosomes and the responses of cells to toxic materials, in *Scientific Basis of Medicine.* London: Athlone Press.

BARNES J.M. & PAGET G.E. (1965) Mechanisms of toxic action, in *Progress in Medicinal Chemistry*, 4, 18. Ed. Ellis G.P. & West G.B. London: Butterworth.

BOYLAND E. & GOULDING R. eds. (1968) *Modern Trends in Toxicology 1.* London: Butterworth.

BROWNING E. (1965) *Toxicity and Metabolism of Industrial Solvents.* Amsterdam: Elsevier.

DAVIES C.N. (1954) *Dust is Dangerous.* London: Faber.

PAGET G.E. & BARNES J.M. (1964) Toxicity tests, in *Evaluation of Drug Activities. Pharmacometrics*, vol. 1, p. 135. Eds. Laurence D.R. & Bacharach A.L. New York: Academic Press.

Poisonous Chemicals used on Farms and Gardens (1969) London: Department of Health and Social Security.

REES K.R. (1968) Cellular injury by drugs, in *Biological Basis of Medicine*, vol. 2. Eds. Bittar E.E. & Bittar N. New York: Academic Press.

Research into Environmental Pollution (1968) Technical Report Series, No. 406. Geneva: World Health Organization.

SCHOENTAL R. (1966) Toxicology of natural products. *Food Cosmet. Toxicol.* 3, 609.

TALALAY P. ed. (1964) *Drugs in our Society.* Baltimore: Johns Hopkins Press.

Chapter 33
Biological effects of radiation

Interest in the biological effects of ionizing radiation was aroused immediately after the discovery of X-rays by Roentgen in 1895. Harmful consequences for those who worked with the new rays were soon evident, as skin ulcers which underwent malignant transformation, and severe anaemia. The first studies were concerned with the protection of scientists and others working with X-rays and with radium which was discovered in 1898. These provided the basis for regulations designed to protect those whose occupations involved exposure to radiation. The first regulations of this kind were enforced in the United Kingdom in 1921. In 1928 an International Committee on Radiological Protection was formed under the auspices of the League of Nations.

Other early work was done by radiotherapists, intent on improving the scope and efficiency of this form of medical treatment, and by geneticists. The capacity of X-rays to induce nondisjunction at meiosis was described by Mavor in 1921 and in 1928 Muller demonstrated their ability to produce point mutations.

World War II increased interest in the effects of radiation. Radioactive isotopes had been used for physiological and other studies before 1939 but only after the war was rapid progress made in this field. Advances in the production and use of radioactive isotopes followed on the development of the atomic bomb. The tragic effects of atomic warfare stimulated interest in the biological effects of radiation. Much work since 1946 has been concerned with the detection of chronic and genetic effects of radiation exposure in the survivors of Hiroshima and Nagasaki and their children. Other studies have been carried out in Britain and the United States in people who have been exposed to radiation by radiotherapy. Further knowledge of the acute effects of high doses of radiation in man has been provided by the outcome of radiation accidents.

Another important aspect of radiation studies in man has been the detection of possible chronic effects of exposure to relatively low doses, such as those resulting from diagnostic radiology, occupational exposure and radioactive fall-out from weapon testing. This is an exacting field of study which has given rise to conflicting results. Retrospective observations have special

difficulties and liability to error and prospective studies may need to be continued for many years. In both, the expected effects may be slight, difficult to detect or affect only a small proportion of those exposed, so that very large numbers of people have to be studied (p. 35.13).

Death from aplastic anaemia soon after high doses, as was experienced at Hiroshima and Nagasaki, stimulated interest in the possibility of treatment by bone marrow homografts. Animal experiments have shown that the immunosuppressive activity of high doses of radiation facilitates successful homografting and that the most serious effects of radiation fall upon tissues which normally have a high rate of cell replacement. As a result radiation exposure has become a useful experimental procedure in the investigation of cell kinetics.

Generalizations about the biological effects of radiation are particularly liable to error. Effects may vary not only with such obvious factors as dose, type of radiation and whether it is applied externally or arises from internally deposited radioactive substances (p. 29.14). Other important aspects of radiation dose are the rate of delivery, whether it is fractionated in time and the duration of the radiation-free periods between doses. Other variables include the actual tissues irradiated, their metabolic and mitotic activity, whether the whole body or only part of it is irradiated, and the age of the irradiated organism.

Types of radiation and their sources

The atom consists of a nucleus surrounded by orbital electrons. The nucleus is composed of protons, each with a net positive charge and a mass of unity, and uncharged neutrons of equal mass. The orbital electrons are of negative charge equivalent to the positive charge of the nucleus, and have negligible mass.

X-rays are electromagnetic radiations of zero mass and charge. They are generally produced by the bombardment of a metallic target by fast electrons. The energy of X-rays so produced is determined mainly by the energy of the bombarding electrons, which in turn depends on the voltage used to accelerate them. Diagnostic X-ray apparatus and conventional sets used for radiotherapy have voltages in the range 50–300 kilovolts. Conventional X-ray apparatus is now being replaced for radiotherapeutic uses by supervoltage equipment producing X-rays of several million volts energy. X-rays may occur naturally in the course of radioactive decay involving the emission of β-particles.

Like X-rays, from which they are distinguished only by their origins, **γ-rays** are electromagnetic radiations. They arise from the nucleus during a nuclear reaction whereas X-rays are of orbital origin. In general, γ-rays are of greater energy than X-rays, but this is not invariably so. The nuclear reactions giving rise to γ-rays may be induced, or occur spontaneously in the course of the radioactive decay of many unstable elements.

α-Particles have a positive charge of 2 and a mass of 4. They are simply the nuclei of helium atoms without orbital electrons and consist of two protons and two neutrons. They penetrate tissues to a depth of less than a millimetre but produce intense irradiation within their limited range. α-Particles result from nuclear reactions produced by high energy radiations and are emitted in the decay of some elements such as radium and uranium.

β-Particles are indistinguishable from ordinary electrons and so have a negative charge of unity and negligible mass. They originate in the nucleus of an atom when a neutron changes into a proton and an electron, as in the decay of some radioactive substances. β-Particles penetrate tissues poorly but may produce significant irradiation of deep tissues if they arise from isotopes deposited internally. Positrons are β-particles of positive charge.

Protons are the nuclei of hydrogen atoms with both mass and positive charge of unity. They are produced by high energy accelerators or in tissues as a consequence of neutron bombardment.

Neutrons are of unit mass and neutral charge. They are short-lived but generally of high energy and penetration, so resembling X- and γ-rays. They result only from nuclear reactions or from the explosion of a nuclear weapon. Slow and fast neutrons are distinguished and differ greatly in their biological effects. Slow neutrons are of relatively little biological importance, but fast neutrons make an important contribution to the harmful effects of nuclear weapons.

Fundamental effects of radiations in tissues

X-rays and γ-rays behave similarly in tissues. Since they are uncharged, interaction occurs only with tissue electrons which they actually meet. Accordingly, they are less likely to interact than are the charged α- and β-particles and their paths in tissues are longer. Interactions commonly result in the release of ionizing electrons which are similar to β-particles; unlike primary β-radiation, however, the electrons produced by X- and γ-rays arise deep in the tissues.

By virtue of their charges, α- and β-particles may repel or attract orbital electrons of tissue atoms without actually hitting them. Consequently, they produce relatively dense primary ionization along their short paths through tissues. Some of the orbital electrons they eject from target atoms may themselves produce ionization.

Protons are similar to α- and β-particles as regards their behaviour in tissues. Their chief biological interest arises from their production, by the stripping of the nuclei of hydrogen atoms, along the paths of fast neutrons. These protons are intermediate between α- and β-particles in both the density of ionizations along their paths and the length of the paths.

Neutrons, whether fast or slow, are not strictly speaking ionizing radiations. The only ionizations they produce result from the secondary charged particles which are released from target nuclei when they acquire an extra neutron. All the biological effects of slow neutrons are produced in this way. Fast neutrons cause the release of protons from the stripped nuclei of hydrogen atoms they meet, as already mentioned.

Natural sources of radiation

External radiations to which man is subject include cosmic radiation and radiation from the air, ground and building materials. The intensity of cosmic radiation varies with altitude and geographical location. The dose rate is of the order of 24 millirads (mrads)/year at sea level, but about three times that rate at altitudes of 3000 m. Its penetration is such that the dose rate for different organs of the human body is about the same. This is also true of radiation from radioactive elements in soil and rocks and in some building materials, notably granite. Because of the radioactivity of granite the mean dose-rate in Aberdeen granite houses is 85 mrads/year, compared with 60 mrads/year in sandstone houses in Edinburgh.

Dose-rates for external radiation from all natural sources vary from 50 to 200 mrads/year. A very small contribution is made by the inhalation of the radioactive gases, radon, thoron and other decay products diffusing into the atmosphere from the earth. Some is inhaled directly by man, some is incorporated in plants and animal foodstuffs and later ingested by man; and some is deposited in the environment and contributes to natural external radiation.

Apart from the inhaled and ingested radon, thoron and their decay products, most natural **internal radiation** is derived from the radioactive isotopes of carbon and potassium. ^{14}C results from the action of cosmic radiation on nitrogen and reaches the earth from the stratosphere. Thereafter it is progressively distributed through all living tissues. ^{40}K is also widely distributed in the human body and is a much more important source of natural internal radiation yielding about 15 mrads/year to the gonads compared with 1 mrad from ^{14}C.

Man-made sources of radiation

MEDICAL RADIOLOGY
The most important artificial source of radiation exposure for man is medical radiology. In the United States it may provide a higher average gonad dose than natural background radiation. In Britain it has been estimated to be responsible for about one-fifth as much. Most of the total is attributable to diagnostic radiology, with radiotherapy, and the diagnostic use of radioactive isotopes providing lesser doses.

The need to reduce exposure to man-made radiation to a minimum (p. 35.13) has resulted in improved practices in medical radiology. Higher standards of medical care would have resulted in increased doses from diagnostic radiology but for improved apparatus and techniques. Radiotherapy for nonmalignant disease is used less than formerly. Only radiation from the use of radioactive isotopes in the diagnosis of disease seems likely to increase. Reduction in radiation exposure may be effected by the use of more sensitive apparatus and smaller doses, and of isotopes of very short half-life.

OCCUPATIONAL EXPOSURE
Before 1939 almost all occupational radiation exposure was sustained by medical and other personnel concerned with diagnostic radiology and radiotherapy. Notable exceptions were the ingestion of radium and mesothorium by dial painters using luminous paints and inhalation of radioactive substances by miners at Schneeberg in Saxony and Jackymov in Bohemia. Some of the dial painters developed bone necrosis and bone tumours while the miners acquired cancers, notably of the respiratory tract (p. 28.16).

The occupational exposure of workers in medical radiology was closely controlled in most countries soon after the potential hazard was appreciated. Control takes the form of measuring the dose rate in the vicinity of a source of radiation. If it exceeds about one-tenth of the maximum permissible dose for occupational exposure, monitoring of individual workers is carried out. This is done by requiring them to wear a badge containing photographic film which blackens on exposure to radiation. Excessive occupational exposure can be reduced by improvements in the apparatus or process. When excessive personal exposure is detected despite these measures, the individual workers may be restricted as to the time they spend in exposed situations.

The use of X-ray fluoroscopy in shoe fitting, widely practised for a few years, was shown to be a potential source of exposure to harmful radiation, and these devices have now been declared illegal in many countries.

The increasing use of radioactive isotopes and of radiography in industry creates new and potentially dangerous situations. These can only be detected and the dangers reduced or eliminated by the constant vigilance of a professional protection service. An extreme example of a new hazard may be provided by the development of space exploration and travel. It seems likely that excessive doses of highly penetrant cosmic radiation may at times be encountered in the Van Allen belt.

NUCLEAR EXPLOSIONS AND ACCIDENTS
It is probable that most of the casualties at Hiroshima and Nagasaki were due to blast, burns and falling buildings rather than to harmful effects of radiation. The Hiroshima bomb produced γ-rays and neutrons while the Nagasaki bomb released relatively fewer neutrons. Although both bombs produced radioactive fall-out of products of nuclear fission, this fall-out made only a slight contribution to the total radiation of those exposed. In contrast, the accident at Bikini in 1954 resulted in heavy fall-out of radioactive isotopes, mainly of iodine and strontium.

^{131}I and ^{90}Sr are important atmospheric contaminants after weapon testing and accidents at nuclear reactors. Much of their importance lies in their biological properties whereby the ^{131}I is concentrated in the thyroid gland (p. 6.8) and ^{90}Sr in bone. Where the effects of a radioactive isotope are liable to fall particularly on one organ or tissue it is sometimes called the **critical organ.**

The half-life of ^{131}I is 8 days and that of ^{90}Sr, 28 years. ^{90}Sr and some other long-lived isotopes are thus still very active when they return to the earth's surface over a very wide area after having been distributed through the stratosphere. ^{137}Cs and ^{14}C are similarly produced and disseminated. Such fall-out is estimated to have resulted in an average yearly dose of 2·4 mrads in the period 1954–9. This dose is to be compared with the estimated 50–200 mrads/year from natural external radiations.

Biological effects of radiation
The basic mechanisms of the biological effects of radiation are only imperfectly understood. It was formerly believed that all or most of the effects of radiation on cells were due to **direct interaction** between the ionizing radiation and the structure or substance affected. While this kind of interaction probably occurs it is now regarded as less important than an **indirect effect** mediated by the cell water (p. 25.12). The primary radiochemical effect on tissues appears to be the liberation of uncharged H atoms and OH radicals. These are highly reactive and are often called hot radicals. They can combine in various ways to produce equally reactive groups, such as HO_2, H_2O_2 and O_2. It is likely that many reactive organic peroxides are also produced.

This basic radiochemical reaction probably determines the influence of Po_2 in determining radiosensitivity. In general, increased Po_2 at the time of radiation increases sensitivity. This effect has been used in radiotherapy to increase the sensitivity of some tumours by treating the patient while in an atmosphere of increased O_2 pressure. Conversely, radiation sensitivity is reduced by hypoxia.

A great many substances confer partial protection against the biological effects of radiation. These include glutathione, nitrite, *p*-aminopropiophenone, cysteine, cysteamine and cystamine. It is believed that all these compounds are protective by virtue of their hypoxic effect. Substances with sulphydryl groups probably have a special affinity for binding oxygen.

EFFECTS OF RADIATION ON MITOSIS
Replication of DNA is an essential prerequisite for cell division. Although cells already in mitosis at times of radiation may complete their division, one of the most important effects of radiation is to inhibit mitosis. This effect is dose dependent. Some cells may be lethally damaged by radiation and others already in mitosis at the time of radiation may continue DNA synthesis without completing mitosis. The overall effect is a reduction in mitotic index. Although the question of relative sensitivity of different cells to radiation is complex the greatest effects are seen in tissues which normally have a high mitotic index and the effects of cell death without replacement are especially obvious in the bone marrow, gastrointestinal mucosa and skin. Cellular aspects of injury by ionizing radiations are described on p. 25.12.

CHROMOSOMAL ABNORMALITIES AND MUTATIONS
Apart from inhibition of mitotis, radiation has other effects which profoundly influence normal cell division. Radiations have been shown to be mutagenic in every plant and animal species in which they have been adequately tested. Furthermore, there is a strong correlation between the induction of mutations by radiation and their capacity to produce gross and visible chromosomal aberrations. Reference has already been made to the early demonstration of more frequent occurrence of meiotic nondisjunction after radiation exposure (p. 31.15).

In man chromosomal changes following irradiation have been studied mainly in the peripheral blood lymphocytes and, to a lesser extent, in the bone marrow. Lymphocytes are amongst the most radiosensitive of cells. Nevertheless, although the degree of chromosomal damage by any radiation dose may be greater for lymphocytes than for other cells, the type of chromosomal aberration is unlikely to differ between cells. These aberrations include deletions, acentric fragments, dicentric chromosomes, ring chromosomes and other chromosomal rearrangements. All seem to depend on the breakage of chromosomes by radiation, with or without the joining of the broken ends of one or two chromosomes.

These abnormalities have been most studied after exposure to higher doses of radiation, such as are used in radiotherapy or encountered in radiation accidents. Nevertheless, similar aberrations have been found after therapeutic doses of radioiodine and after diagnostic X-irradiation involving doses in the range 12–35 rads. Some of the more stable chromosomal abnormalities have been found in the peripheral blood lymphocytes of irradiated survivors at Hiroshima and Nagasaki, 20 years after exposure.

It is not known what relation these chromosomal abnormalities found in apparently healthy people have to the harmful late effects of irradiation to which they are prone. The common occurrence of similar chromosomal aberrations in leukaemic and in other neoplastic cells occurring in people with and without significant radiation exposure is interesting but inconclusive.

The same chromosomal changes have been found after external exposure to X-rays, γ-rays and fast neutrons and after internal radiation by β- and γ-rays. Where the effect of dose has been studied quantitatively, it is found that the frequency of chromosomal damage is, generally speaking, proportional to the radiation dose.

Radiation dose

The measurement of radiation dose for biological purposes is inherently difficult. These difficulties have led to use of a variety of units and even to the use of several different definitions of the same unit at different times. The details of these definitions need not concern us here but certain basic concepts are important.

The **roentgen** is a unit of exposure dose in air applicable only to X- and γ-rays. It can be measured directly. In contrast, the **rad** is a unit of absorbed dose in a particular medium, commonly a tissue. It cannot readily be measured directly. The same exposure (in roentgens) may result in different absorbed doses (in rads) in different tissues. Another unit of radiation dose is the **rem** (roentgen equivalent for man). This takes into account the relative biological efficiency of the absorbed energy. For β-, γ- and X-rays the dose in rems is equal to that in rads. For α-particles and neutrons it may be many times higher.

DOSE-RATE AND FRACTIONATION
In general, the biological effects of radiation are directly proportional to the total dose received. Nevertheless, the effects may be greatly influenced by the time taken to deliver a particular dose. If the radiation is not delivered continuously but in fractions, the duration and number

of the radiation-free intervals may be as important as the dose-rate while exposure is actually going on. The radiation-free intervals may reduce the severity of effects by permitting some repair and recovery to occur.

Repair processes in tissues damaged by radiation are complex and vary from one tissue to another. Two of the more important processes involved are the removal of lethally damaged cells and their replacement by new ones. Much remains unknown about the potential of repair to influence the delayed somatic and genetic effects of radiation.

THE CONCEPT OF A DOSE THRESHOLD
There is great difficulty in deciding whether there are levels of radiation dose below which no harmful effect results. The difficulty is particularly great as regards delayed somatic effects and genetic effects in man. The latent period of such somatic effects may well be many years, and in the case of genetic effects, several generations. If the expected effects are detectable in only a small proportion of those exposed, very large numbers must be studied.

In deciding on so-called permissible doses of radiation, whether for the population as a whole or for particular groups, it is generally assumed that there is no dose threshold.

PERMISSIBLE DOSES OF RADIATION
In deciding an acceptable dose of radiation for man it is necessary to weigh the possible harmful against the beneficial effects. The overall benefits of medical radiology, for example, which constitute the largest man-made source of exposure, have to be balanced against its possible hazards.

All attempts to arrive at permissible doses of radiation involve assumptions and extrapolations. Nevertheless, certain general principles have been followed in addition to the assumption of no dose threshold. Calculations err in favour of safety. It is usually accepted that a dose level permissible for adults in particular occupations is not suitable for children whose tissues may be more sensitive to harmful effects. Furthermore, as regards the higher doses acceptable for small groups engaged in special occupations, it is usually required that these groups should not constitute more than a certain proportion of the general population. While allowing for the greater exposure of small groups, the dose is often expressed as an average for the whole population in a generation of 30 years.

An example of a permissible dose is that arrived at for the whole population by the International Commission on Radiation Protection and endorsed by the Medical Research Council in the United Kingdom. It is recommended that the gonadal dose to the whole population from all sources other than natural background radiation and medical radiology should not exceed 5 rem/generation of 30 years, and that medical exposure should be kept to the lowest practicable level.

THE MEDIAN LETHAL DOSE (LD 50)
This is the dose of radiation that will, on average, kill 50 per cent of an exposed population within 30 days of exposure. The median lethal dose for whole-body irradiation is of the order of 500 rem. If only part of the body is exposed the effects are much less severe. At a dose of 600 rem to the whole body almost all those exposed will die. This is LD 100 for whole body irradiation in man but for obvious reasons it cannot be accurately determined.

Clinical consequences of radiation

THE ACUTE RADIATION SYNDROME
Direct information on the syndrome in man has emerged from observations on Japanese exposed at Hiroshima and Nagasaki and from accidents at nuclear reactors.

Cerebral effects which are invariably fatal occur soon after very high doses of radiation. The onset of symptoms occurs within a few hours and death generally follows within 2 days. They include lethargy, tremors, ataxia and convulsions. These may be related to arteritis, oedema, and pyknotic changes, especially in cerebellar cells. Nausea and vomiting also occur, particularly after the exposure of any considerable volume of tissue to a high dose.

At lower dose levels, or if recovery from the cerebral syndrome should occur, gastrointestinal symptoms predominate. Nausea, vomiting and severe diarrhoea are associated with histological evidence of necrosis of the intestinal mucosa. If the dose is sufficiently small to allow regeneration of the bare villi, replacement of losses of fluid and electrolytes may be followed by recovery. The gastrointestinal features occur in 3–5 days and, if untreated, death may occur soon after onset of symptoms or up to ten days later. If regeneration of the intestinal mucosa does not occur, localized and generalized infection may follow. The occurrence of granulocytopenia makes bacterial infection of the denuded mucosa almost certain.

After lower doses of the order of 500 rads to the whole body, anorexia, nausea and vomiting may subside without the occurrence of diarrhoea. In that event, the haemopoietic effects follow in two to three weeks.

The effects of whole body irradiation on the peripheral blood are secondary to effects on bone marrow and lymphoid tissue. These take time to develop and initially are clinically silent. Many Japanese victims of the atomic bombs were able to return to work after transient anorexia, only to die of haemorrhage or infection complicating aplastic anaemia several weeks later.

Lymphocytolysis begins immediately after exposure

and lymphopenia is maximal 24 hours later. Effects in the bone marrow are slower to evolve. Mitosis and DNA synthesis are arrested at once but the marrow becomes hypocellular only when maturing cells are delivered to the peripheral blood and not replaced by fresh divisions. The granulocytes in the peripheral blood may show an initial transient rise only to fall thereafter and reach a minimum 6 weeks following exposure. Platelet levels behave similarly but reach a minimum in the fourth week when spontaneous haemorrhage may occur. Death may occur in this period from a combination of haemorrhage, gastrointestinal ulceration and infection. Hypogammaglobulinaemia resulting from lymphocytolysis probably increases the liability to infection.

Significant anaemia occurs later than either granulocytopenia or thrombocytopenia, unless its onset is hastened by haemorrhage or infection. If these do not occur, haemoglobin levels below 7 g/100 ml are reached about 2 months after the total cessation of erythropoiesis. If haemorrhage or infection does not supervene recovery is likely.

The accepted treatment is aimed at protecting the victim from infection by nursing in a sterile room with filtered air. Food is sterilized and losses of fluid and electrolyte must be replaced. Preparations of IgG prepared from pooled human plasma have been given in an attempt to prevent infection. When infection occurs, antibiotic therapy is indicated. Anaemia and thrombocytopenia may be controlled by transfusion of packed red blood cells and platelet concentrates. Successes have also been claimed for bone marrow homografts in the victims of some nuclear reactor accidents.

Radiation exposure in pregnancy

High doses of radiation such as were encountered at Hiroshima and Nagasaki may result in abortion or foetal death. Lower doses before the eighteenth week may have resulted in an increased number of microcephalic children born subsequently.

Only essential diagnostic radiation should be carried out in pregnancy, and particular care taken to avoid direct exposure of the foetus.

Delayed somatic effects of radiation

Cataracts

These occur only after exposure to relatively high doses of radiation, as in reactor accidents and Japanese atom bomb survivors. Neutron radiation is particularly liable to be followed by the occurrence of these lenticular opacities.

Leukaemias

An increased incidence of leukaemias has been found in many groups of individuals as a late consequence of heavy radiation exposure. The most carefully studied have been patients who have received X-ray therapy for ankylosing spondylitis and Japanese survivors at Hiroshima and Nagasaki. In both these groups the incidence of leukaemias bears a direct relationship to the dose of radiation. The types are chronic myeloid and acute leukaemia with various kinds of cellular differentiation. No increase was noted amongst the Japanese survivors until 2 years after radiation and the peak incidence occurred in the sixth to eighth year afterwards. A second peak incidence of acute

TABLE 33.1. Average annual rate of leukaemias per 100,000 of population in a sample of exposed persons in Hiroshima and Nagasaki. After Bizzozero O.J. *et al.* (1966) *New Engl. J. Med.* **274**, 1095.

Type	Year of onset			
	1946–9	1950–4	1955–9	1960–4
Exposed at 0–1500 metres from the hypocentre				
Acute	2·07	28·21	26·24	9·24
Chronic granulocytic (myeloid)	4·15	19·91	10·50	9·54
Exposed at 1501–10,000 metres from the hypocentre				
Acute	0	1·32	3·46	1·46
Chronic granulocytic (myeloid)	1·24	0·66	0·69	0·73

leukaemia only, occurred thirteen years after exposure. Twenty years after radiation the number of new cases of acute leukaemia and chronic myeloid leukaemia amongst the heavily exposed survivors was still higher than in members of the general Japanese population of the same ages. For less heavily exposed survivors the rates have not differed from those for the Japanese population as a whole since 1946.

Acute leukaemia and chronic myeloid leukaemia also occur in other individuals including radiologists, children irradiated *in utero* (p. 35.13) and patients receiving radiotherapy for both malignant and nonmalignant diseases. The mode of induction of leukaemia by radiation is not known. The occurrence of chromosomal changes in blood and bone marrow cells after radiation exposure, and the finding of similar changes in leukaemic cells in the minority of individuals who subsequently develop leukaemia, is only suggestive. The Philadelphia chromosome (p. 28.12), which is specific for chronic myeloid leukaemia, occurs in postradiation cases of the disease. It has not been demonstrated with certainty in irradiated persons who have not developed chronic myeloid leukaemia.

Radiation exposure has been used as a means of inducing leukaemias in laboratory animals in which its effect is additive to those of leukaemogenic viruses and inherited predisposition.

Other neoplasms

The first instance of skin cancer in a radium worker was described in 1902. Since then there have been innumerable instances of tumours of skin, thyroid, bone, larynx, pharynx and lung following both occupational and therapeutic radiation exposure. Because of their generally longer latent period, their occurrence among patients irradiated for ankylosing spondylitis and in Japanese survivors was not recognized as quickly as the increased occurrence of leukaemias in the same groups.

An increase in the occurrence of carcinoma of the breast was recently found among women who had had repeated fluoroscopy for the control of artificial pneumothorax used many years previously in the treatment of tuberculosis. These women had received very high total doses, of the order of 90 rads.

Aplastic anaemia

The status of aplastic anaemia as a late effect of radiation exposure is uncertain. It undoubtedly occurs as an acute effect and at high dose levels it may prove fatal; many cases of anaemia that occur as a late effect of radiation exposure are in fact due to acute leukaemia.

Sterility

Radiation doses sufficient to cause amenorrhoea may be followed by resumption of normal ovulation. In cases where recovery is slow, premature ovarian involution may occur with permanent sterility.

Doses of up to 300 rads to the human testes may be followed by ultimate recovery of normal spermatogenesis, as judged by the number of sperm. Even after doses of 100 rads or more, oligospermia may be of slow onset and complete recovery may follow after months of no effective spermatogenesis.

Accelerated nonspecific ageing

The evidence for a nonspecific reduction in lifespan after radiation exposure in man and animals is unconvincing. At higher doses, life expectation is reduced but there is insufficient evidence to enable any nonspecific ageing effect to be distinguished from the numerous harmful effects of radiation, both acute and chronic, on various tissues (p. 36.12).

Other delayed somatic effects in man

Myocarditis, pericarditis, pneumonitis and a form of chronic nephritis may all occur as late consequences of high doses of radiation. These effects are relatively uncommon but occur in patients who have received some forms of radiotherapy without appropriate shielding of the organs in question.

The inflammatory response

With high doses, cell necrosis and a polymorph response are seen but these changes develop more slowly than after other forms of injury and may not reach a maximum until several weeks after exposure. In other respects the histological appearances of the tissue are those of a nonspecific inflammatory response although some features suggest specifically a radiation injury. Some blood vessels are dilated while in others there is marked thickening and hyalinization of the vessel walls. Cells with ballooned cytoplasm showing pyknosis are sometimes seen (p. 25.26). In the healing phase fibroblasts assume unusual forms. As in other forms of chronic inflammation, healing is by the formation of a fibrous scar, but this scar lacks the usual toughness and is readily damaged by further radiation. A radiation ulcer of the skin often fails to heal as the epithelium does not readily grow over the fibrous tissue in the base.

Genetic effects of radiation in man

There is a tantalizing lack of direct evidence in man bearing on this important question. That harmful mutations may result from radiation seems almost certain. They have been found in every other species studied, and the demonstration of microscopic radiation damage to human chromosomes makes the occurrence of finer damage almost beyond question. The difficulty in man is to detect and measure the effects of these mutations.

All but a few genetic mutations are certain to be harmful. In other species, harmful recessives are much more common after radiation exposure than are mutant genes which behave as dominants or intermediates. As a consequence, few are detectable in the first generation after radiation exposure. In man, the detection of such harmful recessives is further complicated by the impossibility of the kind of controlled breeding used by experimental workers, and by the longer human generation time.

The most likely human populations for the detection of radiation-induced mutations are the offspring of survivors of the atomic bombs exploded at Hiroshima and Nagasaki. These have been studied by what is known as the **population characteristic method**. In this approach, the offspring of the irradiated individuals are compared with the offspring of controls or the population as a whole as regards such features as stillbirths, neonatal deaths, sex ratio, birth weight, congenital malformations and postnatal development. It is reasonable to assume that this method may detect the summation of harmful mutations occurring at many genetic loci. The only positive finding is a significant change in the sex ratio of children born to exposed parents, whether the irradiated parent was the father or the mother or both. These findings are in agreement with the results of several smaller studies on the sex ratio of children born to radiologists, X-ray technicians and patients who have received radiotherapy. All these findings are in keeping with the induction of harmful mutations in human subjects, both male and female, exposed to radiation. Part of the observed effects on the sex ratio of children may be due to the induction of meiotic nondisjunction by radiation. This seems as likely to be demonstrable in man as in other species. The best direct evidence of this is an excess of stillbirths and trisomic children born to women who have had diagnostic abdominal radiation before the pregnancy in question. Apart from the population characteristic technique used at Hiroshima and Nagasaki it might be possible to detect harmful effects of radiation in man by what is known as the **specific phenotype method**. This requires the measurement of the occurrence of known and readily detected dominant effects in the children of irradiated parents. No convincing evidence of such effects has yet been found but they are likely to be very difficult to detect.

An ingenious approach was made to the question of the occurrence of genetic effects of radiation in a part of the state of Kerala in South India. There, the occurrence of thorium-bearing minerals makes for a very high natural background radiation. Gruneberg and his colleagues trapped a number of wild rats in the area of high background and in a neighbouring area of normal radiation background. No difference was found between the two groups of rats in respect of a number of skeletal and dental measurements. Both groups of rats included a number of pregnant females. Their litters *in utero* were compared to provide data on fertility and embryonic mortality and no difference was found. It thus seems less urgent to organize the difficult and expensive study of human subjects which was once contemplated, although possible effects in man cannot be excluded.

FURTHER READING

CRONKITE E.P. & BOND V.P. (1960) *Radiation Injury in Man.* Springfield: Thomas.

The Hazards to Man of Nuclear and Allied Radiations (Cmnd. 9780) (1956) London: H.M.S.O.

The Hazards to Man of Nuclear and Allied Radiations. (Cmnd. 1225) (1960) London: H.M.S.O.

MEREDITH W.J. & MASSEY J.B. (1968) *Fundamental Physics of Radiology.* Bristol: Wright.

NEEL J.V. (1963) *Changing Perspectives on the Genetic Effects of Radiation.* Springfield: Thomas.

OUGHTERSON A.W. & WARREN S. (1956) *Medical Effects of the Atomic Bomb in Japan.* New York: McGraw-Hill.

PURDOM C.E. (1963) *Genetic Effects of Radiations.* London: Newnes.

Reports of the United Nations Scientific Committee on the Effects of Atomic Radiation. (1958 & 1964) New York: United Nations.

RUBIN P. & CASARETT G.W. (1968) *Clinical Radiation Pathology.* Philadelphia: Saunders.

WARREN S. (1961) *The Pathology of Ionizing Radiation.* Springfield: Thomas.

Chapter 34
Demography, vital and health statistics

The Romans invented the idea of a periodic census of the people and resources of their empire; Jesus of Nazareth was born in Bethlehem because his family had travelled there for a Roman census, the purpose of which was to provide information about the number of people who could be taxed. Like the Romans, the British imperialists took much trouble to number the people and introduced censuses in their overseas colonies and dominions. Other colonial powers did likewise, so there are some records of the population in many parts of the world for about the last 100 years. Recording of baptisms and marriages was obligatory in many mediaeval European countries where parish registers helped to prevent violation of ecclesiastic laws proscribing marriages between kin; burials were also recorded in these registers. Repeated outbreaks of plague led to an ordinance in England in 1532, requiring weekly completion of 'Bills of Mortality', and this in a much modified form is still enforced. Using these early records Graunt published in London in 1662 the first book on vital statistics, the *Natural and Political Observations upon the Bills of Mortality, With Reference to the Government, Religion, Trade, Growth, Air, Diseases, and the Several Changes of the Said City*. Graunt was one of the first Fellows of the Royal Society and this book was an important contribution to the development of science at that time. He calculated age-specific death rates (p. 34.2) and so was among the first to document the very high mortality of infants and young children; he also observed that death rates were higher in towns than in rural areas.

Accurate and comprehensive records of births, marriages and deaths, with age and cause of death, which are essential data of modern vital statistics have been refined and improved since then. Sweden has had an Official Statistical Commission since 1758; and the **General Register Office** (GRO) was established in London in 1839, two years after the Births, Marriages and Deaths Registration Act, which provided for the registration of these events. Farr, the first **medical statistician** to the GRO and Graham, the first **Registrar-General**, did much in England and Wales to establish the reputation for precision of the records. These records have been of great value for many purposes, not least of which has been the development of **demography**, the scientific study of factors that influence population. Similar systems of recording are used in many other nations and have been introduced with varying degrees of success in many developing countries. Computers, used increasingly to expedite processing of data, may eventually allow annual reports to be published within weeks rather than years of the end of the period to which they refer; it may soon be possible to obtain at short notice a tabulation of complex statistical data which might once have required years of clerical work.

Value of vital and health statistics

These statistics reflect the health of the community in much the same way as records of temperature, pulse and respiration reflect the health of the individual. Quantitative knowledge of the effects of diseases upon the community is essential for planning countermeasures and for evaluating their effectiveness. Attempts to foresee trends in the pattern of disease are valuable in planning future medical and social services; future needs for trained persons, for accommodation and for equipment can be estimated and appropriate budgetary and other arrangements can be made. Statistical records are also a valuable tool of the research worker, enabling him to identify causes of disease and to distinguish related diseases with different distributions or natural histories. The scope of such statistics has been greatly enlarged in the last two decades. Statistical data on nonfatal illnesses are collected both from the health services and directly from the population by sample surveys based on interviews and examinations. Statistics relating to hospital patients are collected in many countries; data have been collected from general practitioners and other community-based services in a few places. In Britain available morbidity statistics refer mostly to patients discharged from hospitals and to data on specific diseases notifiable by law. In addition, many general practitioners (through the Royal College of General Practitioners), medical officers of health, and research workers in medical schools have compiled morbidity data about conditions of special interest. **Record linkage** involves collation of several items of information about the same person. For example hospital and public health records may be linked with data from register offices so that individual health dossiers covering a lifetime can be compiled. This has great potential value for long-term studies of the natural history of disease.

INDICATORS OF COMMUNITY WELLBEING

A study group of the World Health Organization defined twelve components of the level of living of a community as follows, health including demographic conditions, food and nutrition, education including literacy and skills, conditions of work, employment situation, aggregate consumption and savings, transportation, housing including household facilities, clothing, recreation and entertainment, social security, and human freedoms. Others besides the first of these are associated with health, though their relative importance differs. All can be measured or counted, with varying degrees of precision. The study group gave pride of place to health as a component of the level of living, and in this chapter only health and those components with obvious close relevance are considered.

DEFINITIONS AND METHODS

A **census** is an enumeration of the people. A good census is needed by almost every branch of government, not least by the health department. Census soon becomes obsolete, so it is customary to repeat the enumeration at intervals of 10 years. In countries where many of the people are illiterate or follow a nomadic way of life the information collected can give little more than the numbers of both sexes and a rough estimate of age. In more highly developed countries a more detailed assessment is possible, covering age, sex, marital status, number of dependants, nature of habitation, occupation and many other facts. Information is usually collected by enumerators, who obtain information from heads of households about every individual present in the locality for which they are responsible on the day of census. Save when interrupted by war in 1941 the census has been held in Britain in the first year of every decade since 1801. It is now realized that 10-year intervals are inadequate for some purposes, and additional data were collected in 1966 from a 10 per cent sample of the population.

The 1966 sample census showed that about 10 per cent of the population had changed their home town in the previous 12 months. This is a higher figure than in earlier estimates and it reflects increasing mobility of the population. Among the problems raised by this internal migration is the provision of continuity of medical care; efficient storage and retrieval of medical records is essential if continuing care is to be achieved for a mobile population.

Population figures obtained by census or estimate provide the denominators for the calculation of vital rates.

Vital rates are an expression of the frequency of events such as births, marriages and deaths, in proportion to the total population in which they occur. The numbers of these events are obtainable from registrations. Rates are calculated by dividing the number of relevant events in a given time by the total population midway through the period. This population (the denominator) is called the **population at risk**. The resulting fractions are multiplied, usually by a round number (thousand, hundred thousand, million), so that the rates can be expressed as manageable numbers. For example, in England and Wales in 1966 there were 849,823 live births and the mid-year population was 48,188,700. Therefore the **live birth rate** per thousand was

$$\frac{849,823}{48,188,700} \times 1000 = 17 \cdot 6 \text{ per 1000.}$$

In the same year there were 563,624 deaths, so the **crude death rate** per thousand was

$$\frac{563,624}{48,188,700} \times 1000 = 11 \cdot 7 \text{ per 1000.}$$

Crude death rates do not allow for the age structure of the population or for other factors which may influence mortality, and are a relatively insensitive indicator of community health and level of living. To compare the mortality experience of populations separated by time or place or social structure, age-specific, sex-specific and cause-specific death rates are calculated. For age-specificity it is usual to divide the population into 5-year age groups, 0–4 years, 5–9 years, and so on; because these divisions are too small for some purposes, they are combined in various ways, commonly 0–14 (years of infancy and childhood) 15–44 (years of reproductive life) 45–64 (years of middle age) and 65 and over (years of retirement). Other age divisions are often used for special purposes; one of considerable utility is the first year of life, age 0–1. The **infant mortality rate** is defined as the

$$\frac{\text{number of deaths in a year of infants under 1 year of age}}{\text{number of live births in the year}} \times 1000.$$

The infant mortality rate is a sensitive indicator of community health, for when standards of hygiene and sanitation are low, a high proportion of babies die in the first year of life, from gastroenteritis and respiratory infections (table 34.1).

Other important rates of mortality in early life are the **neonatal mortality rate**, i.e.

$$\frac{\text{number of deaths in a year of infants aged up to 28 days}}{\text{number of live births in the same year}} \times 1000$$

the **postneonatal mortality rate**, i.e.

$$\frac{\text{number of deaths of infants in the period 28 days to 12 months after birth}}{\text{number of live births in the same year}} \times 1000,$$

and the **perinatal mortality rate,** i.e.

$$\frac{\text{stillbirths} + \text{deaths in first week of life}}{\text{total live and still births in the same year}} \times 1000.$$

Deaths in the first month of life are mostly associated with prenatal and intranatal factors, congenital malformations, prematurity and birth injury; in the remainder of the first year of life, these conditions are of less importance, but infections and accidents are relatively common, reflecting environmental living conditions. The perinatal mortality rate is a sensitive indicator of the standard of antenatal and obstetric care because most of the deaths in this group are associated with prematurity or birth injury, and so are to some extent preventable if medical care is adequate.

The **maternal mortality rate** is another useful indicator of living conditions, reflecting standards of maternal health and medical care around the time of childbirth. It is expressed as the

$$\frac{\substack{\text{annual number of deaths associated with preg-}\\ \text{nancy, childbirth and the puerperium}}}{\text{number of live and still births in the same year}} \times 1000.$$

Comparisons between countries or regions and at different periods of time can be facilitated by **standardization of death rates,** which allow for differences in population structure. The procedure in Britain is to calculate a **Standardized Mortality Ratio (SMR)** which shows the number of deaths observed (i.e. registered) in the year of experience as a percentage of the number which would have been expected in that year, had the sex/age mortality rates of a standard population operated on the actual population in the year of experience. Death rates in different social, regional or occupational groups within the same country can be accurately compared in this way. For example, Bournemouth, a haven of retired people, had a crude death rate of 17·0 per 1000 in 1966, one of the highest rates in Britain. In Bootle, Lancashire, in the same year, the crude death rate was only 9·2 per 1000, not because Bootle was healthier than Bournemouth, but because it contained a smaller proportion of elderly and retired people. The SMR of Bootle in 1966 was 130 and of Bournemouth 89; thus the SMR provides a more acceptable indication of the comparative levels of health in these two towns than do their crude death rates. Cause-specific and age-specific SMRs are also used.

TABLE 34.1. Birth rate per 1000, infant mortality rate per 1000, percentage of population aged 0–14 years, annual percentage rate of increase, and expectation of life at birth. The upper list is of industrially developed countries and the lower list is of countries in the process of becoming or yet to become industrialized. Japan is in a mid-position on the table, having moved very rapidly into an advanced industrial and technological era.

This table contains much important information. Note the decline in birth rate in industrial countries over the past 40 years and their smaller proportion of children in relation to the total population, when compared to non-industrialized nations; this means that their rate of increase will be less than in the latter group of countries in the next as well as in the present generation.

	Birth rate			Infant mortality rate			Aged 0–14 1964–6 (%)	Annual rate of increase 1964–6 (%)	Life expectation at birth (years) latest available	
	1920–4	1945–9	1964–6	1920–4	1945–9	1964–6			Male	Female
Sweden	20	19	16	61	26	13	22	0·7	71	75
Denmark	23	21	18	82	41	19	24	0·8	70	75
Netherlands	26	23	19	74	40	14	29	1·4	71	76
England & Wales	21	19	18	77	39	19	23	0·8	68	74
Scotland	24	20	19	92	51	23	26	0·2	66	72
U.S.A.	23	23	19	77	33	23	31	1·5	67	74
Australia	23	23	19	61	28	18	30	2·0	68	74
Japan	35	27	14	165	67	19	30	1·0	65	70
Ceylon	39	39	33	192	111	56	41	2·6	62	61
India*	33	27	38	187	177	73	41	2·4	42	41
Philippines	33	N.A.	25	157	115	73	47	3·3	47	48
Mexico	31	45	45	226	105	54	44	3·4	55	58
Jamaica	36	31	39	175	90	35	41	2·0	56	59
Venezuela	28	39	47	155	98	48	45	3·6	N.A.	N.A.
Chile	41	34	36	241	150	107	40	2·3	50	54
Nigeria*	N.A.	N.A.	49	N.A.	110	70	N.A.	2·0	N.A.	N.A.
Ghana	N.A.	N.A.	50	N.A.	82	38	45	2·7	38	38

* Some figures available for registration districts only, not necessarily representative of whole country. N.A. = not available.

Life tables are a further refinement of mortality statistics; they were first used by actuaries, interested in the individual's chances of survival, or of dying before his next birthday. A life table begins with a hypothetical population of 100,000 at birth. Arithmetical methods are used to calculate numbers of survivors at the end of each successive year of age, assuming the hypothetical population has the same mortality experience at each age as the real population, whose age-specific mortality rates are known. Further calculations are made to obtain the **probability of dying** before the next birthday, and the **expecta-**

tectomy combined with radiotherapy in the management of carcinoma of the breast. Comparisons are best made by life table analysis of large numbers of patients treated by these methods; due allowance is then made for the effects of other causes of death on the number of survivors at the end of each year after the completion of treatment. The results of the two methods are similar, i.e. the proportion of cases alive at the end of each successive year after completion of treatment is about the same in both groups. Life table analysis has also been used to compare survival rates of patients with breast cancer

TABLE 34.2. Abridged life tables showing years of expectation of life at birth and subsequent ages, based on the mortality experience of England and Wales in the stated periods.
   Note the relatively small increase in life expectation at age 45 and 65, especially of males, in comparison to the increase in life expectation at birth over the last 120 years.

Expectation of life at age	1838–54		1891–1900		1920–2		1950–2		1964–6	
	Male	Female	Male	Female	Male	Female	Male	Female	Male	Female
0	39·9	41·7	44·1	47·8	55·6	59·6	66·4	71·5	68·4	74·7
15	43·2	43·9	45·2	47·6	50·1	53·1	54·4	59·0	55·4	61·3
25	36·1	37·0	37·0	39·4	41·6	44·5	45·0	49·4	46·0	51·5
45	22·8	24·1	22·2	24·2	25·2	27·7	26·5	30·8	27·1	32·5
65	10·8	11·5	10·3	11·3	11·4	12·9	11·7	14·3	12·0	15·7

tion of life of a hypothetical individual in the life table population at each age from birth onward. Expectations of life at birth or at some other convenient age are sometimes used to compare the state of health of different countries (see table 34.1), or of the same country at different periods of time. The expectation of life at birth and at different ages of males and females in England and Wales during the last 150 years are shown in table 34.2. The figures are calculated from life tables using data mostly from years close to a census. It can be seen that there has been a large increase in expectation of life at birth since 1838–54, but after middle age the increase has been much smaller; people who reach middle age are not living much longer than in Victorian times, but a higher proportion are surviving to middle age. Female experience has been more favourable than male, mainly because of a smaller mortality from ischaemic heart disease and lung cancer in middle aged women, discussed more fully below.

Life tables are useful when analysing the mortality from occupational diseases, e.g. pneumoconiosis or industrial malignant diseases. This method is also used to compare survival rates of patients treated in different ways for cancer and to assess the efficacy of different treatments. For example, there has been much discussion about the relative merits of radical mastectomy and of simple mas-

before and after radical mastectomy became available; before 1900, less than 20 per cent of patients remained alive five years after the condition had been diagnosed; today the proportion is slightly more than 50 per cent. A less happy picture emerges when life table analysis is carried out in relation to the clinical stage (i.e. severity) of the disease when it is first diagnosed; this suggests that whatever form of treatment is used, it has little effect on the ultimate fate of the patient. Patients whose disease is detected at a very early stage have, on average, a longer remaining life span than patients whose disease is far advanced when it is first detected; but this longer time is about equal to the time it would take the disease to progress from an early to an advanced stage.

Ageing of the population describes the condition when an increasing proportion of older people are present. Its most common cause is a simultaneous decline in birth and death rates.

Epidemiologists may express the burden of a particular disease in a population in two ways. The number of new cases arising within a given period divided by the population at risk gives the **incidence rate** for that period. The number of cases existing at a point in time divided by the population at risk gives the **point prevalence rate**, or simply **prevalence rate**.

SOCIAL CLASS

All men are not equal. From earliest times the efficient operation of human communities has required specialization of work and a hierarchical social structure has been an inevitable consequence. In mediaeval Europe, ability, aggressiveness, chance and family connections sorted the people into the aristocracy who had all the land, wealth and power, and the serfs who had none. Between the two there developed a middle class of merchants, bankers, doctors, lawyers and priests; this class retained its name while replacing partially the aristocracy at the upper end of the social ladder. The industrial revolution created much greater complexity of manufacturing industries and so added to the diversity of occupations and opportunities for individual advancement. Difficult tasks demanding great skill, responsibility and prolonged training are usually rewarded with prestige and high income while unskilled jobs offer lower income and status. The citizens of an industrial state can be graded socially in terms of educational level and specialized skills acquired by training, income or wealth, rateable value of property or dwellings, and prestige or status in society. The correlation between all these is close, though there are some obvious exceptions; bookmakers, professional footballers and pop singers for example may not advance in the educational system as far as clergymen or university teachers but they often have larger incomes. There are also important, if ill-defined, differences in attitudes or sense of values, not necessarily related to income or education, distinguishing philistines from aesthetes, puritans from hedonists, and those who value health from those who take no care to husband it. As most people have a definite occupation, this is a

useful criterion in constructing a scale of social status; the economic value of the occupation is probably the most important of several factors which relate social class to experience of health and sickness. T.H.C. Stevenson, Chief Medical Officer of the General Register Office in 1911, devised the **Registrar-General's Occupation Classification** which is given in table 34.3.

TABLE 34.3. The Registrar-General's classification of occupations with examples of each social class and the proportions of the male employed population in each at the 1961 census. Figures for 1951 in parenthesis.

Class	Description, examples	Percentage
I	Higher professional and administrative: medical practitioners, lawyers, managers of large commercial organizations	3·6 (3·3)
II	Minor professions and businessmen: school teachers, pharmacists, farmers	14·5 (14·5)
III	Skilled occupations: (1) clerical, e.g. bank-teller (2) manual, e.g. occupations requiring apprenticeship training	48·6 (52·9)
IV	Intermediate and semiskilled workers: factory operatives, agricultural workers	19·8 (16·1)
V	Unskilled workers: labourers, domestic servants	8·7 (13·1)
Unclassified		4·8 (—)

This has proved a useful epidemiological tool; there are significant associations between social class and many diseases (fig. 34.1). Although useful to the epidemiologist,

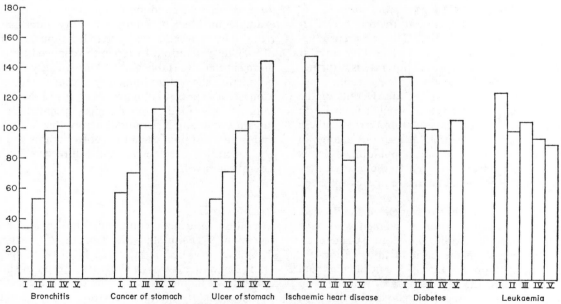

FIG. 34.1. Social class and mortality: SMRs for specific diseases of males aged 20–64, England and Wales 1949–53.

the Registrar-General's classification of occupations has several defects. It takes no account of the status of those not working and can give a misleading impression of the social or economic importance of certain occupational groups in the community. At the 1961 census, a socio-economic classification was used for the first time. This divided the population into seventeen economically active (wage-earners, salaried and self-employed persons) and nine economically inactive categories. Reallocation of the former into one of the five social classes is possible but the latter group of categories, which includes students, housewives, inmates of institutions and retired persons, has no precise equivalent, although it makes up for this by being a more accurate designation. A classification into twenty-six is cumbersome for statistical analysis but correlation of socioeconomic groups with health and sickness experience might prove to be at least as close as social class.

FERTILITY

An important indicator of the wellbeing of a society is its capacity to reproduce itself and so perpetuate its existence. Birth rates are an inaccurate indicator of fecundity as they do not allow for the age distribution of the population or for mortality in infancy or childhood before the newborn have reached reproductive life. The **fertility-rate** allows for the former, by expressing live births as a proportion of the female population of child-bearing age (15–44 years). The legitimate fertility rate is the number of legitimate live births divided by the total number of married women aged 15–44 (per 1000). The **reproduction rate** allows for differences in fertility at age periods throughout the reproductive years of life. It can be calculated separately for the two sexes, i.e. male births in proportion to the number of males aged 15–19, 20–24 and so on to 40–44, and female births in proportion to the number of females aged 15–19, 20–24, . . ., 40–44. The gross reproduction rate is calculated from the sum of fertility rates at single years of age; the net reproduction rate is a further refinement which allows for deaths in the age range 0–14, i.e. before the reproductive years of life. Details of the methods of calculation are given in specialist works on demography and interested readers are referred to these for further information. A simple measure of change in numbers is the **rate of increase** of a population, which is the percentage change from one year to the next; it may be positive or negative. Some illustrative figures are given in table 34.1.

Another measure of fertility is **completed family size**, the number of live-born children of women who have completed their reproductive life, i.e. aged 45 and over. This can be computed on the basis of information obtained at a census. Completed family size in England and Wales has declined in the last 100 years, from 6·16 in 1861–9 to 3·30 in 1900–9 and (estimated) 2·15 in 1951.

The population has increased despite this diminution in completed family size, partly because a larger proportion of children survive long enough to marry and reproduce in their turn. For this reason another useful indicator, this time of potential fertility, is the proportion of the population aged under 15 years. If this is high and rising, a sharp increase in numbers of the population will follow if the majority of these children survive into the reproductive years. This has been happening in many developing countries which have recently emerged from an era of high infant and childhood mortality. Some relevant figures are given in table 34.1.

Trends in fertility and reproduction rates can be interpreted best in the context of data on other sociological changes. Thus in Britain the age at which women marry has progressively fallen, the ages of bride and groom have approached closer to equality, and higher proportions of young married couples have been starting married life in homes away from the parents, than in the early part of the twentieth century. These changes, which reflect increasing affluence, greater emancipation of young people (especially young women), and perhaps less readily measurable changes in attitudes to marriage, might have been expected to lead to increasing fertility and reproduction rates. That they have not done so is due primarily to family planning.

Until recently, population increased relatively slowly in most tropical countries. Malaria, gastroenteritis, acute respiratory disease, tuberculosis and parasitic infestations combined to cause very high mortality in infancy, childhood and adolescence, so that in some places only one in four or five of all who were born stayed alive long enough to reproduce themselves. The main effect of introducing public health measures in these countries has been to reduce infant and childhood mortality very rapidly. For example in Mexico, infant mortality rates have been reduced from over 200 per 1000 to less than 60 in the space of a single generation. In Japan the change has been even more spectacular (table 34.1). Consequently the graph of population shows that humanity appears to have entered a phase of exponential increase (fig. 34.2). Mankind will outgrow his food supply unless population growth rates are contained. Unquestionably this is the greatest and the gravest public health problem of this and the next few generations. It deserves and will receive further consideration in vol. 3.

MIGRATION

Migration influences community health and the interpretation of health statistics. Generally it is the young, fit and fertile who migrate. The birth rate falls and the crude death rate rises as a short-term result of substantial emigration; immigration has the opposite effect. Migration has slightly altered the ethnic composition of the

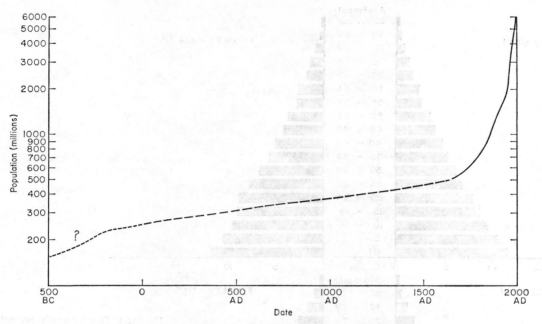

FIG. 34.2. World population from early history to 2000 A.D. (logarithmic scale).

population in Britain in the last decade. In the period 1960–66, about 582,000 immigrants entered England and Wales on passports from 'new' Commonwealth countries, i.e. predominantly non-European by ethnic origin, and 549,000 emigrants departed on UK passports; these were mostly Anglo-Saxon stock. In the same period, 192,000 people entered England and Wales on foreign passports, 49,000 entered on passports from 'old' Commonwealth countries (Australia, New Zealand and Canada) and 220,000 entered from the Irish Republic. This is a massive population movement by any standards, and is part of the world-wide turbulence of population which has been produced primarily by disproportion between population growth rates and availability of natural resources in various parts of the world since the middle of the nineteenth century. Like the Irish and the central Europeans who crossed the Atlantic to North America in the nineteenth and early twentieth centuries, the West Indians and Pakistanis who came to Britain recently had a simple choice, migrate or sink into deeper poverty. Many who have settled permanently in Britain are materially better off than their contemporaries who stayed at home, and it is likely that the better nutritional standards will be reflected in greater average heights and weights of the next generation, compared to those who did not migrate. Such changes have been observed among Japanese in Hawaii and California. The short-term economic and social consequences of these massive migrations are considerable, but it is possible that the ultimate genetic effects, which will not be apparent for several centuries may be even greater. Antagonism between migrant and settler is often aggravated by visible differences between

them; it is to be hoped that in time the ethnic groups will intermingle and the visible differences, like the social, economic and cultural differences, will become less obvious, perhaps disappear altogether.

Internal migration is constantly changing the population distribution within Britain. Scotland has been exporting people to England for several hundred years. After a long period of movement into SE England, the balance began to shift in the mid-1960s to East Anglia and the W. Midlands. These population movements have obvious implications for decisions about major capital investment, e.g. on new hospitals.

Population changes in Britain

Statistics of the size of the population in England and Wales were not systematically available until the introduction of the census in 1801, but there is no reason to doubt the accuracy of estimates in the eleventh century and towards the end of the seventeenth century. The population of England and Wales was about 1·5 million in 1086 and 5·5 million in 1695. At the time of the census in 1801 it was 9 million; by 1851 it had doubled to 18 million and by 1911 it had doubled again to 36 million. In 1966 it had increased by a further third to 48 million, and no doubt would have been much greater were it not for considerable emigration. It is evident that after several centuries of gradual growth the population increased more rapidly during the eighteenth century and this increase continued throughout the nineteenth and into the early twentieth century. Over the same period the age composition of the population changed. Today, more than 12

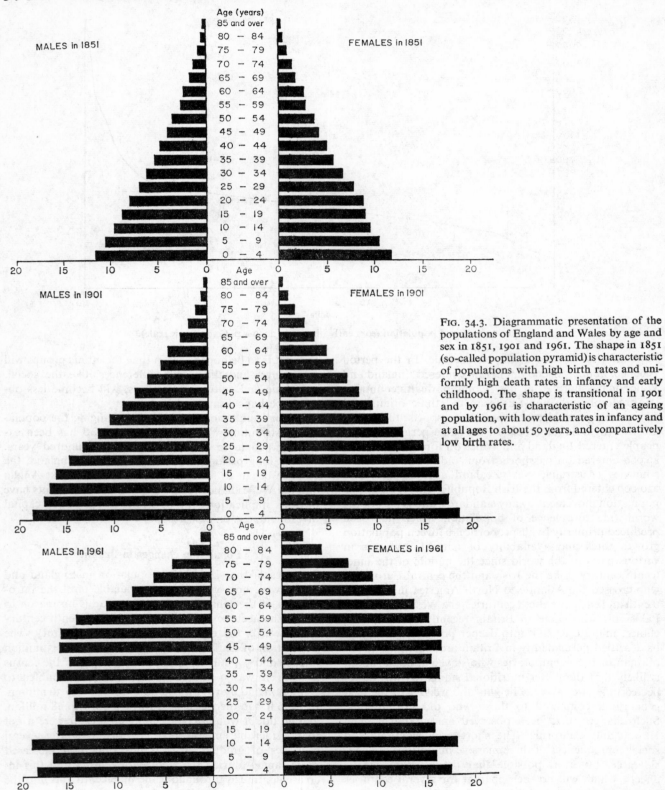

FIG. 34.3. Diagrammatic presentation of the populations of England and Wales by age and sex in 1851, 1901 and 1961. The shape in 1851 (so-called population pyramid) is characteristic of populations with high birth rates and uniformly high death rates in infancy and early childhood. The shape is transitional in 1901 and by 1961 is characteristic of an ageing population, with low death rates in infancy and at all ages to about 50 years, and comparatively low birth rates.

per cent of the population is over 65 years of age and less than 23 per cent is aged under 15, whereas a century ago less than 5 per cent were over 65 and just over 35 per cent were under 15 years of age. The proportion aged 65 and over is expected to increase to about 15 per cent in the next 20 years, and then to remain stable while the proportion aged under 15 will rise again to above 25 per cent.

The exact causes of the sudden increase in the eighteenth century have been the subject of controversy among demographers. The principal cause of population growth was probably a decline in mortality, because the evidence is against the alternative explanation of an increase in the birth rate. Although detailed data are not available it is fairly certain that the birth rate in Britain at the end of the seventeenth century was already high, and could not have risen much further. There is no evidence that the marriage rate increased or that the age at marriage fell. There is no evidence of a change in fertility rate; birth control was almost certainly not practised then or earlier, and there is no evidence of any change in the incidence of diseases which might affect fertility.

The changes in the age composition of the population during the last 100 years have been due first to the fact that both the death rate and the birth rate have been falling, and second to the fact that there have been major changes in the death rate during the first fifty years of life. During the nineteenth century the death rates between ages 3 years and 50 years fell remarkably, and during the twentieth century the death rate in the first three years of life has also fallen. The effects on age distribution of the decline in birth rate and increase in the proportion surviving infancy, childhood and early adult life are shown in fig. 34.3. Death in the first fifty years of life is now relatively uncommon, although intrauterine or foetal death rates and death rates in the later age groups have altered little.

Mortality statistics

The least equivocal indicator of community health is death. The common causes of death, and the ages at which death commonly occurs, are especially useful. Even without precise knowledge of the causes of death, some inferences concerning community health can be drawn if the age groups in which the majority of deaths occur are known. Infant and maternal mortality rates vary inversely with standards of hygiene and sanitation, and are influenced by standards of medical care. Malnutrition and undernutrition also jeopardize the individual child's chances of survival, as do tropical diseases such as malaria. When the majority of deaths occur in old age rather than infancy, the causes are quite different; communicable diseases and malnutrition are then under control and people instead die of degenerative, neoplastic and chronic inflammatory disorders (table 34.4). The sex distribution of deaths has altered in European countries during the past 150 years. Male births exceed female in the ratio of 106:100 and this ratio varies little from country to country.

An excess of male deaths occurs at all ages. Among boys and young men this is especially due to violence whereas at later ages it is mainly due to ischaemic heart disease, chronic bronchitis and carcinoma of the lung. The position was different in the first half of the nineteenth century, when maternal mortality was still considerable. At that time young and middle-aged widowers were much more numerous than young widows.

COMMON CAUSES OF DEATH

The distribution of causes of death differs with age, between the sexes, in relation to environmental factors such

TABLE 34.4. Contribution to mortality of leading causes of death. Scotland 1965.

Age group	Deaths occurring in age group (%)	Leading causes of death	Contribution to mortality in this age group (%)
0–1	4·1	Birth injuries	31·7
		Congenital malformations	20·5
		Diseases of early infancy	18·0
		Bronchitis and pneumonia	12·5
		Other violence	7·0
		Diarrhoea	2·7
1–24	2·0	Traffic accidents	24·2
		Other violence	18·7
		Malignant neoplasms	11·4
		Bronchitis and pneumonia	6·9
		Diseases of nervous system	6·4
		Heart diseases	5·0
25–44	4·0	Malignant neoplasms	24·7
		Heart diseases	22·7
		Diseases of nervous system	9·8
		Other violence	8·8
		Traffic accidents	6·2
		Bronchitis and pneumonia	4·1
45–64	25·9	Heart diseases	35·9
		Malignant neoplasms	29·0
		Diseases of nervous system	11·7
		Bronchitis and pneumonia	6·4
		Other violence	2·5
		Traffic accidents	1·3
65+	64·1	Heart diseases	36·9
		Diseases of nervous system	21·9
		Malignant neoplasms	16·5
		Bronchitis and pneumonia	7·6
		Other violence	2·1
		Senility	0·6
All ages	100·0	Heart diseases	33·9
		Malignant neoplasms	19·3
		Diseases of nervous system	17·7
		Bronchitis and pneumonia	7·2
		Other violence	3·0
		Traffic accidents	1·3

Diseases of nervous system consists mainly of vascular lesions ('stroke').
Other violence comprises domestic and industrial accidents and suicide.

as occupational exposure to noxious substances, and between countries at different levels of health and economic development. Table 34.4 lists the leading causes of death according to age, in Scotland in 1965; the distribution is similar in other industrially developed countries. Only about one death in ten occurs before middle age, in sharp contrast to India and other countries at a similar level of development, where two thirds or more of all deaths occur before the age of 45 years. The leading causes of death in developing countries are infections, the more important being tuberculosis and other respiratory infections, and infectious diarrhoea.

Death certification

Mortality statistics provide much information in addition to the age at which death takes place. In most countries

disease or condition directly leading to death, and the antecedent morbid conditions which contributed directly to this. Other significant conditions contributing to but not related to the disease or condition causing death should also be mentioned (fig. 34.4). Ideally the medical terms and diagnostic labels used on death certificates should be based on an accepted international classification. Unfortunately the *Manual of the International Statistical Classification of Diseases, Injuries and Causes of Death* (*ICD*) which is drawn up and regularly revised by committees of the World Health Organization is sadly inadequate. The precision of death certification is not very great; in hospital practice, where adequate diagnostic aids are most likely to be used, only a little over half of all deaths can be certified accurately without autopsy examination. The accuracy also varies with the cause,

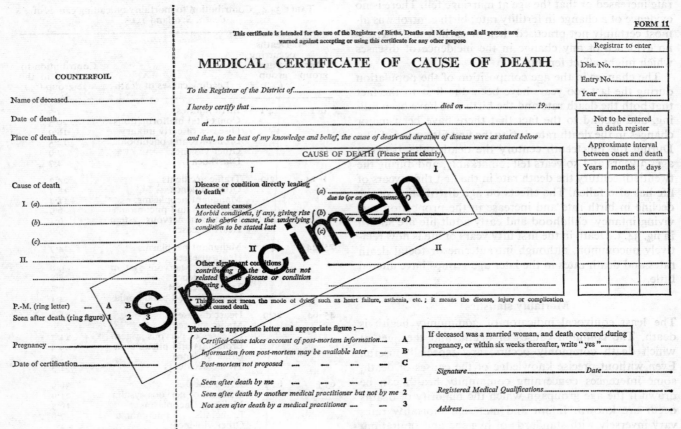

FIG. 34.4. Form of death certificate used in Scotland. The form is similar in most other countries.

doctors have an obligation to certify their opinion as to the cause of death. It is unacceptable to record that death was due to heart failure or asphyxia. The death certificate is both a legal and a statistical document. Its form has been agreed internationally to provide for worldwide comparisons of mortality statistics. The doctor or other authority certifying death is required to name the

being highest when death is due to accidents or to certain forms of malignant disease in young people. Less than 30 per cent of deaths in Britain are preceded by an operative or other diagnostic procedure or followed by autopsy and can thus be certified with precision. Ischaemic heart disease and lung cancer are confirmed by autopsy or before death by appropriate diagnostic procedures in under

50 per cent of cases. The steadily rising mortality rates from these conditions in middle-aged men are however confirmed by epidemiological surveys which indicate that the increasing number of death certificates bearing these diagnoses does in fact parallel a real increase in incidence of death from these diseases.

Mortality changes in Britain

Statistical information on mortality relates principally to cause of death, to age and to sex. Although data on the cause of death must be subject to general reservations about the historical consistency of diagnostic terminology there is no doubt that there has been a remarkable change in the frequency with which infections have been certified as a cause of death and a comparable change in the opposite direction in the frequency of the noninfectious diseases (fig. 34.5). In accounting for these changes it is

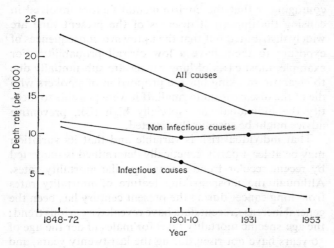

FIG. 34.5. Mean annual death rates, males, England and Wales. From McKeown T. & Lowe C.R. (1966) *Introduction to Social Medicine.* Oxford: Blackwell Scientific Publications.

reasonable to distinguish three groups of diseases, tuberculosis, gastrointestinal infections, and acute infections, such as scarlet fever, diphtheria and smallpox.

During the latter half of the nineteenth century the decline in tuberculosis accounted for almost half of the total decline in mortality. The death rate from tuberculosis has steadily fallen since the earliest period for which we have any useful information (fig. 34.6). Specific therapy played no part in this early fall, nor did specific preventive procedures. The causes of the improvement have been much discussed. Tuberculosis is a disease of poverty and mortality rates fell throughout the period when personal incomes and living standards were rising in the second half of the nineteenth and the first half of the twentieth centuries; the disease waned as people became better housed,

better clad and better fed. Analysis of tuberculosis death rates by generation of birth (cohort analysis, p. 34.16) shows that earlier generations had higher mortality at all ages than those born more recently. Declining death rates from gastrointestinal infections can be explained by improved standards of personal hygiene and environmental sanitation. In the case of the acute infections it is almost certain that a change in the virulence of the streptococcus accounts for reduced mortality from scarlet fever; and introduction of specific immunization procedures helped to reduce the number of deaths from smallpox and diphtheria.

Death in early life is now largely determined by the circumstances of prenatal and intranatal experience. The most common conditions associated with perinatal mortality are prematurity, congenital malformations, asphyxia and birth injury. The circumstance most associated with variation in perinatal mortality in Britain is the social class of the parents. Despite improvements in perinatal mortality over the past twenty-five years, the differences between the classes have been unaffected and, for a wide

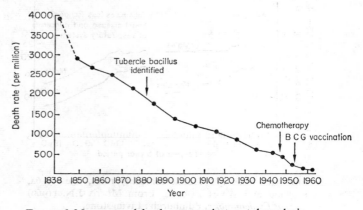

FIG. 34.6. Mean annual death rate, respiratory tuberculosis, England and Wales. From McKeown T. & Lowe C.R. (1966) *Introduction to Social Medicine.* Oxford: Blackwell Scientific Publications.

variety of causes of death, infants whose parents are in social class V experience from two to five times the mortality of those whose parents are in social class I. The reasons for this variation include differences in maternal physique and health, but a substantial part of the variation can be attributed to the quality of medical care. If in Scotland the perinatal mortality rates of social class I births could be achieved for all, more than 1500 lives would be saved each year. This is more than could be saved by the eradication of prematurity and congenital malformations and would represent a gain in years of life similar to that which would be achieved by the elimination of death from cancer.

The increase in noncommunicable diseases as a cause of death is particularly marked at the later ages. At least part of the increase is a consequence of the change in the age structure of the population. Has mortality from non-communicable diseases increased apart from this? Because of difficulties in comparing diagnostic terminology over a long period, certified causes of death in relation to many diseases cannot be interpreted reliably. For example, coronary thrombosis was described only during the present century and it is therefore impossible for us to study its historical trends over a longer period. Changes both in diagnostic fashions and in the precision of diagnostic techniques have undoubtedly contributed to the apparent increase in mortality from the neoplastic and degenerative conditions. Because age and sex have been more consistently recorded on death certificates than has diagnosis, it is useful to interpret mortality statistics in relation to these, rather than to changes in diagnostic patterns.

There have been increasing differences in the sex-specific death rates, both crude and age-specific, over the past 100 years (fig. 34.7). Whereas female death rates have

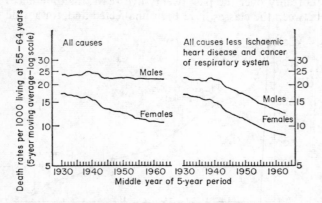

FIG. 34.7. Male and female mortality rates, age 55–64, England and Wales 1930–64. From Morris J.N. (1969) *Uses of Epidemiology*. Edinburgh : Livingstone.

steadily fallen, male rates ceased to fall some twenty-five years ago and have actually begun to rise slightly at later ages. The most important causes are sex differences in mortality from ischaemic heart disease and lung cancer, and it is therefore reasonable to conclude that the total occurrence of these conditions has increased. Another sex difference of considerable interest occurs in mortality from bronchitis. In successive generations there has been a relative increase in mortality among males, affecting all generations since the one whose young men were involved in World War I. The most plausible explanation of this phenomenon is that this was the first generation in which large numbers acquired the habit of cigarette smoking.

In Britain, mortality at the later ages is at present largely attributable to cardiovascular disease, malignant disease and obstructive lung disease. There is an environmental component in the aetiology of these diseases, but

this derives more from individual behaviour than from agents in the physical environment. The possibility that there is also a hereditary component makes it clear that attempts to prevent these diseases by modifying behaviour will pose very different problems from those encountered by the pioneers of public health in the nineteenth century. The features of the environment that needed to be changed in the last century were considered aesthetically undesirable quite apart from any influence they had on health. The behavioural factors that are important in the morbidity of the present time include a wide range of pleasures whose desirability often outweighs the associated long-term risk. It seems unlikely that the human species will develop a genetically determined antipathy to these hazards; the selective effect of a distaste for over-eating, lack of exercise or cigarette smoking will be small, as these habits influence mortality mainly in the post-reproductive period of life.

An additional consideration which at first seems discouraging is that the environmental factors involved in causing the important diseases of the present time are widely distributed but that the untoward consequences of exposure to them have a low overall probability. For example, most cases of lung cancer are substantially due to cigarette smoking but the proportion of smokers who die of the disease is quite small. If it were possible to identify the individuals at especially high risk, preventive advice might be specifically directed.

That individual risk is variable and that its variation may be at least partly genetically determined is suggested by recent secular trends in age-specific mortality rates. Although the most striking feature of mortality rates from lung cancer during the present century has been the general increase, recent data have revealed a curious trend; the age-specific mortality rates for males under the age of 50 years have not risen during the last twenty years, and in the age range 30–34, mortality rates from lung cancer have been falling slightly. At ages over 50 years the rates have risen and the later the age, the greater has been the rise (fig. 34.8).

The possibility that age-specific differences might be due to corresponding differences in the thoroughness of diagnosis is ruled out by the absence of a similar phenomenon in female mortality rates which, at all ages, are much lower than those of males. Almost any reasonable explanation of the phenomenon involves the hypothesis that the age at which lung cancer is contracted reflects individual responsiveness to the aetiological agent. Those who die young are presumably highly susceptible, while those whose death is delayed until a later age are less susceptible. In the first half of the twentieth century, the cigarette smoking habit increased in prevalence to the point where it was almost universal among males. The death rates of those with a rapid response to smoking would be expected to follow the smoking trend after only

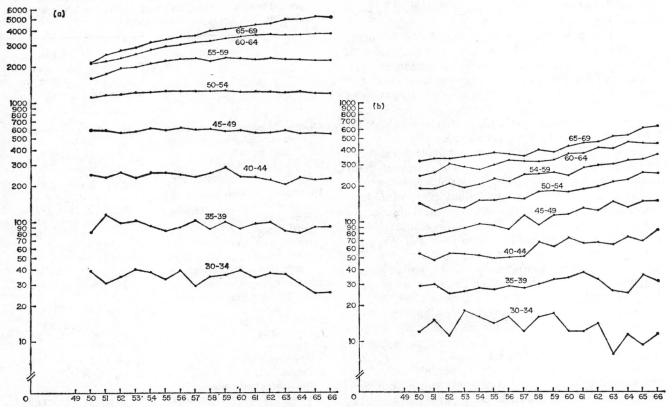

FIG. 34.8. Age-specific mortality rates for lung cancer (a) male (b) female, England and Wales, 1949–66. Small numbers produce rather unstable rates at ages 30–34 in females but rates are rising at all ages over 35 in females, only over 55 in males.

a short interval, while the death rates of those in whom the disease takes longer to appear would follow the smoking trends of a period longer ago. Thus we should expect flattening out of the death rates to occur first among young people and later in older people.

That the postulated variability in responsiveness to the pathogenic stimulus may be genetically determined is suggested by two main considerations. The first is that there is a sex difference in mortality from cancer of the lung at any given level of cigarette consumption. The second consideration is a more general one and is relevant to all conditions which show a sharp rise in mortality after middle age. Many of these diseases, characteristic of the post-reproductive phase of life, may occur at these later ages precisely because individuals genetically disposed to contract them while young have been selectively eliminated from the population. In the case of lung cancer the introduction of cigarette smoking as a reinforcement to selection pressure began two or three generations ago. Its earliest effect might be the presently discernible tendency for lung cancer mortality rates to fall among young adults. This possibility, that high risk is to some extent genetically determined, paradoxically enhances the possi-

bility of control; early identification of individuals at high risk may become feasible. The implication that preventive medicine may in future depend more on the identification and specific education of high risk persons, has social consequences not only relevant to the functions and organization of health services and the training of doctors but also to the general education of the public.

Morbidity statistics

Doctors or other health workers in most countries are required to notify certain illnesses and disabilities whenever they encounter them. The frequency of **notification of communicable diseases** may thus be a reliable indicator of community health. Diagnosed cases of diphtheria and typhoid fever are probably notified in Britain with completeness approaching 100 per cent. However a few cases of whooping-cough or measles may pass unrecognized, and it is unlikely that all are notified, because many doctors do not take very seriously their obligation to notify these diseases. Other important diseases which by statute should be notified to public health or other authorities may not be recognized because of diagnostic difficulties; thus some cases of lead poisoning, a notifiable industrial disease, may not be detected, and some patients may shun medical attention, e.g. some cases of open pulmonary tuberculosis.

Cancer registration has been introduced in many countries in order to obtain data on incidence and survival. In Britain, however, hospital inpatients and outpatients with a diagnosis of cancer are registered on a voluntary basis. Age, sex, diagnosis (site and nature of lesion) and method of treatment are recorded and the information forwarded to the General Register Office for consolidation and statistical tabulation.

Sickness from causes other than notifiable diseases can be ascertained and enumerated by means of sickness certificates, or by the recording of episodes of sickness seen by general practitioners. **Sickness certificates** are variable in quality. Those issued for short-term sickness absence are commonly imprecise, but their utility as a source of information about community health is greater when the disability leads to prolonged absence from work. The possible causes are fewer in number and are often given a precise diagnostic label. Although cancer is rarely specified, ischaemic heart disease and chronic bronchitis are commonly certified causes of chronic disability. Total numbers of sick absences from work or school give some indication of the prevalence of sickness, revealing for instance quite marked seasonal variations.

Morbidity studies in general practice are difficult to mount and to execute, but if properly carried out they can provide valuable information about the sickness experience of a large and probably representative section of the population. In 1955 the General Register Office and the College of General Practitioners cooperated in a morbidity survey in which 171 doctors collected data for 12 months, covering the sickness experience of over 350,000 people in England and Wales. From this survey came much useful information about the nature and frequency of conditions for which people consult their family doctor. Respiratory disorders were first in overall frequency, conditions of the nervous system and sense organs were second, and digestive disorders third (table 34.5). The distribution has been found to be much the same in similar surveys elsewhere. It should be noted that these are not, strictly speaking, surveys of community morbidity or sickness experience; what is recorded is contacts with the doctor; people who are sick but do not see a doctor are not counted.

Hospital statistics

Admission to hospital is dependent upon the availability of beds and on established custom, as well as upon the nature and severity of the condition from which the patient suffers. Virtually all cases of acute appendicitis, intestinal and prostatic obstruction, and perforated peptic ulcer are admitted to hospital. The same is not true of acute ischaemic heart disease, some cases of which die

TABLE 34.5. Frequency of presentation of conditions in general practice. From *Studies on Medical and Population Subjects*, No. 14 (1958) London : H.M.S.O.

	Percentage of patients consulting	Patient consultation rate per 1000
Diseases of respiratory system	23·1	264·2
Acute nasopharyngitis (common cold)		81·1
Bronchitis, all forms		62·3
Influenza, non-epidemic year		38·2
Diseases of nervous system and sense organs	9·5	119·8
Wax in ears		21·4
Otitis media		19·8
Refractive errors		14·3
Conjunctivitis		14·0
Cerebral vascular lesions		4·9
Diseases of digestive system	8·6	107·0
Gastritis and functional disorders		35·4
Gastroenteritis		22·2
Peptic ulcer		9·2
Hernia		7·3
Appendicitis		4·0
Diseases of skin	8·4	105·6
Infections (boils, etc.)		38·5
Dermatitis, impetigo, eczema		34·9
Accidents, poisoning, violence	8·2	102·0
Sprains and strains		26·5
Symptoms and ill-defined conditions	7·5	94·8
Diseases of bones and organs of movement	6·7	86·8
Arthritis and rheumatism		64·9
Diseases of circulatory system	5·3	68·4
Hypertension		15·7
Ischaemic heart disease		7·2
Infective and parasitic diseases		55·0
Diseases of genitourinary system		52·9
Allergic, endocrine, metabolic and nutritional diseases		50·8
Asthma, urticaria, hay fever		27·5
Obesity		11·4
Mental psychoneurotic and personality disorders		50·0
Psychoneurotic disorders		45·7
Pregnancy		16·9
Diseases of blood and blood-forming organs		14·3
Neoplasms		10·7
Congenital malformations and certain diseases of infancy		4·6
Nonsickness (routine medical examinations, etc.)		53·4

within moments of onset, others of which are nursed at home. To this extent hospital admission statistics (or to be more precise, statistics of hospital discharges and deaths) are an unrepresentative sample of community sickness experience; hospital-based doctors who generalize about the frequency of medical conditions on the basis of hospital experience may be guilty of serious error. However, hospitals represent a major part of health services and even if hospital statistics inaccurately reflect life outside, their value is unquestioned. In England and Wales a 10 per cent sample and in Scotland all deaths and discharges from hospitals for acute diseases are subjected to statistical analysis by age, sex, diagnostic category, length of hospital stay, and so forth. The use of computers to process the data makes available a wide range of tabulations in addition to those which are regularly published in the reports from the **Hospital Inpatient Enquiry**. These have shed much light on the working of hospital services. Statistics from mental hospitals (and from the psychiatric wards of general hospitals) are differently based. Because a large proportion of these patients stay for a long time, statistics are based on admissions as well as discharges and periodic censuses are also carried out.

Child health

The health of children is of obvious national importance. Communicable diseases predominantly affect children, and so relevant information about child health is contained in the notifications of these diseases. Further facts are collected at routine medical examinations which are carried out by the school medical services. Children in Britain are mostly examined routinely three times, in their first school year, at about the time of transition from primary to secondary school, and again before leaving. Dental examinations are held more frequently, and so are medical examinations in some schools and in some other countries. Published statistics give the numbers of children found to be suffering from various impairments and diseases. Visual and hearing loss, poor posture and dental caries, and more serious conditions such as congenital heart disease are often first detected at school medical examinations. The annual reports of the school medical services show on the whole a steady improvement in child health, including nutritional status, during the twentieth century.

Community health surveys

More information about sickness experience can be gathered by approaching selected individuals or groups in the general population to ask questions about their health or to carry out physical examinations. An example of a comprehensive investigation of this nature is the United States National Health Survey which has been collecting information by household interviews since 1957,

and by physical examination since 1959. As a result much information is now available about the frequency of acute and chronic illness, duration of disability, consumption of drugs, admissions to hospital, and so forth. Detailed diagnostic data are not available from the household interview survey as the information is collected by lay interviewers but diagnostic data and normal ranges for many biological values have been obtained in the health examination surveys. Numerous smaller surveys have been done, sometimes with especial attention to particular aspects of sickness experience, for example concentrating upon symptoms and signs of cardiovascular disease or mental health. A good example in Britain is the work of Cochrane and others in South Wales.

Measurement of mental health

Mental health is difficult enough to define, and still more difficult to measure. Indicators of the wellbeing of society which are often quoted and can be misleading, include illegitimate birth rates, divorce and separation rates, suicide, delinquency and crime rates, the frequency of chronic alcoholism and convictions for drunkenness and notifications of venereal disease. It is true that some of these provide useful information on social wellbeing, but allowance must be made for factors that can influence the figures. For example suicide might not be certified as a cause of death because of religious sanctions against it or if dependants' claims for insurance would be jeopardized. Moreover, suicide statistics are not a homogeneous category reflecting mental illness exclusively; suicides include the incurably ill seeking early release from suffering, the economically defeated and others whose suicidal act is an expression of social and religious custom. A sudden rise in the rate of convictions for drunkenness or drug addiction, for prostitution or juvenile delinquency, may reflect a change of superintendent of police rather than an increase of the mental or social malaise in the community.

Rates of admission of patients to mental hospitals may similarly mislead for they are influenced by the interaction of supply and demand for beds, by changing fashions in treatment which lead to outpatient rather than institutional care, and, when disease entities are being considered, by diagnostic disagreements. Hospital admission rates also mislead by failing to take into account the proportion of the community who suffer from mental, psychoneurotic and personality disorders, but do not receive care in institutions, if indeed they receive any medical care at all. Morbidity studies in general practice help to fill this hiatus and suggest that each year about 50 persons in every 1000 consult their family doctor because of some psychiatric disorder. Surveys of whole communities have given rather contradictory results because of differences in definition of mental, psychoneurotic and personality disorders. Depending on criteria used to define mental illness, its prevalence lies somewhere between 1 in 20 and 1 in 5 of the general population.

Special surveys

Special surveys have been made for many purposes, e.g., to measure the heights and weights of school children, so that inferences can be made about growth rates and indirectly about nutritional status, to ascertain the prevalence of dental decay and to discover cases of pulmonary tuberculosis.

Special surveys may be integrated with a routine service such as school medical examinations; they may be a separate service in their own right, e.g. mass radiography for the detection of tuberculosis and other chest diseases, or they may be set up as specific research programmes.

Longitudinal or 'cohort' studies

The methods of health measurement so far considered all require the collection and analysis of facts as they exist at a given time. Health may also be studied by following the progress of a group of people over a prolonged period in a longitudinal or cohort study. In this manner Douglas and his colleagues have obtained valuable information about the physical and mental development and health, social wellbeing and educational attainments of a sample of people born in Britain in one week in 1946. Similar methods are used to follow the progress of several groups of adults in selected communities. Detailed information gradually accumulates about every individual in a cohort study, and with some reservations it may be possible to generalize from these observations to the community from which the selected individuals have been drawn. For example, Dawber and others have followed the progress of a random sample of about 5000 people living at Framingham, Massachusetts, and Epstein and others have studied about 8000 inhabitants of the small town of Tecumseh, Michigan. Both studies have been concerned with chronic diseases, especially ischaemic heart disease. Overweight, cigarette smoking, hypertension, elevated serum cholesterol level and left ventricular hypertrophy are among the so-called risk factors which have been demonstrated unequivocally to be associated with significantly higher incidence of ischaemic heart disease.

Mortality statistics can be analysed by cohorts or generations of births, a procedure which has demonstrated what appear to be generation differences in susceptibility to diseases such as tuberculosis (fig. 34.9) and lung cancer (fig. 34.10).

> FIG. 34.10. Male mortality from lung cancer by generation of birth, Scotland. Whereas fig. 34.9 shows a steady decline in mortality from tuberculosis with each successive generation, the reverse has occurred in the case of lung cancer, each generation showing greater mortality than its predecessor. Compare fig. 34.8 which presents similar data in the form of age-specific rates.

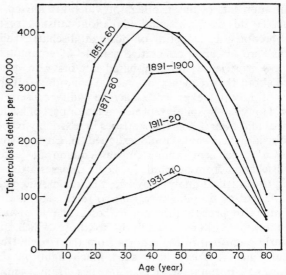

FIG. 34.9. Male mortality from respiratory tuberculosis by cohort or generation of birth, England and Wales. From Springett V.H. (1952) *Lancet* i, 521.

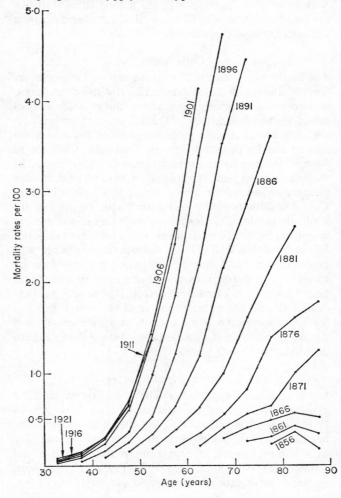

In a cohort or generation analysis the mortality or morbidity experience of successive generations is examined. Thus, the survivors of males born in the last five years of the nineteenth century were aged 0–4 in 1900, 10–14 in 1910, 20–24 in 1920, 30–34 in 1930, 40–44 in 1940, 50–54 in 1950, 60–64 in 1960 and so on. Published tables of mortality statistics provide sex-, age- and cause-specific rates from which the relevant figures for each generation of births can be extracted. In this way the data summarized in figs. 34.9 and 34.10 were compiled. This technique differs from the usual methods of examining mortality statistics, which compare age-specific rates at different ages at a given period, e.g. rates in 1966 of men aged 45–54, 55–64, etc., or compare secular trends in age-specific mortality rates, e.g. mortality of men aged 45–64 in 1926, 1936, 1946, 1956, 1966.

Record linkage

Data relating to the several vital and health events recorded in respect of an individual can be assembled so that the whole body of data for the person can be treated as a statistical unit. If this is then to be extended to include all individuals in a large population, each such individual must be reliably and unambiguously identified on each of the several records relating to him. Thus record linkage depends on the availability of a good identifying system which can be handled by automatic data processing machines. A possible system would assign a unique number to each individual at birth. Such a number might consist of a sequence of digits corresponding to the day, month and year of birth, digits for sex and for registration district of birth, and a further digit sequence corresponding to the individual's order of birth registration in that district. Unfortunately, unless the numbers are known to the individuals their use is limited.

However, use may be made of the variety of names and the relatively small number of births on any one day. The chance of two different persons (not twins) having the same name, sex and date of birth, is very small. There are about 3000 births each day in England; only about fifty of these have the commonest surname (Smith); only twenty-five are of each sex and probably only one has even the commonest forename. Computer-based procedures for using these facts to link records have been well justified in practical trials. Acheson has used such methods successfully in the Oxford Record Linkage Study. When vital statistics have been matched with other data such as clinical records from hospitals or general practice, a treasure house of epidemiology is unlocked. Even in the numerically small-scale Oxford Record Linkage Study, important discoveries have included identification of deficiencies of antenatal care in general practice, and an association between nasopharyngeal carcinoma and occupation in woodworking industries.

Record keeping in clinical practice

Computer workers have a saying, 'garbage in, processed garbage out'. The quality of epidemiological data is only as high as the quality of the records upon which they are based. Mortality statistics are an incomplete indicator of community health at least to the extent that death certification is faulty. Records compiled in clinical practice are often inadequate as a source of epidemiological data. Retrospective record reviews depending on facts recorded in a medical history which might have been taken once only by a young overworked hospital doctor, cannot be expected to yield precise knowledge of the patient's previous occupations or lifetime smoking habits. Even seemingly significant clinical data, results of laboratory investigations, final diagnosis, and details of therapeutic regime, may not have been fully recorded. When a clinician compiles accurate and complete clinical case notes, he makes a lasting and significant contribution to the care of his patients and to the ultimate understanding of disease.

FURTHER READING

ACHESON E.D. (1967) *Medical Record Linkage*. London: Oxford University Press.

BENJAMIN B. (1968) *Health and Vital Statistics*. London: Allen & Unwin.

DAWBER T.R. *et al.* (1962) The epidemiology of coronary heart disease—the Framingham enquiry. *Proc. roy. Soc. Med.* **55**, 265.

DOUGLAS J.W.B. (1968) *The Home and the School*. London: McGibbon & Kee.

EPSTEIN F.H. *et al.* (1965) Epidemiological studies of cardiovascular disease in a total community—Tecumseh, Michigan. *Ann. intern. Med.* **62**, 1170.

SMITH A. (1964) Trends in mortality from respiratory disease 1929–1963. *Ann. Rep. Registrar General Scotland 1963, No. 109.*

SWAROOP S. (1960) *Introduction to Health Statistics*. Edinburgh: Livingstone.

Chapter 35
The epidemiological approach to disease

Disease can be studied at the bedside, in the laboratory and in the community, the three methods complementing one another. The third method is **epidemiology**, the study of the distribution and determinants of disease in populations. Clinical medicine is concerned with the diagnosis and treatment of disease in individual patients; in the laboratory, biochemical, microbiological and pathological aspects are investigated while in epidemiology evidence of disease is studied and measured in a whole population. Although the epidemiological, clinical and laboratory approaches may differ in emphasis, they overlap at many points.

The domain of clinical medicine extends beyond the current state of the individual patient to the environment in which the patient lives, his personal habits, his work, the health of other members of his family, and the changes that may have occurred in these factors in the past. While the good clinician studies as far as possible all the circumstances of a particular patient's disease, the epidemiologist studies, again as far as possible, all the patients in a defined population. Both clinician and epidemiologist increase understanding of disease and both hope to control it. However, the clinician seeks information to help him reach the correct diagnosis and to provide a basis for the successful management of the patient, while the epidemiologist investigates factors implicated in the causation of the disease, hoping to find specific ways of preventing it.

Epidemiology now takes all disease for its brief, but was originally concerned with communicable disease and especially with epidemics. An **epidemic** is defined as the occurrence of numbers of cases of a disease in excess of normal expectations. It follows that normal expectations must be known. Diseases are spoken of as **endemic** if substantial numbers of cases are present at all times.

Every doctor must know something about the epidemiology of the diseases with which he is dealing and should be aware of the possibilities of epidemiology as an investigative technique.

History

Epidemiology is not a new science. Hippocrates appreciated the importance of studying disease in its environmental context, as his title, *Airs, Waters, Places*, implies. The Hippocratic aphorisms could only have been compiled after prolonged and careful observation of many patients. There was often little else the ancient physician could do but observe the progress of disease in individual patients and, on many occasions, the progress of epidemics. In 1546 Fracastorious wrote *De Contagione*, generally regarded as the first treatise on epidemiology; he recognized the contagiousness of epidemic diseases such as typhus, and described the three methods of infection, by direct contact, by 'fomites' or infected clothing, utensils, etc., and at a distance, as in smallpox and plague, i.e. 'droplet infection' in modern parlance. In the next 300 years many distinguished physicians added to epidemiological knowledge. Sydenham, the greatest of the seventeenth century English physicians, advocated careful observation at the bedside, but his *Medical Observations* (1676) include much epidemiological as well as clinical wisdom. Another early epidemiologist was Ramazzini, who identified environmental hazards associated with certain occupations and published his results in 1700; he is regarded as the founder of occupational or industrial medicine.

NINETEENTH CENTURY SANITARY REFORM
Until comparatively recently, the major health problems in every country were epidemic and endemic communicable diseases and little effective treatment was available. A doctor who wanted to influence events could do so only by studying the circumstances in which disease occurred in a community and by trying to alter those circumstances. In Britain, the challenge presented by the spread of disease in the rapidly growing industrial towns during the nineteenth century was met by the emergence of dedicated sanitary reformers. These included many doctors and the whole movement was supported by epidemiological studies. Their work was made possible by the introduction of a complete registration system of births, marriages and deaths (p. 34.1). Two English doctors exemplify the nineteenth century development of epidemiology; one, William Farr, was an exponent of vital statistics and the other, John Snow, adopted the field study or 'shoe-leather' approach. Both studied the

spread of the great cholera epidemics that occurred in Britain between 1832 and 1876.

Farr's annual reports on vital statistics provided evidence of the effects on health of the grim environmental conditions of his time, and formed ammunition for sanitary reform as the following extract from his 1874 report shows.

'Take for example the group of 51 districts called healthy for the sake of distinction, and here it is found that the annual mortality per cent of boys under 5 years of age was 4·246, of girls, 3·501. Turn to the district of Liverpool; the mortality of boys was 14·475, of girls 13·429. Here it is evident that some pregnant exceptional causes of death are in operation in this second city of England. What are these causes? Do they admit of removal? If they do admit of removal, is this destruction of life to go on indefinitely? It is found that of 10,000 children born alive in Liverpool 5396 live five years; a number that in the healthy districts could be provided by 6554 annual births. This procreation of children to perish so soon, the sufferings of the little victims, the sorrows and expenses of their parents, are as deplorable as they are wasteful. In Liverpool the death of children is so frequent and dreadful, that a special system of insurance has been devised to provide them with coffins and burial ceremonies. The mother when she looks at her baby is asked to think of its death, and to provide by insurance not for its clothes but for its shroud and other cerements.'

There can be no doubt that Farr, by this combination of fact and stirring language, stimulated action to improve living conditions and community health.

SNOW ON CHOLERA

Snow, a London anaesthetist, studied epidemics of cholera in the 1840s and became convinced that polluted water was responsible for these. At that time London was supplied by many water companies, most of them drawing from the heavily polluted Thames. From 1849–53 there was no cholera in London; during that time the Lambeth Water Company moved their works upstream to Thames Ditton and so obtained relatively pure water. The parts of London supplied by this company were also supplied by the Southwark and Vauxhall Company who drew from the river at Battersea, a very polluted part of the Thames. These circumstances gave Snow a chance to test his hypothesis about the spread of cholera.

An epidemic of cholera occurred in the summer of 1853, and Snow was able to show that in districts supplied only by the Southwark and Vauxhall Company the death rate was 114 per 100,000 while it was 60 per 100,000 in districts supplied by both companies; but there were no deaths at all in districts supplied exclusively by the Lambeth Company. These results were suggestive but by no means conclusive. The districts with different supplies could have differed in many ways; for example those with the 'good' supply might have been wealthier and less overcrowded, and to a certain extent this was so. The next year Snow sought better evidence. He had discovered that in the districts where both companies supplied water, they had competed for custom in almost every street; so that in every neighbourhood there were some houses supplied by the Southwark and Vauxhall, some by the Lambeth Company. When an epidemic occurred in July 1854, he obtained the addresses of everyone who died from cholera in districts where both water companies were operating and personally visited their houses to discover which supply was taken.

He went on to find out the number of houses supplied by each company and so was able to calculate rates (table 35.1). The rate of cholera deaths per 10,000 houses

TABLE 35.1. Mortality from cholera in London in the 4 weeks ending 5 August, 1854. Adapted from Frost W.H. (1936) *Snow on Cholera*. New York: Commonwealth Fund.

Water company	Houses supplied	Deaths in 4 weeks ending 5.8.54	Rate per 10,000 houses
Southwark and Vauxhall	40,046	286	71
Lambeth	26,107	14	5
All others	287,345	277	9

was 14 times greater among those supplied by the Southwark and Vauxhall Company than among those supplied by the Lambeth Company. Moreover, as the table also shows, the rate in houses supplied by the Lambeth Company (5 per 10,000) was lower than that in the rest of London (9 per 10,000) although the former houses were in the area of greatest incidence of the disease.

Snow's achievement not only showed how cholera could be prevented but illustrated how a careful study of its occurrence and a logical analysis of the evidence could lead to an understanding of a mysterious disease. His conclusion, as paraphrased by Frost (1936): 'that cholera was due to a specific micro-organism, an obligate parasite, propagating only in the human intestinal tract and disseminated by ingestion of excreta', was a remarkable feat thirty years before Koch discovered the cholera vibrio.

Many other studies of the distribution and determinants of communicable diseases were carried out in the nineteenth and early twentieth centuries. Among the most important of these were the studies by Manson of filariasis, Ross of malaria, and Reed of yellow fever. These three physicians not only worked out the complex epidemiology of tropical diseases spread by insect vectors, but also firmly established an understanding of ecology, the interaction between living things, and founded the science of medical entomology.

TAKAKI AND BERIBERI

Towards the end of the nineteenth century, research on conditions thought to be communicable pointed the way towards epidemiological study of noncommunicable disease. One of these was the investigation of beriberi carried out by Takaki, a Japanese naval doctor, in the 1880s. Numerous attempts were made at that time to isolate a causal organism from cases of beriberi; in fact, seventeen different organisms were demonstrated confidently by various investigators. Takaki studied the conditions in which the disease occurred in the Japanese Navy and after detailed investigations of its incidence in relation to many environmental factors, he came to the conclusion that a dietary deficiency was the cause; he thought that when the ratio of protein to carbohydrate was too low, beriberi resulted. About the time Takaki completed his investigations, a naval training ship with a complement of just under 300 men reported 169 cases of beriberi on a voyage lasting 9 months. Takaki tested his dietary hypothesis by sending another ship to repeat the voyage, this time supplying the crew with an improved diet. Only fourteen cases occurred, all in individuals who had refused to take the condensed milk and meat provided. Takaki, now Surgeon General, was able to take the necessary action to improve the diet in the navy, with the result that beriberi virtually disappeared within a year. Although his theory of the precise dietary fault was wrong, his demonstration that the disease was due to the lack of some nutritional substance was quite clear. Nearly 50 years later thiamin, the vitamin concerned, was synthesized (vol. 1, p. 5.13).

Takaki's work illustrated the part epidemiology can play in the investigation of noncommunicable disease. Beriberi was a problem because no successful treatment of the sick person was available and the nature of the disease was not understood. Clinical investigation of individual patients was unable to contribute to this understanding and so attention was focused on the study of the conditions in which the disease flourised. Takaki was able to achieve the ultimate aim of epidemiology, the abolition of the disease, at least in the Japanese Navy. Beriberi is no longer widespread, but is still an important condition in some rural areas in the East, where epidemiological methods have a place in helping to control it. For example, a curious feature of the incidence of beriberi in Malaya during the 1930s was its rise during periods of prosperity and its fall when the economy was depressed. Burgess was able to explain this pattern by an epidemiological study; when the country prospered, small-holders were able to buy milled rice (deficient in thiamin) and in consequence the disease appeared; in hard times they ate their own hand-pounded rice. This was less palatable but contained the essential vitamin. Infant mortality rates similarly increased with prosperity, due to the rise in infantile beriberi.

GOLDBERGER AND PELLAGRA

In much the same way as Takaki, Goldberger investigated pellagra in the Southern United States before World War I. This too was then thought to be a communicable disease. Goldberger observed that it occurred among inmates but not staff of institutions such as prisons and mental hospitals; if it were communicable, staff who were exposed should have become infected. He then showed that it could not be transmitted by any means whatsoever to volunteers, but that isolated volunteers developed the disease when fed on a monotonous diet comparable to that of institutional inmates. He was able to demonstrate that the pellagra-preventing factor was water soluble and heat stable, and occurred in the same foodstuffs as thiamin, but he died before the identification of nicotinic acid (vol. 1, p. 5.14). Takaki and Goldberger were pioneers in the use of epidemiology for the study of diseases that were not infectious.

The studies of epidemic dropsy by Lal and Roy and others in Bengal are another example of epidemiological investigation of a mysterious disease; this was shown to be due to poisoning by Mexican poppy seeds which occurred as a contaminant in mustard oil used to prepare curries.

MODERN TRENDS

In this century, the emphasis of epidemiology in Britain and America has shifted in accordance with changing patterns of disease and attention is concentrated mostly on noncommunicable disorders.

Despite the increasing refinement of epidemiological methods, described below, the investigation of epidemic communicable disease still requires painstaking detective work. The procedures and machinery of notification are the tools of the communicable disease epidemiologist, and a 'shoe-leather approach', collecting information in the field rather than waiting for it to arrive at a desk in the health department, is essential. The work is fascinating and must always remain a vital part of the medical services; although communicable diseases are now much less common in contemporary industrial nations, the defences against them cannot be allowed to fall into disrepair. Explosive outbreaks of food poisoning, epidemic influenza, hospital-acquired infections, venereal diseases, and occasionally imported diseases are always a challenge. In the search for sources and mode of spread of an epidemic, all the evidence must be carefully sifted. The task may be simplified by advances in microbiology and immunology, because laboratory tests can sometimes pinpoint the source of infection, such as a typhoid carrier, or contamination of the sterile water supply in an operating theatre. Computers expedite the processing of data.

Methods

Measurement of disease in populations is the basis of epidemiology. Comparisons almost always must be made between populations by calculating rates. The first step is to define the population which provides the denominator for the calculation of rates (p. 34.2). This may be the whole population of a country or region, or perhaps a specified group. For example in recent years there have been studies on all the children born in Britain in the first week of March 1946, on London busmen, on San Francisco longshoremen, and on all doctors on the *Medical Register* in Britain in 1951. Communities have also been selected for detailed study; Framingham, Massachusetts, and the Rhondda Fach in South Wales have been used as field laboratories.

Since it may be difficult or too expensive to gather information from all the population, reliance must often be placed on the findings in a representative sample. The basis of **probability sampling** is a procedure which ensures that every individual in the population has an equal chance of being selected in the sample which is studied in detail. There are good and bad methods of sampling. It is unacceptable to draw a sample of, say, every hundredth name in the telephone directory. This sample is subject to socioeconomic bias, weighted in favour of the well-to-do in residential suburbs; and a uniform sample based on an alphabetical listing is deficient in people with uncommon names. Sampling names which begin with certain letters of the alphabet can lead either to inclusion or exclusion of disproportionate numbers of Scots (names beginning with Mac) or Irish (names beginning with O'). Voters lists or electoral rolls are a better basis from which to sample. To avoid the bias of uniform regular sampling **a table of random numbers** should be used.

Another method, popular in countries where lists of the population are not available, is **area sampling.** A region is dissected into easily defined localities, each containing approximately equal populations. Areas are then sampled by the use of random numbers. Individuals or households in each sampled area can be investigated, or further sampled in the same way. This is the method used in the United States National Health Survey (p. 34.15). Statistical methods (vol. 1, chap. 3) are applied to ensure the validity of results obtained in sample surveys.

OBTAINING DATA

Existing sources of information such as vital statistical records are a fruitful source, used by many since Farr's time to throw light on health problems and associated environmental factors. Nowadays morbidity data are also used. Medical certificates for sickness absences from work, general practitioners' records, hospital inpatient and outpatient records, and specific notifications such as cancer registrations may have epidemiological importance, either as they are routinely compiled, or after being augmented by specifically collected facts.

If existing sources of information are inadequate, the next step is often to ask questions of medical staff, patients or members of the public who may be approached by postal questionnaire or personal interview. The former is cheaper and larger numbers can be surveyed, but personal interview is often the only way to get detailed information, especially about behaviour or attitudes that might influence health. Although even more expensive, a further method is to conduct medical examinations, e.g. anthropometry, measurement of blood pressure, and biochemical values.

In an enquiry based on sampling, the results are subject to bias if the response rate is low. Steps should be taken to find out whether those who do not respond differ qualitatively in any important respect from the respondents. For example, early results of a mass radiography survey can be misleading, suggesting a somewhat better state of affairs than if the first comers were truly representative of the whole population; it is often found that individuals who shun medical attention include a disproportionate number with chronic respiratory disease including tuberculosis.

INCIDENCE AND PREVALENCE

A distinction must be made between incidence, the occurrence of new disease, and prevalence, the total amount of disease present in a given population (p. 34.4).

The **incidence** of a disease is defined as the number of persons who develop a disease during a given period of time and is commonly expressed as a rate per 1000 of those at risk. In chronic disease, the definition of new development can be difficult. According to circumstances, the measurement of incidence may be based on the first appearance of an abnormality, e.g. in an electrocardiogram, or of a symptom or upon the first absence from work or the first admission to hospital.

Prevalence is defined as the number of persons manifesting a disease, either at a given point in time (point prevalence) or during a given period of time (period prevalence). Both measures are commonly expressed as a rate per 1000 population at risk. As with incidence, prevalence may measure clinical or subclinical disease or precursor abnormalities (p. 35.9).

Incidence and prevalence are related; the prevalence of a disease is determined by its incidence and duration. For acute illnesses, the two measures are similar; for chronic illnesses, prevalence is much higher than incidence. For example, the annual incidence of new cases of malignant disease in Britain is about 160,000; some recover, and those who do not, mostly have the condition for more than a year, so the prevalence of all cases in

Britain is probably at least twice the annual incidence, say 320,000. Each measure has its particular value. Incidence is used in looking for the causes of disease; the comparison of new occurrences in different population groups may suggest environmental or other factors associated with high or low incidence. Prevalence is of special importance in the organization of health services, where knowledge of how much disease is present in a community must be available if resources are to be used properly.

The use of these measurements can be divided arbitrarily into studies of the distribution of disease (descriptive epidemiology) and studies designed to test hypotheses about determinants of disease (analytical epidemiology). There is often overlap but the distinction is useful for explanatory purposes.

OBSERVER VARIATION

The fallacies and fallibility of clinical investigation may be brought to light by measuring symptoms and signs in large numbers of people; this may provide a clearer understanding of the fact that biological values have a **normal range** which shades off into the abnormal, rather than a clear-cut end point between normal and abnormal. The decision between normal and abnormal must often be arbitrary and this may cause an observer difficulty in categorizing correctly.

In recording and interpreting variables such as blood pressure, electrocardiographic changes and opacities on chest radiographs, it is important to take steps to minimize this as well as other possible sources of error. For example, in measuring blood pressure in a survey, allowance must be made for errors due to variation in the sphygmomanometer, to variations in the environmental conditions under which an individual's pressure is being measured, and for variation in the observer's ability to detect the precise end points and to read the scale accurately. On this last point, an observer may claim to be reading to the nearest 5 mm but inspection of the results may show a decided preference for readings ending in 0 rather than 5 (**digit preference**). Variability of a single observer on different occasions, **intra-observer variation**, has been well demonstrated in the interpretation of radiographs; the same picture may be interpreted as normal on one occasion and abnormal on the next. Similarly, two or more observers may disagree on their interpretations of the same radiograph, **inter-observer variation**. Observer variation can be controlled by careful definition of the criteria of abnormality and by training and testing.

Observer variation occurring in the clinical examination of patients is still greater. Experts frequently disagree about a patient's heart sounds, let alone their interpretation. Surgeons asked to estimate the size of an abdominal mass in one test of observer variation offered measure-

ments varying by over 300 per cent. A final fact about observer variation, particularly depressing for the medical student, is that examiners marking students' papers sometimes disagree so widely that the same paper may be given an honours grade by one and failed by another. An elaborate system of safeguards against the consequences of this exists in all good university departments.

In order to evaluate symptoms, questions have had to be designed to elicit **reproducible responses**, i.e. the wording of the question must be so precise that only a limited range of alternative answers are possible (preferably just 'yes' or 'no', or a number, such as the volume of sputum expectorated daily). Questionnaires are available about disorders of the mind and diseases of the respiratory, cardiovascular and musculoskeletal systems, and answers to these are valid, reliable and reproducible. The questions can be translated into other languages so it is possible to compare symptomatology in populations from different geographical, ethnic and cultural backgrounds. These questions are useful in day-to-day clinical practice as well as in epidemiological surveys because they have been carefully designed and tested to ensure that the responses are exact and can be scored or scaled. A chest physician would be wise always to use the Medical Research Council standard questions about the nature of cough and sputum, to obtain meaningful data by which to judge the progress of his patients.

Descriptive epidemiology

Descriptive epidemiology often begins with the analysis of available sources of data, usually published data on mortality and morbidity, and its value is accordingly limited by the nature and accuracy of the facts recorded. Conclusions drawn from such sources are therefore tentative and serve only as a basis for further work. Standard methods were developed for studying epidemics. The spread of the disease was considered under three headings, **time, place** and **persons** or alternatively under the headings host, agent and environment. In an outbreak of communicable disease, the characteristics shown under time, place and persons may indicate quite clearly the mode of spread (table 35.2). These approaches are also useful in the investigation of noncommunicable disease; the pattern shown by descriptive study of a chronic disease may provide clues to its causation and lead to the formulation of hypotheses. More often, it may simply delineate a group in the population at high risk of developing a particular disease and thus requiring special attention from the medical services.

Time

Epidemics of communicable disease are explosive in onset, e.g. when contaminated food or water is consumed simultaneously by large numbers of people. Successive waves of an epidemic can occur if the causative agent or organism is most efficiently transmitted only after a latent interval during which the infected host is non-infectious; this may happen with syphilis and smallpox, but the pattern is rarely clearly defined. Seasonal variation in the pattern of epidemicity is common, sometimes dependent upon the activity of an insect vector, at other times not so

Almost all diseases vary markedly in incidence with age. Communicable diseases such as measles are generally commonest among children but devastating epidemics can occur among adults in a community not previously exposed (measles, smallpox and tuberculosis helped Europeans to conquer the New World in this way). If

TABLE 35.2. Possible epidemic patterns of communicable disease, with some examples. Adapted from Reid D.D. (1962) *Theory and Practice of Public Health*, ed. W. Hobson. London: Oxford University Press.

Epidemiological factors	Mode of spread			
	Direct contact	Airborne infection	Ingestion	Vector
Time	Sporadic	Rapid	Explosive	Usually slow, may be seasonal
Place	Bed, household	Universal	Localized	Confined to vector area
Persons	Family, close personal contact	Children	Common diet or source of supply	Occupational or environmental exposure
Examples	Leprosy, venereal diseases, scabies, puerperal sepsis	Measles, mumps, rubella, influenza	Food poisoning, enteric fever, dysentery, cholera	Malaria, filariasis, trypanosomiasis, yellow fever

easily explained (reasons for the maximum incidence of poliomyelitis in late summer were never found). Variation in incidence over a period of many years is referred to as **secular change**; an example is the steady decline in tuberculosis (fig. 34.6, p. 34.11).

In the chronic diseases, changes are measured in years and, for obvious reasons, interest tends to be concentrated on diseases that are increasing in incidence. These can be identified by examining secular change in age-specific mortality rates (p. 34.13) or by cohort or generation differences in mortality rates (p. 34.16).

Place
Comparisons can be made between countries, for example those with different climates or living standards; or within countries for example between rural and urban areas, or areas distinguished by various geographical features.

Spot maps to plot the location of cases have been much used to study the spread of epidemics, ever since Snow thus followed the course of the Cholera outbreak in Soho in 1854. The technique remains as valuable today, e.g. suggesting the role of an insect vector in Burkitt's lymphoma (p. 28.10); mapping shows that the cases occur only within an altitude, temperature and rainfall range compatible with the activity of an insect such as the mosquito.

Persons
Rates are calculated by age, sex, marital state, occupation or social class; sometimes ethnic or cultural characteristics, religion and family size are relevant.

age incidence is bimodal as with Hodgkin's disease and some forms of leukaemia, the possibility of two sets of aetiological factors is suggested. Sex differences are also observed in incidence and mortality from most diseases, often without obvious explanation. Male incidence and mortality rates exceed female for most communicable diseases (whooping cough is one of the few exceptions) and for most forms of malignant disease (table 28.3, p. 28.17). Striking differences in incidence of many diseases between ethnic, socio-economic and occupational groups have often been related to underlying environmental factors, of which the standard of living is perhaps the most important. Many diseases are significantly associated with poverty or wealth (fig. 34.1, p. 34.5) and some which were formerly thought to be associated with ethnic origin are now believed to be associated more directly with the way of life. For example, carcinoma of the breast is common among women who have not breast-fed their offspring; the higher incidence among western European than Japanese women may not be related to their racial differences, but to the culture: western women, for better or worse, are emancipated from breastfeeding more frequently than the Japanese.

INTERPRETATION
Caution is essential in interpreting the nature of associations disclosed by these analyses. The way in which the relevant population has been constituted must be considered. For example, a particular occupation or geographical area may show a high rate of disease; before assuming that conditions of work or way of life are responsible, it is well to remember that there may have been some form of selection into or out of that popula-

tion. Certain occupations might attract sickly or handicapped individuals; or the fittest individuals might selectively leave the occupation or area. It is important to know the history of how a particular population came to be in a particular place at a particular time.

COMPLETING THE CLINICAL PICTURE
The most interesting part of descriptive epidemiology is concerned with extending knowledge of the distribution of disease beyond the analysis of readily available data. This has been described by Morris as completing the clinical picture and it consists of identifying all the cases in a defined population and sometimes identifying those still in the subclinical or presymptomatic stage. Some examples illustrate how the clinical picture is completed and why this is important.

Ruptured ventricle is a cause of sudden death and is one of the consequences of ischaemic heart disease. Crawford and Morris were impressed by the disagreement in the literature about its incidence. Most papers referred only to hospital patients, and there were conflicting reports on the incidence by sex and age and on an association with anticoagulant therapy. Crawford and Morris wrote:
'The wide differences in the literature on the age and

They searched the post-mortem records of over 95 per cent of the hospitals in the area and obtained records of all the cases occurring in a 65 per cent sample of necropsies carried out in coroners' mortuaries. By scaling up the figures they estimated the total number of cases in the period. Table 35.3 shows that only a small and quite unrepresentative fraction of the total cases were seen in hospital. Teaching hospital experience was particularly unrepresentative; their data indicate that the condition was as common under age 70 as over, and that it was much more common in men than women under 70 with reversal of the sex ratio over 70. A quarter of the male hospital patients under 70 had been given anticoagulant treatment.

When the total figures were related to the population at risk, it was evident that incidence increased sharply with age; below 70, incidence was in fact rather higher in men than in women but over the age of 70, the incidence was similar in both sexes. There are more old women than old men in the population, so the calculation of rates corrects the apparent excess in the numbers of old women affected. In the whole study, only thirteen cases were found who were known to have had anticoagulant therapy. Thus conclusions drawn from the hospital figures alone would be at variance with the true picture in the population.

TABLE 35.3. Number of cases of ruptured ventricle in London 1957–8: estimated total. Adapted from Crawford M.D. & Morris J.N. (1960), *Brit. med. J.* **2**, 1624.

Age	Male				Female			
	Hospitals		Coroners' mortuaries	Total	Hospitals		Coroners' mortuaries	Total
	Teaching	Other			Teaching	Other		
Under 70	15	13	86	114	4	4	60	68
70 & over	4	11	145	160	13	19	240	272
Total	19	24	231	274	17	23	300	340

sex distribution of spontaneous rupture of the ventricle and in the estimates of its frequency are due to selection in the material, to the varying chances of post-mortem examination being made in cases of sudden death, and to bias in the type of hospital studied. The discrepancies must be further aggravated by the use of simple hospital numbers as a basis for estimates of population frequency rates; it is these that are involved in statements that a disease has a different incidence in the two sexes or at different ages.'
Crawford and Morris sought information about deaths from ruptured ventricle in a defined population, the London County Council area of 3¼ million during 1957–8.

This is an example of work done to check the validity of conclusions drawn from the study of hospital patients. The hospital doctor must always keep in mind the possibly unrepresentative nature of the patients and illness seen in hospital; if findings based on hospital patients are to be generalized, enquiries should be carried out in the community to check whether these patients represent an unbiased sample of all persons with the illness.

Chronic glaucoma is a major cause of blindness in the elderly. It has long been believed that raised intraocular pressure precedes and is responsible for the changes in the optic disc and the consequent blindness. It has therefore seemed logical to attempt to prevent the development of chronic glaucoma by identifying individuals with raised intraocular pressure and giving them the appropriate treatment. Examination of large numbers of apparently healthy individuals would produce acceptable results, only if the distribution of intraocular pressure were bimodal, with the characteristic associated defects in the visual field and abnormalities in the optic discs (cupped) occurring only in the right-hand curve (fig. 35.1a).

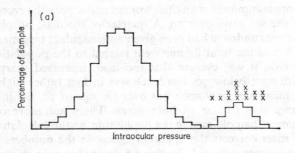

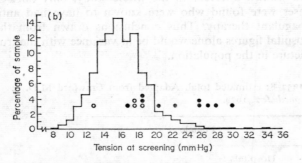

FIG. 35.1. (a) Ideal distribution of pressure and relation to established glaucoma; ×, cases of newly discovered glaucoma. (b) Intraocular pressure in 1920 male right eyes; ○, newly discovered cases with field defect, cupped disc but tension never recorded above 21 mm Hg; ●, newly discovered cases with 'true' glaucoma, field defect, cupped disc and tension known to rise above 21 mm Hg. From Graham P.A. (1968) *The Early Diagnosis of Visual Defects*. London: Office of Health Economics.

In a survey in the Rhondda Fach in South Wales, Hollows and Graham measured intraocular pressure, tested visual fields and examined optic discs. Their results (fig. 35.1b) are very different from fig. 35.1a. As Graham put it:

'Not only is there a smooth transition from the main body of the population to those with higher pressures, but marked glaucoma-like defects in the visual field occur at pressures which would not be regarded as "abnormal" even on the basis of an upper limit of two standard deviations above the mean value. This means that false negatives occur with undesirable frequency when a single measurement of pressure is used. Follow-up studies have shown that some of these patients do at times have pres-

sures above "normal", so that they are false negatives for the fully developed disease with "raised" pressure, field defect and cupped optic disc. Others, however, have never shown higher pressures, and appear to have developed the typical disc and field changes of chronic glaucoma at "normal" levels of pressure. When one also considers the fact that it has been found that there is no apparent correlation between intraocular pressure and the type of field defect usually considered to be the earliest sign of glaucomatous optic atrophy, it becomes clear that we have yet much to learn about the aetiology and early natural history of this disease.'

This is an example of the growing number of epidemiological enquiries stimulated by the search for effective early intervention in chronic disease. In the process of 'completing the clinical picture' fundamental questions about the nature of the disease were raised.

Ischaemic heart disease (IHD) is a major cause of death in the western world (p. 34.9). The incidence of IHD (coronary thrombosis, myocardial infarction, acute angina pectoris, coronary insufficiency are among its names and modes of presentation) has risen rapidly since the 1930s. Among middle-aged men, i.e. age 45–64 years, IHD now accounts for over a quarter of all deaths in Britain, and most other industrially developed nations. The two principal lines on which work is proceeding in an attempt to reduce mortality are prevention and early effective treatment of the acute attack.

Epidemiological studies form the basis for the moves towards prevention and also play a part in attempts to provide better early treatment. The provision of intensive coronary care units in hospital and of mobile units to go to the patient in his home are expensive in the use of money and manpower. It is therefore proper to assess the work of these units and to measure their effects on the mortality and morbidity from IHD in a community.

Since little is known about the total attack rate of the disease, about the proportions of patients treated at home and in hospital in any area and the outcome of treatment, and about the timing of events after symptoms begin, it was decided to record data about every occurrence of acute IHD in Edinburgh over a period of one year.

The study was based on notification by general practitioners of every patient under the age of 70 in whom acute myocardial infarction was suspected. In order to obtain the fullest possible notification, doctors were encouraged to notify any case in which they were at all suspicious of infarction, and form-filling kept to a minimum. At the time of notification, a simple questionary provided a record of the findings on clinical examination. Further clinical details came from the hospital doctor and the case notes, and basic demographic and social data from the patient; information about the times at which events occurred were also recorded. If the patient was kept at home, a doctor from the team visited the patient, usually within 12 hours, recorded an ECG, withdrew blood for the measurement of enzymes that might have been released into the blood as a result of necrosis of heart muscle and obtained the demographic, social and timing information. The general practitioner was informed by telephone of the interpretation of the ECG and the results of enzyme tests. He was then asked to record further brief clinical details of the patient's progress between the second and fourth days.

General practitioners also notified cases of sudden death in their practices; further notifications came from the Police Surgeon. The data collected about each patient fell under four headings:

(1) diagnostic information sufficient to classify the case as one of 'definite infarction' 'probable infarction' 'coronary insufficiency without infarction' (ischaemia), 'insufficient information' or 'any other condition',

(2) clinical information sufficient to classify the severity of the attack under four main grades,

(3) information about the timing of events following the occurrence of symptoms, and

(4) simple demographic and social data.

In the year of the study, 1296 people under the age of 70 were identified as suffering acute episodes of ischaemic heart disease. This is an attack rate of 4·6 per thousand population; 42 per cent died within four weeks of the attack, and of those dying, just over one third died within an hour of the onset of symptoms. These results emphasize the need to consider ways of preventing attacks, since medical care can do almost nothing for patients dying so quickly. Further analysis of this data should show in detail how the disease presents and is treated in a defined population; this information should help in the planning of future services.

When the clinical picture is completed in these ways, cases of previously unrecognized or undetected disease (the **submerged part of the iceberg**) are revealed.

An illustration of the iceberg phenomenon in relation to many forms of disease and disability is by the use of a model of a hypothetical general practice, showing disease recognized by the practitioner (based on data collected by 171 British general practitioners in a 12 month morbidity survey) and the total amount of disease and precursors of disease which could be expected on the basis of surveys in representative populations. The comparison of 'observed' and 'expected' disease in the hypothetical practice (table 35.4) gives some idea of the concealed portion of the iceberg and of the opportunities in the future for early and presymptomatic diagnosis.

Epidemiological intelligence services

No health service can work effectively without an intelligence service. In Britain, in the days when communicable disease was a major problem, notification and

TABLE 35.4. Experience of 1 year in the average general practice. From Last J.M. (1963) *Lancet* ii, 28.

	Patients with disease recognized by the doctor	Total present in practice, including unrecognized and presymptomatic cases, and precursors of disease
Pulmonary tuberculosis	1	2–3
New cases of cancer	7	12
Anaemia,		
Females 15–44	12	114
45–64	7	37
65 +	5	35
Diabetes mellitus, age 45 +	12	26
Glaucoma, age 45 +	3	17
Urinary infections, females		
age 15 +	20	40
Hypertension,		
males age 45 +	8	30
females age 45 +	24	131
Bronchitis,		
males age 45–64	24	47
females age 45–64	19	24
Rheumatoid arthritis,		
age 15 +	11	25
Epilepsy	7	14
Psychiatric disorders,		
males age 15 +	27	58
females age 15 +	62	102

registration fulfilled this function. New methods must be devised to provide essential information about noncommunicable diseases; descriptive epidemiology is developing the techniques for doing so. In addition to the above pilot study of IHD surveillance, cancer registries (p. 34.14) and medical record linkage (p. 34.17) are examples of other uses of descriptive epidemiology to monitor and evaluate the health services.

These and many other applications of epidemiology all add to our knowledge of the natural history of disease. The differing techniques and reasons for applying them outlined above will be increasingly relevant in the medical practice of the future. Identification and definition of precursors and subclinical cases, and efficient management of acute cases make effective control at least a possibility.

EVALUATION OF MEDICAL CARE

Among the determinants of disease in the community, the quality of medical care is increasing in importance. It is natural, therefore, to try to assess medical care. Work so far has been mostly descriptive, even anecdotal, although some of it has been widely quoted and has had some effects on medical policy. For example, a field survey of

American general practice by Peterson and others in 1953–4 has been cited as evidence of inferior standards, despite the fact that the survey only described the doctors' method of work, which was notable mainly for short cuts in the procedures of history-taking and physical examination, traditionally regarded as essential features of patient care in medical schools. No evidence was produced to indicate whether the clinical performance of these doctors made any difference to the welfare of their patients. In fact we can infer from other studies that the welfare of patients may be jeopardized.

Other work has revealed variations in the practice of hospital specialists. The Hospital Inpatient Enquiry (p. 34.15) besides being a source of morbidity data, has produced much useful evidence about the working of hospital services. Among the more important findings are substantial differences between hospitals in length of stay after common surgical procedures like hernia repair (fig. 35.2) and significant differences in case-fatality rates between teaching and nonteaching hospitals in England and Wales (table 35.5); these have been shown not to be

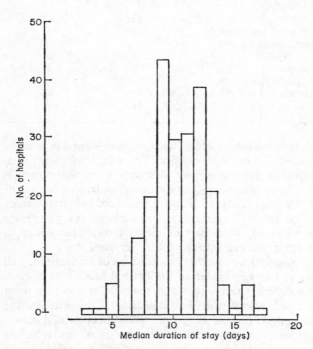

FIG. 35.2. Distribution of median duration of stay in hospital groups of patients with inguinal hernia without mention of obstruction, 1960. (Only those groups with more than ten cases in the sample are included.)

The distribution suggests that duration of stay is decided by fashion or custom (perhaps dependent upon habits of individual consultant surgeons) rather than on any rational basis. Two questions may be asked: does duration of stay influence duration of disability and does it influence recurrence rates? From Heasman M.A. (1964) How long in hospital? *Lancet* ii, 539.

TABLE 35.5 Number of cases of certain diseases, number of deaths, and case-fatalities among patients admitted to teaching and nonteaching hospitals, 1951. From Lee J.A.H., Morrison S.L. & Morris J.N. (1957) *Lancet*, ii, 785.

Diagnosis	Teaching hospitals		Nonteaching hospitals	
	Cases (and deaths)	Case-fatality (%)	Cases (and deaths)	Case-fatality (%)
Acute appendicitus with peritonitis males, all ages	469 (16)	3·4	219 (15)	6·8
Acute appendicitis with peritonitis females, all ages	360 (15)	4·2	171 (14)	8·2
Perforated peptic ulcer males, ages 45–64	393 (30)	7·6	132 (14)	10·6
Hyperplasia of prostate ages 65–74	660 (41)	6·2	280 (48)	17·1

due to case selection. These differences raise important questions about differing standards of medical care with which they are likely to be associated. As epidemiological methods become more sophisticated, the nature of these differences should be identified, and improvement of the quality of medical care should follow.

Analytical epidemiology

This term is used to describe studies specifically designed to test hypotheses, usually about associations between exposure to certain factors and the occurrence of disease. The hypothesis may have arisen from descriptive studies, in which the incidence of the disease has been found to be particularly high in a group in the population with special characteristics, or it may have arisen from clinical observations on a comparatively small number of patients. Diseases may have many causes and there is often a complex interaction between environmental, personal and genetic factors and the development of disease. Epidemiology helps to isolate certain factors that may be involved in this interaction, and to measure their importance. If associated factors can be confirmed, preventive measures can be worked out, even in the absence of complete understanding of the mechanisms involved.

In hypothesis testing two elements must be considered; first, can the postulated association be demonstrated, and second, is the association causal? If experimental studies were possible, both questions could be answered. Since experiment is often impossible, most research in this field must be observational; the answer to the second question depends upon judgement and is often based on the results of multiple testing of the particular hypothesis. One useful test is to see whether there is a consistent quantitative relationship between the postulated cause and its disease effect. Two methods are commonly used, i.e. the case-history or retrospective study and the cohort or prospective study.

CASE HISTORY OR RETROSPECTIVE STUDIES

This approach can be considered as an extension of the clinician's history-taking into the field of population studies. The procedure is to investigate a series of patients suffering from the disease in question and determine their experience of the factor which is thought to be associated with it. This could be past exposure to a particular environment, or a particular kind of behavioural pattern. A suitable control group is selected and similar enquiries made about their experience. Comparisons are then made between the proportions of cases and controls showing the environmental exposure or behaviour patterns. For example, an early test by Doll and Hill of the hypothesis that smoking and carcinoma of the lung were associated gave the results shown in table 35.6.

TABLE 35.6. The association between cigarette smoking and carcinoma of the lung in males. From Doll & Hill (1950) *Brit. med. J.* ii, 739.

	Patients with carcinoma of the lung	Controls
	%	%
Smokers	99·7	95·8
Nonsmokers	0·3	4·2

These indicate that there is some association, but it is not marked. By quantifying the amount smoked, the test became more impressive, as given in table 35.7.

It is now obvious that a higher proportion of patients with carcinoma are heavy cigarette smokers.

The difficulties of retrospective studies lie in collecting adequate numbers of a suitably representative series of cases, selecting an appropriate control group, and collecting reliable historical data from both groups. The aim, as always in epidemiology, is to compare like with like, in other words, to find a control group that appears to differ from the cases only in respect of the disease under study and then to find out whether it also differs in exposure to the postulated associated factor.

There are obvious sources of bias which can invalidate work of this kind. The fact that patients who suffer from a disease are questioned about the past, limits the possibilities and may make it difficult to rely on the findings. When, however, documentary evidence of previous exposure or activity is available, this form of study may be reliable. Retrospective studies are often used as a first test of a hypothesis; if it stands up, then the next test may take the form of a cohort study.

TABLE 35.7. The association between cigarette smoking and carcinoma of the lung in males in relation to the amount smoked. From Doll and Hill (1950) *Brit. med. J.* ii, 739.

	Patients with carcinoma of the lung	Controls
	%	%
Nonsmokers	0·3	4·2
Smokers of 1–4 cigarettes/day	5·1	8·5
5–14	38·5	45·1
15–24	30·2	29·3
25+	25·9	12·9

COHORT OR PROSPECTIVE STUDIES

A cohort or prospective study begins by enquiring into the exposure to a postulated factor in a population group and then follows that group over a period of time, measuring the incidence of the disease in subgroups with different exposures. Thus Doll and Hill went on from their case history study to a cohort study; they chose doctors on the *Medical Register* in Britain in 1951 as their cohort and asked them to record their smoking habits at that time. They then recorded the deaths that occurred in the next few years and calculated the death rates from lung cancer according to the previous data on smoking. Their results are shown in table 35.8.

TABLE 35.8. Annual death rates of British doctors from carcinoma of the lung according to cigarette smoking habits; 5-year follow-up. From Doll & Hill (1956) *Brit. med. J.* ii, 1071.

	Deaths/100,000
Nonsmokers	7
Light smokers	47
Moderate smokers	86
Heavy smokers	166

Doctors are a particularly suitable population for prospective study because they are comparatively easy to follow up, and when sick usually choose leading physicians to care for them. Their death certificate diagnoses are therefore more than usually reliable.

In a cohort study, measurement of the associated factor occurs before the disease has shown itself; a major source of bias in case history studies is, therefore, removed. Moreover, in a cohort study it is possible to estimate the relative risks involved; in the example above, heavy smokers have death rates from carcinoma of the lung twenty-three times greater than those of non-smokers.

In the United States, Hammond and Horn conducted surveys similar to those of Doll and Hill with identical results. There is overwhelming statistical evidence for a causal relationship between cigarette smoking and lung cancer. The incidence is not only directly proportional to the type of tobacco smoked and the number of cigarettes smoked (fig. 35.3) but is reduced among ex-cigarette-smokers in proportion to the duration of their abstention from the habit (fig. 35.4). Full accounts of the evidence

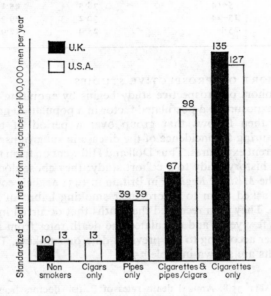

FIG. 35.3. Death rates from carcinoma of the lung in men according to the type of tobacco smoked. These figures are taken from the prospective study of British doctors aged 35 and over by Doll and Hill in 1959, and of American men aged 50–69 by Hammond and Horn in 1958. Only in the U.S.A. were there enough cigar smokers only to estimate their death rate which was the same as for nonsmokers. The similarity of the rates in both studies is impressive. The differences between cigarette smokers and other tobacco smokers may be due to the greater tendency of cigarette smokers to inhale the smoke. From *Smoking and Health* (1962) Report of the Royal College of Physicians. London: Pitman.

can be found in the reports on smoking and health published by the Royal College of Physicians of London, and by the United States Surgeon-General. The evidence associating cancer with atmospheric pollution is less convincing. Lung cancer mortality rates are highest among residents of urban industrial areas, but are also high in some nonindustrial areas, e.g. the Channel Islands. Lung cancer is a rare disease among people who have never smoked at all. Cigarette smoking is harmful to health in several other ways. Ischaemic heart disease and peripheral vascular disease occur significantly more often

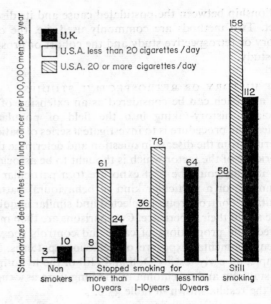

FIG. 35.4. The effect of giving up smoking on death rates from lung cancer. In this figure the death rates given for American men relate only to cases in which the diagnosis was established microscopically, so that these rates are lower than those illustrated from the same source in fig. 35.3. Only in the American study were heavier and lighter smokers separated. There was a similar, much reduced death rate in those who had given up smoking, especially if the period without smoking had been for more than ten years before the beginning of the study; but the heavier smokers who had given up smoking retained a higher mortality than the lighter smokers who continued to smoke. From *Smoking and Health* (1962) Report of the Royal College of Physicians. London: Pitman.

among heavy cigarette smokers, and so do chronic bronchitis and peptic ulcer. Women who smoke cigarettes have smaller (and sometimes premature) babies compared to women who do not smoke.

Although cohort studies look forward in time and can therefore be described as 'prospective', that term can be misleading. It is sometimes possible to reconstruct a population that was exposed to a measured factor in the past (for example, a group of factory workers exposed to occupational hazard, or infants born in hospital with a known exposure to radiation *in utero*) and to find out about their incidence of disease since that time. A cohort or prospective study, therefore, does not necessarily mean waiting for time to pass before results can be obtained. It can even be done so 'retrospectively' that all cases are dead at the time of enquiry. Cohort analysis of mortality statistics (p. 34.16) is perhaps the extreme example of this.

Most often, however, a cohort study requires the investigators to wait for an adequate number of cases to occur and is therefore usually more expensive and time-consuming than a case history study.

TABLE 35.9. Numbers of mothers reporting X-ray examination of the abdomen and other sites in three periods; ratios of case mothers to control mothers. From Stewart A., Webb I. & Hewitt M.A. (1958). *Brit. med. J.* i, 1495.

Period	X-ray examination		
	Abdominal	Other	Any
Before marriage	44/26 = 1·69	335/275 = 1·22	361/296 = 1·22
Between marriage and relevant conception	109/121 = 0·90	213/184 = 1·16	304/285 = 1·07
During relevant pregnancy	178/93 = 1·91	117/100 = 1·17	273/184 = 1·48
Any period	296/215 = 1·38	531/456 = 1·16	692/593 = 1·17

The case/control ratio of 1·91 for abdominal X-ray exposures during the relevant pregnancy
  (1) differs from the 'expected' ratio (1·00) at the level of $P < 10^{-7}$;
  (2) differs from the contemporary ratio for other X-ray exposures (1·17) at the level $P \simeq 0·011$ and from the ratio for other X-ray exposures in any period (1·16) at the level $P < 0·001$;
  (3) differs from the ratio for abdominal X-ray exposures in any period (1·38) at the level $P \simeq 0·012$.

The testing of a particular hypothesis by these different methods is illustrated by their use in the study of the relationship between childhood malignant disease and radiation. In the 1950s, following the upsurge of interest in the effects of radiation after the use of atomic bombs in 1945, Alice Stewart and her colleagues at Oxford developed a hypothesis that foetal irradiation was associated with the later development of leukaemia and other malignant conditions in childhood. They tested this hypothesis by designing a case history or retrospective study. The method was to trace all the children in England and Wales who had died of leukaemia or cancer before their tenth birthday during the years 1953–5 and to compare certain of their prenatal and postnatal experiences with those of a control group of living children. Controls were matched by age, sex and locality (factors in which the investigators were not interested) and selected from local birth registers.

The mothers of cases (dead children) and controls were interviewed and the same questions asked of both groups. Although the interviewing doctors knew into which group a mother fell, they did not know that the greatest interest lay in the questions about radiographic examination during the relevant pregnancy.

The investigators were able to interview the mothers of 1416 out of the total 1694 dead children in the 'case' group (83·6 per cent). After certain exclusions data were available about 1299 mothers in each group (cases and controls). The relevant findings appear in table 35.9.

The authors commented on this table in these words.

'It will be seen that 692 mothers of cases reported at least one diagnostic X-ray exposure compared with only 593 mothers of controls, a case/control ratio of 1·17. Though this case excess is significant, it is not very large, and might perhaps be attributed to relative under-reporting of X-ray exposures on the control side. If, however, under-reporting by control mothers was the only reason for the case excess one would expect to find similar case/control ratios for each type of examination and for each period of life. In fact the ratio is higher for abdominal (1·38) than for other types of examination (1·16), and higher for all examinations during the relevant pregnancy (1·48) than during earlier periods (1·22 and 1·07). In particular, the ratio for abdominal X-ray examinations during the relevant pregnancy is outstandingly high (1·91). The chance probability of obtaining so high a ratio is less than one in ten million. Moreover, as the footnote (table 35.9) shows, this ratio is significantly higher than the ratio for X-ray examinations of other sites in this period, and than the ratio for abdominal X-ray examinations as a whole. Hence there is *prima facie* evidence that abdominal X-ray examinations during pregnancy—the only type of examination involving direct exposure of the foetus—can contribute to the aetiology of malignant disease in children.'

Stewart and her colleagues also presented data on the dose–response relationship (table 35.10). With the exception of the drop in ratio for three films, there does appear to be a consistent relationship.

TABLE 35.10. Distribution of cases and controls irradiated *in utero* according to the numbers of abdominal films reported taken during the relevant pregnancy. From Stewart *et al.* (1958).

No. of films	Cases	Controls	Ratio
0	1121	1206	0·93
1	37	27	1·37
2	60	26	2·31
3	23	18	1·28
4 or more	32	10	3·20
(Unknown number)	(26)	(12)	(2·17)
Total	1299	1299	1·00

After full discussion the authors concluded that children who had been X-rayed *in utero* were twice as likely as other children to die of a malignant disease before their tenth birthday.

The results were clearly of concern to obstetricians and radiologists and were also of major interest in suggesting that small doses of ionizing radiation were carcinogenic. Many criticisms were made of the case history or retrospective study, with its possibilities of bias in mothers' memory and interviewers' technique, and in the selection of controls. Court Brown, Doll and Hill carried out a cohort or prospective study to check the findings.

They used the technique of reconstructing a cohort, comprising approximately 40,000 live-born children whose mothers had been X-rayed during pregnancy between 1945 and 1956. Using death registration data they identified all children in this cohort who had died of leukaemia. These 'observed' numbers were compared with those which would be 'expected' in the same population if it had experienced the nationally occurring death rates from leukaemia in the relevant age and sex groups. In all, nine deaths from leukaemia were observed among children whose mothers had been irradiated, compared to an expected 10·5 deaths. Thus this test of the hypothesis that irradiation enhanced the risk of malignancy produced a negative result. However, the number of cases of leukaemia that were observed was small and chance factors alone may have resulted in a fairly substantial risk being overlooked. If the effect of irradiation *in utero* were to raise the incidence of leukaemia by 50 per cent the expected number of cases would have been $\frac{150}{100} \times 10\cdot5$, or 15·8. In these circumstances it would not be unreasonable to attribute to chance the fact that only nine cases were observed ($P=0\cdot04$); but it is unlikely that the effect of irradiation could be much more. Had the effect been to double the risk, the probability of obtaining only nine

observed cases (or less) would have been less than 1 in 300.

The position at this point, then, was that the original case history study might have overestimated a real risk but that if so, the subsequent cohort study was based on too small numbers to provide a satisfactory test. Clearly a much larger scale cohort study was required and this was carried out by MacMahon; he obtained records from maternity hospitals in the north-eastern United States using much larger numbers, in fact 734,243 children. He was able to show that the excess risk of leukaemia and other malignant conditions in childhood after foetal irradiation was of the order of 40 per cent (table 35.11).

This example illustrates some of the ways in which a causal hypothesis can be tested. It shows the huge numbers that may have to be studied in order to demonstrate one factor in the multiple causation of disease and the need for careful statistical analysis. These studies did not discover 'the cause' of childhood malignancies but they did show that a particular diagnostic procedure in obstetrics carried a definite risk; this knowledge not only points the way towards minimizing the risk but provides new information about the effects of small doses of radiation. It is appropriate here only to describe the general lines on which hypothesis testing of this kind is carried out. The careful attention to detail necessary in such investigations and the minutiae of the methods employed must be studied in the original papers.

THE INDIVIDUAL'S CHANCES

Most of the uses of epidemiology defined by Morris have been described and discussed in this and the preceding chapter. Epidemiology can be used to study the historical changes in disease, to assess the state of community health, to evaluate the working of health services, to identify syndromes, to search for causes of disease, to 'complete the clinical picture' and to estimate the indi-

TABLE 35.11. Observed and expected numbers of children dying from leukaemia and other childhood malignant diseases who were exposed to prenatal diagnostic irradiation, by age at death. From MacMahon B. (1962) *J. nat. Cancer Inst.* **28**, 1173.

Age	Leukaemia			Cancer of nervous system and other sites			Total of all malignant diseases		
	Observed	Expected	Ratio	Observed	Expected	Ratio	Observed	Expected	Ratio
0–2	9	8·1	1·1	15	10·0	1·5	24	18·1	1·3
3–4	17	11·1	1·5	9	7·3	1·2	26	18·4	1·4
5–7	21	10·4	2·0	12	6·3	1·9	33	16·7	2·0
8+	0	2·9	—	2	2·9	0·7	2	5·8	0·3
Total	47	32·5	1·4	38	26·5	1·4	85	59·0	1·44

The ratio of observed to expected can also be expressed as a percentage risk. Thus the ratio of observed cases of all malignant diseases at all ages, to the expected number is 1.44 (bottom row last column in the table); this means that the excess risk of malignant disease following foetal irradiation is 44 per cent.

vidual's chances of getting or of dying from various diseases. The last of these deserves further mention because of its value in the consulting room and at the bedside.

It is a matter of simple arithmetic to estimate the individual's chances from the available data on incidence or mortality rates in the population from which he comes; it is of course merely an 'average' chance or risk. For example, as table 34.4 (p. 34.9) shows, approximately 20 per cent of the deaths in Scotland are due to malignant neoplasms. Put another way, this is the same as saying that in Scotland the individual's chances of dying of cancer are about 1 in 5. Cancer registry data make it possible to calculate age-specific incidence rates for cancer and so to work out the individual's chances of getting cancer; it is closer to one in four than one in five. From Doll and Hill's studies of British doctors it is possible to calculate that the chance of a 35-year-old male doctor dying before reaching the age of 45 is 1 in 90 if he is a nonsmoker, 1 in 23 if he is a heavy cigarette smoker. Many other examples are given by Morris, to whose book the reader is referred. The facts are useful to doctors seeking to persuade their patients to adopt a more healthy way of life.

Applied epidemiology

Describing a disease as unrecognized implies that symptoms and/or physical signs could be elicited by appropriate methods. An example is sputum-positive pulmonary tuberculosis; the patient usually has symptoms (cough, sweats, etc.) often has physical signs (wasting, abnormal respiratory sounds) and the diagnosis can be confirmed by bacteriology and radiology. Presymptomatic or subclinical disease remains concealed from the patient because it is not accompanied by perceptible departure from normal health; a good example is carcinoma *in situ* of the cervix (see below). A precursor of disease is an abnormal state which is commonly associated with the subsequent development of disease. For example, elevated serum cholesterol is a precursor of IHD.

Screening is the procedure of surveying a population for unrecognized or presymptomatic disease or for precursors. Doctors approach members of the public, rather than waiting to be approached. The aim is early detection of as many cases as possible at a stage when treatment can reverse, halt or at least retard the progress of the disease. It is pointless to screen for a disease if no treatment is available. After the success of mass miniature radiography in screening large populations for pulmonary tuberculosis, there was much enthusiasm for screening to detect other serious chronic diseases. Methods were developed to screen for diabetes mellitus, chronic glaucoma, phenylketonuria, carcinoma of the cervix, carcinoma of the breast, haemolytic disease of the newborn, bacteriuria and a number of other conditions. Initial enthusiasm has somewhat waned. The pitfalls of glau-

coma screening have already been mentioned. There is not much evidence that early detection of some chronic diseases materially influences their course although the incidence of complications may be reduced (e.g. carcinoma of the breast, diabetes). Economic aspects cannot be ignored. If the screening test is expensive and the condition rare, the cost of finding a case may be prohibitive; however, it has to be set against the cost of caring for advanced cases which might otherwise have been prevented, and against lost years of life and productivity.

Carcinoma of the cervix illustrates some of the problems of assessing the value of screening. This is a common malignant disease of women and the emotional and political appeal of mass campaigns for its early detection is considerable. The method is cervical cytology, i.e. histopathological examination of stained smears from the cervix or vaginal vault. When abnormal cells are detected, the next step is cone biopsy of the cervix, i.e. excision of a cone of tissue with the base on the vaginal surface of the cervix, the apex at or near the internal os of the cervical canal (vol. 1, fig. 37.4). When examination of the excised cone shows no extension of the lesion beyond the basement membrane, the condition is called carcinoma *in situ*. Early experience with cervical cytology and cone biopsy were favourable. In British Columbia the incidence of clinically invasive carcinoma of the cervix fell from 28 per 100,000 in 1955 to 13 per 100,000 in 1966. However, the condition is commonest among women of high parity and poor hygiene, and the decline at least partly reflects changing social conditions. The improvement cannot necessarily be ascribed to the effect of mass screening. The natural history of carcinoma *in situ* is unknown. Is it a presymptomatic disease or a precursor, not necessarily always followed by invasive carcinoma? Since cone biopsy removes the lesion, its natural history cannot be studied. Another difficulty is disagreement among pathologists as to the interpretation of microscopic appearances, and this has helped to preclude calculation of observer error rates. There is no agreement about optimum timing and frequency of screening the individual women. Two further points on the debit side are that the most vulnerable women are least likely to attend cancer detection clinics and that cone biopsy may render a young woman sterile. Despite these uncertainties and disadvantages, cervical cytology has been widely adopted in many countries; well over a million women are examined each year in Britain. Knox has pointed out that the only way to resolve the uncertainties is by epidemiological survey of a large population; at least 100,000 women would have to be enrolled, examined, and re-examined; the interval between examination and re-examination should be varied in order better to study the natural history; the whole survey could be done in about five years. Unless this kind of evaluation is done, we may never know whether cervical cytology is of any value.

After reviewing the evidence on screening for some common conditions, McKeown and others drew up a scheme for the evaluation of screening procedures, which may be partly paraphrased as follows:

Definition of the problem. What abnormality is to be detected? What can be done about it? Who is to be screened? When? How?

Review of position before screening. What is the evidence (and how adequate is it) on prevalence, natural history and medical significance of the abnormality? How effective were previous methods of preventing and treating it?

Review of evidence concerning the screening procedure. What is the evidence on the effectiveness of the proposed diagnostic method (applicability to the group whose investigation is proposed, error rates, comparison with traditional diagnostic methods, availability of resources, cost, etc.)? What is the evidence on the effectiveness of the proposed treatment?

Conclusions concerning the state of the evidence on the problem as a whole. What conclusions emerge from consideration of all existing evidence? What are the medical advantages and disadvantages, compared to other approaches to the problem? How do costs compare?

Acquisition of further evidence, if necessary.

Initial applications. What application is justified? For what scale and duration should it be planned? How should it be supervised, and what resources should be committed? Is screening to be conducted on a service or research basis? If the latter, with what objectives?

The reader is referred to the essays on screening (Further Reading at the end of this chapter) for full details on this application of epidemiology.

Relevance of epidemiology

The design and execution of epidemiological studies usually requires specialists; but the knowledge gained from them and the application of that knowledge are part of medicine as a whole. Some understanding of the principles and methods is required by all doctors so that

epidemiological evidence can be studied in an informed and critical way. A clear appreciation that the established disease presented by patients represents only the tip of the iceberg may suggest the possibilities of population studies to complement clinical and laboratory research. Much of the best work in epidemiology has been done by teams including clinicians and epidemiologists; the latter often depend upon an approach from a clinician with an idea suggested by study of individual patients. Clinicians who are aware of the possibilities and who occasionally adopt the epidemiological approach may stimulate the most fruitful work.

At a practical level, it is clear that much chronic disease presents clinically at a late stage in the pathological process. The condition may then be irreversible and treatment only palliative. The control of such disease depends upon the development of procedures to find those affected at an early, presymptomatic stage and to intervene effectively at that time. Now, and increasingly in the future, good medical practice needs the epidemiological as well as the clinical approach.

FURTHER READING

FROST W.H. (1936) *Snow on Cholera*. New York: The Commonwealth Fund.

CLARK D.W. & MACMAHON B. eds. (1967) *Preventive Medicine*, London: Churchill.

MORRIS J.N. (1964) *Uses of Epidemiology*. Edinburgh: Livingstone.

PAUL J.R. (1966) *Clinical Epidemiology*. Chicago: University of Chicago Press.

Screening in Medical Care (1968) (a collection of essays). London: Oxford University Press.

WILSON J.M.G. & JUNGNER G. (1968) *Principles and Practice of Screening For Disease*. Geneva: World Health Organization.

WITTS L.J., ed. (1964) *Medical Surveys and Clinical Trials*. London: Oxford University Press.

Chapter 36
Ageing

'To love playthings well as a child, to lead an adventurous and honourable youth, and to settle when the time arrives into a green and smiling age, is to be a good artist in life'

R. L. Stevenson

The slowing down of physiological functions at the end of the period of youth brings a need to 'settle' that leads ultimately to death. This process of ageing is common to all animals and its scientific study is known as **gerontology** (Greek, *Geron*, an old man).

While most men and women may be judged as 'good artists in life', some unfortunately find old age is far from green and smiling. As life advances, both physical and psychological disorders become more common and severe and difficulties in adjusting to the social environment increase. **Geriatrics** is that branch of medicine devoted to the problems of old age and it has sociological, pathological, psychological and clinical aspects. In 1870, 5 per cent of the British people were over 65 years old; in 1966, this proportion was just over 12 per cent and it will increase to 15 per cent over the next 20 years (p. 34.8). Geriatrics is thus an increasing part of medical practice.

Life span

The concept of life span is that there is a limit beyond which an individual cannot survive. For man 'the days of our years are three score and ten; and if by reason of strength they be fourscore years, yet it is their strength, labour and sorrow; for it is soon cut off and we fly away'. The psalmist's statement is essentially correct, but a few survive longer. Some 250 people in Britain celebrate their hundredth birthday each year. There are well authenticated cases of persons living to 110, but reports of longer survival have not been supported on full investigation. Women have a life span about five years more than men and about five times as many women as men reach 100 years.

A curious feature of the life span is that it differs greatly between species. Man is the longest living mammal, but some reptiles have longer life spans and a tortoise has been reported to have died at the age of 176 years. Swans are traditionally able to outlive man and

there have been many elderly parrots, but most birds, like small mammals, have a life span of less than 10 years. Insects have much shorter life spans and a mayfly survives for only one day. It is not easy to account for such wide variation and this constitutes a fundamental problem of gerontology.

The limit to the life span arises from the fact that there is an increasing likelihood of death as age advances. The increase in the mortality rate with age in many species including man is approximately exponential. This relationship was first noted by Gompertz in 1825 and can be expressed as follows:

$$R_t = R_0 e^{at} + A$$

Where R_0 is the mortality rate at time t_0, and R_t the rate at time t, A is Makehams' constant which allows for age-independent causes of death. The size of the exponential constant determines the life span.

Mortality is least at about 12 years. In industrial countries this is followed by a period of slowly increasing mortality until age 30 or so, after which the chances of dying increase progressively.

FACTORS AFFECTING THE LIFE SPAN
Many have sought for the secrets of longevity, but they remain for the most part hidden. There are, however, three factors which are known to alter the life span of animals, but the extent to which they apply to man is uncertain.

Heredity
The old advice that, if you wish to have a long life, you should choose your parents carefully is sound. It is, however, difficult to obtain evidence that life span in man is genetically determined, though studies in monovular twins strongly support this view. There are a few remarkable examples of elderly monovular twins dying from identical illnesses within a few days of each other, despite having lived in very different circumstances for many years.

Diet
Many years ago McCay at Cornell University showed that it was possible to prolong the life span of rats by

delaying their growth and development by underfeeding and this has been confirmed in many species, but there is no evidence that this is true for man. However, the age of puberty in girls and boys is two years earlier than it was one hundred years ago. The average age of the menarche was 15·3 years in 1845, 14·8 years in 1890, and 12·9 years in 1962. This change is probably due to better feeding. It is not impossible that by feeding our children too well we are shortening their lives.

Life expectation at birth has increased remarkably over the past hundred years (table 34.2, p. 34.4); this has been due mainly to control of infant and child mortality from infections. Life expectation beyond middle age has hardly altered in the past hundred years and probably over a much longer time. The leading cause of death in middle-aged men is ischaemic heart disease, and this is more likely to affect the overfed.

Ionizing radiation
Exposure of experimental animals to ionizing radiation reduces their life span. Some of this reduction is due to the direct effect of radiation, e.g. the acute radiation syndrome and increased liability to cancer. Exposure to radiation may also accelerate the changes of ageing and hence lead to premature death. For obvious reasons there is no conclusive evidence on this point in humans.

However, recent reports from the Atomic Bomb Casualty Commission reveal that A-bomb survivors of Hiroshima and Nagasaki are now showing the signs of ageing at much earlier ages than is usual.

The changes associated with ageing in man

A major difficulty in describing the manifestations of ageing in humans is the problem of distinguishing the effects of ageing from those of disease. The older the person, the more likely is disease present. This is not to say that disease is an inescapable accompaniment of ageing, as is shown by the occasional finding of nonagenarians with little evidence of atherosclerosis or other degenerative processes.

There is much evidence to support the view that ageing is accompanied by diminishing powers of adaptation and increased vulnerability to stress; ageing humans show diminished power to survive trauma and to resist and overcome infections. Stress of any kind produces a more profound effect upon the ageing body, which also takes longer to restore the normal internal environment. Medawar has expressed this succinctly by defining ageing as 'that change of the bodily faculties, sensibilities and energies which renders the individual progressively more likely to die from accidental causes'.

Clinically, the characteristic feature of disability in the aged is that multiple pathological processes are commonly present. In one study patients admitted to a geriatric hospital were found to have an average of six pathological conditions each, and in another survey of the general (not sick) population aged 65 and over, the mean number of conditions causing disability was rather more than three.

From the point of view of clinical medicine it is justifiable to ask how important it is to study and diagnose these multiple diseases since many of them are degenerative and the sufferers have only a limited expectation of life. Such a question, however, displays a failure to understand the nature of disability in old people. Although some serious diseases such as malignant neoplasia are more likely to occur in older than in younger age groups, many conditions from which old people suffer are amenable to cure or considerable alleviation, e.g. various forms of anaemia, malnutrition, some endocrine dysfunctions, psychiatric states such as depression and some confusional psychoses, and congestive cardiac failure which in the elderly is commonly associated with mild myocardial disease. Even for conditions which cannot be improved directly, e.g. osteoarthrosis of the hips, exercises to restore lost muscle power and mechanical aids may greatly increase the functional capacity. These multiple pathological processes often produce a vicious circle and lead to total dependency. An example is the obese old lady, whose obesity aggravates degenerative arthrosis in her knees and hips so that she becomes less and less mobile. This in turn may aggravate her obesity and lead to difficulties in securing a proper diet; shopping and cooking are disrupted. In addition the sedentary life, which she is obliged to lead, produces urinary stagnation and predisposes to urinary tract infection. Thus the combination of conditions, each relatively benign, may result in total dependency. If in addition loneliness, social isolation and apathy are added, it is apparent how serious the situation may become.

ORGAN AND TISSUE CHANGES
Some pathological changes are commonly found in aged individuals during life or at autopsy and may be properly regarded as characteristic of the ageing process. The skin, especially on exposed parts of the body, becomes atrophic and loses its elasticity; it becomes wrinkled and eventually deep furrows may form. Contrary to the claims of the cosmetic industry, this is an inexorable and irreversible process; it is associated with histological changes which include atrophy of the rete pegs, the epidermal processes which project downwards between the dermal papillae, and degeneration of the dermal collagen and elastic fibres. This degeneration is prominent in the upper part of the dermis, and is exhibited by fragmentation of the fibres, the short fragments becoming curled up and thickened. The degenerated collagen fibres acquire a basophilic appearance.

Most individuals begin to develop **atherosclerosis** at an

early age, e.g. in their twenties, but it is of minor degree and usually present as a few small plaques in the aorta. The condition increases in severity with age, and affects other vessels, e.g. the coronary and cerebral arteries. This process is, however, usually very slow and gradual, and may never reach clinical significance. In others, it progresses so as to interfere with the blood flow through the affected vessel, sometimes to an extent sufficient to cause a myocardial or cerebral infarct (p. 25.4). In old people, autopsy usually reveals a significant degree of atherosclerosis, although this may be minimal or absent in the coronary arteries, and indeed such a finding may be causally associated with the individual's longevity; when mental confusion occurs in old age it can often be accounted for by the presence of arterial disease in the cerebral arteries, with resultant cerebral ischaemia.

Another vascular change which may be seen in old age is a hyaline or structureless type of thickening of the arterioles, particularly in spleen and kidney. Indeed, this thickening occurs commonly in splenic arterioles and is present often from middle age onwards. Such **hyaline arteriolosclerosis**, as it is called, is the morphological accompaniment of hypertension at other ages and in other organs.

Old people sometimes exhibit retardation of the healing process; for example fractures may not unite easily. This, however, may be due to local ischaemia, resulting from arterial disease, rather than to any more generalized abnormality.

The organs in very old people often appear atrophic at autopsy. This is usually associated with an increase of the pigment lipofuscin in the cells; when this involves the heart, it is known as **brown atrophy** (p. 36.5). In bone the decrease in the amount of the osteoid matrix known as osteoporosis tends to develop and the bones of old people break more easily than those of the young. There is always atrophy of the gonads in old age; in women, the uterus and ovaries atrophy after the menopause.

Psychological aspects of ageing

Workers in geriatrics never fail to be impressed by the overriding importance of psychological factors in determining how an ageing person copes with increasing physical and social problems. Many old people are severely disabled with physical disease and yet, they are well preserved mentally, have 'strong' personalities, are anxious to preserve their independence and manage their lives with skill and competence. On the other hand others who are physically well preserved, rosy-cheeked, well-muscled and free from physical disability, cannot cope with the ordinary task of daily living because of mental impairment. They end up as permanent institutional patients, unless they are fortunate enough to have willing and competent relatives.

Until recently it was assumed that ageing meant an overall loss of mental function and all aspects of intellectual function were progressively and irretrievably lost. Recent studies have shown that the ageing mind is not affected in this simple way and it would be surprising if it were. Much of the evidence suggests that the ageing mind is more resilient than was formerly believed.

SENSORY AND MOTOR PERFORMANCE
The older person is slow to recognize a signal and to respond to it. At one time this was thought to be due mainly to defective sense organs such as eyes and ears, or to slowness of conduction of impulses to effector organs. Although such changes occur, the main delay is in the brain. The aged brain takes longer to appreciate a stimulus, to identify its nature and to select the most appropriate response.

MEMORY
There is a failure of short term retention of data in the aged. This is not due to diminution in the capacity to hold or store information but to increased distractability of the older subject, whose attention is more easily drawn away from the problem under consideration by irrelevant stimuli. This is the factor which probably accounts for the elderly person's increased difficulty with problem solving tests.

Another feature of the ageing person's memory is the greater difficulty in recalling information. This is shown by a tendency to 'rigidity' in the elderly person who is asked to identify an object related to a previously identified one. This is explained in psychological terms by comparing the memory to a vast store in which items are kept in pigeonholes. If the elderly person has found one item of information in a particular pigeonhole, he tends to look in nearby pigeonholes for the next item, although this may be concerned with an entirely different subject.

LEARNING AND WORK
The learning difficulties experienced by the elderly are due to impaired short-term retention and comprehension. If an older subject is given enough time and is undisturbed he succeeds in registering information and learning can be achieved successfully.

This ability has considerable practical importance in societies in which older workers are under pressure to learn new skills and techniques, as traditional trades disappear in the new industrial revolution.

While speed of movement is lost in older workers, overall function may be more than compensated by increased accuracy. Thus in some circumstances there may be little or no falling off in overall performance with ageing, but in certain industries, especially in modern production lines, it may not be possible to compensate for loss of speed. This may lead to serious deterioration in achievement and morale and in reduced employability.

In a similar way the value of past experience (what passes for 'wisdom') enables an older, experienced person to produce satisfactory answers to complex problems more rapidly than a younger, inexperienced person. This of course is the case only where previous experience is relevant and the problems are in some degree familiar. Where the older person is confronted with problems requiring new solutions outside his previous range of experience, then there is either delay in providing a solution or the solution is inappropriate. Thus, depending on whether experience is appropriate to a new problem, the older tycoon of industry is hailed as either very wise or is accused of rigidity of mind.

It is interesting to speculate upon the relevance of these facts to different trades and professions. At one end of the scale there is the research worker in pure science whose main value is his ability to see new solutions to old or new problems. At the other end we have the learned judge or ecclesiastic whose main contribution may be to produce similar answers to similar questions over many years and in whom rigidity may be hailed as a virtue.

PERSONALITY

How an individual reacts under different circumstances depends upon his personality, his past experience, his anticipation of future events, his sociocultural background and conditioning and upon his intellectual capacity. Thus an old lady who has been inclined to have a suspicious nature is apt to misconstrue what people are saying in her vicinity or to misinterpret gestures as being hostile or antagonistic especially if she becomes deaf. Another common finding is that older persons show a heightened emotional tone as a result of which tears flow more readily.

MOTIVATION

It is not sufficient to possess the wit to tackle problems; the willingness to do so is equally important. In other words, sufficient interest must be stimulated or aroused. 'Getting going' is of practical importance in old people, many of whom feel out of things and have difficulty in occupying mind and body. This leads to a chronic underactivity of brain which breeds apathy and lack of interest. The garrulousness or even querulousness of some old people may represent an attempt to raise their brain activity to a level nearer the optimum. A similar explanation may underlie the increased physical activity or restlessness seen in some old people. In these individuals, failing ability to cope with intellectual problems may lead to physical overactivity, often manifesting itself as ineffectual and fruitless behaviour, i.e. substitution of work for thought.

Physiological changes

Of the many morphological changes occurring with age, the important ones are those which decrease the functional capacity of the tissues and increase the likelihood of death.

Fig. 36.1 shows the changes with age in resting functional rates of many tissues and gives a measure of body

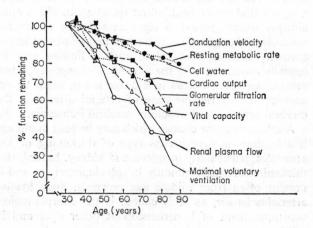

FIG. 36.1. The average per cent of various human functional capacities or values remaining at different ages taking 30 years as 100%. Data from Shock N.W. *et al.* (1957) *Geriatrics*, **12**, 40.

decline; however it does not reflect the balance which must exist between the declining demands on a tissue by an aged body and the declining capacity of ageing tissues to meet them. Most tissues have a large functional reserve and its erosion with time impairs resting functional levels relatively late in life. As a result, changes in

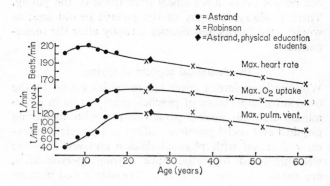

FIG. 36.2. Effects of exercise on maximum O_2 uptake, heart rate and maximum pulmonary ventilation of men at various ages. All values obtained over a 5- or 6-min period during maximal work on a treadmill or bicycle ergometer. From Asmussen E. (1958) *Handbook of Respiration*, ed. Dittmer D. & Grebe R. Nat. Acad. Sciences Nat. Research Council, p. 146.

the resting functional rates give an inadequate indication of the true extent of ageing or when it starts. For such purposes, changes in peak functional capacity with age are better indices, since they reflect more closely the overall effects of age. Of the scanty data available, changes in the maximal rates of various measurements connected with exercise are the best documented (fig. 36.2). An added complication is the difficulty in deciding whether a decline in the functional capacity of a tissue is due to ageing of the tissue itself, or whether it represents secondary ageing, due to changes in other tissues.

TISSUE DECLINE

Whether primary or secondary, a decline in the functional capacity of a tissue must be due to either a depletion of cell numbers or a decline in the function of individual cells, or both. Functional decline may arise in many ways. In those tissues in which cells are either not replaced during life or to only a limited extent e.g. brain, kidney, ovary, skeletal and heart muscle, the rate of cell loss determines the functional life span of the tissue. The human brain weighs 1500g at the age of 30, but on average only 1360g at 90. Similarly, the kidneys during this period lose almost 50 per cent of their nephrons; both these changes are due largely to cell loss. It is estimated that on average 30 brain cells die every minute. The body, thus dies a little every day.

Ageing is much less obvious in tissues in which mitosing cells continue to be seen and mitosis itself may have a rejuvenatory effect. In tissues in which regular cell replacement is a normal occurrence e.g. gut epithelium, epidermis, blood cells, cell depletion is not a threat so long as mitotic ability is retained. If some stem cells in these tissues lose their mitotic ability with age, multiplication of other stem cells could compensate adequately. However, changes in the pattern of mitosis occur in many tissues with age. In some, the rate of mitosis decreases with age e.g. liver; in others it is said to increase e.g. mouse skin. In the mouse colon, the transit time of cells from the stem cell sites in the crypts of glands to the tips of the villi, where they are exfoliated, increases with age, although the distance travelled remains constant. The stem cell cycle gradually lengthens and the rate of cell production decreases. Similar evidence exists for the mouse duodenum, and the turnover time of human stomach parietal cells increases from 30 to 40 days between maturity and old age. These changes may reflect an intrinsic wearing out of stem cells, or they may be secondary to changes in vascular, nervous or humoral factors affecting the gut wall.

The suggestion that regularly mitosing cells, e.g. stem cells of gut epithelium, may age more slowly than post-mitotic cells, e.g. brain cells, arises from the observation that accumulation of the pigment lipofuscin, which is closely correlated with age (fig. 36.3), is lower in mitosing

cells. Lipofuscin may arise as a breakdown product of lysosomes since they have certain enzymes and lipid components in common; the presence of fewer lysosomes in mitosing cells may explain the slower accumulation of

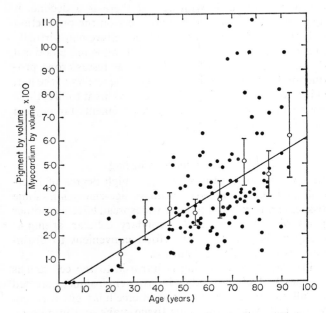

FIG. 36.3. Relationship between age and pigment in the human myocardium. From Strehler B.L. *et al.* (1959) *J. Geront.* **14**, 430.

pigment, but it remains uncertain whether there is any causal relationship between lipofuscin and ageing or between lysosomes and ageing. It is naturally difficult to say whether cells which are renewed regularly, age markedly during their lifespans, since it is not certain whether they die from ageing, from environmental causes e.g. desiccation in skin, abrasion in gut or whether they are recognized as 'old' and destroyed, as may be so with red blood cells. All that can be said is that gut epithelial cells, for example, have a greater opportunity to deteriorate as their turnover gradually falls with age.

The suggestion that mitosis might have a rejuvenatory effect on cells arises from the possibility that 'accumulated cell errors' may not be passed on during mitosis, or that certain cell processes may be lost due to cell ageing and be renewable at mitosis. Do 'new cells' replace the old and dying, or are the progeny of old stem cells inferior in some respects to those of young stem cells? The qualitative differences between the red blood cells of young and old persons are very minor; slight increases in mean cell diameter and in osmotic fragility occur between 50 and 70 years, but neither has any effect on their life span.

Although cell depletion may be less serious and cellular ageing slower in mitosing tissues, such tissues do age.

Decline occurs in the secretory capacity of many parts of the gut, associated with decrease in mucosal thickness and cell numbers. The epidermis becomes thinner, contains fewer cells, and rete pegs are lost (p. 36.2). There are conflicting reports concerning a possible fall in the number of marrow cells with age. If there is a decline, it appears to be small and has no effect on the production of blood cells. The numbers of blood cells remain virtually unchanged with age except for a fall in the red blood cell count in the male to female levels, as testosterone production falls. Despite these changes, the ageing of the gut, skin and blood-forming cells poses no threat to life; these tissues are capable of meeting requirements far beyond the life span of the body.

Mechanisms of ageing

In a metazoan organism, where a high degree of intercellular integration exists, primary age-changes in some tissues can hardly fail to have widespread effects on other parts of the body, and secondary cellular ageing is easily envisaged. It is, therefore, convenient to distinguish two possible mechanisms.

Primary cellular ageing is intrinsic to the cell and is independent of the body's internal environment created by all the tissues and of the intercellular environment which cells within the same tissue make and impose on each other. The only valid method of demonstrating primary cellular ageing is by separating cells from the body environment and from each other by cell culture.

Secondary cellular ageing is a result of changes in other tissues of the body or of a change in the state of the intercellular environment within the tissue. The main techniques of investigating this type of ageing involve tissue transplantation.

PRIMARY CELLULAR AGEING

That ageing is an intrinsic phenomenon of individual cells is suggested by studies in protozoa, malignant cells and cell cultures.

Protozoa

Maupas compared the behaviour of protozoan populations to the ageing of metazoan cells. Such populations should mimic metazoan cells in their life cycles, and undergo a similar phase of ageing and death, unless nuclear reorganization by sexual reproduction or autogamy allows rejuvenation of the genetic material. A comparison between metazoan and protozoan ageing is an attractive idea, in that it helps us to look on metazoa as a composite of mortal protozoa-like cells, each cell ageing independently of the others and each with a definitely limited life span under asexual conditions. However, it is complicated and possibly robbed of its usefulness by Sonnebonn's demonstration of the immortality of some strains of paramecia in that they appear to be capable of indefinite life by asexual reproduction alone. Such evidence suggests the possibility that all cells may be potentially immortal, given a suitable environment; other protozoa however require periodic sexual reproduction to survive.

Malignant cells

Hela cells, a strain of carcinoma cells used for culturing viruses, and other tumour cells display an apparent immortality in tissue culture, but these cells have chromosomes which are abnormal in size, staining properties and number. As a result their properties cannot be compared with normal cells; nevertheless it is intriguing to ponder how these cells become immortal and in what way this is related to their chromosome abnormality. Normal metazoan cells of many types in culture may undergo a spontaneous transformation which allows them to divide indefinitely. They also show abnormal chromosomes and behave as tumour cells if implanted into animals. What happens? Is there a breakdown of ageing, as well as other cell controls, or are the possible ageing effects of genetic deterioration within cells postponed by having multiple chromosome replicas in such cells?

Mammalian cells in culture

Despite exceptions, asexual reproduction in many cells cannot be carried out indefinitely. Ageing paramecia show a marked reduction in the asexual fission rate, abnormal cell types appear and a reduction in the number of viable progeny from asexual fission occurs. Strikingly similar is Hayflick's demonstration that embryonic lung fibroblasts are capable of only 50 ± 10 mitoses in culture before they die (fig. 36.4). After a period of active multiplication, there is a gradual decrease in mitotic activity, chromosome aberrations appear and cell death becomes imminent. Like mouse colon cells *in vivo* these cells also show an increased generation time *in vitro*.

Hayflick's experiments also suggest that there is a correlation between the number of potential divisions remaining and the age of the donor tissue. While fibroblasts from human embryos may divide 50 ± 10 times, those from persons 0–20 years divide only 30 ± 10 times, and from people over 20, only 20 ± 10 times. Furthermore, the cells of shorter-lived animals are capable of fewer mitotic divisions; Hayflick claims that fibroblasts from chickens and various rodents (rats, mice, hamsters and guinea-pigs) usually do not divide more than 15 times in culture.

Is the significant link the one between ageing and mitosis, or between ageing and metabolic activity? Hayflick found that cell division interrupted by freezing in liquid nitrogen to $-190°C$ could be restarted without a change in the number of potential divisions still remaining.

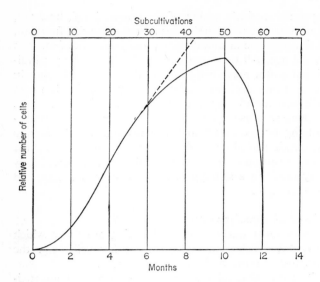

FIG. 36.4. Life span of human cells determined by allowing a population to multiply until it has doubled in size. After a culture of cells from embryonic tissue has grown to a particular point, it is divided in two. Cell division ceases after about fifty such subcultivations. It is possible at any time (although it is rare) for a spontaneous change to occur after which the cells multiply indefinitely (broken line). From Hayflick L. (1968) *Sci. Amer.*, **218**, 3, 32.

Nevertheless, skin grafts and blood cells deteriorate gradually when stored at $-78°C$, a temperature at which both mitotic and metabolic activity are nil. Since glycerol improves the 'keeping properties' of cells, the diffusion of molecules from their previously ordered state may also play a part in ageing.

Hayflick's experiments have been subject to a good deal of criticism. His control observations fail to exclude possible environmental effects of the culture on life span; in addition Puck has managed to culture rabbit fibroblasts for 600 mitotic divisions without abnormal chromosomes appearing. While Puck made daily subculturings, Hayflick divided his cultures every 4 days.

The mortality of cells is therefore still open to question. Cells may well prove to be immortal, if the correct culture conditions can be found. At present there is a stronger case for ageing being due to a decline in cellular integration, rather than to intrinsic cell mortality.

SECONDARY CELLULAR AGEING

'Death is the price paid by higher organisms for differentiation and specialization of function.' Besides the unlikely hypothesis that all ageing in metazoa is the result of primary cellular ageing, there are three other distinct possibilities, all of which involve secondary cellular ageing.

(1) Ageing may consist of a group of processes occurring partly as a result of primary ageing in several tissues and also because of secondary cellular age changes in other tissues, the latter arising as a result of the former.

(2) Ageing may be due to a single process occurring in one tissue, which results in secondary changes in other tissues. This would imply that one tissue is responsible for the ageing of the whole body.

(3) The third possibility denies the existence of primary cellular ageing. It is conceivable that the body may age by secondary cellular ageing alone. Overcrowding of cells within a tissue leads to competition for nutrients and accumulation of waste products; an eventual breakdown of integration between cells occurs, and in this way the cells and tissue age secondarily.

AGEING AT TISSUE LEVEL

Organ transplantation has been used to determine whether the ageing of a tissue is dependent on the tissue itself, or secondary to changes in other tissues. By transplanting young tissues into old animals and old tissues into young animals, tissue can be separated from what may be a tissue-ageing environment. Do old animals prematurely age young tissues? Can young animals rejuvenate old tissues? The best tissues for such experiments are those least dependent on nerve supply.

Probably no tissue ages completely independently of the rest of the body. Some tissues do so to a large extent, e.g. ovary, while for others, e.g. skin and muscle, ageing is markedly influenced by the body environment.

The ovary

This is an organ with an intrinsic life span. Krohn found that if old ovaries are transplanted into young mice, they are not rejuvenated and oestrus cycles do not reappear. However, if young ovaries are transplanted into old mice oestrus cycles continue. However, ovaries from old mice which have been hypophysectomized when young, unlike normal old ovaries, are still sensitive to gonadotrophins and produce ova which develop into normal embryos when transplanted into young mice. It seems that the ovary has an intrinsic life span but is dependent on being driven by a normal pituitary gland. When the pituitary gland is removed, the life span is interrupted but not prolonged.

The functional life span of the ovary is bound up with its initial number of oocytes and their rate of release. This number declines with age and the menopause occurs when few oocytes are left. The cessation of menstrual cycles is due to failure of the ovaries to respond to stimulation by pituitary gonadotrophins.

Tissues may also be taken from a young animal, kept in suspended animation at low temperatures and later transplanted back into the same animal when it has aged, so avoiding the hazards of possible rejection. Naturally this method cannot be used to graft old tissues into young animals, and there are also difficulties in storing tissues at low temperatures for long periods without deterioration. Parkes, however, has succeeded in restarting oestrus cycles in rats by giving them back their own ovaries in old age. An ovary can thus be aged by the body only in terms of its gradual depletion of oocytes; in terms of the rate of depletion of ova it is not aged by an old body more than it is by a young one.

Significant ageing of oocytes does not seem to occur, as 'old' ovaries from hypophysectomized mice can still produce normal embryos. Finally, if oocyte depletion is solely a function of the numbers lost in each cycle, might the artificial suppression of ovulation by the contraceptive pill delay the menopause and as a result permit women to have children well into their 80s?

While the ovaries are not essential to life, and their removal neither prolongs nor shortens the life span, ovarian decline is associated with a number of changes which are commonly recognized as features of ageing, and also with a rise in the serum cholesterol. While this may have no marked effect on life span, it is significant that following the menopause, whether natural or brought about prematurely by ovariectomy, the female death rate from ischaemic heart disease begins to rise and approaches the male levels. Oestrogens have plasma lipid-lowering properties and also influence the activity of many enzymes within the arterial walls, which may protect the vessel against the deposition of lipids.

The skin
This tissue is largely aged by other tissues at a very slow rate; it has a potential life span far beyond that of the individual. A piece of ear skin grafted from flank to flank of young mice of the same genetic strain may be kept alive for 6 years, or more than twice the age normally attained by this strain of mice. Grafts of young and old skin appear to be equally vigorous. Ageing skin transplanted into a young mouse acquires some of the properties of the younger host, such as the hair regrowth cycle. The rate at which plucked hair regrows is slowed down in young skin transplanted into old hosts; the new rate is the same as host skin beside the graft. Skin appears to age not because it is old but because it is in an old animal, i.e. secondary ageing.

Skeletal muscle
Ageing is possibly inherent in the tissue, but it is influenced by other tissues. No transplantation data exist, and furthermore none is likely since muscle depends on its nerve supply for its continued survival. Between the ages of 30 and 90 muscle weight and strength fall by about 30 per cent, due mainly to irreversible loss of some muscle cells and atrophy of others. This decline may represent intrinsic ageing of the muscle itself; however, it is influenced by declining nerve and endocrine function, and a decrease in blood supply and use made of muscles in old age. All these parameters decline with age; individual motor nerve cells die and the number of fibres in nerve trunks decreases; testosterone production in males falls and blood supply to all tissues, including muscle, decreases. Muscle atrophy can be induced experimentally by nerve transection or orchidectomy, and is seen in ischaemic atrophy and disuse atrophy. In addition, the administration of testosterone and cortisol to the elderly may result in a striking increase in muscle weight and grip strength.

The cardiovascular system
Tissues most likely to control ageing are those which have the greatest influence over other cells, e.g. the vascular, nervous and endocrine systems.

The fact that all the age changes occur at approximately the same rate favours a single process. However, according to Maynard–Smith, natural selection would also ensure synchrony by selecting out vulnerable factors in living systems that tend to cause death before or during the reproductive period. Age changes may represent merely those instabilities of tissues which occur after the reproductive period and therefore have no opportunity of being eliminated.

It is an attractive idea that the cardiovascular system may be the origin of ageing for the whole body. By starving cells of oxygen and nutrients and leaving them with accumulations of carbon dioxide and other waste products, the resulting environment might bring about ageing. Cardiac output begins to decrease after the third decade, and blood flow to all tissues falls as a consequence. The decrease in resting cardiac output is largely due to a decline in stroke volume of about 0·7 per cent/year, but heart rate also falls. Resting O_2 consumption and CO_2 production both fall, probably by about 0·5 per cent/year. It might therefore be conjectured that cellular perfusion declines more than O_2 consumption, thus effectively producing tissue ischaemia. Evidence however, for increases in A–V oxygen differences is conflicting. While peripheral resistance increases for all tissues, it is most marked in the kidneys and approximately half the annual reduction in cardiac output consists of reduced renal flow; thus blood flow and oxygen consumption may well run parallel in other tissues. Resting O_2 consumption/litre of intracellular water has been reported to remain unchanged as age advances. It is also difficult to demonstrate whether the decline in cardiac output is the primary cause of decline in oxygen consumption or vice versa. When sensitive methods become available for detecting tissue ischaemia, it may be possible to assess more accurately the role of the vascular system in ageing.

The nervous system

Brain cells die and are not replaced, but it is doubtful whether the loss is ever great enough to be lethal. Central reaction times are increased and the average speed of conduction in peripheral nerves falls about 15 per cent between the ages of 30 and 90; this is due to either loss of fast fibres or to reduction in the conduction speed of all fibres. The number of fibres in a nerve trunk falls 30 per cent between the ages of 30 and 90.

As Comfort says, old people are less likely to react fast enough to seeing a car, as well as being less likely to recover after a car accident. It has been suggested that presenile and senile dementia may represent an intensification of the normal ageing of the nervous system; senile plaques and fibrillary changes readily seen in the neurones in these diseases are present in a mild form in most old people. The proneness to accidents and the poor response to infection in the elderly and particularly in people with these diseases may have a common origin in changes in the nervous system.

The endocrine system

The reproductive hormones were once regarded as a possible source of everlasting life. However, they cannot prolong life, although they may prevent or delay a few of the changes associated with ageing. Testosterone secretion declines with age in males and this may account in part for muscle atrophy and also for the drop in red blood cell count which occurs late in life. Eunuchs do not die prematurely, nor does testosterone treatment reverse ageing or prolong life. It may, however, restore libido and muscle strength. The decline in testosterone output without significant changes in plasma corticoid concentration has been blamed for the predominance of catabolic processes in old people.

Although adrenocorticosteroid production falls slightly with age, plasma corticosterone and cortisol concentrations remain essentially unchanged. This may be due to a decrease in either utilization or inactivation. Decreased inactivation may be responsible as excretion of corticosteroid metabolites (11 deoxy 17-corticosteroids) falls and plasma concentrations of these substances do not rise. While decreased inactivation explains their longer half-life in the plasma with age, it is also possible that there is decreased utilization.

Radioactive iodine studies in old age show a decrease in the uptake of ^{131}I as well as in its turnover rate. The concentration of circulating protein-bound iodine and the sensitivity to TSH are unchanged.

Theories of ageing

Despite large investments of manpower, money and time devoted to elucidate the ageing processes at the cellular level, understanding is still extremely limited. This is due mainly to ignorance of cellular dynamics and control. In general, theories of ageing fall into two broad categories, deteriorative and programmed.

Deteriorative theories

Ageing may be in large part the result of deterioration in the integratory homeostasis which exists between cells of the same tissue and of other tissues. Such deterioration might follow ischaemia, the accumulation of toxic substances, undernutrition and various forms of disuse due to decline in nervous or endocrine control, or in functional demands. All these may result in a form of atrophy with increasing years which we recognize as ageing. In addition there are the effects of intrinsic deterioration within the cells themselves.

CHANGES IN CELL ORGANELLES WITH AGE

Changes observed in various cell organelles have frequently been proposed as possible causes of ageing. The only constituents of cells that can age, however, are those which are not turned over regularly. These include substances and structures which survive for a significant period before being broken down and replaced, and also structures and substances which accumulate in cells because mechanisms for their breakdown either do not exist or are inadequate. Changes in mitochondria and ribosomes could cause ageing, the former by starving the cell of energy, the latter by failing to synthesize essential proteins or by synthesizing defective ones. Both are turned over too rapidly in many cells to be a primary cause of ageing, but if the mechanisms for their synthesis or breakdown deteriorate, ageing might be expressed through them. Ribosomes are synthesized in the nucleus; mitochondria, it is thought, are to some extent self-synthesized by mitochondrial DNA and partly by nuclear DNA. Ageing beginning in such DNA could be expressed through these organelles.

The turnover of lysosomes is not well understood but it is not believed to be rapid. They have enormous potential to wreak havoc in cells should they deteriorate with age and release their enzymes. The age-pigments found in many cells of elderly animals contain enzymes (cathepsins and acid phosphatase) similar to those found in lysosomes. In addition, they contain the fluorescent component lipofuscin, similar in composition to various autooxidized lipids, which may have come from lysosomal membranes. It has therefore been suggested that these pigments are the incomplete breakdown products of lysosomes. What has drawn so much attention to age-pigments is their apparently linear accumulation with age in many cells (fig. 36.3, p. 36.5). It seems that they accumulate faster in non-mitosing cells, where lysosomes tend to be more numerous. Accumulation is particularly prominent in adrenocortical cells, myocardial cells, nerve cells, interstitial cells of Leydig in the testis, kidney proximal tubule cells and ovarian interstitial cells.

In human myocardial cells age-pigment may occupy 6–10 per cent of the cell volume at advanced ages. Cardiac lipofuscin accumulates five times faster in dog myocardial cells than in those of man; it is interesting that man lives approximately five times longer. This oxidized lipid would seem to result from a time-dependent process, which may or may not be linked to the synthesis or breakdown of lysosomes. The question of whether such pigment is harmful remains unanswered. A clinkering of essential cell processes has been suggested but harmful effects remain to be demonstrated despite the large volumes often occupied by these intracellular pigments.

MOLECULAR AGEING OF STABLE PROTEINS

All proteins with a slow turnover rate have, in theory, the opportunity to deteriorate significantly before they are replaced. It is possible that the existence within the body of such protein in differing degrees of deterioration might have a harmful effect on function and contribute to ageing.

Collagen

Collagen, which has a particularly long half life in many tissues and represents approximately 25 per cent of the total protein mass of the body, may well be a significant factor in ageing. X-ray diffraction studies of collagen fibrils suggest an increase in crystalline alignment of the molecules with age, and an increasing degree of cross-linkage of collagen molecules may also occurr. This is now under experimental test as a possible 'life-shortening' factor, using lathyrogen substances which prevent cross linkages. The shrinkage properties of the collagen in rat tail tendon when placed in a warm water bath have been shown by Verzar to be characteristic of age (fig. 36.5). Rat collagen ages forty times faster than human collagen as judged by the Verzar test; man also lives something like forty times longer.

However, it is difficult to demonstrate that molecular ageing of collagen has any harmful effects. The tensile strength of tendons is actually increased. The amount of collagen present in skin increases with age, but with no apparent harmful effects. Intimal thickening in blood vessels consists predominantly of collagen deposition and increases with age. Atherosclerosis is often seen in association with intimal thickening, and in some vessels arises as a more or less inevitable accompaniment of old age. It has been postulated that increasing amounts of intercellular matrix around cells, including collagen, might affect diffusion into and out of cells and thus cause them to age.

Enzymes

Ageing of proteins can occur also when the normal mechanisms existing for their replacement, i.e. nucleus, ribosomes, etc., deteriorate. Then the proteins remain

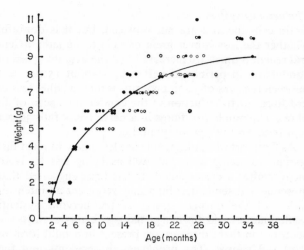

FIG. 36.5. Weight required to prevent thermal contraction of rat-tail tendon collagen versus age: ●, healthy animals; ○, animals died spontaneously. There is no difference between the two groups. From Verzar F. *et al.* (1960) *Gerontologia* (*Basel*), **49**, 12.

without replacement and age *in situ*, and may also decrease in quantity if the mechanism existing for their breakdown still remains functional. In human and rabbit red blood cells, in which nuclei and ribosomes (and therefore protein synthetic ability) have been lost, the activity of glucose-6-phosphate dehydrogenase declines with age. This enzyme is essential to the red cell for the production of energy via the hexose monophosphate pathway. With ageing of the cell, the enzymes' affinity for its co-enzyme NADP and for its substrate glucose-6-phosphate decreases, suggesting a structural change. Other changes in activity of the enzyme such as increased sensitivity to NADPase inhibition and increased thermolability also occur with age. It will be remembered that the activity of this enzyme is closely associated with NADP and therefore any change in its affinity for this substance is of prime importance with regard to its function. Similarly, hexokinase and lactic dehydrogenase show modifications with age which are reflected in decreased catalytic activity. Changes in the electrophoretic pattern with disappearance or modification of the isoenzymes are deduced as evidence for the structural modifications of the enzymes.

The relevance of such changes is not just that they demonstrate functional effects of structural changes with age. They also illustrate that the life span of a cell may be given a finite limit by a decline of intracellular enzymes, for which the replacement mechanism either does not exist or has deteriorated. In red blood cells, there is much evidence to suggest that G6PD may protect cell proteins and the cell membrane against oxidative denaturation; gradual decline in enzyme activity is possibly a factor controlling red blood cell life span.

AGEING THEORIES INVOLVING DNA

Theories of cellular ageing which explain it as the end result of changes in DNA are numerous; in contrast the available data of changes in DNA are scanty. DNA content increases in many ageing cells due to increasing polyploidy (vol. 1, p. 12.16).

The observations on which theories of DNA ageing are based are that increased chromosomal aberrations are seen with age in mouse liver cells, barley seeds and cultured leucocytes. Jacob, Court-Brown and Doll, in 1961, found that the proportion of human leucocytes with abnormal chromosomes rises from 4 per cent at 10 years of age to 13–15 per cent at 80.

Increased somatic mutation theory

Of the various cellular theories of ageing, this is the most popular; it proposes that ageing is due to mutations in the DNA of somatic cells, random in time and similar to the damage which causes abnormal progeny if it occurs in germ cells.

If mutations accumulate in cells with age, one can envisage changes in the proteins synthesized by cells as a result of gene changes, or complete lack of certain proteins if the changes are too marked for the genes to remain functional. Essential proteins within the cell such as key-enzymes might be changed and lose their specific steric configurations, resulting in upsets in the dynamic intracellular state and cellular ageing. Proteins for extra-cellular use might be altered or their production diminished, e.g. digestive enzymes, hormones or neuro-transmitter substances. The possibilities are legion. Cell surface antigens are other proteins which might be changed, thus sparking off autoimmune phenomena; on the other hand, it is conceivable that changes might sweep in the opposite direction. In specialized differentiated cells, the majority of genes are repressed. Genetic mutations, giving rise to faulty repressors or lack of synthesis of repressors, would lead to de-differentiation of cells with age. De-differentiation may be in fact one form of atrophy which does occur in many cells with age.

So far only chromosome breaks and chromosome polyploidy and aneuploidy have been shown to occur. There is no direct evidence that mutations occur as people age or that mutations cause ageing. Radiation used as an experimental tool may, however, mutate genes and also shorten life, but there is doubt whether such shortening constitutes an acceleration of ageing and whether it occurs as a result of mutation.

DNA fragmentation theory

DNA in the cell is known to have two functions:

(1) self-duplication for mitosis, and

(2) synthesis of mRNA and control over protein synthesis.

In bacteria, one break in the circular DNA molecule prevents mitosis, whereas RNA synthesis is still possible when there are many breaks; DNA is still able to act as a template for RNA synthesis because the strands of DNA are long enough to transcribe 'protein codes' to mRNA. On the same principle, it is postulated that if cells age by gradual DNA fragmentation, either spontaneously or as a result of harmful factors in the cell environment, mitotic ability is lost first and then the ability to synthesize mRNA and thus form proteins. It has been shown that ageing cells do in fact lose these abilities in this order, but fragmentation of DNA may not be the reason. The changes one can envisage in ageing cells as a result of gradual failure of protein synthesis are just as great as for mutations; failure to synthesize gene-repressors and other proteins would give the whole spectrum of possible changes.

Alexander has postulated that DNA repair mechanisms may exist in mammalian cells and that ageing of DNA begins when these mechanisms deteriorate. This modification is based on observations of DNA repair mechanisms in bacteria, and evidence of DNA turnover in non-mitosing mammalian cells.

Cross-linking theory

This postulates that cell proteins and DNA spirals in the chromosomes may be immobilized by the formation of covalent cross-links between adjacent peptide bonds or adjacent DNA spirals. On the one hand, such changed proteins might resist 'turnover' or the mechanisms responsible might not recognize them, with the result that they accumulate in the cell (age-pigments?); on the other hand, DNA cross-linkage would impair or possibly change the pattern of protein synthesis in a cell.

Abnormal binding of histone

The abnormal binding of histone could lead to permanent repression of the genes for synthesizing essential proteins and so cause cell death. However, histone repression of genes is not firmly established.

EVALUATION OF POSSIBLE CAUSATIVE FACTORS OF AGEING

A few of the main factors which have been postulated are:

(1) radiation,
(2) free radicals,
(3) thermal accidents,
(4) viruses, and
(5) autoimmune reactions.

In assessing these factors, the aim is generally to demonstrate that they (1) shorten life span, (2) shorten life span equally for all causes of death, and (3) effect morphological changes similar to those seen in aged animals.

It is worth bearing in mind that an agent may fulfil all of these criteria and still not be a cause of normal ageing.

Radiation causes increased chromosome aberrations in cells and can induce mutations. It also leads to shortening of life if given in doses which do not cause immediate radiation damage and death. What is doubtful is whether chromosome aberrations can be used as a valid index of mutations induced with radiation, and whether the life shortening caused by radiation represents an acceleration of ageing.

Free radicals are molecular groupings possessing an unpaired electron and thus a strong oxidizing tendency. They occur transiently in oxidation-reduction reactions in the tissues and their reactivity may cause cell damage and ageing. Harman reports prolongation of life in mice by feeding antioxidants such as 2-mercaptoethylamine (2MEA), butylated hydroxytoluene (BHT), cysteine hydrochloride and ascorbic acid.

Thermal accidents through small amounts of heat liberated accidentally from chemical reactions, either by controlled enzyme or uncatalysed reactions, might denature cell proteins and adversely affect DNA.

Perhaps death is due to an accumulating infection with viruses, which gradually take over more and more cells with age. Viruses certainly cause malignant changes which apparently can endow cells with indefinite life; they might also damage or change the genes in a different way to cause early ageing.

Walford has postulated that ageing may be a generalized, mild and long continued autoimmune phenomenon. In a cell population which is becoming more and more diverse, lymphocytes might suffer mutation in their 'immunological memory' and begin reacting against self-antigens. So far this is purely speculative.

Programmed theories of ageing

It may seem logical that ageing, a process itself consisting largely of deterioration, should be due to deterioration of the systems responsible for normal cell control, rather than to an extension of cell control in the form of a pre-set programme for cell ageing. Deterioration theories, however, have to explain the following facts,

(1) the wide variation found in life span between species, and

(2) the inheritance of life span within a species.

Why do different species vary so widely in their instability that a mayfly lives only for one day, and a tortoise for 176 years?

This wide variation in life span might be explained on the grounds that natural selection prevents ageing from beginning until the reproduction period is over (p. 36.8). The inheritance of life span may be no more than inheritance of a particular tendency for instability in the species.

Programming and the life span of some species
The life cycle of *Paramecium aurelia* shows characteristics which strongly suggest programming in the form of a phased shift in the genome. This may involve the sequential switching 'on' and 'off' of particular genes as they are required. The successive stages of the life cycle, sexual immaturity, maturity and senescence, are each characterized by three different responses to starvation; first there is neither autogamy nor conjugation, secondly only conjugation and then lastly only autogamy. The argument for a definite life cycle is that the ciliate always goes through these stages in the same order whether the environment is good, bad or indifferent. In *Paramecium bursaria*, the onset of maturity can be delayed though never prevented by suboptimal feeding. Similar phenomena exist for insects, rotifers and rats. Insects can be prevented from metamorphosing and do not begin to age before being allowed to undergo metamorphosis. Worker bees born near the end of the summer live to the following spring, although their normal life span is much shorter. It seems that phases in their existence can be held up under certain conditions.

Senescence as a controlled body characteristic
So many factors connected with development, growth and maintenance of structure seem to be controlled. The programmed cell death occurring in the tadpole tail in frog metamorphosis encourages the view of lysosome-mediated programmed ageing; lysosome concentrations are markedly raised in the tadpole's tail at this period and are thought to be involved in cell resorption. The inheritance of body size and the feedback controls existing to maintain liver size and marrow stem-cell numbers give additional support to the proposition that controls may also exist to govern life span.

Differences in the rates of ageing of similar structures in different animals
Large differences in rates of ageing of similar structures in different animals are difficult to explain by deterioration theory. For example, it is difficult to believe that tissue environment is much more deleterious in some animals than in others. The idea that such differences in rates of ageing are present is suggested by the following observations:

(1) chromosome aberrations accumulate more rapidly in the livers of short-lived mice than in those of longer lived strains,

(2) cardiac lipofuscin accumulates five times faster in dogs than in men, and

(3) rat collagen ages forty times more rapidly than human collagen.

If ageing is programmed, it is interesting to consider just how this could be achieved. Three theories exist.

(1) Development involves a gradual and increasing repression of genes, a process known as differentiation. The primitive cell is capable of synthesizing any protein of the species; the differentiated cell can synthesize rela-

tively few. Senescence may be characterized by a diminishing ability to synthesize proteins. If senescence is merely an extension of development, it becomes easy to understand how the diminishing ability to synthesize certain proteins could arise from a sequential continuation of gene repression until vital proteins were repressed; cell death would then occur as the cell 'ran out of programme'.

(2) A suggestion of Medvedev's is that instead of mutations arising haphazardly, certain genes might be responsible for making them. In this way the genetic material might decline with age. Mutator genes which determine mutation frequencies are known to occur in micro-organisms and plants. Studies by McClintock have demonstrated genes controlling the occurrence of somatic mosaicism in maize.

(3) Cell deterioration could be programmed in the genes but be mediated in lysosomal action. Examples of programmed cell death exist in development. The resorption of tadpoles' tails during metamorphosis involves a local increase in the lysosomal enzyme concentration in the tail, and this is believed to be controlled by the thyroid. Similarly a group of cells exists in the body of the developing chick embryo whose death is necessary for the release of the wing for subsequent movement. These cells still die on schedule when transplanted to the back.

Conclusions

THE AGEING LOCI

It is difficult to decide whether ageing has one or many causes. Each tissue may age independently at its own rate and according to its own built-in programme, but the actual process may be the same for all tissues. On the other hand, a **single ageing locus** may control the secondary ageing of all other tissues, so that all tissues age together but by different processes. When the number of possible combinations of loci and processes is so great, there are bound to be common factors in any mechanism which attempts to account for overall ageing.

AGEING AND DEATH

The most significant association of ageing is with death. The functional decline of ageing is not only important because of the limitations it places on mental and physical capacities, but also because of the limitation it places on life. Ageing is probably the factor which makes death inevitable. By retarding ageing we can hope not only to prolong the adult period of maximum vigour, but perhaps also to prolong total life span. All age changes do not result in functional decline and all changes resulting in functional decline do not necessarily cause death, e.g. testosterone restores muscle strength, libido and the secondary sexual characteristics in the ageing male

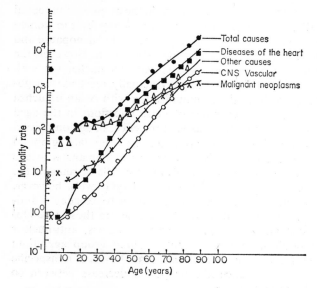

FIG. 36.6. Gompertz plot of cause-specific human mortality rates. From Strehler B.L. & Mildvam A.S. (1960) *Science*, **132**, 14.

but it does not prolong life. Testicular decline does not limit it either. If age changes contribute to death, then they must either predispose to or cause death in old age.

The age distribution of the diseases of old age and the Gompertzian increase in mortality rate from them suggest a cumulative factor (fig. 36.6). Such a factor may be ageing, or alternatively it may be the cumulative effects of the environment. In some circumstances ageing may be due to the environment (i.e. wear and tear), in others it is possibly spontaneous and wholly inevitable.

There are three ways in which ageing can be claimed indirectly or directly to cause death in old age.

(1) The body's ability to cope with stress, and to control deviations from homeostatic 'set-points' of the internal environment decreases with age. This is due to a decrease in the maximal rates of many processes, as a result of age-related decline in the total functional capacities of tissues. Such decline limits the body's compensatory mechanisms to 'set-point' deviations.

(2) The body's ability to cope with infection decreases with age. Despite certain inconsistencies, the available information suggests a decline in the immunological system with age, with the consequence that the elderly become more vulnerable to infection. Diminished resistance to infection may be related to a reduction in lymphoid tissue; this starts in adolescence and is marked in old age, when lymph nodes are converted to nodules of fat with only a rim of lymphoid tissue. Experimental animals show a decreased production and impaired maintenance of adequate antibody levels, and a decreased vigour in both immediate and delayed hypersensitivity reactions. In mice, the decline in the immune system is

believed to be due to a decrease in the number of potential antibody-forming cells. Symptoms of hay fever in women are reported to abate or disappear at the menopause and to become less severe in middle-aged men. However, the response to typhoid vaccine remains unchanged with age, and people over 40 may actually react more vigorously to single dose immunization with Asian influenza vaccine. The occurrence of more infections in the aged tends to complicate studies of the effect of age on plasma globulin, because such infections stimulate globulin formation. IgG levels tend to rise in humans with age while the concentration of albumin falls or remains the same. Despite an increase in total IgG levels, however, there may be a decrease in antibodies to exogenous antigens. The antibodies which increase are those to endogenous antigens (e.g. rheumatoid factors, anti-nuclear antibodies). Anti-A and anti-B blood group agglutinin decrease with age after a peak at 30. Levels of nonspecific immune substance like properdin decrease between 60 and 90 years of age.

While the ability to form antibodies seems to decline, studies with mice indicate that homograft reactions do not decline with age as judged by rejection time. As a result tissue transplantation is not likely to be easier in the elderly.

(3) Some of the diseases of old age may be due directly to age changes. While environmental aspects are important, malignancy and many age-related autoimmune diseases may be due to random mutations accumulating with age. According to Burch, the age distribution of many diseases, e.g. cancer, rheumatoid arthritis, systemic lupus erythematosus, systemic sclerosis and chronic thyroiditis, can be described by multiple exponential equations. He has recently also included such age changes as greying of hair and the loss of permanent teeth with age. The initiation of each of these changes may depend on the accumulation of a small number (generally less than ten) of specific random mutations in predisposed individuals.

As already mentioned, atherosclerosis may arise in part as a consequence of a normal age change in the form of intimal thickening. This might lead to ischaemia, causing loss of lipid-mobilizing substances from the vessel wall, with consequent accumulation of lipids including cholesterol. Cholesterol is sclerogenic and the resulting atherosclerosis is a major factor in ischaemic heart disease and cerebrovascular accident, two leading causes of death in old age. However, the common criticism levelled against such a proposal is that atherosclerosis is not inevitable. In the majority of people, atherosclerosis appears to progress steadily after middle life, but in a few development is very slow; these may reach an advanced age with atherosclerosis present to a degree insufficient to cause any clinical symptoms. Yet it should be remembered that one of the most striking features of age changes is their great variation between individuals and in nature.

FURTHER READING

HAYFLICK L. (1968) Human cells and ageing. *Sci. Amer.*, **218**, 3, 32.

MAYNARD SMITH J. (1963) The causes of ageing. *Proc. roy. Soc. B.* **157**, 115.

STREHLER B.L. (1962) *Time, Cells and Ageing*. New York: Academic Press.

WELFORD, A.T. (1958) *Ageing and Human Skill*. London: Oxford University Press.

The term glycosaminoglycan was suggested by Jeanloz for polysaccharides which contain amino sugars, superseding the name 'mucopolysaccharide'. This nomenclature is now frequently used in the biochemical literature and the revised names of the individual compounds are given in the following table.

Former name	New name
Mucoprotein	Protein-polysaccharide or proteoglycan
Acidic mucopolysaccharide	Glycosaminoglycuronoglycan
Amino sugar-containing polysaccharide	Glycosaminoglycan
Chondroitin sulphate A	Chondroitin-4-sulphate
Chondroitin sulphate C	Chondroitin-6-sulphate
Chondroitin sulphate B	Dermatan sulphate
Keratosulphate	Keratan sulphate
Heparitin sulphate	Heparan sulphate
Heparin	Heparin

For individual proteoglycans the type of glycosaminoglycan precedes the word protein, e.g. chondroitin-4-sulphate-protein.

Index

For each reference the first number is the chapter and the second the page within the chapter.